Bend your knees.	**Doble las rodillas.** *__Doh__-bleh lahs roh-__dee__-yahs.*
Do you have pain here?	**¿Tiene dolor aquí?** *Tee-__eh__-neh doh-__lohr__ ak-__kee__?*
Breathe deeply.	**Respire profundo.** *Rehs-__pee__-reh proh-__foon__-doh.*
Drink clear liquids.	**Tome líquidos claros.** *__Toh__-meh __lee__-kee-dohs __klah__-rahs.*
Can you give us a stool sample?	**¿Puede darnos una muestra de excremento?** *__Pweh__-deh __dahr__-nohs __oo__-nah __mwehs__-trah deh eks-kreh-__mehn__-toh?*
When was the last time you had a bowel movement?	**¿Cuándo fue la última vez que obró (que usó el baño)?** *__Kwahn__-doh fweh lah __ool__-tee-mah behs keh oh-__broh__ (keh oo-__soh__ ehl __bah__-nyoh)?*
Drink eight glasses of water a day.	**Tome ocho vasos de agua al día.** *__Toh__-meh __oh__-choh __bah__-sohs deh __ah__-gwah ahl __dee__-ah.*
Do you have sexual relations with men (women, prostitutes)?	**¿Tiene usted relaciones sexuales con hombres (mujeres, prostitutas)?** *Tee-__eh__-neh oos-__tehd__ rel-lah-see-__oh__-nehs sek-soo-__ah__-lehs kohn __ohm__-brehs (moo-__heh__-rehs, prohs-tee-__too__-tahs)?*
Are you allergic to any medicine or food?	**¿Es alérgica a alguna medicina o alimento?** *Ehs ah-__lehr__-hee-kah ah aho-__goo__-nah meh-dee-__see__-nah oh ah-lee-__mehn__-toh?*
Do you take medicine?	**¿Toma usted medicina?** *__Toh__-mah oos-__tehd__ meh-dee-__see__-nah?*
Do you have the medicine with you?	**¿Trae la medicina con usted?** *__Trah__-eh lah meh-dee-__see__-nak kohn oos-__tehd__?*
Take your medication.	**Tome su medicina.** *__Toh__-meh soo meh-dee-__see__-nah.*
I am going to give you pain medicine.	**Le voy a day medicina para el dolor.** *Leh __boh__-ee ah dahr med-dee-__see__-nah __pah__-rah ehl doh-__lohr__.*
Do you have shortness of breath?	**¿Tiene falta de aire?** *Tee-__ehn__-eh __fahl__-tah deh __ah__-ee-reh?*
We need a urine sample.	**Necesitamos una muestra de orina.** *Neh-seh-see-__tah__-mohs __oo__-nah __mwehs__-trah deh oh-__ree__-nah.*
You need a catheter in your bladder.	**Usted necesita una sonda en la vejiga.** *Oos-__tehd__ neh-seh-__see__-tah __oo__-nah __sohn__-dah ehn lah beh-__hee__-gah.*
Have you lost weight?	**¿Ha perdido peso?** *Ah pehr-__dee__-doh __peh__-soh?*
How long have you had the discharge?	**¿Cuánto tiempo tiene con el deshecho/flujo?** *__Kwahn__-toh tee-__ehm__-poh tee-__eh__-neh kohn ehl dehs-__eh__-choh/__floo__-hoh?*
What do you use to prevent pregnancy?	**¿Qué clase de anticonceptivo usa para prevenir el embarazo?** *Keh __klah__-seh heh ahn-tee-kohn-sept-__tee__-boh __oo__-sah __pah__-rah preh-beh-__neer__ ehl ehm-bah-__rah__-soh?*
When was your last period?	**¿Cuándo fue su última regla/menstruación?** *__Kwahn__-do fweh soo __ool__-tee-mah __reh__-glah/mehns-troo-ah-see-__ohn__?*

(Spanish Phrases appear in their entirety in Appendix F)

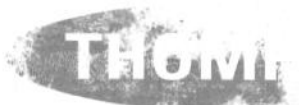

Introduction to

THOMPSON'S

Introduction to Maternity and Pediatric Nursing

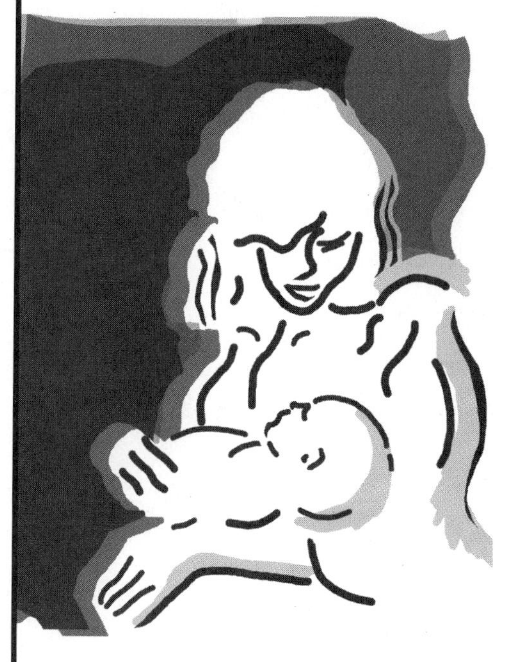

Edition 3

Gloria Leifer, MA, RN
Associate Professor
Obstetrics, Pediatrics, and Orthopedic Nursing
Riverside Community College
Riverside, California

W.B. SAUNDERS COMPANY
A Division of Harcourt Brace & Company
Philadelphia London Toronto Montreal Sydney Tokyo

W.B. SAUNDERS COMPANY
A Division of Harcourt Brace & Company

The Curtis Center
Independence Square West
Philadelphia, PA 19106

Library of Congress Cataloging-in-Publication Data

Thompson's introduction to maternity and pediatric nursing. — 3rd ed.
/ edited by Gloria Leifer.
p. cm.
Rev. ed. of: Introduction to maternity and pediatric nursing /
Eleanor Dumont Thompson, 2nd ed. c1995.
Includes bibliographical references and index.
ISBN 0-7216-7557-3
1. Maternity nursing. 2. Pediatric nursing. I. Leifer, Gloria.
II. Thompson, Eleanor Dumont. Introduction to maternity and
pediatric nursing.
[DNLM: 1. Maternal-Child Nursing—methods. 2. Pediatric Nursing-
-methods. WY 157.3T478 1999]
RG951.T46 1999
610.73′62—dc21
DNLM/DLC 98-38331

THOMPSON'S INTRODUCTION TO MATERNITY AND PEDIATRIC NURSING, 3rd edition ISBN 0-7216-7557-3

Printed in the United States of America 9 8 7 6 5 4 3 2 1

Dedicated to

Sarah Masseyaw Leifer

A nurse, humanitarian, and mother

and

Daniel Peretz Hartston, M.D.

A pediatrician, husband, and father

Special Contributor

Emily Slone McKinney, MSN, RN, C
Education Coordinator
Women's Pavilion of Health
Baylor Medical Center at Irving
Irving, TX

Human Reproductive Anatomy and Physiology • Prenatal Development • Prenatal Care and Adaptations to Pregnancy • Nursing Care of Women with Complications during Pregnancy • Nursing Care during Labor and Birth • Nursing Management of Pain during Labor and Birth • Nursing Care of Women with Complications during Labor and Birth • The Family after Birth • Nursing Care of Women with Complications Following Birth • The Nurse's Role in Women's Health Care

Preface

THE TRANSFORMING ROLE OF THE LICENSED PRACTICAL/ VOCATIONAL NURSE

Depth with **simplicity** is the theme of the revision of this text. This theme is based upon current health care reform and the need to adapt to the changes that are occurring in order to maintain quality patient care. The role of the nurse at every level is changing. The curriculum of educational programs preparing the LPN/LVN must also change in order to adequately prepare their graduate for entry level positions. Because of cost containment, more LPN/LVN nurses are working in home health and assuming some leadership responsibilities in nursing homes, with unlicensed staff. Critical thinking skills become essential and are reflected in this text by the inclusion of detailed rationales. In past years the LPN/LVN was considered a terminal certificate. Today, however, many LPN/ LVN programs are considered "ladders" into the ADN program. Vocational nurses progressing to the ADN program often do not repeat maternity and pediatric content. The theme of this edition *depth* with *simplicity* provides basic information for the LPN/LVN while adding just enough depth to meet the needs of the "ladder" student. There are several LPN/LVN to BSN educational programs in the United States that are supported by nursing leaders and by the National League for Nursing (NLN). Several studies have recommended the upgrading of knowledge at the LPN/LVN level. A quality educational program at the LPN/LVN level will improve the performance of the pool of LPN/LVN's in health care practice as well as enhance their mobility.

The information incorporated into this text is based upon the philosophy of most nursing education programs that prepare the LPN/LVN student for entry level positions. Curriculums are focused on medical-surgical nursing of adults. Maternity-pediatric nursing is presented at an introductory level with emphasis on how infants and children differ from adults. This edition emphasizes how techniques of care may differ based upon anatomical, physiological and psychological differences between the infant, child or pregnant adult and the traditional adult medical-surgical client. In order to limit the size of this book and make it more useful as a reference tool, some content common to medical-surgical nursing is not included, making this a maternity/pediatric content specific text. Careful consideration of the LPN/LVN Nurse Practice Acts have guided the inclusion of skills and techniques in this text. This organization facilitates the use of this text in a combined maternity/pediatric course, a separate maternity course followed by an independent pediatric course, or a medical-surgical course that integrates the maternity and pediatric client throughout the curriculum.

Pediatric health is closely related to obstetrical care and maternal risk factors. For this reason, maternity and pediatric nursing are often studied together, as some preventable pediatric disorders stem from conditions before or at conception. There has been an explosion of information concerning obstetrics and pediatrics combined with a very limited amount of classroom time to discuss this information in most curriculum across the country. For these reasons, and for cost containment in student education, a mandate was apparent for a combined text. This combined text provides comprehensive discussions of family centered care, health promotion and illness prevention, woman's health issues and growth and development of the child *and the parent.* In this combined text, the information forms one continuum of knowledge flowing from conception to adulthood. The concept of studying simple-to-complex and health-to-illness is retained. The systems approach is maintained in presenting physiological illness (other than congenital anomalies that are present at birth and communicable diseases of children).

In their 1991 publication "Healthy American; Practitioners for 2005: An Agenda for Action for US Health Professional Schools" the PEW Health Professions Commission recommended that nursing graduates must "meet the evolving health care needs" of clients and possess the "ability to deal with a racially and culturally diverse society" (p. 18). These recommendations are reflected in this text as detailed discussions and explanations of diverse cultural health care practices relating to maternity and pediatric care. The LPN/LVN education includes tasks and technology based in acute care hospitals. However, the modern trend of health care reform moves the focus from the institution to the population. Recognition of the interdisciplinary health care team that works with this population is essential and referred to throughout this edition with emphasis on the nurses role. A section concerning health care practices and herbal medicine is presented to provide the student with an understanding of the practices within the community that may impact the care provided by the nurse. An understanding of techniques to promote compliance and healthy, safe self-care practices are reviewed.

Managed care gave birth to the clinical pathway and LPN/LVN's must understand their role in that plan of care. Sample nursing care plans are presented throughout the text and the student is introduced to the clinical pathway that is also known as the "critical pathway" or "care map."

This book, with the theme of **depth** with **simplicity** is designed both to prepare the LPN/LVN student for mobility in the profession and to enable the LPN/LVN to provide quality maternity and pediatric nursing care to a diverse population in a rapidly changing world.

STUDENT LEARNING FOCUS

Several user friendly features incorporated into this edition facilitate learning and enhance review. They include *chapter outlines* at the beginning of each chapter that focuses the student on the scope of the content. *Vocabulary terms* are provided to aid the reader in assessing their reading comprehension. The vocabulary words are italicized in the text as they are defined and used. The *objectives* of the chapter are identified to help the student focus on the topics to be studied. *Tables and boxes* present facts, comparisons and summaries in outline form to increase reader understanding. *Nursing tips* within each chapter enhance retention by emphasizing important concepts. *Key points* at the end of each chapter summarize concepts and serve as a study guide or review for the student. *Multiple choice review questions* at the end of each chapter test comprehension and application of knowledge learned from the chapter. *Color* is utilized to enhance visual appeal, clarify concepts and maintain interest. *New line drawings* are used to identify and emphasize details often hidden in photographs. Each photograph provides specific information. An *updated bibliography* or reference list validates content and refers the reader to sources for in-depth study of specific topics.

Study Guide

The **Study Guide for Thompson's Introduction to Maternity and Pediatric Nursing,** Third Edition, written by Emily Slone McKinney, MSN, RN, C, and Jean Weiler Ashwill, MSN, RN, CPNP, has been revised to correspond with this new edition. It is intended to help the student master the content of the textbook. Every chapter in the Study Guide coincides with the chapter of the same name in the text.

Matching and completion *Learning Activities* help reinforce factual material related to maternity and pediatric nursing. In addition, *Thinking Critically* exercises, *Case Studies,* and *Other Learning Activities* help the student apply factual material to the clinical setting.

Multiple choice *Review Questions* appear at the end of each chapter in the study guide. The questions have a dual purpose: to help students review chapter content and to help them become more comfortable in answering typical test items.

An *Answer Key* for the Learning Activities and Review Questions is provided in the **Instructor's Manual for Thompson's Introduction to Maternity and Pediatric Nursing,** Third Edition. Rationales are included with the answers to the Review Questions.

INSTRUCTIONAL PACKAGE

A revised **Instructor's Manual,** written by Christine M. Rosner, PhD, RN, is available to qualified adopters of the text. Selected objectives, course outlines, lesson plans, resources for audiovisual supplements, and a test bank are included.

New to This Edition

Also available to qualified adopters of the text are **Transparencies** and an **ExaMaster.** The transparencies contain additional full-color figures that supplement the figures in the textbook. The ExaMaster is the computerized version of the test bank from the Instructor's Manual.

Notice

Nursing is an ever-changing field. Standard safety precautions must be followed, but as new research and clinical experience broaden our knowledge, changes in treatment and drug therapy become necessary or appropriate. Readers are advised to check the product information currently provided by the manufacturer of each drug to be administered to verify the recommended dose, the method and duration of administration, and contraindications. It is the responsibility of the treating physician relying on experience and knowledge of the patient to determine dosages and the best treatment for the patient. Neither the Publisher nor the editor assumes any responsibility for any injury and/or damage to persons or property.

The Publisher

Acknowledgments

Reader confidence in earlier editions of *Introduction to Maternity and Pediatric Nursing* provided the enthusiasm and encouragement for the scope of this revision. I want to thank Ilze Rader, former Senior Nursing Editor at W.B. Saunders Company, for believing in my ability to accomplish this task, for providing insight and inspiration, and for nurturing the creativity necessary for a text that enters a new century of learning.

My first text published by W.B. Saunders Company, *Principles and Techniques in Pediatric Nursing,* was originally published in 1965. Subsequent revisions and the ANA "Book of the Year" award nourished my interest in writing. I have published several journal articles but I am happy to return to the textbook arena.

As a parent, I recognize the value and have experienced the joys of a happy, healthy, loving family. Guiding the growth and development of four tiny children who are now grown and productively contributing to society, is an experience that is unique. I would like to express my gratitude to my children, Heidi Barnet, Amos, and Eve and David Fleck for their encouragement and patience. They have taught me firsthand what it means to be an anxious parent, thus in a sense providing a basis for including content that may enable the student to lessen the anxieties of other parents. My past travels with my husband made it possible for me to personally investigate the cultural practices and problems of maternity and pediatric clients in developed and undeveloped areas of Africa, the Far East, the Middle East, and Europe as well as many parts of the United States, including Alaska. My appreciation is extended to the many members of the medical and nursing professions in these countries for their time and cooperation.

I would also like to thank the medical and nursing staff of Riverside County Regional Medical Center and the Southern California Kaiser Permanente Medical Center in Fontana, California, for their assistance in obtaining current information.

I want to thank Eleanor Dumont Thompson for providing a solid basis on which the revision is built. Emily Stone McKinney, MSN, RN, C, is a special contributor who brings expertise in maternity nursing and experience in textbook publication.

Marie Thomas, Senior Editorial Assistant at W.B. Saunders worked wonders with all of the fine details essential to successful publication. She is a key link to the publisher and a supportive friend to the author. Terri Wood, Editor, Nursing Books, and Terri Ward, the Developmental Editor, encouraged me to incorporate new trends while maintaining traditional concepts. The blending into one text of traditional, current, and future practices necessary for LPN/LVNs to function in the next century was a challenge that required cooperation and compromise. It was a pleasure to work on this team where simple exposition was allowed to develop into a hearty feast of knowledge that will hopefully serve to educate and whet the appetite of the reader for continued education. Also thanks to Tony and Maria Caruso, production editors, for fusing various portions into a finished product.

I would also like to acknowledge the efforts of my research consultant, Trena L. Rich RN, MSN, ANP, who provided valuable assistance in assuring currency of research, equipment, and resources. I could not have ventured into this project without the able assistance of Carolyn Boyd, who provided computer expertise with critical manuscript proofing and competent, constructive suggestions.

Finally, and most important, I would like to thank my students from Fordham School of Nursing, Hunter College, California State College at Los Angeles, and Riverside Community College for helping me apply and redefine concepts of teaching and learning.

Gloria Leifer Hartston

Reviewers

I would like to thank the following educators and clinicians who carefully reviewed manuscript and offered many excellent suggestions for improvement.

Sylvia C. Austin, RN, MEd
Okaloosa Applied Technical Center
Ft. Walton Beach, Florida

Genie M. Bartlett, MSN, RN
University of Texas at Tyler
Tyler, Texas

Veronica K. Casey, RNC, MA
Norwalk Community-Technical College
Norwalk, Connecticut

Jeannine Charest, BSN, RN
Lehigh Carbon Community College
Schnecksville, Pennsylvania

Jeanne S. Clow, RN, BSN, MsEd
Coordinator
Otsego Area School of Practical Nursing
Oneonta, New York

Tammy M. Collier, RN, NREMT-A
Delta Technical Institute
Jonesboro, Arkansas

Anne M. Comiskey, RN, BSN
Nassau BOCES
Westbury, New York

Susan C.F. Cook, RN, BS, RD
Arkansas State University
Mountain Home, Arkansas

Mattie T. DuBose, RN
Drake State Technical College
Huntsville, Alabama

Sherry J. Goff, BSN, RN, EMT
Blinn College
Bryan, Texas

Phyllis M. Graves, RN
Waynesville Technical Academy
Waynesville, Missouri

Sheila F. Guidry, DNS, MSN, RN
Director/Chair, Practical Nursing Program
Wallace Community College
Selma, Alabama

Lois Harrion, RN, MS, BA
Director, Vocational Nursing Program
Simi Valley Adult School
Simi Valley, California

Daphene Heern, RN
Delta Technical Institute
Jonesboro, Arkansas

Judith Ryan Higel, JD, RN, MS
Tri-Rivers Center for Adult Education
Ohio State University at Marion
Marion, Ohio

Patricia Laing-Arie, RN
Meridian Technology Center
Stillwater, Oklahoma

Laura LeAnne Massey, BSN, RN
University of Arkansas Community College
Hope, Arkansas

Sibyl Linonis McNelly, BSN, RN
Somerset County Area Vocational Technical School
Somerset, Pennsylvania

Victoria Lynne Oxner, BSN, RN
Arkansas State University
Mountain Home, Arkansas

Kim I. Smith, MSN, RN, MA
Shelton State Community College
Tuscaloosa, Alabama

Margie F. Smith, BSN, RN
IVY Technical State College
Greencastle, Indiana

Sherri L. Smith, RN
Delta Technical Institute
Jonesboro, Arkansas

Margaret E. Souders, RNS, MS
Phoenix College
Phoenix, Arizona

Kathleen G. Stilling, RN, C, MS
Johnston School of Practical Nursing
Baltimore, Maryland

Anita Webb, RN, BSE
Northwest Technical Institute
Springdale, Arkansas

Contents

Color plates follow pages 328 and 776

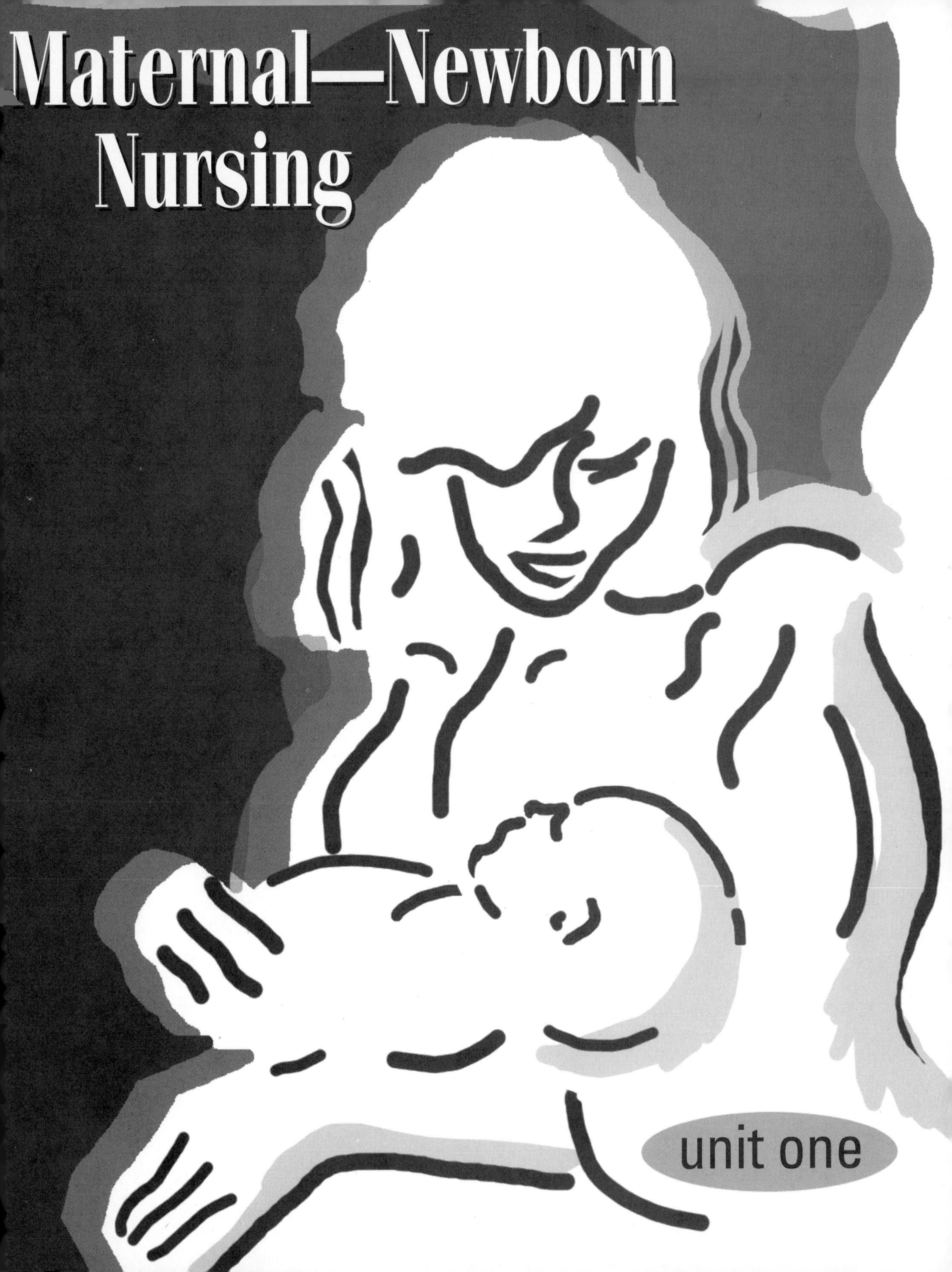
Maternal—Newborn
Nursing
unit one

chapter 1

The Past, the Present, and the Future of Maternity and Pediatric Nursing

Outline

Objectives

On completion and mastery of Chapter 1, the student will be able to:

- Define each vocabulary term listed.
- Contrast present-day concepts of maternity and child care with those of the past.
- List three environmental stresses on the childbearing family.
- List four reasons why statistics are important.
- Discuss how one's culture affects childbirth and child care.
- List the five steps of the nursing process.
- Recall the contributions of persons in history in the field of maternity and pediatric care.
- Name two international organizations concerned with maternity and child care.
- List three federal programs that assist mothers and infants.
- Define the role of the community-based nurse as a provider of health care to mothers and children.
- List the organizations concerned with setting standards for nursing care of maternity and pediatric clients.
- State the influence of the federal government on maternity and pediatric care.
- Discuss common terms used in expressing vital statistics.
- Contrast a nursing care plan with a clinical pathway.
- Describe types of alternative health care practices.
- Illustrate the role of the nurse in alternative health care.
- Discuss the roles and functions of a school nurse.
- Describe the role of the community health nurse as a provider of health care.

Vocabulary

acupuncture
advanced practice nurse
advocate
allopathic
alternative health care
aromatherapy
birthing centers
clinical nurse specialist
clinical pathway
cost containment
documentation
DRG
empowerment
family care plan
full inclusion
Healthy People 2000
herbal medicine
HMO
LDR room
mainstream
midwife
nurse practitioner
nursing care plan
nursing process
obstetrics
obstetrician
osteopath
paperless charting
Pediatric Nurse Practitioner
pediatrics
podalic version
PPO
puerperium
rolfing
statistics

INTRODUCTION

The word *obstetrics* is derived from the Latin term *obstetrix,* which means "midwife." It is the branch of medicine that pertains to care of women during pregnancy, childbirth, and the postpartum period *(puerperium).* Maternity nursing is the care given by the nurse to the expectant family before, during, and following birth.

A physician specializing in the care of women during pregnancy, labor, birth, and the postpartum period is an *obstetrician.* These physicians perform cesarean deliveries and treat women with known or suspected obstetric problems as well as attend normal deliveries. Many family physicians and certified nurse-midwives also deliver babies. The skill and knowledge related to obstetrics have evolved over centuries.

Pediatrics is defined as the branch of medicine that deals with the child's development and care and the diseases of childhood and their treatment. The word is derived from the Greek *pais, paidos* "child" and *iatreia* "cure."

Family-centered care recognizes the strength and integrity of the family as the core of planning and implementing health care. The family as caregivers and decision makers are an integral part of both obstetric and pediatric nursing. The philosophy, goals, cultural, and ethnic practices of the family contribute to their ability to accept and maintain *control* over the health care of its members. This control is called *empowerment.* The nurse's role in maternity and pediatric family-centered care is to enter a contract or partnership with the family to achieve the goals of health for its members.

THE PAST

Europe

The earliest records concerning childbirth are in the Egyptian papyruses (circa 1550 BC). Later advances were made by Soranus, a Greek physician who practiced in 2nd-century Rome and who is known as the father of obstetrics. He instituted the practice of podalic version, a procedure used to rotate a fetus to a breech, or feet-first, position. Podalic version is important in delivering the second baby in a set of twins. In this procedure, the physician reaches into the uterus and grasps one or both of the baby's feet to facilitate delivery. Planned cesarean birth is safer and used more often today. Such scientific exploration halted with the decline of the Roman Empire and the ensuing Dark Ages.

During the 18th century, Karl Credé (1819–1892) and Ignaz Semmelweis (1818–1865) made contributions that improved the safety and health of mother and child during and after childbirth. In 1884 Credé recommended instilling 2% silver nitrate into the eyes of newborns to prevent blindness caused by gonorrhea. This procedure has basically stayed the same, except that 1% silver nitrate is administered or antibiotic ointments are used. Credé's innovation has saved the eyesight of incalculable numbers of babies.

The classic story of Semmelweis is interesting and tragic. In the 1840s, he worked as an assistant professor in the maternity ward of the Vienna general hospital. There he discovered a relationship between the incidence of puerperal fever (or "childbed fever"), which caused many deaths among women in lying-in wards, and the examination of new mothers by student doctors who had just returned from dissecting cadavers. Semmelweis deduced that puerperal fever was septic, contagious, and transmitted by the *unwashed hands* of physicians and medical students. Semmelweis's outstanding work, written in 1861, is titled *The Causes, Understanding, and Prevention of Childbed Fever.* Not until 1890 was his teaching finally accepted.

Louis Pasteur (1822–1895), a French chemist, confirmed that puerperal fever was caused by bacteria

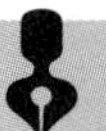

Nursing Tip

Two nursing journals focusing on maternal and child health are the *Journal of Obstetric, Gynecologic, and Neonatal Nursing (JOGNN)* and the *American Journal of Maternal Child Nursing (MCN).*

and could be spread by improper handwashing and contact with contaminated objects. The simple, but highly effective, procedure of handwashing continues to be one of the most important means of preventing the spread of infection in the hospital and home today. Joseph Lister (1827–1912), a British surgeon influenced by Pasteur, experimented with chemical means of preventing infection. He revolutionized surgical practice by introducing antiseptic surgery.

The United States

The immigrants who reached the shores of America brought a wide variety of practices and beliefs about the birth process. Many practices were also contributed by the Native American nations. Most deliveries in the early United States were attended by a midwife or relative. One midwife, Samuel Bard, who was educated outside the United States, is credited with writing the first American textbook in obstetrics.

Oliver Wendell Holmes (1809–1894), when a young Harvard physician, wrote a paper detailing the contagiousness of puerperal fever, but he, like Semmelweis, was widely criticized by his colleagues. Eventually, the "germ theory" became accepted, and more mothers and babies began to survive childbirth in the hospital.

Before the 1900s most babies were born at home. Only very ill patients were cared for in lying-in hospitals. Maternal and child morbidity and mortality rates were high in such institutions because of crowded conditions and unskilled nursing care. Hospitals began to develop training programs for nurses. As the medical profession grew, physicians developed a closer relationship with hospitals. This, along with the advent of obstetric instruments and anesthesia, caused a shift to hospital care during childbirth. By the 1950s hospital practice in obstetrics was well established. By 1960 more than 90% of births in the United States occurred in hospitals.

However, hospital care did not embrace the family-centered approach. Often the father waited in a separate room during the labor and birth of his child. The mother was often sedated with "twilight sleep" and participated little during labor and delivery. After birth, the infant was not reunited with the parents for several hours. Parent–infant bonding was delayed.

Organizations concerned with setting standards for maternity nursing developed. These include the American College of Nurse-Midwives (ACNM), the Association of Women's Health, Obstetric, and Neonatal Nurses (AWHONN), formerly the Nurses Association of the American College of Obstetricians and Gynecologists (NAACOG), and the Division of Maternal Nursing within the American Nurses Association.

Abraham Jacobi (1830–1919) is known as the father of pediatrics because of his many contributions to the field. The establishment of pediatric nursing as a specialty paralleled that of departments of pediatrics in medical schools, the founding of children's hospitals, and the development of separate units for children in foundling homes and general hospitals.

In the Middle Ages, the concept of childhood did not exist. Infancy lasted until about the age of 7, at which time the child was assimilated into the adult world. The art of that time depicts the child wearing adult clothes and wigs. Most children did not attend school.

Methods of child care have varied throughout history. The culture of a society has a strong influence on standards of child care. Many primitive tribes were nomads. Strong children survived, whereas the weak were left to die. This practice of infanticide (French and Latin *infans,* "infant," and *caedere,* "to kill") helped to ensure the safety of the group. As tribes became settled, more attention was given to children, but they were still frequently valued for their productivity. Certain peoples, such as the Egyptians and the Greeks, were advanced in their attitudes. The Greek physician Hippocrates (460–370 BC) wrote of illnesses peculiar to children.

Christianity had a considerable impact on child care. In the early 17th century, several children's asylums were founded by Saint Vincent de Paul. Many of these eventually became hospitals, although their original concern was for the abandoned. The first children's hospital was founded in Paris in 1802. In the United States, numerous homeless children were cared for by the Children's Aid Society, founded in New York City in 1853. In 1855 the first pediatric hospital in the United States, The Children's Hospital of Philadelphia, was founded.

By the 1960s a separate pediatric unit in hospitals was commonplace. However, parents were restricted by rigid visiting hours that allowed parent–

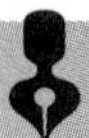

Nursing Tip

Cultural beliefs today, as in the past, affect how a family perceives health and illness. Holistic nursing includes being alert for cultural diversity and incorporating this information into nursing care plans.

infant contact for only a few hours each day. When medically indicated, nursing mothers were allowed to enter the pediatric unit for one hour at a time to breastfeed their infant.

Government Influences in Maternity and Pediatric Care

The high mortality rate of mothers and infants motivated action by the federal government to improve care. The Sheppard-Towner Act of 1921 provided funds for state-managed programs for maternity care. Since then, Title V of the Social Security Act has also been providing funds for maternity care. The National Institutes of Health (NIH) support maternity research and education. The Title V amendment of the Public Health Services Act established Maternal-Infant Care Centers in public clinics. Title XIX of the Medicaid program increases access to care by indigent women. Head Start programs were established to increase educational exposure of preschool children. The National Center for Family Planning provides contraceptive information and the Women's, Infant's and Children's (WIC) program provides supplemental food and education for the poor.

The Children's Bureau

Lillian Wald, a nurse who was interested in the welfare of children, is credited with suggesting the establishment of a federal children's bureau.

Once the Children's Bureau was established in 1912, it focused its attention on the problems of

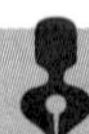

Nursing Tip

Innovative community programs such as foster grandparents, home health or parent aides, and Phone a Friend (a call-in program for children home alone after school), are of particular value to dysfunctional or isolated families.

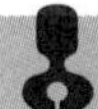

Nursing Tip

Today the Children's Bureau is administered under the auspices of the Department of Health and Human Services.

infant mortality. This study was followed by one that dealt with maternal mortality. This study eventually led to birth registration in all states. In the 1930s the Children's Bureau investigations led to the development of hot lunch programs in many schools.

The Fair Labor Standards Act, passed in 1938, established a general minimum working age of 16 (Fig. 1–1) and a minimum working age of 18 for jobs considered hazardous. More important, this act paved the way for the establishment of national minimum standards for child labor and provided a means of enforcement.

White House Conferences

The First White House Conference on Children and Youth was called by President Theodore Roosevelt in 1909. It gathered every 10 years.

In the White House Conference on Child Health and Protection (1930), the Children's Charter was drawn up (Box 1–1). This is considered to be one of the most important documents in child care history. It lists 17 statements related to the needs of children

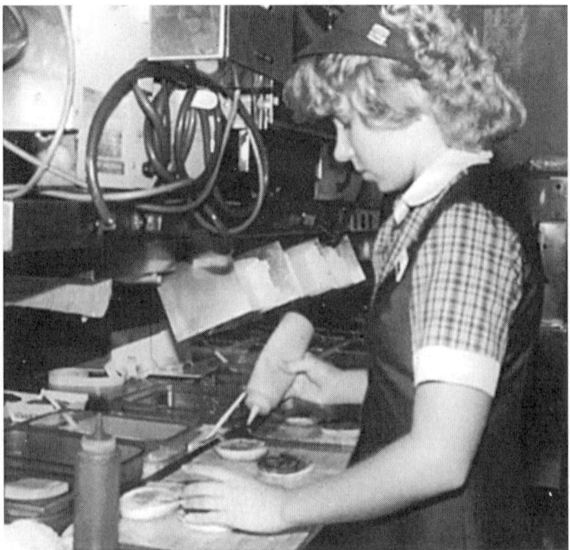

Figure 1–1. • The Fair Labor Standards Act of 1938 stipulates a minimum working age of 16 years.

BOX 1–1

THE CHILDREN'S CHARTER OF 1930

I. For every child spiritual and moral training to help him or her to stand firm under the pressure of life.

II. For every child understanding and the guarding of personality as a most precious right.

III. For every child a home and that love and security which a home provides; and for those children who must receive foster care, the nearest substitute for their own home.

IV. For every child full preparation for the birth, the mother receiving prenatal, natal, and postnatal care; and the establishment of such protective measures as will make child-bearing safer.

V. For every child protection from birth through adolescence, including: periodical health examinations and, where needed, care of specialists and hospital treatment; regular dental examinations and care of the teeth; protective and preventive measures against communicable diseases; the ensuring of pure food, pure milk, and pure water.

VI. For every child from birth through adolescence, promotion of health, including health instruction and health programs, wholesome physical and mental recreation, with teachers and leaders adequately trained.

VII. For every child a dwelling-place safe, sanitary, and wholesome, with reasonable provisions for privacy; free from conditions which tend to thwart development; and a home environment harmonious and enriching.

VIII. For every child a school which is safe from hazards, sanitary, properly equipped, lighted, and ventilated. For younger children nursery schools and kindergartens to supplement home care.

IX. For every child a community which recognizes and plans for needs; protects against physical dangers, moral hazards, and disease; provides safe and wholesome places for play and recreation; and makes provision for cultural and social needs.

X. For every child an education which, through the discovery and development of individual abilities, prepares the child for life and through training and vocational guidance prepares for a living which will yield the maximum of satisfaction.

XI. For every child such teaching and training as will prepare him or her for successful parenthood, home-making, and the rights of citizenship and, for parents, supplementary training to fit them to deal wisely with the problems of parenthood.

XII. For every child education for safety and protection against accidents to which modern conditions subject the child—those to which the child is directly exposed and those which, through loss or maiming of the parents, affect the child directly.

XIII. For every child who is blind, deaf, crippled, or otherwise physically handicapped and for the child who is mentally handicapped, such measures as will early discover and diagnose his handicap, provide care and treatment, and so train the child that the child may become an asset to society rather than a liability. Expenses of these services should be borne publicly where they cannot be privately met.

XIV. For every child who is in conflict with society the right to be dealt with intelligently as society's charge, not society's outcast; with the home, the school, the church, the court, and the institution when needed, shaped to return the child whenever possible to the normal stream of life.

XV. For every child the right to grow up in a family with an adequate standard of living and the security of a stable income as the surest safeguard against social handicaps.

XVI. For every child protection against labor that stunts growth, either physical or mental, that limits education, that deprives children of the right of comradeship, of play, and of joy.

XVII. For every rural child as satisfactory schooling and health services as for the city child, and an extension to rural families of social, recreational, and cultural facilities.

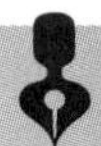

Nursing Tip

Two international organizations concerned with children are the United Nations Children's Fund (UNICEF) and the World Health Organization (WHO).

in the areas of education, health, welfare, and protection. This declaration has been widely distributed throughout the world.

The 1980 White House Conference on Families focused on involving the states at the grass-roots level. A series of statewide hearings was held to identify the most pressing problems of families in the various localities. A tremendous range of viewpoints on many subjects was shared, and specific recommendations were made.

In 1974 and 1975 the government passed the "Child Abuse Prevention and Treatment" Act. The "Education for All Handicapped Children" Act provides for support and public education of handicapped children. In 1982 the Community Mental Health Center was funded, and the "Missing Children's" Act was passed, providing a nationwide clearinghouse for missing children.

International Year of the Child

The year 1979 was designated as the International Year of the Child (IYC). Its purpose was to focus attention on the critical needs of the world's 1.5 billion children and to inspire the nations, the organizations, and the individuals of the world to consider how well they are providing for children (U.S. Commission of the International Year of the Child, 1980). At this time the United Nations reaffirmed the Declaration of the Rights of the Child (Box 1–2).

Public Health Department

The public health department assumes a great deal of responsibility for the prevention of disease and death during childhood. This is done on national, state, and local levels. The water, milk, and food supplies of communities are inspected. Maintenance of proper sewage and garbage disposal is enforced. Epidemics are investigated, and when necessary, persons capable of transmitting diseases are isolated. The public health department is also concerned with the inspection of housing.

Laws requiring the licensing of physicians and pharmacists indirectly affect the health of children and of the general public. Protection is also afforded by the Pure Food and Drug Act, which controls medicines, poisons, and the purity of foods. Programs for disaster relief, care and rehabilitation of handicapped children, foster child care, family counseling, family day care, protective services for abused or neglected children, and education of the public are maintained and supported by govern-

BOX 1–2

THE UNITED NATIONS DECLARATION OF THE RIGHTS OF THE CHILD

The general assembly proclaims that the child is entitled to a happy childhood and that all should recognize these rights and strive for their observance by legislative and other means:

1. All children without exception shall be entitled to these rights regardless of race, color, sex, language, religion, politics, national or social origin, property, birth, or other status.
2. The child should be protected so that he or she may develop physically, mentally, morally, spiritually, and socially in freedom and dignity.
3. The child is entitled at birth to a name and nationality.
4. The child is entitled to healthy development which includes adequate food, housing, recreation, and medical attention. He or she shall receive the benefits of Social Security.
5. The child who is handicapped physically, mentally, or emotionally shall receive treatment, education, and care according to his or her need.
6. The child is entitled to love and a harmonious atmosphere, preferably in the environment of his or her parents. Particular love, care, and concern need to be extended to children without families and to the poor.
7. The child is entitled to a free education and opportunities for play, recreation, and to develop his or her talents.
8. The child shall be the first one protected in times of adversity.
9. The child shall be protected against all forms of neglect, cruelty, and exploitation. He or she should not be employed in hazardous occupations or before the minimum age.
10. The child shall not be subjected to racial or religious discrimination. The environment should be peaceful and friendly.

Nursing Tip

The American Academy of Pediatrics (AAP), made up of pediatricians from across the nation, has established a position of leadership in setting health standards for children.

mental and private agencies. State licensing bureaus control the regulation of motor vehicles. Car seats for infants and children are currently mandatory. Protection of the public by law enforcement agencies is important because automobile accidents rank among the leading causes of injury and death in children.

THE PRESENT

Maternity Care

Significant changes have occurred in maternity care. In family-centered childbearing, the family is recognized as a unique system. Every family member is affected by the birth of a child. Family involvement during pregnancy and birth is seen as constructive and, indeed, necessary for bonding and support. To accommodate family needs, alternative birth centers, birthing rooms, rooming-in units, and mother–baby coupling have been developed. The whole sequence of events may take place in one suite of rooms. These arrangements are alternatives to the previously standard separate areas of labor and delivery, which made it necessary to transport a mother from one area to another and fragmented her care.

The three separate sections of the maternity unit have merged. The Labor-Delivery, Postpartum, and Newborn Nursery have become *Labor, Delivery, and Recovery (LDR) rooms.* The patient is not moved from one area to another, but receives care during labor and delivery and then remains in the same room to recover and care for her new infant. The rooms are often decorated to look homelike. Freestanding birthing centers outside the traditional hospital setting are popular with low-risk maternity patients. The birthing centers provide comprehensive care, including antepartum, labor-delivery, postpartum, mother's classes, lactation classes, and follow-up family planning. *Home births* utilizing midwives is not a current widespread practice because malpractice insurance is expensive and emergency equipment for unexpected complications is not available.

Cost containment has influenced maternity care by requiring the discharge of mother and newborn in 24 hours or less. As a result of problems that occurred, recent legislation mandates a 48-hour hospital stay for vaginal deliveries and 4 days for a cesarean section.

Clinical pathways, also known as critical pathways or care maps (multidisciplinary action plans), are collaborative guidelines that define multidisciplinary care in terms of outcomes within a timeline. A *variance* in the clinical pathway is the difference between the outcome expected and the outcome achieved. The patient may be discharged early or later than expected because of the variance. The care plan is adjusted accordingly. Sample clinical pathways are presented throughout the chapters.

Current maternity practice focuses on a high-quality family experience. *Childbearing is seen as a normal and healthy event.* Parents are prepared for the changes that take place during pregnancy, labor, and delivery. They are also prepared for the changes in family dynamics. Treating each family according to their individual needs is considered paramount.

During the 1950s the hospital stay for labor and delivery was 1 week. The current stay in uncomplicated cases is 2 days. Routine follow-up of the newborn takes place in about 2 weeks. A nurse visits the homes of infants and mothers who appear to be at high risk.

Procedural modifications for the nurse include the institution of universal (standard) precautions during delivery (see Appendix A), during umbilical cord care, and in the nursery. More emphasis on data entry and retrieval makes it necessary for personnel to be computer-literate.

Sociologically, families have become smaller, the number of single parents is increasing, child and spouse abuse is rampant, and more mothers must work to help support the family. These developments present special challenges to maternal and child health nurses. Careful assessment and documentation to detect abuse are necessary, and nurses must be familiar with community support services for women and children in need. Nurses must also be flexible and promote policies that make health care more available for working parents. Teaching

Nursing Tip

According to standards recommended by the American College of Obstetricians and Gynecologists (ACOG), pregnant women should ideally make about 13 prenatal visits over the course of a normal, full-term pregnancy.

must be integrated into care plans and individually tailored to the family's needs and its cultural and ethnic background.

Midwives

Throughout history, women have played an important role as birth attendants or *midwives.* The first school of nurse-midwifery opened in New York City in 1932. There are many accredited programs across the United States, all located in or affiliated with institutions of higher learning. The certified nurse-midwife (CNM) is a registered nurse who has graduated from an accredited midwife program and is nationally certified by the American College of Nurse-Midwives (Fig. 1–2). The CNM provides comprehensive prenatal and postnatal care and attends uncomplicated deliveries. Each patient must have a back-up physician who will accept her should a problem occur.

Role of the Consumer

Consumerism has played an important part in family-centered childbirth. In the early 1960s the natural childbirth movement awakened expectant parents to the need for education and involvement. Prepared childbirth, La Leche League (breastfeeding advocates), and Lamaze classes gradually became accepted. Parents began to question the routine use of anesthesia and the exclusion of fathers from delivery.

Today, a father's attendance at birth is commonplace. Visiting hours are liberal, and extended contact with the newborn is encouraged. The consumer continues to be an important instigator of change.

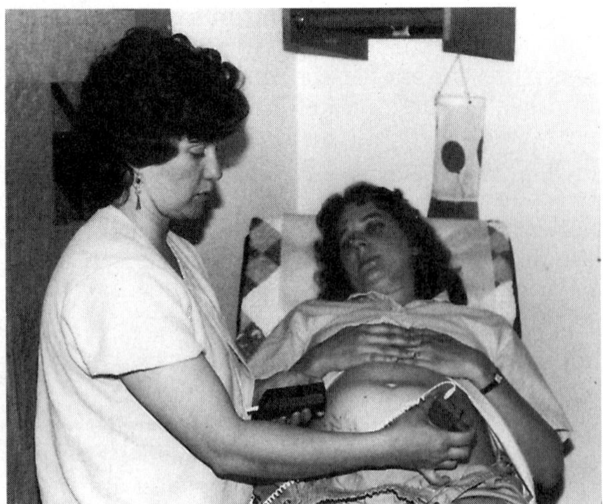

Figure 1–2. • The certified nurse-midwife provides comprehensive maternity care for her clients.

Consumer groups, with the growing support of professionals, are helping to revise restrictive policies once thought necessary for safety. It has been demonstrated that informed parents can make wise decisions about their own care during this period if they are adequately educated and given professional support.

Cross-Cultural Considerations

The cultural background of the expectant family strongly influences its adaptation to the birth experience. Nursing Care Plan 1–1 lists nursing interventions for selected diagnoses that pertain to cultural diversity. One way in which the nurse gains important information about an individual's culture is to *ask the pregnant woman* what she considers normal practice. A summary of assessment questions might be:

- How does the woman view her pregnancy (as an illness, a vulnerable time, or a healthy time)?
- Does she view the birth process as dangerous? Why?
- Is birth a public or private experience for her?
- In what position does she expect to deliver (i.e., squatting, lithotomy, or some other position)?
- What type of help does she need before and after delivery?
- What role does her immediate or extended family play in relation to the pregnancy and birth?

Such information helps to promote understanding and individualizes patient care. It also increases the satisfaction of patient and nurse with the quality of care provided. Cultural influences on nursing care are discussed in Chapter 21.

Child Care

The Pediatric Nurse as an Advocate

Pediatric nurses are increasingly assuming a role as child advocates. An advocate is a person who intercedes or pleads on behalf of another. Advocacy may be required for both the child's physical and emotional health and may include other family members. Hospitalized children frequently cannot determine or express their needs. When nurses feel that the child's best interests are not being met, they must seek assistance. This usually involves taking the problem through the normal chain of command. Nurses need to document their efforts to seek instruction and direction from their head nurse, supervisors, or the physician.

NURSING CARE PLAN 1–1

Selected Nursing Diagnoses: Care of Childbearing Families Related to Potential or Actual Stress Caused by Cultural Diversity

Nursing Diagnosis: Communication, impaired verbal related to language barriers

Goals	Nursing Interventions	Rationale
The woman will have an opportunity to share information and states she understands what is explained to her	1. Arrange for a family or staff member interpreter as needed	1. Interpreter can provide support for woman and help to lessen her anxieties; poor communication can result in time delays, errors, and misunderstanding of intent
	2. Clearly define instructions in woman's language of origin	2. A shared language is necessary for communication to take place
	3. Provide written instructions in woman's language wherever possible	3. Written instructions can be reviewed at a less stessful time by client; in some cases it is necessary to determine if person can read
	4. Explain the use and purpose of all instruments and equipment, along with the effects or possible effects on the mother and fetus	4. Education of family lessens anxiety and provides family with a sense of control
	5. Provide opportunities for clarification and questions	5. Learning takes time; repetition of important material promotes learning; nurse can determine woman's understanding of information and clarify misconceptions

Nursing Diagnosis: Family coping; compromised related to isolation, different customs, attitudes, or beliefs

Goals	Nursing Interventions	Rationale
Family members will state that they feel welcome and safe in the environment provided	1. Encourage prenatal classes and a visit to the maternity unit before delivery	1. Families who have clear, accurate information can better participate in labor and delivery; viewing the delivery setting before using it decreases anxiety about the unknown
	2. Inform families about routines, visiting hours, significant persons who can assist in labor and delivery, and location of newborn after delivery	2. Families have different expectations of the health care system; they may hesitate to ask questions because of shyness or fear of "losing face"
	3. Determine and respect practices and values of family and incorporate them into nursing care plans as much as possible	3. Clarification of culturally specific values and practices will avoid misunderstanding and conflict with the nurse's value system; nursing care plans promote organization of care and communication among staff members

Statistics

Statistics refers to the process of gathering and analyzing numeric data. Statistics concerning birth, death, and illness (morbidity) provide valuable information for determining or projecting the needs of a population or subgroup and for predicting trends. In the United States, vital statistics are compiled for the country as a whole by the National Center for Health Statistics and are published in its annual report, *Vital Statistics of the United States,* and in the pamphlet *Monthly Vital Statistics.* Reports in this field are also issued by the various state bureaus of vital statistics. Other independent agencies also supply statistics on various specialties.

A maternity nurse may use statistical data to become aware of reproductive trends, to determine populations at risk, to evaluate the quality of prenatal care, or to compare relevant information from state to state and country to country. Box 1–3 lists some terms used in gathering vital statistics.

Table 1–1 shows statistics that reveal more than half of all infant deaths were due to congenital anomalies, preterm status, sudden infant death syndrome (SIDS), and respiratory distress syndrome

BOX 1–3

COMMON VITAL STATISTICS TERMS

Birth rate: The number of live births per 1000 population in one year

Fertility rate: The number of births per 1000 women ages 15 to 44 yr in a given population

Maternal mortality rate: The number of maternal deaths per 100,000 live births that occurs as a direct result of pregnancy (includes the 42-day postpartum period)

Neonatal mortality: The number of deaths of infants less than 28 days of age per 1000 live births per year

Fetal mortality: The number of fetal deaths (fetuses weighing 500 g or more) per 1000 live births per year

Perinatal mortality: Includes both fetal and neonatal deaths per 1000 live births per year

Infant mortality rate: The number of deaths of infants under 1 year of age per 1000 live births per year

(RDS). The statistics show that the death rate from all causes has declined more than 44% between 1979 and 1996.

Table 1–2 shows the international infant mortality rates from various countries between 1993 and 1995. The statistics reveal that although the mortality rates for the United States have declined, the United States does *not* have the lowest death rate.

Table 1–3 shows the rate of low birth weight (LBW) newborns and infant mortality rates for states within the United States. These statistics reveal that the states with the highest LBW also have the highest infant mortality rates.

Technology

Technological advances have enabled many infants to survive that may have died some years ago. High-risk prenatal clinics and the neonatal intensive care unit enable the 1-pound preemie to have an opportunity to survive. Children with heart problems are now treated by a pediatric cardiologist. Much of the complex surgery needed by the newborn with a congenital defect is provided by the pediatric surgeon. Emotional problems are managed by pediatric psychiatrists. Many hospital laboratories are well equipped to test pediatric specimens. Chromosomal studies and biochemical screening have made identification and family counseling more significant than ever. The field of perinatal biology has advanced to the forefront of pediatric medicine.

The medical profession and allied agencies work as a team for the total well-being of the patient. Children with defects previously thought to be incompatible with life are taken to special diagnostic and treatment centers where they receive expert attention. Following discharge, many of these children are being cared for in their homes. The number of chronically disabled children is growing. Some are dependent on sophisticated hospital equipment such as ventilators and home monitors. The nursing care at home may require the suctioning of a tracheostomy, central line care, and other highly technical skills. Parents must be carefully educated and continually supported. Although this type of care is cost-effective and psychologically sound for the child, respite care is extremely important, because 24-hour-a-day care is extremely taxing for the family, both physically and psychologically.

The American Nurses Association (ANA) develops standards of care that serve as a guide to meet some current challenges. These standards are used when policies and procedures are established. Also, each state has a nurse practice act that determines the scope of practice for the registered nurse, practical nurse, and certified nurse assistant. These descriptions vary from state to state, so nurses must keep informed about the laws in the state where they are employed.

Health Care Delivery Systems

Cost containment is a major motivation in current health care, especially when health costs rise without decreases in morbidity and mortality. Many hospitals are merging to increase their buying power and reduce duplication of services.

Insurance reimbursement has become an important consideration in health care. The federal government has had to revise its Medicare and Medicaid programs. Among other changes it instituted *diagnosis-related groupings (DRGs).* These refer to a Medicare system that determines payment for a hospital stay based on the patient's diagnosis. This mandate has had a tremendous impact on health care delivery. Patients are being discharged earlier, and more care is being given in skilled nursing facilities and in the home. Some insurance companies are employing nurses in the role of case managers. Nurses remaining in institutions also may be required to assume the role of case managers and to become more flexible through cross training. Nurses are expected to be concerned with keeping hospital costs down while maintaining quality care. Many suggest that the future of nursing may depend on how well nurses can demonstrate their value and cost-effectiveness.

Health maintenance organizations (HMO) and *preferred provider organizations (PPO)* have emerged as alternative medical care delivery systems. Insurers and providers of care have united to hold costs down and yet remain competitive. A two-tiered system has evolved: one tier serves the more financially stable people (private insurance, HMO/PPO), and the other serves the less financially stable people (Medicare and Medicaid). In addition, a large percentage of persons are uninsured or underinsured. This presents problems in access and quality of health care. Box 1–4 defines managed care systems.

Health promotion continues to assume increased importance. Preventing illness or disability is cost-effective; more important, it saves the family from stress, disruptions, and financial burden. Healthy children are spending fewer days in the hospital. Many conditions are treated in same-day surgery, ambulatory settings, or emergency rooms. Rather than being distinct, hospital and home care have become interdependent.

Chronically ill children are living into adulthood, creating the need for more support services. Medically fragile and technology-dependent children may change the profile of chronically ill children. The nurse is often the instigator of support services to these patients through education and referral. Ideally these services will assist the child to become as independent as possible, to lead a productive life, and to be integrated into society. In the past, the term *mainstream* was used to describe the process of integration of a physically or mentally challenged child into society. The term *full inclusion,* an expansion of the mainstream policy, is being used more frequently today. Early infant intervention pro-

Table 1–1

INFANT DEATHS AND INFANT MORTALITY RATES FOR THE 10 LEADING CAUSES OF INFANT DEATH IN 1996, UNITED STATES, 1979, 1995, AND 1996

		1996			1995			1979			Percent Change
Cause of Death	Rank*	Number	Percent	Rate†	Number	Percent	Rate†	Number	Percent	Rate†	1979–1996
All causes	—	28245	100.0	721.5	29583	100.0	758.6	45665	100.0	1306.8	–44.8
Congenital anomalies	1	6463	22.9	165.1	6554	22.2	168.1	8923	19.5	255.4	–35.4
Disorders relating to short gestation and unspecified low birth weight	2	3706	13.1	94.7	3933	13.3	100.9	3495	7.7	100.0	–5.3
SIDS	3	2906	10.3	74.2	3397	11.5	87.1	5279	11.6	151.1	–50.9
Respiratory distress syndrome	4	1368	4.8	34.9	1454	4.9	37.3	5458	12.0	156.2	–77.7
Newborn affected by maternal complications of pregnancy	5	1212	4.3	31.0	1309	4.4	33.6	1621	3.5	46.4	–33.2
Newborn affected by complications of placenta, cord, and membranes	6	892	3.2	22.8	962	3.3	24.7	970	2.1	27.8	–18.0
Accidents and adverse effects	7	772	2.7	19.7	787	2.7	20.2	1080	2.4	30.9	–36.2
Infections specific to the perinatal period	8	747	2.6	19.1	788	2.7	20.2	981	2.1	28.1	–32.0
Pneumonia and influenza	9	485	1.7	12.4	492	1.7	12.6	1129	2.5	32.3	–61.6
Intrauterine hypoxia and birth asphyxia	10	429	1.5	11.0	475	1.6	12.2	1393	3.1	39.9	–72.4

*Rank based on number of deaths.
†Rate per 100,000 live births.
Note: 1996 data are preliminary; 1995 and 1979 data are final. In 1995, infections specific to the perinatal period was ranked seventh; accidents and adverse effects was eighth. In 1979, respiratory distress syndrome was ranked second; disorders relating to short gestation and unspecified low birth weight, fourth; newborn affected by complications of placenta, cord, and membranes, eleventh; accidents and adverse effects, ninth; infections specific to the perinatal period, tenth; pneumonia and influenza, seventh; and intrauterine hypoxia and birth asphyxia, sixth.
From American Academy of Pediatrics. (1997). Annual summary of vital statistics, 1996. *Pediatrics, 100*(6), 913.

Table 1–2

LIVE BIRTHS AND BIRTH RATES FOR 1995 OR 1996 AND INFANT MORTALITY RATES FOR 1993, 1994, AND 1995 FOR COUNTRIES OF 2,500,000 POPULATION AND WITH INFANT MORTALITY RATES EQUAL TO OR LESS THAN THE UNITED STATES IN 1993, 1994, OR 1995

			Infant Mortality Rate		
	Number of Births 1995 or 1996	Birth Rate 1995 or 1996	1993	1994	1995
Sweden	95,158	10.8	4.8	4.4	3.7
Finland	60,196	11.7	4.4	4.7	3.9
Singapore	48,738	16.0	4.7	4.3	4.0
Japan	1,203,000	9.6	4.3	4.2	4.3
Hong Kong	64,599	10.2	4.8	4.5	4.6
Switzerland	82,805	11.7	5.6	5.1	4.8*
France	734,000	12.6	6.5	6.1	4.9
Norway	60,664	13.8	5.0	5.2	—
Denmark	67,675	12.9	5.4	5.7	5.3
Germany	765,221†	9.4†	5.8	5.6	5.3
Netherlands	184,000	11.9	6.3	5.6	5.4*
Austria	87,823	10.8	6.5	6.3	5.5
Spain	352,200	9.0	6.7	7.2	5.6
Australia	256,190†	14.2†	6.1	5.9	5.7
Canada	375,680	12.5	6.3	6.2	6.1
Belgium	115,638†	11.4†	7.9	7.6	6.1
United Kingdom	732,049†	12.5†	6.3	6.2	6.2
Italy	521,346†	9.1†	7.2	6.6	6.2
Ireland	48,530†	13.5†	6.0	5.9	6.4
New Zealand	57,795†	16.3†	7.2	—	6.7
United States	3,914,953	14.8	8.4	8.0	7.6
Greece	101,500	9.7	8.5	7.9	7.9

*Rate reported is for 1996; no 1995 rate was located.
†Figures are for 1995.
Sources: United Nations Demographic Yearbook for 1996; United Nations Population and Vital Statistics Report, April 1, 1997, Series A Vol. XLIX, No. 2; and Population Reference Bureau (1994 figures for Norway and France).
From American Academy of Pediatrics. (1997). Annual summary of vital statistics, 1996. *Pediatrics, 100*(6), 914.

grams for children with developmental disabilities attempt to reduce or minimize the effects of the disability. These services may be provided in a clinic or in the home. The need for in-home family-centered pediatric care will continue to grow with the number of children with chronic illness who survive.

Quality of life is particularly relevant. Organ transplants have saved some children; however, the complications, limited availability, and expense of these transplants create moral and ethical dilemmas. Older children with life-threatening conditions need to be included in planning modified advance directives with their families and the medical team.

These developments, along with the explosion of information, emphasis on individual nurse accountability, new technology, and the use of computers in medicine, make it especially desirable for nurses to maintain their knowledge and skills at a level necessary to provide safe care. Employers

BOX 1–4

MEDICAL CARE DELIVERY SYSTEM

Managed care. Integrates financing with health care for members. For a monthly "capitation" fee, contracts with physicians and hospitals to provide health care with strict utilization review for cost containment
HMO. A health maintenance organization that offers health services for a fixed premium
PPO. A preferred provider organization contracts with providers for services on a discounted fee-for-service basis for members
Utilization review. Reviews appropriateness of health care services and guidelines for doctors for treatment of illness, controlling management of care to achieve cost containment

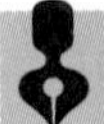

Nursing Tip

Expanded nursing roles include the clinical nurse specialist, the pediatric nurse practitioner, the school nurse practitioner, the family practitioner, and the certified nurse-midwife.

Table 1–3
INFANT MORTALITY RATES AND PERCENT OF LOW BIRTH WEIGHT (LBW) BY RACE FOR THE UNITED STATES AND EACH STATE, 1995

	LBW*			Infant Mortality		
State	All Races†	White	Black	All Races†	White	Black
United States	7.3	6.2	13.1	7.6	6.3	15.1
Alabama	9.0	7.1	13.0	9.8	7.1	15.2
Alaska	5.3	5.1	12.4	7.7	6.1	‡
Arizona	6.8	6.6	13.1	7.5	7.2	17.0
Arkansas	8.2	6.8	13.1	8.8	7.2	14.3
California	6.1	5.5	12.0	6.3	5.8	14.4
Colorado	8.4	8.0	15.9	6.5	6.0	16.8
Connecticut	7.1	6.3	12.7	7.2	6.5	12.6
Delaware	8.4	7.0	12.9	7.5	6.0	13.1
District of Columbia	13.4	5.6	15.9	16.2	‡	19.6
Florida	7.7	6.4	12.1	7.5	6.0	13.0
Georgia	8.8	6.5	13.1	9.4	6.5	15.1
Hawaii	7.0	5.3	11.1	5.8	‡	‡
Idaho	5.9	5.8	‡	6.1	5.8	‡
Illinois	7.9	6.1	14.5	9.4	7.2	18.7
Indiana	7.5	6.9	13.0	8.4	7.3	17.5
Iowa	6.0	5.8	11.1	8.2	7.8	21.2
Kansas	6.4	5.9	12.2	7.0	6.2	17.6
Kentucky	7.6	7.1	12.8	7.6	7.4	10.7
Louisiana	9.7	6.7	14.0	9.8	6.2	15.3
Maine	6.1	6.0	‡	6.5	6.3	‡
Maryland	8.5	6.2	13.5	8.9	6.0	15.3
Massachusetts	6.3	5.9	10.4	5.2	4.7	9.0
Michigan	7.7	6.3	14.0	8.3	6.2	17.3
Minnesota	5.9	5.5	12.1	6.7	6.0	17.6
Mississippi	9.8	7.0	13.0	10.5	7.0	14.7
Missouri	7.6	6.5	14.1	7.4	6.4	13.8
Montana	5.8	5.9	‡	7.0	7.0	‡
Nebraska	6.3	6.0	12.0	7.4	7.3	‡
Nevada	7.4	6.7	13.6	5.7	5.5	‡
New Hampshire	5.5	5.5	‡	5.5	5.5	‡
New Jersey	7.6	6.2	13.1	6.6	5.3	13.3
New Mexico	7.5	7.7	10.5	6.2	6.1	‡
New York	7.6	6.4	12.4	7.7	6.2	13.9
North Carolina	8.7	6.8	13.8	9.2	6.7	15.9
North Dakota	5.3	5.1	‡	7.2	6.7	‡
Ohio	7.6	6.5	13.9	8.7	7.3	17.5
Oklahoma	7.0	6.4	12.5	8.3	8.0	15.1
Oregon	5.5	5.4	10.3	6.1	5.9	‡
Pennsylvania	7.4	6.2	14.2	7.8	6.2	17.6
Rhode Island	6.8	6.3	11.3	7.2	7.0	‡
South Carolina	9.3	6.8	13.7	9.6	6.7	14.6
South Dakota	5.6	5.5	‡	9.5	7.9	‡
Tennessee	8.7	7.2	14.0	9.3	6.8	17.9
Texas	7.1	6.4	12.2	6.5	5.9	11.7
Utah	6.3	6.2	10.7	5.4	5.3	‡
Vermont	5.4	5.4	‡	6.0	6.2	‡
Virginia	7.7	6.1	12.9	7.8	5.7	15.3
Washington	5.5	5.2	11.1	5.9	5.6	16.2
West Virginia	7.9	7.6	16.5	7.9	7.6	‡
Wisconsin	6.0	5.1	13.7	7.3	6.3	18.6
Wyoming	7.4	7.3	‡	7.7	6.8	‡

*Percent of births less than 2500 g.
†Includes races other than white and black.
‡Figure does not meet standards of reliability or precision.
Note: Rates per 1000 live births in specified group. Live births based on race of mother.
Source: National Center for Health Statistics, National Vital Statistics System, 1995. From American Academy of Pediatrics. (1997). Annual summary of vital statistics, 1996. *Pediatrics, 100*(6), 915.

often offer continuing education classes for their employees. Most states require proof of continuing education for renewal of nursing licenses.

Advanced Practice Nurses

In keeping with the current practice of focusing on prevention of illness and maintenance of health rather than the treatment of illness, the specialty of *pediatric nurse practitioner (PNP)* was born. The PNP provides ambulatory and primary care for clients. The school nurse, oncology nurse, or child life specialist expands the accessibility of preventative health care to the well child.

Clinical nurse specialists (CNS) provide care in the hospital or community to specific specialty patients, such as cardiac, neurologic, or oncologic care. They conduct primary research and facilitate necessary changes in health care management. Often the PNP and the CNS are called *advanced practice nurses,* and they have an RN as well as an advanced degree. Advance practice nurses can specialize in OB or pediatrics.

Nursing Process

The nursing process was developed in 1963 and referred to a series of steps describing the systematic problem-solving approach nurses used to identify, prevent, or treat actual or potential health problems. In 1973 the American Nurses Association (ANA) developed standards relating to this nursing process that have been nationally accepted and include:

- *Assessment.* Collection of patient data, both subjective and objective
- *Diagnosis.* Analysis of data in terms of North American Nursing Diagnosis Association (NANDA) Nursing Diagnoses (Appendix C)
- *Outcome identification.* Identification of individualized expected patient outcomes
- *Planning.* Preparation of a plan of care designed to achieve stated outcomes
- *Implementation.* Carrying out of interventions identified in the plan of care
- *Evaluation.* Evaluation of outcome progress and redesigning plan if necessary

The nursing process is a framework of action designed to meet the individual needs of patients. It is problem oriented and goal directed and involves the use of critical thinking, problem solving, and decision making. The nursing process is expressed in an individualized nursing care plan. Diagnoses approved by NANDA are found in Appendix C. Table 1–4 differentiates between medical and nursing diagnoses.

Table 1–4
COMPARISON OF MEDICAL AND NURSING DIAGNOSES

Medical Diagnosis	Nursing Diagnosis
AIDS	Nutrition: less than body requirements related to anorexia and evidenced by weight loss
Gestational diabetes	Knowledge deficit related to effects of diabetes mellitus on pregnant woman and fetus, manifested by crying, anxiety
Cystic fibrosis	Ineffective airway clearance related to mucus accumulation manifested by rales, fatigue

Nursing Care Plans

The nursing care plan is developed as a result of the nursing process. It is a written instrument of communication among staff members that focuses on individualized patient care. Sample care plans for maternity and pediatric nursing are provided throughout the text.

THE FUTURE

Health Care Reform

The federal government is working to provide a health care reform plan that will reduce the cost of health care while making it more accessible to all. Nurses are involved in the health care reform movement as patient advocates, to ensure that the patient receives quality care. Health insurance plays an important role in health care delivery. Having health insurance does not ensure access to expensive care, as the insurance company often must "approve" the expenditure before the test or care is provided. Those families who cannot afford health insurance often do not seek preventative health care, such as prenatal care, or infant immunizations, and well-baby check-ups. These problems must be dealt with as health care reform evolves. Managed care and utilization review committees who review the appropriateness of health care services impact the management of patients by physicians. Continued study is needed to determine the effect of managed care on quality and cost containment of health care.

The future role of the nurse will involve providing health care in a variety of settings and working closely with the multidisciplinary health care team. The nurse will function as a caregiver, teacher, collaborator, advocate, manager and researcher. Competence in care and accountability to the patient, family, community, and profession are core responsibilities of the nurse entering the twenty-first century.

The revolution in medical care involves the conflict between cost containment and quality care. When health care became big business, cost containment was born and managed care was the result. Managed care openly evaluates care given and, in the right environment, can result in increased quality. Quality assurance committees are investigating the routine management of patients, especially in the area of preventative care and tests. Nurses will take a key role in the forming the health care picture of tomorrow.

Healthy People 2000

Healthy People 2000 is a statement of national health promotion and disease prevention objectives facilitated by the federal government. The objectives are designed to utilize the vast knowledge and technology of health care that was developed in the 20th century to improve the health and quality of life of Americans in the 21st century. The report identifies objectives in broad categories of effort: health promotion, health protection, preventative services, and the development of surveillance and data systems. The specific goals include increasing the span of healthy life, reducing health disparities among Americans, and achieving access to preventative care for all Americans. Some priority areas include maternal and infant health, immunizations, prevention of sexually transmitted diseases, oral health, nutrition, and physical fitness. It is a "vision for the new century" to achieve a nation of healthy people. An example of the specific contribution of the school nurse to the concept of *Healthy People 2000* is described in Box 1–5.

BOX 1–5

AN EXAMPLE OF THE SPECIFIC CONTRIBUTIONS OF THE SCHOOL NURSE TO THE CONCEPT OF HEALTHY PEOPLE 2000

The expanding role of the school nurse will include:

1. Reviewing participation in and effectiveness of physical education programs for normal and disabled students
2. Providing nutritional education and guidance
3. Supervising school nutrition programs
4. Participating in maintaining a drug- and tobacco-free environment for students
5. Providing education in prevention of sexually transmitted diseases
6. Providing guidance to students and staff concerning prevention of injuries
7. Providing oral health education
8. Providing age-appropriate HIV education
9. Reviewing immunization laws and records
10. Assessing the community needs in relation to the child population and reassessing/revising roles in relation to prevention, screening, monitoring, teaching, and follow-up of health needs or problems

Documentation

Documentation, or charting, has always been a legal responsibility of the nurse. When a medication is given or a treatment is performed, it is accurately documented on the patient's chart. Charting responsibilities also include head-to-toe assessment of the patient and a recording of data pertinent to the diagnosis and response to treatment. There have been many forms of charting required by different hospitals in different areas of the country that guide the nurse toward comprehensive charting. A traditional problem has been with several members of the multidisciplinary health care team accessing the chart at the same time. When the nurse was recording a medication administered, the medication record was "tied-up" until the recording was complete. When a doctor was reviewing the chart and progress of the patient, the records were "tied-up" until the conference was completed. With the advent of computers, computerized charting will shortly be fine-tuned and utilized by all hospitals in the country. Computerized charting is a paperless method of charting that may be accomplished with a wireless pad and an electronic pen. Security features are usually built-in and prompts encourage accurate and comprehensive charting by "forcing" certain entries before the user can progress through the system. Critical ranges can be programmed into the computer so the nurse is "alerted" to deviations from the norm as information is recorded. Using computerized charting, all caregivers have access to patient records on all patients at all times from a variety of locations. The adaptation and application of computerized programs to the hospital setting should motivate all nurses to become *basically* computer literate.

Community-Based Nursing

Nursing care within the community and in the home is not a new concept in maternal child nursing. The work of Lillian Wald, founder of the Henry Street Settlement, brought home health care to poor children. Margaret Sanger's work as a Public Health Nurse accessed care for poor pregnant women and was the seed for the development of modern planned parenthood programs. The community is now the major health care setting for all clients, and the challenge is to provide safe, caring, cost-effective, quality care to mothers, infants, and families. This challenge involves the nurse as a patient advocate to influence government, business, and the community to recognize the need for supporting preventative care of maternal-infant clients to ensure a healthy population for the future. The nurse must work with the interdisciplinary health care team to identify needs within the community and create cost-effective approaches to comprehensive preventative and therapeutic care. The role of the nurse as an educator within the community is facilitated by the use of schools, churches, health fairs, computer web sites, and the media. Some registered nurses are branching out into the community as private practitioners, such as lactation consultants for new mothers. The nursing care plan is expanding to become a *family care plan* as the nurse is providing care to the client in the home. Creativity; problem solving; coordination of multidisciplinary caregivers; case management; assessment and referral are just some of the essential skills required of a nurse providing community-based care to maternal-infant clients.

Preventative care is only one aspect of current and future home care–community-based nursing. Therapeutic care is also provided in the home setting, and the nurse must educate the family concerning the monitoring, care and need for professional referral when necessary. Specialized care such as fetal monitoring of high-risk pregnant women, apnea monitoring of high-risk newborns, diabetic glucose monitoring, heparin therapy, and total parenteral nutrition can be safely accomplished in the home setting often with computer or telephone accessibility to a nurse manager.

The home health care team, as advocated by the American Academy of Pediatrics Committee on Children with Disabilities includes a pediatrician, nurses, occupational, physical and respiratory therapists, speech therapists, home teachers, social workers, and home health aids. The American Academy of Home Health Care Physicians demonstrates a medical commitment to the concept of home care for the future.

Alternative Health Care Practices

The 1990s have brought a change in the focus of health care, moving the patient from the hospital into the home. As nurses enter this new health care environment within the community, they will no longer be surrounded by familiar equipment, practices, and support personnel. Instead, nurses will encounter some *alternative health care* practices involving clients that want increasing control over their health problems, need to be a part of the decision-making process, and want to incorporate cultural beliefs and traditions in their care. The client, in addition to accepting treatment prescribed by a traditional medical doctor, may also be consulting other healing authorities, such as holistic practitioners, naturopaths, and nutritional consultants (Fig. 1–3). Food therapy, vitamin and mineral supplements, herbal therapy, and acupressure are common forms of alternative therapies practiced in many homes. Box 1–6 lists popular folk healers.

Recent studies have shown that 34% of adults in the United States have used alternative health care therapies. Of 2055 children attending an ambulatory clinic, 11% had previously been treated by alternative health care practitioners. Nurses need to be well informed about the use and validity of alternative health care therapies. Although nurses do not advocate or discourage the use of such health care practices, knowledge of various types of alternative therapies can aid the nurse in identifying a contraindication or an interaction with traditional medicine that may be prescribed for the child. The hospital setting is somewhat of a controlled environment, but nursing care in the home brings new challenges.

Overview of Common Alternative Health Care Practices

An underlying premise of alternate healing techniques is that symptoms are the result of a problem in the body that may not be related to the

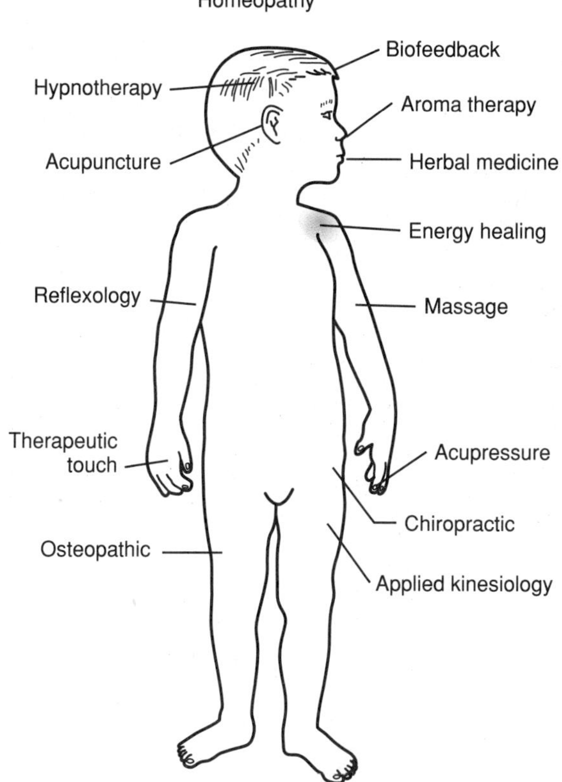

Figure 1–3. • Alternative health care.

specific symptom manifested. The body is thought to have a self-healing ability that can be aided by spinal manipulation or energy manipulation. Soft-tissue massage is thought to bolster the immune response. Fascia pressure, stretching and manipulation *(rolfing)* is thought to improve muscle and bone function. Neuromuscular massage relieves muscle tension and trigger points of pain and generally improves circulation.

Osteopaths combine manipulative therapy with traditional (allopathic) medicine. Pressure point therapy is based on the theory that certain areas of the body are connected to specific identified pressure points on the feet, hands, ears, and others. It is believed that channels conduct vital energy through the body.

Energy healing involves the belief that an electromagnetic flow emerges from the therapist's hands and can funnel energy into the patient. Some believe that repatterning a patient's own energy field can aid in healing. The body, mind, spirit, and emotions are usually involved in this type of therapy. Massage therapy is often used for children with asthma, arthritis, and eating disorders. Gentle touch massage therapy has been shown to have positive effects on premature infants.

Massage and manipulative therapy is contraindicated in patients with cancer, osteoporosis, localized infection, and cardiac and circulatory disorders. Children with Down's syndrome are particularly prone to cervical spine anomalies and may be injured by manual therapy. Children who have a history of sexual abuse do not usually respond favorably to touch therapy.

The role of the nurse in counseling a patient who demonstrates an interest in alternative therapies is to determine that no obvious contraindications exist and discuss positive and negative aspects. Alternative medical treatment does have the ability to increase the patient's sense of self-control over their bodies. As long as the alternative treatment does not replace proven traditional methods of treatment, the patient can be encouraged to try a combined approach. Some herbal remedies (e.g., St. John's wort) are currently undergoing structured medical trials to prove or disprove their medical value.

Homeopathy. Homeopathy accounts for approximately 25% of pediatric visits to alternative health practitioners. Homeopathy uses plants, herbs, and earth minerals that are thought to stimulate the body's immune system to deal with specific health problems. Only one remedy is administered at a time, and minimum dosage is the principle of most practitioners. The homeopathic philosophy involves belief that disease is an energy imbalance and remedies prescribed assist the body to reestablish correct balance. Homeopathic remedies are taken sublingually and should not be combined with caffeine, alcohol, or traditional medications. Some homeopathic medicines are alcohol-based and some contain mercury or arsenic bases that can cause toxicity or allergic responses in children.

Ayurveda. *Ayurveda* is an ancient Indian healing regime that deals with biological rhythms of nature and can include music, herbs, massage, aromatherapy and a diet tailored to the specific body type.

Aromatherapy. *Aromatherapy* is an ancient practice involving condensed fluid or essence of specific

BOX 1–6

POPULAR CULTURAL FOLK HEALERS

Mexican. Curanderos
African-American. Root doctor
Asian and Chinese. Herbalist
Puerto Rican. Espiritistas or santiguadoras
Navajo. Singers

BOX 1–7

COMMON HERBS, THEIR USES AND CAUTIONS

Aloe vera has been widely researched and has proven antibacterial and antiinflammatory topical effects. However it can cause gastrointestinal upset if taken internally. An aloe extract is currently under study for use in HIV and other viral illnesses.

Bilbery is an antioxident that is thought to lower cholesterol and treat nightblindness. The leaves may be toxic with prolonged use.

Chamomile, or manzanilla, tea is used worldwide to calm infants with colic. It has antiinflammatory and sedative effects and is used widely in aromatherapy. Chamomile has also been shown to have mood-elevating effects. Use cautiously if allergic to ragweed.

Chaparral, or greasebush, is used to retard aging and improve skin conditions. The herb is toxic to the liver and should not be used for children.

Coltsfoot is used for coughs but is toxic to the liver.

Echinacea boosts the immune system, has an antiinflammatory effect and enhances wound healing. It is used extensively for snakebites. The product is currently being researched and appears harmless.

Ephedra (Ma Huang) is used for asthma, as a decongestant, and central nervous system stimulant. It is also sold as "ecstasy" and used with other illegal stimulants to create a euphoric feeling. It can cause hypertension, anxiety, and toxic psychosis. Overdoses can be deadly. Ephedra can cause uterine contractions in pregnant women.

Feverfew is used to treat migraine headaches and arthritis. Rebound headaches can occur if it is stopped suddenly. Tachycardia and dermatitis can occur.

Ginko is thought to improve blood flow, but should not be taken with blood thinners, warfarin, vitamin E, or fish oils.

Golden seal is used to treat acne, conjunctivitis, dehydration, skin rashes, colds, diarrhea, and Giardia infections. It can increase cardiac output and cause hypertension and uterine contractions. In infants less than 1 month old, hyperbilirubinemia may result.

Jin Bu Huan is used to relieve pain. It depresses the heart rate and can cause respiratory problems.

Kombucha, or kargasok tea, is a fungus that can cause metabolic acidosis. Used for children with cancer, multiple sclerosis, and to prevent aging.

Licorice is used to treat asthma and stomach maladies. It can cause water retention and potassium depletion and should not be used if kidney, heart disease, or hypertension exists.

Melatonin is used as a sleep aid. It may have side effects such as headaches, depression, and hypothermia.

Osha is used to treat colds and flu. It should not be used during pregnancy and lactation due to antispasmodic effect.

St. John's wort is used as an antidepressant. Some recent studies may implicate photosensitivity or ileus as a complication of long-term use.

Siete Jarabes is a combination of sweet almond, castor oil, licorice, honey, and other ingredients that have a cathartic and expectorant effect. It is often used for asthma and congestion. May have laxative or hypertensive side effects.

Tea tree oil is used to treat wounds and skin infections but can cause muscle incoordination if taken internally or irritate tissue if applied to open wounds.

Yohimbe is considered to be an aphrodisiac and a body builder. It can cause seizures and kidney failure.

herbs that are combined with steams or baths to inhale or bathe the skin. Essential oils are concentrated and, if undiluted, are usually used in 2- to 5-drop doses. Often a few drops of the herbal oil is added to soaps or regular lotions immediately before use. Concentrated oils are volatile and must be freshly prepared. Eucalyptus oil, peppermint oil, and aloe vera are the most commonly used preparations for various physical and psychological benefits.

Hypnotherapy. The patient enters a hypnotic trance and under the guidance of the practitioner specific suggestions are given to the patient that can be long-lasting. Smoking cessation and pain control have been successfully achieved using this method. Some patient's resist the trance state and are not candidates for hypnotherapy.

Guided Imagery. The ancient Greeks believed the mind could influence the body and asking the patient to focus on a specific image can result in reduction of stress and increased performance.

Biofeedback. *Biofeedback* is a type of relaxation therapy that enables the patient to recognize tension in the muscles via responses on an electronic machine and visual electromyography responses. The process is used by traditional medical doctors for drug addiction and chronic pain control.

Reflexology. *Reflexology* deals with reflex points in the hands and feet that are thought to correspond to every organ or part of the body. Massaging these reflex points can relieve specific problems.

Acupuncture/Acupressure. *Acupuncture* is an ancient oriental practice that works on the principle that the body has complex meridians that are pathways to specific organs or parts of the body. "Chi" energy is thought to regulate proper body function, and acupuncture or acupressure is applied to restore a balance of chi energy. In acupuncture, hair-thin needles are applied to specific meridians and may stimulate nerve cells to release endorphins.

Acupressure uses finger pressure and massage on the meridian sites rather than needles. Acupuncture and acupressure have achieved popularity in the Western world, and many doctors, as well as patients, advocate combining these practices with conventional medicine, especially for chronic pain or maladies.

Herbal Remedies. The World Health Organization (WHO) reports that herbal remedies are frequently used worldwide and are first-line treatment for most children in Third World countries. *Herbal medicine* has been used for thousands of years in many countries. Herbs are powerful nutritional agents, and most are safe to ingest. Occasionally an allergic-type reaction is encountered, possibly because of differences in processing or storing the product. Herbal products are sold in stores, but the growth, processing, storage, and prescription are not regulated as they are for traditional drugs. There are general guidelines for their use, however, including dosages and recommendations that herbal mixtures are preferred to single-herb products.

Many current medications are related to herbal remedies. Digitalis originates from foxglove, opiates from poppy flowers, and quinine from the chin chova trees. However, some herbs can be fatal to children (Ephedra). Herbal remedies consumed during pregnancy can reach the fetus. Breastfeeding mothers who use herbal remedies can pass the substance to their nursing infants. Home-grown herbs, such as chamomile used for tea, can be contaminated with botulism. Taking time to elicit an accurate history from parents may reveal their practice of using herbal remedies for the family. Box 1–7 lists common herbs popular in the United States, their uses and cautions.

Herbal capsules are about four times stronger than herbal teas, and *herbal extracts* are about four to eight times stronger than capsules. Most extracts should not be taken longer than 6 consecutive days. *Herbal tinctures* contain a high amount of alcohol and are not often recommended. *Herbal baths* are relaxing and soothing, and herbal salves, oils, compresses, and poultices use the skin as the body's organ of ingestion. Most practitioners emphasize that herbal dosage is determined by body weight and that mega doses can be harmful.

Chiropractic Care. Chiropractors account for 36% of pediatric alternative medical care visits. The chiropractor works on the belief that as almost every nerve in the body enters the spinal canal, varied illnesses can be the result of spinal subluxation. Manipulation of the spine via a handheld "activator" delivers a controlled thrust to a problem area and re-aligns the spine. Most chiropractors also use massage, diet, nutritional, and enzyme therapy for a more comprehensive approach. Chiropractors offer well baby care by preventative manipulation. Its effectiveness has not been proven by research studies.

Sauna/Heat Therapy. Overheating the body has long been used to speed up metabolism and inhibit replication of viruses and bacteria. The sweating that results from the sauna is thought to help eliminate body waste. Patient should monitor their pulse during treatment. Some conditions can inhibit the ability to perspire and heat can adversely affect the cardiac status of some clients. Therefore, medical guidance should be sought before using this type of therapy.

Nursing Tip

Some Herbal Products That Can Be Dangerous to infants

Chaparral
Germander (lamiaceae)
Pennyroyal oil
Ephedra
Goldenseal

KEY POINTS

- In 1840 Ignaz Semmelweis suggested that handwashing was an important concept in preventing infection. This simple procedure is still a cornerstone of nursing care.
- The cultural background of the expectant family plays an important role in their adaptation to the birth experience.
- The educational focus for the childbearing family is that childbirth is a normal and healthy event.
- *Statistics* refers to gathering and analyzing numeric data.
- *Birth rate* refers to the number of live births per 1000 population in 1 year.
- In the United States vital statistics are compiled for the country as a whole by the national Center for Health Statistics.
- The nursing process consists of five steps: assessment, nursing diagnosis, planning, implementation, and evaluation. It is an organized method of nursing practice and a means of communication among staff members.
- The culture of a society has a strong influence on family and child care.
- Lillian Wald, a nurse, is credited with suggesting the establishment of the Children's Bureau.
- The Fair Labor Standards Act, passed in 1938, controls child labor.
- The White House Conferences on Children and Youth investigated and reported on matters pertaining to children and their families among all classes of people.
- The Children's Charter of 1930 is considered one of the most important documents in child care history.
- The United Nations Declaration of the Rights of the Child calls for freedom, equality of opportunity, social and emotional benefits, and enhancement of each child's potential.
- The American Nurses Association (ANA) has written standards of maternal-child health practices.
- Diagnosis-related groups (DRG), a form of cost containment, continue to affect nursing practice.
- Advanced practice nurses are registered nurses with advanced degrees who specialize, manage care, and conduct research.
- LDR rooms provide family-centered birthing and promote early parent–infant bonding.
- Clinical pathways are collaborative guidelines that define multidisciplinary care in terms of outcomes within a timeline.
- The nursing care plan is a written instrument of communication that uses the nursing process to formulate a plan of care for a specific patient. It utilizes nursing diagnosis and involves critical thinking and problem solving.
- *Healthy People 2000* is a statement of national health promotion that is a vision for the new century. The objectives are designed to utilize 20th-century technology and knowledge to improve health care and quality of life in the 21st century.
- Charting is the legal responsibility of the nurse and includes a head-to-toe assessment and data pertinent to the diagnosis and response of the patient to treatment.
- Home health care involves therapy, monitoring, teaching, and referral.
- The nurse must understand the culture and tradition of the family and their influence on health practices.
- Nurses need to be well informed about the use and validity of alternative health care therapies and understand potential interactions with prescribed medication and treatments.
- Utilization Review Committees, Quality Assurance Committees, the American Academy of Pediatrics Committee on Children with Disabilities, the American Academy of Home Care Physicians, and the Association of Women's Obstetric and Neonatal Nurses (AWHONN) are some of the organizations that set and maintain standards of maternity and pediatric care.

MULTIPLE-CHOICE REVIEW QUESTIONS

Choose the most appropriate answer.

1. The number of deaths of infants younger than 28 days of age per 1000 live births is termed
   a. birth rate.
   b. neonatal birth rate.
   c. neonatal morbidity rate.
   d. neonatal mortality rate.
2. The man known as the father of pediatrics is
   a. Benjamin Spock.
   b. Hippocrates.
   c. John Semmelweis.
   d. Abraham Jacobi.
3. An organization that sets standards of care for maternity and pediatric nursing is the
   a. American Medical Association.
   b. American Nurses Association.
   c. Utilization Review Committee.
   d. American Academy of Pediatrics.
4. One of the most important documents in child care history formulated by the White House Conference was the
   a. Fair Labor Practice Act.
   b. The Children's Charter.
   c. Missing Children's Clearinghouse.
   d. Education for Handicapped Children Act.
5. The nurse should communicate to parents that herbal medicines sold over-the-counter
   a. are harmless to children.
   b. are effective substitutes for traditional medication.
   c. can interact with prescribed medications and produce adverse effects.
   d. should never be given to children.

BIBLIOGRAPHY AND READER REFERENCE

Alschuler, L., & Benjamen, S. (1997). Herbal medicine: What works, what's safe. *Patient Care, 31*(16), 48.

Bakerink, J., Gaspe, S., Jr., Dimand, R., et al. (1996). Multiple organ failure after ingestion of pennyroyal oil from herbal tea in two infants. *Pediatrics, 98,* 944.

Behrman, K., Kleigman, K., & Arvin, A. (1996). *Nelson's textbook of pediatrics.* Philadelphia: Saunders.

Berkowitz, C. (1996). *Pediatrics: A primary care approach.* Philadelphia: Saunders.

Bower, P., Rubik, B., & Weiss, S. (1997). Manual therapy: Hands-on healing. *Patient Care,* 69(31).

Committee on Children with Disabilities. (1995). Guidelines for Home Care of Infants, Children and Adolescents with Chronic Disease. *Pediatrics,* (1995) *96*(1), 161.

Cookfair, J. (1996). *Nursing care in the community* (2nd ed.) St Louis, MO: Mosby.

Goldberg, A., Gardner, H. E., & Gibson, L. E. (1994). Home care: The next frontier of pediatric practice. *Journal of Pediatrics, 125,* 686.

Gray, M. (1996). Herbs: Multicultural folk medicines. *Orthopaedic Nursing, 15*(2), 49.

U.S. Department Health and Human Services (1991). *Healthy People 2000.* DHHS Publication # (PHS) 91-50213. Washington, DC: Government Printing Office.

Keegan, L. (1998). Getting comfortable with alternative and complementary therapies. *Nursing* 98, *28*(4), 50.

Kemper, K. J. (1996). *The holistic pediatrician comprehensive guide to safe and effective therapies for the 25 most common childhood ailments.* New York: Harper Perennial.

Kemper, K. J. (1996). Seven herbs every pediatrician should know. *Contemporary Pediatrics, 13*(12), 79.

Kornfeld, J. (1997). Managed care from my perspective. *Hospital Practice, 32*(6), 45–52.

Murray, M. (1995). *The healing power of herbs.* Rocklin, CA: Prima Publisher.

National Association for Home Care. (1995). *Basic statistics about home care.* Washington, DC: NAHC.

Pachter, L. (1997). Practicing culturally sensitive pediatrics. *Contemporary Pediatrics, 14*(9), 139.

Rector-Page, L. (1996). *Healthy healing, an alternative healing reference,* 10th ed. Sierra, CA: Healthy Healing Publications.

Samson, W., & London, W. (1995). Analysis of homeopathic treatment of childhood diarrhea. *Pediatrics, 96,* 961.

Schuman, A. (1997). Home sweet home: The best place for pediatric care. *Contemporary Pediatrics, 14*(3), 79–104.

Spigelblatt, L. (1997). Alternative medicine, a pediatric conundrum. *Contemporary Pediatrics, 14*(8), 57.

Wilkinson, J. (1996). *Nursing process, a critical thinking approach.* Reading, MA: Addison-Wesley.

chapter 2

Human Reproductive Anatomy and Physiology

Outline

PUBERTY

MALE REPRODUCTIVE SYSTEM
- External Genitalia
- Internal Genitalia

FEMALE REPRODUCTIVE SYSTEM
- External Genitalia
- Internal Genitalia
- Female Pelvis
- Breasts
- Female Reproductive Cycle and Menstruation

Objectives

On completion and mastery of Chapter 2, the student will be able to:

- Define each vocabulary term listed.
- Describe changes of puberty in males and females.
- Identify the anatomy of the male reproductive system.
- Explain the functions of the external and internal male organs in human reproduction.
- Describe the influence of hormones in male reproductive processes.
- Identify the anatomy of the female reproductive system.
- Explain the functions of the external, internal, and accessory female organs in human reproduction.
- Explain the menstrual cycle and the female hormones involved in the cycle.

Vocabulary

climacteric
dyspareunia
menarche
ovulation
ovum
rugae
semen
smegma
spermatogenesis

The nurse needs a foundation in reproductive anatomy and physiology to better understand the processes involved in human reproduction. This chapter addresses the anatomy and physiology of the male and female reproductive systems.

PUBERTY

Puberty is a period of rapid change in the lives of boys and girls during which the reproductive systems mature and become capable of reproduction. This transition from childhood to adulthood has been identified and often celebrated by various rites of passage. Some cultures have required demonstrations of bravery, such as hunting wild animals or displays of self-defense. Ritual circumcision has been another rite of passage. In the United States today, some adolescents participate in religious ceremonies such as bar/bat mitzvah or confirmation, but for others, these ceremonies are unfamiliar. The lack of a "universal rite of passage" to identify adulthood has led to confusion for some contemporary adolescents.

Boys

Male hormonal changes begin between 10 and 13 years of age, but outward changes are not apparent until 13 to 16 years of age, when the penis and testes increase in size. Testosterone, the primary male hormone, causes the boy to grow taller and to become more muscular. Growth in height continues longer in boys than in girls, causing men to be generally taller than women at maturity. Pubic, axillary (armpit), chest, and facial hair appear, although there are racial differences in the quantity and distribution of body hair. Nocturnal emissions ("wet dreams") may occur, and the boy should be prepared for them. His voice deepens, but is often characterized by squeaks or cracks before reaching its final pitch.

Girls

Female hormonal changes begin about 6 months earlier than the boy's. However, her growth in height occurs sooner, making it seem that she begins puberty about 2 years before boys of the same age. The first outward change of puberty in the girl is development of the breasts at about 10 to 11 years (Fig. 20–5). The first menstrual period *(menarche)* occurs 2 to 2½ years later (12 to 13 years). Her reproductive organs mature to prepare for sexual activity and childbearing. The girl experiences a growth spurt, but hers ends earlier than the boy's. Her hips broaden as her pelvis assumes the wide basin shape needed for birth. Pubic and axillary hair appear. The quantity varies, as it does in males.

MALE REPRODUCTIVE SYSTEM

The male reproductive system is made of external and internal organs (Fig. 2–1).

External Genitalia

The penis and the scrotum are the male external genitalia.

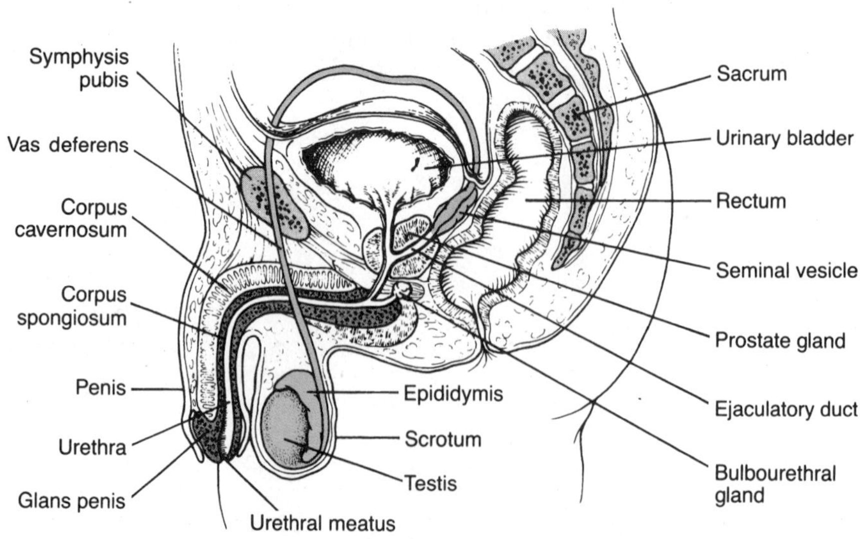

Figure 2–1. • The male reproductive organs.

Penis. The penis has two functions:

- To provide a duct to expel urine from the bladder
- To deposit sperm in the female's vagina to fertilize an ovum

The penis is comprised of the glans and the body. The glans is the round, distal end of the penis. It is visible on a circumcised penis but is hidden by the foreskin on an uncircumcised one. At the tip of the glans is an opening called the urethral meatus. The body of the penis contains the urethra (the passageway for sperm and urine) and erectile tissue (the corpus spongiosum and two corpora cavernosa). During sexual stimulation, blood is trapped within the spongy erectile tissue allowing the usually flaccid penis to become erect. The erection allows the man to penetrate the woman's vagina during sexual intercourse.

Scrotum. The scrotum is a sac that contains the testes. The scrotum is suspended from the perineum, keeping the testes away from the body and thereby lowering their temperature. This cooling is necessary for normal sperm production (spermatogenesis).

Internal Genitalia

The internal genitalia include the testes, ducts, and accessory glands.

Testes. The testes (testicles) are a pair of oval organs housed in the scrotum. They have two functions:

- Manufacture male germ cells (spermatozoa, or sperm).
- Secrete male hormones *(androgens).*

Sperm are made in the convoluted seminiferous tubules that make up the 250 to 400 lobules of the testes. Sperm production begins at puberty and continues throughout the life span of the male.

The production of *testosterone,* the most abundant male hormone, begins with the anterior pituitary gland. Under the direction of the hypothalamus, the anterior pituitary gland secretes follicle-stimulating hormone (FSH) and luteinizing hormone (LH). FSH and LH initiate the production of testosterone in the Leydig cells of the testes. Testosterone has several effects not directly related to reproduction:

- Increases muscle mass
- Promotes strength
- Promotes growth of long bones
- Enhances production of red blood cells

These effects result in the greater strength and stature and a higher hematocrit level in males than in females. Testosterone also increases production of sebum, a fatty secretion of the sebaceous glands of the skin and may contribute to the development of acne. Male hormonal activity continues throughout life.

Ducts. The epididymis, one from each testicle, store and carry the sperm to the penis. The sperm may remain in the epididymis for 2 to 10 days where they mature and then move on to the vasa deferens. Each vas deferens passes upward into the body, goes around the symphysis pubis, circles the bladder, and passes downward to form, with the ducts from the seminal vesicles, the ejaculatory ducts. The ejaculatory ducts then enter the back of the prostate gland and connect to the upper part of the urethra.

Accessory Glands. The accessory glands produce secretions (seminal plasma) to protect the sperm and promote its motility. The accessory glands are the *seminal vesicles,* the *prostate gland,* and the *bulbourethral glands,* also called *Cowper's glands.* The secretions of these glands:

- Nourish the sperm
- Protect the sperm from the acidic environment of the woman's vagina
- Enhance the motility (movement) of the sperm

The seminal plasma and sperm together are called *semen.* Semen may be secreted during sexual intercourse before ejaculation. Therefore, pregnancy may occur even if ejaculation takes place outside the vagina.

FEMALE REPRODUCTIVE SYSTEM

The female reproductive system consists of external genitalia, internal genitalia, and accessory structures, namely the bony pelvis and mammary glands (breasts).

External Genitalia

The female external genitalia are collectively called the *vulva.* They include the mons pubis, labia majora, labia minora, fourchette, clitoris, vaginal vestibule, and perineum (Fig. 2–2).

Mons Pubis. The mons pubis (mons veneris) is a pad of fatty tissue covered by coarse skin. It protects the symphysis pubis and contributes to the rounded contour of the female body.

Labia Majora. The labia majora are two folds of fatty tissue on each side of the vaginal vestibule.

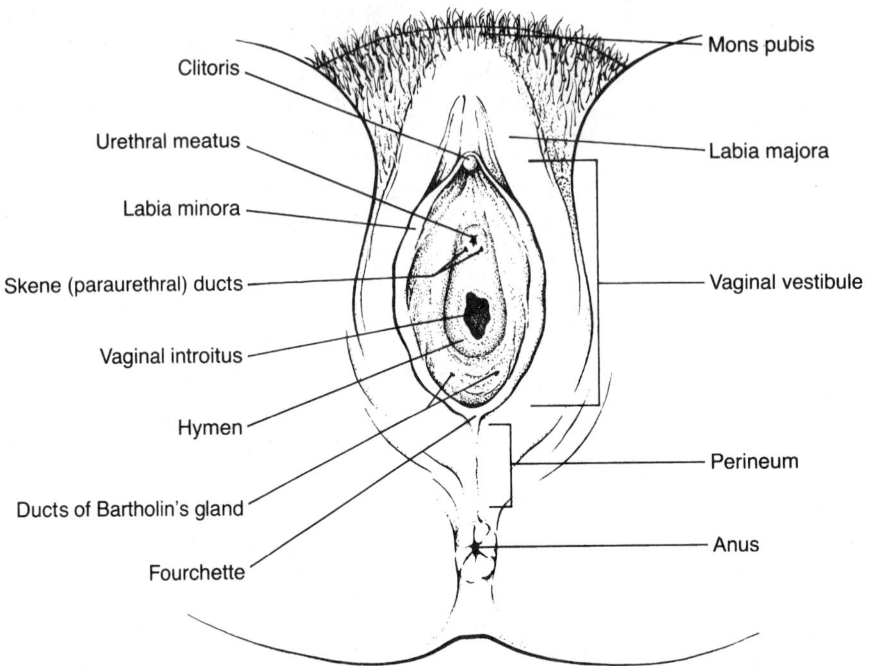

Figure 2–2. • The external female reproductive organs.

Many small glands are located on the moist interior surface. Short curly pubic hair develops on the mons pubis and labia majora at puberty.

Labia Minora. The labia minora are two thin, soft folds of erectile tissue that are seen when the labia majora are separated. Secretions from sebaceous glands in the labia are bactericidal to reduce infection and also lubricate and protect the skin of the vulva.

Fourchette. The fourchette is a fold of tissue just below the vagina, where the labia majora and the labia minora meet. Lacerations during childbirth often occur in that area.

Clitoris. The clitoris is a small erectile body in the most anterior portion of the labia minora. It is similar in structure to the penis. Functionally, it is the most erotic, sensitive part of the female genitalia, and it produces *smegma.* Smegma is a cheeselike secretion of the sebaceous glands in the area.

Vaginal Vestibule. The vaginal vestibule is the area seen when the labia minora are separated. There are five openings:

- The *urethral meatus* is approximately 2 cm below the clitoris. It has a foldlike appearance with a slit-type opening, and it serves as the exit for urine.
- *Skene's ducts* (paraurethral ducts) are on each side of the urethra and provide lubrication for the urethra. They may be sites for infection.
- The *vaginal introitus* is the external portion of the vagina.
- The *hymen* is a thin elastic membrane that closes the vagina from the vestibule to various degrees.
- The *ducts of Bartholin glands* (vulvovaginal glands) provide lubrication for the vaginal introitus during sexual arousal.

Perineum. The perineum is a strong, muscular area between the vaginal opening and the anus. The elastic fibers and connective tissue of the perineum allow stretching to permit the birth of a full-term infant. The perineum is the site of the episiotomy (incision) or tears during birth. Pelvic weakness or painful intercourse *(dyspareunia)* may result if the damage does not heal properly.

Internal Genitalia

The internal genitalia are the vagina, uterus, fallopian tubes, and ovaries. Figure 2–3 illustrates the side view of these organs, and Figure 2–4 illustrates the frontal view.

Vagina. The vagina is a tubular structure made of muscle and membrane tissue that connects the external genitalia to the uterus. Because it meets at a right angle with the cervix, the anterior wall is about 2.5 cm (1 inch) shorter than the posterior wall, which varies from 7 to 10 cm (approximately

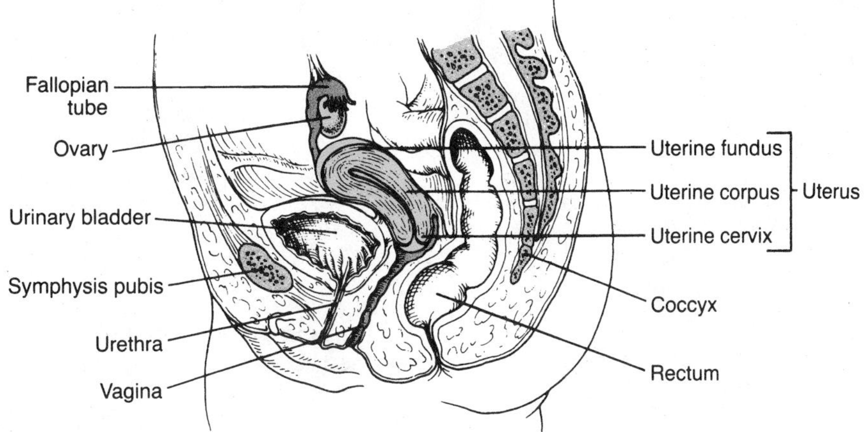

Figure 2–3. • Side view of the internal female reproductive organs.

2.8 to 4 inches). The marked stretching of the vagina during delivery is made possible by the *rugae,* or transverse ridges of the mucous membrane lining. The vagina is self-cleansing and during the reproductive years maintains a normal acidic pH of 4 to 5. The self-cleansing activity may be altered by antibiotic therapy, by frequent douching and excessive use of vaginal sprays, or by deodorant sanitary pads or deodorant tampons.

The functions of the vagina are:

- To act as an organ for intercourse
- To allow drainage of menstrual fluids and other secretions
- To provide a passageway for the baby's birth

Uterus. The uterus (womb) is a hollow muscular organ in which a fertilized ovum is implanted, an embryo develops, and a fetus develops. It is shaped like a pear or light bulb. In a mature, nonpregnant female, it weighs approximately 60 g (2 ounces) and is 7.5 cm (3 inches) long, 5 cm (2 inches) wide, and 1 to 2.5 cm (0.4 to 1 inch) thick. The uterus lies between the bladder and the rectum. It is supported by ligaments, two major pairs being the round and broad ligaments.

Blood and Nerve Supply. The main blood supply to the uterus is carried by

- Uterine arteries, which branch off the hypogastric (internal iliac) arteries

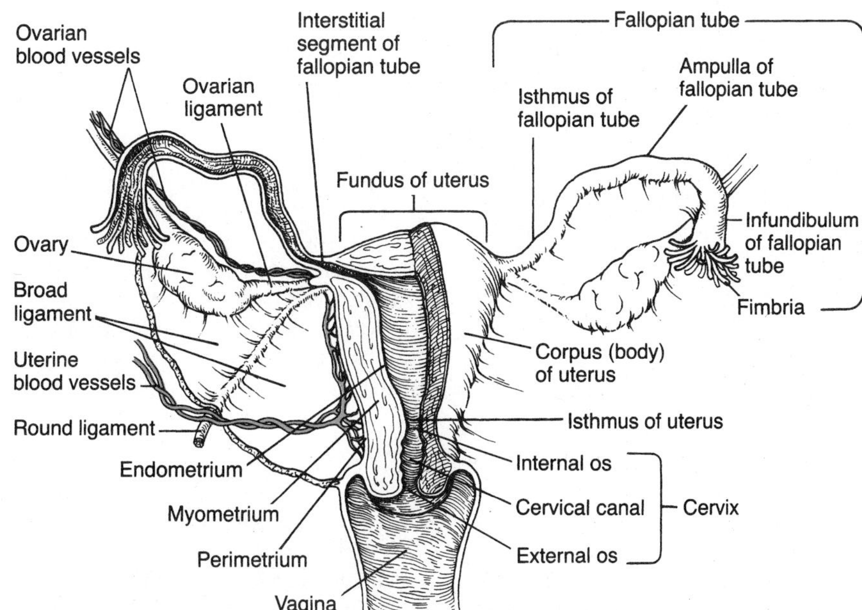

Figure 2–4. • Frontal view of the internal female reproductive organs.

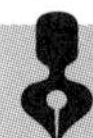

Nursing Tip

The self-cleansing function of the vagina is emphasized in teaching women about feminine hygiene. An excellent opportunity for the nurse to reinforce women's learning about the protective functions of the cervix is during examinations such as the Papanicolaou (Pap) smear and while discussing family planning.

- Ovarian arteries, which branch off the descending aorta

The autonomic nervous system innervates the reproductive system, meaning that its functions are not under voluntary (conscious) control. Sensory and motor nerves enter the spinal cord at the lower thoracic and upper lumbar levels of the spinal cord (T-12 through L-2). Sensory innervation is important to labor pain management.

Anatomy. The uterus is separated into three parts: fundus, corpus, and cervix. The *fundus* (upper part) is broad and flat. The fallopian tubes enter the uterus on each side of the fundus. The *corpus* (body) is the middle portion, and it plays an active role in menstruation and pregnancy.

The fundus and corpus have three distinct layers:

- The *perimetrium* is the outermost or serosal layer that envelops the uterus.
- The *myometrium* is the middle muscular layer that functions during pregnancy and birth. It has three involuntary muscle layers: a longitudinal outer layer, a figure-eight interlacing middle layer, and circular inner layer that forms sphincters at the fallopian tube attachments and at the internal opening of the cervix.
- The *endometrium* is the inner or mucosal layer that is functional during menstruation and implantation of the fertilized ovum. It is governed by cyclical hormonal changes.

The cervix is a tubular structure that connects the vagina and the uterus.

The *cervix* (lower part) is narrow and tubular and opens into the upper vagina. The portion of the uterus that joins the corpus to the cervix is called the isthmus and during pregnancy is referred to as the lower uterine segment. The cervix consists of a cervical canal with an internal opening near the uterine corpus, called the internal os, and an opening into the vagina called the external os. The mucosal lining of the cervix has four functions:

- Lubricates the vagina
- Acts as a bacteriostatic agent
- Provides an alkaline environment to shelter deposited sperm from the acidic pH of the vagina
- Produces a mucous plug in the cervical canal during pregnancy

Fallopian Tubes. The fallopian tubes, also called uterine tubes or oviducts, extend laterally from the uterus, one to each ovary (Fig. 2–4). They vary in length from 8 to 13.5 cm (3 to 5.3 inches). Each tube has four sections:

- The *interstitial* portion runs into the uterine cavity and lies within the wall of the uterus.
- The *isthmus* is a narrow area near the uterus.
- The *ampulla* is the wider area of the tube and is the usual site of fertilization.
- The *infundibulum* is the funnel-like enlarged distal end of the tube. Fingerlike projections from the infundibulum called *fimbriae* hover over each ovary and "capture" the ovum (egg) as it is released by the ovary at ovulation.

The four functions of the fallopian tubes are to provide:

- A passageway in which sperm meet the ovum
- A site of fertilization
- A safe, nourishing environment for the ovum or zygote (fertilized ovum)
- A means of transporting the ovum or zygote to the corpus of the uterus

Cells within the tubes have *cilia* (hairlike projections) that beat rhythmically to propel the ovum toward the uterus. Other cells secrete a protein-rich fluid to nourish the ovum after it leaves the ovary.

Ovaries. The ovaries are two almond-shaped glands, each about the size of a walnut. They are in the lower abdominal cavity, one on each side of the uterus. Ovarian ligaments connect the ovaries to the lateral uterine walls. The ovaries have two functions:

- Production of hormones, chiefly estrogen and progesterone
- Maturation of an ovum during each reproductive cycle

At birth, every baby girl has all the ova (oocytes) that will be available during her reproductive years (approximately 2 million cells). These degenerate significantly so that by adulthood her remaining oocytes number in the thousands. Of these, only a small percentage are actually released (about 400 during the reproductive years). *Oogenesis* (formation of the immature ova) does not occur after fetal development. Any ova that remain after the *climacteric* (the period surrounding menopause) no longer respond to hormone stimulation to mature.

Female Pelvis

The bony pelvis occupies the lower portion of the trunk of the body. It is formed by four bones attached to the lower spine:

- Two innominate bones
- Sacrum
- Coccyx

Each innominate bone is made up of an ilium, pubis, and ischium, which are separate during childhood but fused by adulthood. The ilium is the lateral, flaring portion of the hip bone; the pubis is the anterior hip bone. These two bones join to form the symphysis pubis. The ischium is below the ilium. Its significant feature is the ischial spine (Fig. 2–5). An ischial spine, one from each ischium, juts inward to varying degrees. The posterior pelvis consists of the sacrum and coccyx. Five fused, triangular vertebrae at the base of the spine form the sacrum. Below the sacrum is the coccyx, the lowest part of the spine.

The functions of the pelvis are to

- Support and distribute body weight
- Support and protect pelvic organs
- Form the birth passageway

Strong pelvic floor muscles stabilize and support the internal and external reproductive organs. The most important of these muscles is the levator ani, which supports the three structures that penetrate it: the urethra, vagina, and rectum.

Types of Pelves. There are four basic types of pelves (Fig. 2–6). Most women have a combination of pelvic characteristics rather than having one pure type.

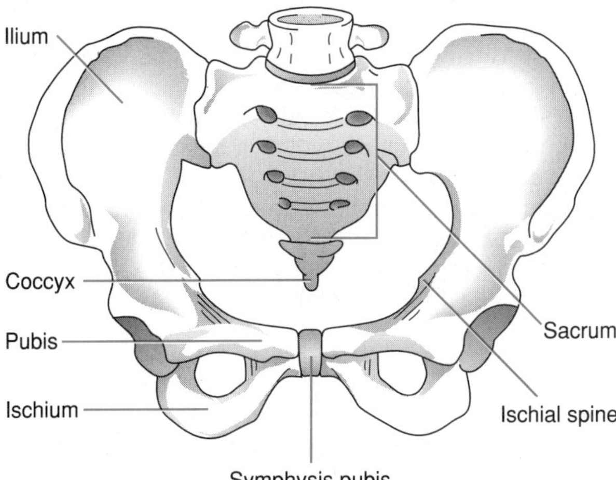

Figure 2–5. • Frontal view of the female pelvis.

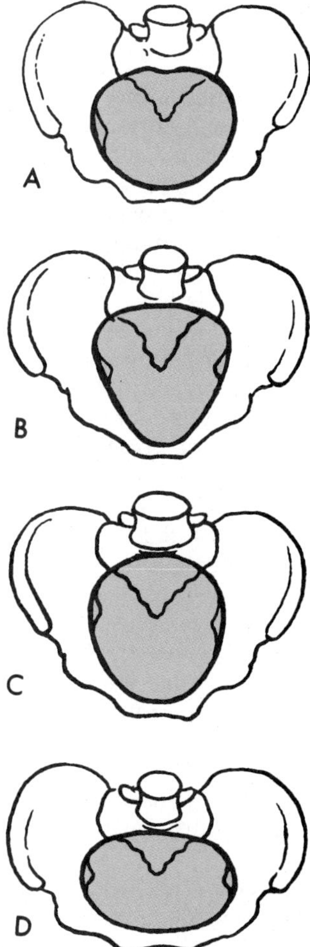

Figure 2–6. • Four types of pelves. **A,** Gynecoid. **B,** Android. **C,** Anthropoid. **D,** Platypelloid. (Modified from Moore, M. [1983]. *Realities in childbearing* [2nd ed.]. Philadelphia: Saunders.)

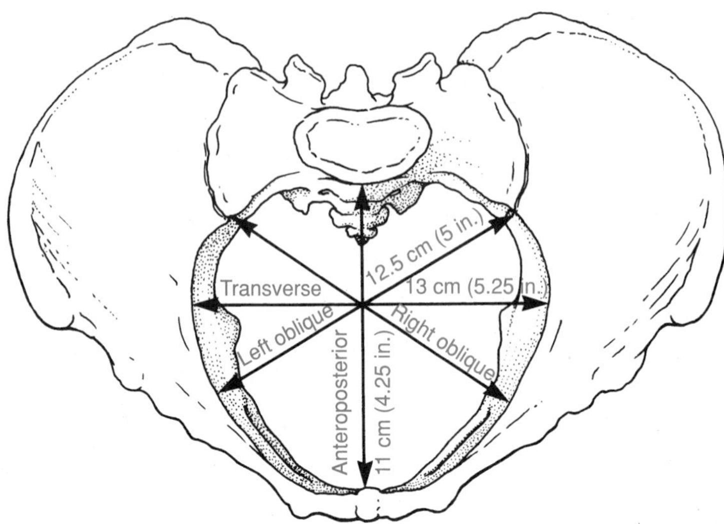

Figure 2–7. • Four important pelvic inlet diameters are the anteroposterior, the transverse, and the right and left oblique diameters. (Modified from *Illustrated Stedman's medical dictionary* [1990]. [25th ed.]. Baltimore: Williams & Wilkins.)

- The *gynecoid* pelvis is the typical female pelvis, with rounded anterior and posterior segments. This type is most favorable for vaginal birth.
- The *android* pelvis has a wedge-shaped inlet with a narrow anterior segment; it is typical of the male anatomy.
- The *anthropoid* pelvis has an anteroposterior diameter that equals or exceeds its transverse diameter. The shape is a long, narrow oval. Women with this type of pelvis can usually deliver vaginally, but their baby is more likely to be born in the occiput posterior (back of the fetal head toward the mother's sacrum) position.
- The *platypelloid* pelvis has a shortened anteroposterior diameter and a flat, transverse oval shape. This type is unfavorable for vaginal birth.

True and False Pelves. The pelvis is divided into the false and true pelves by an imaginary line, called the linea terminalis, that proceeds from the sacroiliac joint to the anterior iliopubic prominence. The upper, or false, pelvis supports the enlarging uterus and guides the fetus into the true pelvis. The lower, or true, pelvis consists of the inlet, pelvic cavity, and outlet. The true pelvis is most important during birth.

Pelvic Diameters. The diameters of the pelvis are important to consider for a successful vaginal delivery (Fig. 2–7).

Pelvic Inlet. The pelvic inlet, just below the linea terminalis, has three obstetrically important diameters: anteroposterior, transverse, and right and left oblique. The anteroposterior diameter is between the symphysis pubis and the sacrum and is the shortest inlet diameter. The transverse diameter is measured across the linea terminalis and is the largest inlet diameter. The right oblique diameter is measured from the right sacroiliac joint to the prominence of the linea terminalis. The left oblique diameter is measured in the same way on the other side.

Pelvic Cavity. The pelvic cavity has a number of diameters, the most important being the interspinous (or bispinous) transverse diameter. The distance between the ischial spines should be at least 10.5 cm (4.13 inches) and is the shortest pelvic diameter.

Pelvic Outlet. The diameters of the pelvic outlet are the anteroposterior, intertuberous transverse, and anterior and posterior sagittal diameters. The anteroposterior diameter can change as the fetus passes if the coccyx is easily moveable. The intertuberous transverse diameter is measured between the ischial tuberosities ("sit bones") and is the shortest outlet diameter. The sagittal diameters are measured from the middle of the transverse diameter to the suprapubic bone anteriorly and to the sacrococcygeal joint posteriorly.

Breasts

Female breasts (mammary glands) are accessory organs of reproduction. They produce milk following birth to provide nourishment and maternal antibodies to the infant (Fig. 2–8). The nipple, in the center of each breast, is surrounded by a pigmented areola. Montgomery's glands (Montgomery's tubercles) are small sebaceous glands in the areola that secrete a substance that lubricates and protects the breasts during lactation.

Each breast is made of 15 to 24 lobes arranged like the spokes of a wheel. The lobes are separated by adipose (fatty) and fibrous tissues. The adipose tissue affects size and firmness and gives the breasts a smooth outline. Breast size is primarily determined by the amount of fatty tissue and is unrelated to a woman's ability to produce milk.

Alveoli (lobules) are the glands that secrete milk. They empty into about 20 separate lactiferous (milk-carrying) ducts. Milk is stored briefly in widened areas of the ducts, called ampullae or lactiferous sinuses.

Female Reproductive Cycle and Menstruation

The female reproductive cycle consists of regular changes in secretions of the anterior pituitary gland, the ovary, and the endometrial lining of the uterus (Fig. 2–9). The anterior pituitary gland, in response to the hypothalamus, secretes follicle-stimulating hormone (FSH) and luteinizing hormone (LH). The FSH stimulates maturation of a follicle, a spherical cavity on an ovary that contains a single ovum. Several follicles start maturing during each cycle, but only one usually reaches final maturity. The maturing ovum and corpus luteum (the empty follicle after the ovum is released) produce increasing amounts of estrogen and progesterone, which leads to a buildup of the endometrium. A surge in LH stimulates final maturation and the release of an ovum.

Ovulation occurs when a mature ovum is released from the follicle. The corpus luteum turns yellow (luteinizing) immediately after ovulation and secretes increasing quantities of progesterone to prepare the uterine lining for a fertilized ovum. About 12 days after ovulation, the corpus luteum degenerates if fertilization has not occurred, and progesterone and estrogen levels decrease. The fall in estrogen and progesterone causes the endometrium to break down, resulting in menstruation. The anterior pituitary gland secretes more FSH and LH, beginning a new cycle.

The beginning of menstruation, called *menarche*, occurs at about 12 to 13 years of age. Early cycles are often irregular and may be anovulatory. Regular cycles are usually established within 6 months to 2 years of the menarche. In an average cycle, the flow (menses) occurs every 28 days, plus or minus 5 to 10 days. Stress, fatigue, or illness may interfere with the cycle. The flow itself lasts from 2 to 8 days with a blood loss of 50 to 100 ml.

The *climacteric* is a period of years during which the woman's ability to reproduce gradually declines. *Menopause* refers to the final menstrual period, although the terms *menopause* and *climacteric* are often casually used interchangeably.

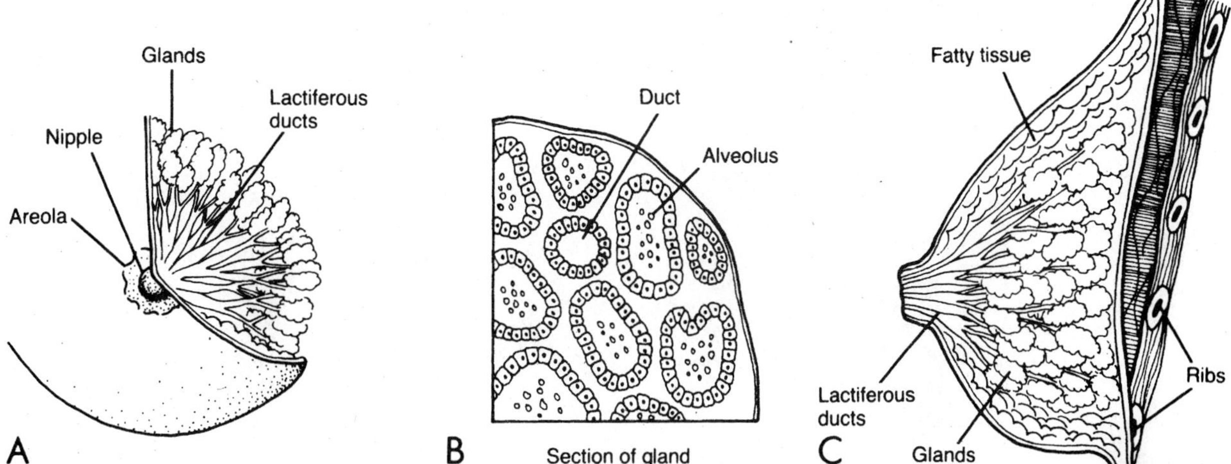

Figure 2–8. • Structures in the breast. **A,** Milk-producing glands and ducts are arranged around the nipple like the spokes of a wheel. **B,** Microscopic cross-section of a milk-producing gland. **C,** Side view of the breast, illustrating glands, lactiferous ducts, and fatty tissue. (From O'Toole, M., ed. [1997]. *Miller-Keane Encyclopedia & dictionary of medicine, nursing, & allied health* [6th ed.]. Philadelphia: Saunders.)

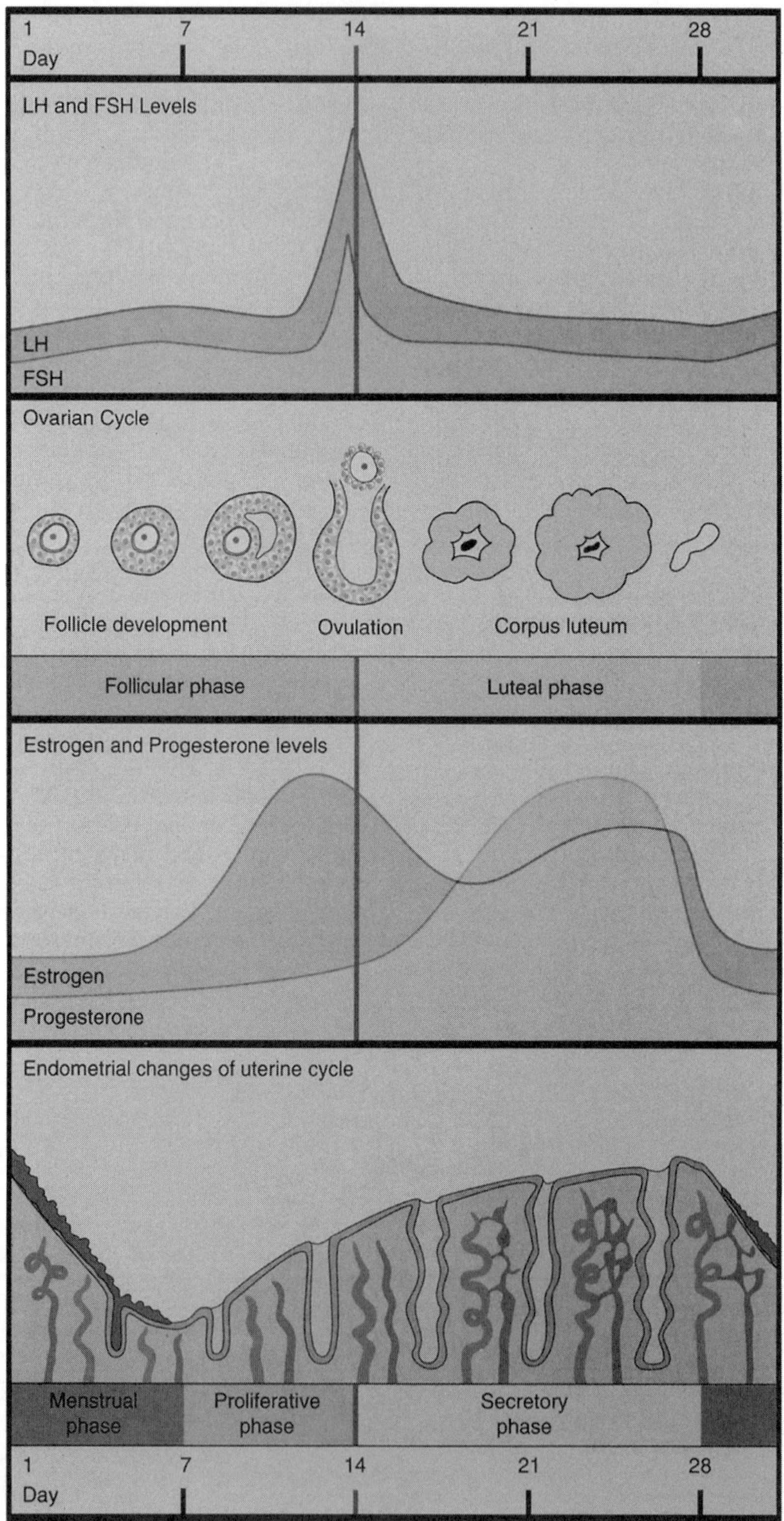

Figure 2–9. • Menstrual cycle. Note hormonal control of the menstrual cycle and the effects on ovaries *(center)* and endometrium *(bottom)*. (From Polaski, A.L., Tatro, S.E. [1996]. *Luckmann's core principles and practice of medical-surgical nursing*. Philadelphia: Saunders.)

KEY POINTS

- Puberty begins about six months earlier in girls, but the girl's early growth spurt makes it seem that she begins puberty much earlier than the boy.
- Testosterone is the principal male hormone. Estrogen and progesterone are the principal female hormones. Testosterone secretion continues throughout a man's life, but estrogen and progesterone secretion are very low after a woman reaches the climacteric.
- The penis and scrotum are the male external genitalia. The scrotum keeps the testes cooler than the rest of the body, promoting normal sperm production.
- The two main functions of the testes are to manufacture sperm and to secrete male hormones (androgens), primarily testosterone.
- The myometrium (middle muscular uterine layer) is functional in pregnancy and labor. The endometrium (inner uterine layer) is functional in menstruation and implantation of a fertilized ovum.
- There are four basic pelvic shapes, but women often have a combination of characteristics. The gynecoid pelvis is the most favorable for vaginal birth.
- The pelvis is divided into a false pelvis above the linea terminalis and the true pelvis below this line. The true pelvis is most important in birth. The true pelvis is further divided into the pelvic inlet, pelvic cavity, and pelvic outlet.
- The female breasts are composed of fatty and fibrous tissue and of glands that can secrete milk. The size of a woman's breasts is determined by the amount of fatty tissue and does not influence her ability to secrete milk.
- The female reproductive cycle consists of regular changes in hormone secretions from the anterior pituitary gland and the ovary, maturation and release of an ovum, and buildup and breakdown of the uterine lining.

MULTIPLE-CHOICE REVIEW QUESTIONS

Choose the most appropriate answer.

1. Spermatozoa are produced in the
   a. vas deferens
   b. seminiferous tubules
   c. prostate gland
   d. Leydig cells
2. Production of estrogen from the ovaries occurs under the influence of
   a. luteinizing hormone
   b. growth hormone
   c. adrenocorticotropic hormone
   d. follicle-stimulating hormone
3. The typical male pelvic type is the
   a. gynecoid
   b. android
   c. anthropoid
   d. platypelloid
4. The muscular layer of the uterus that is the functional unit in pregnancy and labor is the
   a. perimetrium
   b. myometrium
   c. endometrium
   d. cervix

BIBLIOGRAPHY AND READER REFERENCE

Black, J. M., & Matassarin-Jacobs, E. (1997). *Luckmann and Sorensen's medical-surgical nursing: Clinical Management for Continuity of Care* (5th ed.). Philadelphia: Saunders.

Gorrie, T. M., McKinney, E. S., & Murray, S. S. (1998). *Foundations of maternal-newborn nursing* (2nd ed.). Philadelphia: Saunders.

Guyton, A. C., & Hall, J. E. (1996). *Textbook of medical physiology* (9th ed.). Philadelphia: Saunders.

chapter 3

Prenatal Development

Outline

CELL DIVISION

GAMETOGENESIS

FERTILIZATION
- Sex Determination

DEVELOPMENT
- Tubal Transport of the Zygote
- Implantation of the Zygote
- Cell Differentiation
- Accessory Structures of Pregnancy
- The Embryo
- The Fetus

MULTIFETAL PREGNANCY

Objectives

On completion and mastery of Chapter 3, the student will be able to

- Define each vocabulary term listed.
- Describe the process of gametogenesis in human reproduction.
- Explain human fertilization and implantation.
- Describe embryonic development.
- Describe fetal development and maturation of body systems.
- Describe the development and functions of the placenta, umbilical cord, and amniotic fluid.
- Compare fetal circulation to circulation after birth.
- Explain similarities and differences in the two types of twins.

Vocabulary

amniotic sac
autosome
chorion
decidua
diploid
embryo
fertilization
fetus
gametogenesis
germ layers
haploid
placenta
surfactant
teratogen
zygote

Each human being is unique, even though each has the same organ systems functioning in more or less the same manner. One's uniqueness results from the interaction of genetic and environmental factors. First, the 46 chromosomes contained in each cell of the body determine a person's particular combination of features. Chromosomes are composed of genes, which are the units of heredity and contain the information necessary for expression of specific features, traits, and body functions. The familial traits carried on the 46 chromosomes are uniquely blended when male and female reproductive cells (ovum and sperm) form in *gametogenesis* and unite to make a new person.

The intrauterine environment also influences the developing baby. The intrauterine environment promotes optimum prenatal growth if the mother is well nourished, has no chronic diseases or infections, and avoids exposure to harmful substances such as alcohol. However, the mother who gains insufficient weight or ingests toxic substances such as illicit drugs, tobacco, or alcohol may deprive her fetus of needed nutrients or expose the baby to damaging substances *(teratogens).* Therapeutic drugs may also be teratogenic, so a woman should inform her caregivers if she thinks she is pregnant.

CELL DIVISION

Cell division is the basic mechanism of human growth and regeneration. The division of a cell begins in its nucleus, which contains the gene-bearing chromosomes. The two types of cell division are mitosis and meiosis.

Mitosis occurs in somatic (body) cells and is chiefly responsible for the body's growth, development, and replenishment throughout its life. The number of chromosomes in a somatic cell is 46, known as the *diploid number.* A cell divides mitotically by first replicating each chromosome in its nucleus; each of the 46 pairs of chromosomes then separates to form two identical daughter cells, each having 46 single chromosomes with the same genetic material as the parent cell.

Meiosis is a special reduction division that occurs only during the formation of *gametes* (sex cells). In gametogenesis, there are two successive meiotic divisions that result in four cells, each containing half the total number of chromosomes (23); this is known as the *haploid number* of chromosomes. The male gamete is called a *sperm;* the female gamete is an *ovum.*

GAMETOGENESIS

Gametogenesis is the process in which cells divide by meiosis to form gametes. Male gametogenesis is called *spermatogenesis* and occurs in the seminiferous tubules of the testes (see p. 27). This process involves two meiotic divisions and results in four sperm from each primary spermatocyte, each with 22 *autosomes* (non-sex chromosomes) and either an X or a Y sex chromosome, for a total of 23.

Female gametogenesis, called *oogenesis,* also involves two meiotic divisions of a primary oocyte but results in one ovum and two small nonfunctional polar bodies. Oogenesis begins during prenatal life when oocytes multiply by mitosis, like all other body cells. The female fetus does not make more ova after the 30th week of gestation. The first meiotic division of the oocyte occurs shortly before ovulation. The second meiotic division is completed if the ovum is fertilized by a sperm.

The mature ovum also contains the haploid number of chromosomes: 22 single chromosomes and an X sex chromosome. In oogenesis, the extra chromosomes produced by each meiotic division are contained in the polar bodies, which eventually disintegrate. This process is illustrated in greater detail in Figure 3–1.

FERTILIZATION

Fertilization occurs when a sperm penetrates an ovum and unites with it and the total number of chromosomes is restored to 46. The time during which fertilization can occur is brief because of the short lifespan of mature gametes. The ovum is estimated to survive for up to 24 hours after ovulation. The sperm remains capable of fertilizing the ovum for 48 to 72 hours after being ejaculated in the area of the cervix. However, one study (Wilcox, Weinberg, & Baird, 1995) found that fertilization was sometimes possible when intercourse occurred as long as 5 days before ovulation.

The amount of semen in a normal ejaculation is 2 to 5 ml, and the number of sperm ranges from 200 million to 600 million. The sperm pass through the cervix and uterus and into the fallopian tubes by means of the flagellar (whiplike) activity of their tails.

Fertilization occurs in the outer third of the fallopian tube, near the ovary (Fig. 3–2). High estrogen levels at ovulation facilitate movement of the ovum through the fallopian tube and promote secretion of cervical mucus that is favorable for the passage of sperm.

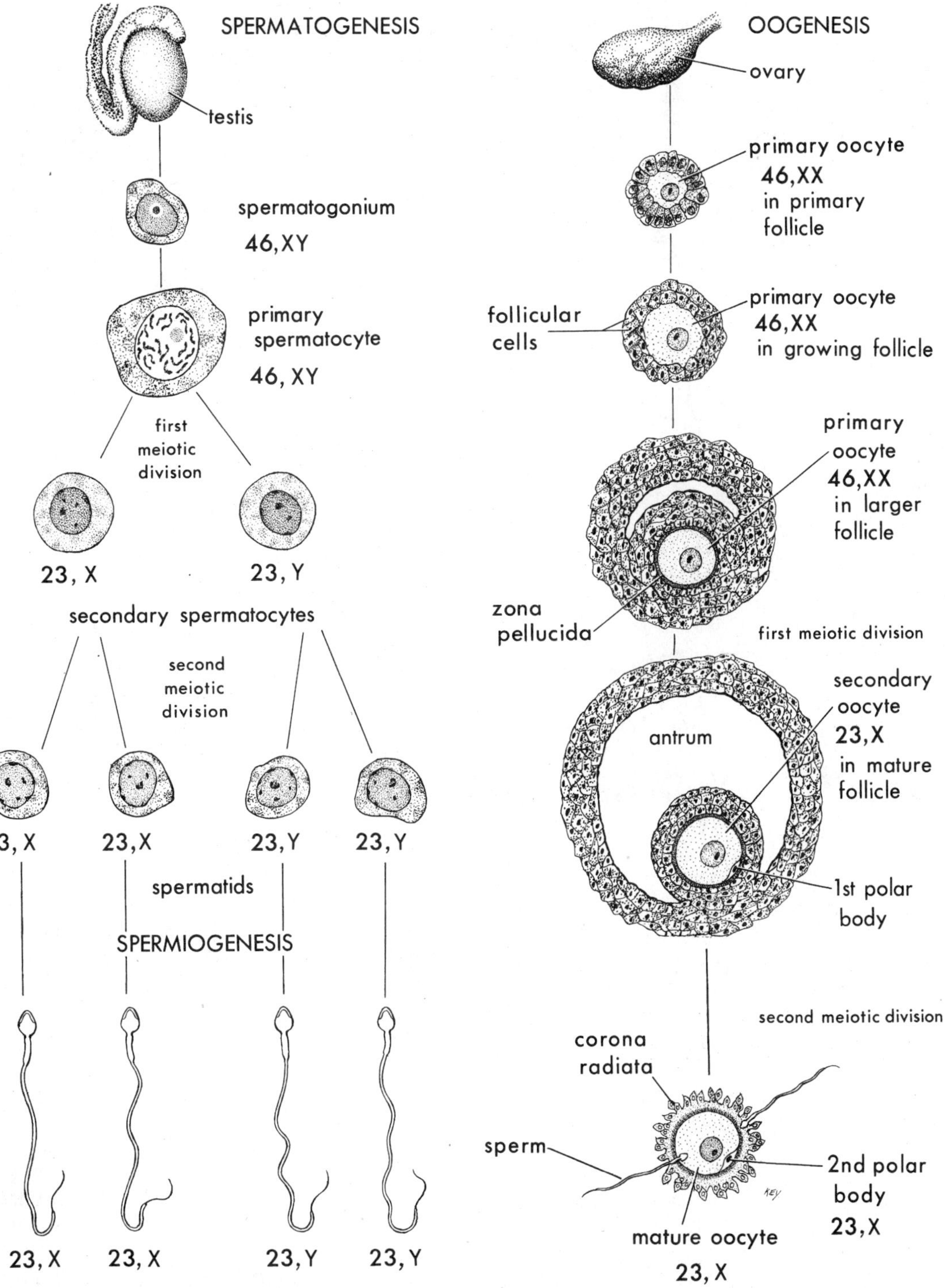

Figure 3–1. • Normal gametogenesis, consisting of spermatogenesis and oogenesis. Four sperm develop from one primary spermatocyte, but only one mature oocyte (ovum) results from maturation of a primary oocyte. (From Moore, K. L., & Persaud, T. V. N. [1998]. *The developing human: Clinically oriented embryology* [6th ed.]. Philadelphia: Saunders.)

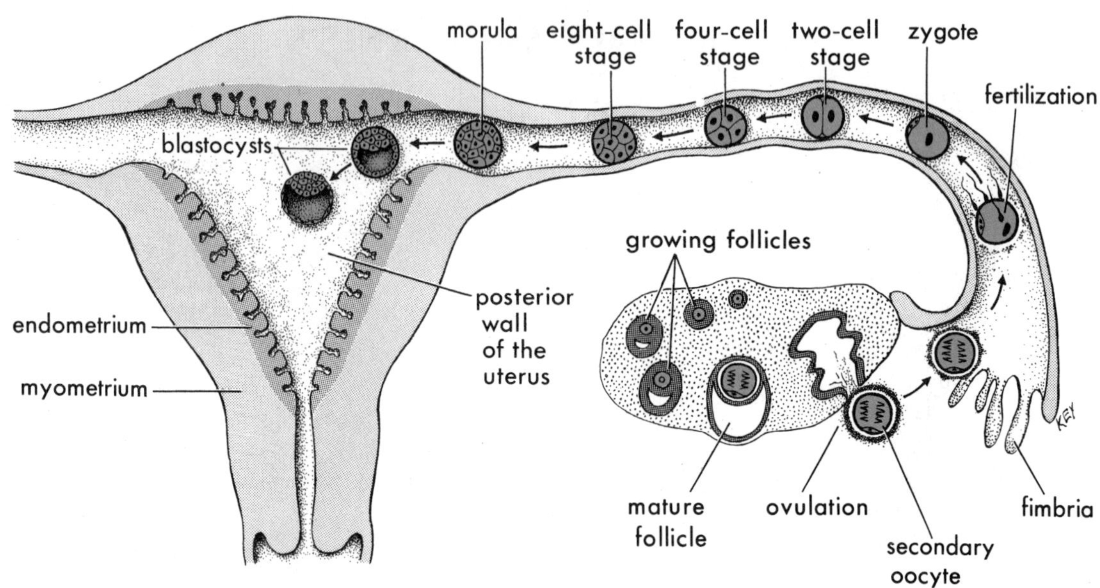

Figure 3–2 • Ovulation and fertilization, which initiate human development. The zygote passes through the fallopian tube and enters the uterus in the blastocyst stage, where normally it implants in the center of the posterior uterine wall. (From Moore, K. L., & Persaud, T. V. N. [1998]. *The developing human: Clinically oriented embryology* [6th ed.]. Philadelphia: Saunders.)

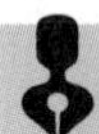

Nursing Tip

During sexuality counseling, the nurse should emphasize that the survival time of sperm ejaculated into the area of the cervix may be up to 72 hours and that pregnancy has occurred with intercourse as long as 5 days before ovulation.

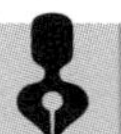

Nursing Tip

Both mother and father influence the sex of their offspring, although the father contributes the actual sex chromosome. This fact may reduce blame when the child is not of the desired sex.

Sex Determination

The sex of human offspring is determined at fertilization. The ovum always contributes an X chromosome, whereas the sperm can carry an X *or* a Y chromosome. When a sperm carrying the larger X chromosome fertilizes the X-bearing ovum, a female child (XX) results. When a smaller, Y-bearing sperm fertilizes the ovum, a male child (XY) is produced.

Because his sperm can carry either an X or a Y chromosome, the male partner determines the gender of the child. However, the pH of the female reproductive tract and the estrogen levels of the woman's body affect the survival rate of the X- and Y-bearing sperm and the speed of their movement through the cervix and fallopian tubes. Thus, the mother has some influence on which sperm fertilizes the mature ovum.

DEVELOPMENT

Three basic stages characterize prenatal development. The *zygote* is the cell formed by the union of the sperm and ovum. Between 3 and 8 weeks after conception is the stage of the *embryo.* From the 9th week after conception until birth, the developing baby is called a *fetus.*

Tubal Transport of the Zygote

A chemical change in the membrane surrounding the zygote causes it to become impenetrable to other sperm as soon as fertilization occurs. The zygote is transported through the fallopian tube and into the uterus. During transport through the fallopian tube, the zygote undergoes rapid mitotic division, or *cleavage.* Cleavage begins with two cells, which subdivide into four and then eight cells to form the *blastomere.* The size of the zygote does not increase; rather, the individual cells become smaller as they divide and eventually form a solid ball called the *morula* (Fig. 3–2).

The morula enters the uterus on the 3rd day and floats there for another 2 to 4 days. The cells form a cavity, and two distinct layers evolve. The inner layer is a solid mass of cells called the *blastocyst* (Fig. 3–2), which develops into the embryo and embryonic membranes. The outer layer of cells, called the *trophoblast,* develops into an embryonic membrane, the *chorion* (Fig. 3–3). Occasionally, the zygote does not move through the fallopian tube and instead becomes implanted into the lining of the tube, resulting in a tubal ectopic pregnancy (see p. 85).

Implantation of the Zygote

The zygote usually implants in the upper section of the posterior uterine wall. The cells burrow into the prepared lining of the uterus, called the endometrium, until the entire blastocyst is covered by 10 days after conception. The endometrium is now called the *decidua.* The decidua over the blastocyst is called the decidua capsularis; the area under the blastocyst is called the decidua basalis and gives rise to the maternal part of the placenta; the remaining uterine lining is called the decidua vera (parietalis).

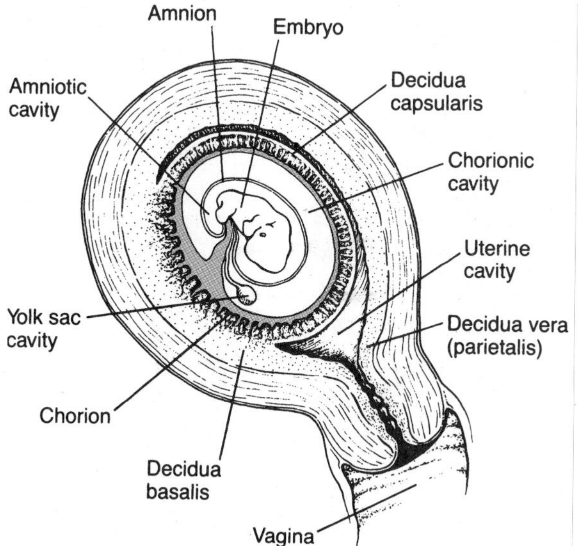

Figure 3–3 • After implantation, the endometrial lining of the uterus is known as the decidua. The cells of the zygote begin to differentiate into the chorion, amnion, yolk sac, and embryo.

Cell Differentiation

From fertilization to implantation, the cells within a zygote are identical to one another. After implantation, the cells begin to differentiate and develop special functions. The chorion, amnion, yolk sac, and primary germ layers appear.

Chorion. The chorion develops from the trophoblast (outer layer of embryonic cells) and envelops the amnion, embryo, and yolk sac. It is a thick membrane with fingerlike projections called *villi* on its outermost surface. The villi immediately below the embryo extend into the decidua basalis on the uterine wall and form the embryonic/fetal portion of the placenta (see pp. 42–43).

Amnion. The amnion is the second membrane and is a thin membrane that envelops and protects the embryo. It forms the boundaries of the amniotic cavity, and its outer aspect meets the inner aspect of the chorion.

The chorion and amnion together form an amniotic sac filled with fluid (bag of waters) that permits the embryo to float freely. Amniotic fluid is clear, has a mild odor, and often contains bits of vernix (fetal skin covering) or lanugo (fetal hair on the skin). The volume of amniotic fluid steadily increases from about 30 ml at 10 weeks of pregnancy to 350 ml at 20 weeks (Moore & Persaud, 1993). The volume of fluid is about 1000 ml at 37 weeks. In the latter part of the pregnancy, the fetus may swallow up to 400 ml of amniotic fluid per day and normally excretes urine into the fluid. The functions of amniotic fluid are to:

- Maintain an even temperature
- Prevent the amniotic sac from adhering to the fetal skin
- Allow symmetrical growth
- Allow buoyancy and fetal movement
- Act as a cushion to protect the fetus from injury

Yolk Sac. On the 9th day after fertilization, a cavity called the yolk sac forms in the blastocyst. It functions only during embryonic life and initiates the production of red blood cells. This function continues for about 6 weeks, until the embryonic liver takes over. The umbilical cord then encompasses the yolk sac, and the yolk sac degenerates.

Germ Layers. After implantation the zygote in the blastocyst stage transforms its *embryonic disc* into three primary *germ layers* known as *ectoderm, mesoderm,* and *endoderm.* Each germ layer develops into a different part of the growing embryo. The specific body parts that develop from each layer are listed in Box 3–1.

BOX 3–1

BODY PARTS THAT DEVELOP FROM THE PRIMARY GERM LAYERS

Ectoderm
Outer layer of skin
Oil glands and hair follicles of skin
Nails and hair
External sense organs
Mucous membrane of mouth and anus

Endoderm
Lining of trachea, pharynx, and bronchi
Lining of digestive tract
Lining of bladder and urethra

Mesoderm
True skin
Skeleton
Bone and cartilage
Connective tissue
Muscles
Blood and blood vessels
Kidneys and gonads

Accessory Structures of Pregnancy

The placenta, umbilical cord, and fetal circulation support the fetus as it completes prenatal life and prepares for birth.

Placenta

The *placenta* (afterbirth) is a temporary organ for fetal respiration, nutrition, and excretion. It also functions as an endocrine gland. Early maternal-placental-fetal circulatory structures are in place at 22 days after conception, when the embryonic heart begins to beat.

The placenta forms when the chorionic villi of the embryo extend into the blood-filled spaces of the mother's decidua basalis. The maternal part of the placenta arises from the decidua basalis, and has a beefy red appearance. The fetal side of the placenta develops from the chorionic villi and the chorionic blood vessels. The amnion covers the fetal side and umbilical cord and gives them a grayish, shiny appearance at term.

Placental Transfer

A thin membrane separates the maternal and fetal blood, and the two blood supplies do not normally mix. However, separation of the placenta at birth may allow some fetal blood to enter the maternal circulation, which can cause problems with fetuses in subsequent pregnancies if the blood types are not compatible. The placenta is divided into 15 to 20 segments called *cotyledons*. Some placentas have a small accessory lobe attached to the main placenta. Placental structures and blood circulation patterns are shown in Figure 3–4.

Fetal deoxygenated blood and waste products leave the fetus through the two umbilical arteries and enter the placenta through the branch of a main stem villus, which extends into the intervillous space. Oxygenated, nutrient-rich blood from the mother spurts into the intervillous space from the spiral arteries. The fetal blood releases carbon dioxide and waste products and takes in oxygen and nutrients before returning to the fetus through the umbilical vein.

The thin placental membrane provides some protection but is not barrier to most substances ingested by the mother. Many harmful substances, such as drugs (therapeutic and abused), nicotine, and viral infectious agents, are transferred to the fetus and may cause fetal drug addiction, congenital anomalies, and fetal infection. However, the placenta can also be used to deliver therapeutic medications to the fetus, such as to deliver digitalis to the fetus with heart failure (Gorrie, McKinney, & Murray, 1998).

Nursing Tip

The placenta is much larger than the developing baby during early pregnancy, but the fetus grows faster. At term, the placenta weighs about one-sixth the weight of the infant.

Placental Metabolism

During early pregnancy the placenta makes glycogen, cholesterol, and fatty acids to nourish the embryo/fetus. These substances are also needed for the placenta's own functions.

Placental Hormones

Four hormones are produced by the placenta: progesterone, estrogen, human chorionic gonadotropin (hCG), and human placental lactogen (hPL).

Progesterone. Progesterone is first produced by the corpus luteum and later by the placenta. It has several functions during pregnancy:

- Maintains uterine lining for implantation of the zygote
- Reduces uterine contractions to prevent spontaneous abortion
- Prepares the glands of the breasts for lactation

Estrogen. Estrogen also has several important functions during pregnancy:

- Stimulates uterine growth
- Increases the blood flow to uterine vessels
- Stimulates development of the breast ducts to prepare for lactation

Estrogen's other effects are not directly related to pregnancy. These include:

- Increased skin pigmentation (such as the "mask of pregnancy")
- Vascular changes in the skin and the mucous membranes of the nose and mouth
- Increased salivation

Human Chorionic Gonadotropin. Human chorionic gonadotropin (hCG) is the hormone "signal" sent to the corpus luteum that conception has occurred. The hCG causes the corpus luteum to persist and to continue production of estrogen and progesterone. hCG is detectable in maternal blood as soon as implantation occurs, usually 8–10 days after fertilization and is the basis for most pregnancy tests.

Human Placental Lactogen. hPL is also known as human chorionic somatomammotropin (hCS). The hPL stimulates adjustments in the mother's metabolism, making more glucose available to meet fetal energy needs.

Umbilical Cord

The umbilical cord develops with the placenta and fetal blood vessels; it is the lifeline between mother and fetus. Two arteries carry blood away

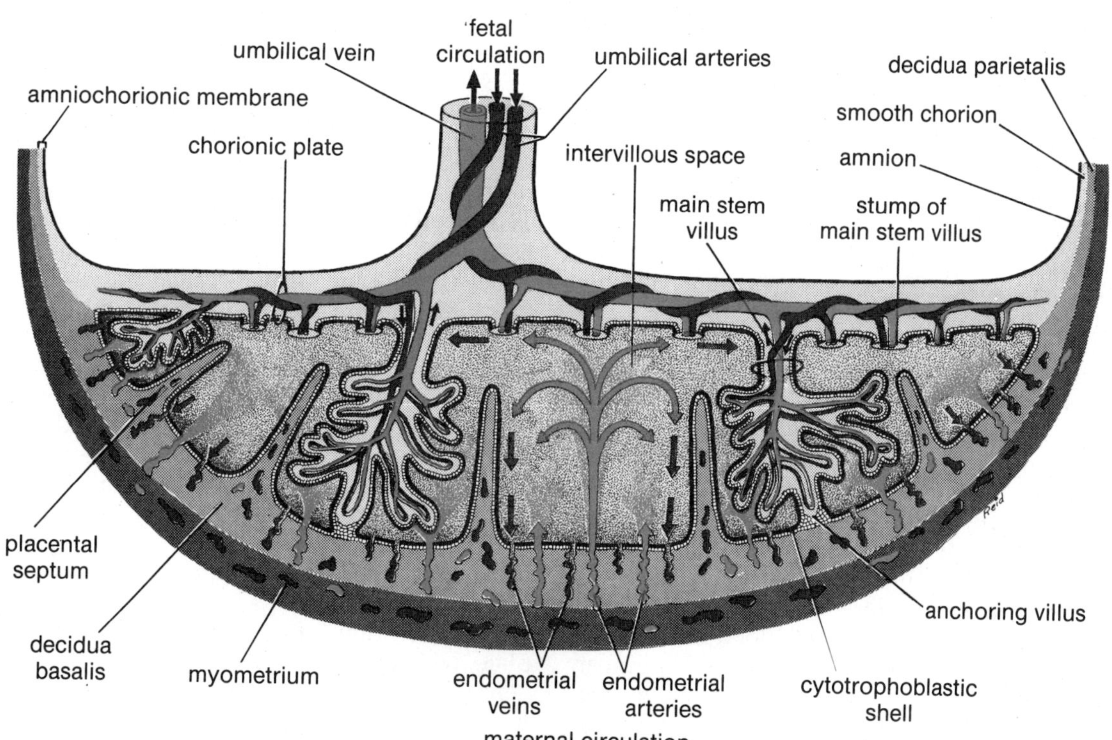

Figure 3–4 • Arrangement of the placental blood vessels. The blood of the fetus flows through the umbilical arteries into the fetal capillaries in the villi and then back to the fetal circulation through the umbilical vein. Maternal blood is transported by the uterine spiral arteries to the intervillous space, and it leaves by the uterine veins to return to the maternal circulation. (From Moore, K. L., & Persaud, T. V. N. [1998]. *The developing human: Clinically oriented embryology* [6th ed.]. Philadelphia: Saunders.)

Nursing Tip

An easy way to remember the number and type of umbilical cord vessels is the woman's name AVA, which stands for "artery-vein-artery."

from the fetus and one vein returns blood to the fetus. *Wharton's jelly* covers and cushions the cord vessels and keeps the three vessels separated. The vessels are coiled within the cord to allow movement and stretching without restricting circulation. The normal length of the cord is 30 to 90 cm (12 to 36 inches).

The umbilical cord is usually inserted near the center of the placenta. Insertion of the cord into the edge of the placenta is known as battledore insertion. A rare insertion, called velamentous insertion, is the insertion of the umbilical cord along the membranes that cover the placental surface. Reduced fetal blood supply or fetal hemorrhage are possible results of these abnormalities.

Fetal Circulation

After week 4 of gestation, circulation of blood through the placenta to the fetus is well established (Fig. 3–5). Because the fetus does not breathe and the liver does not have to process most waste products, several diversions in the post-birth circulatory route are needed. The three fetal circulatory shunts are the:

- Ductus venosus, which diverts some blood away from the liver as it returns from the placenta
- Foramen ovale, which diverts most blood from the right atrium directly to the left atrium, rather than circulating it to the lungs
- Ductus arteriosus, which diverts most blood from the pulmonary artery into the aorta

Circulation before Birth. Oxygenated blood enters the fetal body through the umbilical vein. About half the blood goes to the liver through the portal sinus; the remainder enters the inferior vena cava through the *ductus venosus.* Blood in the inferior vena cava enters the right atrium, where most passes directly into the left atrium through the *foramen ovale.* A small amount of blood is pumped to the lungs by the right ventricle to nourish them. The rest of the blood from the right ventricle joins that from the left ventricle through the *ductus arteriosus.* After circulating through the fetal body, blood having a lower oxygen saturation and containing waste products is returned to the placenta through the umbilical arteries.

Circulation after Birth. Fetal shunts are not needed after birth after the infant breathes and blood is circulated to the lungs. The foramen ovale closes because pressure in the right side of the heart falls as the lungs become fully inflated and there is now little resistance to blood flow through them. The infant's blood oxygen level rises, causing the ductus arteriosus to constrict. The ductus venosus closes when the flow from the umbilical cord stops.

Closure of Fetal Circulatory Shunts. The foramen ovale closes functionally (temporarily) within 2 hours after birth and permanently by 3 months of age. The ductus arteriosus closes functionally within 15 hours and closes permanently in about 3 weeks. The ductus venosus closes functionally when the cord is cut and closes permanently in about 1 week. After permanent closure, the ductus arteriosus and ductus venosus become ligaments.

Because they are functionally closed rather than permanently closed, some conditions may cause the foramen ovale or ductus arteriosus to reopen after birth. A condition that impedes full lung expansion, such as respiratory distress syndrome, can increase resistance to blood flow from the heart to the lungs, causing the foramen ovale to reopen. Similar conditions often reduce the blood oxygen levels and can cause the ductus arteriosus to remain open. See Chapters 12, 13, and 14 for further discussion of newborn changes and problems.

The Embryo

The developing baby is called an embryo from the third through the end of the eighth week after fertilization. The number of weeks refers to the number since fertilization of the ovum (fertilization age). Gestational age is calculated from the date of the woman's last menstrual period and is about 2 weeks longer than fertilization age.

Week 3. The developing baby measures 1.5 mm (0.06 inch) from crown to rump (CRL, or crown–rump length), and its weight is negligible. The embryonic disc is pear-shaped, having a wide cephalic (head) end and a narrow caudal (tail) end. The future brain and spinal cord are a flat neural plate, which begins closing in the middle to form a neural tube. The gastrointestinal tract is developing from the endoderm and is near the yolk sac. The heart is single-chambered and tubular at this stage, and begins beating.

Week 4. The embryo is about 4 mm (0.16 inch) CRL. The neural tube closes to form the brain and spinal cord. The primitive structure of the eyes,

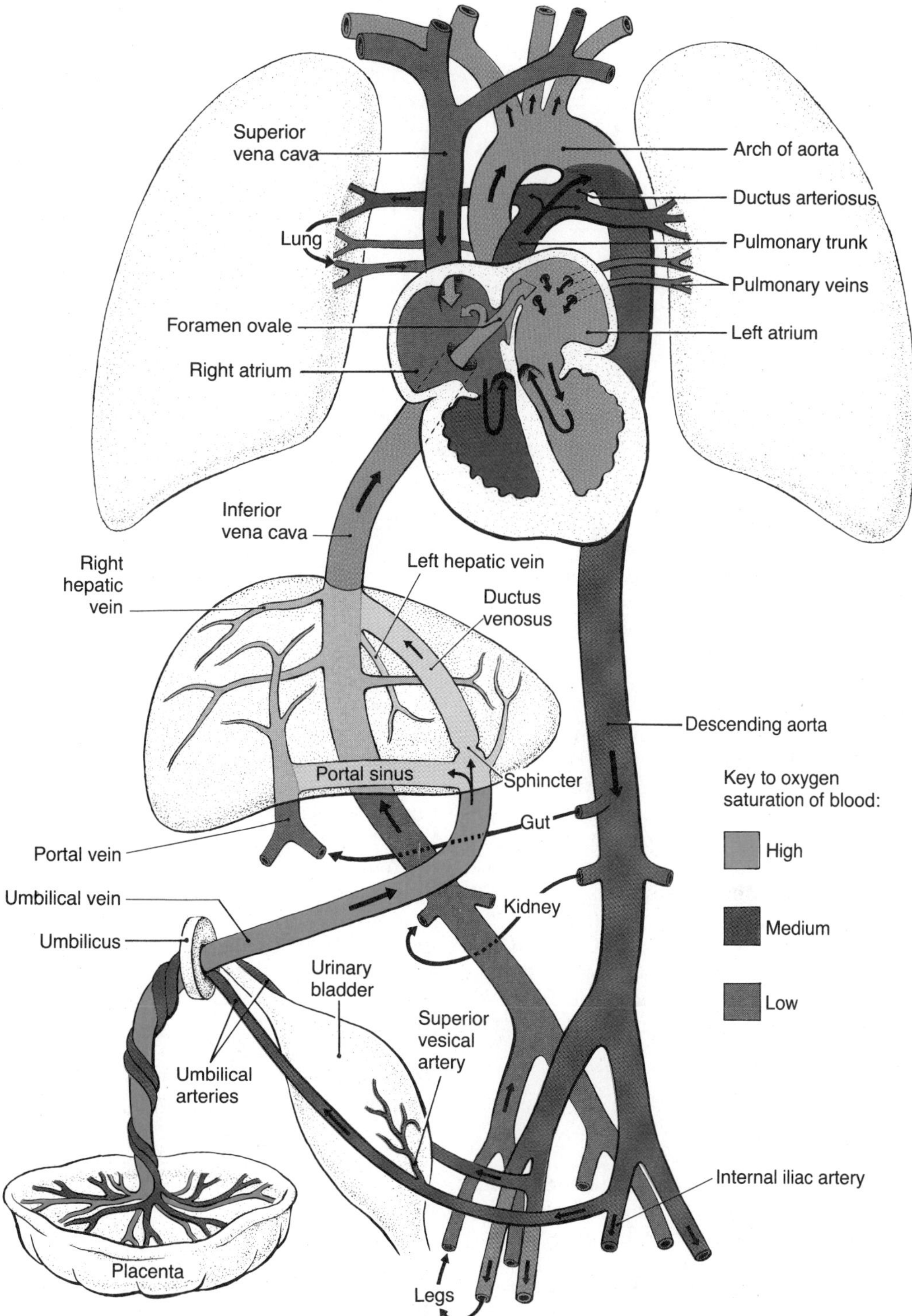

Figure 3–5 • Fetal circulation. (From Moore, K. L., & Persaud, T. V. N. [1998]. *The developing human: Clinically oriented embryology* [6th ed.]. Philadelphia: Saunders.)

ears, jaws, limb buds, and kidneys is established. The esophagus and trachea start as one tube, but begin dividing into separate structures. At day 28, the heart pumps fetal blood. Small buds appear on the side of the embryo and will form the arms and legs.

A major feature of the 4th week is the formation of 42 *somites.* Somites are paired segments along the neural tube, formed by the thickened mesoderm, that develop into the vertebral column and muscles of the body.

Week 5. During the 5th week, the embryo grows to 8 mm (0.3 inch) CRL. The eyes and nose continue noticeable development. The embryo assumes a C-shape, and a large head and a tail are seen. The heart has two atrial chambers. The developing intestines are mostly contained within the umbilical cord. The arms and legs are paddle-shaped.

Week 6. The embryo is now 13 mm (0.5 inch) CRL. The limb buds are extending and the joints are becoming noticeable. The primitive skeletal and muscle systems are developing. The beating heart now has all four chambers and is pumping blood that the liver is beginning to produce. The external, middle, and internal ears appear. The trachea, bronchi, and lung buds of the respiratory system are evolving. The upper lip along with the oral and nasal passages is forming.

Week 7. At 7 weeks, the embryo is 18 mm (0.7 inch) CRL. The face is formed, the tongue is a separate structure within the mouth, and the palate closes. The diaphragm separates the thoracic cavity from the abdominal cavity. The optic nerve is formed, and fused eyelids are apparent. Differentiation of internal male and female reproductive organs begins. Male and female embryos look alike from outward appearances until after 10 weeks.

Week 8. The embryo's length is 30 mm (1.2 inches) CRL. The basic structure of all body systems is established by the end of the eighth week. Fingers and toes are formed, as is the structure of the ear. The neural tube closes.

The Fetus

At the beginning of the 9th week, the developing baby is called a fetus (Table 3–1). The body form is easily recognized as human, with all the necessary external features and internal organ systems in place. Measurements of the fetal body length in this section are also for the crown–rump length rather than including the length of the legs and thus will be shorter than the total fetal length.

Week 10. The fetus is now about 61 mm (2.4 inches) CRL and weighs 14 g (0.5 oz). Fingernails and toenails begin growing, the intestines are enclosed in the abdomen, urine forms and enters the bladder, and the lacrimal (tear) ducts have developed. The fetal heart beat may be detected by a Doppler transducer.

Week 12. The fetus is now 87 mm (3.5 inches) CRL and weighs 45 g (1.6 ounces). The fetal liver gradually decreases production of red blood cells as the spleen begins to produce them. Bile begins to form in the liver, and the gallbladder starts to form. Lungs have a definite shape, and the skin is a delicate pink. Bones and muscles continue growing and developing. The fetus has been moving for 4 weeks, although the mother will not feel it for another 4 weeks.

Week 16. The length of the fetus has increased to 140 mm (5.6 inches) CRL, and weight is about 200 g (7 ounces). Fetal heart tones may be heard with a *fetoscope,* which is a specially adapted stethoscope for listening to the fetal heart. Teeth begin to form, and the digestive tract begins to function with the collection of *meconium,* which is a mixture of amniotic fluid and secretions of the intestinal glands. Scalp and lanugo hair appear, and sweat glands develop. Blood vessels are visible through the delicate skin. The sex of the fetus is externally discernible. Most women begin feeling fetal movements (quickening) about this time.

Week 20. The fetus reaches the midpoint of the gestational period, a time that is often referred to as the point of *viability* because the fetus may survive briefly if born at this time. The length is about 160 mm (6.4 inches) CRL and weight is about 460 g (about 1 pound). Incisors, canine, and first molar teeth are all developing. The fetus can suck its thumb and swallow amniotic fluid. The cellular structure of the alveoli of the lungs is complete. By the end of week 20, lanugo hair covers the fetal body except for the palms of the hands and soles of the feet. Fetal movements are readily felt by the pregnant woman and an experienced examiner.

Brown fat has a dark brown hue that is due to its density, enriched blood supply, and abundant nerve supply. It forms around the kidneys, adrenals, and neck; between the scapulae; and behind the sternum. Because it generates more heat than normal fat, brown fat is the primary source of heat for the newborn.

Week 24. Rapid growth continues, with the fetus measuring 230 mm (9.2 inches) CRL and weighing about 820 g (1.8 pounds). Vernix caseosa is a cheese-like secretion from the fetal sebaceous glands and dead epidermal cells that protects the delicate fetal skin from abrasions, chapping, and hardening that could result from the constant immersion in amniotic fluid.

Table 3–1
EMBRYONIC AND FETAL DEVELOPMENT

Age	Length (crown to rump)	Weight	Body Systems
Embryo			
Week 3 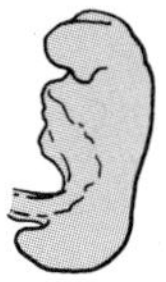	1.5 mm (0.06 in)	*	*Cardiovascular:* single tubular heart and major blood vessels appear *Nervous:* embryonic disc and primitive spinal cord and brain appear *Gastrointestinal:* GI tract is close to yolk sac
Week 4 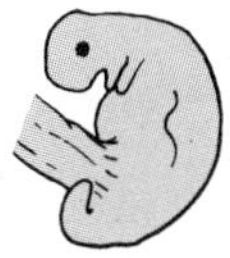	4 mm (0.16 in)	*	*Musculoskeletal:* somites (42) appear along neural tube (will develop into vertebral column and muscles); primitive jaw and limb develop *Nervous:* neural tube closes *Gastrointestinal:* esophagus and trachea division occurs *Genitourinary:* primitive kidney appears *Skin/senses:* primitive eyes and ears appear
Week 5 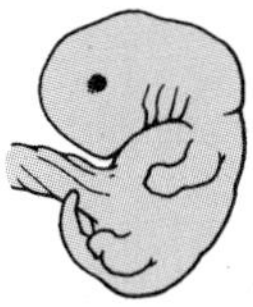	8 mm (0.3 in)	*	*Musculoskeletal:* limbs begin to lengthen *Cardiovascular:* heart has two atrial chambers and pumps its own blood *Nervous:* five distinct areas of brain exist, and 10 pairs of cranial nerves *Skin/senses:* eyes and nose are noticeable
Week 6 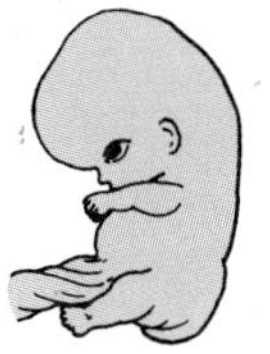	13 mm (0.5 in)	*	*Musculoskeletal:* limbs continue to extend; primitive skeleton, skull, and jaws begin to ossify *Cardiovascular:* heart has all four chambers *Gastrointestinal:* oral and nasal cavities and upper lip are forming *Genitourinary:* sex glands appear *Respiratory:* trachea, bronchi, and lung buds are evolving *Skin/senses:* external, middle, and internal ear is forming
Week 7 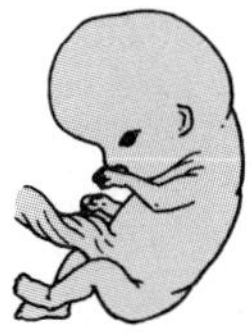	18 mm (0.7 in)	*	*Musculoskeletal:* limbs continue to extend *Cardiovascular:* heart continues to pump fetal blood, which liver begins to make *Nervous:* optic nerve is formed *Gastrointestinal:* abdominal cavity separates from thoracic cavity; tongue is separate in mouth; palate folds *Genitourinary:* male and female reproductive organs differentiate, but external appearance is similar *Skin/senses:* face is formed; eyelids fuse
Week 8 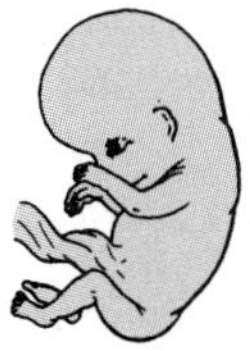	30 mm (1.2 in)	*	*Musculoskeletal:* fingers and toes are formed *Cardiovascular:* heart function and fetal circulation are complete *Skin/senses:* ears are complete

Table continued on following page

Table 3-1
EMBRYONIC AND FETAL DEVELOPMENT *(Continued)*

Age	Length (crown to rump)	Weight	Body Systems
Fetus			
Week 10 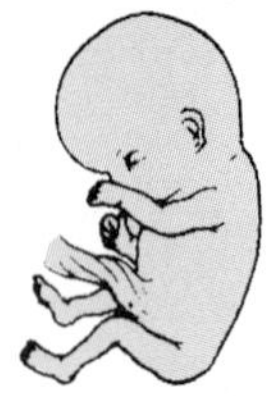	61 mm (2.4 in)	14 g (0.5 oz)	*Musculoskeletal:* growth continues *Cardiovascular:* fetal circulation is functioning *Nervous:* fetus moves about *Gastrointestinal:* intestines are enclosed in abdomen *Genitourinary:* urine forms and enters bladder *Skin/senses:* tear ducts form; fingernails and toenails grow
Week 12	87 mm (3.5 in)	45 g (1.6 oz)	*Musculoskeletal:* growth and development continue *Cardiovascular:* fetal liver produces red blood cells *Gastrointestinal:* bile is stored in gallbladder *Respiratory:* lungs have definite shape *Skin/senses:* skin is delicate pink
Week 16 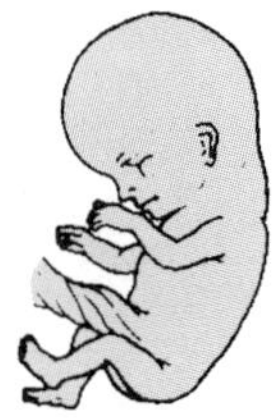	140 mm (5.6 in)	200 g (7 oz)	*Musculoskeletal:* acceleration of growth *Cardiovascular:* fetal heart is heard with fetoscope; blood vessels are visible under skin *Nervous:* mother feels movement of fetus *Gastrointestinal:* teeth form; digestive tract begins to function and collects meconium *Genitourinary:* sex of fetus is externally apparent *Skin/senses:* scalp hair, lanugo hair, and sweat glands develop
Week 20 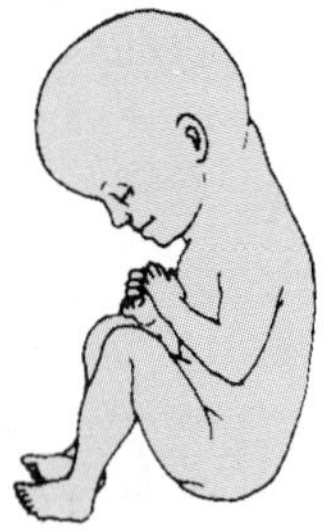	160 mm (6.4 in)	460 g (1 pound)	*Musculoskeletal:* brown fat begins to form *Nervous:* fetus is able to suck thumb *Gastrointestinal:* incisors, canine, and first molar teeth are developing; fetus swallows amniotic fluid *Respiratory:* structure of alveoli of lungs is complete
Week 24	230 mm (9.2 in)	820 g (1.8 pounds)	*Respiratory:* nostrils open; respiratory movements occur *Skin/senses:* eyes are complete; skin is red and wrinkled; vernix caseosa is present
Week 28	270 mm (10.8 in)	1300 g (3 pounds)	*Musculoskeletal:* adipose tissue increases *Nervous:* regulatory function noted *Genitourinary:* testes descend into scrotum in male *Skin/senses:* eyebrows and eyelashes are present; eyelids are open
Week 32	300 mm (11.8 in)	2100 g (4.6 pounds)	*Musculoskeletal:* skeletal system is fully developed and flexible for passage at birth *Nervous:* continues to mature; fetus regulates body temperature *Respiratory:* rhythmic respirations

Table 3–1
EMBRYONIC AND FETAL DEVELOPMENT *(Continued)*

Age	Length (crown to rump)	Weight	Body Systems
Week 38	360 mm (14.4 in)	3400 g (7 pounds)	*Musculoskeletal:* many creases are seen over soles of feet *Genitourinary:* rugae in scrotum (males) or labia majora (females) are well developed *Skin/senses:* skin is pink and smooth; vernix caseosa remains only in skin folds; lanugo hair remains on shoulders and upper back; ear lobes are firm

*Negligible.
From Moore, K. L., & Persaud, T. J. M. (1998). *Before we are born: Essentials of embryology and birth defects* (5th ed). Philadelphia: Saunders.

Also during week 24, the nostrils open, respiratory movements occur, and alveoli begin to produce *surfactant.* Surfactant is a mixture of lipids that covers the internal walls of the alveoli of the lungs; it enables the alveoli to stay open so that adequate lung expansion will occur.

Week 28. Fetal CRL increases to 270 mm (10.8 inches) CRL and fetal weight increases to 1300 g (about 3 pounds). Eyebrows and eyelashes are present, and the eyelids are open. The nervous system begins some regulatory functions, and in males the testes descend into the scrotum.

Week 32. Fetal CRL is 300 mm (11.8 inches) and the weight is about 2100 g (4.6 pounds). The fetal nervous system continues to mature, so that rhythmic respirations and regulation of body temperature are possible if birth occurs at this time. The fully developed skeletal system is soft and flexible, permitting the fetus to position itself for passage through the pelvis. Muscle and fat accumulate.

Week 38. The fetus has now filled out its wrinkled skin with subcutaneous fat, so that its length is about 360 mm (14.4 inches) CRL and its weight is about 3400 g (7 pounds). The skin is pink and smooth with vernix caseosa present only in skin folds. Some lanugo may persist on the shoulders and upper back. Characteristics of the mature fetus include firm ears, many creases over the soles of the foot, and either rugae in the scrotum or well-developed labia majora.

MULTIFETAL PREGNANCY

Twins occur once in every 90 pregnancies in North America. When hormones are given to assist with ovulation, twinning and other multifetal births (triplets, quadruplets, and quintuplets) are more likely to occur. The first set of septuplets to survive were born in the United States in 1997.

Dizygotic (DZ) twins (Fig. 3–6), also called fraternal twins, may or may not be of the same sex and develop from two separate ova fertilized by two separate sperm. Dizygotic twins always have two amnions, two chorions, and two placentas, although their chorions and placentas sometimes fuse. Dizygotic twins tend to repeat in families, and the incidence increases with maternal age. They are about as much alike as any siblings. Different races have varying incidences of dizygotic twinning.

- African: 1 in 20 births
- Asian: 1 in 150 births
- United States white: 1 in 80 births

Monozygotic (MZ) twins (Fig. 3–7), often called identical, are genetically identical, have the same sex, and look alike because they develop from a single fertilized ovum. Physical differences between monozygotic twins are caused by prenatal environmental factors involving variations in the blood supply from the placenta. Most monozygotic twins begin to develop at the end of the 1st week after fertilization. The result is two identical embryos, each with its own chorion but with a common placenta and some common placental vessels. Monozygotic twins normally have a single amnion (inner sac). If the embryonic disc does not divide completely, various types of conjoined (formerly called Siamese) twins may form. They are named according to the regions that are joined (e.g., thoracopagus indicates an anterior connection of

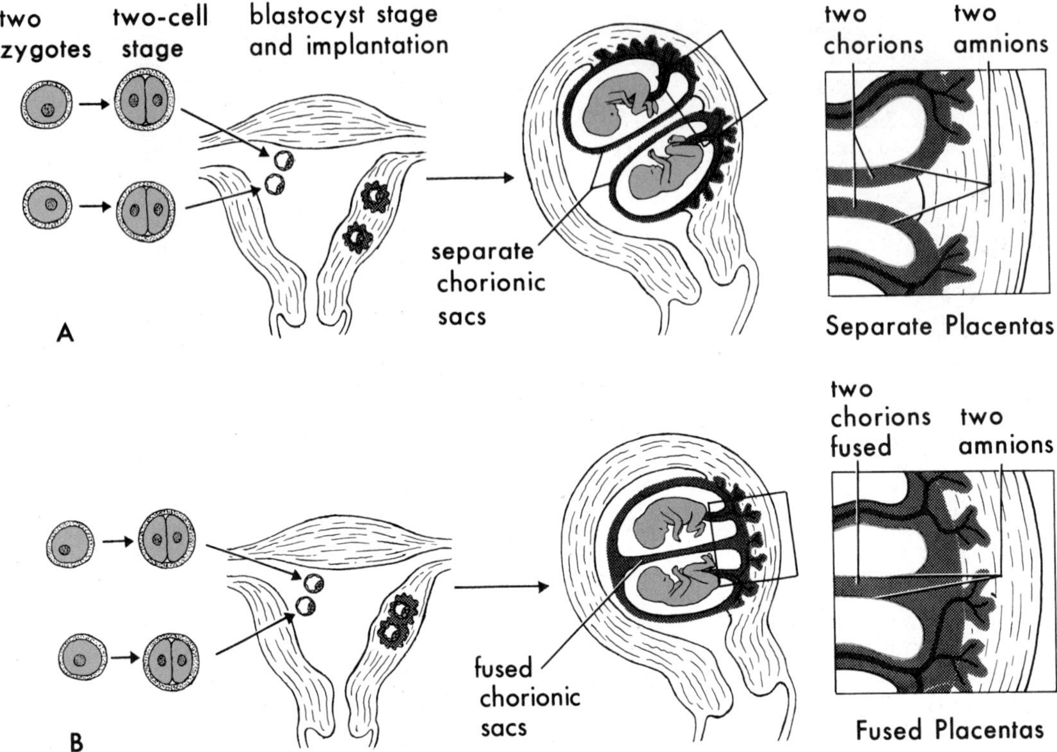

Figure 3–6 • Development of dizygotic twins from two zygotes. The relations of the fetal membranes and placentas are shown. **A,** The blastocysts implant separately. **B,** The blastocysts implant close together. In both cases there are two amnions and two chorions, and the placentas may be separate or fused. (From Moore, K. L., & Persaud, T. V. N. [1998]. *The developing human: Clinically oriented embryology* [6th ed.]. Philadelphia: Saunders.)

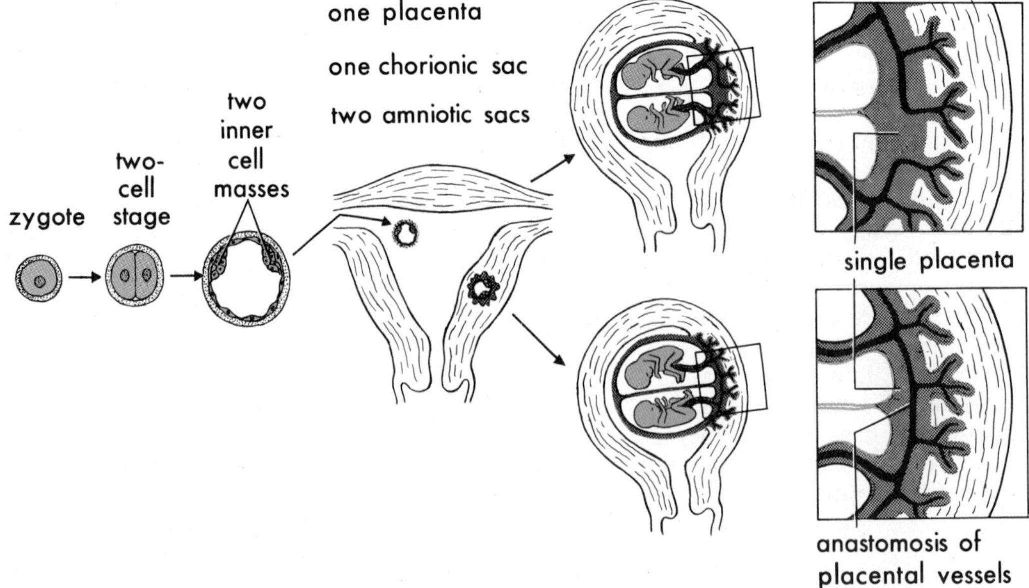

Figure 3–7 • Development of about 65% of monozygotic twins: one zygote undergoes division of its inner cell mass (embryoblast) toward the end of the first week. Such twins have separate amnions, a single chorion, and a common placenta. (From Moore, K. L., & Persaud, T. V. N. [1998]. *The developing human: Clinically oriented embryology* [6th ed.]. Philadelphia: Saunders.)

the thoracic regions). These twins have a single amnion.

Many twin or higher multiples are born prematurely, because the uterus becomes overdistended. The placenta may not be able to supply sufficient nutrition to both fetuses, resulting in one or both twins being smaller than expected. Birth defects are more common in monozygotic twins.

KEY POINTS

- The uniqueness of each individual results from the blending of genes on the 46 chromosomes contained in each body cell and the environment of the embryo and fetus during development.
- Gametogenesis in the male is called spermatogenesis and occurs in the seminiferous tubules of the testes. Each mature sperm has 22 autosomes plus either an X or a Y sex chromosome, for a total of 23. Gametogenesis in the female is called oogenesis. It begins in the graafian follicle, continues at ovulation, and is not completed until fertilization occurs. The mature ovum has 22 autosomes plus the X sex chromosome, for a total of 23. At conception, the total number of chromosomes is restored to 46.
- When the ovum is fertilized by an X-bearing sperm, a female results; when it is fertilized by a Y-bearing sperm, the child will be male.
- After fertilization in the fallopian tube, the zygote enters the uterus, where implantation is complete by 10 days after fertilization. If the zygote fails to move through the tube, implantation occurs there and a tubal ectopic pregnancy results.
- When implantation occurs in the uterine lining, the cells of the zygote differentiate and develop into the following structures: chorion, amnion, yolk sac, and primary germ layers. The chorion develops into the embryonic/fetal portion of the placenta; the amnion encloses the embryo and the amniotic fluid; the primary germ layers develop into different parts of the growing fetus; and the yolk sac, which functions only during embryonic life, begins to form red blood cells.
- The three germ layers of the embryo are the ectoderm, mesoderm, and endoderm. From these, all the structures of the individual will develop.
- All body systems are formed and functioning in a simple way by the end of the 8th week.
- The accessory structures of pregnancy are the placenta, umbilical cord, and fetal circulation. These structures continuously support the fetus throughout prenatal life in preparation for birth.
- The placenta is an organ for fetal respiration, nutrition, and excretion. It is also a temporary endocrine gland that produces progesterone, estrogen, human chorionic gonadotropin (hCG), and human placental lactogen (hPL).
- Fetal circulation transports oxygen and nutrients to the fetus and disposes of carbon dioxide and other waste products from the fetus. The temporary fetal circulatory structures are the foramen ovale, ductus arteriosus, and ductus venosus. They divert most blood from the fetal liver and lungs because these organs do not fully function during prenatal life.

MULTIPLE-CHOICE REVIEW QUESTIONS

Choose the most appropriate answer.

1. The child's sex is determined by the
   a. dominance of either the X or the Y chromosome
   b. number of X chromosomes in the ovum
   c. ovum, which contributes either an X or a Y chromosome
   d. sperm, which contains either an X or a Y chromosome
2. A woman who wants to become pregnant should avoid all medications unless prescribed by a physician who knows she is pregnant because
   a. the placenta allows most medications to cross into the fetus
   b. medications often have adverse effects when taken during pregnancy
   c. fetal growth is likely to be slowed by many medications
   d. the pregnancy is likely to be prolonged by some medications
3. The umbilical cord normally contains
   a. one artery, one vein
   b. two arteries and two veins
   c. two arteries, one vein
   d. two veins
4. The purpose of the foramen ovale is to
   a. increase fetal blood flow to the lungs
   b. limit blood flow to the liver
   c. raise the oxygen content of fetal blood
   d. reduce blood flow to the lungs
5. Twins are often born early because the
   a. distended uterus becomes irritable
   b. amnion and chorion fuse permanently
   c. woman's body cannot tolerate the weight
   d. fetuses become too large to deliver vaginally

BIBLIOGRAPHY AND READER REFERENCE

Blackburn, S. T., & Loper, D. L. (1992). *Maternal, fetal, and neonatal physiology: A clinical perspective.* Philadelphia: Saunders.

Glass, R. H. (1994). Gamete transport, fertilization, and implantation. In R. K. Creasy and R. Resnick (Eds.), *Maternal-fetal medicine: Principles and practice* (pp. 89–95). Philadelphia: Saunders.

Gorrie, T., McKinney, E., & Murray, S. (1998). *Foundations of maternal newborn nursing* (2nd ed.). Philadelphia: Saunders.

Guyton, A. (1996). *Textbook of medical physiology* (9th ed.). Philadelphia: Saunders.

Moore, K. L., & Persaud, T. V. N. (1998). *The developing human: Clinically oriented embryology* (6th ed.). Philadelphia: Saunders.

Moore, K. L., & Persaud, T. V. N. (1998). *Before we are born: Essentials of embryology and birth defects* (5th ed.). Philadelphia: Saunders.

Moore, K. L., Persaud, T. V. N., & Shiota, K. (1994). *Color atlas of clinical embryology.* Philadelphia: Saunders.

Wilcox, A. J., Weinberg, C. R., & Baird, D. D. (1995). Timing of sexual intercourse in relation to ovulation. *New England Journal of Medicine, 333*(23), 1517–1521.

chapter 4

Prenatal Care and Adaptations to Pregnancy

Outline

Objectives

On completion and mastery of Chapter 4, the student will be able to

- Define each vocabulary term listed.
- Calculate the expected date of delivery and duration of pregnancy.
- Differentiate among the presumptive, probable, and positive signs of pregnancy.
- List the goals of prenatal care.
- Discuss prenatal care for a normal pregnancy.
- Explain the nurse's role in prenatal care.
- Describe the physiologic changes during pregnancy.
- Identify nutritional needs for pregnancy and lactation.
- Revise nursing care related to care of the pregnant adolescent.
- Describe client education related to common discomforts of pregnancy.
- Discuss nursing support of emotional changes that occur in a family during pregnancy.

Vocabulary

antepartum
Braxton Hicks' contractions
Chadwick's sign
Goodell's sign
gravida
Hegar's sign
lightening
para
pica
trimester

Pregnancy is a temporary, physiologic (normal) process that affects the woman physically and emotionally. All systems of her body adapt to support the developing baby. The focus of nursing care during pregnancy is to teach the mother how to maintain good health or, in the case of a mother with a condition that places her or her fetus at risk, to improve her health as much as possible. This chapter reviews prenatal care, the physiologic and psychological changes of pregnancy, and nursing care to meet the needs of women and families.

GOALS OF PRENATAL CARE

Early and regular prenatal care is the best way to ensure a healthy outcome for both mother and baby. Obstetricians, family practice physicians, certified nurse-midwives (CNMs), and nurse practitioners provide prenatal care. Unlike the other health care providers, the nurse practitioner does not usually attend the woman at birth. The office or clinic nurse assists the health care provider, helps to evaluate the expectant family's physical, psychological, and social needs, and teaches the woman self-care.

The major goals of prenatal care are to

- Ensure a safe birth for mother and baby by promoting good health habits and reducing risk factors
- Teach health habits that may be continued after pregnancy
- Educate in self-care for pregnancy
- Provide physical care
- Prepare parents for the responsibilities of parenthood

To achieve these goals, professionals must do more than offer physical care. They must work as a team to create an environment that allows for cultural and individual differences and is supportive of the entire family.

Nursing Tip

The major role of the nurse during prenatal care includes performing a physical assessment of the pregnant woman, identifying and reevaluating risk factors, educating in self-care, providing nutrition counseling, and promoting the family's adaptation to pregnancy.

Prenatal Visits

Ideally, health care for childbearing begins before conception. Preconception care identifies risk factors that may be changed before conception to reduce their negative impact on the outcome of pregnancy. For example, the woman may be counseled about how to improve her nutritional state before pregnancy or may receive immunizations to prevent infections that would be harmful to the developing baby. Some risk factors cannot be eliminated, such as preexisting diabetes, but preconception care helps the woman to begin pregnancy in the best possible state of health.

Prenatal care should begin as soon as a woman suspects that she is pregnant. A complete history and physical examination identify problems that may affect the woman or her fetus. The history should include:

- Obstetric history: number and outcomes of past pregnancies, problems in the mother or infant
- Menstrual history: usual frequency of menstrual cycles and duration of flow; first day of the last normal menstrual period (LNMP); any "spotting" since the last normal menstrual period
- Contraceptive history: type used; whether an oral contraceptive was taken before the woman realized she might be pregnant; whether an intrauterine device is still in place
- Medical and surgical history: infections such as hepatitis or pyelonephritis; past surgical procedures; trauma that involved the pelvis or reproductive organs

Nursing Tip

The nurse listens to concerns and answers questions from the expectant family during each prenatal visit. This is a prime time for teaching good health habits, as most women are highly motivated to improve their health.

- Family history of the woman and her partner to identify genetic or other problems that may pose a risk for the pregnancy
- Woman's and partner's health history to identify risk factors, such as genetic defects or use of alcohol, drugs, or tobacco, and possible blood incompatibility between the mother and fetus
- Psychosocial history to identify stability of lifestyle and ability to parent a child; significant cultural practices or health beliefs that affect the pregnancy

The woman has a complete physical examination on her first visit to evaluate her general health, determine her baseline weight and vital signs, evaluate her nutritional status, and to identify current problems such as infections. A pelvic examination is done to evaluate the size, adequacy, and condition of the pelvis and reproductive organs and to assess signs of pregnancy (see p. 57). Her estimated date of delivery (EDD) is calculated based on the LNMP. An ultrasound examination may be done at this visit or at a later visit to confirm the EDD. Assessment for risk factors that may affect the pregnancy is done during the first visit and updated at subsequent visits.

Several laboratory tests are done on the first or second prenatal visit. Others are done at specific times during pregnancy and may be repeated at specific intervals. Several tests are done for all pregnant women; others are based on the presence of specific risk factors. Standard precautions are used when handling body fluids (see Appendix A). Table 4–1 lists common prenatal laboratory tests.

The recommended schedule for prenatal visits in an uncomplicated pregnancy is as follows:

- Conception to 28 weeks—every 4 weeks
- 29 to 36 weeks—every 2 to 3 weeks
- 37 weeks to birth—weekly

If complications arise, the pregnant woman will be seen more often. Routine assessments made at each prenatal visit include

- Review of known risk factors and assessment for new ones.
- Vital signs. The woman's blood pressure should be taken in the same arm and in the same position each time for accurate comparison with her baseline.
- Weight to determine if the pattern of gain is normal. Low prepregnant weight or inadequate gain are risk factors for preterm birth, a low-birthweight infant, and other problems. A sudden rapid weight gain is associated with pregnancy-induced hypertension.
- Urinalysis for protein, glucose, and ketones.
- Glucose screening between 24 and 28 weeks. Additional testing is done if the result of this screening test is 140 mg/dl or higher.
- Fundal height to determine if the fetus is growing as expected and the volume of amniotic fluid is appropriate.
- Leopold's maneuvers to assess the presentation and position of the fetus by abdominal palpation.

Table 4–1
COMMON PRENATAL LABORATORY TESTS

Test	Purpose
Blood grouping	Determine blood type
Rh factor and antibody screen	Determine risk for maternal–fetal blood incompatibility
Complete blood count	Detect anemia, infection, or cell abnormalities
Hemoglobin (Hgb) and/or hematocrit	Detect anemia at later prenatal visits
VDRL or rapid plasma reagin (RPR)	Syphilis screen
Rubella titer	Determine immunity
Tuberculin skin test	Screening test for tuberculosis
Hemoglobin electrophoresis	Identify presence of sickle cell trait or disease (women of African or Mediterranean descent)
Hepatitis B screen	Identify carriers of hepatitis B
Human immunodeficiency virus (HIV) screen	Offered to detect HIV infection
Urinalysis	Detect infection, renal disease, or diabetes
Pap test	Screen for cervical cancer
Cervical culture	Detect sexually transmissible diseases such as gonorrhea, chlamydia, or group B streptococci
Maternal serum alpha-fetoprotein (MSAFP)	Screen for fetal anomalies such as neural tube defects or chromosome abnormalities
Maternal blood glucose	To screen for gestational diabetes

From Gorrie, T. M., McKinney, E. S., & Murray, S. M. (1998). *Foundations of maternal-newborn nursing* (2nd ed). Philadelphia: Saunders.

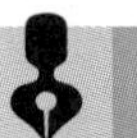

Nursing Tip

Early and regular prenatal care is important in reducing the number of low-birth-weight babies born and in reducing mortality and morbidity rates for mothers and newborns.

- Fetal heart rate. During very early pregnancy the fetal heart rate is taken with a Doppler transducer; in later pregnancy, it may also be heard with a fetoscope. Beating of the fetal heart can be seen on ultrasound examination as early as 8 weeks after the LNMP.
- Review of nutrition for adequacy of calorie intake and specific nutrients.
- Discomforts or problems that have arisen since the last visit.

The nurse establishes rapport with the expectant family by conveying interest in their needs, listening to their concerns, and directing them to appropriate resources. The health care team must show sensitivity to the family's cultural and health beliefs and incorporate as many as possible into care. For example, Muslim laws of modesty dictate that a woman be covered (hair, body, arms, and legs) when in the presence of an unrelated male. A female health care provider is often preferred. Latino families expect a brief period of conversation during which pleasantries are exchanged before "getting to the point" of the visit. An Asian woman may nod her head when the nurse teaches her, leading the nurse to believe that she understands and will use the teaching. However, the woman may be showing respect to the nurse rather than agreement with what is taught. Eye contact, which is valued by many Americans, is seen as confrontational in some cultures.

Definition of Terms

The following terms are used to describe the obstetric history of a woman:

- **Gravida:** Any pregnancy, regardless of duration; also, the number of pregnancies, including the one in progress, if applicable.
- **Nulligravida:** A woman who has never been pregnant.
- **Primigravida:** A woman who is pregnant for the first time.
- **Multigravida:** A woman who has been pregnant before, regardless of the duration of the pregnancy.
- **Para:** A woman who has given birth to one or more children who reached the age of viability (20 weeks of gestation), regardless of the number of fetuses delivered and regardless of whether those children are now living; also, the number of pregnancies that ended at or after the age of viability.
- **Primipara:** A woman who has given birth to her first child (past the point of viability), regardless of whether the child was alive at birth or is now living. The term is also used informally to describe a woman before the birth of her first child.
- **Multipara:** A woman who has given birth to two or more children (past the point of viability), regardless of whether the children were alive at birth or are presently alive. The term is also used informally to describe a woman before the birth of her second child.
- **Nullipara:** A woman who has not given birth to a child who reached the point of viability.
- **Abortion:** The end of pregnancy before 20 weeks of gestation, either spontaneously or induced.
- **Gestational Age:** Prenatal age of the developing baby calculated from the first day of the woman's last normal menstrual period.
- **Fertilization Age:** Prenatal age of the developing baby calculated from the date of conception; about 2 weeks shorter than the gestational age.

The gravida number increases by one each time a woman is pregnant, whereas the para number increases only when a woman delivers a fetus of 20 weeks of gestation or more. For example, a woman who has had two spontaneous abortions (miscarriages) at 12 weeks of gestation, has a 3-year-old son, and is now 32 weeks pregnant would be described as gravida 4, para 1, abortions 2. The TPAL system (Box 4–1) is a standardized way to describe the outcomes of a woman's pregnancies on her prenatal record.

Determining the Estimated Date of Delivery

The average duration of a term pregnancy is 40 weeks (280 days) after the last menstrual period, plus or minus 2 weeks. Nägele's rule is used to determine the EDD. To calculate the EDD, one identifies the first day of the LNMP, counts

BOX 4–1
TPAL SYSTEM TO DESCRIBE PARITY

T—number of *term* infants born (infants born after at least 37 weeks of gestation)
P—number of *preterm* infants born (infants before 37 weeks of gestation)
A—number of pregnancies *aborted* (spontaneously or induced)
L—number of children now *living*

Example:

Name	Gravida	Term	Preterm	Abortions	Living
Katie Field	3	1	0	1	1
Anna Luz	4	1	1	1	2

Katie Field: gravida 3, para 1011
Anna Luz: gravida 4, para 1112

BOX 4–2
NÄGELE'S RULE TO DETERMINE THE EDD

- Determine first day of the last normal menstrual period (LNMP).
- Count backward 3 months.
- Add 7 days.
- Correct the year if needed.

Example:

1st day of LNMP: January 27
Count backward 3 months: October 27
Add 7 days: November 3 is EDD

backward 3 months, and then adds 7 days (Box 4–2). The year is updated if applicable. The EDD is an *estimated* date, as many normal births occur before and after this date. The EDD may also be determined with a wheel (Fig. 4–1), an electronic calculator for this purpose, physical examination, ultrasound, or a combination of these methods.

Pregnancy is divided into three 13-week parts called *trimesters.* Predictable changes occur in the woman and the fetus in each trimester. Understanding these developments helps to better provide anticipatory guidance and identify deviations from the expected pattern of development.

INDICATIONS OF PREGNANCY

The indications of pregnancy are divided into three general groups: presumptive, probable, and positive, depending on how likely they are to be caused by factors other than pregnancy.

Presumptive Indications

The presumptive indications of pregnancy are those from which a definite diagnosis of pregnancy cannot be made. These signs and symptoms are common during pregnancy, but often can have other causes as well. The presumptive indications include the following:

Amenorrhea, the cessation of menses, in a healthy, sexually active woman is often the first sign of pregnancy. However, strenuous exercise, changes in metabolism and endocrine dysfunction, chronic disease, certain medications, early menopause, or serious psychological disturbances may be the cause.

Nausea and sometimes *vomiting* occur in at least half of all pregnancies. "Morning sickness" describes the symptoms, although they may occur at any time of day. A distaste for certain foods or even their odors may be the main complaint. The nausea begins about 6 weeks after the LNMP and usually improves by the end of the first trimester. Emotional problems or gastrointestinal upsets may also cause nausea and vomiting.

Breast changes include tenderness and tingling as hormones from the placenta stimulate growth of the ductal system in preparation for breastfeeding. Similar breast changes also occur premenstrually in many women.

Pigmentation changes occur primarily in dark-skinned women. They include increased pigmentation of the face (chloasma, or "mask of pregnancy"), breasts (darkening of the areolae), and abdomen (linea nigra, a line extending in the midline of the

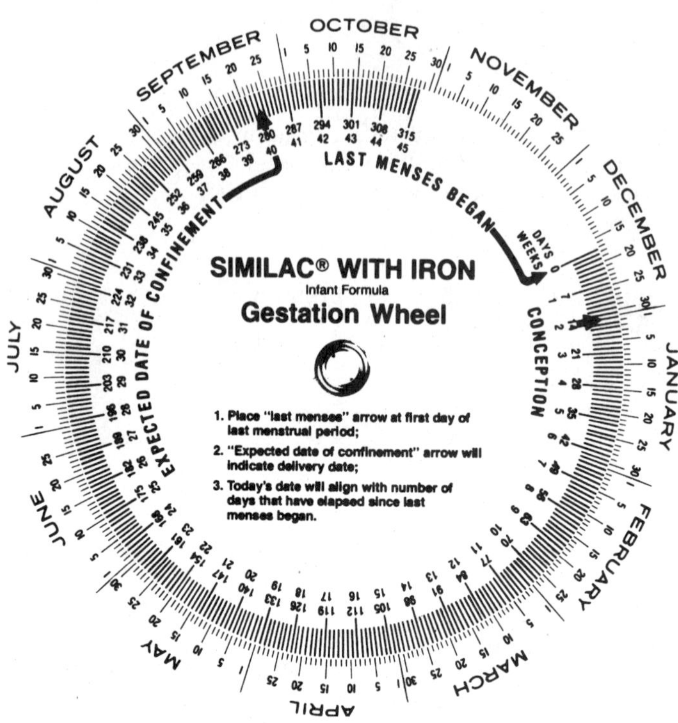

Figure 4–1. • A gestation wheel can be used to calculate the estimated date of delivery (EDD), or *due date.* The arrow labeled "Last menses began" is placed on the date the woman's last menstrual period began. The estimated date of delivery, also called estimated date of confinement (EDC) is read at the arrow labeled "40." (Courtesy of Ross Laboratories, Columbus, OH.)

abdomen from just above the umbilicus to the symphysis pubis). See Fig. 4–2 for illustration of common skin changes of pregnancy.

Frequency and *urgency of urination* are common in the early months of pregnancy. The enlarging uterus, along with the increased blood supply to the pelvic area, exerts pressure on the bladder. Urinary frequency occurs in the 1st trimester until the uterus expands and becomes an abdominal organ in the 2nd trimester. Again in the 3rd trimester, the pregnant woman experiences frequency of urination when the presenting part descends in the pelvis in preparation for birth. Causes of urinary disturbances other than pregnancy are urinary tract infections and pelvic masses.

Fatigue and *drowsiness* are early symptoms of pregnancy. Fatigue is believed to be caused by increased metabolic needs of the woman and fetus. In an otherwise healthy young woman, it is a significant sign of pregnancy. However, illness, stress, or sudden changes in life-style may also cause fatigue.

Quickening, fetal movement felt by the mother, is first perceived at 16 to 20 weeks of gestation as a faint fluttering in the lower abdomen. Women who have previously given birth often report quickening earlier than women who have not. This is an im-

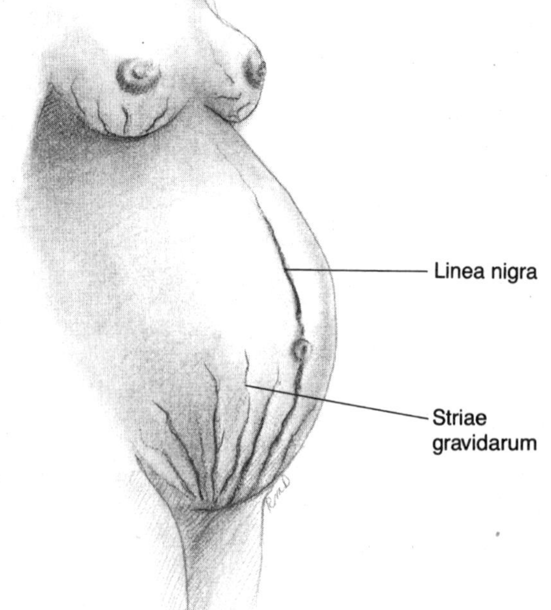

Figure 4–2. • Abdominal striae are pinkish-white or purple-gray lines that may occur in pregnancy. They may be found on the breasts, abdomen, and thighs. The dark line at the midline is the linea nigra, an area of increased pigmentation most noticeable in dark-skinned women.

portant event to record, because it marks the approximate midpoint of the pregnancy and is another reference point to verify gestational age. Abdominal gas, normal bowel activity, or false pregnancy (pseudocyesis) are other possible causes.

Probable Indications

The probable indications of pregnancy provide stronger evidence of pregnancy. However, these also may be caused by other conditions.

Goodell's sign is the softening of the cervix and the vagina caused by increased vascular congestion. *Chadwick's sign* is the purplish or bluish discoloration of the cervix, vagina, and vulva caused by increased vascular congestion. Hormonal imbalance or infection may also cause both Goodell's and Chadwick's signs. *Hegar's sign* is a softening of the lower uterine segment. Because of the softening it is easy to flex the body of the uterus against the cervix *(McDonald's sign).*

Abdominal and uterine enlargement occur rather irregularly at the onset of pregnancy. By the end of the 12th week, the uterine fundus may be felt just above the symphysis pubis, and it extends to the umbilicus between the 20th and 22nd weeks (Fig. 4–3). Uterine or abdominal tumors may also cause enlargement.

Braxton Hicks' contractions are irregular, painless uterine contractions that begin in the 2nd trimester. They become progressively more noticeable as term approaches and are more pronounced in multiparas. They may become strong enough to be mistaken for true labor. Uterine fibroids (benign tumors) may also cause these contractions.

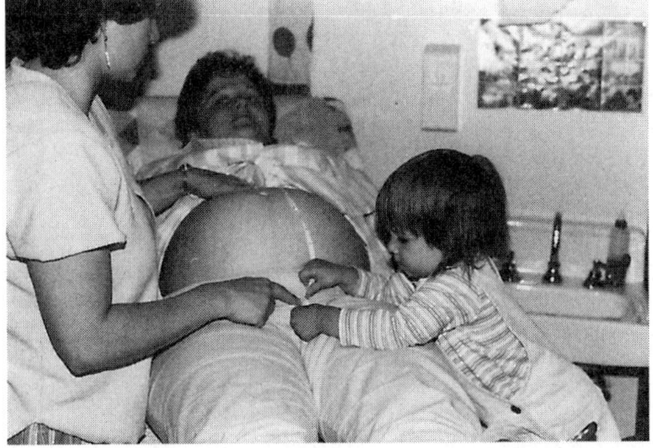

Figure 4–3. • The height of the fundus is measured to evaluate fetal growth. Siblings are encouraged to participate actively in prenatal care of the expanding family. Here, "big sister" holds the tape measure. (Courtesy of Woman-Care, Des Moines Birth-Place, Des Moines, IA.)

Ballottement is a maneuver by which the fetal part is displaced by a light tap of the examining finger on the cervix and then rebounds quickly. Uterine or cervical polyps (small tumors on a stem) may cause the sensation of ballottement on the examiner's finger.

Fetal outline may be identified by palpation after the 24th week. It is possible to mistake a tumor for a fetus.

Abdominal striae (stretch marks) are fine, pinkish-white or purplish-gray lines that some women develop when the elastic tissue of the skin has been stretched to its capacity (Fig. 4–2). Increased amounts of estrogen cause a rise in adrenal gland activity. This change plus the stretching are believed to cause a breakdown and atrophy of the underlying connective tissue in the skin. Striae are seen on the breasts, thighs, abdomen, and buttocks. After pregnancy the striae lose their bright color and become thin, silvery lines. Striae may occur with skin stretching from any cause, such as weight gain.

Pregnancy tests use maternal urine or blood to determine the presence of hCG, a hormone produced by the chorionic villi of the placenta. Home pregnancy tests based on presence of hCG in the urine are capable of greater than 97% accuracy, but the instructions must be followed *precisely* to obtain this accuracy. Professional pregnancy tests are based on urine or blood serum and are more accurate. A highly reliable pregnancy test is the *radioimmunoassay (RIA).* The RIA accurately identifies pregnancy as early as 1 week after ovulation. Pregnancy tests of all types are probable indicators because several factors may interfere with their accuracy: medications such as antianxiety or anticonvulsant drugs, blood in the urine, malignant tumors, or premature menopause.

Positive Indications

Positive signs of pregnancy are caused only by a developing fetus. They include demonstration of fetal heart activity, fetal movements felt by an examiner, and visualization of the fetus with ultrasound.

Fetal heartbeat may be detected as early as 10 weeks of pregnancy by using a Doppler device (Fig. 4–4). The examiner can detect the fetal heartbeat using a fetoscope between the 18th and 20th weeks of pregnancy. The time when the fetal heartbeat is heard with a fetoscope is important because it provides another marker of the approximate midpoint of gestation. When assessing the fetal heart-

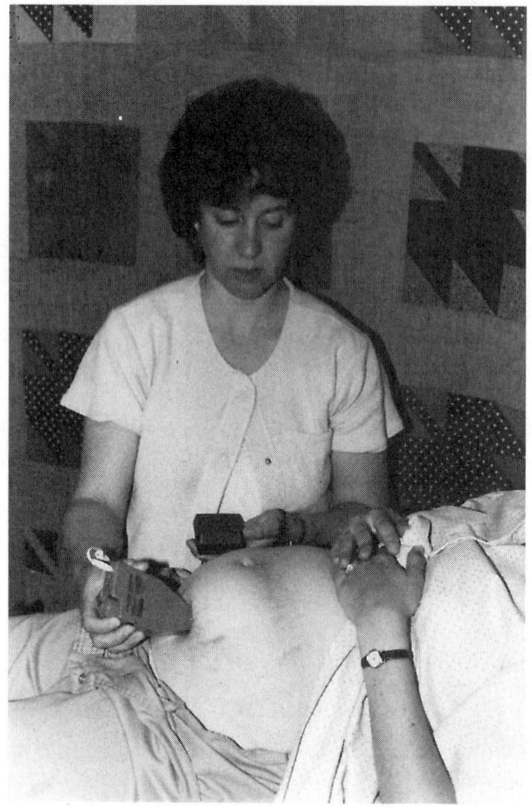

Figure 4–4. • The fetal heart rate is checked at each prenatal visit. Hearing the baby's heartbeat is reassuring to the expectant mother and helps her accept the reality of her pregnancy. (Courtesy of Woman-Care, Des Moines BirthPlace, Des Moines, IA.)

beat with a Doppler or fetoscope, the woman's pulse must be assessed at the same time to be certain that fetal heart action is what is actually heard. The fetal heart rate at term ranges between a low of 110 to 120 beats/min and a high of 150 to 160 beats/min (NAACOG, 1990, Menihan, 1996). The rate is higher in early gestation and slows as term approaches.

Additional sounds that may be heard while assessing the fetal heartbeat are the uterine and funic souffles. *Uterine souffle* is a soft blowing sound heard over the uterus during auscultation. The sound is synchronous with the mother's pulse and is caused by blood entering the dilated arteries of the uterus. The *funic souffle* is a soft swishing sound heard as the blood passes through the umbilical cord vessels.

Fetal movements can be felt by a trained examiner in the 2nd trimester. Fetal activity must be distinguished by the examiner, because to a prospective mother, normal intestinal movements can appear similar to the faint fetal movements typical of early pregnancy. Fetal movements can be seen with ultrasonography.

Identification of the embryo or fetus by means of ultrasound observation and photography of the gestational sac is possible as early as 4 to 5 weeks of gestation with 100% reliability. This noninvasive method is the earliest positive sign of a pregnancy.

NORMAL PHYSIOLOGIC CHANGES IN PREGNANCY

The woman's body undergoes dramatic changes as she houses and nourishes her growing baby. Most of these changes reverse shortly after birth. Nursing Care Plan 4–1 lists interventions for selected nursing diagnoses pertaining to normal physiologic changes during pregnancy.

Reproductive System

Uterus

The uterus undergoes the most obvious changes in pregnancy. Before pregnancy it is a small, muscular, pear-shaped pelvic organ that weighs about 60 g (2 ounces) and measures 7.5 cm (3 inches) × 5 cm (2 inches) × 2.5 cm (1 inch) and has a capacity of about 10 ml (one-third of an ounce). The uterus expands gradually during pregnancy by increasing both the number of myometrial (muscle) cells during the 1st trimester and the size of individual cells during the 2nd and 3rd trimesters. The uterus becomes a temporary abdominal organ at the end of the 1st trimester. At term, the uterus reaches the woman's xiphoid process and weighs about 1000 g (2.2 pounds). Its capacity is about 5000 ml (5 quarts), enough to house the term fetus, placenta, and amniotic fluid.

Cervix

Soon after conception the cervix changes in color and consistency. Chadwick's and Goodell's signs appear. The glands of the cervical mucosa increase in number and activity. Secretion of thick mucus forms a *mucous plug* that seals the cervical canal. The mucous plug prevents ascent of vaginal organisms into the uterus. With the beginning of cervical thinning *(effacement)* and opening *(dilation)* near the onset of labor, the plug is loosened and expelled.

NURSING CARE PLAN 4–1

Selected Nursing Diagnoses for Normal Physiologic Changes During Pregnancy

Nursing Diagnosis: Health-seeking behaviors related to client's desire for a healthy pregnancy outcome

Goals	Nursing Interventions	Rationale
The woman will state her understanding of expected body changes during pregnancy The woman will state danger signals during pregnancy and what actions to take if they occur	1. Encourage woman to write down questions to ask her health-care provider at each visit	1. Many women are nervous during prenatal visits, and they may forget to ask questions
	2. Answer questions during prenatal visits. Arrange for an interpreter if necessary	2. Answering her questions and reassuring her about expected changes reduce anxiety. Teaching in her primary language helps to ensure her understanding
	3. Clearly teach the woman problems she should promptly report (see Box 5–1)	3. Not all changes during pregnancy are normal, and the woman should clearly understand danger signals that require immediate attention
	4. Provide printed material in the woman's primary language for reference and for her to share with significant other if he or she does not attend prenatal visits	4. Printed material provides reference if woman forgets and/or for review later if questions arise. It helps to reinforce both the expected changes of pregnancy and danger signs to report

Nursing Diagnosis: Knowledge deficit related to common discomforts of pregnancy

Goals	Nursing Interventions	Rationale
Woman identifies causes of discomfort and appropriate measures to alleviate them	1. Provide suggestions for self-help measures to reduce discomforts	1. Woman will not interpret normal discomforts as dangerous; she is able to distinguish between normal and abnormal
Nasal stuffiness and epistaxis	a. Raise humidity in house by cool-air vaporizer during very dry weather	a. Humidity keeps the nasal mucosa moist, reducing nosebleeds.
	b. Blow nose gently	b. Prevents trauma to membranes and vessels of nose
	c. If bleeding occurs, apply pressure to nostrils and place ice over nose; call health care provider if bleeding continues for longer than 5 minutes	c. Pressure and ice compresses promote vasoconstriction to slow bleeding. If ordinary measures do not stop bleeding, the woman may require nasal packing
Faintness when lying on back (supine hypotensive syndrome)	a. Explain that dizziness, a clammy feeling, and rapid heartbeat may occur when lying flat on the back because the heavy uterus presses on the major blood vessels in the abdomen	a. Being prepared for symptoms and their cause helps the woman promptly to relieve them rather than interpreting them as abnormal
	b. Teach her to avoid the supine position when lying down. Placing a small pillow under one hip relieves this discomfort and maintains blood flow to the uterus	b. Supine hypotensive syndrome is promptly relieved by moving the heavy uterus off the aorta and inferior vena cava
Constipation	a. Teach woman to maintain a fluid intake of at least 8 glasses of water, excluding caffeinated drinks	a. Progesterone slows intestinal peristalsis during pregnancy, allowing time for more water to be reabsorbed and making the stool drier. Increasing the fluid intake replaces some of the reabsorbed fluids. Caffeinated drinks act as a diuretic, which counteracts their fluid benefit

Continued on following page

NURSING CARE PLAN 4–1 *continued*

Selected Nursing Diagnoses for Normal Physiologic Changes During Pregnancy

Nursing Diagnosis: Knowledge deficit related to common discomforts of pregnancy

Goals	Nursing Interventions	Rationale
Constipation *continued*	b. Teach women to eat a well-balanced diet with whole grains, raw fruits, and vegetables	b. Foods high in fiber add bulk to the stool, keeping it softer and easier to pass
	c. Encourage her to respond promptly to the urge to defecate	c. Delaying the urge to defecate promotes additional drying of the stool
Heartburn	a. Teach woman to eat several small meals throughout the day	a. The cardiac sphincter of stomach relaxes, causing gastric contents to enter esophagus; small meals prevent further upward pressure
	b. Advise her to sit up for 30 minutes following meals	b. Sitting up may prevent reflux of gastric contents into the esophagus
Frequency in urination	a. Explain to woman that bladder pressure during first trimester is due to expansion of uterus in pelvic area; in third trimester, pressure is due to fetal descent into pelvis	a. Understanding the pattern of normal urinary frequency helps the woman to identify better if problems occur
	b. Teach woman signs and symptoms of urinary tract infection, i.e., burning and pain on urination, flank pain, and/or fever	b. Early detection of urinary tract infections allows prompt treatment and prevents complications such as preterm labor
	c. Advise woman to drink at least 8 glasses of noncaffeinated liquids each day	c. Adequate fluid intake helps to keep the urine acid and keeps urine flushed out, reducing the chance for urinary tract infection to occur
Skin changes	a. Reassure woman that darkened skin areas are temporary and will gradually disappear after giving birth	a. Although they are not a true discomfort, the skin changes of pregnancy may distress some women. Knowing that most are temporary helps them to accept the changes
	b. Advise woman that creams and lotions have not been clearly shown to prevent striae (stretch marks)	b. If the woman knows that these preparations are not guaranteed to prevent striae, she can save money
	c. Tell woman to consult her health care provider if itching of the striae becomes a problem	c. Antipruritic ointments may relieve the itching that accompanies striae in some women
Backache	a. Advise woman to wear low-heeled shoes	a. Relaxation of the pelvic joints promotes lordosis. High-heeled shoes further exaggerate the lordosis and add to the backache, especially as the uterus becomes heavier
	b. Teach good posture and body mechanics to the woman: • Maintain an erect posture when sitting or standing, with the head up and shoulders back • Use foot supports if legs are short and a pillow behind back • Do not bend over to pick up heavy objects. Squat, bring object near you, and lift with the strong muscles of the legs • Exercises that may help backache include tailor sitting, shoulder circling, and pelvic rock	b. Good posture and good body mechanics prevent additional strain

Ovaries

The ovaries do not produce ova (eggs) during pregnancy. The *corpus luteum* (empty graafian follicle; see p. 32) remains on the ovary and produces progesterone to maintain the *decidua* (uterine lining) during the first 6 to 7 weeks of the pregnancy until the placenta can perform this function.

Vagina

The vaginal blood supply increases, causing the bluish color of Chadwick's sign. The vaginal mucosa thickens and rugae (ridges) become prominent. The connective tissue softens to prepare for distention as the baby is born. Secretions of the vagina increase. In addition, the vaginal pH becomes more acidic to protect the vagina and uterus from pathogenic microorganisms. However, the vaginal secretions also have higher levels of glycogen, a substance that promotes the growth of *Candida albicans,* the organism that causes yeast infections.

Breasts

Hormone-induced breast changes occur early in pregnancy. High levels of estrogen and progesterone prepare the breasts for lactation. The areolae of the breasts usually become deeply pigmented, and sebaceous glands in the nipple called tubercles of Montgomery become prominent. The tubercles secrete a substance that lubricates the nipples.

In the last few months of pregnancy, thin yellow fluid called *colostrum* can be expressed from the breasts. This "premilk" is high in protein, fat-soluble vitamins, and minerals, but low in calories, fat, and sugar. Colostrum contains the mother's antibodies to diseases and is secreted for the first 2 to 3 days after birth in the breastfeeding woman.

Respiratory System

The pregnant woman breathes more deeply, although her respiratory rate increases only slightly, if at all. These changes increase oxygen and carbon dioxide exchange because she moves more air in and out with each breath. The expanding uterus exerts upward pressure on her diaphragm, causing it to rise about 4 cm (2 inches). To compensate, her rib cage flares, increasing the circumference of the chest about 6 cm (2.5 inches). Dyspnea may occur until the fetus descends into the pelvis *(lightening),* relieving upward pressure on the diaphragm.

Increased estrogen levels during pregnancy cause edema or swelling of the mucous membranes of the nose, pharynx, mouth, and trachea. The woman may have nasal stuffiness, epistaxis (nosebleeds), and changes in her voice. A similar process occurs in the ears, causing a sense of fullness or earaches.

Cardiovascular System

The growing uterus displaces the heart upward and to the left. The blood volume gradually increases *(hypervolemia)* about 45% over that of the prepregnant state by 32 to 34 weeks, at which time it levels off or declines slightly. This increase provides added blood for

- Exchange of nutrients, oxygen, and waste products in the placenta.
- Needs of expanded maternal tissue.
- Reserve for blood loss at birth.

Cardiac output increases because more blood is pumped from the heart with each contraction and the pulse rate increases by 10 to 15 beats/min.

Blood pressure does not increase with the higher blood volume because resistance to blood flow through the vessels decreases. A blood pressure of 140/90 or a significant elevation above the woman's baseline requires attention. *Supine hypotension,* also called *aortocaval compression,* may occur if the woman lies on her back. This position allows the heavy uterus to compress her inferior vena cava, reducing the amount of blood returned to the heart. Circulation to the placenta may be reduced by pressure on the aorta, resulting in fetal hypoxia. Symptoms of supine hypotension include faintness, lightheadedness, dizziness, and agitation. Displacing the uterus to one side by turning the client is all that is needed. If the woman must remain flat for any reason, a small towel roll placed under one hip accomplishes the same thing.

Orthostatic hypotension may occur whenever a woman stands from a recumbent position, resulting in faintness or lightheadedness. Cardiac output decreases because venous return from the lower body suddenly falls. *Palpitations* (sudden increase in heart rate) may occur from increases in thoracic pressure, particularly if the woman moves suddenly.

Although both plasma (fluid) and red blood cells (erythrocytes) increase during pregnancy, they do not increase by the same amount. The fluid part of the blood increases more than the erythrocyte component. This leads to a *dilutional* or *pseudoanemia* (false anemia). As a result, the normal prepregnant hematocrit level of 36% to 48% may fall to 33% to

Table 4–2
NORMAL BLOOD VALUES IN NONPREGNANT AND PREGNANT WOMEN

Value	Nonpregnant	Pregnant
Hemoglobin (g/dl)	12–16	11–12
Hematocrit (%)	36–48	33–46
Red blood cells (million/mm^3)	3.8–5.1	4.5–6.5
White blood cells	5000–10,000/mm^3	5000–12,000/mm^3 Rises during labor and postpartum up to 25,000/mm^3
Platelets	150,000–400,000/mm^3	Slight decrease during pregnancy; marked increase 3–5 days after birth
Fibrinogen (mg/dl)	200–400	300–600

46%. Although this is not true anemia, the hematocrit count is reevaluated to determine if it falls lower. The white blood cell (leukocyte) count also increases (Table 4–2).

Gastrointestinal System

The growing uterus displaces the stomach and intestines toward the back and sides of the abdomen. Increased salivary secretions *(ptyalism)* sometimes affect taste and smell. The mouth tissues may become tender and bleed more easily because of increased blood vessel development caused by a high estrogen level. Teeth are not affected by pregnancy, contrary to popular beliefs.

The demands of the growing fetus increase the woman's appetite and thirst. The acidity of gastric secretions is decreased; emptying of the stomach and motility (movement) of the intestines are slower. Women often feel bloated and may experience constipation and hemorrhoids. *Pyrosis* (heartburn) is caused by the relaxation of the cardiac sphincter of the stomach, which permits reflux (backward flow) of the acid secretions into the lower esophagus.

Urinary System

The urinary system excretes waste products for both the mother and fetus during pregnancy. The glomerular filtration rate of the kidneys rises. The renal tubules increase reabsorption of substances that the body needs to conserve, but may not be able to keep up with the high load of some substances that the glomeruli filter, such as glucose. Therefore, glycosuria and proteinuria are more common during pregnancy. Water is retained because it is needed for increased blood volume and for dissolving nutrients for the fetus.

The relaxing effects of progesterone cause the renal pelvis and ureters to lose tone, resulting in decreased peristalsis to the bladder. The diameter of the ureters and bladder capacity increase because of the relaxing effects of progesterone, causing urine stasis. The combination of urine stasis and nutrient-rich urine makes the pregnant woman more susceptible to urinary tract infection. Consuming at least 8 glasses of water each day reduces the risk for urinary tract infection. Although the bladder can hold up to 1500 ml of urine, the pressure of the enlarging uterus causes frequency of urination, especially in the 1st and 3rd trimesters.

Integumentary and Skeletal Systems

The high levels of hormones produced during pregnancy cause a variety of temporary changes in the integument (skin) of the pregnant woman. In addition to the pigmentary changes discussed under the presumptive signs of pregnancy, the sweat and sebaceous glands of the skin become more active to dissipate heat from the woman and fetus. Small red elevations of skin with lines radiating from the center, called *spider nevi,* may occur. The palms of the hands may become deeper red. Skin changes are reversed shortly after giving birth.

The woman's posture changes as her baby grows within the uterus. The anterior part of her body becomes heavier with the expanding uterus, and the curve in her lumbar spine becomes more pronounced. The woman often experiences low backaches, and in the last few months of pregnancy, rounding of the shoulders may occur along with aching in the cervical spine and upper extremities.

The pelvic joints relax with hormonal changes during late pregnancy and entry of the fetal presenting part into the pelvic brim in the last trimester. A woman often has a "waddling" gait in the last few weeks of pregnancy because of a slight separation of the symphysis pubis.

NUTRITION FOR PREGNANCY AND LACTATION

Good nutrition is essential to establish and maintain a healthy pregnancy and to give birth to a

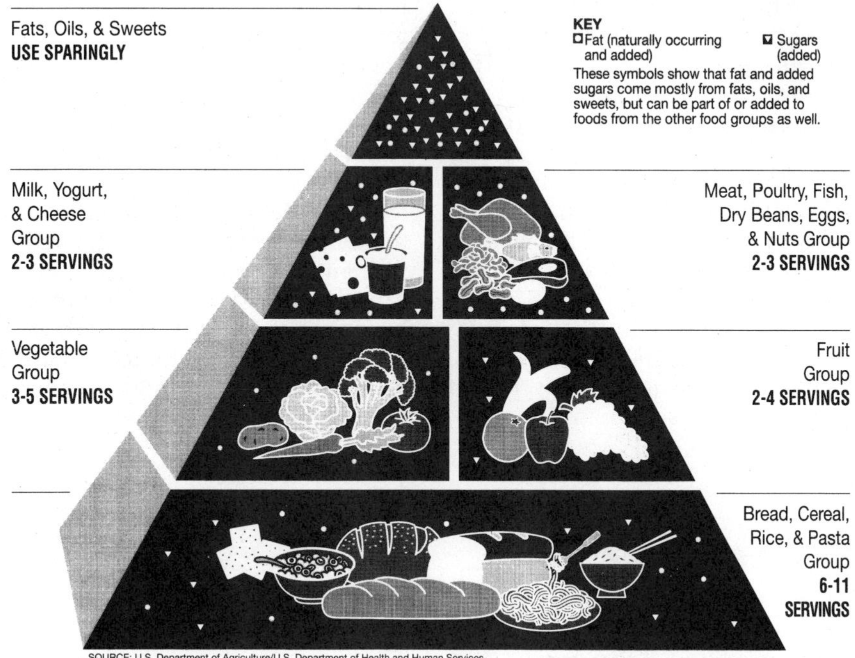

Figure 4–5. • The food guide pyramid is a daily guide to healthful eating for all people. Pregnant and lactating women can base their diet on the same pyramid. (Courtesy of U.S. Department of Agriculture and U.S. Department of Health and Human Services).

healthy baby. Good nutritional habits begun before conception and continued during pregnancy promote adaptation to the maternal and fetal needs. The food guide pyramid is a guide for healthy daily food choices for the public (Fig. 4–5). Women who follow this guide before pregnancy will be well nourished at the time of conception. Nursing Care Plan 4–2 lists common nursing diagnoses and interventions for nutrition during pregnancy and lactation.

The woman should read food labels carefully to promote intake of calories that are nutrient dense rather than empty. The Food and Drug Administration (FDA) along with the U.S. Department of Agriculture has developed uniform food labels that inform consumers of the contents of packages and canned goods (Fig. 4–6).

Weight Gain

In the past a woman's weight gain was restricted during pregnancy. Rickets, caused by a deficiency of vitamin D caused deformity of women's pelves many years ago. It was thought that minimal weight gain would keep the fetus small and therefore easier to deliver. More recently low weight gain was thought to reduce the risk for pregnancy-induced hypertension, a theory that has been disproved.

Low maternal weight gain is associated with complications such as preterm labor, and recommendations for weight gain during pregnancy have gradually increased. Current recommended weight gains during pregnancy are

- Women of normal weight: 25 to 35 pounds (11.5 to 16 kg)
- Underweight women: 28 to 40 pounds (12.5 to 18 kg)
- Overweight: 15 to 25 pounds (7 to 11.5 kg)

Women with multiple fetuses should gain more weight. The adolescent should gain in the upper

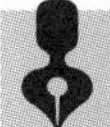

Nursing Tip

There is a high correlation between maternal diet and fetal health. To ensure that deficiencies do not occur during the critical first weeks of pregnancy, the nurse explains to women of childbearing age the value of eating well-balanced meals so they may start pregnancy in a good nutritional state.

part of the range currently recommended for adult women.

The pattern of weight gain is also important. The general recommendation is that a woman gain 3.5 pounds (1.6 kg) during the 1st trimester and just under 1 pound per week (0.44 kg) during the rest of pregnancy. Nausea and vomiting and some transient food dislikes often limit weight gain or cause weight loss during the 1st trimester, but the weight is usually regained when the gastrointestinal upsets subside.

Women often want to know why they should gain so much weight when their baby only weighs 7 or 8 pounds. The nurse can use the distribution of weight gain during pregnancy shown in Table 4–3 to teach women about all the factors that contribute to weight gain.

Nutritional Requirements

A calorie increase of 300 kcal/day is recommended to provide for the growth of the fetus, placenta, amniotic fluid, and maternal tissues. Three hundred calories is not a large increase. A banana, a carrot, a piece of whole wheat bread, and a glass of low-fat milk total about 300 kcal. Caloric intake must be nutritious to have beneficial effects on pregnancy. Four important nutrients that are

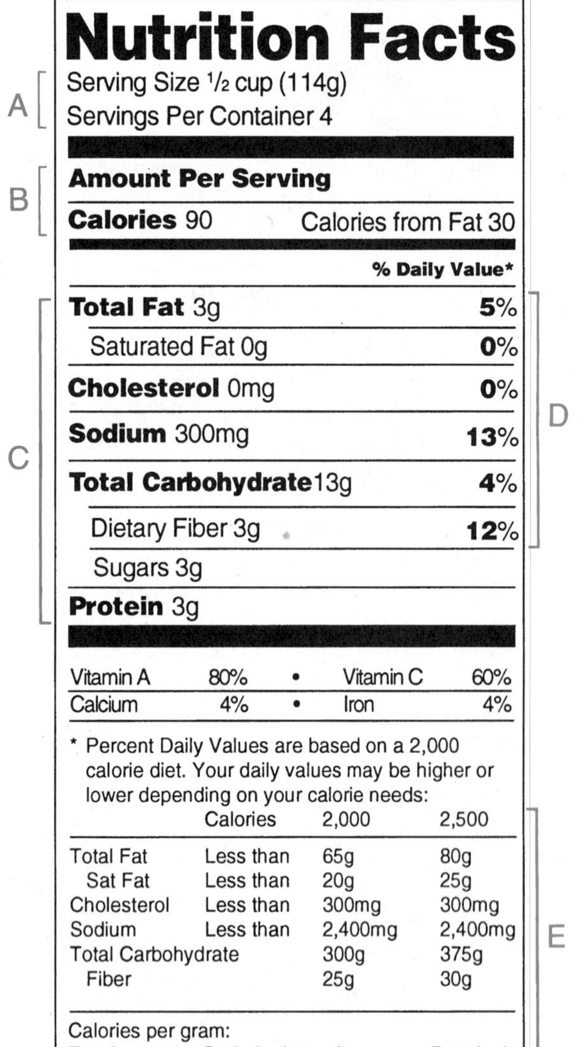

Figure 4–6. • The standard food label is headed "Nutrition Facts." **A,** Serving sizes are standardized for varying products and are given in common measures. **B,** Calories from fat should be under 30% of one's total caloric intake. **C,** Nutrients are listed. **D,** Percentage of daily value is given for each nutrient. This can be used to compare foods for a balanced diet. **E,** Daily values are listed for people who eat 2000 calories (most women, children, and men over 50 years of age) and 2400 calories (most teenage boys, younger men, and very active people). (Courtesy of Food and Drug Administration, U.S. Department of Agriculture).

NURSING CARE PLAN 4–2

Selected Nursing Diagnoses for Nutrition During Pregnancy and Lactation

Nursing Diagnosis: Knowledge deficit related to importance of nutrition in pregnancy and lactation

Goals	Nursing Interventions	Rationale
Woman verbalizes need for good nutrition in pregnancy and lactation.	1. Assess age, parity, present weight, prepregnant nutritional status, food preferences and dislikes, food intolerances and general health of pregnant woman	1. Many factors influence nutritional status of woman during pregnancy and lactation; nutrition teaching must be individualized to best meet her pregnancy nutritional needs
	2. Assess socioeconomic and cultural factors that may influence food choices. Make recommendations to fit specific needs. Consult with a dietitian if the woman's nutritional needs are complex	2. Socioeconomic and cultural factors affect the woman's food choices. These factors must be considered to increase the chance that a woman will adhere to dietary recommendations. The assessment may identify the need for referral to programs such as the Women, Infants, and Children (WIC) nutrition program
	3. Review specific nutritional needs and food sources for optimum outcome of pregnancy and successful lactation	3. If woman understands specific nutritional needs of pregnancy and food sources, she is more likely to choose foods that meet these needs
	4. Provide written information in the woman's primary language on nutrition and food preparation. Modify the information to incorporate cultural practices or food dislikes or intolerances	4. Written information reinforces verbal teaching and helps woman to recall forgotten information. Recommendations must fit within a woman's individualized needs to increase the chance that she will adhere to them
	5. Encourage questions and provide appropriate answers	5. Allows nurse to identify and correct areas of inadequate knowledge or misunderstanding
Woman implements good nutrition during pregnancy and lactation, as evidenced by a 24-hour diary	1. Teach the woman the purpose of and how to maintain a 24-hour food diary. Teach the woman to eat normally and to write down everything she eats and drinks, including approximate amounts, for one day	1. A 24-hour food diary helps the nurse to evaluate a woman's usual diet, likes, dislikes, and how her diet can be improved. It may identify the need for referral to a dietitian
	2. Review the 24-hour intake from the diary and make appropriate recommendations for improvement. Refer to a dietitian if nutritional assessment reveals complex needs	2. Analysis of usual meals and snacks enables the nurse to identify adequate and inadequate intake of specific nutrients. The 24-hour diary allows the nurse to reinforce areas of adequate intake and concentrate on areas of deficient nutrients
	3. Teach the woman about the food guide pyramid and how to read food labels	3. Choices on food guide pyramid provide essential nutrients on a daily basis. Reading labels helps the woman to select more nutritious items from those available
Woman demonstrates a gradual weight gain appropriate for her during pregnancy (25–35 pounds for most women)	1. Maintain a chart to show the actual weight of woman at each visit	1. Weight chart identifies both the amount and the pattern of weight gain to identify inadequate or excessive gain
	2. Review progress of weight with woman at each visit and compare it with the recommended amount of gain for that point in pregnancy	2. Identifies if the woman's weight gain is normal and if additional teaching or exploration of her needs are required

Table 4–3

DISTRIBUTION OF WEIGHT GAIN IN PREGNANCY

Source of Weight Gain	Weight Gain in Pounds
Uterus	2.5 (1.1 kg)
Fetus	7.0–7.5 (3.2–3.4 kg)
Placenta	1.0–1.5 (0.5–0.7 kg)
Amniotic fluid	2.0 (0.9 kg)
Breasts	1.5–3.0 (0.7–1.4 kg)
Blood volume	3.5–4.0 (1.6–1.8 kg)
Extravascular fluids	3.5–5.0 (1.6–2.3 kg)
Maternal reserves	4.0–9.5 (1.8–4.3 kg)
Total	25.0–35.0 (11.4–15.9 kg)

From Gorrie, T. M., McKinney, E. S., & Murray, S. S. (1998). *Foundations of maternal-newborn nursing* (2nd ed). Philadelphia: Saunders.

especially important in pregnancy are protein, calcium, iron, and folic acid. The amounts are specified in Table 4–4.

The pregnant woman should use the same food guide pyramid to choose her daily diet. Servings that will supply enough of the additional nutrients needed are presented in Table 4–5. A sample menu for a pregnant woman is shown in Box 4–3.

Protein. Added protein is needed for metabolism and to support the growth and repair of maternal and fetal tissues. An intake of 60 g/day is recommended during pregnancy. The best sources of protein are meat, fish, poultry, and dairy products. Beans, lentils, and other legumes; breads and cereals; and seeds and nuts, combined with another

Table 4-5

DAILY FOOD PATTERN FOR PREGNANCY

Food	Amount
Milk, nonfat or low fat, yogurt, cheese	3 to 4 cups
Meat (lean), poultry, fish, egg	2 servings (total of 4–6 oz)
Vegetables, cooked or raw: dark green/deep yellow; starchy, including potatoes, dried peas, and beans; all others	3 to 5 servings, all types, often
Fruits, fresh or canned, dark orange including apricots, peaches, cantaloupe	2 to 4 servings, all types, often
Whole grain and enriched breads and cereals	7 or more servings
Fats and sweets	In moderate amounts
Fluids	8 to 10 glasses (8 oz)

Adapted from Mahan, L. K., & Escott-Stump, S. (1996), *Krause's food, nutrition, & diet therapy* (9th ed). Philadelphia: Saunders.

Table 4–4

RECOMMENDED DIETARY ALLOWANCES FOR WOMEN

					Lactating	
	15–18 Years	19–24 Years	25–50 Years	Pregnant	First 6 Months	Second 6 Months
Energy (kcal)	2200	2200	2200	+0 1st trimester +300 2nd trimester +300 3rd trimester	+500	+500
Protein (g)	44	46	50	60	65	62
Vitamin A (mg RE)	800	800	800	800	1300	1200
Vitamin D (mg)	10	10	5	10	10	10
Vitamin E (mg a-TE)	8	8	8	10	12	11
Vitamin K (mg)	55	60	65	65	65	65
Vitamin C (mg)	60	60	60	70	95	90
Thiamin (mg)	1.1	1.1	1.1	1.5	1.6	1.6
Riboflavin (mg)	1.3	1.3	1.3	1.6	1.8	1.7
Niacin (mg NE)	15	15	15	17	20	20
Vitamin B_6 (mg)	1.5	1.6	1.6	2.2	2.1	2.1
Folate (mg)	180	180	180	400	280	260
Vitamin B_{12} (mg)	2	2	2	2.2	2.6	2.6
Calcium (mg)	1200	1200	800	1200	1200	1200
Phosphorus (mg)	1200	1200	800	1200	1200	1200
Magnesium (mg)	300	280	280	320	355	340
Iron (mg)	15	15	15	30	15	15
Zinc (mg)	12	12	12	15	19	16
Iodine (mg)	150	150	150	175	200	200
Selenium (mg)	50	55	55	65	75	75

Adapted with permission from, *Recommended Dietary Allowances* (10th ed). Copyright 1989 by the National Academy of Sciences. Courtesy of the National Academy Press, Washington, D.C.

RE, retinol equivalent; TE, tocopherol equivalent; NE, niacin equivalent.

BOX 4–3

SAMPLE MENU FOR A PREGNANT WOMAN

Breakfast
Orange juice, ½ cup
Oatmeal, ½ cup
Whole grain or enriched toast, 1 slice
Peanut butter, 2 tsp
Decaffeinated coffee or tea

Midmorning
Apple
High bran cereal, ¼ cup
Nonfat Yogurt, ½ cup

Lunch
Turkey (2 oz) sandwich on rye or whole-grain bread with lettuce and tomato and 1 tsp mayonnaise
Green salad
Salad dressing, 2 tsp
Fresh peach
Nonfat or low-fat milk, 1 cup

Midafternoon
Nonfat or low-fat milk, 1 cup
Graham crackers, 4 squares

Dinner
Baked chicken breast, 3 oz
Baked potato with 2 tbsp sour half-and-half
Peas and carrots, ½ cup
Green salad
Salad dressing, 2 tsp
Fresh pear

Evening
Nonfat frozen yogurt, 1 cup
Fresh strawberries

This menu assumes that the woman is of normal prepregnancy weight, that her weight gain is appropriate, that her activity is moderate, and that she is carrying only one fetus. Changes would be needed for the underweight or overweight woman, the teenager, or a woman with a multifetal pregnancy.

Adapted from Mahan, L. K., & Escott-Stump, S. (1996). *Krause's food, nutrition, and diet therapy* (9th ed.). Philadelphia: Saunders.

plant or animal protein, can provide all the amino acids (components of protein) needed.

Examples of complementary plant protein sources are corn and beans, lentils and rice, and peanut butter and bread. Plant proteins are also complemented with animal proteins, for example, in grilled cheese sandwiches, cereal with milk, and chili made of meat and beans. The complementary foods must be eaten together, because all the amino acids necessary for building tissues (essential amino acids) must be present at the same time.

Information about non-meat sources of protein should be given to women who are vegetarians, to ensure that their protein needs are met. The information can also help reduce the family's food budget, because many plant protein sources are less expensive than animal sources.

Calcium. Pregnancy and lactation increase calcium requirements by nearly 50%. The recommended daily allowance of calcium for pregnant women is 1200 mg. Dairy products are the single most plentiful source of this nutrient. Other sources of calcium include enriched cereals, legumes, nuts, dried fruits, broccoli, green leafy vegetables, and canned salmon and sardines that contain bones. Calcium supplements are necessary for women who do not drink milk (or eat sufficient amounts of equivalent products). Supplements are also necessary for women under 25 years because their bone density is not complete. Calcium supplements should be taken separately from iron supplements for best absorption. Nondairy alternatives for women with lactose intolerance are given on page 71.

Iron. Pregnancy causes a heavy demand for iron, because the fetus must store an adequate supply to meet the needs of the first 4 to 6 months after birth. In addition, the pregnant woman increases her production of erythrocytes. The recommended dietary allowance (RDA) is 15 mg/day for nonpregnant adult women and 30 mg/day for pregnant women. Women who have iron deficiency may need more.

It is difficult to obtain this much iron from the diet alone, and most health care providers prescribe iron supplements of 30 mg/day beginning in the 2nd trimester, after morning sickness decreases. Taking the iron on an empty stomach improves absorption, but many women find it difficult to tolerate it without food. It should not be taken with high-calcium foods such as milk, or with coffee or tea. Vitamin C (ascorbic acid) may enhance absorption (Mahan & Escott-Stump, 1996).

Iron comes in two forms, *heme,* found in red and organ meats, and *nonheme,* found in plant products. Heme iron is best absorbed by the body. Nonheme plant foods that are high in iron include molasses, whole grains, iron-fortified cereals and breads, dark-green leafy vegetables, and dried fruits.

Folic Acid. Folic acid (folacin or folate) is a water-soluble B vitamin essential for the formation and maturation of both red and white blood cells in bone marrow. This vitamin can also reduce the incidence of neural tube defects such as spina bifida and anencephaly. The RDA for a pregnant woman is 400 µg (0.4 mg). Food sources of folic acid are liver; kidney and lima beans; fresh, dark-green leafy vegetables; lean beef; potatoes; whole-wheat bread; dried beans; and peanuts.

Because adequate intake of folic acid *from conception* has shown to have a large impact on reducing the incidence of neural tube defects, the Centers for Disease Control and Prevention recommends that all fertile American women consume 400 µg (0.4 mg) of folic acid daily. A higher level of 4 mg per day is recommended for women who have previously had an infant with a neural tube defect and plan to become pregnant again (Mitchell, 1997).

Fluids. The woman should drink 8 to 10 glasses (8-ounce) of fluids each day. Water should compose most of this intake. Drinks high in sugar should be limited, as should caffeinated drinks. Caffeine acts as a diuretic, counteracting some of the benefit of the fluid intake. The woman should limit her daily caffeine consumption to two cups of coffee or its equivalent.

Special Nutritional Considerations

Pregnant Teenager. *Gynecologic age* is the number of years between the onset of menses and the date of conception. The teenager who conceives soon after having her first period has greater nutritional needs than one who is more sexually mature. The nurse must consider the teenager's characteristics of resistance, ambivalence, and inconsistency when planning nutritional interventions. The nurse must also remember that the girl's peer group is of utmost importance to her and help her find nutritious foods that allow her to fit in with her friends.

Inadequate pregnancy weight gain and nutrient deficits are more likely in the pregnant teen. The girl's continuing growth plus the growth of the baby may make it difficult for her to meet her nutritional needs. Also, a body image in which she sees herself as "fat" at a time when appearance is a high priority combined with peer pressure to eat "junk" foods places the pregnant adolescent at special risk. Childbearing teenagers are more likely to be poor and to have closely spaced pregnancies, further adding to their nutritional risk.

Even a moderate positive change in diet helps and the nurse should give the girl positive reinforcement for her efforts. Fast foods with poor nutritional content are often the teenager's foods of choice. However, the nurse can tell the teenager that many fast food restaurants offer salads, muffins, chicken, tacos, baked potatoes, and pizza. These foods provide many important nutrients and allow her to socialize with her peers at mealtime.

Nutritional intervention is necessary early in prenatal care to ensure a healthy mother and baby. Many communities offer programs for adolescents that provide social support, education about prenatal care, and nutritional advice. Teenagers often respond well in peer groups. The nurse often refers these young women to programs such as Women, Infants, and Children and food stamps if needed.

Sodium Intake. The sodium intake of pregnant women was restricted in the past in an attempt to prevent edema and pregnancy-induced hypertension. It is now known that sodium should not be restricted during pregnancy. Sodium intake is essential for maintaining normal sodium levels in plasma, bone, brain, and muscle because both tissue and fluid expand during the prenatal period. However, foods high in sodium should be taken in moderation during pregnancy.

Diuretics to rid the body of excess fluids are not recommended for the healthy pregnant woman because they reduce fluids necessary for the fetus. The added fluid during pregnancy supports the mother's increased blood volume.

Pica. The craving for and ingestion of nonfood substances such as clay, starch, raw flour, and cracked ice is called *pica.* Ingestion of small amounts of these substances may be harmless, but frequent ingestion in large amounts may cause problems. Starch can interfere with iron absorption, and large amounts of clay may cause fecal impaction. Any other nonfood substance ingested in large quantities may be harmful because necessary nutrients for healthy development will not be available.

Pica is a difficult habit to break, and the nurse often becomes aware of the practice when discussing nutrition, food cravings, and myths with the pregnant woman. The nurse should educate the pregnant woman in a nonjudgmental way about the importance of good nutrition, so that the pica habit can be eliminated or at least decreased.

Lactose Intolerance. Some women cannot digest milk or milk products, which increases their risk for calcium deficiency. Intolerance to lactose is caused by a deficiency of lactase, the enzyme that digests the sugar in milk. Native Americans, Latinas, and persons of African, Middle Eastern, and Asian descent have a higher incidence of lactose intolerance than whites. Signs and symptoms include abdominal distention, nausea, vomiting, and loose stools after ingestion of dairy products. In such cases a daily calcium substitute can be taken.

Substitutes for dairy products are listed in the section on calcium. Lactose-intolerant women may tolerate cultured or fermented milk products, such as aged cheese, buttermilk, and yogurt. The enzyme lactase (LactAid) is available in tablet form or as a liquid to add to milk. Lactase-treated milk is also available commercially and can be used under a physician's direction.

Gestational Diabetes. Gestational diabetes is first diagnosed during pregnancy rather than being present before pregnancy (see p. 103). Calories should be evenly distributed during the day among three meals and three snacks to maintain adequate and even blood glucose levels. Pregnant diabetic women are susceptible to hypoglycemia (low blood glucose) during the night, because the fetus continues to use glucose while the mother sleeps. It is suggested that the final bedtime snack be one of protein and a complex carbohydrate to provide more blood glucose stability. Dietary management may be supervised by a registered dietitian.

Nutrition during Lactation

The intake during lactation should be about 500 cal more than the nonpregnant woman's RDA. A guide to adequate caloric intake is a stable maternal weight and a gradually increasing infant weight.

The protein intake should be 65 mg/day, so that the growing baby will have adequate protein. Calcium and iron intake is the same as that during pregnancy to allow for the infant's demand on the mother's supply. Vitamin supplements are often continued during lactation.

Fluids sufficient to relieve thirst should be taken. Eight to ten glasses of liquids other than those containing caffeine are adequate. Very large quantities of liquids are not necessary.

Some foods should be omitted during lactation if they cause gastric upset in the mother or baby. The mother will often identify foods that seem to upset her baby. Caffeine should be restricted to the equivalent of two cups of coffee each day. Lactating mothers should be instructed that drugs she takes are secreted in varying amounts in the breast milk. Drugs should be taken only with the doctor's advice. Alcohol intake should be restricted to an occasional single glass for breastfeeding women.

COMMON DISCOMFORTS IN PREGNANCY

Various discomforts occur during normal pregnancy as a result of physiologic changes. The nurse should teach the woman measures to relieve these discomforts. The nurse should also explain signs of problems that can be confused with the normal discomforts. Providing information written in the woman's primary language gives her a reference if she has questions later.

Nausea is a problem chiefly in the 1st trimester. Persistent nausea with vomiting that significantly interferes with food and fluid intake is not normal and should be reported. Relief measures include the following:

- Eat dry toast or crackers before getting out of bed in the morning.
- Drink fluids between meals instead of with meals.
- Eat small, frequent meals.
- Avoid fried, greasy, or spicy foods and foods with strong odors, such as cabbage and onions.

Vaginal discharge is more noticeable because of the increased blood supply to the pelvic area. A discharge that is yellow or has a foul odor or is accompanied by itching and inflammation suggests vaginal infection and should be reported. Measures to manage the discharge and reduce the risk for infection include the following:

- Bathe or shower daily.
- Powder with dry cornstarch if desired.
- Wear loose-fitting cotton panties.
- Do not douche unless specifically ordered by the health care provider.
- Wipe the perineal area from front to back after toileting.

Fatigue may be difficult in the early months of the pregnancy if the mother is working or has other small children. Measures to cope with fatigue include the following:

- Try to get at least 8 to 10 hours of sleep at night.
- Take a nap during the day if possible.
- Use measures such as relaxation techniques, meditation, or a change of scenery.

The extreme exhaustion usually diminishes in the 2nd trimester, and often women then feel exhilarated and full of energy. The tired feeling may return again during the last 4 to 6 weeks of the pregnancy. Again, daytime naps and as much restful nighttime sleep as possible help to provide the energy needed for labor.

Backache occurs because of the spine's adaptation to the back's changing contour as the uterus grows. Relief measures include the following:

- Maintain correct posture with the head up and the shoulders back. Avoid exaggerating the lumbar curve. Wearing low-heeled shoes helps the woman maintain better posture.
- Squat rather than bend over when picking up objects.
- When sitting, support the arms, feet, and back with pillows as needed.
- Exercises include tailor sitting, shoulder circling, and pelvic rocking.

Constipation occurs because of slowed peristalsis, use of iron supplements, and pressure of the growing uterus on the large intestine. Relief measures include the following:

- Drink at least eight glasses of water each day, not counting coffee, tea, or carbonated drinks.
- Add dietary fiber in foods, such as unpeeled fresh fruits and vegetables, whole-grain cereals, bran muffins, oatmeal, potatoes with skins, and fruit juices.
- Limit cheese consumption if this tends to be constipating.
- Limit sweet foods if they cause flatulence.
- Consult the health care provider if iron supplements cause constipation. Do not stop taking the iron because a change in the supplement may help.
- Get plenty of exercise. A brisk 1-mile walk is good to stimulate peristalsis.
- Establish a regular time each day for having a bowel movement. Defecate as soon as the urge occurs rather than delaying.
- Take laxatives or enemas only under the direction of the health care provider.

Varicose veins are common in the pregnant woman because the large uterus slows venous return, causing the blood to pool in her veins. This pooling may eventually break down the competence of the valves within the veins, resulting in varicosities. Varicose veins are seen most often on the back of the calves and behind the knees. Excessive weight gain and genetic predisposition affect the occurrence of varicosities and their persistence after the pregnancy. Varicosities may occur on the vulva, especially after the 20th week of pregnancy. They are usually temporary and subside after the delivery. Measures to relieve the discomfort of varicosities include the following:

- Avoid constricting clothing or crossing the legs at the knees.
- Elevate the legs above the hip level when resting.
- Support hose or elastic stockings increase venous blood flow. For best results they should be applied before getting out of bed each morning.
- Avoid standing in one position for prolonged periods. Walk around for a few minutes every 2 hours.

Hemorrhoids are varicosities of the rectum and anus that become more severe with constipation and with descent of the baby's head into the pelvis. They generally decrease or disappear after birth, when pressure is relieved. Relief measures include the following:

- Anesthetic ointments, witch hazel pads, or rectal suppositories
- Sitz baths (see p. 226)
- Measures to avoid constipation as previously discussed

Heartburn causes discomfort mainly in late pregnancy, when the uterus presses against the esophagus where it enters the stomach. This pressure may cause a reflux of gastric acids into the esophagus, resulting in a burning feeling in the chest and a bitter taste in the mouth. Suggestions to reduce heartburn include the following:

- Eat small, frequent meals and avoid fatty foods.
- Reduce smoking and caffeine intake.
- Sit upright and sleep with an extra pillow under the head.
- Deep breathing and sips of water may relieve the burning.

- Use antacids if recommended by the health care provider. Those high in sodium (Alka-Seltzer, baking soda) should be avoided.

Dyspnea is often encountered in late pregnancy as the uterus exerts pressure on the diaphragm. Even with mild exercise, many women are unable to breathe deeply. Most women notice improvement in dyspnea with lightening (about 2 weeks before birth with the first baby). Suggestions for relief include the following:

- Rest with the upper torso propped up.
- Avoid exertion.

Leg cramps may occur in the first 6 weeks of pregnancy but are more often experienced during the 3rd trimester. The superficial calf muscles of the legs involuntarily contract, causing severe pain. Increased uterine weight, increased circulatory load, inadequate rest, and imbalance of the calcium-to-phosphorus ratio are implicated as causes. Intake of phosphorus may exceed the calcium intake, resulting in a calcium-to-phosphorus imbalance. Measures to relieve leg cramps include the following:

- Extend the affected leg, keep the knee straight, and flex the foot. Stand and apply pressure on the affected leg to stretch the muscles in spasm.
- Elevate the legs periodically during the day to improve circulation.
- Consult the health care provider about reduction of milk intake or use of aluminum hydroxide capsules to restore an ideal calcium-to-phosphorus ratio.

Edema of the lower extremities is common, especially after the 20th week of pregnancy. It is caused by the increased circulatory load and slower venous return of blood from the legs. Edema in the face and hands may be a sign of pregnancy-induced hypertension and should be reported to the health care provider. Temporary relief measures for lower extremity edema include the following:

- Elevate the legs when sitting.
- Avoid tight restrictive bands around the legs.
- Relieve varicosities to reduce edema.

PSYCHOLOGICAL ADAPTATIONS TO PREGNANCY

Pregnancy creates a variety of confusing feelings for all members of the family, whether or not the pregnancy was planned. Both parents may feel ambivalence about having a child and being a parent. First-time parents may be anxious about how the new baby will affect their relationship as a couple. Parents who already have a child may wonder how they can stretch their energies and love to another child and how the new baby will affect their older child or children. The nurse who provides prenatal care helps families to work through this crisis in their lives. Nursing Care Plan 4–3 lists interventions for some nursing diagnoses that apply to common emotional changes of pregnancy.

Impact on the Mother

Reva Rubin (1984) noted four maternal tasks that the woman accomplishes during pregnancy as she becomes a mother. The four tasks are:

- Seeking safe passage for herself and her fetus. This involves both health care by a professional and adhering to important cultural practices.
- Securing acceptance of herself as a mother and for her fetus. Will her partner accept the baby? Does her partner or family have strong preferences for a child of a particular sex? Will a baby be accepted even if he or she does not fit the ideal?
- Learning to give of self and to receive the care and concern of others. The woman will never again be the same carefree girl she was before her baby's arrival. She depends on others in ways she has not experienced before.
- Committing herself to the child as she progresses through pregnancy. Much of the emotional work of pregnancy involves protecting and nurturing the fetus.

Pregnancy is more than a physical event in a woman's life. During the months of pregnancy, she first accepts the fetus as part of her self and gradually moves to acceptance of the child as an independent person. She moves from being a pregnant woman to being a mother. The woman's responses change as pregnancy progresses. They will be discussed here in the framework of the three trimesters of pregnancy.

NURSING CARE PLAN 4-3

Selected Nursing Diagnoses for Emotional Changes During Pregnancy

Nursing Diagnosis: Family coping: Potential for growth

Goals	Nursing Interventions	Rationale
Couple identifies their concerns about becoming parents.	1. Assess the woman and her partner for their emotional reactions to the pregnancy. Reassure them if their reactions are normal	1. Many women and men feel ambivalence during early pregnancy and may be reluctant to discuss it. Many people are relieved to know that reactions such as ambivalence are common even in highly desired pregnancies
	2. Teach couple the expected emotional changes that most women have during pregnancy, such as: • Mood swings • Focus on herself • A sense of vulnerability and dependence as labor approaches	2. Understanding these expected changes that occur in pregnancy helps the couple to realize that they are temporary and do not reflect emotional problems
	3. Refer mother and partner to prenatal and parenting classes	3. Prenatal classes help to develop an accurate picture of developing fetus, provide support and socialization with other expectant parents, and educate parents in responsibilities in care of a newborn and growing child
Parents identify strengths in their family relationships. Parents seek guidance for relationship problems they identify.	1. Assess family relationships at prenatal visits. Determine the usual roles of family members.	1. Determining family structure and relationships helps the nurse to individualize any needed interventions.
	2. Determine if there are cultural practices or health beliefs that are important to the couple or that dictate their family roles	2. Parents are more likely to follow the advice of health care professionals if their individualized needs are considered
	3. Determine sources of emotional support for the family, such as grandparents or other relatives, and friends	3. Support from significant others helps the couple to adapt to the changes of pregnancy and the challenges of parenthood. Support sources also helps them cope with crises that may arise

First Trimester

The woman may have difficulty believing that she is pregnant during early pregnancy because she may not feel much different. If a home pregnancy test was positive, the woman often feels "more pregnant" after a professional confirms it, even though her pregnancy is only a few minutes older than it was before that confirmation. Early sonography examination helps the woman to see the reality of the developing baby within her. Women (and their partners) often show off their sonogram photos to anyone who will look, just as they show their baby pictures later.

Nursing Tip

Ambivalence about becoming a mother is normal in early pregnancy, and mood swings are common throughout pregnancy. Fathers often experience ambivalence.

Most women have conflicting feelings about being pregnant *(ambivalence)* during the early weeks. Many, if not most, wanted pregnancies are unplanned. The parents may have wanted to wait longer so they could achieve career or educational goals or to have longer spacing between children. Women who have planned their pregnancies, or even worked hard to overcome infertility, also feel ambivalence. They wonder if they have done the right thing and at the right time. Moreover, the woman often feels that she should not have these conflicting feelings. The nurse can help the woman to express these feelings of ambivalence and reassure her that they are normal.

The woman focuses on herself during this time.

She feels many new physical sensations, but none of them seem related to a baby. These physical changes and the higher hormone levels cause her emotions to be more unstable *(labile)*. The nurse can reassure the woman and her partner, who is often confused by her moods, about their cause and that they are normal.

Second Trimester

The fetus now becomes real to the woman. Her weight increases and the uterus becomes obvious as it rises up into the abdomen. If she has not already heard the fetal heartbeat or seen it beating on a sonogram, the woman usually hears it early in the second trimester. She feels fetal movement, and this is a powerful aid to helping her to distinguish the fetus as a separate person.

The second trimester is a more stable time during pregnancy for most women. They have resolved many of their earlier feelings of ambivalence. They take on the role of an expectant mother wholeheartedly. The mother becomes totally involved with her developing baby and her changing body image *(narcissism)*. She often devotes a great deal of time to selecting just the right foods and the best environment to promote her health and that of her baby. She welcomes the solicitous concern of others, when they caution her not to pick up a heavy package or work too hard. She may lose interest in work or other activities as she devotes herself to the project of nurturing her fetus. The nurse can take advantage of her heightened interest in healthful living to teach good nutrition and other habits that can benefit the woman and her family long after pregnancy ends.

The woman "tries on" the role of mother by learning what babies are like. She wants to hear stories of what she and her mate were like when they were infants. She often fantasizes about how her baby will look and behave or what sex the baby will be. She may or may not want to know the sex of the baby if it is apparent on a sonogram, sometimes preferring to be surprised at the birth. The woman who has had a baby before undergoes a similar transition as she imagines what this specific baby will be like and how he or she will compare to siblings.

The body changes of pregnancy are now evident. The woman may welcome them as a sign to all that her fetus is well protected and thriving. But these same changes may be unwelcome to her because they are perceived as unattractive and cause her discomfort.

The body changes may alter her sexual relationship with her partner as well. Both partners may fear harming the developing baby, particularly if they have previously lost a pregnancy. Her increasing size, discomforts, and the other changes of pregnancy may make one or both partners have less interest in intercourse. The nurse can assure them that these changes are temporary and help them explore other expressions of love and caring.

Third Trimester

As her body changes even more dramatically, a mother alternates from feeling "absolutely beautiful" and "productive" to feeling "as big as a house" and "totally unloved" by her partner. These mood swings reflect her sense of increased vulnerability and dependence on her partner. She becomes introspective about the challenge of labor that is ahead and its outcome. Her moods may again be more labile.

The mother begins to separate herself from the pregnancy and to commit herself to the care of an infant. She and her partner begin making concrete preparations for the baby's arrival. They buy clothes and equipment the baby will need. Many take childbirth preparation classes. The woman's thinking gradually shifts from "I am pregnant" to "I am going to be a mother."

The minor discomforts of pregnancy become tiresome during the last weeks. It seems that pregnancy will never end. A woman benefits from the gentle understanding of the people near and dear to her. With the support of her family and health care professionals, she can develop inner strength to accomplish the tasks of birth.

Impact on the Father

Responses of fathers vary widely. Some want to be fully involved in the physical and emotional aspects of pregnancy. Others prefer a management role, helping the woman adhere to recommendations of her physician or nurse-midwife. Some fathers want to "be there" for the woman, but prefer not to take an active role during pregnancy or birth. Cultural values influence the role of fathers, because pregnancy and birth are viewed exclusively as women's work in some cultures. The nurse should not assume that a father is disinterested if he takes a less active role in pregnancy and birth.

Fathers go through similar processes as expectant mothers. Initially they may also have difficulty perceiving the fetus as real. Ambivalence and self-questioning about their readiness for fatherhood are typical. Fathers who attend prenatal appointments with the woman can see the fetus on ultrasound or hear the fetal heartbeat, making the baby seem more like a real person.

The father is often asked to provide emotional support to his partner while struggling with the issue of fatherhood himself. Too often, he receives the message that his only job is to support the pregnant woman rather than being a parent who is also important and has needs. The nurse should explore the father's feelings and encourage him during prenatal appointments, childbirth preparation classes, and during labor and birth. He is trying to learn the role of father, just as the woman is trying to learn the role of mother.

Impact on Grandparents

Prospective grandparents have different reactions to a woman's pregnancy as well. They may eagerly anticipate the announcement that a grandchild is on the way, or they may feel that they are not ready for the role of grandparent, which they equate with being old. The first grandchild often causes the most excitement in grandparents. Their reaction may be more subdued if they have several grandchildren, which may hurt the excited pregnant couple.

Grandparents have different ideas of how they will be involved with their grandchildren. Distance from the younger family dictates the degree of involvement for some. They may want to be fully involved in the plans for the new baby and help with child care, often traveling a great distance to be there for the big event. Other grandparents want less involvement because they welcome the freedom of a childless life again. Most grandparents are in their 40s and 50s, a time when their own career demands and care of their aging parents often competes with their ability to be involved with grandchildren.

If grandparents and the expectant couple have similar views of their roles, little conflict is likely. However, if the pregnant couple and the grandparents have significantly different expectations of their role and involvement, disappointment and conflict may occur. The nurse can help the young couple understand their parents' reactions and help them to negotiate solutions to conflicts that are satisfactory to both generations.

Impact on the Single Mother

The single mother may still be an adolescent or she may be a mature woman. She has special emotional needs, especially if the father has left her, does not acknowledge the pregnancy, or if she does not care to have a relationship with the father. Some single mothers can turn to their parents, siblings, or close friends for support. Other single women are homosexual and have the support of their female partner. Women who do not have emotional support from significant others will have more difficulty completing the tasks of pregnancy. Their uncertainty in day-to-day living competes with mastering the emotional tasks of pregnancy.

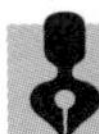

Nursing Tip

The nurse must anticipate resistive behavior, ambivalence, and inconsistency in the adolescent. The nurse must consider the girl's developmental level and the priorities typical of her age, such as the importance of her peer group, focus on appearance, and difficulty considering the needs of others.

Impact on the Single Father

The single father may take an active interest in and financial responsibility for the child. The couple may plan marriage eventually, but it is often delayed a few years. A single father may provide emotional support for the mother during the pregnancy and birth. He often has strong feelings of surprise and accomplishment when he becomes aware of his partner's pregnancy. He may want to participate in plans for the new baby and take part in infant care after birth. His participation is sometimes rejected by the woman, however.

Impact on the Adolescent

Pregnant adolescents often have to struggle with feelings they find difficult to express. They are fraught with conflict about how to handle an unplanned pregnancy. Initially, they must face the anxiety of breaking the news to their parents. Denial of the pregnancy until late in gestation is not uncommon. There may be financial problems, shame, guilt, relationship problems with the baby's father, and feelings of low self-esteem. Alcoholism and substance abuse may be part of the complex picture.

The nurse must assess the girl's developmental and educational level and her support system to best provide care for her. A critical variable is the girl's age. Young adolescents have difficulty considering the needs of others, such as the fetus. The nurse helps the teenage girl to complete the developmental tasks of adolescence while assuming the new role of motherhood. Ideally, separate prenatal classes tailored to their needs help adolescent girls to learn to care for themselves and assume the role of mother.

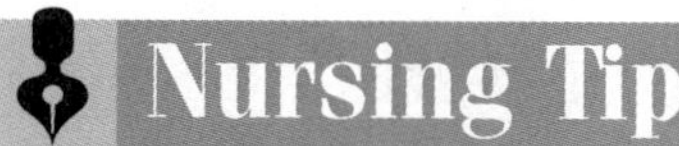

The pregnant teenager has to cope with two of life's most stress-laden transitions simultaneously, adolescence and parenthood.

KEY POINTS

- Early and regular prenatal care promotes the healthiest possible outcome for mother and baby.
- Determination of the woman's estimated date of delivery is calculated from her last normal menstrual period. Other methods to confirm gestational age include dates of hearing the fetal heartbeat with a Doppler.
- The length of a pregnancy is 40 weeks after the last normal menstrual period plus or minus 2 weeks. The expected date of delivery is determined by using Nägele's rule. Other ways to determine this date include a gestation wheel, a special electronic calculator, physical examination, date of quickening, or ultrasound.
- Presumptive indications of pregnancy often have other causes. Probable indications more strongly suggest pregnancy, but can still be caused by other conditions. Positive indications have no other cause except pregnancy. The three positive indications of pregnancy include detection of a fetal heartbeat, fetal movements felt by a trained examiner, and visualizing the embryo or fetus on ultrasound.
- Quickening, a presumptive indicator of pregnancy that occurs at 16 to 20 weeks, marks the first half of the pregnancy, and is a good reference point for identifying the gestational age of the developing fetus.
- The uterus undergoes the most obvious changes in pregnancy: it increases in weight from approximately 60 g (2 ounces) to 1000 g (2.2 pounds); it increases in capacity from about 10 ml (one-third of an ounce) to 5000 ml (5 quarts).
- The mother's blood volume increases about 45% over her prepregnant volume to perfuse the placenta and extra maternal tissues. Her blood pressure does not rise because resistance to blood flow in her arteries decreases. The fluid portion of her blood increases more than the cellular portion, resulting in a pseudoanemia.
- Supine hypotension, or aortocaval compression, may occur if the pregnant woman lies on her back. Turning to one side or placing a small pillow under one hip can relieve this hypotension.
- To provide for the growth of the fetus and maternal tissues, the mother needs 300 extra, high-quality calories daily. Important nutrients that must increase are protein, calcium, iron, and folic acid. Five hundred extra calories are needed for lactation.
- Adequate folic acid intake from conception can reduce the incidence of neural tube defects such as anencephaly or spina bifida. The Centers for Disease Control and Prevention recommend that all fertile American women consume 400 µg (0.4 mg) of folic acid daily.
- The nurse should teach pregnant women the expected discomforts of pregnancy and relief measures. Abnormal signs and symptoms should also be reviewed.
- The pregnant woman must accept the fetus as part of her self in preparation to accept the newborn as a separate person.
- Fathers should be included in prenatal care to the extent they and the woman desire.

MULTIPLE-CHOICE REVIEW QUESTIONS

Choose the most appropriate answer.

1. A woman is having a prenatal visit at 18 weeks of pregnancy. Why is it important to ask her about fetal movement?
   a. Absence of fetal movement at this time suggests that the pregnancy is more advanced than her dates indicate.
   b. Denial of fetal movement at this stage in pregnancy may indicate that the woman is not accepting her pregnancy.
   c. If she has started feeling fetal movement, the fetal heartbeat will be checked with a fetoscope to confirm that the fetus is living.
   d. Fetal movement is first felt by the mother about this time and provides a marker for approximate gestational age.
2. A pregnant woman complains that she has a large amount of vaginal secretions. The next most appropriate nursing action is to
   a. consult her nurse-midwife for a cream or douche.
   b. ask her if the discharge is irritating or causes itching.
   c. advise her to change cotton panties twice daily.
   d. tell her to reduce sexual intercourse for a few weeks.
3. During a prenatal exam at 30 weeks' gestation, a woman is lying on her back. She suddenly complains of dizziness and faintness. These symptoms are most likely caused by
   a. anxiety about what will happen during the impending prenatal exam.
   b. low blood glucose because she skipped breakfast to avoid excessive weight gain.
   c. anemia secondary to poor iron intake and limited erythrocyte production.
   d. compression of the inferior vena cava and aorta by the heavy uterus.
4. A woman is being seen for her first prenatal care appointment. Her pregnancy has been confirmed by a blood test, and she had a positive home pregnancy test as well. She tells the nurse, "I always wanted a baby, but maybe now is just not the right time. I'm so confused!" The nurse should respond by
   a. reassuring her that having conflicting feelings about the baby and being a parent are common in early pregnancy.
   b. asking her if she would be willing to attend group counseling sessions to help to analyze her feelings about motherhood.
   c. notifying the baby's father about the woman's ambivalence about pregnancy and motherhood.
   d. telling her that all women feel this way from time to time and that the feeling will eventually go away.
5. Prenatal nursing care for the father should emphasize
   a. giving him tools so he can help the mother get through pregnancy.
   b. involving him in the pregnancy as much as he and the mother desire.
   c. encouraging him to attend all prenatal visits with the mother.
   d. making the fact of fatherhood as real as possible to him.

BIBLIOGRAPHY AND READER REFERENCE

American Academy of Pediatrics & American College of Obstetricians and Gynecologists. (1997). Maternal and newborn nutrition. In *Guidelines for perinatal care* (4th ed.). Elk Grove Village, IL: American Academy of Pediatrics.

Bishop, B. E. (1992). Congratulations Reva! [Editorial]. *MCN: American Journal of Maternal-Child Nursing, 17.*

Carpenito, L. (1993). *Handbook of nursing diagnosis* (6th ed.). Philadelphia: Lippincott.

Cunningham, F. G., MacDonald, P. C., Gant, N. F., Leveno, K. J., Gilstrap, L. C., Hankins, G. D. V., & Clark, S. L. (1997). *Williams obstetrics* (20th ed.). Norwalk, CT: Appleton & Lange.

Driscoll, J. W. (1996). Psychosocial adaptation to pregnancy and postpartum. In K. R. Simpson & P. A. Creehan (Eds.), *AWHONN's perinatal nursing* (pp. 61–71). Washington, DC: Association of Women's Health, Obstetric, and Neonatal Nurses.

Fallon, M. K. (1996). Physiologic changes of pregnancy. In K. R. Simpson & P. A. Creehan (Eds.), *AWHONN's perinatal nursing* (pp. 45–59). Washington, DC: Association of Women's Health, Obstetric, and Neonatal Nurses.

Gorrie, T. M., McKinney, E. S., & Murray, S. S. (1998). *Foundations of maternal-newborn nursing* (2nd ed.). Philadelphia: Saunders.

Kendig, S., & Barron, M. L. (1996). Antenatal care and risk assessment strategies. In K. R. Simpson & P. A. Creehan (Eds.), *AWHONN's perinatal nursing* (pp. 73–107). Washington, DC: Association of Women's Health, Obstetric, and Neonatal Nurses.

Mahan, L. K., & Escott-Stump, S. (1996). *Krause's food, nutrition & diet therapy* (9th ed.). Philadelphia: Saunders.

Menihan, C. A. (1996). Intrapartum fetal monitoring. In K. R. Simpson & P. A. Creehan (Eds.), *AWHONN's perinatal nursing* (pp. 187–225). Washington, DC: Association of Women's Health, Obstetric, and Neonatal Nurses.

Mitchell, M. K. (1997). *Nutrition across the life span.* Philadelphia: Saunders.

Nichols, F. H., & Zwelling, E. (1997). *Maternal-newborn nursing: Theory and practice.* Philadelphia: Saunders.

Rubin, R. (1984). *Maternal identity and the maternal experience.* New York: Springer.

chapter 5

Nursing Care of Women with Complications during Pregnancy

Outline

Objectives

On completion and mastery of Chapter 5, the student will be able to

- Define each vocabulary term listed.
- Describe each antepartum complication and its treatment.
- Identify methods to reduce a woman's risk for antepartum complications.
- Discuss management of concurrent medical conditions during pregnancy.
- Describe environmental hazards that may adversely affect the outcome of pregnancy.
- Describe how pregnancy affects care of the trauma victim.
- Explain nursing care for each antepartum complication.
- Describe psychosocial nursing interventions for the woman who has a high-risk pregnancy and her family.
- Explain use of fetal diagnostic tests in women with complicated pregnancies.

Vocabulary

abortion
disseminated intravascular coagulation (DIC)
eclampsia
erythroblastosis fetalis
hydramnios
incompetent cervix
macrosomia
preeclampsia
products of conception
teratogen
tonic-clonic seizure

Most women have uneventful pregnancies that are free of complications. However, others have complications that threaten their well-being and that of their babies. Many problems can be anticipated during prenatal care and thus prevented or made less severe. Others occur without warning.

Early and regular prenatal care allows the physician or nurse-midwife to identify a woman's risk factors and to detect complications quickly. Women who have no prenatal care or begin care late in pregnancy may have complications that are severe because they were not identified early. Box 5–1 describes the danger signs that should be taught to every pregnant woman and reinforced at each prenatal visit. The woman should be taught to notify her physician or nurse-midwife if any of these danger signs occur.

Complications during pregnancy can have any of three etiologies:

- They may relate to the pregnancy itself.
- They may occur because the woman has a medical condition or injury that complicates the pregnancy.
- They may result from environmental hazards that affect her or her fetus.

BOX 5–1

DANGER SIGNALS IN PREGNANCY

Sudden gush of fluid from vagina
Vaginal bleeding
Abdominal pain
Persistent vomiting
Epigastric pain
Edema of face and hands
Severe, persistent headache
Blurred vision or dizziness
Chills with fever over 38.3°C (101°F)
Painful urination or reduced urinary output

PREGNANCY-RELATED COMPLICATIONS

Complications of pregnancy that will be covered include hyperemesis gravidarum, bleeding disorders, hypertension, and blood incompatibility between the woman and fetus.

Hyperemesis Gravidarum

Mild nausea and/or vomiting are easily managed during pregnancy (see p. 71). In contrast, the woman with hyperemesis gravidarum has excessive nausea and vomiting that significantly interfere with her food intake and fluid balance. Fetal growth may be restricted resulting in a low-birth-weight baby. Dehydration impairs perfusion of the placenta, reducing the delivery of oxygen and nutrients to the fetus.

Manifestations. Hyperemesis gravidarum differs from "morning sickness" of pregnancy in one or more of these ways:

- Persistent nausea and vomiting, often with complete inability to retain food and fluids
- Significant weight loss
- Dehydration, evidenced by a dry tongue and mucous membranes, by decreased turgor (elasticity) of the skin, scant and concentrated urine, and a high hematocrit
- Electrolyte and acid–base imbalances
- Psychological factors, such as unusual stress, emotional immaturity, passivity, or ambivalence about the pregnancy

Treatment. The physician will rule out other causes for the excessive nausea and vomiting, such as gastroenteritis or liver, gallbladder, or pancreatic disorders, before making this diagnosis. The medical treatment for hyperemesis gravidarum is to correct dehydration and electrolyte or acid–base imbalances with oral or intravenous fluids. Antiemetic drugs such as promethazine (Phenergan) may be prescribed after the physician informs the woman about any potential harm to the developing baby. An occasional woman needs total parenteral nutrition. The woman may need hospital admission, sometimes several times, to correct dehydration and inadequate nutrition if home measures are not successful. The condition is self-limiting in most women, although it is quite distressing to the woman and her family.

Nursing Care. Nursing care focuses on client teaching because most care occurs in the home. The woman should reduce factors that trigger nausea and vomiting. She should avoid food odors, such as meal preparation areas and tray carts if she is hospitalized. If she becomes nauseated when her food is served, remove the tray promptly and offer it again later. Foods should be served at their most appetizing temperature.

Intake and output are kept to assess fluid balance. Frequent, small amounts of food and fluid keep the stomach from becoming too full, which can trigger vomiting. Easily digested carbohydrates, such as crackers or baked potatoes, are tolerated best. Foods with strong odors should be eliminated. Taking liquids between meals of solid foods helps to reduce gastric distention. Food should be served attractively and without negative comments such as "I hope you will be able to hold this down." Sitting upright after meals reduces gastric reflux (backflow).

The emesis basin is kept out of sight so that it is not a visual reminder of vomiting. It should be emptied at once if the woman vomits.

Stress may contribute to hyperemesis gravidarum; stress may also result from this complication. The nurse should provide support by listening to the woman's feelings about pregnancy, childrearing, and living with constant nausea. Although psychological factors may play a role in some cases of hyperemesis gravidarum, the nurse should not assume that every woman with this complication is adjusting poorly to her pregnancy.

Bleeding Disorders of Early Pregnancy

Several bleeding disorders can complicate early pregnancy, such as spontaneous abortion, ectopic pregnancy, or hydatidiform mole. Induced abortion is covered in Chapter 11.

Spontaneous Abortion

Abortion is the intentional or nonintentional ending of a pregnancy before 20 weeks' gestation, the point of viability. Spontaneous abortion occurs in at least 15% of pregnancies. Many early spontaneous abortions no doubt occur before the woman is aware of being pregnant. Lay people often use the word *miscarriage* to describe spontaneous abortion and to distinguish it from induced abortion. In most cases the developing baby or placenta (products of conception) is abnormal. Maternal factors may also contribute to spontaneous abortion:

- Infections
- Endocrine disorders
- Abnormalities of the reproductive organs
- Immune factors

Manifestations. There are six categories of spontaneous abortion. Four are based on the extent of cervical dilation and amount of tissue passed (Fig. 5–1). Two others describe special situations related to spontaneous abortion.

Threatened Abortion. The woman has intermittent light bleeding ("spotting"). The cervix is closed, and no tissue is passed. In about half of the women with threatened abortion, inevitable abortion develops. Usually cramping or backache accompany the light bleeding.

Inevitable Abortion. The woman has increased bleeding and cramping and the cervix dilates. The membranes (bag of waters) may rupture, but no tissue is passed.

Incomplete Abortion. Signs and symptoms are similar to those of inevitable abortion, but some tissue is passed.

Complete Abortion. All products of conception are expelled. Bleeding and cramping decrease, and the cervix closes.

Missed Abortion. The fetus dies within the uterus during the first half of pregnancy, but is not expelled for several weeks. The changes of early pregnancy (nausea, breast changes, and uterine growth) cease.

Recurrent Abortion. Three or more consecutive spontaneous abortions are a commonly recognized standard. An older term for recurrent abortion is *habitual abortion.* Possible causes include the following:

- Genetic or chromosomal abnormalities
- Structural abnormalities of the reproductive tract such as an incompetent cervix that does not remain closed until the end of pregnancy
- Inadequate progesterone levels to maintain the placenta
- Immunologic factors
- Medical conditions such as diabetes mellitus or infections

Treatment. A vaginal ultrasound examination is done to determine if the embryo or fetus is living. If the process has not advanced beyond threatened abortion, the woman is advised to stop sexual activity until the bleeding has stopped for 2 weeks. Bed rest at home may be recommended.

If the woman has an inevitable abortion, treatment is to await natural evacuation of the uterus. If natural evacuation is not effective or if the woman has an incomplete abortion, her uterus is emptied by vacuum (suction) aspiration or by dilation and curettage (D&C). See Table 5–1 for description of these procedures.

Missed abortion may be managed by awaiting spontaneous expulsion of the fetus for 3 to 5 weeks.

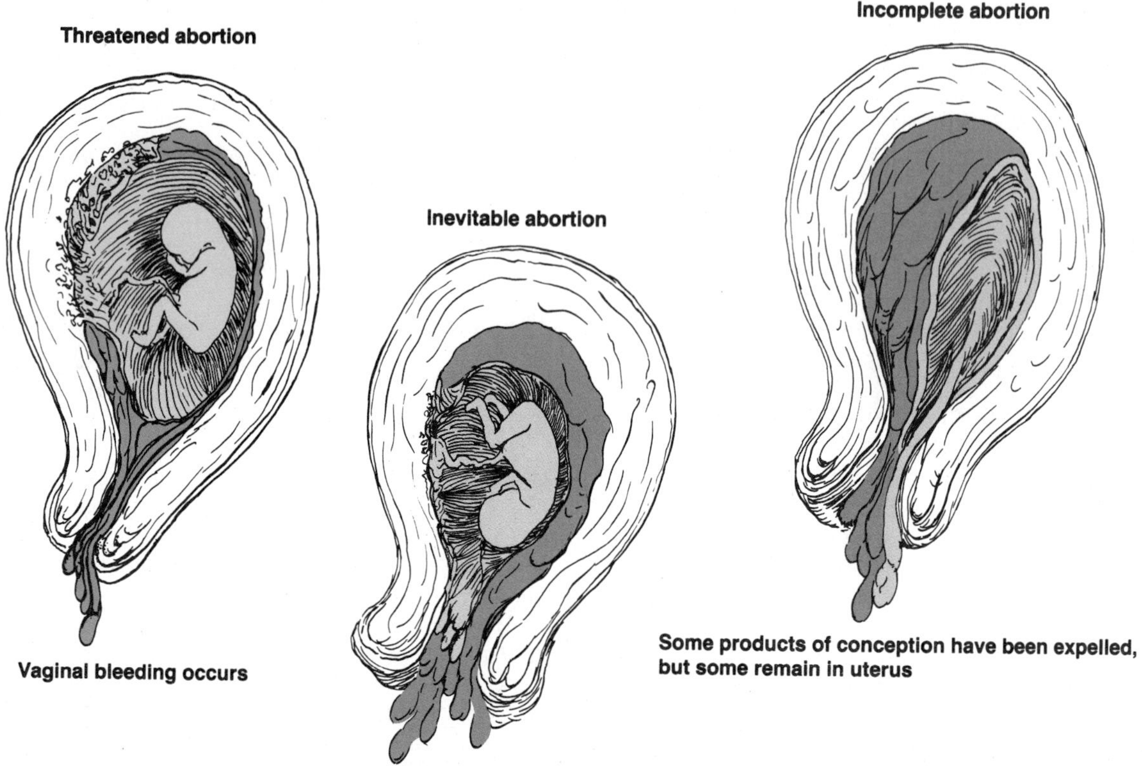

Figure 5–1. • Three types of spontaneous abortion.

Infection or clotting abnormalities are potential complications of a missed abortion. If spontaneous expulsion does not occur, uterine contractions are induced with prostaglandins. Curettage or vacuum aspiration may be needed to empty the uterus.

Therapy for the woman who has recurrent spontaneous abortion depends on whether a treatable cause is identified. Incompetent cervix is managed with a surgical procedure (cerclage) to reinforce the cervix with a pursestring suture. Improved control of diabetes and treatment of infections may allow the woman to carry her fetus to maturity.

Oxytocin (Pitocin) controls blood loss before and after curettage, much as the drugs do after term birth. Rh immune globulin (RhoGAM [300 μg] or the lower-dose MICRhoGAM [50 μg]) is given to Rh-negative women after any abortion to prevent development of antibodies that might harm the fetus during a subsequent pregnancy. The dose ordered depends on duration of gestation.

Nursing Care

Physical Care. The nurse documents the amount and character of bleeding and saves anything that

Table 5–1

PROCEDURES USED IN SPONTANEOUS AND INDUCED ABORTION

Procedure and Description	Comments
Vacuum aspiration (vacuum curettage). Cervical dilation with metal rods or laminaria (a substance that absorbs water and swells, thus enlarging the cervical opening) followed by controlled suction through a plastic cannula to remove all products of conception (POC)	Used for 1st-trimester abortions; also used to remove remaining POC following spontaneous abortion; may be followed by curettage (see dilation and curettage); paracervical block (local anesthesia of the cervix) or general anesthesia needed; conscious sedation with midazolam (Versed) may be used
Dilation and curettage (D&C). Dilation of the cervix as in vacuum curettage followed by gentle scraping of the uterine walls to remove POC	Used for 1st-trimester abortions and to remove all POC following a spontaneous abortion; greater risk of cervical or uterine trauma and excessive blood loss than with vacuum curettage; paracervical block or general anesthesia needed

looks like clots or tissue. A pad count and an estimate of how much each is saturated (e.g., 50%, 75%) more accurately documents blood loss. The woman with threatened abortion who remains at home is taught to report increased bleeding or passage of tissue.

The nurse should check the hospitalized woman's bleeding and vital signs to identify hypovolemic shock resulting from blood loss. She should remain NPO if she has active bleeding. Lab tests, such as a hemoglobin and hematocrit, are ordered.

After vacuum aspiration or curettage, the amount of vaginal bleeding is observed. The blood pressure, pulse, and respirations are checked every 15 minutes for 1 hour, then every 30 minutes until discharge from the postanesthesia care unit. Her temperature is checked on admission to the recovery area and every 4 hours until discharge to identify infection.

Most women are discharged directly from the recovery unit to their home after curettage. Rh immune globulin is given to the Rh-negative woman before she leaves. Guidelines for self-care at home include:

- Report increased bleeding. Do not use tampons, which may cause infection.
- Take temperature every 8 hours for 3 days. Report signs of infection (temperature of 38°C [100.4°F] or higher; foul odor or brownish color of vaginal drainage).
- Take oral iron supplement if prescribed. See Chapter 4 for information about taking iron supplements.
- Resume sexual activity as recommended by the physician (usually after the bleeding has stopped).
- Return to the physician at the recommended time for a checkup and contraception information.
- *Pregnancy can occur before the first menstrual period.*

Emotional Care. Our society often underestimates the emotional distress spontaneous abortion causes the woman and her family. Even if the pregnancy was not planned or not suspected, they often grieve for what might have been. Their grief may last longer and be deeper than they or other people expect. The nurse listens to the woman and acknowledges the grief she and her partner feel. Table 5–2 contains information about communicating with the family experiencing pregnancy loss. Spiritual support of the family's choice and community support groups may help the family work through the grief of spontaneous abortion. Nursing Care Plan 5–1 suggests interventions for families experiencing early pregnancy loss.

Ectopic Pregnancy

Ectopic pregnancy occurs when the fertilized ovum (zygote) is implanted outside the uterine cavity (Fig. 5–2). Of all ectopic pregnancies, 95% occur in the fallopian tube (tubal pregnancy). An obstruction or other abnormality of the tube prevents the zygote from being transported into the uterus. Scarring or deformity of the fallopian tubes or inhibition of normal tubal motion to propel the zygote into the uterus may result from:

- Hormonal abnormalities
- Inflammation

Table 5–2
COMMUNICATING WITH A FAMILY EXPERIENCING PREGNANCY LOSS

Effective Techniques	Ineffective Techniques
Keep the family together	Do not give the woman/family any information
Wait quietly with family: "being there"	Separate family members
Say "I'm sorry," or "I'm here if you need to talk"	Discourage expressions of sadness; for example, expecting the father to be strong for the mother's sake
Touch (may not be appreciated by some people or in some cultures)	Avoid interacting with the family and talking about their loss
Refer to spontaneous abortion as "miscarriage" rather than the harsher sounding "abortion"	Act uncomfortable with the family's expressions of grief
Provide mementoes as appropriate (lock of hair, photograph, footprint); save keepsakes for later retrieval if the family does not want them immediately	Minimize the importance of the pregnancy by comments such as, "You're young—you can always have more children," "At least you didn't lose a real baby," "It was for the best, the baby was abnormal," or "You have another healthy child at home"
Alert other hospital personnel to the family's loss to prevent hurtful comments or questions	Say, "I know how you feel;" self-disclosure of your similar experience must be used carefully and only if it is likely to be therapeutic to the client
Allow the family to see the fetus if they wish; prepare them for the fetus's appearance	Encourage the family not to cry
Reduce the number of staff with whom the family must interact	
Summon a chaplain, minister, or rabbi	
Make referrals to support groups in the area	

NURSING CARE PLAN 5–1

Selected Nursing Diagnoses for the Family Experiencing Early Pregnancy Loss

Nursing Diagnosis: Grieving related to loss of anticipated infant

Goals	Nursing Interventions	Rationale
The woman and family will express grief to significant others The woman and family will complete each stage of the grieving process within individual time frames	1. Promote expression of grief by providing privacy, eliminating time restrictions, allowing support persons of choice to visit, and recognizing individualized grief expressions and cultural norms	1. Grief is an individual process and people react to it in different ways; these measures encourage woman and family to express grief and begin resolving it
	2. Use the four stages of grief as a basis for nursing interventions: a. Stage 1: shock and disbelief at loss; characterized by numbness, apathy, impaired decision making b. Stage 2: seeking answers for why loss happened; characterized by crying, tears, guilt, loss of appetite, insomnia, blame placing c. Stage 3: disorganization; characterized by feelings of purposelessness and malaise; gradual resumption of normal activities d. Stage 4: reorganization; characterized by sad memories, but daily functioning returns	2. Knowledge of normal stages of grieving helps nurse identify whether it is progressing normally or if there is dysfunctional grieving in any family member; stages help nurse better interpret clients' behavior; for example, blame placing is a normal part of grieving and is not necessarily directed at the nurse or caregivers; allows nurse to reassure client that feelings are normal without diminishing intensity of their feelings
	3. Use open communication techniques, such as a. Quiet presence b. Expression of sympathy ("I'm sorry this happened") c. Open-ended statements ("This must be really sad for you") d. Reflection of client's expressed feelings ("You feel guilty because you didn't stay in bed constantly?")	3. These examples of open communication encourage family to express feelings about the loss, which is the first step in resolving them
	4. Reinforce explanations given by the physicians or others (e.g., what the problem was, why it occurred); use simple language	4. Grieving people often do not hear or understand explanations the first time they are given because their concentration is impaired

- Infection
- Adhesions
- Congenital defects
- Endometriosis (uterine lining outside the uterus)

Use of an intrauterine device for contraception may contribute to ectopic pregnancy because these devices promote inflammation and infection within the uterus. Smoking at the time of conception has also been associated with ectopic pregnancy (Cunningham et al., 1997). A woman who has had a previous tubal pregnancy or a failed tubal ligation is also more likely to have an ectopic pregnancy.

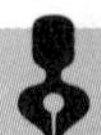

Nursing Tip

Supporting and encouraging the grieving process in families that suffer a pregnancy loss, such as a spontaneous abortion or ectopic pregnancy, allow them to resolve their grief.

A zygote that is implanted in a fallopian tube cannot survive for long because the blood supply and size of the tube are inadequate. The zygote or embryo may die and be reabsorbed by the woman's body, or the tube may rupture with bleeding into the abdominal cavity.

Manifestations. The woman often complains of lower abdominal pain, sometimes accompanied by light vaginal bleeding. If the tube ruptures, she may have sudden severe lower abdominal pain, vaginal bleeding, and signs of hypovolemic shock (Box 5–2). The amount of vaginal bleeding may be minimal because most blood is lost into the abdomen rather than externally. Shoulder pain is a symptom

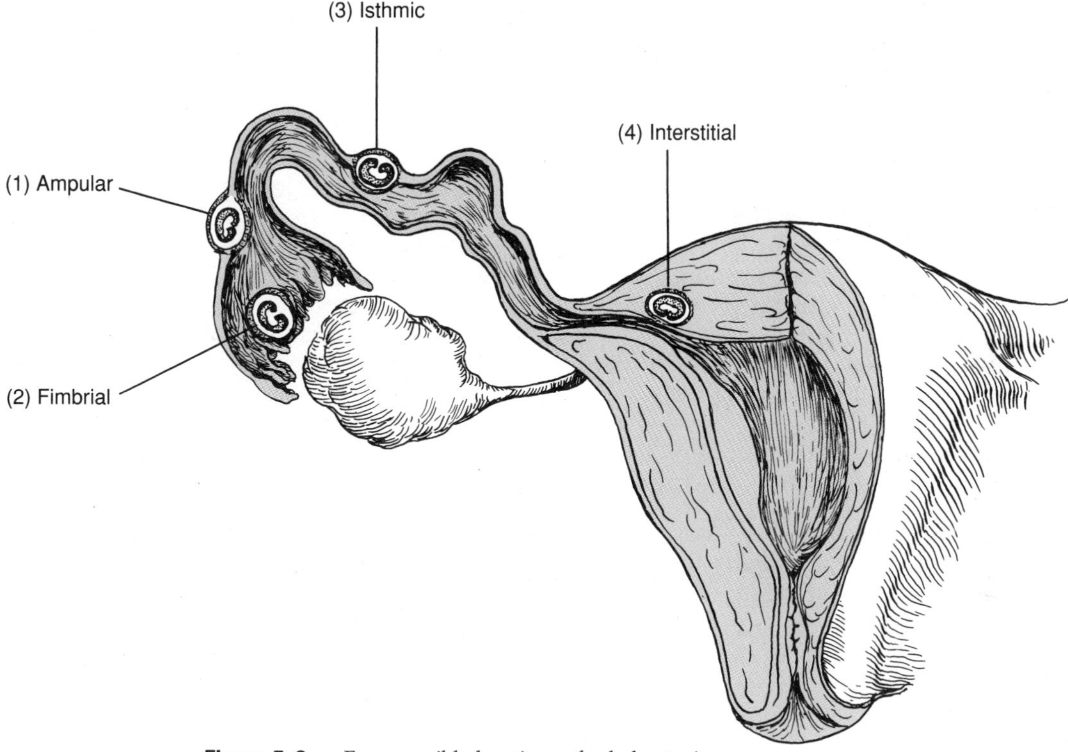

Figure 5–2. • Four possible locations of tubal ectopic pregnancy.

that often accompanies bleeding in the abdomen (referred pain).

Treatment. A sensitive pregnancy test for human chorionic gonadotropin (hCG) is done to determine if the woman is pregnant. Transvaginal ultrasound examination determines whether the embryo is growing within the uterine cavity. Culdocentesis (puncture of the upper posterior vaginal wall with removal of peritoneal fluid) may occasionally be done to identify blood in the woman's pelvis, which suggests tubal rupture. A laparoscopic examination may be done to view the damaged tube with an endoscope (lighted instrument for viewing internal organs).

The physician attempts to preserve the tube if the woman wants other children, but this is not always possible. The priority medical treatment is to control blood loss. Blood transfusion may be required for massive hemorrhage. One of three courses is chosen, depending on the gestation and the amount of damage to the fallopian tube:

- No action if the pregnancy is being reabsorbed by the woman's body
- Medical therapy with methotrexate, which inhibits cell division in the embryo and allows it to be reabsorbed, if the tube is not ruptured
- Surgery to remove the pregnancy from the tube if damage is minimal; severe damage requires removal of the entire tube and occasionally the uterus

Nursing Care. Nursing care includes observing for hypovolemic shock as in spontaneous abortion.

BOX 5–2

SIGNS AND SYMPTOMS OF HYPOVOLEMIC SHOCK

Fetal heart rate changes (increased, decreased, less fluctuation)
Rising, weak pulse (tachycardia)
Rising respiratory rate (tachypnea)
Shallow, irregular respirations; air hunger
Falling blood pressure (hypotension)
Decreased (usually less than 30 ml/hr) or absent urine output
Pale skin or mucous membranes
Cold, clammy skin
Faintness
Thirst

Vaginal bleeding is assessed, although most lost blood may remain in the abdomen. The nurse should report increasing pain, particularly shoulder pain, to the physician.

If the woman has surgery, pre- and postoperative care is similar to that for other abdominal surgery:

- Vital signs to identify hypovolemic shock; temperature to identify infection
- Assessment of lung and bowel sounds
- Intravenous fluid; blood replacement will be ordered if loss was substantial
- Antibiotics as ordered
- Pain medication, often with patient-controlled analgesia (PCA) after surgery
- NPO preoperatively. Oral intake usually resumes after surgery beginning with ice chips, then to clear liquids and is advanced as bowel sounds resume.
- Indwelling catheter as ordered. Urine output is a significant indicator of fluid balance and will fall or stop if the woman hemorrhages. The minimal urinary output is 25 to 30 ml/hour.
- Bed rest before surgery; progressive ambulation postoperatively. The nurse should have adequate assistance when the woman first ambulates because she is more likely to faint if she lost a great deal of blood.

The actual frequency of assessments such as vital signs will depend on the woman's hemodynamic stability and the length of time since surgery.

In addition to physical pre- and postoperative care, the nurse provides emotional support because the woman and her family may experience grieving similar to that accompanying spontaneous abortion. Loss of a fallopian tube threatens future fertility and is another source of grief. In addition, the woman who has one tubal pregnancy is more likely to have another one because the condition that favored its occurrence in one tube is likely to affect the other tube.

Hydatidiform Mole

Hydatidiform mole (gestational trophoblastic disease) occurs when the chorionic villi (fringelike structures that form the placenta) abnormally increase and develop vesicles (small sacs) that resemble tiny grapes (Fig. 5–3). The mole may be

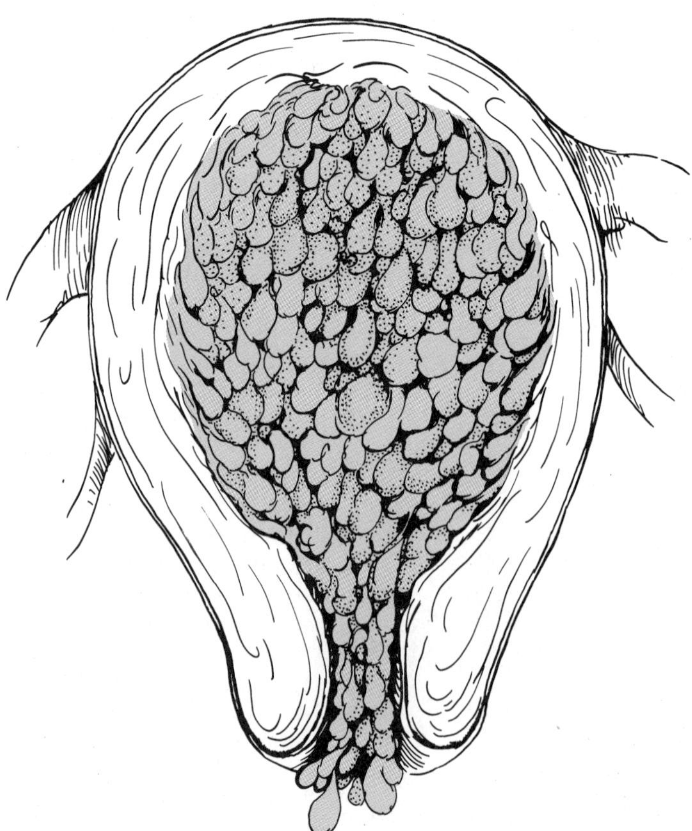

Figure 5–3. • Hydatidiform mole of gestational trophoblastic disease.

Nursing Tip

The nurse should teach the woman to report any danger signs that occur during pregnancy promptly.

complete, with no fetus present, or partial, in which only part of the placenta has the characteristic vesicles. A fetus develops and may be born alive, depending on the extent of the problem. Hydatidiform mole may cause hemorrhage, clotting abnormalities, hypertension, and later development of cancer (choriocarcinoma). Chromosome abnormalities are found in many cases of hydatidiform mole. It is more likely to occur in women at the age extremes of reproductive life, and a woman who has had one molar pregnancy is more likely to have another.

Manifestations. Signs associated with hydatidiform mole appear early in pregnancy and include the following:

- Bleeding, which may range from spotting to profuse hemorrhage; cramping may be present
- Rapid uterine growth and a uterine size that is larger than expected for the gestation
- Failure to detect fetal heart activity
- Signs of hyperemesis gravidarum (see p. 82)
- Unusually early development of pregnancy-induced hypertension (see p. 92)
- Higher than expected levels of hCG
- A distinctive "snowstorm" pattern on ultrasound but with no developing baby in the uterus
- Signs of a pulmonary embolism if the vesicles enter the venous circulation

Treatment. The uterus is evacuated by vacuum aspiration and sharp curettage (D&C). The level of hCG is tested until it is undetectable and the levels are followed for at least one year. Persistent or rising levels suggest that vesicles remain or that malignant change has occurred. The woman should delay conceiving until follow-up care is complete because a new pregnancy would confuse tests for hCG. Rh immune globulin is prescribed for the Rh-negative woman.

Nursing Care. The nurse observes for bleeding and shock; care is similar to that given in spontaneous abortion and ectopic pregnancy. If the woman also experiences hyperemesis or preeclampsia, the nurse incorporates care related to those conditions as well. The woman has also lost a pregnancy, so the nurse should provide care related to grieving, similar to that for a spontaneous abortion. The need to delay another pregnancy may be another concern if the woman is nearing the end of her reproductive life and wants a child.

The need for follow-up examinations is reinforced, as is the need to avoid pregnancy during this time. Rh immune globulin is administered to the Rh-negative woman. The woman is taught how to use contraception (see Chapter 11).

Bleeding Disorders of Late Pregnancy

Bleeding in late pregnancy is often caused by placenta previa or abruptio placentae (Table 5–3).

Placenta Previa

Placenta previa occurs when the placenta develops in the lower part of the uterus rather than in the upper part. There are three degrees of placenta previa, depending on the location of the placenta in relation to the cervix (Fig. 5–4):

- Marginal: placenta reaches the edge of the cervical opening
- Partial: placenta partly covers the cervical opening
- Total: placenta completely covers the cervical opening

A low-lying placenta is implanted near the cervix, but it does not cover any of the opening. This variation is not a true placenta previa and may or may not be accompanied by bleeding. The low-lying placenta may be discovered during a routine ultrasound examination in early pregnancy. It also may be diagnosed during late pregnancy, because the woman has signs similar to those of a true placenta previa.

Manifestations. Painless vaginal bleeding, usually bright red, is the main characteristic of placenta previa. The woman's risk of hemorrhage increases as term approaches and the cervix begins to *efface* (thin) and *dilate* (open). These normal prelabor changes disrupt the placental attachment. Diagnosis is made by ultrasound examination, which reveals the abnormal placement of the placenta. The fetus is often in an abnormal presentation, such as breech or transverse lie, because the placenta occupies the lower uterus, which prevents the fetus from assuming the normal head-down presentation.

The fetus or neonate may have anemia or hypovolemic shock because some of the blood lost may be fetal blood. Fetal hypoxia may occur if a large

Table 5-3
COMPARISON OF PLACENTA PREVIA AND ABRUPTIO PLACENTAE

Placenta Previa	Abruptio Placentae
Abnormal implantation of the placenta in the lower uterus Marginal. Approaches, but does not reach, the cervical opening Partial. Partially covers the cervical opening Total. Completely covers the cervical opening	Premature separation of the normally implanted placenta Partial. Detachment of part of the placenta Total. Complete detachment of the placenta Marginal. Detachment at the edge of the placenta Central. Detachment of the center surface of the placenta; edges stay attached
Bleeding	
Obvious vaginal bleeding, usually bright; may be profuse	Visible dark vaginal bleeding and/or concealed bleeding within the uterus; enlargement of uterus suggests that blood is accumulating within the cavity
Pain	
None, other than from normal uterine contractions if in labor	Gradual or abrupt onset of pain and uterine tenderness; possibly low-back pain
Uterine consistency	
Uterus soft; no abnormal contractions or irritability	Uterus firm and boardlike; may be irritable, with frequent, brief contractions
Fetus	
Fetus may be in an abnormal presentation, such as breech or transverse lie (see pp. 131–132)	Fetal presentation usually normal
Blood clotting	
Normal	Often accompanied by impaired blood clotting More likely to occur if the woman recently ingested cocaine
Postpartum complications	
Infection. Placental site is near the nonsterile vagina	Infection: bleeding into uterine muscle fibers predisposes to bacterial invasion
Hemorrhage. Lower uterine segment does not contract as effectively to compress bleeding vessels	Hemorrhage: bleeding into uterine muscle fibers damages them, inhibiting uterine contraction after birth
Signs of fetal compromise if maternal shock or extensive placental detachment occur	Signs of fetal compromise, depending on amount and location of the placental surface that is disrupted
Fetal/neonatal anemia may occur because some lost blood may be fetal	Fetal/neonatal anemia may occur because some lost blood may be fetal

disruption of the placental surface reduces transfer of oxygen and nutrients.

The woman with placenta previa is more likely than others to have an infection or hemorrhage after birth.

- Infection is more likely to occur because vaginal organisms can easily reach the placental site, which is a good growth medium for microorganisms.
- Postpartum hemorrhage may occur because the lower segment of the uterus, where the placenta was attached, has fewer muscle fibers than the upper uterus. Weak contraction of the lower uterus does not compress open vessels at the placental site as effectively.

Treatment. Medical care depends on the gestation and amount of bleeding. The goal is to maintain the pregnancy until the fetal lungs are mature enough that respiratory distress is not likely (about 34 weeks). Delivery will be done if bleeding is sufficient to jeopardize the mother or fetus, regardless of gestation.

Bed rest reduces downward pressure on the cervix, which might increase bleeding. The woman should lie on her side or have a pillow under one hip to avoid supine hypotension. If bleeding is extensive or the gestation is near term, cesarean delivery is done for partial or total placenta previa. The woman with a low-lying placenta or marginal placenta previa may be able to deliver vaginally unless blood loss is excessive.

Nursing Care. The priorities of nursing care include observation of vaginal blood loss and of signs and symptoms of shock. Vital signs are taken every 15 minutes if the woman is actively bleeding and oxygen is often given to increase the amount delivered to the fetus. Vaginal examination is *not* done by the nurse because it may precipitate bleeding if the placental attachment is disrupted. The fetal heart rate is monitored. The nurse implements care for cesarean delivery, as needed (see p. 195). Postpartum care is routine, although the nurse is espe-

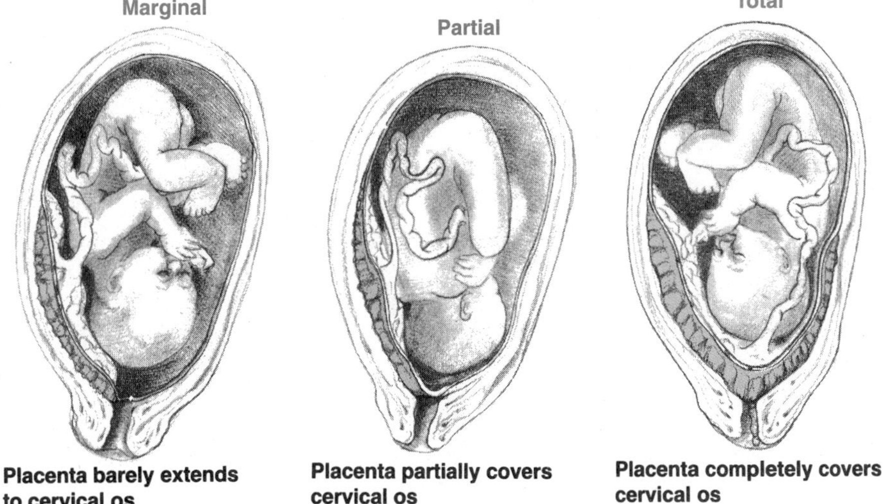

Figure 5–4. • Placenta previa may be marginal, partial, or total, depending on the placental position in relation to the cervical opening.

cially watchful for hemorrhage or infection (see Chapter 10). The parents of the infant are often fearful for their child, particularly if a preterm delivery is required.

Abruptio Placentae

Abruptio placentae is the premature separation of a placenta that is normally implanted. It usually accompanies other complications rather than occurring alone:

- Hypertension
- Cocaine or alcohol use
- Cigarette smoking
- Rupture of the membranes when the uterus was overdistended with fluid (hydramnios, also called polyhydramnios)
- Blows to the abdomen, as might occur in battering or accidental trauma
- Short umbilical cord, which pulls the placenta from the uterine wall as the fetus descends during late pregnancy or labor

Abruptio placentae may be partial or total (Fig. 5–5); it may be marginal (separating at the edges) or central (separating in the middle). Bleeding may be visible or concealed behind the partially attached placenta.

Manifestations. Bleeding accompanied by abdominal or low back pain is the typical characteristic of abruptio placentae. Unlike bleeding in placenta previa, most or all of the bleeding may be concealed behind the placenta. Obvious dark-red vaginal bleeding occurs when blood leaks past the edge of the placenta. The woman's uterus is tender and unusually firm (boardlike) because blood leaks into its muscle fibers. Frequent cramplike uterine contractions often occur (uterine irritability).

The fetus may or may not have problems, depending on how much placental surface is disrupted. As in placenta previa, some of the blood lost may be fetal, and the fetus or neonate may have anemia or hypovolemic shock.

Disseminated intravascular coagulation (DIC), also called consumptive coagulopathy, is a complex disorder that may complicate abruptio placentae.

Nursing Tip

Positioning patient on her side during bed rest helps to improve blood flow to the placenta and more effectively provides oxygen and nutrients to the fetus.

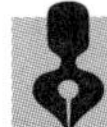

Nursing Tip

If a vaginal examination is done when placenta previa is suspected, the *physician* will do it with preparations for both vaginal and cesarean delivery (a double setup) in place.

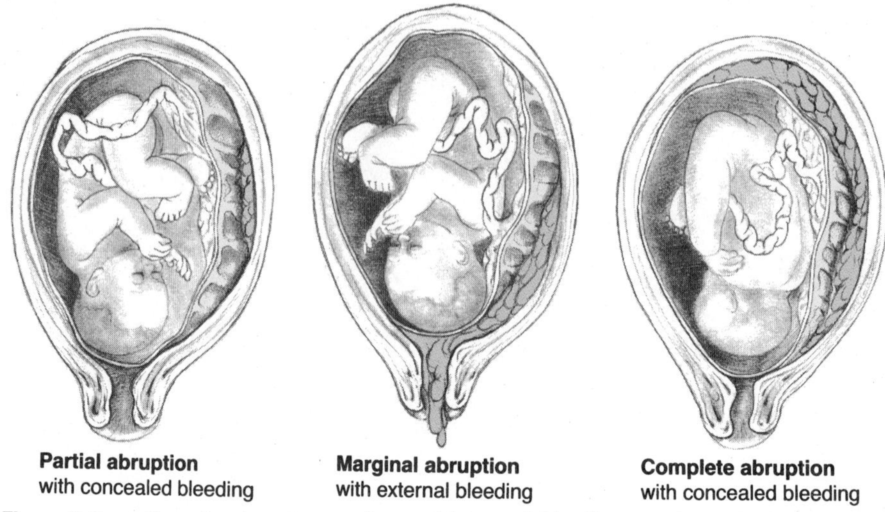

Figure 5–5. • Abruptio placentae may be partial or total; bleeding may be visible or concealed.

The large blood clot that forms behind the placenta consumes clotting factors, leaving the rest of her body deficient in these factors. Clot formation and anticoagulation (destruction of clots) occur simultaneously throughout the body in the woman with DIC. She may bleed from her mouth, nose, incisions, or venipuncture sites because her clotting factors are depleted.

Postpartum hemorrhage may occur because the injured uterine muscle does not contract effectively to control blood loss. Infection is more likely to occur because the damaged tissue is susceptible to microbial invasion.

Treatment. In most cases, immediate cesarean delivery is done because of the risk for maternal shock, clotting disorders, and fetal death. Blood and clotting factor replacement may be needed because of DIC. The mother's clotting action quickly returns to normal after birth because the source of the abnormality is removed.

Nursing Care. The nurse observes for and reports signs and symptoms of abruptio placentae, especially if a woman has any of the conditions described. Observation for shock and for bleeding from the nose, gums, or other unexpected sites allows prompt medical intervention. The fetus is monitored, as with placenta previa. Rapid increase in the size of the uterus suggests that blood is accumulating within it. The uterus is usually very tender and hard. Nursing care after birth is similar to that with placenta previa.

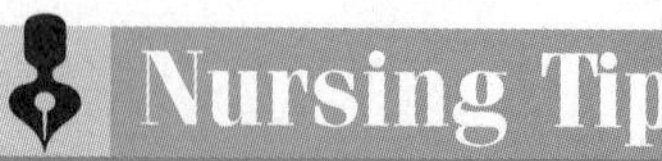

Pain is an important symptom that distinguishes abruptio placentae from placenta previa.

The fetus sometimes dies before delivery (see p. 85 for nursing care related to fetal death [stillbirth] and support of the grieving family). Many therapeutic communication techniques outlined in Table 5–2 are appropriate.

Hypertension during Pregnancy

Hypertension may exist before pregnancy (chronic hypertension), but it usually develops as a pregnancy complication (*pregnancy-induced hypertension* [PIH]). A woman with chronic hypertension may develop PIH in addition to her chronic condition. Table 5–4 compares different types of hypertension during pregnancy. This section focuses on PIH because it is a common complication, occurring in 7% of pregnancies. The term *preeclampsia* may be used when PIH includes proteinuria and edema. Preeclampsia progresses to *eclampsia* when convulsions occur. One sometimes hears the word *toxemia,* an old word for PIH.

The cause of PIH is unknown, but birth is its cure. It usually develops during late pregnancy but can develop during the intrapartum or even the early postpartum period. Vasospasm (spasm of the arteries) is the main characteristic of PIH. Although the cause is unknown, any of several risk factors

Table 5–4
HYPERTENSIVE DISORDERS OF PREGNANCY

Pregnancy-induced hypertension (PIH)	Development of hypertension (BP over 140/90) in a previously normotensive woman after 20 weeks of gestation
Preeclampsia	Renal involvement leads to proteinuria
Eclampsia	Central nervous system involvement causes seizures
HELLP (*h*emolysis, *e*levated *l*iver enzymes, *l*ow *p*latelets)	Liver and coagulation abnormalities dominate the clinical picture
Chronic hypertension	Presence of hypertension before 20 weeks of gestation

From ACOG. (1996). *Hypertension in pregnancy.* Technical bulletin #219. Author.

Table 5–5
MILD VERSUS SEVERE PREECLAMPSIA

	Mild	Severe
Systolic BP	<160 mm Hg	>160 mm Hg
Diastolic BP	<100 mm Hg	>110 mm Hg
Proteinuria	Trace	>5 g/24 hr
Creatinine	Normal	Elevated
Thrombocytopenia	Absent	Present
Oliguria	Absent	<500 ml/24 hr
Liver enzyme elevation	Minimal	Marked
Fetal growth restriction	Absent	Present
Headache, visual disturbances or abdominal pain	Absent	Present

increases a woman's chance of developing PIH (Box 5–3).

Manifestations

Vasospasm impedes blood flow to the mother's organs and placenta, resulting in one or more of these signs: (1) hypertension, (2) edema, and (3) proteinuria (protein in the urine). Severe PIH can also affect the central nervous system, eyes, urinary tract, liver, gastrointestinal system, and blood clotting function. See Table 5–5 for a summary of mild versus severe preeclampsia.

Hypertension. Despite an increase in blood volume and cardiac output, most pregnant women do not have a rise in blood pressure (Fig. 5–6) because they seem to have a resistance to factors that cause vasoconstriction. Also, the resistance to blood flow in their vessels (peripheral vascular resistance) decreases because of the effects of vasodilators. The woman with PIH, however, has a greater sensitivity to vasoconstrictors and a decreased amount of vasodilators. A blood pressure of 140/90 is considered hypertensive in pregnancy. The previous standard, a rise of 30 mm Hg in the systolic or 15 mm Hg in the diastolic blood pressure, is no longer considered valid (ACOG, 1996).

BOX 5–3

RISK FACTORS FOR PREGNANCY-INDUCED HYPERTENSION (PIH)

- First pregnancy
- African American
- Family history of PIH
- Age over 40 years
- Multifetal pregnancy (e.g., twins)
- Chronic hypertension
- Chronic renal disease
- Diabetes mellitus
- Other genetic and immunologic factors
- Low socioeconomic status and young maternal age have been implicated as risk factors, but the actual independent contribution of these factors is uncertain.

From The American College of Obstetricians and Gynecologists. *Hypertension in pregnancy.* Technical bulletin #219. Washington, DC, © ACOG, January 1996.

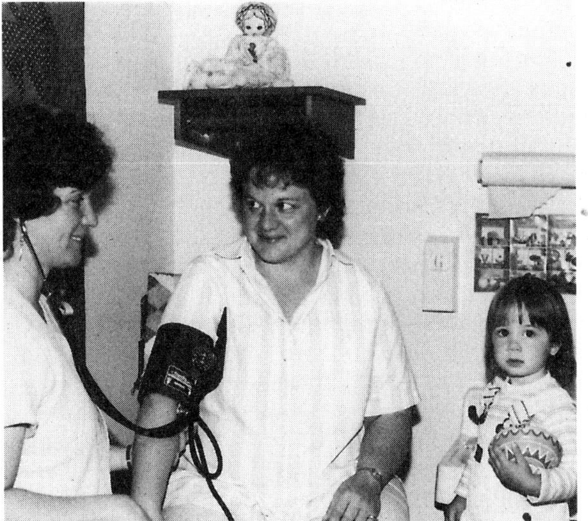

Figure 5–6. • Blood pressure is checked at every prenatal visit to detect early signs of pregnancy-induced hypertension. (Courtesy of WomanCare, Des Moines BirthPlace, Des Moines, IA.)

Edema. Edema occurs because fluid leaves the blood vessels and enters the tissues. Although total body fluid is increased, the amount within the blood vessels is reduced (hypovolemia), further decreasing blood flow to the maternal organs and placenta. It is likely to be the first sign the woman notices.

Sudden excessive weight gain is the first sign of fluid retention. Visible edema follows the weight gain. Edema of the feet and legs is common during pregnancy, but edema above the waist suggests PIH. The woman may notice facial swelling or stop wearing rings because they are hard to remove. Edema is severe ("pitting") if a depression remains after the tissue is compressed.

Edema resolves quickly after birth as excess tissue fluid returns to the circulation and is excreted in the urine. Urine output may reach 6 liters daily and often exceeds fluid intake.

Proteinuria. Proteinuria develops as reduced blood flow damages the kidneys. This damage allows protein to leak into the urine. A clean-catch (midstream) or catheterized urine specimen is used to check for proteinuria, because vaginal secretions might give a false-positive result.

Other Manifestations. Other signs and symptoms occur with severe preeclampsia. All are related to decreased blood flow and edema of the organs involved.

Central Nervous System. A severe, unrelenting headache may occur because of brain edema and small cerebral hemorrhages. The severe headache often precedes a convulsion. Deep tendon reflexes become hyperactive because of central nervous system irritability.

Eyes. Visual disturbances such as blurred or double vision or "spots before the eyes" occur because of arterial spasm and edema of the retina. Visual disturbances often precede a convulsion.

Urinary Tract. Decreased blood flow to the kidneys reduces urine production and worsens hypertension. The kidneys respond to low blood flow as they do to hypovolemia, by releasing substances to raise the blood pressure.

Respiratory System. Pulmonary edema (accumulation of fluid in the lungs) may occur with severe PIH.

Liver. Liver enzymes are elevated because of reduced circulation, edema, and small hemorrhages.

Gastrointestinal System. Epigastric pain or nausea occur because of liver edema, ischemia, and necrosis and often precede a convulsion.

Blood Clotting. HELLP syndrome is a variant of PIH that involves *h*emolysis (breakage of erythrocytes), *e*levated *l*iver enzymes, and *l*ow *p*latelets. Hemolysis occurs as erythrocytes break up when passing through small blood vessels damaged by the hypertension. Obstruction of hepatic blood flow causes the liver enzymes to become elevated. Low platelets occur when the platelets gather at the site of blood vessel damage, reducing the number available in the general circulation. Low platelets cause abnormal blood clotting.

Eclampsia. Progression to eclampsia occurs when the woman has one or more generalized tonic-clonic seizures. Facial muscles twitch; this sign is followed by generalized contraction of all muscles (tonic phase), then alternate contraction and relaxation of muscles (clonic phase). *An eclamptic seizure may result in cerebral hemorrhage, abruptio placentae, fetal compromise, or death of the mother or fetus.*

Effects on Fetus. PIH reduces maternal blood flow through the placenta and decreases oxygen available to the fetus. Fetal hypoxia may result in meconium (first stool) passage into the amniotic fluid or in fetal distress. The fetus may have intrauterine growth restriction and at birth may be long and thin with peeling skin if the reduced placental blood flow has been prolonged. Fetal death sometimes occurs.

Treatment

Medical care focuses on prevention and early detection of PIH and on treatment. Drugs are often needed to prevent convulsions and to reduce a dangerously high blood pressure.

Prevention. Several studies have been done on the safety and effectiveness of preventive measures for women at risk to develop PIH. These involve taking low-dose aspirin (60 to 80 mg/day) or calcium. Research on prevention measures is ongoing.

Correction of some risk factors reduces the risk for PIH. For example, improving the diet, particularly of the adolescent, may prevent PIH and promote normal fetal growth. Other risk factors, such as family history, cannot be changed. However, early and regular prenatal care allows PIH to be diagnosed promptly, so that it is more effectively managed.

Treatment. The treatment for PIH depends on whether it is mild or severe and on the maturity of the fetus. Treatment focuses on (1) maintaining blood flow to the woman's vital organs and the placenta and (2) preventing convulsions. Birth is the cure for PIH. If the fetus is mature, pregnancy is ended by labor induction or cesarean birth. If PIH is severe, the fetus is often in greater danger from being in the uterus than from being born prematurely.

Some women who have mild PIH and a preterm fetus can be managed at home if they can comply with treatment and if home nursing visits are possible. If the woman has severe PIH or cannot comply with treatment, or if home nursing visits are not available, she is usually admitted to the hospital. Conservative treatment, whether at home or in the hospital, includes the following:

- Activity restriction to allow blood that would be circulated to skeletal muscles to be conserved for circulation to the mother's vital organs and the placenta. The woman should remain on bed rest on her side to improve blood flow to the placenta. She can walk to the bathroom if she has mild PIH.
- Maternal assessment of fetal activity ("kick counts"). She should report a decrease in movement or if none occur during a 4-hour period.
- Blood pressure monitoring two to four times per day in the same arm and in the same position. A family member must be taught the technique if the woman will remain at home.
- Daily weight on the same scale, in the same type of clothing, and at the same time of day to observe for sudden weight gain.
- Checking urine for protein with a dipstick, using a first-voided, clean-catch specimen.

Diuretics and sodium restriction are not prescribed for PIH. They are not effective for treatment of PIH and may aggravate it because they further deplete the woman's blood volume. Salt is not restricted, but intake of high-salt foods is discouraged. The woman's diet should have adequate calories, protein, and sodium (see Chapter 4 for prenatal dietary guidelines).

Fetal diagnostic tests (Table 5–6) that may be done are:

- Serial sonography to identify growth restriction or decreased amniotic fluid
- Amniocentesis to determine if the fetal lungs are mature before labor induction or cesarean birth (Fig. 5–7)
- Evaluations of placental function and its ability to provide oxygen and waste removal for the fetus, such as biophysical profile (Fig. 5–8), nonstress test, contraction stress test

Any of several drugs may be used to treat PIH.

Magnesium Sulfate. Magnesium sulfate is an anticonvulsant given to prevent seizures. It may slightly reduce the blood pressure, but its main purpose is as an anticonvulsant. It is usually given by intravenous infusion (controlled with an infusion pump). Administration continues for at least 12 to 24 hours after birth because the woman remains at risk for seizures.

Magnesium is excreted by the kidneys. Poor urine output (less than 25 ml/hr) may allow serum levels of magnesium to reach toxic levels. Excess magnesium first causes loss of the deep tendon reflexes (Fig. 5–9), which is followed by depression of respirations; if levels rise further, collapse and death can occur. *Calcium gluconate* reverses the effects of magnesium and should be available for immediate use when a woman receives magnesium sulfate.

The therapeutic serum level of magnesium is 4 to 8 mg/dl, which would be an abnormal level in a person not receiving this therapy. The woman with this serum level is slightly drowsy but retains all her reflexes and has normal respiratory function; the level is high enough to prevent convulsions.

Magnesium inhibits uterine contractions. Most women receiving the drug must also receive oxytocin to strengthen labor contractions (see p. 189). They are at risk for postpartum hemorrhage because the uterus does not contract firmly on bleeding vessels after birth. This contraction-inhibiting effect of magnesium makes it useful to stop preterm labor.

Antihypertensive Drugs. Antihypertensive drugs reduce blood pressure if it reaches a level that might cause intracranial bleeding, usually higher than 160/100. Severe hypertension can harm the fetus by causing abruptio placentae or placental infarcts (death of placental tissue). Hydralazine (Apresoline), nifedipine (Procardia), verapamil (Calan), or labetalol (Normodyne) may be used.

Diuretics. Diuretics such as furosemide (Lasix) may be required if the woman develops pulmonary edema.

Nursing Care

Nursing care focuses on (1) assisting women to obtain prenatal care, (2) helping them cope with therapy, (3) caring for acutely ill women, and (4) administering medications. Nursing Care Plan 5–2 gives common interventions for women with PIH.

Promoting Prenatal Care. Nurses can promote awareness of how prenatal care allows risk identification and early intervention if complications arise. Nurses can help the woman to feel like an individual, especially in busy clinics, which often seem impersonal, thus encouraging her to return regularly.

Coping with Therapy. Daily weights identify sudden gain that precedes visible edema. The weight should be checked early in the morning, after urination, and in similar clothes each day.

Table 5–6
FETAL DIAGNOSTIC TESTS

Tests and Description	Uses During Pregnancy
Ultrasound examination. Use of high-frequency sound waves to visualize structures within the body; the examination may use a transvaginal probe or an abdominal transducer; abdominal ultrasound during early pregnancy requires a full bladder for proper visualization (have the woman drink 1 to 2 quarts of water before the examination)	Visualize a gestational sac in early pregnancy to confirm the pregnancy Identify site of implantation (uterine or ectopic) Verify fetal viability or death Identify a multifetal pregnancy, such as twins or triplets Diagnose some fetal structural abnormalities Guide procedures, such as chorionic villous sampling, amniocentesis, percutaneous umbilical blood sampling Determine gestational age of the embryo or fetus Locate the placenta Determine the amount of amniotic fluid Observe fetal movements
Doppler ultrasound blood flow assessment. Use of high-frequency sound waves to study the flow of blood through vessels	Determine adequacy of blood flow through the placenta and umbilical cord vessels in women in whom it is likely to be impaired (such as those with pregnancy-induced hypertension or diabetes mellitus)
Alpha-fetoprotein testing. Determining the level of this fetal protein in the pregnant woman's serum or in a sample of amniotic fluid; correct interpretation requires an accurate gestational age	Identify high levels, which are associated with open defects, such as spina bifida (open spine), anencephaly (incomplete development of the skull and brain), or gastroschisis (open abdominal cavity) Identify low levels, which are associated with chromosome abnormalities or gestational trophoblastic disease (hydatidiform mole)
Chorionic villous sampling. Obtaining a small part of the developing placenta to analyze fetal cells at 10 to 12 wk gestation	Identify chromosome abnormalities or other defects that can be determined by analysis of cells. Results of chromosome studies are available 24 to 48 hr later. Cannot be used to determine spina bifida or anencephaly (see alpha-fetoprotein testing). Higher rate of spontaneous abortion following procedure than after amniocentesis. Reports of limb reduction defects in newborns. Rh immune globulin (RhoGAM) is given to the Rh-negative woman
Amniocentesis. Insertion of a thin needle through the abdominal and uterine walls to obtain a sample of amniotic fluid, which contains cast-off fetal cells and various other fetal products; standard genetic amniocentesis is done at 15 to 17 wk gestation; early genetic amniocentesis is done at 11 to 14 wk gestation for some disorders	Early pregnancy. Identify chromosome abnormalities, biochemical disorders (such as Tay-Sachs' disease), and level of alpha-fetoprotein. A fetus cannot be tested for every possible disorder. Spontaneous abortion following the procedure is the primary risk Late pregnancy. Identify severity of maternal–fetal blood incompatibility and assess fetal lung maturity. Rh immune globulin is given to the Rh-negative woman
Nonstress test (NST). Evaluation with an electronic fetal monitor of the fetal heart rate for accelerations of at least 15 beats/min lasting 15 sec in a 20-minute period. Fetal movements do not have to accompany the accelerations.	Identify fetal compromise in conditions associated with poor placenta function, such as hypertension, diabetes mellitus, or postterm gestation. Adequate accelerations of the fetal heart rate are reassuring that the placenta is functioning properly and the fetus is well oxygenated
Vibroacoustic stimulation test. Procedure similar to the NST; in addition, an artificial larynx device is used to stimulate the fetus with sound; expected response is acceleration of the fetal heart rate, as in the NST	Clarify, if the NST is questionable, whether the fetus is well oxygenated, thereby reducing the need for more complex testing Clarify, during labor, questionable fetal heart rate patterns

Table continued on following page

The nurse helps the woman to understand the importance of bed rest and find ways to manage it. Activity diverts blood from the placenta, reducing the baby's oxygen supply, so the nurse must impress upon the woman how important rest is to her baby's well-being. See preterm labor (p. 208) for more information about care related to bed rest.

Caring for the Acutely Ill Woman. The acutely ill woman requires intensive nursing care directed by an experienced registered nurse. A quiet, low-light environment reduces the risk of seizures. The woman should remain on bed rest on her side, often the left side, to promote maximum fetal oxygenation. Side rails should be padded and raised to prevent injury if a convulsion occurs. Stimulation such as loud noises or bumping of the bed should be avoided. Visitors are limited, usually to one or two support persons. An emergency tray (some-

Table 5–6
FETAL DIAGNOSTIC TESTS *(Continued)*

Tests and Description	Uses During Pregnancy
Contraction stress test (CST). Evaluation of the fetal heart rate response to mild uterine contractions by using an electronic fetal monitor; contractions may be induced by self-stimulation of the nipples, which causes the woman's pituitary gland to release oxytocin, or by intravenous oxytocin (Pitocin) infusion. The woman must have at least three contractions of at least 40 seconds duration in a 10-minute period for interpretation of the CST.	Purposes are the same as the NST; the CST may be done if the NST results are nonreasuring (the fetal heart does not accelerate) or if they are questionable
Biophysical profile (BPP). A group of five fetal assessments: fetal heart rate and reactivity (the NST), fetal breathing movements, fetal body movements, fetal tone (closure of the hand), and the volume of amniotic fluid (amniotic fluid index, or AFI). Some centers omit the NST, and others assess only the NST and AFI.	Identify reduced fetal oxygenation in conditions associated with poor placental function, but with greater precision than the NST alone. As fetal hypoxia gradually increases, fetal heart rate changes occur first, followed by cessation of fetal breathing movement, gross body movements, and finally loss of fetal tone Amniotic fluid volume is reduced when placental function is poor
Percutaneous umbilical blood sampling. Obtaining a fetal blood sample from a placental vessel or from the umbilical cord; may be used to give a blood transfusion to an anemic fetus	Identify fetal conditions that can be diagnosed only with a blood sample Blood transfusion for fetal anemia caused by maternal–fetal blood incompatibility, placenta previa, or abruptio placentae
Maternal assessment of fetal movement (kick counts). The mother counts the number of fetal movements in a period of 30 to 60 min three times a day. Other protocols may be used.	Identify, inexpensively and noninvasively, the fetus that may be having slight hypoxia or other compromise.
Tests of fetal lung maturity. Tests a sample of amniotic fluid (obtained by amniocentesis or from the pool of fluid in the vagina) to determine substances that indicate fetal lungs are mature enough to adapt to extrauterine life: Lecithin-to-sphingomyelin (L/S) ratio. A 2:1 ratio indicates fetal lung maturity (3:1 ratio desirable for diabetic mother); fluid usually obtained by amniocentesis Presence of phosphatidylglycerol (PG) Presence of phosphatidylinositol (PI) Foam stability index (FSI, or "shake test"). Persistence of a ring of bubbles for 15 min after shaking together equal amounts of 95% ethanol, isotonic saline, and amniotic fluid	Evaluate whether the fetus is likely to have respiratory complications in adapting to extrauterine life. May be done to determine whether the fetal lungs are mature before performing an elective cesarean birth or inducing labor if the gestational age is questionable. Also used to evaluate whether the fetus should be promptly delivered or allowed to mature further when the membranes rupture and the gestation is less than about 37 wk or if the gestation is questionable

times called a "toxemia tray") containing drugs and emergency equipment is placed in the room. Suction equipment is available for immediate use.

If a seizure occurs, the nursing focus is to prevent injury and restore oxygenation to the mother and fetus. If the patient is not already on her side, the nurse should try to turn her before the seizure begins, when facial twitching begins. The nurse does not forcibly hold the woman's body but prevents her from striking hard surfaces.

Breathing stops during a seizure. An oral airway, inserted *after* the seizure, facilitates breathing and suctioning of secretions. Aspiration of secretions can occur during a seizure, so the physician may order chest radiographs and arterial blood gases. Oxygen by face mask improves fetal oxygenation. The fetus is monitored continuously. The woman is reoriented to the environment when she regains consciousness. Labor may progress rapidly after a seizure, often while the woman is still drowsy (see p. 143 for signs of impending birth).

Administering Medications. Magnesium sulfate is administered by an experienced registered nurse. A practical nurse may assist. Hospital protocols provide specific guidelines for care when magnesium sulfate is given. Common protocols include the following:

- Blood pressure, pulse, respirations hourly; temperature every 4 hours
- Deep tendon reflexes every 1 to 4 hours
- Intake and output (often hourly); an indwelling catheter may be ordered
- Check urine protein with a reagent strip (dipstick) at each voiding
- Laboratory serum levels of magnesium every 4 hours

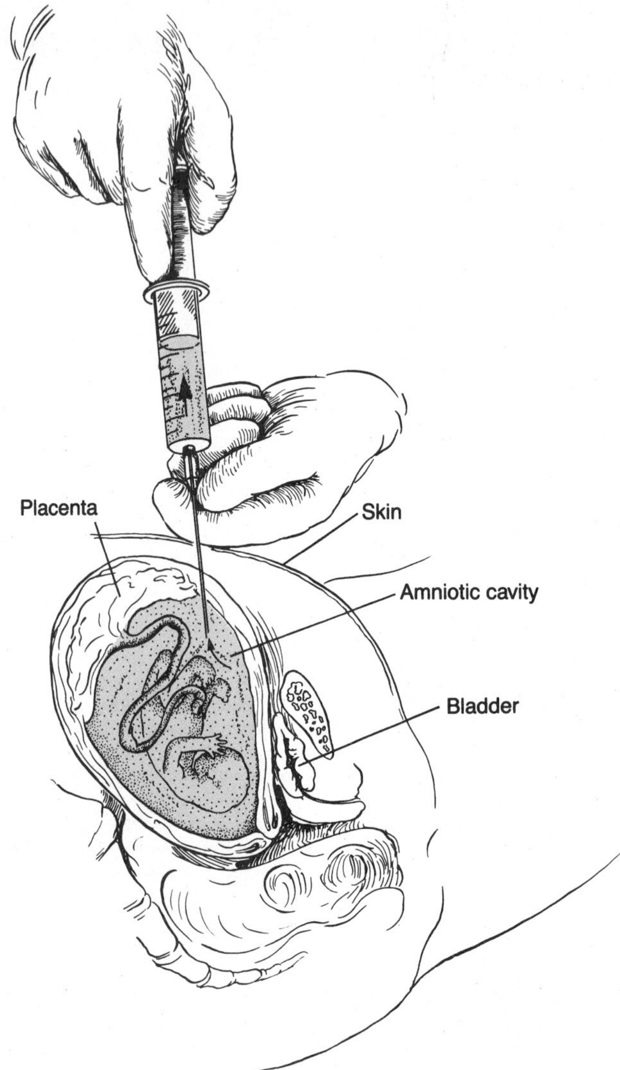

Figure 5–7. • Amniocentesis may be done to obtain a sample of amniotic fluid for a variety of studies, such as genetic studies and tests of fetal lung maturity.

Deterioration of the maternal or fetal condition is promptly reported:

- Increasing hypertension, particularly if blood pressure is 160/100 or higher
- Signs of central nervous system irritability, such as facial twitching or hyperactive deep tendon reflexes
- Decreased urine output, especially if less than 25 ml/hr
- Abnormal fetal heart rates
- Symptoms such as severe headache, visual disturbances, or epigastric pain, which often immediately precede a convulsion

The registered nurse reports signs of possible magnesium toxicity or factors that may cause magnesium toxicity to the physician and prepares calcium gluconate to reverse this toxicity:

- Absent deep tendon reflexes
- Respiration rate of under 12/min
- Urine output less than 25 ml/hr (allows accumulation of excess magnesium in the blood)
- Serum magnesium levels above 8 mg/dL

Assessment for signs and symptoms of PIH must continue for at least 48 hours after birth. Magnesium sulfate is often continued after birth and the nurse must continue to provide care related to this drug. The woman must be carefully observed for postpartum hemorrhage in addition to usual postpartum care.

Blood Incompatibility between the Pregnant Woman and the Fetus

The placenta allows maternal and fetal blood to be close enough to exchange oxygen and waste products without actually mixing (see p. 42). However, small leaks that allow fetal blood to enter the mother's circulation may occur during pregnancy. Larger amounts of fetal blood enter the mother's circulation when the placenta detaches at birth.

If maternal and fetal blood types are compatible, no problem occurs, just as intentional transfusion of compatible blood is not harmful. However, if the maternal and fetal blood types differ, the mother's body will produce antibodies to destroy foreign fetal red blood cells (RBCs, or erythrocytes). Two types of blood incompatibility during pregnancy will be discussed, Rh incompatibility and ABO incompatibility.

Rh Incompatibility

People either have the Rh blood factor on their erythrocytes or they do not. If they have the factor, they are Rh-positive; if not, they are Rh-negative.

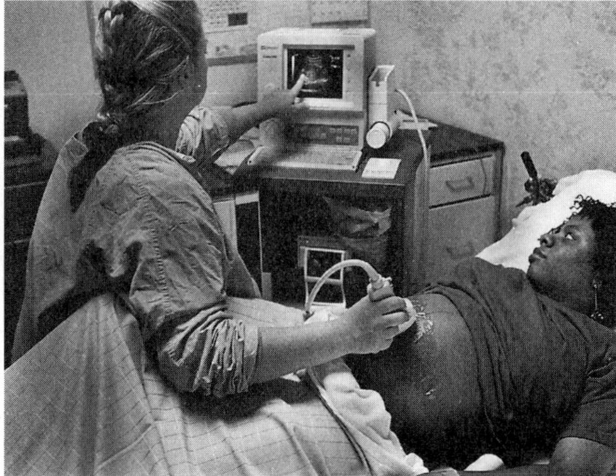

Figure 5–8. • The biophysical profile is done to evaluate the condition of the fetus in the woman who has a problem that may result in impaired placental blood flow.

An Rh-positive person can receive Rh-negative blood if all other factors are compatible because Rh-negative blood is the *absence* of this factor. However, the reverse is not true for the Rh-negative person. Rh incompatibility between the woman and fetus can occur only if the woman is Rh-negative and the fetus is Rh-positive.

The Rh-negative blood type is an autosomal recessive trait, which means that a person must receive a gene for this characteristic from both parents. The Rh-positive blood type is a dominant trait. The Rh-positive person may have inherited two Rh-positive genes or may have one Rh-positive and one Rh-negative gene. This explains why two Rh-positive parents can conceive a baby that is Rh-negative. About 15% of whites are Rh-negative. The incidence is lower in blacks and Asians.

A person with Rh-negative blood is not born with antibodies against the Rh factor and does not immediately react to foreign Rh-positive blood that enters the circulation. However, exposure to Rh-positive blood causes the person to make antibodies to destroy Rh-positive erythrocytes. The antibodies remain ready to destroy any future Rh-positive erythrocytes (sensitization) that enter the circulation.

If fetal Rh-positive blood leaks into the mother's circulation, her body may respond by making antibodies to destroy the Rh-positive erythrocytes. Because this leakage usually occurs at birth, the first Rh-positive baby is rarely affected. However, each time the woman is exposed to more Rh-positive blood (in subsequent pregnancies with Rh-positive fetuses), her body produces antibodies more rapidly. Antibodies against Rh-positive blood are small enough to cross the placenta and destroy the fetal Rh-positive erythrocytes before the baby is born.

Manifestations. The woman has no obvious effects if her body produces anti-Rh antibodies. Increased levels of these antibodies in her blood are revealed by rising antibody titers in laboratory tests.

When these maternal anti-Rh antibodies cross the placenta and destroy fetal erythrocytes, *erythroblastosis fetalis* results. The fetus becomes anemic from destruction of erythrocytes, and accumulated bilirubin from the broken cells causes jaundice that is obvious at birth. In severe cases, the fetus has heart failure and severe edema (hydrops fetalis). A sample of amniotic fluid shows high bilirubin levels. (See Chapter 14 for care of the infant with erythroblastosis fetalis.)

Treatment. The primary management is to prevent manufacture of anti-Rh antibodies by giving Rh immune globulin to the Rh-negative woman at 28 weeks of gestation and within 72 hours after

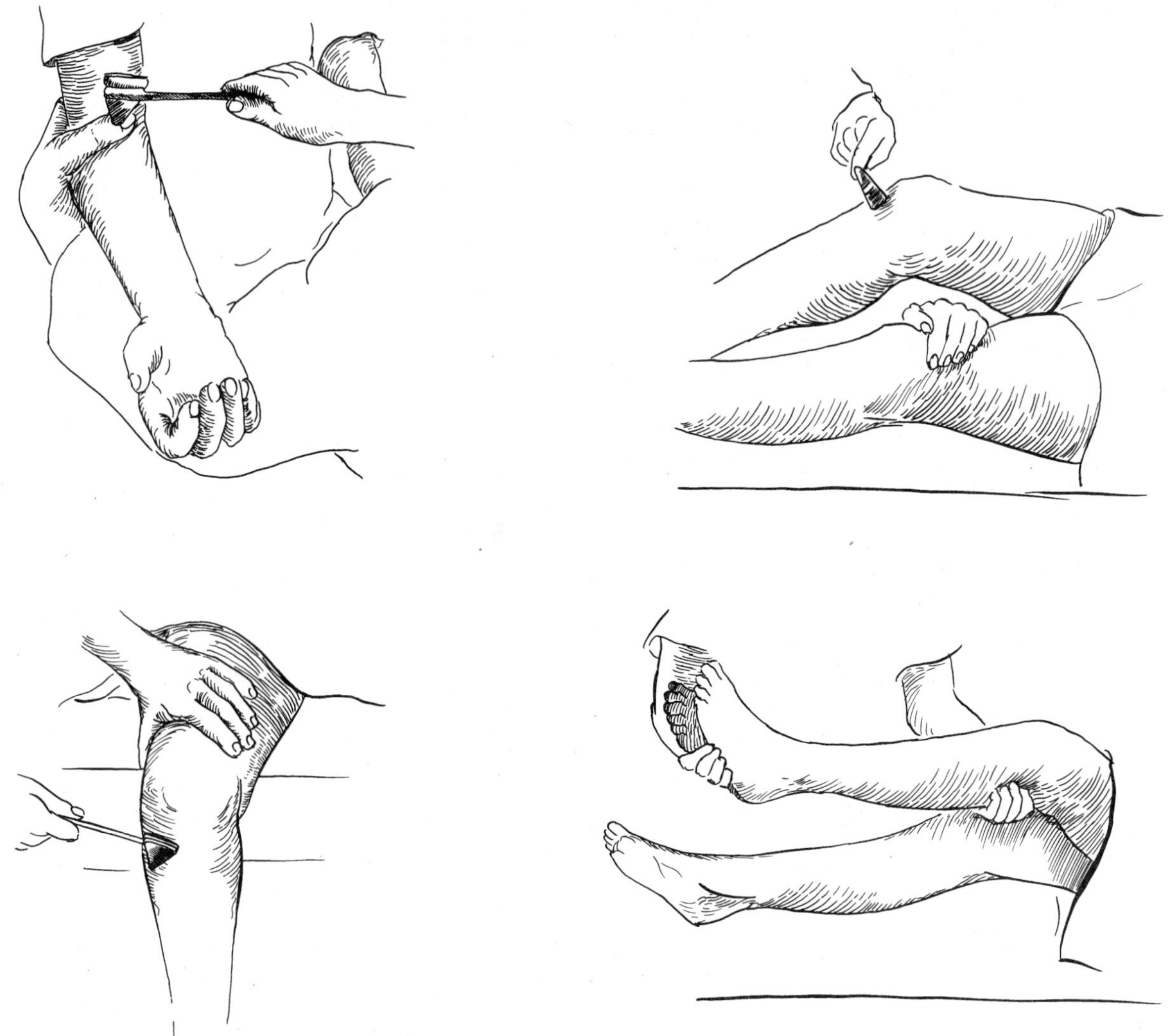

Figure 5–9. • Assessment of the deep tendon reflexes is essential to determine whether the woman is receiving too much or too little magnesium sulfate and to identify the woman likely to have a seizure.

birth of an Rh-positive infant or abortion (see p. 231). It is given after amniocentesis and to women who have bleeding during pregnancy because fetal blood may leak into the mother's circulation at these times. If the fetal blood type is unknown (as in abortion), Rh immune globulin is given. Rh immune globulin has greatly decreased the incidence of infants with Rh incompatibility problems. However, some women are still sensitized, usually because they did not receive Rh immune globulin after childbirth or abortion. Rh immune globulin will not be effective if sensitization has already occurred.

The woman who is sensitized to destroy Rh-positive blood cells is carefully monitored during pregnancy to determine whether too many fetal erythrocytes are being destroyed. Several diagnostic tests may be used, including the Coombs test, amniocentesis, or percutaneous umbilical blood sampling (see Table 5–6).

An intrauterine transfusion may be done for the severely anemic fetus. Group O-negative erythrocytes are injected into the fetal peritoneal cavity, where they are absorbed into the circulation or into one of the fetal umbilical vessels. O-negative blood is transfused because it is compatible with all blood types (universal donor).

The infant is jaundiced at birth because of high blood bilirubin levels. Phototherapy (see Chapter 14) reduces the infant's bilirubin level. In severe cases, exchange transfusion is done to replace the infant's blood with compatible blood that has no

NURSING CARE PLAN 5–2

Selected Nursing Diagnoses for the Woman with Pregnancy-Induced Hypertension

Nursing Diagnosis: Knowledge deficit: home care of mild pregnancy-induced hypertension (PIH)

Goals	Nursing Interventions	Rationale
The woman will restate correct home care measures related to PIH The woman will keep prescribed prenatal appointments	1. Ask woman what she knows about hypertension during pregnancy; include family members if present	1. Allows nurse to build on woman's existing knowledge, reinforcing it and correcting any misunderstandings
	2. Teach woman importance of keeping prenatal appointments, which will be more frequent because she has mild PIH	2. PIH can quickly become more severe between frequent prenatal care visits; many signs of worsening PIH can be detected only at prenatal visits or home visits, and some (such as edema) are considered normal by many women; if woman understands why she should keep appointments, she is more likely to do so
	3. Reinforce prescribed measures to care for herself at home:	3. If woman understands these measures to limit severity of PIH, she may be more motivated to maintain them:
	a. Remain on bed rest, spending most of the time on her side (may walk to the bathroom and eat meals at table in most cases)	a. Bed rest reduces flow of blood to skeletal muscles, thus making more available to placenta; this enhances fetal oxygenation
	b. Eat a well-balanced, high-protein diet; limit high-sodium foods, such as potato chips, salted nuts, pickles, and many snack foods; include high-fiber foods and at least eight glasses of noncaffeine drinks each day; consider food preferences and economic restraints when helping woman choose appropriate foods	b. Women with PIH lose protein in their urine, which must be replaced to maintain nutrition and fluid balance; severe sodium restriction may increase severity of PIH, but a high sodium intake may worsen hypertension and decrease the woman's blood volume; fiber and fluids help to reduce constipation, which is more likely when activity is restricted
	c. Discuss quiet activities the woman enjoys that can be done while she is on bed rest	c. Bed rest can lead to boredom, and the woman may not maintain the prescribed activity if she is bored
	4. Teach woman to report signs that indicate worsening PIH promptly: headache; visual disturbances (blurring, flashes of light, "spots" before the eyes); gastrointestinal symptoms (nausea, pain); worsening edema, especially of the face and fingers; noticeable drop in urine output	4. PIH can worsen despite careful home management and client compliance; if the woman has these symptoms, she needs to be evaluated and hospitalized to prevent progression to eclampsia

Continued on following page

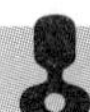

Nursing Tip

Most cases of Rh incompatibility between an Rh-negative mother and an Rh-positive fetus can be prevented with administration of Rh immune globulin (RhoGAM) every time it is indicated.

anti-Rh antibodies and that has a normal bilirubin level.

ABO Incompatibility

ABO incompatibility can occur if the woman has group O blood and the fetus has group A, group B, or group AB blood. Unlike anti-Rh antibodies, anti-A and anti-B antibodies are usually already

NURSING CARE PLAN 5–2 *continued*

Selected Nursing Diagnoses for the Woman with Pregnancy-Induced Hypertension

Nursing Diagnosis: Altered tissue perfusion (maternal vital organs and placenta) related to constriction of small blood vessels

Goals	Nursing Interventions	Rationale
The woman will not have a seizure Rate and pattern of the fetal heart will remain reassuring	1. Assist with fetal heart rate monitoring according to facility's protocol (see p. 145 for more information about fetal heart rate assessments)	1. Generalized vasoconstriction in PIH reduces blood flow to the placenta, thus compromising fetal oxygenation; fetal heart rate patterns may reflect reduced placental blood flow
	2. Keep room quiet and lights dimmed; limit number of personnel and visitors who enter room; side rails should be pulled up and the woman should maintain strict bed rest on her left side; maintain continuous nursing observation	2. Environmental stimulants may precipitate a seizure; if a woman has severe preeclampsia, she could unexpectedly have a seizure, and the nurse must intervene to minimize injury
	3. Keep an emergency tray in her room (sometimes called a "PIH tray" or a "toxemia tray")	3. Contains emergency drugs and equipment that may be needed quickly; equipment often includes airways, Ambu bag, and suction and oxygen equipment; drugs usually include magnesium sulfate, calcium gluconate (to reverse the effects of magnesium sulfate), and hydralazine (for severe hypertension)
	4. Assist the experienced registered nurse with magnesium sulfate administration according to facility protocol; typical care includes a. Deep tendon reflexes (DTRs) b. Maternal blood pressure, pulse, and respirations; report respiration rate of under 12/min c. Urine output; report output of less than 25 ml/hr d. Urine dipstick for ketones e. Monitor serum magnesium levels according to protocol	4. Magnesium sulfate is a central nervous system depressant given to prevent convulsions; inadequate magnesium may not prevent seizures, whereas excess drug levels may cause respiratory depression or cardiopulmonary collapse
	5. Observe for signs that may indicate an imminent seizure; twitching of facial muscles, hyperactive DTRs, epigastric or right upper abdominal quadrant pain, nausea or vomiting; try to prevent injury if woman has a seizure, but do not forcibly restrain her; after seizure, an airway is inserted to facilitate suctioning and oxygen administration; after she awakens following the seizure, reorient her to surroundings	5. Early intervention can reduce maternal injuries if a seizure occurs; forcible restraint may cause greater injury; the woman is likely to be confused and possibly combative after a seizure; continuous oxygenation restores oxygen delivery to the fetus

present in the woman's body. However, fewer of these antibodies cross the placenta than those associated with Rh problems. The fetus does not usually have severe problems. Unlike what occurs with Rh incompatibility, an infant is often affected during the first pregnancy.

The infant may develop jaundice within the first 24 hours, and bilirubin levels may rise rapidly. Phototherapy is usually sufficient to reduce the bilirubin level in ABO incompatibility.

Nursing Care for Pregnancy-Related Blood Incompatibilities

Giving Rh immune globulin every time it is indicated prevents nearly all cases of Rh incompatibility. The chart should be checked for a woman's Rh factor to see if Rh immune globulin is indicated after:

- Birth
- Abortion (spontaneous or induced)
- Episodes of bleeding
- Amniocentesis

The physician or nurse-midwife should be notified if the Rh factor is not documented or if there is no order for Rh immune globulin for an Rh-negative woman when the drug is indicated.

Care of the infant involves observing for jaundice, especially during the first 24 hours of life. Early jaundice or rapidly increasing jaundice is reported to the physician so that serum bilirubin levels can be obtained. (See Chapters 13 and 14 for discussion of nursing care related to neonatal jaundice and phototherapy.)

PREGNANCY COMPLICATED BY MEDICAL CONDITIONS

Medical conditions may require special management during pregnancy. Many become harder to diagnose or control. Others have more adverse effects for the woman or fetus than at other times. Four types of disorders are discussed in this section: (1) diabetes mellitus, (2) heart disease, (3) anemia, and (4) infections.

Diabetes Mellitus

A woman may have either of two types of diabetes mellitus:

- Preexisting diabetes mellitus, which includes insulin-dependent (type I) and non-insulin-dependent (type II) diabetes
- Gestational diabetes mellitus (GDM), which occurs only during pregnancy

Of all pregnant diabetic women, 90% have gestational diabetes mellitus. See a medical-surgical nursing text for a more detailed discussion of diabetes in the nonpregnant person.

Pathophysiology of Diabetes Mellitus

Diabetes mellitus is a disorder in which there is inadequate insulin to move glucose from the blood into body cells. It occurs because the pancreas produces no insulin or insufficient insulin or because cells resist the effects of insulin.

In the woman with diabetes, cells are essentially starving because they cannot use glucose. To compensate, the body metabolizes protein and fat for energy, which causes ketones and acids to accumulate (ketoacidosis). The person loses weight despite eating large amounts of food (polyphagia). Fatigue and lethargy accompany cell starvation. To dilute excess glucose in the blood, thirst increases (polydipsia) and fluid moves from the tissues into the blood. This results in tissue dehydration and excretion of large amounts (polyuria) of glucose-bearing urine (glycosuria).

Effect of Pregnancy on Glucose Metabolism

Pregnancy affects a woman's metabolism, whether or not she has diabetes, to make ample glucose available to the growing fetus. Hormones (estrogen and progesterone) and an enzyme (insulinase) produced by the placenta have two effects:

- Increased resistance of cells to insulin
- Increased speed of insulin breakdown

Most women respond to these changes by secreting extra insulin to maintain normal carbohydrate metabolism while still providing plenty of glucose for the fetus. If the woman cannot increase her insulin production, she will have periods of hyperglycemia as glucose accumulates in the blood.

Women who are diabetic before pregnancy must alter the management of their condition. In the past, the fetuses of women with diabetes often had poor outcomes, such as abnormal fetal growth, stillbirth, and congenital abnormalities. Today, with careful management, most diabetic women can have successful pregnancies and healthy babies. Nevertheless, there are many potential complications of diabetes (Box 5–4).

Gestational Diabetes Mellitus

GDM is common and resolves quickly after birth. Affected women do not have all the classic signs and symptoms of diabetes. They are not usually affected by blood vessel and nerve damage, as are people who have diabetes independent of pregnancy. However, they are more likely to develop overt diabetes within the next 15 years.

Several factors in a woman's history are linked to gestational diabetes:

- Maternal obesity (>90 kg or 198 pounds)
- Large infant, over 4000 g or about 9 pounds (Fig. 5–10)

BOX 5–4
EFFECTS OF DIABETES IN PREGNANCY

Maternal Effects
Spontaneous abortion
Pregnancy-induced hypertension
Preterm labor and premature rupture of the membranes
Hydramnios (excessive amniotic fluid; also called polyhydramnios)
Infections
- Vaginitis
- Urinary tract infections

Complications of large fetal size
- Birth canal injuries
- Forcep-assisted or Cesarean birth

Ketoacidosis

Fetal and Neonatal Effects
Perinatal death
Congenital abnormalities
Macrosomia (large size) or intrauterine growth restriction
Birth injury
Delayed lung maturation
Neonatal hypoglycemia
Neonatal hypocalcemia
Neonatal hyperbilirubinemia and jaundice
Neonatal polycythemia (excess erythrocytes)

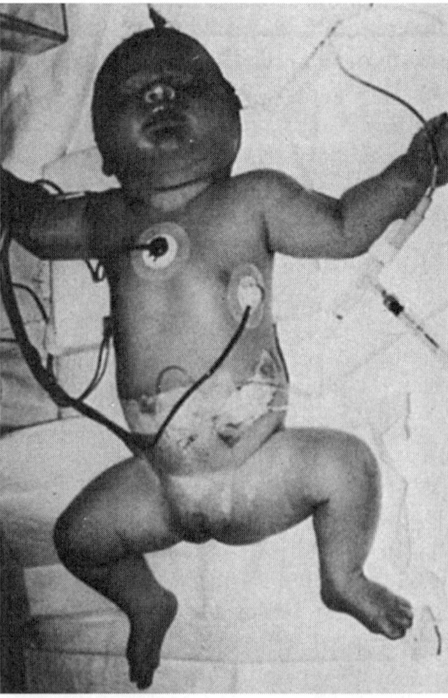

Figure 5–10. • Newborn with macrosomia due to maternal diabetes mellitus during pregnancy. Despite the large size, the infant of a diabetic mother is likely to have problems similar to those of a preterm infant. (From La Franchi, S. [1987]. Hypoglycemia of infancy and childhood. *Pediatric Clinics of North America, 34,* 969.)

- Chronic hypertension
- Maternal age older than 25 years
- Previous unexplained stillbirth or infant having congenital abnormalities
- History of gestational diabetes in a previous pregnancy
- Family history of diabetes

Nursing Care Plan 5–3 lists specific interventions for the pregnant woman with GDM.

Treatment

The nonpregnant person is treated with a balance of insulin or an oral hypoglycemic drug (agent that reduces blood sugar), diet, and exercise. Some people with mild diabetes do not need drugs and control their condition by diet alone. Medical therapy during pregnancy includes identification of gestational diabetes, diet, monitoring of blood glucose levels, insulin, exercise, and selected fetal assessments.

Identification of Gestational Diabetes Mellitus. If the woman does not have preexisting diabetes, a prenatal screening test to identify GDM is done between 24 and 28 weeks of gestation. The woman drinks 50 g of an oral glucose solution (fasting is not necessary). One hour later, a blood sample is analyzed for glucose. If the blood glucose level is 140 mg/dl or higher, a more complex 3-hour glucose tolerance test is done.

Diet. The diet is similar to that for any pregnant woman. Carbohydrate, protein, and fat are balanced to provide for growth and energy needs and to provide adequate calories, vitamins, and miner-

NURSING CARE PLAN 5-3

Selected Nursing Diagnoses for the Pregnant Woman with Gestational Diabetes Mellitus

Nursing Diagnosis: Risk for ineffective management of therapeutic regimen related to lack of knowledge about new diagnosis

Goals	Nursing Interventions	Rationale
The woman identifies appropriate and inappropriate food choices The woman demonstrates correct self-care techniques for assessing blood glucose and administering insulin The woman verbalizes symptoms of hypoglycemia and hyperglycemia, including correct self-care	1. Assess knowledge of diabetes and its management, including family members if appropriate	1. Allows nurse to identify correct and incorrect information and relate new knowledge to what woman already knows, thus promoting individualized teaching
	2. Assist registered nurse to teach prescribed diet; provide written information; have woman identify appropriate foods and the best time to eat them; general guidelines are: a. Avoid simple sugars, such as cakes, candies, and ice creams because they are quickly converted to glucose, causing wide fluctuations in the blood glucose levels b. Eat complex, high-fiber carbohydrates, such as grains, breads, and pasta, because these foods are converted to glucose slowly, thus maintaining stable blood glucose levels c. Eat three meals a day plus at least two snacks to balance insulin and provide sustained release of glucose to prevent hypoglycemia during late afternoon and evening	2. A woman who understands diet requirements is more likely to follow them carefully; written information helps to refresh her memory if she forgets verbal teaching; verbalizing food choices allows the nurse to determine if she has correctly learned the information
	3. Refer woman to a dietitian if she has difficulty accepting or tolerating foods permitted on her diet	3. A dietitian specializes in foods and nutrition and can help the woman to select foods that are acceptable within her dietary limits and that meet her preferences and cultural needs
	4. Assist registered nurse to teach how to perform blood glucose monitoring; have her perform a return demonstration and/or verbalize the regimen; common teaching includes testing frequency, accurate technique, and responses to low or high levels	4. Insulin requirements fluctuate during pregnancy, generally increasing as pregnancy progresses; frequent blood glucose monitoring allows adjustment of insulin, thus maintaining stable blood glucose levels; stable blood glucose levels are associated with better outcomes for mother and baby; return demonstration of skills or verbalizing information helps the nurse determine if the woman has learned information
	5. Assist registered nurse to teach insulin self-administration (see Chapter 30 for additional information); have woman give a return demonstration and/or verbalization of each step; teaching includes when to take insulin and how to administer it	5. Correct insulin administration maintains the most stable blood glucose levels; see #4 for rationale for return demonstration and verbalization

Continued on following page

NURSING CARE PLAN 5–3 *continued*

Selected Nursing Diagnoses for the Pregnant Woman with Gestational Diabetes Mellitus

Nursing Diagnosis: Risk for ineffective management of therapeutic regimen related to lack of knowledge about new diagnosis

Goals	Nursing Interventions	Rationale
	6. Teach signs and symptoms of hypoglycemia and hyperglycemia (see Table 5–7); teach appropriate responses to these signs and symptoms	6. Persistence of low or high blood glucose levels requires adjustment of insulin dose and/or food intake; additionally, hyperglycemia may be an early sign of infection in the diabetic woman; a woman who understands signs, symptoms, and corrective actions is likely to seek care needed to maintain optimal blood glucose levels
	7. Explain that gestational diabetes usually resolves quickly after birth but that it may recur in future pregnancies or in mid-life	7. Short-term nature of gestational diabetes makes its management easier to tolerate; advance information about possible future diabetes improves ongoing health monitoring

Nursing Diagnosis: Knowledge deficit: complications of diabetes during pregnancy

Goals	Nursing Interventions	Rationale
The woman verbalizes correct responses to potential complications of gestational diabetes	1. Teach danger signs in pregnancy (Box 5–1) and reinforce them at each prenatal visit	1. Increases likelihood that woman will seek prompt treatment for all pregnancy complications, including those relating to diabetes
	2. Teach signs and symptoms of urinary tract infection and vaginal infection, especially candidiasis or yeast infection (see p. 116)	2. Candidiasis is common in women with diabetes mellitus; urinary tract infections are common and also can lead to maternal sepsis or preterm labor
	3. Teach woman to report signs of onset or worsening pregnancy-induced hypertension (PIH): severe headache, vision disturbances, abdominal pain; explain importance of keeping prenatal care appointments	3. PIH is more likely to occur in the diabetic pregnant woman; regular prenatal visits at prescribed intervals can prevent or allow early intervention for complications, including PIH
	4. Teach about fetal diagnostic tests done; for example, biophysical profile evaluates how well placenta is delivering oxygen and nutrients to baby	4. Fetal diagnostic tests allow for early identification and prompt intervention for problems; knowledge decreases woman's anxiety related to the unknown; if woman does not understand reason for doing diagnostic tests, she may incorrectly assume that she or her baby is in danger

als. Food intake is divided among three meals and at least two snacks throughout the day to maintain stable blood glucose levels. The timing and content of meals and snacks may require adjustment to avoid early-morning hypoglycemia.

Monitoring of Blood Glucose Levels. To ensure a successful pregnancy, the woman must keep her blood glucose levels as close to normal as possible. For self-monitored glucose, these levels are:

- Fasting: 60–90
- Premeal: 60–105
- 1 hour post-meal: 100–120

The pregnant diabetic woman monitors her blood glucose levels several times a day. Blood glucose self-monitoring is discussed in Chapter 30.

Ketone Monitoring. Urine ketones may be checked to identify the need for more carbohydrate. If the woman's carbohydrate intake is insufficient, she may metabolize fat and protein to produce glucose, resulting in ketonuria. However, ketonuria that is accompanied by hyperglycemia requires prompt evaluation for diabetic ketoacidosis. Ketoacidosis can be rapidly fatal to the fetus. It is more likely to occur in the woman with preexisting diabetes and if she has an infection.

Insulin. Oral hypoglycemics are not used during pregnancy because they can cross the placenta, possibly resulting in fetal birth defects or neonatal hypoglycemia. Insulin is the only drug prescribed to lower blood glucose during pregnancy because it does not cross the placenta. GDM may be controlled by diet and exercise alone, or the woman may require insulin injections. The dose and frequency of insulin injections are tailored to a woman's individual needs. Insulin is often given on a sliding scale, in which the woman varies her dose of insulin based on each blood glucose level.

The woman with preexisting diabetes may need less insulin during early pregnancy because nausea and vomiting reduce her food intake. Insulin needs increase steadily after the 1st trimester in either preexisting diabetes or GDM. After birth, the patient's insulin requirements fall dramatically, usually below prepregnancy needs. GDM resolves promptly after birth, when the insulin-antagonistic (diabetogenic) effects of pregnancy cease.

A combination of short-acting and intermediate-acting insulin is usually prescribed to keep glucose levels stable and near normal throughout the day. Most women with preexisting diabetes need three injections per day to achieve good glucose control. One to two insulin injections daily are typical if a woman with GDM needs insulin. An insulin pump provides a constant level of insulin plus doses at mealtimes to maintain steady blood glucose levels. (See Chapter 30 for discussion of insulin administration and insulin pumps.)

Exercise. Mild exercise, such as walking, is encouraged during pregnancy because it decreases insulin requirements and improves the body's use of glucose. Women who have additional complications may have to stop exercising and stay on bed rest. If so, their insulin requirements may increase. When they resume activity after a period of bed rest, their insulin needs fall and they may have episodes of hypoglycemia.

Fetal Assessments. Assessments (see Table 5–6) may be done to identify fetal growth and the placenta's ability to provide oxygen and nutrients. Ultrasound examinations identify intrauterine growth restriction, macrosomia, and the amount of amniotic fluid that may be excessive in the poorly controlled diabetic woman. However, if placental blood supply is decreased, amniotic fluid may be below normal (oligohydramnios).

Diabetes can affect the blood vessels that supply the placenta, impairing transport of oxygen and nutrients to the fetus and removal of fetal wastes. The nonstress test, contraction stress test, and biophysical profile provide information about how the placenta is functioning. Tests of fetal lung maturity are common if early delivery is considered.

Care during Labor. Labor is work (exercise) that affects the amount of insulin and glucose needed. Some women receive an intravenous infusion of a dextrose solution plus regular insulin as needed. Regular insulin is the *only* type given intravenously. Blood glucose levels are assessed hourly and the insulin dose is adjusted accordingly. The fetus is monitored as in any high-risk pregnancy.

Care of the Neonate. Infant complications after birth may include hypoglycemia, respiratory distress, and injury due to macrosomia. Some infants have growth restriction because the placenta functions poorly. Neonatal nurses and a neonatologist (a physician specializing in care of newborns) are often present at the birth. (See Chapter 14 for discussion of these neonatal problems.)

Nursing Care

Nursing care of the pregnant woman with diabetes mellitus involves helping her to learn to care for herself and providing emotional care to meet the demands imposed by this complication. Care during labor primarily involves careful monitoring for signs that the fetus is not tolerating the stress of labor.

Self-Care. Most women with preexisting diabetes already know how to check their blood sugar and administer insulin. They should be taught why diabetic management changes during pregnancy. The woman with GDM must be taught these self-care skills.

The woman is taught how to select appropriate foods for the prescribed diet. She is more likely to maintain the diet if her caregivers are sensitive to her food preferences and cultural needs. A dietitian can determine foods to meet her needs and find solutions to problems in adhering to the diet.

The woman who takes insulin may experience episodes of hypoglycemia (low blood sugar) or hyperglycemia (high blood sugar). These two conditions are summarized in Table 5–7. The woman is taught to recognize and respond to each condition. A family member is included in teaching, because the woman's thinking and responses may be altered (e.g., confused, combative, lethargic) in either hypoglycemia or hyperglycemia.

Emotional Support. Pregnant women with diabetes often find that living with the close management, diet control, and frequent insulin administration is trying. The expectant mother may be anxious about the outcome for herself and her baby. Therapeutic communication helps her to express her frustrations and fears. For example, to elicit her feelings about her condition the nurse might say, "Many women find that all the changes they have to make are demanding. How has it been for

Table 5–7
COMPARISON OF HYPOGLYCEMIA AND HYPERGLYCEMIA IN THE DIABETIC WOMAN

Hypoglycemia	Hyperglycemia
Caused by excess insulin, excess exercise, and/or inadequate food intake	Caused by inadequate insulin, reduced activity, and/or excessive food intake; more likely if the woman has an infection because this increases her need for insulin
Blood glucose level low (usually under 60 mg/dl)	Blood glucose above normal (greater than 120 mg/dl)
Urine glucose absent	Glucosuria (glucose in the urine); possibly ketonuria (ketones in the urine)
Behavioral and physiologic manifestations: hunger, trembling; weakness; faintness; lethargy; headache; irritability; sweating; pale, cool, moist skin; blurred vision; loss of consciousness	Behavioral and physiologic manifestations: fatigue; headache; flushed, hot skin; dry mouth; thirst; dehydration; frequent urination; weight loss; nausea and vomiting; rapid, deep respirations (Kussmaul's respirations); acetone odor to the breath; depressed reflexes
Measures to correct: drink a glass of milk or juice; eat a piece of fruit or two crackers; recurrent hypoglycemia requires adjustment of insulin or food intake	Measures to correct: evaluate food intake; emphasize that client be honest if she "cheats" to avoid inappropriate adjustment of insulin dose; identify and treat infections; insulin dose often adjusted throughout pregnancy to maintain normal glucose levels

you?" It may help to emphasize that the close management is usually temporary, especially if she has GDM.

As she learns to manage her care, liberal praise motivates the woman to maintain her therapy. The nurse should reinforce when her baby is doing well so she can see the positive effects her efforts are having. She can be encouraged to find alternative exercise or foods to meet her prescribed therapy. Referral to a diabetes management center is often helpful. A woman who is actively involved in her care is more likely to maintain the prescribed therapy.

Heart Disease

Heart disease affects a small percentage of pregnant women. Most heart disease during pregnancy is a result of rheumatic fever or congenital heart defects. Mitral valve prolapse is a common condition in which the leaflets of the mitral valve bulge into the left atrium when the ventricles contract.

Manifestations. If its existence is not known, heart disease is difficult to diagnose during pregnancy, because normal changes mimic cardiac problems. For example, palpitations and heart murmurs are common in uncomplicated pregnancy but may also occur with heart disease.

A woman with heart disease may not tolerate the demands of pregnancy well. Her blood volume and cardiac output increase to supply the placenta and enlarged maternal organs, but these changes impose a greater burden on her impaired heart. Increased levels of clotting factors predispose her to thrombosis (formation of clots in the veins). If her heart cannot meet these demands, congestive heart failure (CHF) results. The fetus suffers from reduced placental blood flow if the mother's heart fails. See Box 5–5 for signs and symptoms of CHF.

During labor, each contraction temporarily shifts 300 to 500 ml of blood from the uterus and placenta into the woman's circulation, possibly overloading her weakened heart. Excess interstitial fluid rapidly returns to the circulation after birth, predisposing the woman to circulatory overload during the postpartum period. She remains at increased risk for CHF after birth until her circulating blood volume returns to normal levels.

Treatment. The pregnant woman with heart disease will usually be under the care of a cardiologist as well as an obstetrician. She needs more frequent antepartum visits to determine how her heart is coping with its increased demands. Excessive weight gain must be avoided because it adds to the

BOX 5–5

SIGNS OF CONGESTIVE HEART FAILURE DURING PREGNANCY

- Persistent cough, often with expectoration of mucus that may be blood-tinged
- Moist lung sounds due to fluid within lungs
- Fatigue or fainting on exertion
- Difficulty breathing on exertion
- Orthopnea (having to sit upright to breathe more easily)
- Severe pitting edema of the lower extremities or generalized edema
- Palpitations
- Fetus: hypoxia or growth restriction if placental blood flow is reduced

Nursing Tip

The nurse should observe the woman with heart disease for signs of congestive heart failure, which can occur before, during, or after birth.

demands on her heart. Sodium is limited to prevent pulmonary edema. Preventing anemia with adequate diet and supplemental iron prevents a compensatory rise in the heart rate, which would add to the strain on the woman's heart. Frequent rest periods decrease the heart's workload. However, a woman on prolonged bed rest for any reason has a greater risk for forming venous thrombi (blood clots).

Drug therapy may include heparin to prevent clot formation. Anticoagulants such as warfarin (Coumadin) may cause birth defects and are not given during pregnancy. Heparin is given if an anticoagulant is needed. Other drugs may include antiarrhythmics to control abnormal heart rhythms. Antibiotics are usually given during the intrapartum period to prevent infection of the heart (bacterial endocarditis) due to organisms that enter the blood during birth. Diuretics such as furosemide (Lasix) may be needed if CHF occurs.

Vaginal birth is preferred over cesarean delivery, because it carries less risk for infection or respiratory complications that would further tax the impaired heart. Forceps or a vacuum extractor may be used to decrease the need for maternal pushing (see Chapter 8).

Nursing Care. A woman with heart disease may be familiar with its management. She should be taught needed changes, such as the change from warfarin anticoagulants to heparin. She is taught to inject the drug and told when to have laboratory studies as ordered. These tests include partial thromboplastin time (PTT), activated partial thromboplastin time (aPTT), and platelets. She should promptly report signs of excess anticoagulation, such as bruising without reason, petechiae (tiny red spots on the skin), nosebleeds, or bleeding from the gums when brushing her teeth.

The woman is taught signs that may indicate CHF, so that she can promptly report them. The nurse helps her to identify how she can obtain rest to minimize the demands on her heart. She should avoid exercise in temperature extremes. She should be taught to stop an activity if she has dyspnea, chest pain, or tachycardia.

The woman may need help to plan her diet, so that she has enough calories to meet her needs during pregnancy but without gaining too much weight. She should be taught about foods that are high in iron and folic acid, such as dark-green vegetables, to prevent anemia. She should avoid foods high in sodium, such as smoked meats, potato chips, and many snack foods.

Stress can also increase demands on the heart. The nurse should discuss stressors in the woman's life and help her to identify ways to reduce them.

Anemia

Anemia is a reduced ability of the blood to carry oxygen to the cells. Hemoglobin levels lower than 10.5 to 11 g/dl indicate anemia during pregnancy (Cunningham et al., 1997; Laros, 1994). Four anemias are significant during pregnancy: two nutritional anemias (iron-deficiency anemia and folic acid–deficiency anemia), and two anemias resulting from genetic disorders, sickle cell disease and thalassemia.

Nutritional Anemias

Most women with anemia have vague symptoms, if any. The anemic woman may fatigue easily and have little energy. Her skin and mucous membranes are pale. Shortness of breath, a pounding heart, and a rapid pulse may occur with severe anemia. The woman who develops anemia gradually has fewer symptoms than the woman who becomes anemic abruptly, such as through blood loss.

Iron-Deficiency Anemia. The pregnant woman needs additional iron for her own increased blood volume, for transfer to the fetus, and for a cushion against the blood loss expected at birth. The red blood cells are small (microcytic) and pale (hypochromic) in iron-deficiency anemia.

Prevention. Iron supplements (30 mg/day) are commonly used to meet the needs of pregnancy and maintain iron stores. Vitamin C may enhance absorption of iron. Iron should not be taken with milk or antacids because calcium impairs absorption.

Treatment. The woman with iron-deficiency anemia needs extra iron to correct the anemia and replenish her stores. She is treated with 200 mg/day of *elemental iron* and continues this dose for about 3 months after the anemia has been corrected.

Folic Acid–Deficiency Anemia. Folic acid (also called folate or folacin) deficiency is characterized by large, immature red blood cells (megaloblastic anemia). Iron-deficiency anemia is often present at the same time. The woman sometimes complains of a sore tongue.

Prevention. Folic acid is essential for normal growth and development of the fetus. Folic acid deficiency has been associated with neural tube defects in the newborn. A supplement of 400 μg (0.4 mg)/day ensures adequate folic acid and is now recommended for all fertile women.

Treatment. Treatment of folate deficiency is with folic acid supplementation, 1 mg/day, over twice the amount of the preventive supplement. The dose of preventive folic acid supplementation may be higher for women who have had a previous child with a neural tube defect. Women with sickle cell disease or thalassemia may need higher doses.

Sickle Cell Disease

Unlike with nutritional anemias, people with sickle cell disease have abnormal hemoglobin that causes their erythrocytes to become distorted in a sickle (crescent) shape during hypoxia or acidosis. The genetic defect is autosomal recessive, meaning that the person receives an abnormal gene from each parent. The abnormally shaped blood cells do not flow smoothly, and they clog small blood vessels. The sickle cells are destroyed faster, resulting in chronic anemia. It is more common in those of African or Mediterranean descent. (See Chapter 26 for further discussion of sickle cell disease.)

Pregnancy may cause a sickle cell crisis with massive erythrocyte destruction and occlusion of blood vessels. Pregnant women with sickle cell disease are more likely to have infections, heart disease, and PIH. The main risk to the fetus is occlusion of vessels that supply the placenta, leading to preterm birth, growth retardation, and fetal death.

The woman will have frequent evaluation and treatment for anemia during prenatal care. Fetal evaluations concentrate on fetal growth and placental function. Oxygen and fluids are given continuously during labor to prevent sickle cell crisis.

Thalassemia

Thalassemia is a genetic trait that causes an abnormality in one of two chains of hemoglobin, the alpha (α) or beta (β) chain. The beta chain is most often encountered in the United States. The person can inherit an abnormal gene from each parent, causing β-thalassemia major, or Cooley's anemia. They usually die in childhood. If only one abnormal gene is inherited, the person will have β-thalassemia minor.

The woman with thalassemia minor usually has few problems other than mild anemia, and the fetus does not appear to be affected. However, administration of iron supplements may cause iron overload in a woman with β-thalassemia minor because the body absorbs and stores iron in higher than usual amounts. Infections can reduce erythrocyte production and accelerate destruction, so should be avoided or treated promptly.

Nursing Care for Anemia during Pregnancy

The woman is taught which foods are high in iron and folic acid (Box 5–6) to prevent or treat anemia. She is taught how to take the supplements so that they are optimally effective. For example, the nurse explains that although milk is good to drink during pregnancy, it should not be taken at the same time as the iron supplement or the iron will not be absorbed as easily. Vitamin C foods may enhance absorption.

The woman is taught that when she takes iron, her stools will be dark-green to black and that mild gastrointestinal discomfort may occur. She should contact her physician or nurse-midwife if these side effects trouble her; another iron preparation may be better tolerated. She should not take antacids with iron.

The woman with sickle cell disease requires close medical and nursing care. She should be taught to seek care for infections promptly, as they may lead to a sickle cell crisis. She is taught about iron and other supplements that are part of her therapy. The woman with β-thalassemia minor is taught to avoid situations where infections are more likely (for example, avoid crowds during flu season) and to report any symptoms of infection promptly.

BOX 5–6

FOODS THAT PREVENT ANEMIAS IN PREGNANCY

Foods High in Iron
Meats, chicken, fish, liver, legumes, green leafy vegetables, whole or enriched grain products, nuts, blackstrap molasses, tofu, eggs, dried fruits, foods cooked in cast-iron pans

Foods High in Folic Acid
Green leafy vegetables, asparagus, green beans, fruits, whole grains, liver, legumes, yeast

Foods High in Vitamin C (may enhance absorption of iron)
Citrus fruits and juices, strawberries, cantaloupe, cabbage, green and red peppers, tomatoes, potatoes, green leafy vegetables

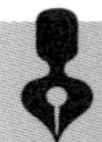

Nursing Tip

To prevent or correct nutritional anemias, such as iron and folic acid deficiencies, the nurse should teach all women good food sources of those nutrients.

Infections

The acronym TORCH has been used to describe infections that can be devastating for the fetus or newborn. The letters stand for the first letters of these four infections and infectious agents: *t*oxoplasmosis, *r*ubella, *c*ytomegalovirus, and *h*erpes simplex virus; the *o* is sometimes used to designate "other" infections. However, there are many more infections that may be devastating for the mother, fetus, or newborn. Some of these are damaging any time they are acquired, while others are relatively harmless except when acquired during pregnancy. Infections that will be covered in this section include the following:

- Viral infections
- Nonviral infections
- Sexually transmissible diseases
- Vaginal infections
- Urinary tract infections

Viral Infections

Viral infections often have no effective therapy and may cause serious problems in the mother and/or fetus or newborn. However, immunizations can prevent some of these infections. Many are sexually transmissible diseases, although they have other routes of transmission.

Cytomegalovirus. Cytomegalovirus, or CMV, is a widespread infection that commonly occurs during the childbearing years. The infection is often asymptomatic in the mother. An infected infant may be asymptomatic or may have serious problems or die:

- Petechiae (often called a "blueberry muffin" rash)
- Deafness
- Blindness
- Mental retardation
- Seizures
- Dental abnormalities

Treatment and Nursing Care. There is no effective treatment for CMV. Therapeutic pregnancy termination may be offered if CMV is discovered during early pregnancy.

Rubella. Rubella is a mild viral disease with a low fever and rash. However, its effects to the developing baby can be destructive. The effects on the embryo or fetus depend on when during pregnancy the infection occurs. Infections occurring in very early pregnancy can disrupt formation of major body systems, while infections acquired later are more likely to damage organs that are already formed. Some effects of rubella on the embryo/fetus include the following:

- Microcephaly (small head size)
- Mental retardation
- Cardiac defects
- Deafness
- Congenital cataracts
- Intrauterine growth restriction (IUGR)

Treatment and Nursing Care. Immunization against rubella infection has been available for some time, but some women of childbearing age are still susceptible. If a woman of childbearing age is immunized, she should not get pregnant for at least 3 months. The vaccine is offered during the postpartum period to nonimmune women. It is *not* given during pregnancy because it is a live attenuated (weakened) form of the virus.

Varicella-Zoster Virus. The varicella-zoster virus causes chickenpox and can become reactivated as shingles later. The infection can cause the pregnant woman to become critically ill. Maternal effects can include the following:

- Preterm labor
- Encephalitis
- Varicella pneumonia, the most serious complication

Effects on the fetus may include:

- Intrauterine infection that occasionally is associated with abnormalities

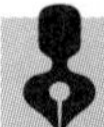

Nursing Tip

Rubella is a cause of birth defects that is almost completely preventable by immunization before childbearing age. The nurse should check each postpartum woman's chart for rubella immunity and notify her physician or nurse-midwife if she is not immune.

- Neonatal infection of varying severity
- Zoster (shingles) appearing months or years after birth

The susceptible woman should be advised to avoid contact with persons having chickenpox and should promptly report any respiratory symptoms if she is infected. Treatment for varicella pneumonia includes full respiratory support, hemodynamic monitoring, and fetal surveillance.

Treatment and Nursing Care. The infant born to a mother is isolated and only immune staff should care for the baby. Immune globulin is recommended for the infant.

Herpesvirus. There are two types of herpesvirus, type 1 and type 2. Type 1 is more likely to cause fever blisters or cold sores. Type 2 is more likely to cause genital herpes. After the primary infection, the virus becomes dormant in the nerves and may be reactivated later as a recurrent (secondary) infection. Initial infection during the first half of pregnancy may cause spontaneous abortion, IUGR, and preterm labor. Most pregnancies are affected by recurrent infections rather than primary infections. The infant is infected by one of these ways:

- The virus ascends into the uterus after the membranes rupture
- The infant has direct contact with infectious lesions

Neonatal herpes infection can be either localized or disseminated (widespread). Disseminated neonatal infection has a high mortality rate and survivors may have neurologic complications.

Treatment and Nursing Care. Neonatal herpes infection can be prevented by avoiding contact with the lesions. If the woman has active genital herpes lesions when the membranes rupture or labor begins, a cesarean delivery is done to avoid fetal contact during birth or ascending infection. Cesarean birth is not necessary if there are no genital lesions. The mother and infant do not have to be isolated as long as direct contact with lesions is avoided. Breastfeeding is safe if there are no lesions on the breasts.

Parvovirus B19. This virus causes *fifth disease* or erythema infectiosum. It is a mild disease that is common in childhood, causing a "slapped cheeks" appearance. During pregnancy, however, maternal infection may cause severe fetal anemia and heart failure. There is no specific treatment.

Hepatitis B. The virus that causes hepatitis B infection can be transmitted by blood, saliva, vaginal secretions, semen, and breast milk, and it can cross the placenta. The person may be asymptomatic or acutely ill with chronic low-grade fever, anorexia, nausea, and vomiting. Some become chronic carriers of the virus. The fetus may be infected transplacentally or by contact with blood or vaginal secretions at birth. The infant is more likely than an adult to become a chronic carrier and a continuing source of infection. Box 5–7 lists those who are at greater risk of having hepatitis B infection.

BOX 5–7

PERSONS AT HIGHER RISK FOR HEPATITIS B INFECTION

Intravenous drug users
Persons with multiple sexual partners
Repeated infection with sexually transmissible diseases
Health care workers with occupational exposure to blood products and needle sticks
Hemodialysis patients
Recipients of multiple blood transfusions or other blood products
Household contact with hepatitis carrier or hemodialysis patient
Persons from areas in Asia and Africa where there is a higher incidence of the disease

Treatment and Nursing Care. All women should be screened for hepatitis B during prenatal care, and the screening should be repeated during the 3rd trimester for women in high-risk groups. Infants born to women who are positive for hepatitis B should receive a single dose of hepatitis B immune globulin (for temporary immunity right after birth) followed by hepatitis B vaccine (for long-term immunity). The Centers for Disease Control and Prevention recommends routine immunization with hepatitis B vaccine for all newborns (those born to carrier mothers and to noncarrier mothers) at birth, 1 to 2 months, and 6 to 18 months. Immunization during pregnancy is contraindicated. If possible, injections should be delayed until after the infant's first bath, so that blood and other potentially infectious secretions are removed to avoid introducing them under the skin. Because they have occupational exposure to blood and other infectious secretions, nurses should be immunized against hepatitis B.

Human Immunodeficiency Virus

The human immunodeficiency virus (HIV) is the causative organism of acquired immunodeficiency syndrome (AIDS). The virus eventually cripples the immune system, making the person susceptible to infections, which eventually result in death. There is no immunization or curative treatment. (See Chapter 31 or a medical-surgical text for further discussion of AIDS, infections associated with the syndrome, and treatment.)

Although first identified in homosexual males, the incidence of HIV infection and AIDS continues to rise in women, particularly African-American and Latino women. HIV infection is acquired one of three ways:

- Sexual contact with an infected person
- Parenteral or mucous membrane exposure to infected blood or tissue
- Perinatal exposure (infants)

Women of childbearing age are most likely to acquire the virus by contaminated needles used in intravenous drug abuse or through heterosexual contact.

The infant may be infected in one of the following ways:

- Transplacentally
- Contact with infected maternal secretions at birth
- Through breast milk

The infected woman has a 20% to 40% chance of transmitting the virus to her fetus perinatally. Infants born to HIV-positive women will be HIV-positive at birth because maternal antibodies to the virus pass through the placenta to the infant. Three to six months are needed to identify the infants who are truly infected.

Treatment and Nursing Care. Pregnant women are questioned about high-risk behaviors for HIV infection (Box 5–8) and offered testing. Testing may also be offered routinely, regardless of a woman's risk status. Women are evaluated for symptoms associated with HIV infection and AIDS, such as weight loss, loss of appetite, nausea, vomiting, diarrhea, fever, night sweats, cough, shortness of breath, and sore throat. Physical examination and laboratory studies are done to determine the status of the woman's immune system, presence of infections associated with AIDS, and presence of sexually transmitted diseases (STDs).

Zidovudine, previously called AZT, is recommended to prolong the woman's life and to reduce vertical transmission of the virus to the fetus. Prevention of and treatment for the various infections that may occur with AIDS are continued during pregnancy. Women may also have complications during pregnancy that are unrelated to their infection, because of adverse social situations such as poverty, malnutrition, and chronic stress. Regular prenatal care identifies these problems as early as possible.

The nurse should assist the woman and her family with anticipatory grieving as needed because the pregnant woman's life is shortened and her baby may not survive. The nurse must anticipate and help the woman to cope with the anxiety that is almost certain about whether the neonate is infected. The woman should be taught to avoid situations where infection with opportunistic microorganisms is likely, such as large crowds, unsanitary conditions, or exposure to people with infections.

Nurses should seize opportunities to educate others about the problem of AIDS and how to prevent it. Prevention involves either avoidance of high-risk behaviors or measures to make transmission of the virus less likely. For example, drug abuse is discouraged because of its many adverse effects; however, if a person continues using intravenous drugs, avoiding shared needles reduces the risk of acquiring HIV infection. Use of a latex condom (not those made from sheep intestines, or "skins") reduces, but does not eliminate, the risk of acquiring the virus through coitus. Oral sex is also a risk factor because infectious secretions can enter small tears in the mucous membranes.

The nurse should maintain standard precautions for contact with potentially infectious body secretions. It is important to wear appropriate protective gear for all situations in which contact with potentially infectious secretions is likely, not just to wear the equipment for those the nurse *thinks* may be infectious. It is impossible to tell what a person is infected with just by looking at them or by their life-style.

BOX 5–8

HIGH-RISK FACTORS FOR HUMAN IMMUNODEFICIENCY VIRUS (HIV)

Intravenous drug abuse
Multiple sexual partners
Prostitution
Blood transfusion before 1985
History of sexually transmitted diseases
Immigration from area where infection is endemic, such as Haiti or Central Africa
Sexual partner in a high-risk group
Sexual partner with HIV infection

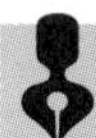

Nursing Tip

The nurse should wear protective equipment, such as gloves, with *every* potential exposure to a patient's body secretions. This practice protects the nurse from many pathogens, not just HIV.

Nonviral Infections

Toxoplasmosis. Toxoplasmosis is a protozoan infection that may be acquired by contact with cat feces, raw meat, or through the placenta. The woman usually has mild symptoms. Congenital toxoplasmosis includes the following possible signs:

- Low birth weight
- Enlarged liver and spleen
- Jaundice
- Anemia
- Inflammation of eye structures
- Neurologic damage

Treatment and Nursing Care. Specific treatment for toxoplasmosis is controversial. Therapeutic abortion may be offered to the woman who contracts the infection during the first half of pregnancy. Nurses can teach women measures to reduce the likelihood of acquiring the infection:

- Cook all meat thoroughly
- Wash hands and all kitchen surfaces after handling raw meat
- Avoid touching the mucous membranes of the eyes or mouth while handling raw meat
- Avoid uncooked eggs and unpasteurized milk
- Wash fruits and vegetables well
- Avoid materials contaminated with cat feces, such as litter boxes, sand boxes, garden soil

Group B Streptococcus Infection. Group B streptococcus (GBS) is a leading cause of perinatal infections that have a high neonatal mortality rate. The organism is found in the woman's rectum, vagina, cervix, throat, and skin. Although she is colonized with the organism, the woman is usually asymptomatic, but the infant may be infected through contact with vaginal secretions at birth. The risk is greater if the woman has a long labor or premature rupture of membranes. It is a significant cause of maternal postpartum infection (endometritis, or infection of the uterine interior), especially after cesarean birth.

GBS can be deadly for the infant. A newborn may have either early-onset or late-onset GBS infection.

- Early-onset GBS infection: within the first 7 days after birth
- Late-onset GBS infection: after 7 days of age

Eighty percent of neonatal GBS infections are early-onset disease, with a mortality rate of 5% to 15%. Early-onset GBS may be manifested in generalized sepsis, pneumonia, or meningitis. Late-onset GBS disease is usually manifested by meningitis. Permanent neurologic impairment may occur with neonatal GBS infection.

Treatment and Nursing Care. The woman can be screened during pregnancy to determine if she is a GBS carrier. However, her carrier status often changes, so she may be negative at the time of the screening, but positive when her membranes rupture. Cultures to screen for GBS should be obtained from the vagina and rectum between 35 and 37 weeks' gestation to increase their accuracy at predicting GBS colonization at birth. If they are positive, or if the woman has the following risk factors for GBS colonization, intravenous intrapartum antibiotics are prescribed:

- Previous infant with GBS infection
- Presence of GBS in urine cultures
- Birth before 37 weeks' gestation (because the woman may not have been screened for GBS)
- Maternal fever during labor
- Membranes ruptured 18 or more hours before birth

Her newborn is usually given antibiotics until infection is ruled out. See Chapter 13 for more information about neonatal GBS infection.

Tuberculosis. The incidence of tuberculosis is rising in the United States, and drug-resistant strains of the bacterium are emerging. Pregnant women are screened as other clients (see Chapter 4 or a medical-surgical nursing text). If the screening test is positive, they should have a chest radiograph (x-ray) with the abdomen shielded. Sputum specimens that are positive for the bacterium confirm the diagnosis.

The adult with tuberculosis experiences fatigue, weakness, loss of appetite and weight, fever, and night sweats. The newborn may acquire the disease by swallowing or inhaling infected amniotic fluid or by contact with an untreated mother after birth.

Congenital tuberculosis is manifested by failure to thrive, lethargy, respiratory distress, fever, and enlargement of the spleen, liver, and lymph nodes.

Treatment and Nursing Care. Isoniazid and rifampin are usually prescribed for 9 months. Ethambutol may be given if drug-resistant tuberculosis is suspected. The infant may have preventive therapy. If the infant's skin test is positive at 3 months, he or she is given a full course of therapy. The healthcare staff, including nurses, must teach the family how the organism is transmitted, and the importance of continuing the anti-tubercular drugs consistently for the full course of therapy. Incompletely treated tuberculosis is a significant cause of drug-resistant organisms.

Sexually Transmissible Diseases

Sexually transmissible diseases (STDs) are those for which a common mode of transmission is sexual intercourse, although several can also be transmitted in other ways. Herpesvirus and HIV infection have been discussed. Five other infections that are typically transmitted sexually are syphilis, gonorrhea, chlamydia, trichomoniasis, and condylomata acuminata (genital warts) (see Table 5–8).

Table 5–8
SEXUALLY TRANSMISSIBLE DISEASES DURING PREGNANCY

Maternal Effect	Fetal and Neonatal Effects	Treatment in Pregnancy and Nursing Considerations
Syphilis. Caused by the bacterium *Treponema pallidum;* a chancre (painless, persistent sore) is the first manifestation; a generalized rash, which appears on the palms and soles as well as on the body, follows 4-6 wk later; low fever may accompany the rash; in untreated patients, syphilis may attack the heart and central nervous system	Transmitted transplacentally; may produce spontaneous abortion, preterm labor, stillbirth, and congenital syphilis; exposure during the 3rd trimester produces milder effects, such as enlarged liver and spleen, rash, and jaundice	Screening during prenatal care is standard; treatment with penicillin before 16 wk can prevent fetal infection because the antibiotic crosses the placenta (the woman is desensitized if she is allergic to penicillin); follow-up visits are essential to be sure the infection has been eradicated; sexual partners should be notified; reinfection during pregnancy is possible
Gonorrhea. Caused by the bacterium *Neisseria gonorrhoeae;* vaginal discharge, which may be profuse and purulent; itching of vulva; painful urination; may be asymptomatic; may cause infertility by blocking the fallopian tubes	Transmitted to the infant during birth by direct contact with the mother's infected birth canal, resulting in eye infection that can cause blindness (ophthalmia neonatorum); may also cause premature rupture of the membranes or preterm birth	Screening during prenatal care is standard; treatment is with ceftriaxone, spectinomycin, or aqueous procaine penicillin (intramuscular); cefixime and ampicillin may be given orally; probenecid is given to increase blood levels of penicillin and ampicillin and effectiveness of treatment; prophylactic eye treatment with erythromycin or tetracycline ointment is standard for all neonates; infected neonates will have additional antibiotics
Chlamydia. Caused by the bacterium *Chlamydia trachomatis;* increased yellow vaginal discharge; painful, frequent urination; patient may be asymptomatic; may cause infertility by blocking the fallopian tubes	Transmitted to the infant's eyes during birth by direct contact with the mother's infected birth canal, resulting in conjunctivitis; may also result in infant pneumonitis; associated with preterm labor, premature rupture of the membranes, growth restriction	Treated during pregnancy with erythromycin; tetracycline is effective but should not be taken during pregnancy; eye prophylactic antibiotic ointment is used as discussed under gonorrhea; silver nitrate eye prophylaxis is not effective against chlamydia
Trichomoniasis. Caused by the protozoon *Trichomonas vaginalis;* frothy, gray-green, foul vaginal discharge; perineal itching; reddened skin	Does not cross the placenta; neonatal infection is short-lived; associated with premature rupture of the membranes and postpartum maternal infection	Avoid treatment until after the 1st trimester to prevent adverse drug effects on fetus; clotrimazole (Gyne-Lotrimin) can be given during the 1st trimester, and systemic metronidazole (Flagyl) can be given during the 2nd and 3rd trimesters; woman taking metronidazole should avoid alcohol for 48 hr after she stops taking the drug
Condylomata acuminata. Caused by the virus, human papillomavirus (HPV); genital warts: cauliflower-like growths accompanied by itching, vulva pain, and vaginal discharge; associated with development of genital cancer	Contact via birth canal can cause laryngeal papillomas resulting in abnormal cry, voice change, hoarseness, or airway obstruction. Symptoms may appear 1 month or more after contact.	Trichloroacetic acid applied topically to the growths, cryotherapy, surgical excision, laser, or electrocautery

All sexual contacts of persons infected with a disease that can be sexually transmitted should be informed and treated; otherwise, the cycle of infection and reinfection will continue. Consistent use of a latex condom, including the female condom, helps to reduce sexual spread of infections.

Vaginal Infections

Vaginal infections besides those discussed in other categories are candidiasis and bacterial vaginosis.

Candidiasis (Monilial Vaginitis). The fungus *Candida albicans* causes most cases of candidiasis, or "yeast infection." Candidiasis is more likely to occur if there is a change in the vaginal environment that favors its growth, such as pregnancy, diabetes mellitus, systemic antibiotic therapy, or oral contraceptive use in the nonpregnant woman. It is more likely if the woman is obese, eats a diet high in sugar, or has impaired immune function. It is sometimes transmitted sexually.

Candidiasis causes intense itching of the vagina, vulva, and rectal area. Urination and sexual intercourse may be painful because of tissue inflammation. The discharge has a curdlike, or "cottage cheese," appearance. Miconazole (Monistat), clotrimazole (Gyne-Lotrimin), and nystatin (Mycostatin) are treatments.

The neonate may acquire the organism in the mouth during passage through the birth canal (thrush). The infant's mouth has white patches that resemble milk curds but that bleed if removal is attempted. Mouth pain makes nursing difficult. Oral nystatin (Mycostatin) is the usual treatment for thrush.

Bacterial Vaginosis. *Gardnerella vaginalis* causes profuse vaginal discharge that has a fishy odor. The fetus is usually unaffected. Metronidazole (Flagyl) is an effective treatment, but it should not be used until after the 1st trimester because of the potential for causing birth defects. Ampicillin is an alternate treatment. Antibiotics for the woman's sexual partner may be prescribed.

Nursing Care for Women with Vaginal Infections. The client is taught measures to reduce the discomfort of vaginal infections. Warm sitz baths followed by dry heat from a hair dryer on a low setting wash away the discharge and are comforting. Cotton underwear promotes air circulation and makes the vaginal environment less favorable for growth of the organisms. Tampons and sanitary pads with plastic backing or deodorant should not be used.

Urinary Tract Infections

The urinary tract is normally self-cleaning, because acidic urine inhibits growth of microorganisms and flushes them out of the body with each voiding. Pregnancy alters the self-cleaning action, because pressure on urinary structures keeps the bladder from emptying completely and because the ureters dilate and lose motility under the relaxing effects of the hormone progesterone. Urine that is retained becomes more alkaline and provides a favorable environment for growth of microorganisms.

Some women have excessive microorganisms in their urine but no symptoms (asymptomatic bacteriuria). The asymptomatic infection may eventually cause cystitis (bladder infection) or pyelonephritis (kidney infection). The woman with cystitis has the following signs and symptoms:

- Burning with urination
- Increased frequency and urgency of urination
- A normal or slightly elevated temperature

If not treated, cystitis can ascend in the urinary tract and cause pyelonephritis. Pyelonephritis is a particularly serious infection in pregnancy and is accompanied by the following signs and symptoms:

- High fever
- Chills
- Flank pain or tenderness
- Nausea and vomiting

Maternal septic shock and preterm birth may occur with pyelonephritis during pregnancy. The high maternal fever is dangerous for the fetus because it increases the fetal metabolic rate, which in turn increases fetal oxygen needs to levels that the mother cannot readily supply.

Treatment. Urinary tract infections (UTIs) are treated with antibiotics, often ampicillin. Asymptomatic bacteriuria is treated with oral antibiotics for 10 days, cystitis for 10 to 14 days. Pyelonephritis is treated with multiple antibiotics, initially administered intravenously.

Nursing Tip

The nurse should teach all women measures to reduce their risk and that of their girls for urinary tract infections.

Nursing Care. All women and girls should be taught how to reduce the introduction of rectal microorganisms into the bladder. For example, a front-to-back direction should be used when wiping after urination or a bowel movement, or when doing perineal cleansing or applying and removing perineal pads. The nurse can begin teaching during the woman's prenatal care and reinforce it during the postpartum stay. The mother should be taught how to clean and diaper a baby girl to avoid fecal contamination of her urethra.

Adequate fluid intake promotes frequent voiding. At least eight glasses of liquid per day, excluding caffeine-containing beverages, helps to flush urine through the urinary tract regularly. Although evidence of its benefit is inconclusive, cranberry juice may make the urine more acidic and therefore less conducive to growth of infectious organisms. In any case, cranberry and other juices add to the woman's fluid intake.

Sexual intercourse mildly irritates the bladder and urethra, which promotes UTI if a woman is prone to it. Urinating before intercourse reduces irritation; urinating afterward flushes urine from the bladder. Using water-soluble lubricant can also reduce periurethral irritation related to intercourse.

Pregnant women should be taught signs and symptoms of cystitis and pyelonephritis, so that they will know to seek treatment at once. Prompt treatment of urinary tract infections reduces the risk for preterm labor and birth.

ENVIRONMENTAL HAZARDS DURING PREGNANCY

Substance abuse is widespread in the United States. It affects every group of people, including pregnant women. The actual prevalence of drug use during pregnancy is difficult to determine because many women hide or underreport it, especially illicit drug use. Women rarely consider legal substances, such as nicotine or alcohol, to be drugs; they may not report them unless specifically asked.

Evaluating the effects of both legal and illicit substances on the woman and fetus is difficult because women often ingest several substances and illicit drugs often contain impurities that alter their properties. The woman and fetus may be affected directly; an example is the vasoconstriction caused by nicotine and cocaine. Indirect effects include inadequate diet, late or absent prenatal care, and infections that are more prevalent in this group, such as STDs, hepatitis B, and HIV.

Several substances are metabolized and eliminated slowly during pregnancy, which prolongs their effects. Many drugs are concentrated in the amniotic fluid, which the fetus drinks. Thus, the substance-exposed fetus, who has a tiny body, is exposed to high levels of the substance for a longer time.

Substances Harmful to the Fetus

It is well established that several legal and illicit substances are harmful to the developing baby. A substance that causes an adverse physical effect on the embryo or fetus is a *teratogen.* The best policy is to abstain from unnecessary substance use during pregnancy, including therapeutic drugs that can be delayed. Many environmental substances are most harmful to the developing baby early in pregnancy, before the woman knows she is pregnant.

Smoking. Smoking, including passive smoking, can cause fetal growth restriction. Tobacco use during pregnancy has been linked to abruptio placentae, preterm birth, stillbirth, increases in neonatal death, and sudden infant death syndrome. Newborns of smoking women tend to be smaller than expected for their gestation because the vasoconstriction that nicotine causes reduces blood flow to the placenta. It is not clear whether smoking causes malformations. Nicotine patches also expose the fetus to this substance.

Alcohol. Alcohol is the most commonly abused drug by women of childbearing age. Fetal alcohol syndrome (FAS) is well documented: prenatal and postnatal growth retardation; mental retardation; and facial abnormalities, including a flat, thin upper lip border and downslanting eyes (Fig. 5–11).

No "safe" level of alcohol intake during pregnancy is known. Women should abstain from alcohol use from conception. A woman who is trying to get pregnant should avoid alcohol because it can damage the fetus before she knows she is pregnant.

Marijuana. Harmful effects of marijuana during pregnancy have not been clearly identified, but they cannot be ruled out. Many marijuana users also ingest other substances that may be harmful or that may exert harmful effects when combined with marijuana.

Cocaine. Cocaine is a local anesthetic and a powerful central nervous system stimulant. It is highly addictive, and it causes euphoria (sense of well-being) and vasoconstriction that may harm the woman and/or the fetus. When the stimulant effects wear off, the woman becomes irritable and depressed and has a strong craving to recapture the euphoria. Adverse maternal effects include tachy-

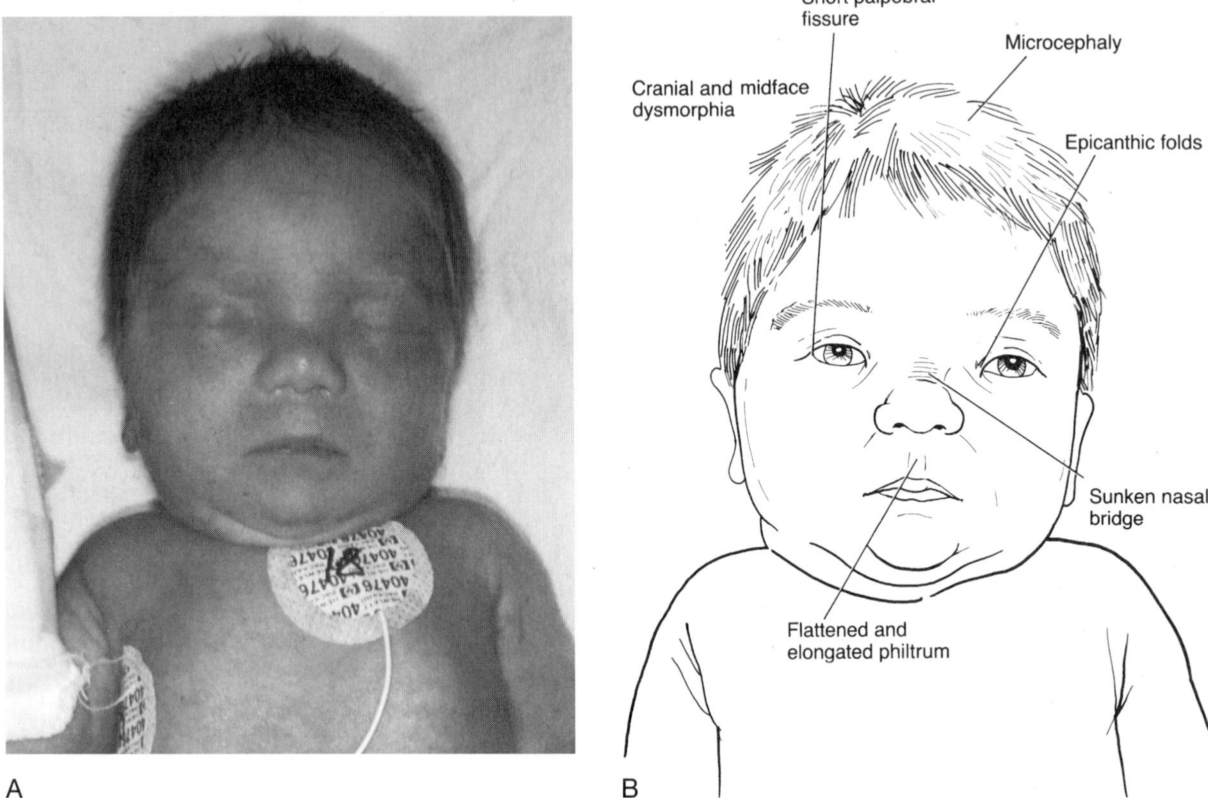

Figure 5–11. • **A,** Infant with fetal alcohol syndrome (FAS). (Courtesy of Trish Beachy, MS, RN, Perinatal Program Coordinator, University of Colorado Health Sciences, Denver, Colorado). **B,** Diagram of facial malformations associated with FAS. (*B* is adapted from Gorrie, T. M., McKinney, E. S., & Murray, S. S. [1998]. *Foundations of maternal–newborn nursing*. Philadelphia: Saunders.)

cardia, hypertension, seizures, stroke, myocardial infarction, and sudden death.

Sudden onset of abnormally strong labor contractions, at term or before term, may occur with maternal cocaine ingestion. The abnormal contractions may lead to spontaneous abortion, preterm rupture of the membranes, preterm birth, or abruptio placentae. Cocaine-induced vasoconstriction interferes with normal exchange of nutrients, oxygen, and waste products in the placenta. Moreover, the fetus receives the drug and cannot effectively excrete it. Fetal effects include tachycardia, nonreassuring electronic fetal monitoring tracings, fetal hyperactivity, and intrauterine growth restriction. The newborn may be very irritable and difficult to console (see also Chapter 16).

Heroin. Heroin is an opiate drug related to morphine. The heroin-addicted woman is likely to be exposed to HIV infection because the drug is taken intravenously. She becomes physically dependent on the drug, and an abstinence syndrome (withdrawal) with the following features results if she does not have it regularly:

- Agitation
- Tearing, rhinorrhea (runny nose)
- Yawning
- Perspiring
- Abdominal and uterine cramps
- Diarrhea
- Muscle pain

Fetal effects include spontaneous abortion in early pregnancy, hyperactivity, hypoxia, passage of meconium into the amniotic fluid, and stillbirth. Neonatal abstinence syndrome occurs within 24 hours of birth: prolonged high-pitched crying, high need for sucking, tremulousness, seizures, hyperactivity, and disrupted sleep-wake cycles. Maintaining the pregnant woman on methadone (another opiate) can prevent serious effects to the fetus during pregnancy and lessen, but not eliminate, neonatal abstinence effects.

Anticonvulsants. Pregnant women with epilepsy have an overall increased rate of pregnancy complications and adverse outcomes (Cunningham et al., 1997). Several anticonvulsants, such as phenytoin, also called diphenylhydantoin (Dilantin), are linked to birth defects during pregnancy. The data from different studies are often contradictory as to whether the specific drug is linked to birth defects. The mother may have seizures if the drug is stopped, which would jeopardize the fetus. The physician prescribes the anticonvulsant that is least teratogenic to the fetus while still controlling the mother's seizures.

Anticoagulants. Heparin cannot cross the placenta to affect the fetus. However, drugs such as warfarin (Coumadin) cross the placenta. Warfarin may cause growth retardation, a small and abnormally shaped head, mental retardation, minor eye abnormalities, depressed bridge of the nose, and hand abnormalities.

Acne Medications. Isotretinoin (Accutane) is a form of vitamin A that can cause serious fetal defects: microcephaly, ear abnormalities, cardiac defects, and central nervous system abnormalities. Acne medications are not essential and a pregnant woman should not take them. The woman of childbearing age must use reliable birth control during isotretinoin therapy and for a time afterward to allow the drug to leave the body. A related drug (etretinate [Tegison]) requires a long time for elimination; it may affect a fetus 11 months after the woman stops using it.

Treatment

Care focuses on identifying the substance-abusing woman early in pregnancy, educating her about their effects and encouraging her to reduce or eliminate their use. Unfortunately, many substance-abusing women first enter care when they are admitted to the hospital in active labor. They often leave the hospital quickly after birth to resume drug ingestion.

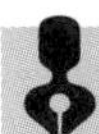
Nursing Tip

When questioning about substance use during pregnancy, focus on how the information will help nurses and physicians to provide the safest and most appropriate care to the pregnant woman and her baby.

Women are screened for infections that are more likely among drug users, such as hepatitis, HIV infection, and STDs. Dietary support and monitoring of their weight gain promote better health for the infant. Methadone may be prescribed for the heroin-dependent woman because it is safer and prevents maternal abstinence syndrome. The infant will also experience withdrawal from methadone, however.

The woman is referred for specific treatment of substance abuse, as indicated. She may have care in outpatient or residential facilities. See a psychiatric text for more information about treatment of substance abuse.

In the case of therapeutic drugs, the woman's need for the drug is weighed against the potential for fetal harm it may cause and the fetal or maternal harm that may occur if the woman is not treated. In general, the physician will choose the least teratogenic drug that is effective and prescribe it in the lowest effective dose.

Nursing Care

Educating women and girls about the effect of drugs on a developing baby is best done before pregnancy, as hazards are often most harmful during early pregnancy. Because drug use is prevalent in schools, preadolescence is not too soon to begin this education. Women should be taught to eliminate use of any unnecessary substance before becoming pregnant. A woman is encouraged to tell any health care provider if she thinks she is pregnant (or is trying to conceive) before having a nonemergency radiograph or being prescribed a drug.

A trusting, therapeutic nurse–client relationship makes it more likely that a woman will be truthful about use of substances, both legal and illicit. The nurse who collects data must use a nonjudgmental approach and treat the problem as a health problem rather than a moral problem.

Screening for drug use begins in a nonthreatening way by questioning about over-the-counter drugs. Next, the nurse asks about regularly taken prescription drugs. Smoking and alcohol use are then assessed. Use of illicit drugs is discussed last. If the woman acknowledges using any substances, legal or illicit, the type, amount, route of ingestion, and frequency of drug use are clarified.

To reduce defensiveness, the nurse might say, "We need to know everything that may affect you or your baby. Some questions may be uncomfortable for you, but we can give you better care if we have honest answers." Reveal an awareness of drugs commonly abused in the community. For example, say, "Do any of your friends have problems with crack cocaine? Is there a lot of drug use in your school or neighborhood?"

If a woman acknowledges using drugs, follow with specific questions about how much she uses and how often. Use terms that are familiar to the illicit drug user. For example, if a woman says she uses cocaine (including "crack"), the nurse might ask these questions:

- How often do you use cocaine?
- Do you snort? Smoke crack? Shoot cocaine? Free-base?
- How many lines or rocks do you use?
- How long do you stay high?
- Do you use other drugs at the same time?
- What do you use to cut your cocaine?

Support the woman who is trying to reduce her drug use. Recognize her efforts to improve her health and that of her baby. For example, acknowledge that avoiding her drug(s) of choice requires great self-control, even if she has been drug-free for only a short time. Avoid adding to her guilt if she relapses.

Praise her efforts to improve her overall health and to have a successful pregnancy. For example, praise her weight gain when it is normal or she reduces her cigarette smoking. Give her positive feedback when she tries to maintain a healthful diet.

The nurse plans care to include problems that often accompany substance abuse. These may include the following:

- Poor diet with inadequate pregnancy weight gain
- STDs because sex is often exchanged for drugs
- Limited choices of pain management during labor
- Nonsupport from significant others and a chaotic life-style

TRAUMA DURING PREGNANCY

There is a high incidence of trauma during the childbearing years. Automobile accidents, homicide, and suicide are the three leading causes of traumatic death. Although pregnant women usually are more careful to protect themselves from harm, increased stress from pregnancy may lead to injury both in and out of the home. Falls are not uncommon owing to the woman's altered sense of balance. The pregnant woman also needs to be especially careful when stepping in and out of the bathtub or when using a ladder or stepstool.

The automobile is another hazard. The woman needs to wear a seat belt every time she is in a car, both as a driver and as a passenger. The lap portion of the belt is placed low, just below her protruding abdomen. The pregnant woman and her fetus are more likely to suffer severe injury or death because of not being restrained during a crash than they are to be injured by the restraint itself. Air bags are a supplemental restraint, intended for use in addition to seat belts. No one should ride with anyone who has been drinking alcohol or whose judgment is impaired for other reasons.

Physical trauma is usually blunt trauma (that caused by falls or blows to the body) but may be penetrating trauma (such as knife or gunshot wounds). Physical abuse against women (battering) is a significant cause of trauma, and the violence often escalates during pregnancy.

The fetus within the enlarged uterus may protect the woman's abdominal organs from some of the trauma. Fetal injuries may be direct, such as a skull fracture, or indirect by disruption of placental blood flow from abruptio placentae, uterine rupture, or maternal hypovolemic shock. Fetal death is related to the severity of maternal injury. The fetus who survives severe maternal trauma may have neurologic deficits.

Battering occurs in all ethnic groups and all social strata. It often begins or becomes worse during pregnancy. The abuser is usually her male partner, but he may be another male, such as the father of a pregnant adolescent. Men who abuse women are also likely to abuse children in the relationship.

Women abused during pregnancy are more likely to have miscarriages, stillbirths, and low-birth-weight babies. They often enter prenatal care late, if at all. The risk of homicide escalates during pregnancy. The time of greatest danger to the abused woman occurs when she leaves her abuser.

Abuse during pregnancy, as at other times, may take many forms. It is not always physical abuse—many women are abused emotionally. Emotional abuse makes leaving the relationship especially difficult, because it lowers the woman's self-esteem and isolates her from sources of help.

Manifestations of Battering

In addition to having late or erratic prenatal care, the battered woman may have bruises or lacerations in various stages of healing. A radiograph may reveal old fractures. The woman tends to minimize injury, or "forget" its severity. She may assume responsibility for the trauma, as evidenced by remarks such as, "If I had only kept the children quiet, he wouldn't have gotten so mad." Her abuser is often unusually attentive after the battering episode.

Treatment of the Pregnant Woman Experiencing Trauma

Pregnancy is a good time to assess the woman for battering, because she may have more regular contact with a health care provider and may also face increased danger at that time. She must be interviewed for possible battering in private, away from the person who may be abusing her. If the woman admits to being battered, further assessment should be done to determine the level of danger to her.

Care of the mother's life-threatening injuries, regardless of their cause, has priority. Management of the fetus depends on the gestational age and whether the fetus is living. Cesarean birth may be done to save the life of a fetus mature enough to survive outside the uterus. If the fetus is too immature to survive or is already dead, cesarean birth is done if it will improve the woman's status or save her life.

Nursing Care

Nurses must be aware that any woman may be in an abusive relationship. Therapeutic, nonjudgmental communication helps establish a trusting relationship. Nonabused women, including nurses, often cannot understand why a woman would stay in a harmful relationship. The abuser has usually isolated the woman by controlling whom she sees, where she goes, and how she spends money. Emotional abuse often supplements physical abuse, making the woman feel that she is "stupid" or "no good" and that she is "lucky that he loves her because no one else would ever love her." She usually feels that she has no choice but to stay in the abusive relationship. She may assume part of the blame, believing that her abuser will stop hurting her if she tries harder.

The woman being assessed for abuse is taken to a private area. The nurse determines whether there are factors that increase the risk for severe injuries or homicide, such as drug use by the abuser, a gun in the house, use of a weapon, or violent behavior by the abuser outside the home. The nurse also determines whether the children are being hurt. *It is vital that the abuser not find out that the woman has reported the abuse or that she intends to leave.*

Nurses can refer women to shelters and other services if they wish to leave the abuser. The decision about whether to end the relationship rests with the woman, however. Abuse of children must be reported to appropriate authorities.

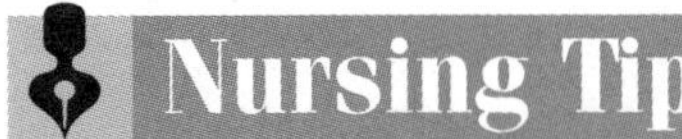

If a woman confides that she is being abused during pregnancy, this information must be kept absolutely confidential. Her life may be in danger if her abuser learns that she has told anyone. She should be referred to local shelters, but the decision to leave her abuser is hers alone.

Nursing care for the acutely injured pregnant woman supplements medical management: the focus is on stabilizing the mother's condition when life-threatening injuries occur. Placing a small pillow under one hip tilts the heavy uterus off the inferior vena cava to improve blood flow throughout the woman's body and to the placenta. An assessment of vital signs and urine output reflects blood circulation to the kidneys. Urine output should average at least 30 ml/hr. Bloody urine may indicate damage to the kidneys or bladder.

The nurse assesses for uterine contractions or tenderness, which may indicate onset of labor or abruptio placentae. Continuous electronic fetal monitoring (see p. 145) is usually instituted if the fetus is viable and near maturity.

EFFECTS OF A HIGH-RISK PREGNANCY ON THE FAMILY

Normal pregnancy is a crisis because it is a time of significant change and growth. The woman with a complicated pregnancy has stressors beyond those of the normal pregnancy. Her family is also affected by the pregnancy.

Disruption of Usual Roles

The woman who has a difficult pregnancy must often remain bed rest at home or in the hospital, sometimes for several weeks. Others must assume her usual roles in the family, in addition to their own obligations. Care of young children is difficult if the woman provides most of their supervision. Placing them in day care may not be an option because the woman must usually stop working.

Nurses can help families adjust to these disruptions by identifying sources of support to help maintain reasonably normal household function. Remind the family that the disruptions in their lives are temporary.

Financial Difficulties

Many women work outside the home, and their salary may stop if they cannot work for an extended period. At the same time, their medical costs are rising. Social service referrals may help the family cope with their expenses. Creditors may extend the time for the family to pay debts or allow them to pay the debt principal only.

Delayed Attachment to the Baby

Pregnancy normally involves gradual acceptance of and emotional attachment to the fetus, especially after the woman feels movement. Fathers feel a similar attachment, although at a slower pace than that of the pregnant woman. The woman who has a high-risk pregnancy often halts planning for the baby and may withdraw emotionally to protect herself from pain and loss if the outcome is poor.

Loss of Expected Birth Experience

Couples rarely anticipate problems when they begin a pregnancy. Most have specific expectations about how their pregnancy, particularly the birth, will proceed. A high-risk pregnancy may result in the loss of their expected experience. They may be unable to attend childbirth preparation classes or to have a vaginal birth. Nurses can help incorporate as many of the couple's plans as possible, particularly at the time of birth.

KEY POINTS

- Hyperemesis gravidarum is persistent nausea and vomiting of pregnancy, often accompanied by weight loss, dehydration, and metabolic imbalances. Psychological factors may play a role in some women.
- The most common reason for early spontaneous abortion is abnormality of the developing baby or placenta.
- If a woman has a rupture from an ectopic pregnancy, the nurse should observe for shock due to hemorrhage into the abdomen. Vaginal blood loss may be minimal, whereas intraabdominal blood loss can be massive.
- The woman who has gestational trophoblastic disease (hydatidiform mole) should have follow-up medical care for 1 to 2 years to detect the possible development of choriocarcinoma. She should not get pregnant during this time.
- Placenta previa is the abnormal implantation of the placenta in the lower part of the uterus. Abruptio placentae is the premature separation of the placenta that is normally implanted.
- The three main manifestations of preeclampsia are hypertension, edema, and proteinuria. The greatest risk to the fetus is reduced blood flow through the placenta, which impairs oxygenation and nutrition. Eclampsia occurs if the woman has one or more generalized seizures.
- Pregnancy promotes the development of diabetes (gestational diabetes) or aggravates preexisting diabetes because it increases resistance to insulin and breaks down insulin more quickly.
- Some infections are mild or even asymptomatic in the nonpregnant woman. Some, such as varicella, can be much more severe during pregnancy. Other infections cause the mother few problems but may be devastating for the fetus or newborn.
- Urinary tract infections are more common during pregnancy because compression and dilation of the ureters result in urine stasis. Preterm labor is more likely to occur if a woman has pyelonephritis.
- The fetus of the woman who takes drugs (legal or illicit) or alcohol is exposed to higher levels of the substance for a longer time because the substances become concentrated in the amniotic fluid and the fetus ingests the fluid.

MULTIPLE-CHOICE REVIEW QUESTIONS

Choose the most appropriate answer.

1. A woman has an incomplete abortion, followed by vacuum aspiration. She is now in the recovery room and is crying softly with her husband. Select the most appropriate nursing action:
   a. leave the couple alone, except for necessary recovery room care
   b. tell the couple that most abortions are for the best because the baby would be abnormal
   c. tell the couple that spontaneous abortion is very common and does not mean they cannot have other children
   d. express your regret at their loss and remain nearby if they want to talk about it
2. A woman is admitted with a diagnosis of "possible ectopic pregnancy." Select the nursing assessment that should be promptly reported:
   a. absence of vaginal bleeding
   b. complaint of shoulder pain
   c. stable pulse and respiratory rate; rise in blood pressure of 10 mm Hg systolic
   d. temperature of 99.6° F (37.6° C)
3. It is important to emphasize that a woman who has gestational trophoblastic disease (hydatidiform mole) continue to have follow-up medical care after initial treatment because
   a. choriocarcinoma sometimes occurs after the initial treatment
   b. she has lower levels of immune factors and is vulnerable to infection
   c. anemia complicates most cases of hydatidiform mole
   d. permanent elevation of her blood pressure is more likely
4. Select the primary difference between the symptoms of placenta previa and abruptio placentae:
   a. fetal presentation
   b. presence of pain
   c. abnormal blood clotting
   d. presence of bleeding
5. The battered pregnant woman is at greatest risk for homicide when she
   a. reports the abuse to the authorities
   b. tells her abuser that she is pregnant
   c. attempts to leave her abuser
   d. goes to prenatal appointments

BIBLIOGRAPHY AND READER REFERENCE

Ament, L. A., & Whalen, E. (1996). Sexually transmitted diseases in pregnancy: Diagnosis, impact, and intervention. *Journal of Obstetric, Gynecologic, and Neonatal Nurses, 25*(8), 657–666.

American Academy of Pediatrics (AAP) and American College of Obstetricians and Gynecologists (ACOG). (1997). *Guidelines for perinatal care* (4th ed.). Washington, DC: Author.

American College of Obstetricians and Gynecologists (ACOG). (1994). *Diabetes in pregnancy.* Technical Bulletin 200. Washington, DC: Author.

American College of Obstetricians and Gynecologists (ACOG). (1996). *Hypertension in pregnancy.* Technical Bulletin 219. Washington, DC: Author.

Anderson, G. (1997). Tuberculosis in pregnancy. *Seminars in perinatology, 21*(4), 328–335.

Barger, M. K., & Fein, E. (1997). High-risk pregnancy. In F. H. Nichols & E. Zwelling (Eds.), *Maternal–newborn nursing: Theory and practice* (pp. 622–700). Philadelphia: Saunders.

Buchanan, T. A., & Coustan, D. R. (1995). Diabetes mellitus. In G. N. Burrow & T. F. Ferris (Eds.), *Medical complications in pregnancy* (4th ed., pp. 29–61). Philadelphia: Saunders.

Burke, M. E., & Poole, J. (1996). Common perinatal complications. In K. R. Simpson & P. A. Creehan (Eds.), *AWHONN'S perinatal nursing* (pp. 109–148). Philadelphia: Lippincott.

Collins, T. M., Saltzman, R. L., & Jordan, M. C. (1995). Viral infections. In G. N. Burrow & T. F. Ferris (Eds.), *Medical complications during pregnancy* (4th ed, pp. 381–403). Philadelphia: Saunders.

Cunningham, F. G., MacDonald, P. C., Gant, N. F., Leveno, K. J., Gilstrap, L. C., Hankins, G. D. V., & Clark, S. L. (1997). *Williams obstetrics* (20th ed). Stamford, CT: Appleton & Lange.

Ferris, T. F. (1995). Hypertension and preeclampsia. In G. N. Burrow & T. F. Ferris (Eds.), *Medical complications in pregnancy* (4th ed., pp. 1–28). Philadelphia: Saunders.

Gorrie, T., McKinney, E., & Murray, S. (1998). *Foundations of maternal–newborn nursing* (2nd ed). Philadelphia: Saunders.

Green, E. M., McFarlane, J., & Watson, M. G. (1997). Vaginal bleeding and abuse: Assessing pregnant women in the emergency department. *MCN: American Journal of Maternal/Child Nursing, 22*(4), 182–186.

Grose, C. (1996). Viral infections in the fetus and newborn. In R. E. Behrman, R. M. Kliegman, A. M. Arvin (Eds.), *Nelson textbook of pediatrics* (15th ed., pp. 523–528). Philadelphia: Saunders.

Kenner, C. (1998). Neonatal acquired immunodeficiency syndrome: Human immunodefiency virus. In C. Kenner, J. W. Lott, & A. A. Flandermeyer (Eds.), *Comprehensive neonatal nursing: A physiologic perspective* (2nd ed., pp. 815–837). Philadelphia: Saunders.

Laros, R. K. (1994). Maternal hematological disorders. In R. K. Creasy & R. Resnik (Eds.), *Maternal–fetal medicine: Principles and practice* (3rd ed, pp. 905–933). Philadelphia: Saunders.

Lee, R. V. (1995). Sexually transmitted infections. In G. N. Burrow & T. F. Ferris (Eds.), *Medical complications in pregnancy* (4th ed., pp. 404–438). Philadelphia: Saunders.

Maiolatesi, C. R., & Peddicord, K. (1996). Methotrexate for nonsurgical treatment of ectopic pregnancy: Nursing implications. *Journal of Obstetric, Gynecologic, and Neonatal Nursing, 25*(3), 205–208.

McAnulty, J. H., Metcalfe ,J., & Ueland, K. (1995). Cardiovascular disease. In G. N. Burrow & T. F. Ferris (Eds.), *Medical complications in pregnancy* (4th ed., pp. 123–154). Philadelphia: Saunders.

McFarlane, J., Parker, B., Soeken, K., & Bullock, L. (1992). Assessing for abuse during pregnancy: Severity and frequency of injuries and associated entry into prenatal care. *JAMA: Journal of the American Medical Association, 267,* 3176–3179.

Mitchell, A., Steffenson, N., Hogan, H., & Brooks, S. (1997). Group B streptococcus and pregnancy: Update and recommendations. *MCN: American Journal of Maternal/Child Nursing,* 22(5), 242–248.

Mitchell, A., Steffenson, N., Hogan, H., & Brooks, S. (1997). Neonatal Group B streptococcal disease. *MCN: American Journal of Maternal/Child Nursing,* 22(5), 249–253.

Montgomery, K. S. (1996). Caring for the pregnant woman with sickle cell disease. *MCN: American Journal of Maternal/Child Nursing, 21*(5), 224–228.

Moore, T. R. (1994). Diabetes in pregnancy. In R. K. Creasy & R. Resnik (Eds.), *Maternal–fetal medicine: Principles and practice* (3rd ed., pp. 934–978). Philadelphia: Saunders.

Persily, C. A. (1996). Relationships between the perceived impact of gestational diabetes mellitus and treatment adherence. *Journal of Obstetric, Gynecologic, and Neonatal Nurses, 25*(7), 601–607.

Polivka, B. J., Nickel, J. T., & Wilkins, J. R. (1997). Urinary tract infection during pregnancy: A risk factor for cerebral palsy? *Journal of Obstetric, Gynecologic, and Neonatal Nurses, 26*(4), 405–413.

Prestige, P. (1997). Domestic violence: Women of all ages. Fourth annual "Women and Children First" conference, Dallas, TX.

Remington, J. S., & Klein, J. O. (1995). *Infectious diseases of the fetus and newborn infant.* Philadelphia: Saunders.

chapter 6

Nursing Care during Labor and Birth

Outline

Objectives

On completion and mastery of Chapter 6, the student will be able to

- Define each vocabulary term listed.
- Describe the four components ("four Ps") of the birth process: the powers, the passage, the passenger, and the psyche.
- Describe how the four Ps of labor interrelate to result in the birth of a baby.
- Explain the normal processes of childbirth: premonitory signs, mechanisms of birth, stages and phases of labor.
- Explain how false labor differs from true labor.
- Compare advantages and disadvantages for each type of childbearing setting: hospital, free-standing birth center, and home.
- Determine appropriate nursing care for the intrapartum client, including the woman in false labor and the woman having a vaginal birth after a cesarean birth (VBAC).
- Explain common nursing responsibilities during the birth.
- Determine nursing care of the mother during the immediate postbirth period.

Vocabulary

amnioinfusion
amniotomy
crowning
episiotomy
fontanel
molding
nuchal cord
station
suture
uteroplacental insufficiency
VBAC

Caring for women and their families during the hours of labor is one of the most challenging of nursing roles. The intrapartum nurse must use many skills in addition to those specific to obstetrical nursing when caring for the family at this time—psychosocial, medical, surgical, and pediatric nursing skills. Good communication skills, effective problem solving, sharp observation, empathy, and common sense are valuable assets for the intrapartum nurse.

Childbirth is a normal process, but one word describes the intrapartum unit: *unpredictable.* The number and status of women needing care can change dramatically in a few minutes. Intrapartum nurses must remain flexible to accommodate these changing client needs.

Nursing students are often apprehensive because intrapartum care seems very different from the nursing care they have given before. For example, pain is an expected and normal part of the birth process, but it may be distressing for the student who had negative experiences related to pain during her own births. Other students feel intrusive because of the intimate nature of intrapartum care.

The nursing student who has no children may feel inadequate when assigned to provide care to these women; yet the same student probably would not hesitate to care for a client whose gallbladder was removed. Men are particularly apprehensive about caring for women in the maternity setting. The ideal approach for both men and women nursing students is a professional approach that emphasizes the nurse's caregiving role. Above all, laboring women need compassionate, competent caregivers, regardless of their previous experience or gender.

COMPONENTS OF THE BIRTH PROCESS

Four interrelated components, often called the "four Ps," make up the process of labor and birth. They are (1) the powers, (2) the passage, (3) the passenger, and (4) the psyche.

The Powers

The powers of labor are forces that cause the cervix to open and that propel the fetus downward through the birth canal. The two powers are (1) the uterine contractions and (2) the mother's pushing efforts.

Uterine Contractions

Uterine contractions are the primary power of labor during the first stage (from onset until full dilation of the cervix). Uterine contractions are involuntary smooth muscle contractions; the woman cannot consciously cause them to stop or start. However, their intensity and effectiveness are influenced by a number of factors, such as walking, drugs, maternal anxiety, and vaginal examinations.

Effect of Contractions on the Cervix. Contractions cause the cervix to *efface* (thin) and *dilate* (open) to allow the fetus to descend in the birth canal (Fig. 6–1). Before labor begins, the cervix is a tubular structure about 2 cm long. Contractions simultaneously push the fetus downward as they pull the cervix upward, an action similar to pushing a ball out the cuff of a sock. This causes the cervix to become thinner and shorter. Effacement is determined with a vaginal examination. It is described as a percentage or as its estimated length in centimeters. Thus, if the cervix is 75% effaced, it is about one-quarter of its original length, or 0.5 cm. When the cervix is 100% effaced, it feels like a thin, slick membrane over the fetus.

Dilation of the cervix is determined during a vaginal examination. Dilation is described in centimeters, full dilation being 10 cm (Fig. 6–2). Both dilation and effacement are estimated by touch rather than being precisely measured.

Phases of Contractions. Each contraction has three phases (Fig. 6–3):

- Increment, the period of increasing strength
- Peak, or acme, the period of greatest strength
- Decrement, the period of decreasing strength

Contractions are also described by their average frequency, duration, intensity, and interval.

Frequency. Frequency is the elapsed time from the beginning of one contraction until the beginning of the next contraction. Frequency is described in minutes and fractions of minutes, such as "contractions every 4½ minutes." *Contractions occurring*

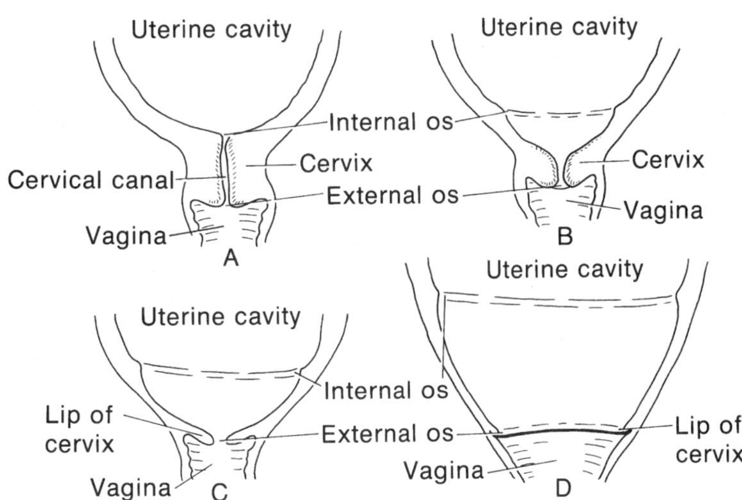

Figure 6–1. • Changes in the cervix during labor. **A,** Before labor the cervix is a tubular structure, about 2 cm long. **B,** The cervix is about 50% effaced (thinned), because it is about half its original length. No cervical dilation has occurred. **C,** The cervix is now completely (100%) effaced and feels like a thin membrane during vaginal examination. Note how the cervix is pulled upward into the lower part of the uterus. Little dilation has occurred. **D,** The cervix is now completely effaced (100%) and dilated (10 cm). (From Moore, M.L. [1983]. *Realities in Childbearing* [2nd ed.]. Philadelphia: Saunders.)

more often than every 2 minutes may reduce fetal oxygen supply.

Duration. Duration is the elapsed time from the beginning of a contraction until the end of the same contraction. Duration is described as the average number of seconds for which contractions last, such as "duration 45–50 seconds." *Persistent contraction durations longer than 90 seconds may reduce fetal oxygen supply.*

Intensity. Intensity is the approximate strength

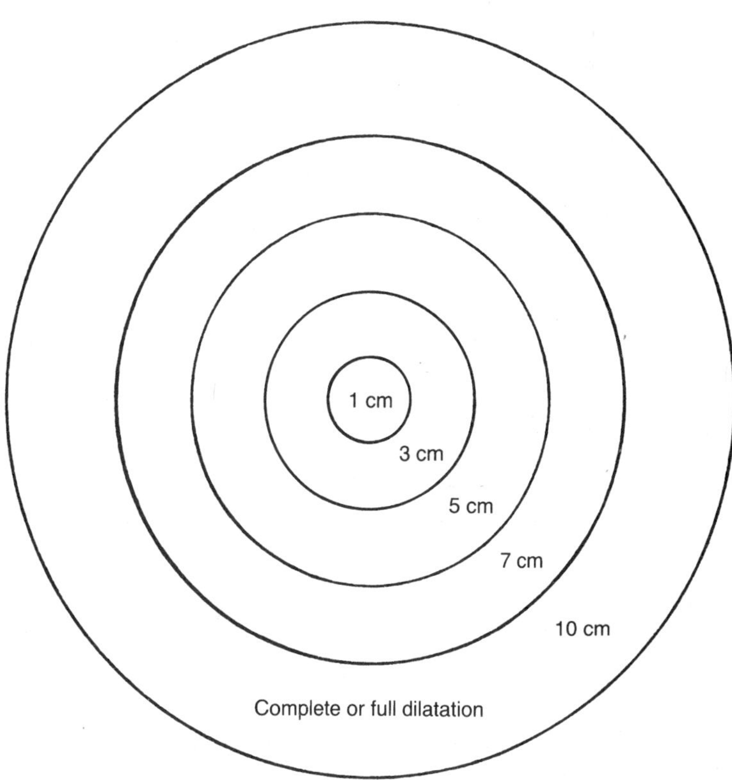

Figure 6–2. • Cervical dilation in centimeters; 10 cm is full dilation.

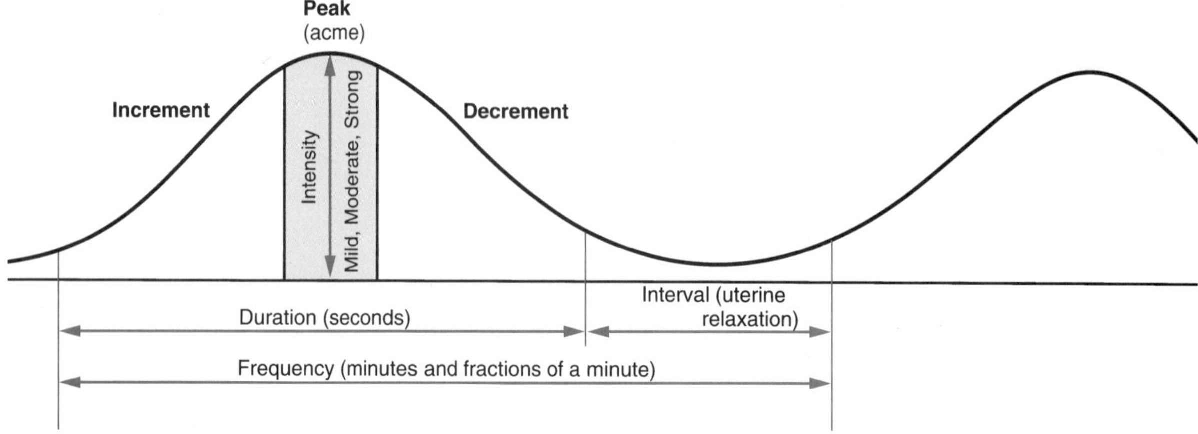

Figure 6–3. • Contraction cycle. Each contraction can be likened to a bell shape, with an increment, peak (acme), and decrement. The frequency of contractions is the average time from the beginning of one to the beginning of the next. The duration is the average time from the beginning to the end of one contraction. The interval is the period of uterine relaxation between contractions.

of the contraction. In most cases, intensity is described in words such as "mild," "moderate," or "strong."

- Mild contractions are easily indented with the fingertips; the uterus feels similar to the tip of the nose
- Moderate contractions can be indented with the fingertips but with more difficulty; the uterus feels similar to the chin
- Firm contractions cannot be readily indented with the fingertips; the uterus feels similar to the forehead

An internal uterine activity monitor (see p. 146) allows recording of the actual pressure within the uterus.

Interval. The interval is the amount of time the uterus relaxes between contractions. Blood flow from the mother into the placenta gradually ceases during contractions and resumes during each interval. The placenta refills with freshly oxygenated blood for the fetus and removes fetal waste products. *Persistent contraction intervals shorter than 60 seconds may reduce fetal oxygen supply.*

Nursing Tip

Report contractions that are more frequent than every 2 minutes, last longer than 90 seconds, or have intervals shorter than 60 seconds to the registered nurse.

Maternal Pushing

When the woman's cervix is fully dilated, she adds voluntary pushing to involuntary uterine contractions. The combined powers of uterine contractions and voluntary maternal pushing propel the fetus downward through the pelvis.

Most women feel a strong urge to push or bear down when the cervix is fully dilated and the fetus begins to descend. However, factors such as maternal exhaustion or sometimes epidural analgesia (see p. 176) may reduce or eliminate the natural urge to push. Some women feel a premature urge to push before the cervix is fully dilated, because the fetus pushes against the rectum.

The Passage

The passage consists of the mother's bony pelvis and the soft tissues (cervix, muscles, ligaments, fascia) of her pelvis and perineum (see p. 31 for a review of the structure of the bony pelvis).

Bony Pelvis. The pelvis is divided into two major parts: (1) the false pelvis (upper, flaring part) and (2) the true pelvis (lower part). The true pelvis is directly involved in childbirth. The true pelvis is further divided into the inlet at the top, the midpelvis in the middle, and the outlet near the perineum. It is shaped somewhat like a curved cylinder or a wide, curved funnel.

Soft Tissues. Women who have had previous vaginal births generally deliver more quickly than women having their first births, because their soft tissues yield more readily to the forces of contractions and pushing efforts. This advantage is not present if the woman's prior births were cesarean. Soft tissue may yield less readily:

- In older mothers
- After cervical procedures that have caused scarring
- After many years between births

The Passenger

The passenger is the fetus, along with the placenta (afterbirth), membranes, and amniotic fluid. Because the fetus usually enters the pelvis head first (cephalic presentation), the nurse should understand the basic structure of the fetal head.

Fetal Head. The fetal head is composed of several bones linked by strong connective tissue, the sutures (Fig. 6–4). A wider area called a fontanel is formed where the sutures meet. Two fontanels are important in obstetrics:

- The anterior fontanel, a diamond-shaped area formed by the intersection of four sutures (frontal, sagittal, and two coronal)
- The posterior fontanel, a tiny triangular depression formed by the intersection of three sutures (the sagittal and two lambdoid)

The sutures and fontanels of the fetal head allow it to change shape as it passes through the pelvis (molding). They are important landmarks in determining how the fetus is oriented within the mother's pelvis during birth.

The main transverse diameter of the fetal head is the biparietal diameter, measured between the points of the two parietal bones on each side of the head. The anteroposterior diameter of the fetal head can vary, depending on how much the head is flexed or extended.

Lie. Lie describes how the fetus is oriented to the mother's spine (Fig. 6–5). The most common one is the longitudinal lie (over 99% of births), in which the fetus is parallel to the mother's spine. The fetus in a transverse lie is at right angles to the mother's spine. The transverse lie may also be called a shoulder presentation. In an oblique lie, the fetus is between a longitudinal and a transverse lie.

Attitude. The fetal attitude is normally one of flexion, with the head flexed forward and the arms and legs flexed. The flexed fetus is compact and ovoid and most efficiently occupies the space in the mother's uterus and pelvis. Extension of the head, arms, and/or legs sometimes occurs.

Presentation. Presentation refers to the fetal part that enters the pelvis first. The cephalic presentation is the most common one. Any of four variations of cephalic presentations can occur, depending on the extent to which the fetal head is flexed (Fig. 6–6).

- The *vertex presentation,* with the fetal head fully flexed, is the most favorable cephalic variation because the smallest possible diameter of the head enters the pelvis. It occurs in about 96% of births.
- The *military presentation* is one in which the fetal head is neither flexed nor extended.
- The *brow presentation* is one in which the fetal head is partly extended. The longest diameter of the fetal head is presenting. This presentation is unstable and tends to convert to either a vertex or a face presentation.
- The *face presentation* is one in which the head is fully extended and the face presents.

The next most common presentation is the breech (about 3%–4% of term births). There are three variations of the breech presentation (Fig. 6–7):

- The *frank breech,* with the fetal legs flexed at the hips and extending toward the shoulders, is the most common.
- The *complete breech* is a reversal of the cephalic presentation, with flexion of the head and extremities.
- The *footling breech* is one in which one or both feet present.

Many women with a fetus in the breech presentation have cesarean births because the head, which is the largest single fetal part, is the last to be born and may be too big to pass through the pelvis. After the fetal body is born, the head must be delivered quickly so that the fetus can breathe, because at this point part of the umbilical cord is outside and the remaining part is subject to compression by the fetal head against the bony pelvis.

When the fetus is in a transverse lie, the fetal shoulder enters the pelvis first. A fetus in this orientation must be born by cesarean delivery because it cannot pass through the pelvis.

Position. Position refers to how a reference point on the fetal presenting part is oriented within the mother's pelvis. The *occiput* is used to describe how the head is oriented if the fetus is in a cephalic vertex presentation. The *sacrum* is used to describe how a fetus in a breech presentation is oriented within the pelvis. The shoulder and back are reference points if the fetus is in a shoulder presentation.

The pelvis is divided into four imaginary quadrants: right and left anterior, and right and left posterior. If the fetal occiput is in the left front quadrant of the mother's pelvis, it is described as left occiput anterior. If the sacrum of a fetus in a breech presentation is in the mother's right posterior pelvis, it is described as right sacrum posterior. See Figure 6–8 for various fetal presentations and positions.

Abbreviations describe the fetal presentation and position within the pelvis (Box 6–1). Three letters are used for most abbreviations:

- *First letter:* Right or left side of the woman's pelvis. This letter is omitted if the fetal reference point is directly anterior or posterior, such as occiput anterior (OA).
- *Second letter:* Fetal reference point (occiput for vertex presentations; mentum [chin] for face presentations; and sacrum for breech presentations).

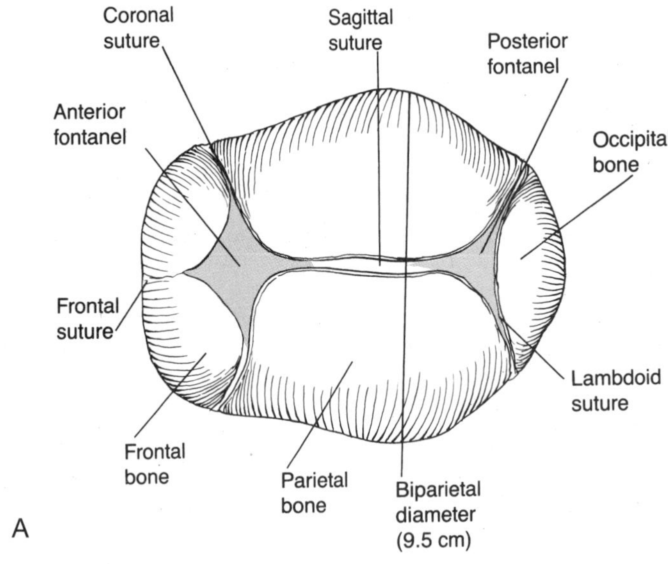

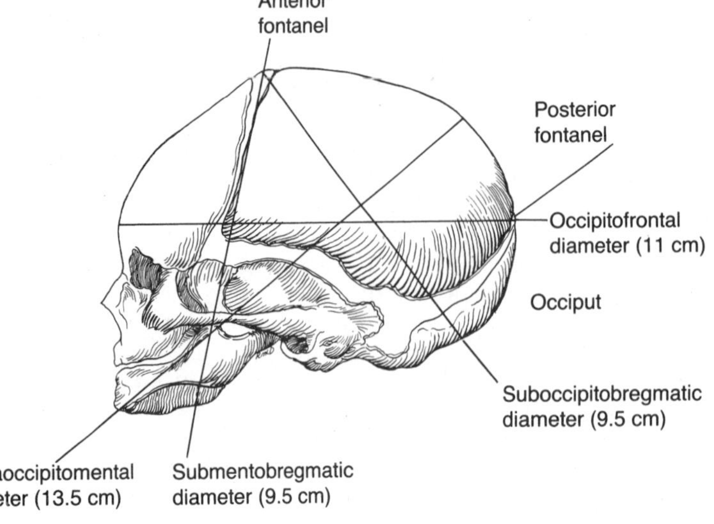

Figure 6–4. • **A,** Bones, sutures, and fontanels of the fetal head. Note that the anterior fontanel has a diamond shape; the posterior fontanel is triangular. **B,** Side view of the fetal head. Note how the anteroposterior diameter will change as the fetal head becomes more or less flexed.

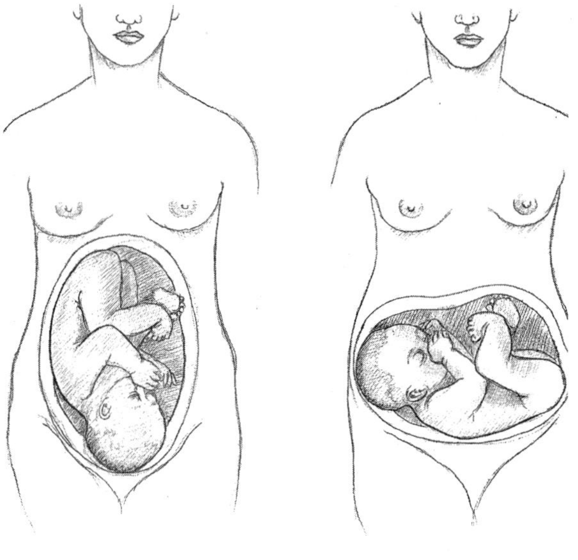

Figure 6–5. • Lie. In the longitudinal lie, the fetus is parallel to the mother's spine. In the transverse lie, or shoulder presentation, the fetus is at right angles to the mother's spine.

- *Third letter:* Front or back of the mother's pelvis (anterior or posterior). Transverse (T) denotes a fetal position that is neither anterior nor posterior.

The bregma (brow) may be specified when the fetal head is partly extended in the brow presentation, but it is not usually important to abbreviate this position because it tends to convert to either a vertex or a face presentation. Four-letter abbreviations exist for shoulder presentations, but they are not used often.

The Psyche

Childbirth is more than a physical process; it involves the woman's entire being. Women do not recount the births of their children in the same manner that they do surgical procedures. They describe births in emotional terms like those they use to describe marriages, anniversaries, religious events, or even deaths. Families are having fewer children, and they often have greater expectations about the birth *experience.* The nurse can promote a positive childbearing experience by incorporat-

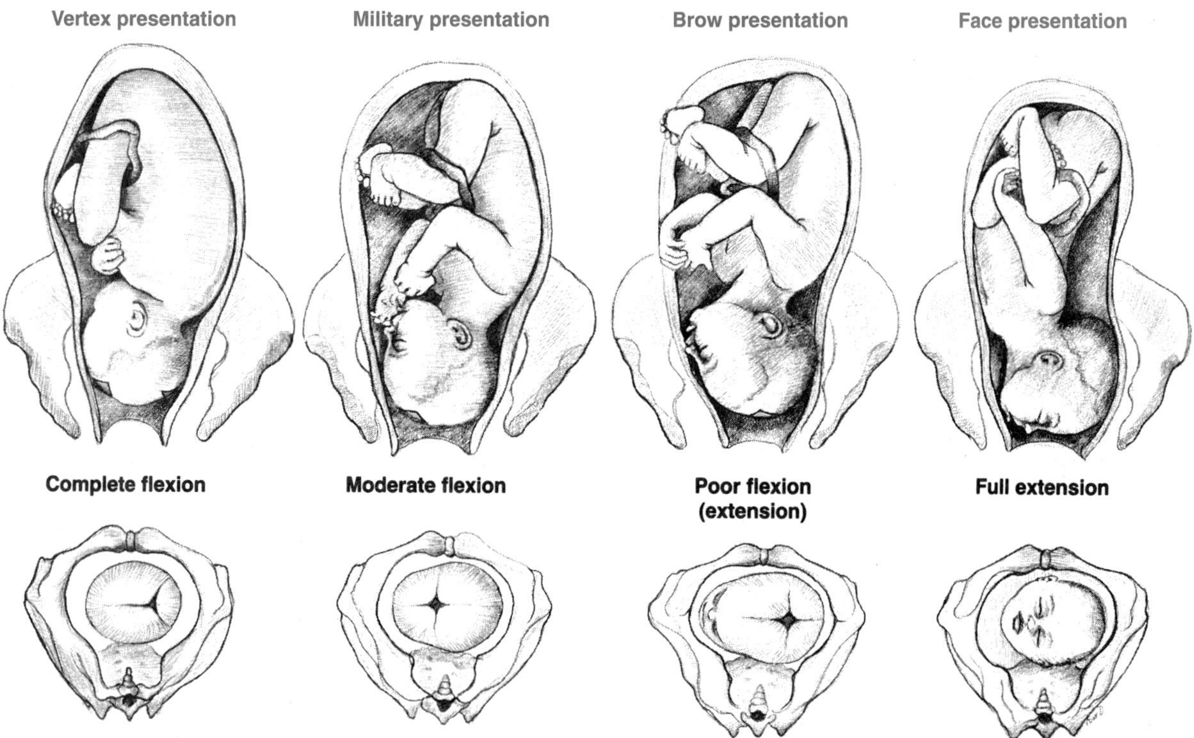

Figure 6–6. • Four types of cephalic presentation. The vertex presentation, in which the fetal chin is flexed on the chest, is the most favorable for vaginal birth because it allows the smallest diameter of the head to go through the pelvis. Note how the anterior and posterior fontanels can be used during vaginal examination to determine the fetal presentation and position in the pelvis.

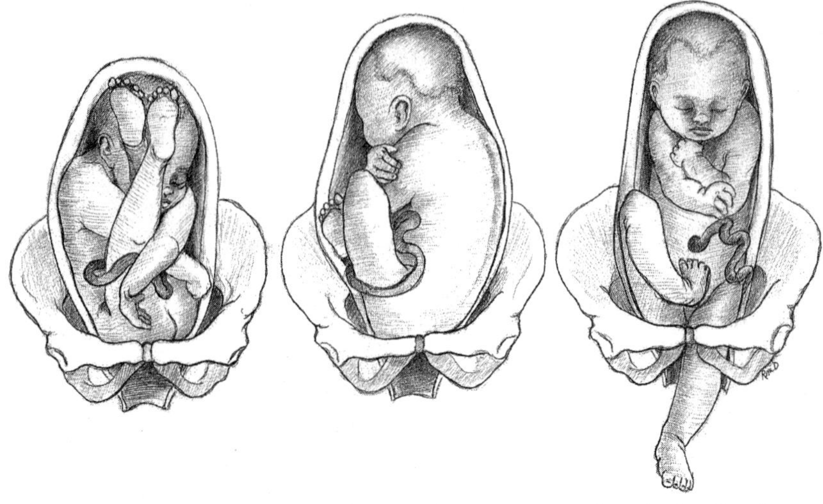

Figure 6–7. • Three variations of the breech presentation. Frank breech is the most common variation. Footling breeches may be single, with one foot presenting, or double, with both feet presenting.

ing as many of the family's birth expectations as possible.

A woman's mental state can influence the course of her labor. For example, the woman who is relaxed and optimistic during labor is better able to tolerate discomfort and work with the physiologic processes. By contrast, marked anxiety can increase her perception of pain and reduce her tolerance of it. Anxiety and fear also cause secretion of stress compounds from the adrenal glands. These compounds, called catecholamines, inhibit uterine contractions and divert blood flow from the placenta.

A woman's cultural and individual values influence how she views and copes with childbirth. For example, the father's presence is encouraged in most birth facilities in the United States. However, if the family's culture is one in which childbirth is truly "woman's work," the father may feel uncomfortable at her side during labor. If they are of the same culture, the woman is unlikely to welcome his nearness at this time either.

Culture influences, but does not dictate, how a woman behaves in labor. For example, in cultures that value stoicism, a woman may quietly endure labor pain without complaint. Other cultural groups express their feelings openly; women from these groups may respond loudly and vigorously to labor.

The nurse must remember that people are individuals within their culture. It is helpful if the nurse knows common cultural beliefs and practices with the populations cared for, but each client or family must be individually assessed. The nurse must think critically when planning care, not simply make assumptions about people.

> **Nursing Tip**
>
> Provide emotional support to the laboring woman so that she is less anxious and fearful. Excessive anxiety or fear can cause greater pain, inhibit progress of labor, and reduce blood flow to the placenta.

NORMAL CHILDBIRTH

The specific event that triggers the onset of labor remains unknown. There are probably many factors that play a part in initiating labor. Labor normally begins when the fetus is mature enough to adjust easily to life outside the uterus yet is still small enough to fit through the mother's pelvis. This point is usually reached between 38 and 42 weeks after the mother's last menstrual period.

Signs of Impending Labor

Signs and symptoms that labor is about to start may occur from a few hours to a few weeks before the actual onset of labor.

Braxton-Hicks Contractions. Braxton-Hicks contractions are irregular contractions that begin dur-

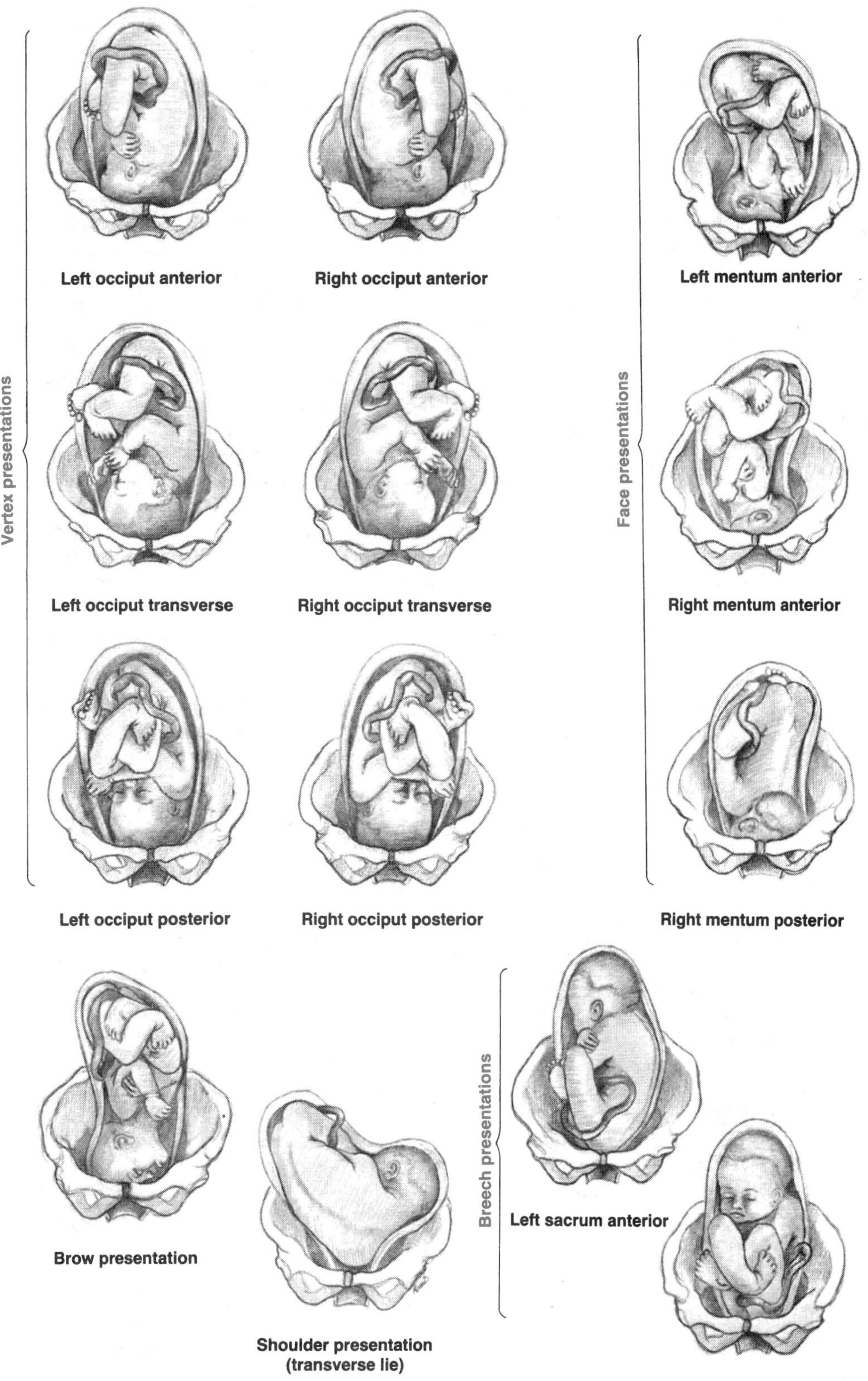

Figure 6–8. • Fetal presentations and positions. The left and right occiput anterior positions are most favorable for normal labor. The occiput posterior positions are often associated with back labor.

BOX 6–1

CLASSIFICATIONS OF FETAL PRESENTATIONS AND POSITIONS

Cephalic Presentations

Vertex	LOA	Left occiput anterior
	ROA	Right occiput anterior
	ROT	Right occiput transverse
	LOT	Left occiput transverse
	OA	Occiput anterior
	OP	Occiput posterior
Face	LMA	Left mentum anterior
	RMA	Right mentum anterior
	LMP	Left mentum posterior
	RMP	Right mentum posterior

Breech Presentations

LSA	Left sacrum anterior
RSA	Right sacrum anterior
LSP	Left sacrum posterior
RSP	Right sacrum posterior

Abbreviations that designate brow, military, and shoulder presentations are not included here because these presentations occur infrequently.

ing early pregnancy and intensify as full term approaches. They often become regular and somewhat uncomfortable, leading many women to believe labor has started (see discussion of true and false labor). Although Braxton-Hicks contractions are often called "false" labor, they play a part in preparing the cervix to dilate and in adjusting the fetal position within the uterus.

Increased Vaginal Discharge. Fetal pressure causes an increase in clear and nonirritating vaginal secretions. Irritation or itching with the increased secretions is not normal and should be reported to the physician or certified nurse-midwife (CNM) because these symptoms are characteristic of infection.

Bloody Show. As the time for birth approaches, the cervix undergoes changes in preparation for labor. It softens ("ripens"), effaces, and dilates slightly. When this occurs, the mucous plug that has sealed the uterus during pregnancy is dislodged from the cervix, tearing small capillaries in the process. Bloody show is thick mucus mixed with pink or dark-brown blood. It may begin a few days before labor, or a woman may not have bloody show until labor is under way. Bloody show may also occur if the woman has had a recent vaginal examination or intercourse.

Rupture of the Membranes. The amniotic sac (bag of waters) sometimes ruptures before labor begins. Infection is more likely if many hours elapse between rupture of membranes and birth, because the amniotic sac seals the uterine cavity against organisms from the vagina. In addition, the fetal umbilical cord may slip down and become compressed between the mother's pelvis and fetal presenting part. For these two reasons, women should go to the birth facility when their membranes rupture, even if they have no other signs of labor.

Energy Spurt. Many women have a sudden burst of energy shortly before the onset of labor ("nesting"). The nurse should teach women to conserve their strength, even if they feel unusually energetic.

Weight Loss. An occasional woman may notice that she loses 1 to 3 pounds shortly before labor begins as hormone changes cause her to excrete extra body water.

True and False Labor

Many women have contractions and other symptoms that make them think they are in labor. However, when they go to the birth facility, their cervix does not efface or dilate within a short observation period (about 1 or 2 hours). If all signs are normal, they usually return home to await true labor.

True labor is characterized by progress (i.e., cervical change). Change in the cervix (effacement and/or dilation) is the key distinction between false labor and true labor. See Table 6–1 for other char-

Table 6–1
COMPARISON OF TRUE LABOR AND FALSE LABOR

False Labor (Prodromal Labor or Prelabor)	True Labor
Contractions are irregular or do not increase in frequency, duration, and intensity	Contractions gradually develop a regular pattern and become more frequent, longer, and more intense
Walking tends to relieve or decrease contractions	Contractions become stronger and more effective with walking
Discomfort is felt in the abdomen and groin	Discomfort is felt in the lower back and lower abdomen; often feels like menstrual cramps at first
Bloody show is usually not present	Bloody show is often present, especially in women having their first baby
No change in effacement or dilation of the cervix occurs	Progressive effacement and dilation of the cervix occur

Engagement, Descent, Flexion

Internal Rotation

External Rotation (Restitution)

Extension Beginning (Rotation Complete)

External Rotation (Shoulder Rotation)

Extension Complete

Expulsion

Figure 6–9. • The mechanisms of labor, also called cardinal movements. The positional changes allow the fetus to fit through the pelvis with the least resistance. (From Ross Laboratories. [1979]. *Clinical education aid no. 13, G169.* Columbus, OH: Author. Reprinted with permission of Ross Laboratories.)

acteristics that distinguish true labor from false labor.

Mechanisms of Labor

As the fetus descends into the pelvis, it undergoes several positional changes so that it adapts optimally to the changing pelvic shape and size. Many of these mechanisms, also called cardinal movements, occur simultaneously (Fig. 6–9).

Descent. Descent is required for all other mechanisms to occur and for the baby to be born. *Station* describes the level of the presenting part, usually the head, in the pelvis. Station is estimated in centimeters from the level of the ischial spines in the mother's pelvis (a zero station). Minus stations are above the ischial spines; plus stations are below the ischial spines (Fig. 6–10). As the fetus descends, the minus numbers get smaller (e.g., –2, –1) and the plus numbers get higher (+1, +2, etc.).

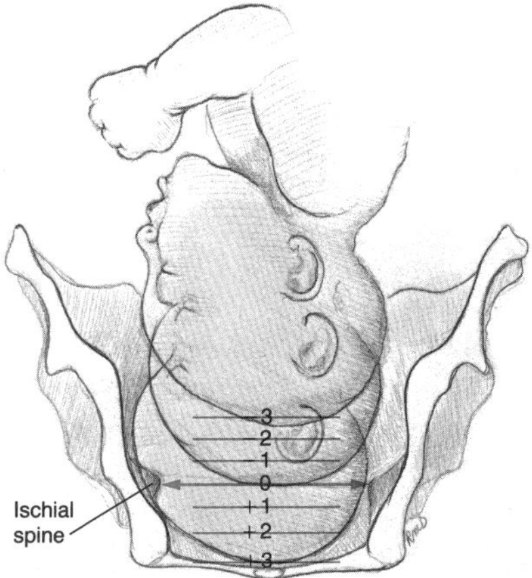

Figure 6–10. • Station describes the level of the fetal presenting part in relation to the ischial spines of the mother's pelvis. It is determined with vaginal examination. "Minus" stations are above the ischial spines; "plus" stations are below the ischial spines.

Engagement. Engagement occurs when the biparietal diameter of the fetal head reaches the level of the ischial spines of the mother's pelvis (presenting part is at a zero station or lower). Engagement often occurs before labor's onset in the woman who has not given birth (a nullipara); it may not occur until well after labor begins if the woman has had prior births (a multipara).

Flexion. To pass most easily through the pelvis, the fetal head should be flexed. As labor progresses, uterine contractions increase the amount of fetal head flexion until the fetal chin is on the chest.

Internal Rotation. When the fetus enters the pelvis, the head is usually oriented so that the occiput is toward the mother's right or left side. As the fetus is pushed downward by contractions, the curved, cylindrical shape of the pelvis causes the head to turn until the occiput is directly under the symphysis pubis (occiput anterior, or OA).

Extension. As the fetal head passes under the mother's symphysis pubis, it must change from flexion to extension so that it can properly negotiate the curve. To do this, the fetal neck stops under the symphysis, which acts as a pivot. The head swings anteriorly as it extends with each maternal push until it is born.

External Rotation. When the head is born in extension, the shoulders are crosswise in the pelvis and the head is somewhat twisted in relation to the shoulders. The head spontaneously turns to one side as it realigns with the shoulders (restitution). The shoulders then rotate within the pelvis until their transverse diameter is aligned with the mother's anteroposterior pelvis. The head turns farther to the side as the shoulders rotate within the pelvis.

Expulsion. The anterior shoulder and then the posterior shoulder are born, quickly followed by the rest of the body.

Stages and Phases of Labor

Women giving birth display common physical and behavioral characteristics in each of four stages of labor. Those who have epidural analgesia during labor may not exhibit the behaviors and sensations associated with each stage and phase. The nurse must also realize that women are individuals and that each responds to labor in her own way. Table 6–2 summarizes the stages and phases of labor.

First Stage

The first stage of labor is the *stage of dilation.* It describes the time from the onset of labor until full dilation of the cervix. The first stage is usually the longest for both nulliparas and for multiparas. Duration of the first stage averages 8 to 10 hours for the nullipara and 6 to 7 hours for the multipara.

Three phases occur within first stage labor: (1) latent phase; (2) active phase; and (3) transition phase. The exact amount of cervical dilation that characterizes each phase is variable. However other important characteristics, such as contraction frequency, duration and intensity, or maternal behavior, distinguish each phase from the other two.

Latent Phase. The latent phase of labor is often completed before the woman enters the birth facility. It comprises about the first 3 cm of cervical dilation. The cervix effaces almost completely during the latent phase of a nullipara's labor; the multipara's cervix often remains thicker, even during advanced labor.

During the latent phase of labor, contractions gradually increase in strength and intensity. They are mild and infrequent in the early part of this phase, increasing to moderate intensity with a frequency of about 5 minutes during the later part.

The woman is usually sociable and excited. She is cooperative but somewhat anxious. She is relatively comfortable, although many women describe sensations similar to menstrual cramps or lower back discomfort.

Active Phase. Active labor is well-named because the pace of labor picks up as the cervix dilates from about 4 to 7 cm. Effacement is completed during the active phase. Contractions intensify until they are about 3 minutes apart, last about 45 seconds or longer, and are moderate to firm.

The expectant mother becomes less sociable, although she is still cooperative. Mentally, she turns inward and concentrates on the task of giving birth. Most women who take analgesia request it during this phase.

Transition Phase. Transition is an intense, shorter phase of labor during which the cervix dilates from 8 to 10 cm. Contractions are firm, 2 to 3 minutes apart; the duration of some may be as long as 90 seconds.

The mother often feels as if she is losing control and thinks that labor will never be over. She often becomes uncooperative and even hostile to her partner and caregivers. The partner and nurse should not be offended by the mother's irritability because it is normal behavior during this phase and means that labor will soon end.

Second Stage

The second stage of labor is the *stage of expulsion,* from the time of full cervical dilation (10 cm) until

Table 6–2
STAGES AND PHASES OF LABOR

Stage	Characteristics	Nursing Care
First Stage (stage of dilation)	Average duration: nullipara, 8–10 hr; multipara, 6–7 hr; onset of labor until full dilation of cervix	
Latent Phase	Onset of labor until about 3 cm of cervical dilation Cervix effaces almost completely in the nullipara; may remain thick in the multipara Contractions mild and infrequent at first; gradually increase to moderate intensity, about every 5 min Woman is usually relatively comfortable Woman is sociable and excited, although somewhat anxious	Orient woman and her partner to the labor area Review parents' birth plan, if they have made one; ask if they have any specific requests about how labor and birth are conducted Monitor fetus by intermittent auscultation or with electronic fetal monitoring (continuous or intermittent) Monitor woman's vital signs (temperature every 4 hr, or every 2 hr after membranes rupture); assess pulse, respirations, and blood pressure hourly Teach or review coping skills, such as breathing techniques Encourage walking if there is no contraindication Initiate procedures such as laboratory examinations, signing permits
Active Phase	Cervix dilates from 4 to 7 cm; effacement is completed Membranes may rupture Contractions intensify until about 3 min apart, duration 45 sec or longer; intensity is moderate to firm Woman concentrates inwardly, although still cooperative May need analgesia or epidural block during this phase	Continue fetal and maternal assessments Observe amniotic fluid for color, quantity, and odor when the membranes rupture Provide general comfort measures, such as attention to her environment, hygiene Encourage changes of position about every half hour; avoid the supine position Watch for bladder distention Assist the woman to use breathing and relaxation techniques (see Chapter 7) Provide reassurance, praise, and support for both the laboring woman and her partner
Transition Phase	Cervix dilates from 8 to 10 cm Intense contractions, firm, 2–3 min apart; duration of some may be as long as 90 sec Woman may become uncooperative and irritable	Continue maternal and fetal assessments Continue comfort measures, but do not disturb the woman unnecessarily Reassure woman and her partner that this is a short, intense phase and that she will regain control

Table continued on following page

the baby's birth. The average duration of the second stage is 50 minutes in the nullipara, although it may last 2 hours or longer. The multipara usually has a second stage averaging 20 minutes. As in the first stage, there is a wide variation in duration of the second stage of labor. Contractions are firm, although they may be slightly less frequent and slightly shorter than during transition.

The woman often describes an involuntary urge to push, or to bear down, with each contraction as the fetal presenting part presses on her rectum. She may say, "I have to push," or "I need to have a bowel movement" when this occurs. Epidural analgesia can prolong the second stage of labor if it depresses the woman's natural urge to push. However, many women who have epidural analgesia can feel the urge to push, although not as intensely as the woman who did not choose this form of pain management. (See p. 176 for further discussion of epidural analgesia.)

The mother usually regains control during the second stage and often says that pushing feels good or makes her feel useful. She may push intensely during contractions yet seem oblivious to her surroundings when each contraction ends. She is simultaneously tired and excited as the second stage ends with her baby's birth.

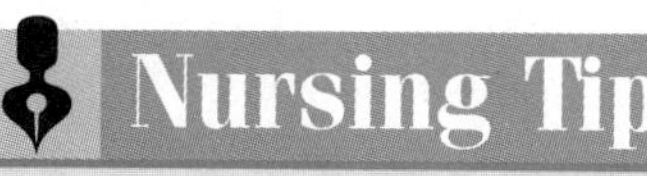

If a woman suddenly loses control and becomes irritable, suspect that she has progressed to the transition phase of labor.

Table 6–2
STAGES AND PHASES OF LABOR *(Continued)*

Stage	Characteristics	Nursing Care
Second Stage (stage of expulsion)	Average duration: nullipara, 50 min; multipara, 20 min; duration varies among women Cervix fully dilated (10 cm) Rectal pressure as fetus descends results in urge to push with contractions; women with epidural block may not have strong urge to push Contractions are still intense but may be slightly less so than in transition phase	Continue comfort measures, reassurance, support, maternal and fetal assessments Observe for perineal bulging and crowning of the fetal head Coach woman in effective pushing techniques; advise her to exhale while pushing or hold her breath for no longer than 4–6 sec Make final preparations for birth (multiparas are prepared earlier than nulliparas)
Third Stage (placental stage)	Average duration: 5–10 min; up to 30 min Woman may feel a slight cramp when placenta detaches Uterus must contract firmly to control bleeding Woman is fatigued and excited; wants to see baby	Give medications such as oxytocin (Pitocin) or put baby to mother's breast to facilitate uterine contraction Observe for blood loss Give initial care to the infant, focusing on respirations and temperature maintenance
Fourth Stage (immediate postbirth recovery)	First 1–4 hr after birth Uterus should remain firmly contracted, about halfway between the woman's umbilicus and symphysis pubis (higher if infant was large) Bleeding (lochia rubra) should saturate no more than one pad per hour Afterpains (uterine cramping) may occur	Assess woman's temperature at beginning of recovery period, then hourly Assess pulse, respirations, blood pressure every 15 min the first hour, every 30 min the second hour, then hourly Assess uterine fundus for firmness, height, and deviation from the midline with each blood pressure check; massage if not firm Have woman urinate if bleeding is excessive or if the uterus is high or not in the midline of the abdomen; catheterize her if she cannot urinate Provide analgesia if needed; place ice compresses to her perineum as needed

Third Stage

The third stage of labor is the *placental stage,* extending from the birth of the baby until the placenta detaches and is expelled. It is the shortest stage, lasting an average of 5 to 10 minutes, although 30 minutes is also normal.

The placenta may be expelled in one of two ways. If the shiny fetal side of the placenta exits first, the placenta is expelled in the more common *Schultze mechanism.* The *Duncan mechanism* describes the exit of the placenta with the rough maternal side presenting (see Fig. 6–11). The birth attendant will examine the placenta to be certain that all of it was expelled. Small bits of placenta that remain in the uterus interfere with uterine contractions that control bleeding.

The uterus must promptly contract and remain contracted after placental expulsion, to control bleeding from the vessels that supplied the placenta before birth. Oxytocin (Pitocin) stimulates the uterus to contract firmly. Oxytocin is usually added to the intravenous infusion or can be given by intravenous push or intramuscularly. The infant's suckling at the mother's breast stimulates uterine contractions because it causes her posterior pituitary gland to release natural oxytocin. External massage also stimulates uterine contraction to control blood loss.

Pain is usually minimal during the third stage. The mother feels brief cramping as the placenta detaches and is expelled. She is tired and excited and wants to see her baby.

Fourth Stage

The fourth stage of labor is the first 1 to 4 hours following birth. The uterus should be easily felt through the abdominal wall as a round, firm object about the size of a grapefruit. It should be centered in the midline, about halfway between the umbilicus and the symphysis pubis. The actual fundal height depends on the size of the infant, and will be higher if a large baby was born. It will appear higher in a short woman, as well.

The woman often has a chill for about 20 to 30 minutes after birth. The cause is unknown, but it stops spontaneously. Discomfort is usually minimal during the fourth stage. Perineal discomfort from bruising, lacerations, or an episiotomy (surgical opening to enlarge the vaginal outlet) is usually felt as a burning or throbbing pain. Some women, especially multiparas or those who had a large baby, have afterpains, or cramping, as the uterus alternately contracts and relaxes.

The woman's bladder fills rapidly after birth because of intravenous fluids given during labor and because fluid retained in her tissues during pregnancy quickly returns to her circulation for excretion. A full bladder can cause excessive bleeding because it pushes the uterus upward and interferes with contraction. The uterus is often displaced to one side when the bladder is full.

The woman is tired, but eager to see and hold her baby. The fourth stage of labor is an ideal time to promote bonding between the family and the new baby.

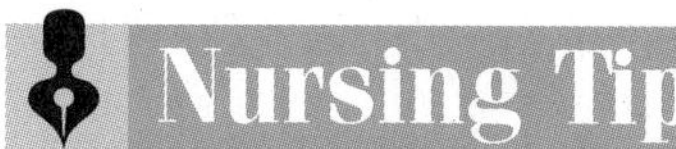

The woman who is having a vaginal birth after cesarean delivery needs special emotional support. She is often anxious, and a cesarean may seem like the easiest way to end her pregnancy.

Vaginal Birth after Cesarean Birth

It was once thought that a woman who had a cesarean delivery for one infant must have a surgical birth for every subsequent infant. Today, physicians carefully select women who are appropriate candidates for *vaginal birth after cesarean (VBAC)*. Of women who have previous cesarean births, 60% to 80% can deliver vaginally (ACOG, 1995a; Cunningham et al., 1997). See pp. 195–198 for more information about cesarean birth and subsequent vaginal births.

Nursing care for women who plan a VBAC is similar to that for women who have had no cesarean births. The main concern is that the uterine scar will rupture (see p. 211), which can disrupt the placental blood flow and cause hemorrhage. Observation for signs of uterine rupture should be part of the nursing care for all laboring women, regardless of whether they have had a cesarean birth.

Women having VBAC often need more support than other laboring women. They are often anxious about their ability to cope with labor's demands

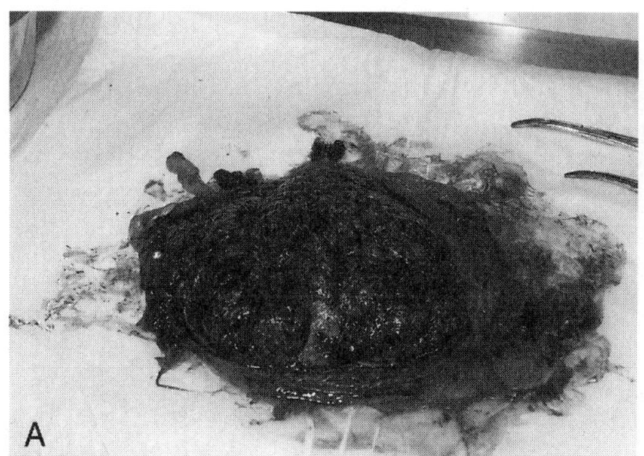

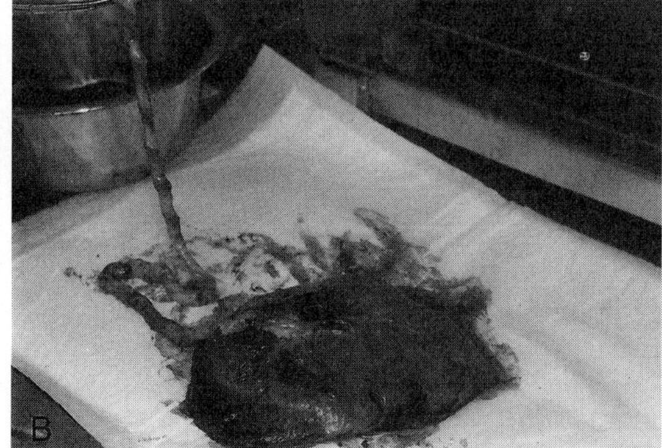

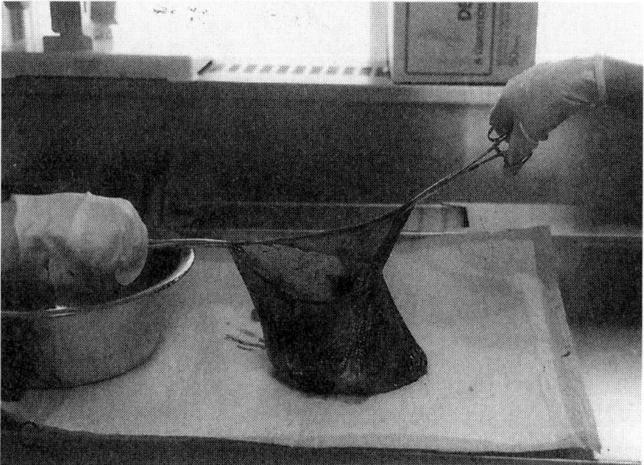

Figure 6–11. • The placenta after delivery. **A,** Maternal side (Duncan delivery). **B,** Fetal side (Schultze delivery). **C,** The amniotic sac, which housed the fetus during intrauterine life.

and to deliver vaginally, especially if they have never done so. If their cesarean birth occurred during labor, rather than before labor started, they may become anxious when they reach the same point in the current labor. The nurse must provide empathy and support to help the woman to cross this psychological barrier. However, the nurse cannot promise the woman that a repeat cesarean birth will not be needed because one may be required for many reasons.

SETTINGS FOR CHILDBIRTH

Depending on facilities available in their area and whether complications are likely, a woman can choose among three settings in which to deliver her baby. Most women give birth in the hospital, whereas others choose free-standing birth facilities. A few women choose home.

Hospitals

Hospital births can take place in a traditional setting, in a birthing room, or in a single-room maternity care setting. The woman who chooses a hospital birth may have a "traditional" setting, in which she labors, delivers, and recovers in three separate rooms. After the recovery period, she is transferred to the postpartum unit.

A more common setting for hospital maternity care is the birthing room, often called an LDR (labor-delivery-recovery) room. The woman labors, delivers, and recovers in this room. She is then transferred to the postpartum unit for continuing care.

The birthing room has a more homelike than institutional appearance. The fully functional birthing bed has wood trim that hides its utilitarian purpose (Fig. 6–12). The beds have receptacles for various fittings, such as a "squat bar," which facilitates squatting during second stage labor. The foot of the bed can be detached or rolled away to reveal foot supports or stirrups. They can be used as operating tables in an emergency, although they are wider than conventional operating room tables. A birthing chair is available in some settings. The mother's position is similar to that in a birthing bed when using a squat bar.

Another hospital birth setting is a single-room maternity care arrangement, often called an LDRP (labor-delivery-recovery-postpartum) room. It is similar to the LDR, but the mother and infant remain in the same room until discharge.

Advantages of hospital-based birth settings include the following:

- Easy access to sophisticated services and specialized personnel if complications develop
- Ability to provide family-centered care to the woman who has a complicated pregnancy

Disadvantages include the following:

- Higher overall costs because the hospital must provide expensive services such as emergency, anesthesia, and critical care departments as well as care for uncomplicated labor

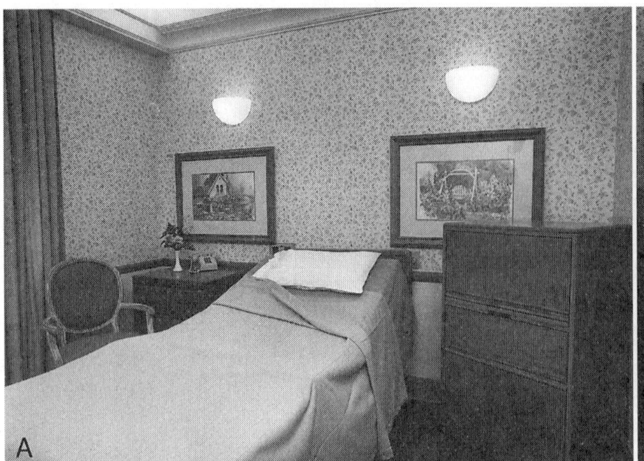

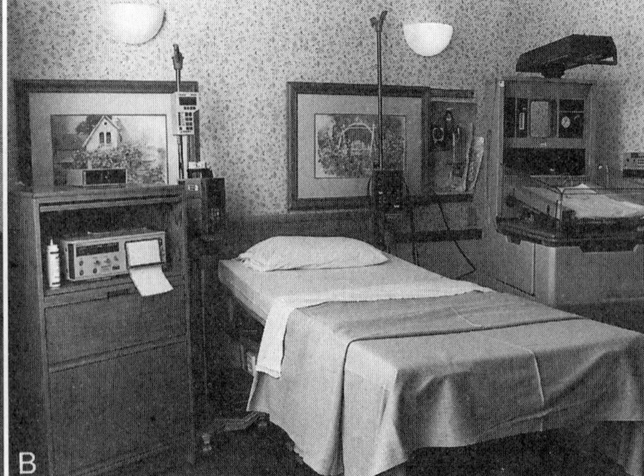

Figure 6–12. • **A,** A typical labor, delivery, and recovery room. **B,** Homelike furnishings can be quickly adapted to provide essential equipment for the birth. (From Gorrie, T.M., McKinney, E.S., & Murray, S.S. [1994]. *Foundations of maternal newborn nursing.* Philadelphia: Saunders.)

- Limited choice of birth attendants (i.e., physician or CNM)

Free-Standing Birth Centers

Some communities have birth centers that are separate from, although usually nearby, hospitals. These settings are similar to outpatient surgical centers. Many birth centers are operated by full-service hospitals and are close enough for easy transfer if the mother, fetus, or newborn develops complications. CNMs often attend the births.

Advantages of free-standing birth centers include the following:

- A homelike setting for the low-risk woman
- Lower costs because the free-standing center does not require expensive departments, such as emergency or critical care

Disadvantages include the following

- A slight, but significant, delay in emergency care if the mother or baby develops life-threatening complications

Home

Some women have their babies at home. Many factors enter their decision, and most families have carefully weighed the pros and cons of their choice.

Advantages of a home birth include the following:

- Control over persons who will or will not be present for the labor and birth, including children
- No risk of acquiring pathogens from other clients
- A low-technology birth, which is important to some families

Disadvantages may include the following and vary with the area of the country:

- Limited choice of birth attendants. Most physicians will not attend home births, and many nurse-midwives will not, either. In many communities, only lay midwives, whose training and abilities vary widely, attend home births. Lay midwives may not operate legally in every state.
- Significant delay in reaching emergency care if the mother or baby develops life-threatening complications
- No preestablished relationship with a physician if the woman or newborn must be transferred to the hospital

ADMISSION TO THE HOSPITAL OR BIRTH CENTER

Intrapartum nursing care begins before admission by educating the woman about the appropriate time to come to the facility. Nursing care includes admission assessments and initiation of needed procedures. Many women have false labor and are discharged after a short observation period; nursing care of these clients is included.

When to Go to the Hospital or Birth Center

During late pregnancy the woman should be instructed about when to go to the hospital or birth center. This is not an exact time, but general guidelines are as follows:

- *Contractions.* The woman should go to the hospital or birth center when the contractions have a pattern of increasing frequency, duration, and intensity. The woman having her first baby is usually advised to enter the facility when contractions are regular (every 5 minutes) for 1 hour. Women having second or later babies should go sooner, when regular contractions are 10 minutes apart for a period of 1 hour.
- *Ruptured membranes.* The woman should go to the facility if her membranes rupture or if she thinks they may have ruptured.
- *Bleeding, other than bloody show.* Bloody show is a mixture of blood and thick mucus. Active bleeding is free-flowing, bright red, and not mixed with thick mucus.
- *Decreased fetal movement.* If the fetus is moving less than usual, the woman should be evaluated. Many fetuses become quiet shortly before labor, but decreased fetal activity can also be a sign of fetal compromise or fetal demise (death).
- *Any other concern.* Because these guidelines cannot cover every situation, the woman should go to the birth facility for evaluation if she has any other concerns.

Infection Control in the Intrapartum Area

The nurse must observe appropriate infection control measures when providing care in any clinical area. Standard precautions apply to several potentially infectious body fluids and many of these are encountered during childbirth: blood, amniotic fluid, and vaginal secretions. In addition, many drugs are parenterally (intramuscularly or intravenously) administered, and sharp instruments are used, thus increasing the nurse's risk for injury and infection. General guidelines for wearing protective gear in the intrapartal area include the following:

- Wear clean gloves (or sterile ones, if appropriate) when contact with any body substance is anticipated. Examples of these situations would be when doing shave preps or enemas, changing disposable underpads or linens, giving perineal care, and changing perineal pads. The newborn infant should be handled with gloves until after the first bath.
- Wear a water-repellent cover gown when exposure to larger amounts of body substances is likely. The nurse wears a water-repellent cover garment during birth to avoid contamination when handling the infant.
- Wear mask and eye shields if splashing of mucous membranes is likely, such as when "scrubbed in" for vaginal or cesarean birth, or if working near an area where blood splashing might occur. When the cord is cut, blood can spurt a surprising distance from the cut end.

See Appendix A for more information about standard precautions.

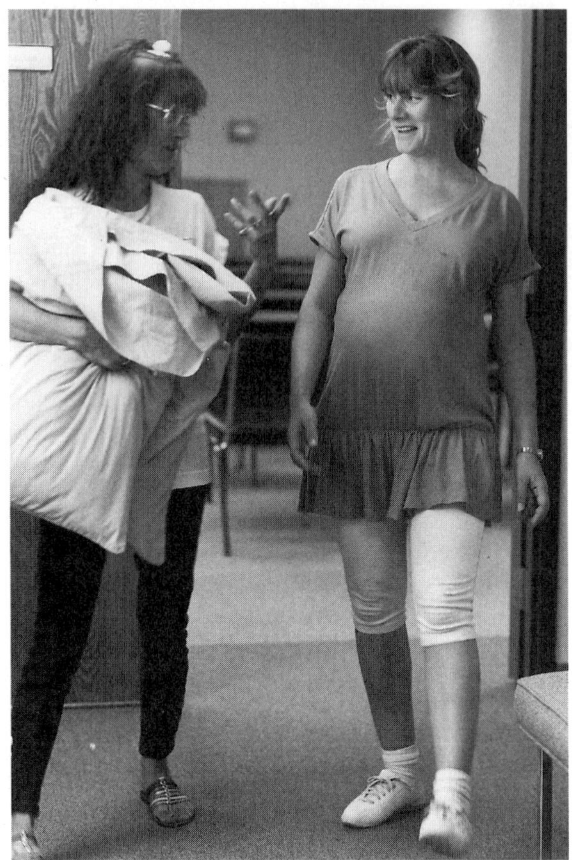

Figure 6–13. • This expectant mother arrives at the birth facility with her friend who is her labor partner. (From Gorrie, T.M., McKinney, E.S., & Murray, S.S. [1994]. *Foundations of maternal newborn nursing*. Philadelphia: Saunders.)

Admission Assessments

When a woman is admitted, the nurse establishes a therapeutic relationship by welcoming her and her family members (Fig. 6–13). The nurse continues developing the therapeutic relationship during labor by determining her expectations about birth and trying to help her to achieve these expectations. Some women have a written birth plan that they have discussed with their birth attendant and the facility personnel. Her partner and other family members whom she wants to be part of her care are included. From the first encounter, the nurse conveys confidence in the woman's ability to cope with labor and give birth to her baby.

Three major assessments are done promptly on admission: (1) fetal condition, (2) maternal condition, and (3) nearness to birth.

Fetal Condition. The fetal heart rate (FHR) is assessed with a fetoscope (stethoscope for listening to fetal heart sounds), a hand-held Doppler transducer, or the external fetal monitor (see p. 145). An older guideline for a normal FHR in a term baby was 120 to 160 beats/min. The newer guidelines (ACOG, 1995b; Menihan, 1996; Murray, 1997) for the normal FHR at term are:

- Lower limit of 110 to 120 beats per minute (BPM)
- Upper limit of 150 to 160 BPM

A preterm fetus usually has a faster FHR. The FHR is somewhat irregular, fluctuating within a range of about 5 to 15 beats/min. It may slow during contractions but should return to its baseline by the end of each contraction. The mature fetus may have a rate slightly slower than 110 BPM with no nonreassuring signs.

When the amniotic membranes are ruptured, the color, amount, and odor of the fluid are assessed. Amniotic fluid should be clear, possibly with flecks of white vernix (fetal skin protectant). Green-stained fluid means that the fetus passed the first stool (meconium) before birth, a situation sometimes associated with fetal compromise or newborn respiratory problems after birth. The amount of fluid expelled is variable, ranging from a small, intermittent trickle to a large gush. The odor is distinctive but not offensive. Foul- or strong-smelling amniotic fluid suggests infection, as does cloudy or yellow fluid.

If it is not clear whether the mother's membranes have ruptured, a Nitrazine or a fern test may be done. Nitrazine paper is a pH paper; alkaline amniotic fluid turns it dark blue-green or dark blue. In the fern test, a sample of amniotic fluid is spread on a microscope slide and allowed to dry. It is then viewed under the microscope; the crystals in the fluid look like tiny fern leaves.

Maternal Condition. The temperature, pulse, respirations, and blood pressure are assessed for signs of infection or hypertension. A temperature over 38°C (100.4°F) is to be reported. Blood pressure elevations of 140 mm Hg systolic or 90 mm Hg diastolic suggest pregnancy-induced hypertension (PIH; see p. 92).

Impending Birth. The nurse constantly observes the woman for behaviors that suggest she is about to give birth. Examples of these behaviors include the following:

- Sitting on one buttock
- Making grunting sounds
- Bearing down with contractions
- Stating "The baby's coming"
- Bulging of the perineum or the fetal presenting part visible at the vaginal opening

If it appears that birth is imminent, the nurse does not leave the woman but summons help with the call bell. Gloves (clean is sufficient to just catch a baby) should be applied in case the infant is born quickly. Emergency delivery kits (called "precip trays" for "precipitous birth") containing essential equipment are in all delivery areas. The student should locate this tray early in the clinical experience because one cannot predict when it will be needed. See Box 6–2 for emergency birth procedures.

Additional Assessments. If the maternal and fetal conditions are normal and if birth is not imminent, other data can be gathered in a more leisurely way. Most birth facilities have a preprinted form to guide admission assessments. Women who have had prenatal care should have a prenatal record on file for retrieval of that information. Examples of assessment data needed are as follows:

- Basic information, such as the woman's reason for coming to the facility, the name of her physician or CNM, medical and obstetric history, allergies, food intake, any recent illness, and medications (including illicit substances).

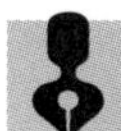

Nursing Tip

It is unlikely that a nursing student must "catch" a baby during an unexpected birth, but the process should be reviewed in case it does occur.

- Woman's plans for birth.
- Status of labor: a vaginal examination is done by the registered nurse, CNM, or physician to determine cervical effacement and dilation, fetal presentation, position, and station; contractions are assessed for frequency, duration, and intensity by palpation and/or with an electronic fetal monitor.
- General condition: a brief physical examination is done to evaluate this; any edema, especially of the fingers and face, and abdominal scars should

BOX 6–2

ASSISTING WITH AN EMERGENCY BIRTH

Get the emergency delivery tray ("precip tray").

Priorities of nursing care are to prevent injury to the mother and baby.

Do not leave the woman if she exhibits any signs of imminent birth, such as grunting, bearing down, perineal bulging, or a statement that the baby is coming. Summon the experienced nurse with the call bell and try to remain calm.

Put on gloves. Either clean or sterile is acceptable because no invasive procedures will be done. Gloves are used primarily to protect the nurse from secretions while catching the baby.

Support the infant's head and body as it emerges. Wipe secretions from the face. Use a bulb syringe to remove secretions from the mouth and nose.

Dry the infant quickly and wrap in blankets or place in skin-to-skin contact with the mother to maintain the infant's temperature.

Observe the infant's color and respirations. The cry should be vigorous and the color pink (bluish hands and feet are acceptable).

Observe for placental detachment and bleeding. After the placenta detaches, observe for a firm fundus. If the fundus is not firm, massage it. The infant can suckle at the mother's breast to promote the release of oxytocin, which causes uterine contraction.

be further explored; fundal height is measured (or estimated by an experienced nurse) to determine if it is appropriate for her gestation; reflexes are checked to identify hyperactivity that may occur with PIH.

Admission Procedures

Several procedures may be done when a woman is admitted to a birth facility. Some common ones are described.

Permits. The mother signs permits for care of herself and her infant during labor, delivery, and the postbirth period. Permission for emergency cesarean delivery is usually included.

Laboratory Tests. Blood for hematocrit and a midstream urine specimen for glucose and protein are common. The hematocrit is often omitted if a woman has had regular prenatal care and a recent evaluation. The woman who did not have prenatal care will have additional tests, which may include a complete blood count, urinalysis, a drug screen, tests for sexually transmitted diseases, and others as indicated.

Intravenous Infusion. An intravenous (IV) line allows administration of fluids and drugs. The woman may have a constant fluid infusion, or venous access may be maintained with a saline lock to permit greater mobility.

Shave Prep. A perineal shave prep is occasionally done to remove pubic hair that would interfere with the repair of a laceration or episiotomy. Its use has declined because it does not prevent infection, as once thought. If done, it is restricted to a small area of the perineum (a "mini-prep"). Clipping the longer perineal hair may be done rather than shaving. The woman who has a cesarean birth will have an abdominal shave prep.

Enema. An enema is sometimes administered if the woman has been constipated or if the nurse notes a significant amount of stool in the rectum when doing a vaginal examination. Small-volume enemas, such as the Fleets, are typical. Extra lubrication of the enema tip avoids irritating hemorrhoids (varicose veins in the rectum), which are common in pregnant and postpartum women.

Nursing Care of the Woman in False Labor

A better term for false labor might be prodromal labor because these contractions help prepare the woman's body and the fetus for true labor. Many women are observed for a short while (1–2 hours) if their initial assessment suggests that they are not in true labor and their membranes are intact. The mother and fetus are assessed during observation as if labor were occurring. Most facilities run an electronic fetal monitor strip of at least 20 minutes to document fetal well-being (see p. 146). The woman can usually walk about when not being monitored. If she is in true labor, walking often helps to intensify the contractions and to cause cervical effacement and dilation.

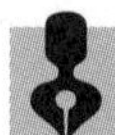

Nursing Tip

Encourage the woman in false labor to return when she thinks she should. It is better to have another "trial run" than to wait at home until she is in advanced labor.

After the observation period, the woman's labor status is reevaluated by doing another vaginal examination. If there is no change in the cervical effacement or dilation, the woman is usually sent home to await true labor. Sometimes, if it is her first baby and she lives nearby, the woman in very early labor is sent home because the latent phase of most first labors is quite long.

Each woman in false labor (or early latent-phase labor) is evaluated individually. Factors to be considered include

- Number and duration of previous labors
- Distance from the facility
- Availability of transportation

If her membranes are ruptured, she is usually admitted even if labor has not begun because of the risk for infection or a prolapsed umbilical cord (see p. 210).

The woman in false labor is often frustrated because she believes pregnancy is almost over, only to be told this is not the real thing after all. She needs generous reassurance that her symptoms will eventually change to true labor. No one stays pregnant forever, although it sometimes feels that way to a woman who has had several false alarms and is tired of pregnancy. Guidelines for coming to the facility should be reinforced before she leaves. Some women gradually make the transition from false labor to true labor and are reluctant to return. They should be reassured that they are not foolish for coming to the facility to be examined, no matter how many times they do so.

CONTINUING NURSING CARE DURING LABOR

After admission, nursing care consists of the following elements:

- Observing the fetus
- Observing the laboring woman
- Helping the woman to cope with labor

Observing the Fetus

Intrapartum care of the fetus includes assessment of FHR patterns and the amniotic fluid. In addition, several observations of the mother's status, such as vital signs and contraction pattern, are closely related to fetal well-being because they influence fetal oxygen supply.

Fetal Heart Rate Assessment

The FHR can be assessed by intermittent auscultation, using a fetoscope or Doppler transducer, or with continuous electronic fetal monitoring. See the procedure for assessing fetal heart rate. Electronic fetal monitoring is more widely used in the United States, but intermittent auscultation is a valid method of intrapartum fetal assessment when performed according to established intervals and a 1:1 nurse–patient ratio (ACOG, 1995b).

Intermittent Auscultation. Intermittent auscultation allows the mother greater freedom of movement, which is helpful during early labor. It is the only method possible if the mother is using a whirlpool or shower during labor and is the method used during home births and in most birth centers. However, intermittent auscultation can be used to collect data about the fetus during a small part of labor. It does not provide a written recording as continuous monitoring does.

Intermittent auscultation of the FHR should be performed as noted in Box 6–3. Figure 6–14 shows the approximate location of the fetal heart sounds when the fetus is in various presentations and positions. *Any FHR outside the normal limits or slowing of the FHR that persists after the contraction ends is promptly reported.*

Continuous Electronic Fetal Monitoring. Continuous electronic fetal monitoring (EFM) allows the nurse to collect more data about the fetus than intermittent auscultation. Except during periods of ambulation, the FHR and uterine contraction pattern are continuously recorded. Most hospitals use continuous EFM because more data are obtained and because the permanent written recording becomes part of the mother's chart.

One disadvantage of EFM is that it hampers ambulation. Some monitors have telemetry, allowing the woman to walk while a transmitter sends the data back to the monitor at her bedside for recording (like a cordless telephone). Intermittent

Procedure for Assessing Fetal Heart Rate

1. *Location.* Identify where the fetal heart sounds will most likely be found, over the fetal back and usually in the lower abdomen. (The nurse may use a procedure called Leopold's maneuvers to feel the approximate location of the fetal head, back, arms, and legs.)
2. *Fetoscope.* Place the head attachment (if there is one) over your head and the earpieces in your ear. Place the bell in the approximate area of the fetal back and press firmly while listening for the muffled fetal heart sounds. When they are heard, count the rate for 1 min. Count the rate in 6-second increments for at least 1 minute. Multiply the low and high numbers by 10 to compute the average range of the rate (for example, 130–140/min). Assess rate before, during, and after at least 1 full contraction cycle. Check the mother's pulse at the same time if uncertain whether the fetal heart sounds are being heard; the rates and rhythms will be different.
3. *Doppler transducer.* Put water-soluble gel on the head of the hand-held transducer. Put the earpieces in your ear, or connect the transducer to a speaker. Turn the switch on and place the transducer head over the approximate area of the fetal back. Count as instructed in step #2. If earpieces are used, let the parents hear the fetal heartbeat.
4. *External fetal monitor.* Read manufacturer's instructions for specific procedures. Connect cable to correct socket on monitor unit. Put water-soluble gel on the transducer and apply as instructed in step #3. Either belts, a wide band of stockinette, or an adhesive ring are used to secure the transducers for external fetal monitoring. The rate is calculated by the monitor and displayed on an electronic panel. The displayed number will change as the machine recalculates the rate.
5. *Chart the rate.* Promptly report rates below 110 beats/min or above 160 beats/min for a full-term fetus. Report slowing of the rate that lingers after the end of a contraction. Report lack of variability in the rate.

BOX 6–3

WHEN TO ASSESS AND DOCUMENT THE FETAL HEART RATE

Use these guidelines for charting the fetal heart rate when the woman has intermittent auscultation or continuous electronic fetal monitoring.

Low-Risk Women

Every hour in latent phase
Every 30 min in active phase
Every 15 min in second stage

High-Risk Women

Every 30 min in latent phase
Every 15 min in active phase
Every 5 min in second stage

Other Assessment Time

When the membranes rupture (spontaneously or artificially)
Before and after ambulation
Before and after medication or anesthesia administration or change in medication
At time of peak action of analgesic drugs
After vaginal examination
After expulsion of enema
After catheterization
If uterine contractions are abnormal or excessive

Adapted from NAACOG (now AWHONN). (1990). *Fetal heart rate auscultation.* Washington, DC: Author. With permission of the Association of Women's Health, Obstetric and Neonatal Nurses. ACOG (1995b), *Technical Bulletin Number 207: Fetal heart rate patterns: Monitoring, interpretation, and management.* Washington, DC: Author.

monitoring is a variation that promotes walking during labor. An initial recording of at least 20 minutes is obtained, then the fetus is remonitored for 15 minutes at regular intervals of 30 to 60 minutes.

EFM can be done with external or internal devices (Fig. 6–15). Internal devices require that the membranes be ruptured and the cervix be dilated 1 to 2 cm to insert the devices. External and internal devices may be combined, usually as an internal FHR sensor and an external uterine contraction sensor. Internal devices are disposable to reduce transmission of infection.

External fetal heart monitoring is done with a Doppler transducer, which uses sound waves to detect motion of the fetal heart and calculate the rate, just as the hand-held model does. A small spiral electrode applied to the fetal presenting part allows internal FHR monitoring.

Contractions are sensed externally with a tocotransducer (a "toco"), which has a pressure-sensitive button. The toco is positioned over the mother's upper uterus (fundus), about where the nurse would palpate contractions by hand. When a toco is used, contractions should be assessed by palpation periodically because the apparent strength of contractions on the monitor varies with her fat layer, the size and position of the fetus, and her position in bed.

Either of two types of devices is used for internal contraction monitoring. One uses a fluid-filled catheter connected to a pressure-sensitive device on the monitor. The other uses a solid catheter with an electronic pressure sensor in its tip.

Evaluating Fetal Heart Rate Patterns. The FHR is recorded on the upper grid of the paper; the uterine contraction pattern is recorded on the lower

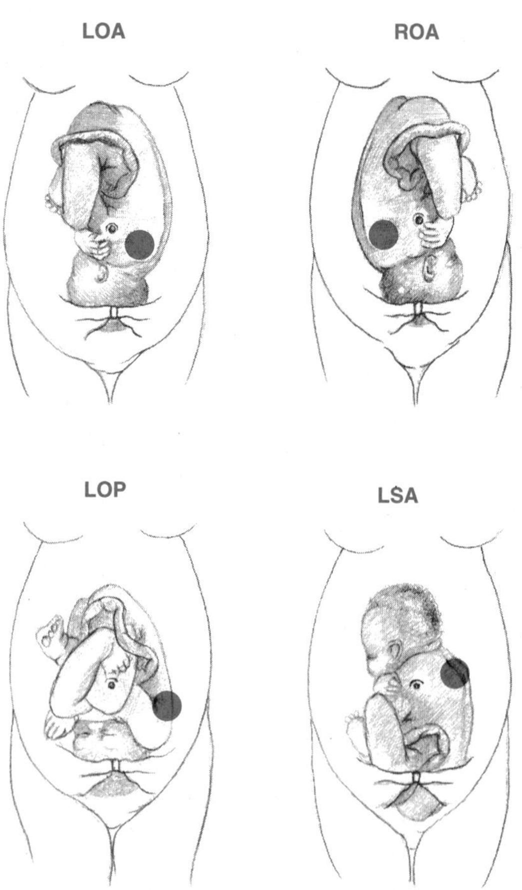

Figure 6–14. • Approximate the location of the fetal heart sounds when the fetus is in various presentations and positions. Note that the fetal heart sounds in breech presentations are higher on the mother's abdomen. (LOA, left occiput anterior; ROA, right occiput anterior; LOP, left occiput posterior; LSA, left sacrum anterior.)

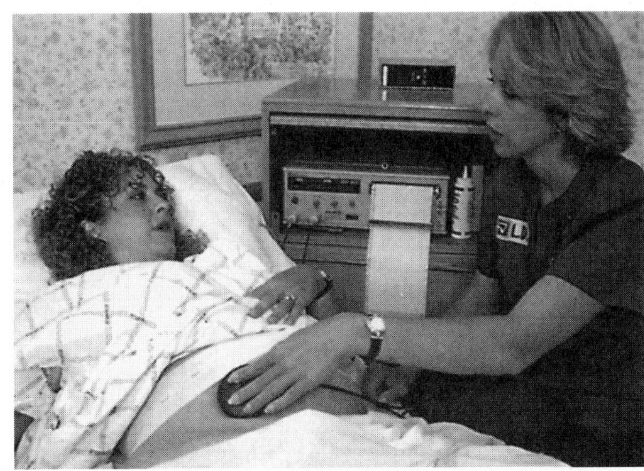

Figure 6–15. • The nurse explains the external electronic fetal monitor to the woman. The uterine activity sensor is placed on her upper abdomen, over the uterine fundus. The Doppler transducer is placed over her lower abdomen, or wherever the fetal heart rate is clearest. (From Gorrie, T.M., McKinney, E.S., & Murray, S.S. [1998]. *Foundations of maternal newborn nursing.* (2nd ed.). Philadelphia: Saunders.)

grid (Fig. 6–16). Both grids must be evaluated together for accurate interpretation of FHR patterns.

The FHR is evaluated for baseline, variability, and periodic changes. The *baseline rate* is the rate between contractions and between periodic changes. *Variability* describes fluctuations, or constant changes, in the baseline rate (Fig. 6–17). Variability causes the recording of the FHR to have a fine sawtooth appearance with larger, undulating wavelike movements. Variability is desirable, but it may be depressed by narcotics given to the woman and may normally be absent if the fetus is preterm.

Periodic changes are temporary changes in the baseline rate. Periodic changes include *accelerations* (rate increases) or one of three types of *decelerations* (rate decreases).

Accelerations. Accelerations are rate increases over the baseline rate of at least 15 beats/min lasting for at least 15 seconds. They suggest a fetus that is well oxygenated.

Early Decelerations. Early decelerations are rate decreases during contractions; they always return

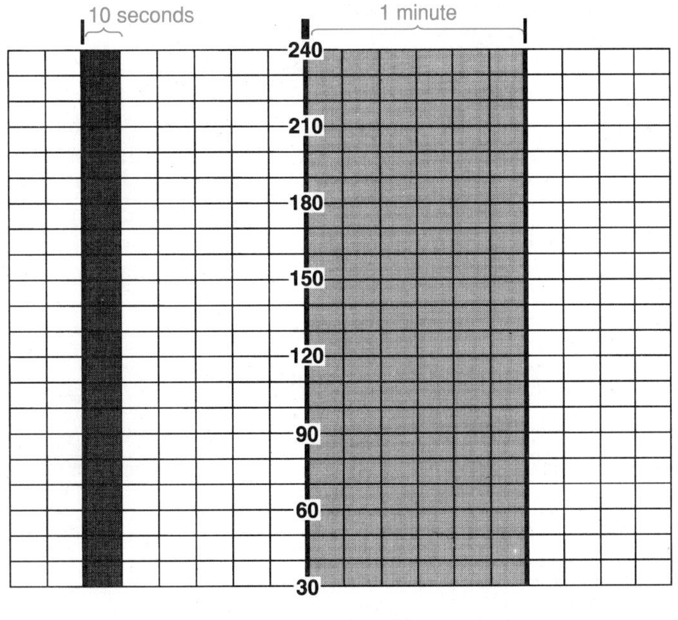

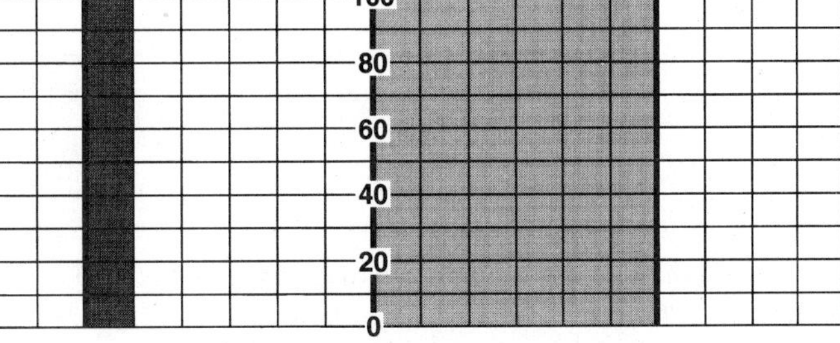

Figure 6–16. • Paper strip for recording electronic fetal monitoring data. Each dark vertical line represents 1 minute. Each lighter vertical line represents 10 seconds.

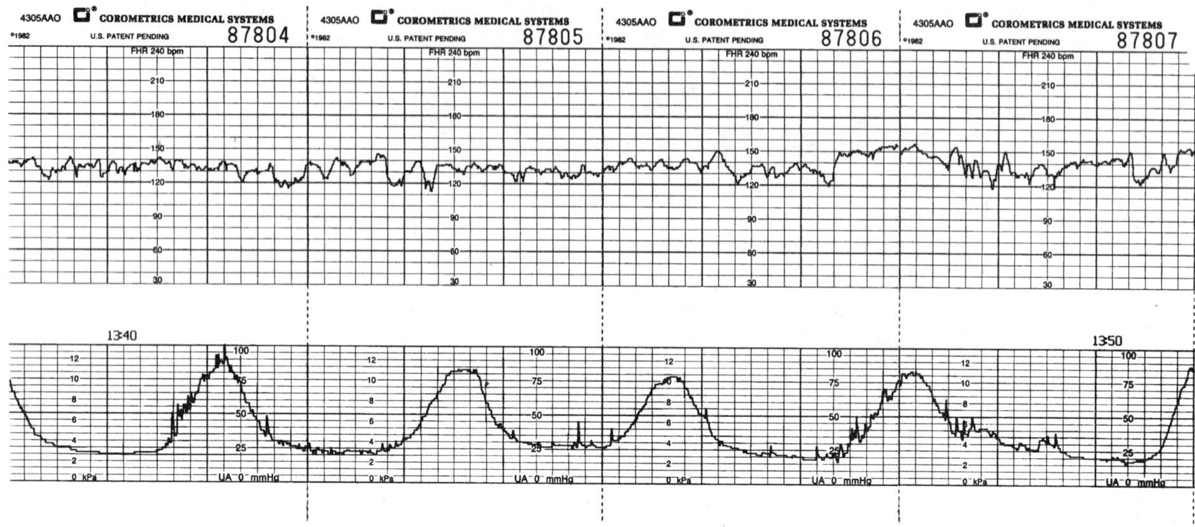

Figure 6–17. • Recording of the fetal heart rate in the upper grid and the uterine contractions in the lower grid. Note the sawtooth appearance of the fetal heart rate tracing due to the constant changes in the rate (variability). (Courtesy of Corometrics Medical Systems, Inc., Wallingford, CT. Redrawn with permission.)

to the baseline rate by the end of the contractions. They result from compression of the fetal head and are reassuring of fetal well-being.

Variable Decelerations. Variable decelerations begin and end abruptly; they are V-, W-, or U-shaped (Fig. 6–18). They do not always exhibit a consistent pattern in relation to contractions. Variable decelerations suggest that the umbilical cord is being compressed, often because it is around the fetal neck (a *nuchal cord*) or because there is inadequate amniotic fluid to cushion it well.

Late Decelerations. Late decelerations look similar to early decelerations, except that they do not return to the baseline FHR until after the contraction ends (Fig. 6–19). Late decelerations suggest that the placenta is not delivering enough oxygen to the fetus *(uteroplacental insufficiency)*.

Nursing Response to Monitor Patterns. An experienced registered nurse with additional education directs the nursing response to EFM patterns. The nursing response depends on the pattern identified (Box 6–4). Accelerations and early decelera-

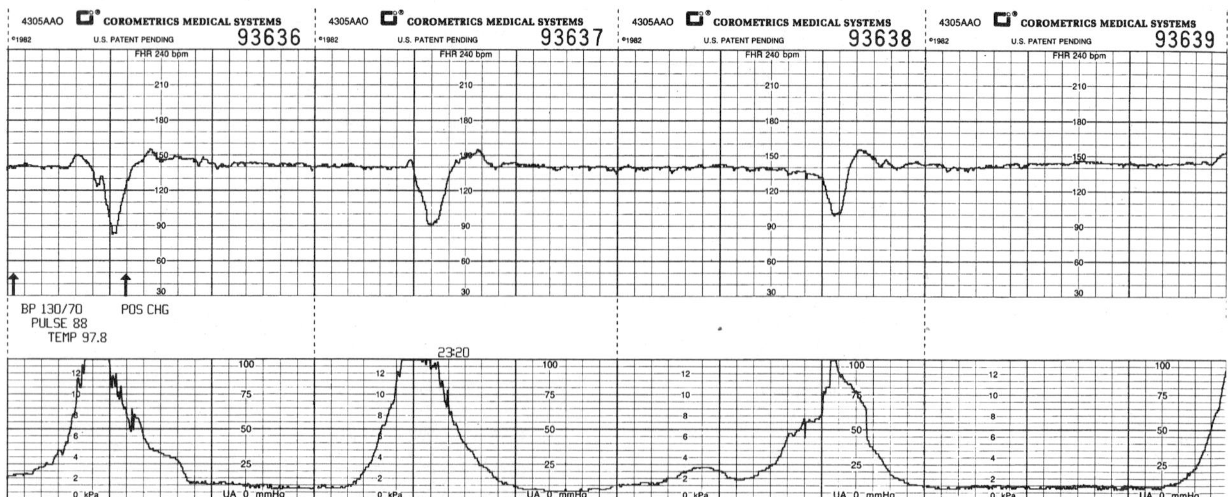

Figure 6–18. • Variable decelerations, showing their typically abrupt onset and offset. They are caused by umbilical cord compression. The first response to this pattern is to reposition the mother to relieve pressure on the cord. (Courtesy of Corometrics Medical Systems, Inc., Wallingford, CT. Redrawn with permission.)

tions are reassuring and thus require no intervention other than continued observation.

Repositioning the woman is usually the first response to a pattern of variable decelerations. Changing the mother's position relieves pressure on the umbilical cord and improves blood flow through it. The woman is turned to her side, or to the other side if she is already on her side. Other positions, such as the knee-chest or a slight Trendelenburg (head-down) may be tried if the side-lying positions do not restore the pattern to a reassuring one. *Amnioinfusion,* a technique in which intravenous fluid is infused into the amniotic cavity through the intrauterine pressure catheter, may be done to add a fluid cushion around the cord.

Late decelerations are initially treated by measures to increase maternal oxygenation and blood flow to the placenta. The specific measures depend on the most likely cause of the pattern, but may include:

- Repositioning to prevent supine hypotension (see p. 63)
- Giving oxygen by face mask to increase the amount in the mother's blood
- Increasing the nonadditive IV fluid to expand the blood volume and make more available for the placenta; this is often needed if regional analgesia or anesthesia causes hypotension
- Stopping oxytocin (Pitocin) infusion because the drug intensifies contractions and reduces placental blood flow
- Giving tocolytic drugs to decrease uterine contractions

The CNM or physician is notified of any nonreassuring pattern after initial steps are taken to correct it.

Assessment of Amniotic Fluid

The membranes may rupture spontaneously or the physician or CNM may rupture them artificially in a procedure called an *amniotomy.* The color, odor, and amount of fluid are charted. The amount of amniotic fluid is usually estimated as scant (only a trickle), moderate (about 500 ml), or large (about 1000 ml or more). Green-stained, cloudy, or yellowish amniotic fluid and fluid that has a strong odor should be reported.

The FHR should be assessed for at least one full minute after the membranes rupture and must be charted. Marked slowing of the rate or variable decelerations suggest that the fetal umbilical cord may have come down with the fluid gush and is being compressed.

Observing the Woman

Intrapartum care of the woman includes assessing her vital signs, contractions, progress of labor, intake and output, and responses to labor.

Vital Signs. The temperature is checked every 4 hours and every 2 hours if it is elevated or if the membranes have ruptured (frequency varies among facilities). A temperature of 38°C (100.4°F) or higher should be reported. If the temperature is elevated, the amniotic fluid is assessed for signs of infection, as noted in fetal assessments. Intravenous

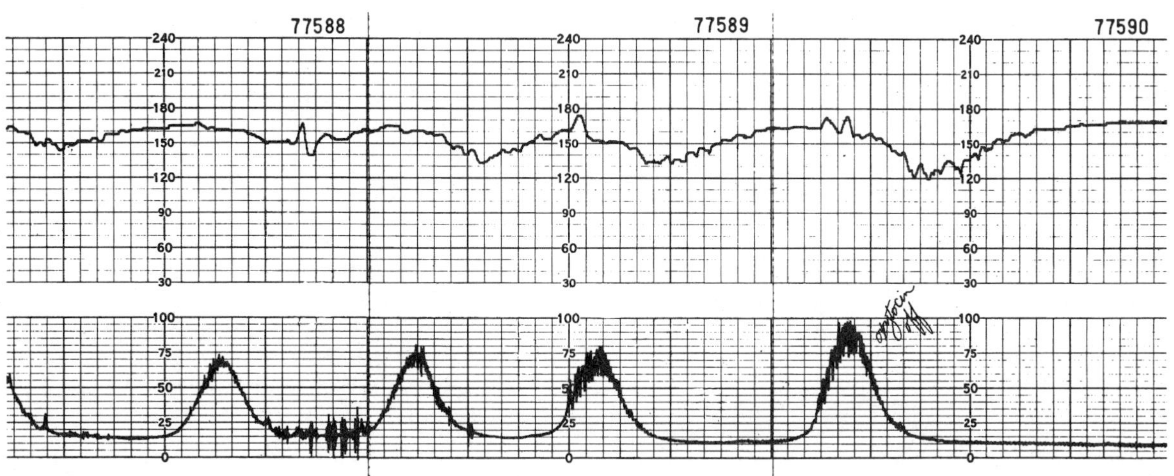

Figure 6–19. • Late decelerations, showing their pattern of slowing, which persists after the contraction ends. The usual cause is reduced blood flow to the placenta (uteroplacental insufficiency [UPI]). Measures to correct this include repositioning the woman, giving oxygen, increasing the nonmedicated intravenous fluid, stopping administration of oxytocin if it is being given, and giving drugs to reduce uterine contractions. (Courtesy of Corometrics Medical Systems, Inc., Wallingford, CT. Redrawn with permission.)

BOX 6–4

REASSURING AND NONREASSURING FETAL HEART RATE AND UTERINE ACTIVITY PATTERNS

Reassuring Patterns

Stable rate with a lower limit of 110 to 120 beats/min and an upper limit of 160 beats/min (term fetus)
Variability present
Accelerations of rate
Contraction frequency greater than every 2 min; duration less than 90 sec; relaxation interval of at least 60 sec

Nonreassuring Patterns

Tachycardia: rate over 160 beats/min for 10 min or longer
Bradycardia: rate under 110 beats/min for 10 min or longer
Decreased or absent variability: little fluctuation in rate
Late decelerations: begin after the contraction starts, and persist after the contraction is over
Variable decelerations: rate abruptly falls when deceleration occurs, returns abruptly to the baseline; may or may not occur in a consistent relationship with contractions.
Absence of variability

antibiotics are usually given to a woman who has a fever because of the risk that the infant will acquire group B streptococcus (GBS) infection. The pulse, blood pressure, and respirations are assessed every hour. Maternal hypotension, particularly if below 90 mm Hg systolic, or hypertension can reduce blood flow to the placenta.

Contractions. Contractions can be assessed by palpation and/or by continuous EFM. Some women have sensitive abdominal skin, especially around the umbilicus. When palpation is used to evaluate contractions, the fingers are placed lightly on her uterine fundus. They should not be palpated for longer than required. The nurse should keep the fingers still when palpating contractions. Moving the fingers over the uterus can stimulate contractions and give an inaccurate idea of their true frequency.

Progress of Labor. The registered nurse or birth attendant does a vaginal examination periodically to determine how labor is progressing. The cervix is evaluated for effacement and dilation. The descent of the fetus is determined in relation to the ischial spines (station). There is no set interval for doing vaginal examinations. The observant nurse watches for physical and behavioral changes associated with progression of labor to reduce the number of vaginal examinations needed. Vaginal examinations are limited to prevent infection, especially if the membranes are ruptured. They are also uncomfortable.

Intake and Output. Women in labor do not usually need strict measurement of intake and output, but the time and approximate amount of each urination are recorded. The woman may not sense a full bladder; she should be checked every 1 or 2 hours for a bulge in front of her uterus. A full bladder is a source of vague discomfort and can impede fetal descent. It often causes discomfort that persists after an epidural block has been initiated.

Policies about oral intake vary among birth facilities. Ice chips are usually allowed to moisten the

Nursing Tip

Report any questionable fetal heart rate or contraction pattern to the experienced labor nurse for complete evaluation.

Procedure for Assessing Contractions by Palpation

1. Place fingertips of one hand lightly on the upper uterus. Keep the fingers relatively still, but move them occasionally so that mild contractions can be felt.
2. Palpate at least three to five contractions for an accurate estimate of their average characteristics.
3. Note the time when each contraction begins and ends. Calculate the frequency by counting the elapsed time from the beginning of one contraction to the beginning of the next. Calculate the duration by determining the number of seconds from the beginning to end of each contraction.
4. Estimate the intensity by trying to indent the uterus at the contraction's peak. If it is easily indented (like the tip of the nose), the contraction is mild; if it is harder to indent (like the chin), it is moderate; if nearly impossible to indent (like the forehead), it is firm.
5. Chart the average frequency (in minutes and fractions), duration (in seconds), and intensity.
6. Report contractions more frequent than every 2 min or lasting longer than 90 sec or intervals of relaxation shorter than 60 sec.

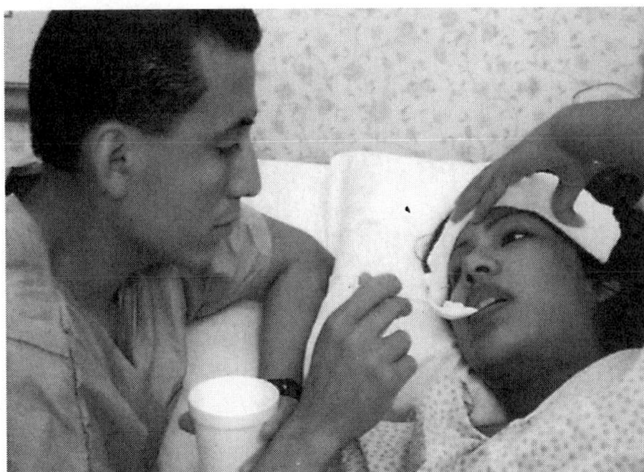

Figure 6–20. • Most laboring women welcome ice chips to ease their dry mouth and a cool damp washcloth on their head. (From Gorrie, T.M., McKinney, E.S., & Murray, S.S. [1998]. *Foundations of maternal newborn nursing* [2nd ed.]. Philadelphia: Saunders.)

mouth, unless it is likely that the woman will have a cesarean birth (Fig. 6–20). Many facilities allow fruit juices, Popsicles, or hard sugarless candy.

Response to Labor. The nurse assesses the woman's response to labor, including her use of breathing and relaxation techniques, and supports adaptive responses. Nonverbal behaviors that suggest difficulty coping with labor include a tense body posture and thrashing in bed. The physician or CNM is notified if the woman requests added pain relief, such as epidural analgesia.

Signs that suggest rapid labor progress are promptly addressed. Bloody show may increase markedly, and the perineum may bulge as the fetal head stretches it. The student or inexperienced nurse should summon an experienced nurse with the call signal if bloody show or perineal bulging increases or if the woman exhibits behaviors typical of imminent birth that were listed earlier. *Do not leave the woman if birth is imminent!*

Helping the Woman Cope with Labor

In addition to consistent assessment of the fetal and maternal conditions, the nurse helps the woman to cope with labor by comforting, positioning, teaching, and encouraging her. Another aspect of intrapartum nursing is care of the woman's partner. Nursing Care Plan 6–1 lists selected nursing diagnoses and interventions for the woman in uncomplicated labor.

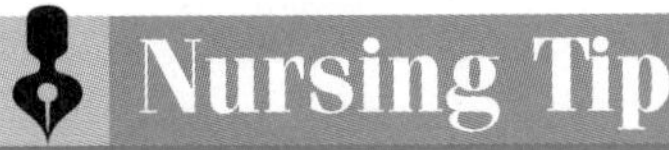

Nursing Tip

If a laboring woman says her baby is coming, *believe* her.

Promoting Comfort. In addition to specific nonpharmacologic and pharmacologic comfort measures discussed in Chapter 7, attention to her environment and hygiene reduces irritants that contribute to the woman's overall discomfort. Positioning makes her more comfortable and helps the progress of labor.

Making the Environment More Comfortable. The nurse adjusts the temperature for comfort. Many women are hot during labor, and a fan circulates the air. Although they are hot, their feet are often cold, so they may want to wear socks. If they are cold, a warmed blanket relieves this discomfort. Soft, indirect lighting, or even semidarkness, promotes relaxation. Bright overhead lights are annoying to anyone who is trying to relax. Soft relaxing music can promote relaxation and reduce distractions from environmental noise.

Hygienic Measures. Bloody show and amniotic fluid constantly leak from the woman's vagina. Regularly changing disposable underpads keeps her somewhat dry. Several underpads are placed beneath her hips at one time so that they can be removed one by one as they are soiled. A folded towel absorbs large amounts of fluids. The absorbent pads should be placed from her mid-back to her knees.

Oral fluids are provided, as permitted. If oral intake is prohibited, a lemon-glycerine swab is used to moisten the woman's mouth. Lip balm makes her lips more comfortable when they become dry from mouth breathing. A moist washcloth placed over her mouth can relieve some of the mouth dryness.

If there is no contraindication, a bath or a shower promotes relaxation and comfort. To avoid overheating the mother, which increases fetal oxygen needs, the water should not be too hot.

Positioning. The woman should regularly change position, avoiding the supine position. In the supine position, the heavy uterus may compress the large blood vessels that supply the placenta and return blood to the woman's heart. Any reduction in placental blood flow reduces fetal oxygen supply.

Upright positions, such as walking or sitting in a chair or rocker, add the force of gravity to uterine contractions (Fig. 6–21). Upright positions are good during early labor because they promote pressure of the fetal presenting part against the cervix.

Leaning forward while sitting or standing helps make the woman who has "back labor" more

NURSING CARE PLAN 6–1

Selected Nursing Diagnoses for the Woman in Uncomplicated Labor

Nursing Diagnosis: Anxiety related to unfamiliarity with hospital birth environment

Goals	Nursing Interventions	Rationale
The woman will express reduced anxiety after interventions The woman will have a relaxed body posture and facial expression after interventions	1. Greet woman and her partner/family warmly on arrival, and escort them to the assigned birthing room	1. Makes family feel welcome and that staff will be considerate of their needs and desires
	2. Briefly orient woman/couple to birthing room; place call signal within easy reach and tell her how to use it; explain any equipment that is used; including its purpose and how it will feel and sound	2. Teaching helps to decrease anxiety related to the unknown and increases a sense of personal control over the situation
	3. Talk with woman/couple about what they expect of the birth experience; for example, ask whom they plan on having present at (or immediately after) birth and type of medications or pain management they anticipate	3. Enables nursing staff to help woman/couple to achieve their expected experience more closely, which promotes their satisfaction; even if all their expectations are not met, they will probably be less anxious if they believe staff cares about their desires

Nursing Diagnosis: Altered comfort related to effect of uterine contractions and pressure from fetal descent

Goals	Nursing Interventions	Rationale
The woman will state that she is able to manage and tolerate the discomfort of labor	1. Encourage woman to assume any position she finds comfortable, other than supine	1. Promotes comfort; supine position can reduce placental blood flow and compromise fetal oxygenation
	2. Assist woman to assume specific positions for special situations in labor: a. Upright positions (sitting, walking, standing) facilitate fetal pressure against cervix, favoring effacement, dilation, and descent b. Back labor may be lessened by sitting or standing while leaning forward, kneeling and leaning forward with support, or by hands-and-knees position because they shift fetal head away from mother's back c. Squatting can increase the pelvic diameters slightly, straighten the pelvic curve, and promote fetal descent by gravity	2. Many woman are not aware that position can significantly improve comfort during labor; position can also facilitate normal processes of labor. Although any position except supine is usually acceptable, these positions may be more comfortable for the mother in the situations described
	3. Adjust temperature with a fan if woman is hot or a warm blanket if she is cool; have her wear socks if her feet are cold	3. Environmental comfort promotes relaxation, which decreases pain perception and increases pain tolerance
	4. Change disposable underpads when they become wet or soiled; use a folded towel between her legs if a large quantity of amniotic fluid is draining	4. Hygienic measures promote comfort and make the environment less favorable for growth of microorganisms
	5. Give woman ice chips, Popsicles, sugarless hard candy, or fruit juices as permitted; if she must remain NPO, use lemon-glycerin swabs or a wet washcloth to moisten her mouth	5. Relieves discomfort of a dry mouth; fruit juices, hard candies, and Popsicles also provide some calories for energy

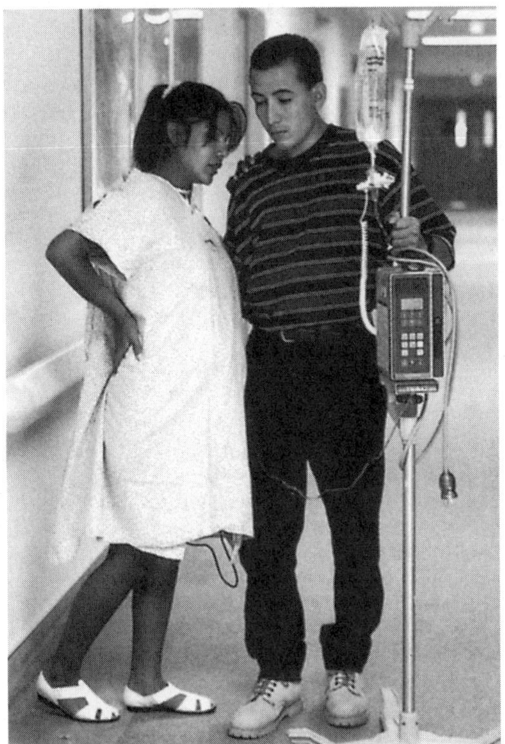

Figure 6–21. • Standing and walking during early labor use gravity to aid fetal descent, reduce back pain, and stimulate contractions. (From Gorrie, T.M., McKinney, E.S., & Murray, S.S. [1998]. *Foundations of maternal newborn nursing* [2nd ed.]. Philadelphia: Saunders.)

comfortable, because it shifts the fetus away from her lower spine. A variation is to kneel on the bed facing the raised head end. The hands-and-knees position has the same effect of shifting the fetus away from her spine; it also favors internal rotation to a more optimal position.

The side-lying position is favored by many women who stay in bed. The woman should regularly change sides to reduce pressure and constant strain on her muscles. Her back and extremities are supported with pillows as she desires. A side-lying position can be used when she is pushing during second-stage labor. The woman who remains in bed may prefer the semisitting position. This position can also be useful when she pushes during the second stage.

> **Nursing Tip**
>
> Regular changes of position make the laboring woman more comfortable and promote the normal processes of labor.

Squatting while being supported by two people on either side or gripping a "squat bar" improves the ability to push because it makes use of gravity and straightens the pelvic curve. Squatting increases the pelvic diameters slightly, which may provide the extra room needed to push the baby out.

Teaching. Teaching the laboring woman and her partner is an ongoing task of the intrapartum nurse. Even women who had prepared childbirth classes often find that the measures they learned are inadequate or that they need to be adapted. Positions or breathing techniques different from those learned in class can be tried. A woman should usually try a change in technique or position for two or three contractions before abandoning it.

Many women are discouraged when their cervix is about 5 cm dilated, because it took many hours to reach that point. They think that they are only halfway through labor (full dilation is 10 cm). However, 5 cm signifies that about two-thirds of the labor is over, because the rate of progress increases. Laboring women often need support and reassurance to overcome their discouragement at this point.

The nurse must often help the woman avoid pushing before her cervix is fully dilated. She can be taught to blow out in short puffs when the urge to push is strong before the cervix is fully dilated. Pushing before full dilation can cause the cervix to swell if it does not yield readily to the pressure, thus slowing progress rather than speeding it.

The nurse teaches or supports effective pushing techniques when the cervix is fully dilated. If the woman is pushing effectively and the fetus is tolerating labor well, the nurse should not interfere with her efforts. The woman takes a deep breath and exhales at the beginning of a contraction. She takes another deep breath and pushes with her abdominal muscles while exhaling. Prolonged breath-holding while pushing can impair blood circulation (the Valsalva maneuver). She should push about 4 to 6 seconds at a time. If she is in a semi-sitting position in bed, she should pull back on her knees, behind her thighs, or using handholds on the bed.

Providing Encouragement. Encouragement is a powerful tool for intrapartum nursing care, because it helps the woman to summon inner strength and gives her courage to continue. After a vaginal examination, she is told of progress in cervical change or fetal descent. Liberal praise is given if she successfully uses techniques to cope with labor. Her partner needs encouragement as well; labor coach-

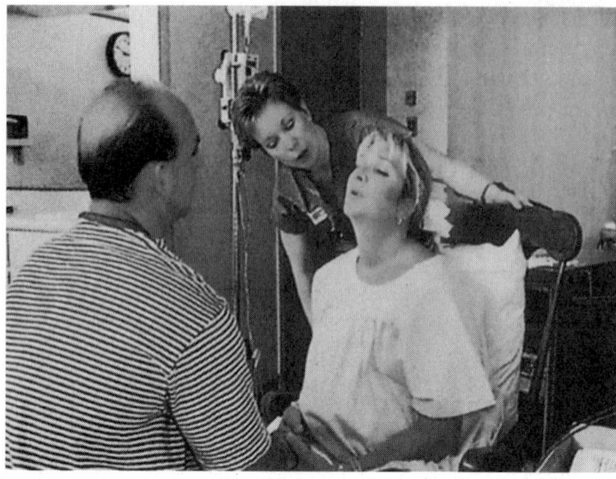

Figure 6–22. • The nurse helps this couple to maintain control during the transition phase of labor. The nurse praises their efforts and suggests new measures to control pain if needed. (From Gorrie, T.M., McKinney, E.S., & Murray, S.S. [1998]. *Foundations of maternal newborn nursing* [2nd ed.]. Philadelphia: Saunders.)

ing is a demanding job. Some women may employ a *doula*, a person whose only job is to support and encourage the woman in the demanding task of giving birth.

The nurse's caring presence cannot be overlooked as a source of support and encouragement for the laboring woman and her partner (Fig. 6–22). Many women feel dependent during labor and are more secure if the nurse is in their room or nearby. Just being present helps, even if no specific care is given because they see the nurse as the expert.

Supporting the Partner. Partners, or coaches, vary considerably in how much involvement they are comfortable with. The labor partner is most often the baby's father but may be the woman's mother or friend. Some partners are truly coaches and take a leading role in helping the woman cope with labor. Others are willing to assist if they are shown how, but they will not take the initiative. Still other couples are content with the partner's encouragement and support but do not expect him or her to have an active role. The partner should be permitted to provide the kind of support comfortable for the couple. The nurse does not take the partner's place but remains available as the couple needs.

The partner should be encouraged to take a break and periodically eat a snack or meal. Many are reluctant to leave the woman's bedside, but they may faint during the birth if they have not eaten. The partner is laboring, too, and needs energy to do so. A chair or stool near the bed allows the partner to sit down as much as possible.

NURSING CARE DURING BIRTH

As birth draws near, the nurse must decide when to make final preparations for birth. Specific nursing responsibilities during and immediately after the birth promote the safety and well-being of the mother and baby.

Making Final Preparations for Delivery

There is no exact time when the woman should be prepared for birth. It depends on the number of babies the woman has had, the length of previous labors, and the overall speed of labor and rate of fetal descent. In general, the woman having her first baby is prepared when about 3 to 4 cm of the fetal head is visible *(crowning)* at the vaginal opening. The multipara is usually prepared when her cervix is fully dilated but before crowning has occurred. If the woman must be transferred to a delivery room rather than give birth in a birthing room, she should be moved early enough to avoid a last-minute rush.

The risk for muscle strains is reduced by moving the woman's legs to foot supports or stirrups simultaneously and not separating her legs too widely. The area behind the knee should be well padded if stirrups are used to avoid compression, which might result in development of a blood clot. These measures are especially important if she has a regional anesthetic, such as an epidural, because she does not have full sensation and may not have normal movement. She should be in a semi-sitting position if foot supports or stirrups are used.

A woman can give birth in many different positions. The "traditional" position, semi-sitting and using foot supports or stirrups, improves access to her perineum but may not be the most comfortable for her or the best one to expel the baby. She may give birth in a side-lying position, squatting, standing, or other positions.

Nursing Responsibilities during Birth

During the birth, physicians or CNMs do not usually need a scrub nurse. The registered nurse

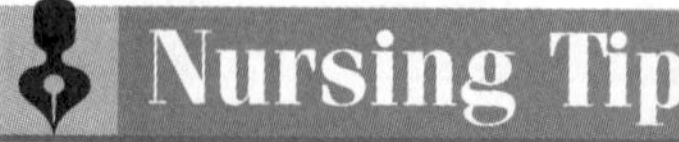

Nursing Tip

Support the woman's partner so that he or she can be the most effective coach possible during labor.

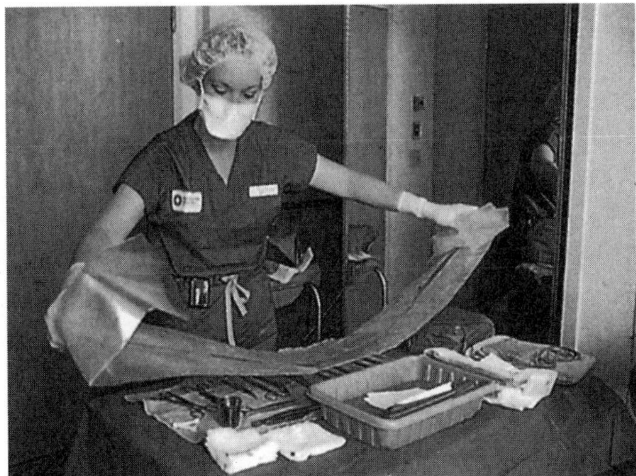

Figure 6–23. • The nurse prepares the sterile instruments that the physician or CNM will use for the birth. (From Gorrie, T.M., McKinney, E.S., & Murray, S.S. [1998]. *Foundations of maternal newborn nursing* [2nd ed.]. Philadelphia: Saunders.)

who cares for the woman during labor usually continues to do so in a "circulating" capacity in the birthing room. Typical delivery and birthing room responsibilities include the following:

- Preparing the delivery instruments and infant equipment (Fig. 6–23)
- Doing the perineal scrub prep (Fig. 6–24)
- Giving drugs to the mother or infant
- Providing initial care to the infant, such as suctioning the airway with a bulb syringe, drying the skin, and placing the infant in a radiant warmer to maintain body heat
- Assessing the infant's Apgar score (see p. 240, Table 9–2)
- Assessing the infant for obvious abnormalities; a note is made if the infant has a stool or urinates
- Identifying the mother and infant with like-numbered identification bands; the father or other support person usually receives a band as well; infant footprints and the mother's fingerprints are often done
- Promoting parent–infant bonding by encouraging parents to hold and explore the infant while maintaining the temperature; observe for eye contact, fingertip or palm touch of the baby, and talking in high-pitched tones, all of which are associated with initial bonding; these observations continue throughout the postpartum period

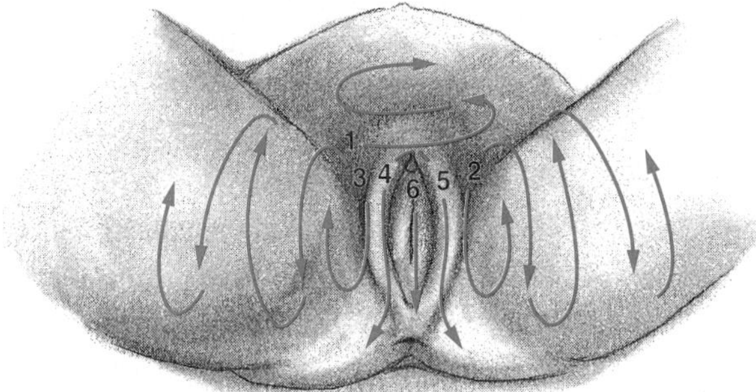

Figure 6–24. • Perineal scrub prep, which is done just before birth. Numbers and arrows indicate the order and direction of each stroke.

Figure 6–25 shows an infant being born in the vertex presentation in a spontaneous vaginal birth. Note that the mother has a right mediolateral episiotomy (from her vagina toward her right buttock). This episiotomy provides more room for a large infant to be born than does the median, or midline, episiotomy (from the vagina directly toward, but not into, her rectum). See Chapter 8 for more information on operative procedures.

NURSING CARE IMMEDIATELY AFTER BIRTH

During the immediate post-birth period (fourth stage), the nurse is responsible for observing the mother's condition and promoting her comfort. If the infant remains with her, the nurse also maintains the infant's safety and observes for complications. This is a good time for the parents to get acquainted with their new baby (Fig. 6–26).

Care of the Mother

Care of the mother in the recovery phase includes observation for hemorrhage and promotion of comfort (see Chapter 9 for additional postpartum care).

Observing for Hemorrhage. The new mother is assessed for signs associated with hemorrhage, which may occur if the uterus relaxes or if lacerations bleed. A common schedule for these assessments is every 15 minutes for 1 hour, every 30 minutes during the second hour, then hourly until she is stable and her recovery period ends.

The uterine fundus is assessed for firmness, height in relation to the umbilicus, and position (midline or deviated to one side). Refer to p. 221 for assessment of the fundus. Vaginal bleeding should be dark red (lochia rubra). No more than one pad should be saturated within an hour, and she should not pass large clots. A continuous trickle of bright red blood suggests a bleeding laceration. The blood pressure, pulse, and respirations are taken to identify a rising pulse or falling blood pressure, which suggest shock. An oral temperature is taken hourly,

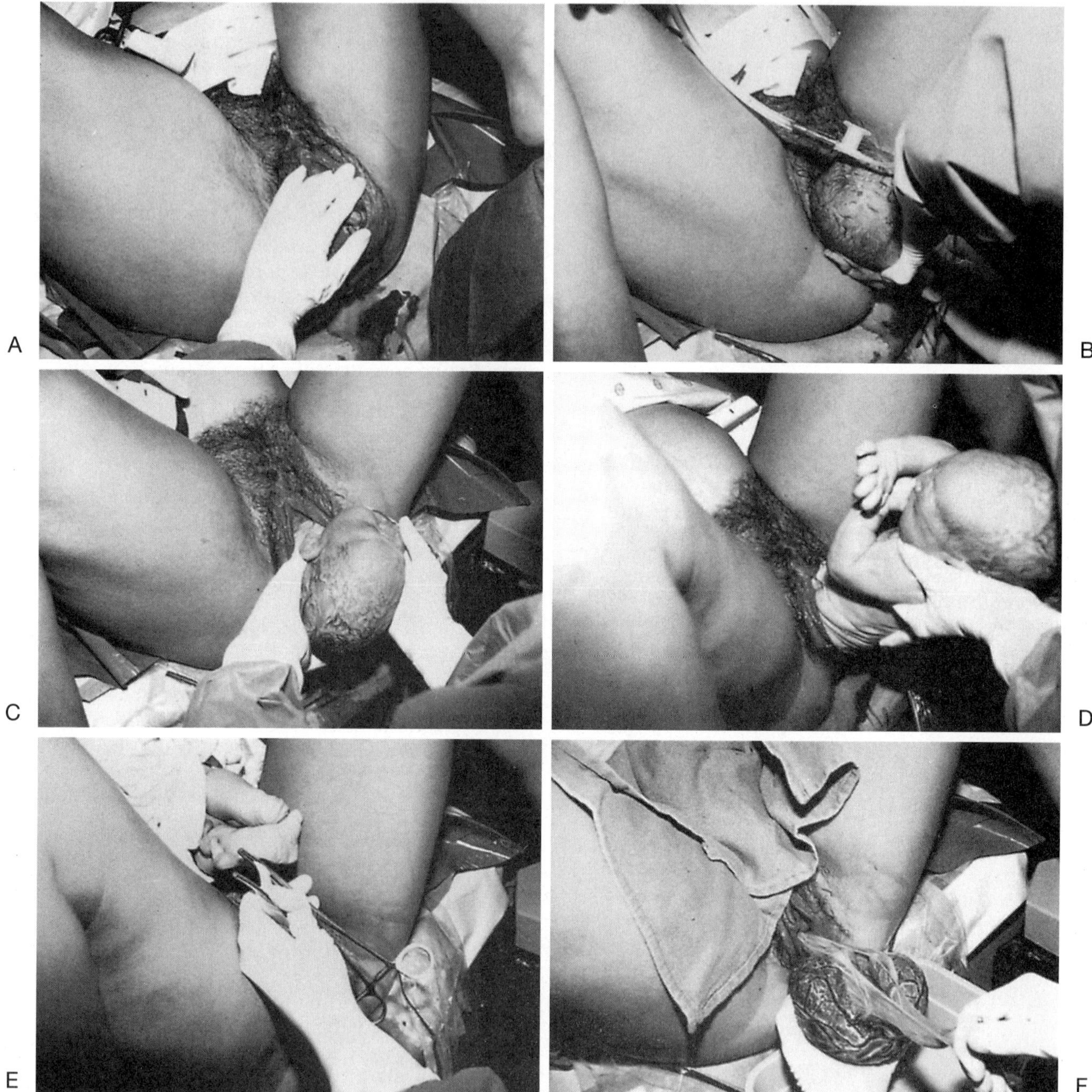

Figure 6–25. • Vaginal birth of a fetus in a vertex presentation. **A,** The fetal head is crowning and distends the labia and perineal tissues. The birth attendant is controlling the exit of the fetal head to minimize maternal trauma. **B,** As the head emerges, the birth attendant prepares to suction the nose and mouth to avoid aspiration of secretions when the infant takes the first breath. **C,** The fetal shoulders are born. **D,** The attendant supports the fetus during expulsion. Note that the fetus has excellent muscle tone as evidenced by facial grimacing and flexion of the arms and hands. **E,** While the infant is in skin-to-skin contact with the mother's abdomen, the attendant doubly clamps the umbilical cord and cuts the cord between the two clamps. Samples of cord blood for analysis are collected after it is cut. **F,** The placenta is born in the more common Schultze delivery, with the shiny fetal side and membranes emerging. The blood vessels that branch from the umbilical cord are visible on the surface. (From Gorrie, T.M., McKinney, E.S., & Murray, S.S. [1998]. *Foundations of maternal newborn nursing* [2nd ed.]. Philadelphia: Saunders.)

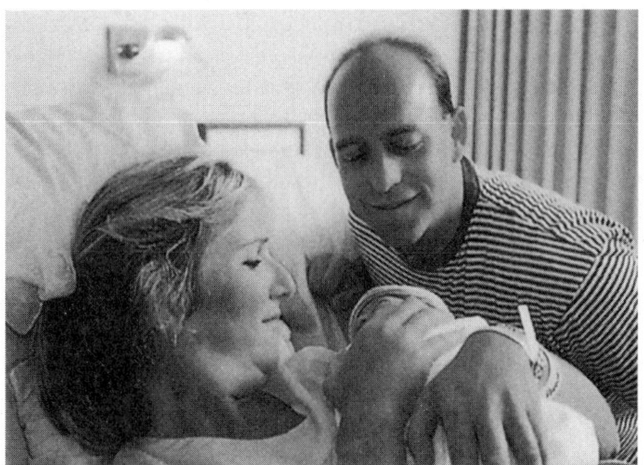

Figure 6–26. • The mother, father, and newborn are brought together as soon as possible after birth to promote bonding. (From Gorrie, T.M., McKinney, E.S., & Murray, S.S. [1998]. *Foundations of maternal newborn nursing* [2nd ed.]. Philadelphia: Saunders.)

unless it is elevated to 38°C (100.4°F) or higher or if the woman has a higher risk for infection.

The bladder is assessed for distention, which may occur soon after birth. The woman often does not feel the urge to urinate because of anesthesia effects, perineal trauma, and loss of fetal pressure against the bladder. If her bladder is full, the uterus will be higher than expected and often displaced to one side. A full bladder inhibits uterine contraction and can lead to hemorrhage. Catheterization will be needed if the woman cannot urinate.

Promoting Comfort. Many women have a shaking chill after birth. They may be shaking yet deny that they are cold. A warm blanket or portable radiant warmer over the woman makes her feel more comfortable until the chill subsides. The warm blanket or radiant warmer also maintains the infant's warmth while parents get acquainted.

An ice pack is placed on the mother's perineum to reduce bruising and edema. A glove can be filled with ice and wrapped in a wash cloth. Perineal pads that incorporate a chemical cold pack are often used. These pads do not absorb as much lochia as those without the cold pack, which must be considered in evaluating the quantity of bleeding. Cold applications are continued for at least 12 hours. A warm pack pad may be used after the first 12 to 24 hours to encourage blood flow to the area. Women who do not have an episiotomy or perineal laceration should be assessed for the need for cold and warm applications.

Afterpains, rhythmic uterine contractions that feel like menstrual cramps, are common in women who have had several babies or whose babies are large. They are worse if the mother's bladder is full. Afterpains increase during breastfeeding because infant suckling stimulates the mother's pituitary gland to secrete oxytocin, causing uterine contractions. Analgesics effectively reduce afterpains, which diminish after the first few days.

Mild oral analgesics are prescribed for postbirth discomfort. The birth attendant will prescribe analgesics that are safest for the breastfeeding mother. Aspirin should not be used for analgesia because it interferes with blood clotting.

Care of the Infant

The infant usually stays with the parents during recovery if there are no complications. The priority care involves promoting respiratory function and maintaining the temperature. (See Chapter 9 for information about care of the infant at birth.)

KEY POINTS

- The four components, or "four Ps," of the birth process are the powers, the passage, the passenger, and the psyche. All interrelate during labor to either facilitate or impede birth.
- True labor and false labor have several differences. However, the conclusive difference is that true labor results in cervical change (effacement and/or dilation).
- The woman should go to the hospital if she is having persistent, regular contractions (every 5 minutes for nulliparas, every 10 minutes for multiparas), if her membranes rupture, if she has bleeding other than normal bloody show, if fetal movement decreases, or for other concerns not covered by the basic guidelines.
- The woman having false labor is usually sent home after a short observation period. The nurse reassures her that she is not foolish for coming to the birth facility and emphasizes guidelines for returning.

- Three key assessments on admission are fetal condition, maternal condition, and nearness to birth.
- Four stages of labor have different characteristics. The first stage is the stage of dilation, lasting from labor's onset to full (10 cm) cervical dilation. First-stage labor is subdivided into three phases: latent, active, and transition. Second-stage labor, the stage of expulsion, extends from full cervical dilation until birth of the baby. The third stage, the placental stage, is from the birth of the baby until the birth of the placenta. The fourth stage is the immediate postbirth recovery period and includes the first 1 to 4 hours after placental delivery.
- The main fetal risk during first- and second-stage labor is fetal compromise due to interruption of the fetal oxygen supply. The main maternal risk during fourth-stage labor is hemorrhage due to uterine relaxation.
- Nursing care during the first and second stages focuses on observing the fetal and maternal conditions and on assisting the woman to cope with labor.
- Continuous electronic fetal monitoring is most common in hospital births, but intermittent auscultation is a valid method of fetal assessment.
- Laboring women can assume many positions. Upright positions add gravity to promote fetal descent. Hands-and-knees or leaning-forward positions promote normal internal rotation of the fetus if "back labor" is a problem. Squatting facilitates fetal descent during the second stage. The supine position should be discouraged because it causes the heavy uterus to compress the mother's main blood vessels, which can reduce fetal oxygen supply.

MULTIPLE-CHOICE REVIEW QUESTIONS

Choose the most appropriate answer.

1. To determine the frequency of uterine contractions, the nurse should note the time from the
   a. beginning to end of the same contraction
   b. end of one contraction to the beginning of the next contraction
   c. beginning of one contraction to the beginning of the next contraction
   d. contraction's peak until the contraction begins to relax
2. Excessive anxiety and fear during labor may result in
   a. an ineffective labor pattern
   b. abnormal fetal presentation or position
   c. release of oxytocin from the pituitary gland
   d. rapid labor and uncontrolled birth
3. A woman who is pregnant with her first baby phones an intrapartum facility and says her "water broke." The nurse should tell her to
   a. wait until she has contractions every 5 minutes for 1 hour
   b. take her temperature every 4 hours and come to the facility if it is over 38°C (100.4°F)
   c. come to the facility promptly, but safely
   d. call an ambulance to bring her to the facility
4. A laboring woman suddenly begins making grunting sounds and bearing down during a strong contraction. The student nurse should initially
   a. ask the experienced nurse to assess the woman
   b. look at her perineum for increased bloody show or perineal bulging
   c. ask her if she needs pain medication
   d. tell her that these are common sensations in late labor
5. To assess contractions by palpation, the nurse should palpate the
   a. fetal head
   b. mother's cervix
   c. uterine fundus
   d. lower abdomen

BIBLIOGRAPHY AND READER REFERENCE

American Academy of Pediatrics (AAP) & American College of Obstetricians and Gynecologists (ACOG). (1997). *Guidelines for perinatal care* (4th ed.). Elk Grove Village, IL, and Washington, DC: Authors.

American College of Obstetricians and Gynecologists. (1995a). *ACOG practice patterns: Vaginal delivery after previous cesarean birth.* Washington, DC: Author.

American College of Obstetricians and Gynecologists. (1995b). *ACOG technical bulletin number 207: Fetal heart rate patterns: Monitoring, interpretation, and management.* Washington, DC: Author.

Bachman, J., & Kendrick, J. M. (1996). Childbirth. In K. R. Rice & P. A. Creehan (Eds.), *Perinatal nursing* (pp. 151–186). Philadelphia: Lippincott.

Burpo, R. H. (1995). The pushing ritual of second stage labor. *Journal of Perinatal Education, 4*(2), 1–5.

Callister, L. C. (1995). Cultural meanings of childbirth. *Journal of Obstetric, Gynecologic, and Neonatal Nursing, 24*(4), 327–331.

Cunningham, F. G., MacDonald, P. C., Gant, N. F., Leveno, K. J., Gilstrap, L. C., Hankins, G. D. V., & Clark, S. L. (1997). *Williams' obstetrics* (20th ed.). Stamford, CT: Appleton & Lange.

Evans, S., & Jeffrey, J. (1995). Maternal needs during labor and delivery. *Journal of Obstetric, Gynecologic, and Neonatal Nursing, 24*(3), 235–240.

Gagnon, A. J., & Waghorn, K. (1996). Supportive care by maternity nurses: A work sampling study in an intrapartum unit. *Birth, 23*(1): 1–6.

Gorrie, T. M., McKinney, E. S., & Murray, S. S. (1998). *Foundations of maternal–newborn nursing* (2nd ed.). Philadelphia: Saunders.

Hodnett, E. (1996). Nursing support of the laboring woman. *Journal of Obstetric, Gynecologic, and Neonatal Nursing, 25*(3), 257–264.

Menihan, C. A. (1996). Intrapartum fetal monitoring. In K. R. Rice & P. A. Creehan (Eds.), *Perinatal nursing* (pp. 187–225). Philadelphia: Lippincott.

Murray, M. (1997). *Antepartal and intrapartal fetal monitoring* (2nd ed.). Albuquerque, NM: Learning Resources International.

NAACOG (now AWHONN). (1990). *OGN Nursing practice resource: Fetal heart rate auscultation.* Washington, DC: Author.

Supplee, R. B., & Vezeau, T. M. (1996). Continuous electronic fetal monitoring: Does it belong in low-risk births? *MCN: American Journal of Maternal and Child Nursing, 21*(6), 301–306.

Tomlinson, P. S., & Mattson-Bryann, A. A. (1996). Family centered intrapartum care: Revisiting an old concept. *Journal of Obstetric, Gynecologic, and Neonatal Nursing, 25*(4), 331–337.

chapter 7

Nursing Management of Pain during Labor and Birth

Outline

CHILDBIRTH AND PAIN
- How Childbirth Pain Differs from Other Pain
- Factors That Influence Labor Pain

EDUCATION FOR CHILDBEARING
- Types of Classes Available
- Preparation for Childbirth

NONPHARMACOLOGIC PAIN MANAGEMENT
- Advantages of Nonpharmacologic Methods
- Limitations of Nonpharmacologic Methods
- Nonpharmacologic Techniques

PHARMACOLOGIC PAIN MANAGEMENT
- Advantages of Pharmacologic Methods
- Limitations of Pharmacologic Methods
- Analgesics and Adjunctive Drugs
- Regional Analgesics and Anesthetics
- General Anesthesia

THE NURSE'S ROLE IN PAIN MANAGEMENT
- The Nurse's Role in Nonpharmacologic Techniques
- The Nurse's Role in Pharmacologic Techniques

Objectives

On completion and mastery of Chapter 7, the student will be able to

- Define each vocabulary term listed.
- Describe factors that influence a woman's comfort during labor.
- List common types of classes offered to childbearing families.
- Describe methods of childbirth preparation.
- Discuss advantages and limitations of nonpharmacologic methods of pain management during labor.
- Discuss advantages and limitations of pharmacologic methods of pain management.
- Explain nonpharmacologic methods of pain management for labor, including the nursing role for each.
- Explain each type of pharmacologic pain management, including the nursing role for each.

Vocabulary

aspiration pneumonitis
blood patch
cleansing breath
cricoid pressure
effleurage
endorphin
focal point
opioid
pain threshold
pain tolerance
systemic drug

Pregnant women are usually interested in how labor will feel and want to know how they can manage the experience, especially the pain they expect. Women manage labor pain by using nonpharmacologic (nondrug) methods or by using pharmacologic (drug) methods. Most women use a combination of the two. Because preparation for childbirth is an important part of nonpharmacologic pain management, it is also discussed in this chapter. General labor comfort measures, such as adjustment of the environment and maternal positioning, were discussed in Chapter 6.

CHILDBIRTH AND PAIN

Pain is an unpleasant and distressing symptom that is personal and subjective. No one can feel another's pain, but empathic nursing care helps to alleviate pain and helps the client to cope with it.

How Childbirth Pain Differs from Other Pain

Childbirth pain differs from other types of pain in several ways:

- It is part of a normal body process.
- The woman has several months to prepare for pain management.
- The pain is self-limiting and rapidly declines after birth.
- The pain of labor ends with the birth of a baby.

Pain is usually a symptom of injury or illness; yet pain during labor is almost a universal part of the normal process of birth. Although excessive pain is detrimental to labor processes, pain can be beneficial, too. It may cause a woman to feel vulnerable and seek shelter and help from others. Pain often motivates her to assume different body positions, which can facilitate the normal descent of the fetus. Birth pain lasts for hours, as opposed to days or weeks. Labor ends with the birth of a baby, followed by a rapid and nearly total cessation of pain.

Factors That Influence Labor Pain

Several factors cause pain during labor and influence the amount of pain a woman experiences. Other factors influence a woman's response to and ability to tolerate labor pain.

Pain Threshold and Pain Tolerance

Two terms are often used interchangeably to describe pain, although they have different meanings. *Pain threshold,* also called pain perception, is the least amount of sensation that a person perceives as painful. Pain threshold is fairly constant, and it varies little under different conditions. *Pain tolerance* is the amount of pain one is willing to endure. Unlike the pain threshold, one's pain tolerance can change under different conditions. A primary nursing responsibility is to modify as many factors as possible so that the woman can tolerate the pain of labor.

Sources of Pain during Labor

Four physical factors contribute to pain during labor:

- Dilation and stretching of the cervix
- Reduced uterine blood supply during contractions
- Pressure of the fetus on pelvic structures
- Stretching of the vagina and perineum

See Chapter 6 for discussion of the physiologic effects of labor on the woman's body. Additional physical and psychosocial factors alter the sensations a woman feels during labor and modify her pain.

Physical Factors That Modify Pain

Several physical factors influence the amount of pain a woman feels or is willing to tolerate during labor.

Central Nervous System Factors

Gate Control Theory. The gate control theory explains how pain impulses reach the brain for interpretation. It supports several nonpharmacologic methods of pain control. According to this theory, pain is transmitted through small-diameter

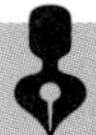

Nursing Tip

Stroking or massage, palm or foot rubbing, pressure, or gripping a cool bed rail stimulate nerve fibers that interfere with transmission of pain impulses to the brain.

nerve fibers. However, stimulating large-diameter nerve fibers temporarily interferes with conduction of impulses through small-diameter fibers. Techniques to stimulate large-diameter fibers and "close the gate" to painful impulses include massage, palm and fingertip pressure, and heat and cold applications.

Endorphins. Endorphins are natural body substances that are similar to morphine. Levels of endorphins increase during pregnancy and reach a peak during labor. Endorphins may explain why laboring women often need smaller doses of analgesia or anesthesia than might be expected in a similarly painful experience.

Maternal Condition

Cervical Readiness. The mother's cervix normally undergoes prelabor changes that facilitate effacement and dilation in labor (see p. 126). If her cervix does not make these changes (ripening), more contractions are needed to cause effacement and dilation.

Pelvis. The size and shape of the pelvis significantly influence how readily the fetus can descend through it. Pelvic abnormalities can result in a longer labor and greater maternal fatigue. In addition, the fetus may remain in an abnormal presentation or position, which interferes with the mechanisms of labor.

Labor Intensity. The woman who has a short, intense labor often experiences more pain than the woman whose birth process is more gradual. Contractions are intense and frequent, and their onset may be sudden. The cervix, vagina, and perineum stretch more abruptly than in a gentler labor. Contractions come so fast that the woman cannot recover from one before another begins. In addition, a rapid labor limits the woman's choices for pharmacologic pain control.

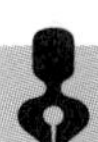

Nursing Tip

Laboring women often tolerate more pain than usual because they have high levels of endorphins and because they are concerned about the baby's well-being.

Fatigue. Fatigue reduces pain tolerance and a woman's ability to use coping skills. Many women are tired when labor begins because sleep during late pregnancy is difficult. The active fetus, frequent urination, and shortness of breath when lying down all interrupt sleep.

Fetal Presentation and Position

The fetal presenting part acts as a wedge to efface and dilate the cervix as each contraction pushes it downward. The fetal head is a smooth, rounded wedge that most effectively causes effacement and dilation of the round cervix. The fetus in an abnormal presentation or position applies uneven pressure to the cervix, resulting in less effective effacement and dilation.

The fetus usually turns during early labor so that the occiput is in the front left or right quadrant of the mother's pelvis (occiput anterior positions; see p. 129). If the fetal occiput is in a posterior pelvic quadrant, each contraction pushes it against the mother's sacrum, resulting in persistent and poorly relieved back pain (back labor). Labor is often longer with this fetal position.

Interventions of Caregivers

Although they are intended to promote maternal and fetal safety, several common interventions may add to pain during labor. Some examples include the following:

- Intravenous lines
- Continuous fetal monitoring, especially if it hampers mobility
- Amniotomy (artificial rupture of the membranes)
- Vaginal examinations or other interruptions

Psychosocial Factors That Modify Pain

Several psychosocial variables alter the pain a woman experiences during labor. Many of these variables interrelate with one another and with physical factors.

Culture. Culture influences how a woman feels about pregnancy and birth and how she reacts to pain during childbirth. Some cultures encourage loud and vigorous expressions of distress as a way of coping with pain, whereas others value stoicism and silent suffering. The nurse must accept each woman's individual expression of pain and realize that some women labor loudly.

Nursing Tip

It is easy to miss important cues about impending birth or development of a complication if a laboring woman is either very stoic or very vocal.

Anxiety and Fear. Moderate anxiety can motivate a woman to learn techniques that increase her pain tolerance. However, excessive anxiety or fear raises her sensitivity to pain and reduces her ability to tolerate it. In addition, excessive anxiety reduces uterine blood flow, makes uterine contractions less effective, and results in muscle tension that counteracts the expulsive power of contractions and maternal pushing. The woman who learns about expected sensations of labor is less likely to interpret them as dangerous or as a symptom of something wrong.

Previous Experiences. Labor is not a woman's first painful experience. During other painful experiences she may have learned skills that increase her ability to cope with labor, including the first labor.

Experience with previous births influences a woman's reactions to her current labor. A woman who had a normal birth before is less likely to interpret the intense sensations with injury or abnormality. The woman who had an epidural block (see p. 176) may have little experience in coping with labor pain. If an epidural is not possible during a subsequent labor, she may be distressed because she compares the painful labor with the "painless" one.

The woman who had a long and difficult labor is often apprehensive during the next labor. If her difficult labor required a cesarean delivery, she may be uneasy about attempting vaginal birth. Repeat cesarean birth may seem like the easier and quicker option. If a repeat cesarean birth is planned and she begins labor before the surgery, she may be upset because she did not expect to experience labor at all.

Childbirth Preparation. Women who prepare for labor through classes, self-study, or other means usually have less anxiety and fear about the unknown. They learn a variety of skills for coping with labor pain. The preparation should be realistic, promoting reasonable expectations about pain and the effectiveness of both nonpharmacologic and pharmacologic pain relief methods.

Support of Significant Others. A woman's labor partner is usually her husband or the baby's father, although the partner may be her mother or a friend. A well-prepared partner is a valuable teammate during labor, encouraging the woman and helping her to use different coping skills.

Friends and family members with children can provide support to the expectant mother if they convey accurate information about the discomfort of labor. It is most distressing to hear that labor is intolerable, but it is equally damaging for others to lead the woman to expect a painless labor. Every labor is different, even in the same woman.

A *doula* is a person hired by the woman to provide support during labor. The doula's only responsibility is to support the laboring woman. The doula does not replace, but supplements, the care of the intrapartal nurse. The nurse retains responsibility for nursing care of the laboring woman.

EDUCATION FOR CHILDBEARING

A variety of classes are offered by most hospitals and free-standing birth centers to help women to adjust to pregnancy, cope with labor, and prepare for life with a baby (Fig. 7–1). Women who plan home birth usually prepare intensely because they want to avoid medications and other interventions associated with hospital births.

Types of Classes Available

Classes during pregnancy focus on topics that contribute to good outcomes for the mother and baby (Box 7–1). Special classes prepare other family members for the birth and new infant. Other classes are sometimes available, such as classes for the woman who has diabetes in pregnancy. Examples of classes that may be available include the following:

- Early pregnancy classes
- Exercise classes for pregnant women
- Sibling classes
- Grandparent classes
- Breastfeeding classes
- Infant care classes

Because this chapter focuses on pain management during labor, techniques of prepared childbirth are discussed most extensively.

Preparation for Childbirth

The time to prepare for labor is before it begins. Prepared childbirth classes teach the woman and her partner a variety of skills to use during labor. Related classes prepare women planning a vaginal birth after cesarean (VBAC) or those expecting a cesarean birth. Separate classes for adolescents may be available, sometimes in their school.

Methods of Childbirth Preparation

Most childbirth preparation classes are based on one of several methods The basic method is often modified to meet the specific needs of the women who attend.

Dick-Read Method. Grantly Dick-Read was an English physician who introduced the concept of a fear-tension-pain cycle during labor. He believed that fear of childbirth contributed to tension, which resulted in pain. His methods include education and relaxation techniques to interrupt the cycle.

Bradley Method. This method was originally called "husband-coached childbirth" and was the first to include the father as an integral part of labor. It emphasizes slow abdominal breathing and relaxation techniques.

Lamaze Method. The Lamaze method, also called the psychoprophylactic method, is the basis of most prepared childbirth classes in the United States. It uses mental techniques that condition the woman to respond to contractions with relaxation rather than tension. Other mental and breathing techniques occupy her mind and limit the brain's ability to interpret labor sensations as painful.

Content of Prepared Childbirth Classes

Regardless of the specific method taught, most classes are similar in basic content. Because the Lamaze method is popular in most areas of the United States, it is the focus of this chapter. Box 7–2 highlights several techniques that may be taught in childbirth classes. Many of the techniques can be

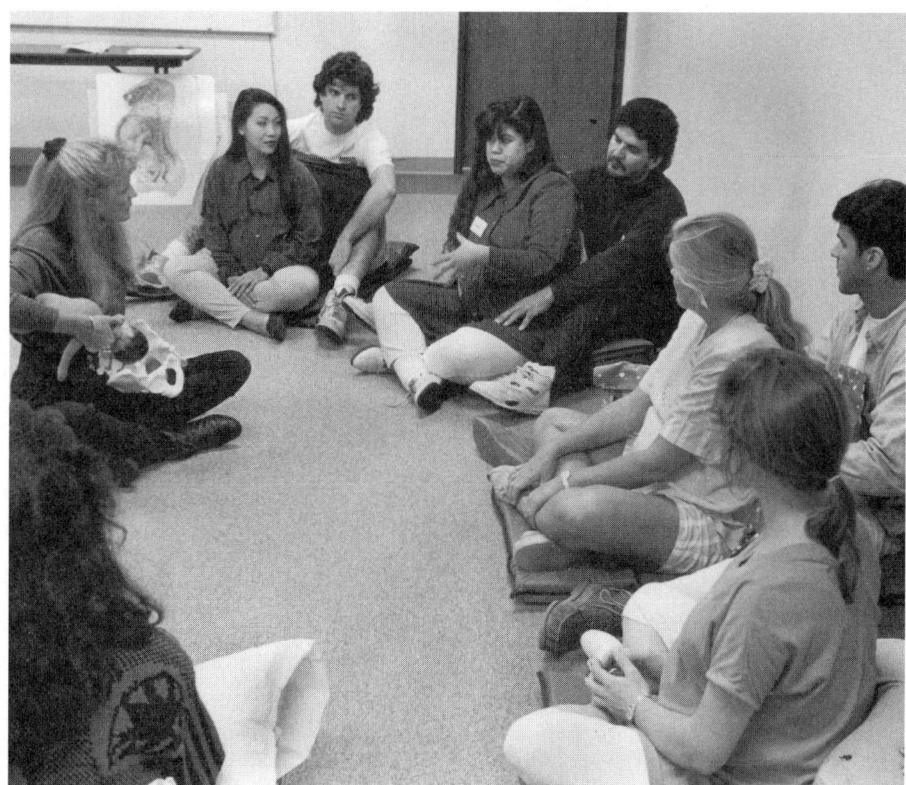

Figure 7–1. • The nurse teaching this class discusses movement of the fetus through the pelvis. (From Gorrie, T.M., McKinney, E.S., & Murray, S.S. [1994]. *Foundations of maternal newborn nursing.* Philadelphia: Saunders.)

BOX 7–1

TYPES OF PRENATAL CLASSES

Early Pregnancy Classes
Changes of pregnancy
Fetal development
Prenatal care
Hazardous substances to avoid
Good nutrition for pregnancy
Relieving common pregnancy discomforts
Working during pregnancy and parenthood
Care of the new baby, such as feeding methods, choosing a pediatrician, and selecting clothing and equipment
Early growth and development

Exercise Classes
Maintaining the woman's fitness during pregnancy
After birth for toning and fitness
Special considerations for exercise during pregnancy:
- Exercises should be low impact
- Heart rate should be no faster than 140 beats/min; her temperature should be no higher than 38° C (100.4° F)
- Woman should not lie in supine position or use the Valsalva maneuver

Sibling Classes
Helping children to prepare realistically for their new brother or sister
Helping children to understand that feelings of jealousy and anger are normal
Giving parents tips about helping older children adjust to the new baby after birth

Grandparent Classes
Changes in childbirth and parenting
Importance of grandparents to a child's development
Reducing conflict between the generations

Breastfeeding Classes
Processes of breastfeeding
Feeding techniques
Solving common problems
Some classes continue after birth

Infant Care Classes
Care of new baby
Needed clothing and equipment

Specialized Classes
Adolescent classes for birth and parenthood preparation
Management of diabetes during pregnancy

used to help the unprepared woman during labor as well.

Education. The woman who learns about changes during pregnancy and childbirth is less likely to respond with fear and tension to labor. Information about cesarean birth is usually included, since 20% to 25% of births in the United States occur by this method.

Exercises. Conditioning exercises, such as the pelvic rock, tailor sitting, and shoulder circling, prepare the woman's muscles for the demands of birth (Fig. 7–2). These exercises also relieve the back discomfort common during late pregnancy.

The Kegel exercise increases control of the muscles that support the pelvic organs It reduces stress incontinence (loss of urine during straining), improves control of pelvic muscles during birth, recovers pelvic muscle tone after birth, and increases sexual sensitivity. To do the Kegel exercise, the woman contracts the muscles that would stop her urine flow in the middle of voiding. The exercise is repeated five times; she gradually works up to about 100 repetitions each day. She should not actually stop her urine flow while voiding to avoid urinary stasis that can lead to infection.

Relaxation Techniques. The ability to release tension is a vital part of the expectant mother's "tool kit." Relaxation techniques require concentration, thus occupying the mind while reducing muscle tension. All require practice to be most effective during labor (Fig. 7–3).

Pain Control Methods for Labor. The woman and her partner learn a variety of techniques that may be used during labor as needed. Examples of these include the following:

- Skin stimulation, such as effleurage or heat
- Mental stimulation
- Breathing techniques

These techniques are most effective if learned before labor begins. They can also be used by the woman who has not attended classes and are discussed with nonpharmacologic pain management (see p. 170).

BOX 7–2

NONPHARMACOLOGIC PAIN RELIEF MEASURES

Progressive Relation

The woman contracts and then consciously releases different muscle groups.

Helps the woman to distinguish tense muscles from relaxed ones.

Woman can assess and then release muscle tension throughout her body.

Must be practiced before labor to be effective.

Neuromuscular Dissociation (Differential Relaxation)

The woman contracts one group of muscles strongly and consciously relaxes all others. Coach checks for unrecognized tension in muscle groups other than the one contracted.

Prepares the woman to relax the rest of her body while the uterus is contracting. Must be practiced before labor to be effective.

Touch Relaxation

The woman contracts a muscle group and then relaxes it when her partner strokes or massages it.

The woman learns to respond to touch with relaxation.

Must be practiced before labor to be effective.

Relaxation against Pain

The woman's partner exerts pressure against a tendon or large muscle of the arm or leg, gradually increasing the pressure and gradually decreasing pressure to simulate the gradual increase, peak, and decrease in contraction strength.

The woman consciously relaxes in spite of this deliberate discomfort.

Gives the woman practice in relaxation against pain.

Must be practiced before labor to be effective.

Effleurage

Massage of the abdomen or other area during contractions.

Interferes with transmission of pain impulses, but prolonged continuous use reduces effectiveness (habituation). The pattern or area massaged should be changed when it becomes less effective.

Massaging in a specific pattern (such as circles or a figure 8) also provides distraction.

Other Massage

Massage of the temples or shoulders often helps relaxation.

Firm massage of hands or feet is often very effective during labor.

Habituation may occur in any type of massage. Change the area massaged if it occurs.

Sacral Pressure

Helps to reduce pain of back labor.

Get the woman's input about the best position. Moving the pressure point a fraction of an inch or changing the amount of pressure may significantly improve effectiveness.

Pressure may also be applied by tennis balls in a sock, a warmed plastic container of intravenous solution, or other means.

Thermal Stimulation

Stimulates temperature receptors that interfere with pain transmission.

Either heat or cold applications may be beneficial. Examples are cool cloths to the face, ice in a glove to the lower back, a warm bath or shower.

A warm bath can slow labor progress during the latent phase of labor. A warm bath, and especially stimulation of the nipples with water currents, can accelerate labor in the active phase.

Do not apply heat or cold to an anesthetized area.

Positioning

Any position except the supine is acceptable if there is no need for a specific position.

Upright positions favor fetal descent.

Hands-and-knees positions help to reduce pain of back labor.

Change positions about every 30 to 60 minutes to relieve pressure and muscle fatigue.

Mental Stimulation

Increase mental concentration on something besides the pain.

May take many forms:

- Focal point: concentrating on a specific object or other point
- Imagery: creating an imaginary mental picture of a pleasant environment or visualizing the cervix opening and the baby descending
- Avoid using mental pictures of actual childbirth until labor's onset
- Music: provides a distraction or provides "white noise" to obscure environmental sounds

Shoulder circling

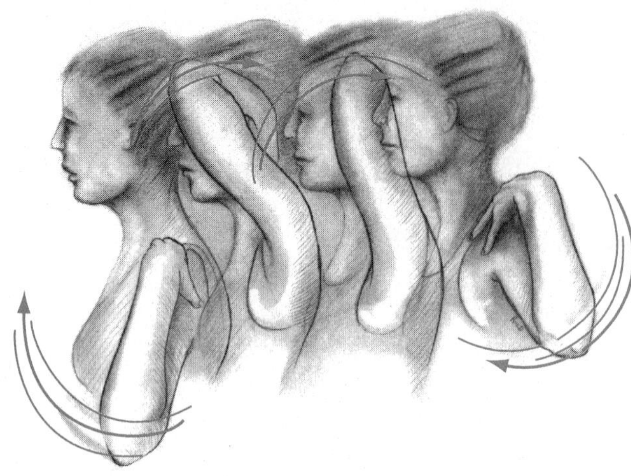

The fingertips are placed on the shoulders, then brought forward and up during inhalation, back and down during exhalation. Repeat 5 times.

Tailor sitting

The woman uses her thigh muscles to press her knees to the floor. Keeping her back straight, she should remain in the position for 5 to 15 minutes.

Pelvic tilt or pelvic rocking

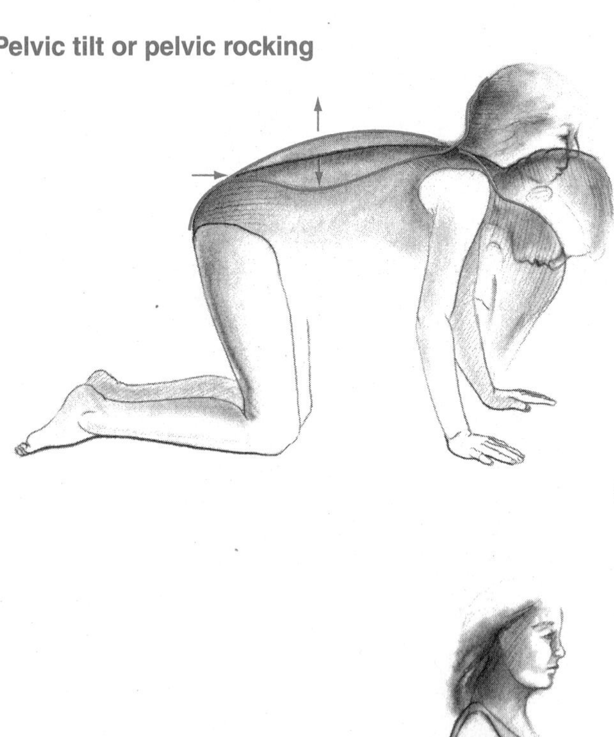

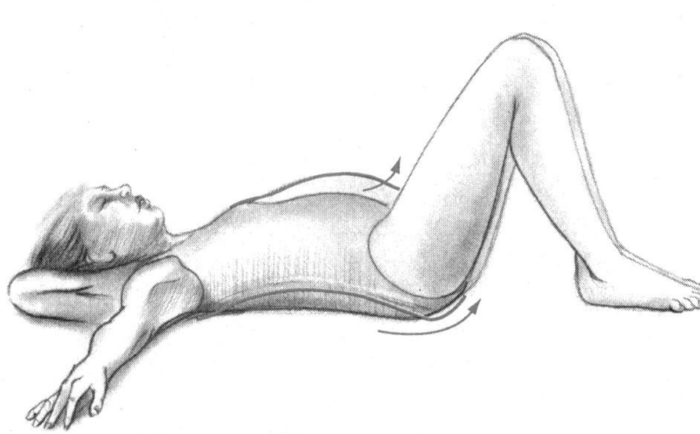

This exercise can be performed on hands and knees, with the hands directly under the shoulders and the knees under the hips. The back should be in a neutral position, not hollowed. The head and neck should be aligned with the straight back. The woman then presses up with the lower back and holds this position for a few seconds, then relaxes to a neutral position. Repeat 5 times. The exercise may also be done in a standing or lying position.

Figure 7–2. • These conditioning exercises prepare the woman's muscles for labor and relieve some of the discomforts of late pregnancy. (From Gorrie, T.M., McKinney, E.S., & Murray, S.S. [1994]. *Foundations of maternal newborn nursing.* Philadelphia: Saunders.)

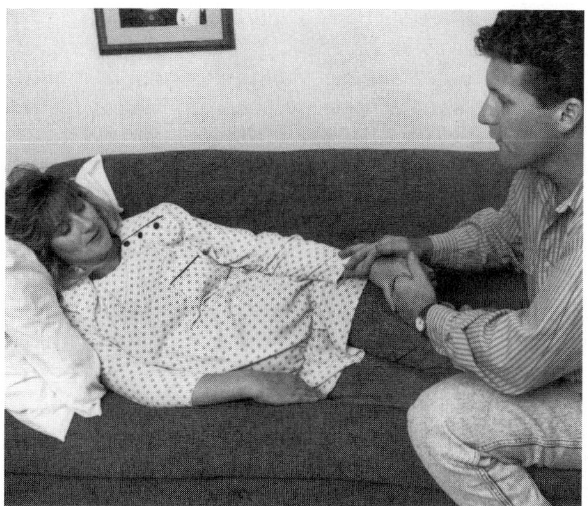

Figure 7–3. • The coach checks for areas of tension while the woman practices relaxation techniques for labor. (From Gorrie, T.M., McKinney, E.S., & Murray, S.S. [1994]. *Foundations of maternal newborn nursing*. Philadelphia: Saunders.)

Variations of Basic Prepared Childbirth Classes

Refresher Classes. Refresher classes consist of one to three sessions to review material learned during a previous pregnancy. Ways to help siblings adjust to the new baby and a review of infant feeding are often included.

Cesarean Birth Classes. Classes for women who expect cesarean birth help the woman and her support person to understand the reasons for this method of delivery and anticipate what is likely to occur during and after surgery. Women who had previous cesarean births may recall little of their experience if it was done after a prolonged and exhausting labor or under emergency conditions. They may need to express their feelings about their past experiences so they can resolve them and better deal with the present pregnancy.

Vaginal Birth after Cesarean Classes. VBAC is desirable whenever it is possible. Women in VBAC classes may need to express unresolved feelings about their previous cesarean birth. Depending on the reason for the cesarean delivery, they may be more anxious about the forthcoming labor. In addition to teaching techniques for coping with labor, these women and their partners need ample time to discuss their experiences and feelings.

Adolescent Prepared Childbirth Classes. A pregnant adolescent's needs are different from those of an adult. Adolescents are therefore usually uncomfortable in regular prepared childbirth classes. They are often single mothers and have a more immature perception of birth and childrearing. Some are not old enough to drive or do not have access to a car and cannot attend classes that target working adults. The content of classes for adolescents is tailored to their special needs. Because acceptance by their peer group is important to teenagers, the girls are a significant source of support to each other. Classes may be held during school. Expectant fathers may be included.

NONPHARMACOLOGIC PAIN MANAGEMENT

Nonpharmacologic pain control methods are important, even if the woman has medication or anesthesia. Most pharmacologic methods cannot be instituted until labor is well established, because they tend to slow progress. Nonpharmacologic methods help the woman to cope with labor before it has advanced far enough to give her medication. Also, most medications for labor do not *eliminate* pain, and the woman will need nonpharmacologic methods to manage discomfort that remains. Nonpharmacologic methods are usually the only realistic option if the woman comes to the hospital in advanced labor.

Advantages of Nonpharmacologic Methods

There are several advantages to nonpharmacologic methods *if pain control is adequate.* Poorly relieved pain increases fear and anxiety, thus diverting blood flow from the uterus and impairing the normal labor process. It also reduces the pleasure of this extraordinary experience.

Nonpharmacologic methods do not harm the mother or fetus. They do not slow labor if they provide adequate pain control. They carry no risk for allergy or adverse drug effects.

Limitations of Nonpharmacologic Methods

For best results, nonpharmacologic methods should be rehearsed before labor begins. They can be taught to the unprepared woman, preferably during early labor, when she is anxious enough to be interested but comfortable enough to learn.

Many women will not have adequate pain control by using these methods alone. No matter how much a woman has practiced, the many factors that influence labor pain often require drug intervention.

Nonpharmacologic Techniques

The nurse may help the woman to use several techniques of nondrug pain control during labor. They include relaxation, skin stimulation, mental stimulation, and breathing techniques. If the woman and her partner attended prepared childbirth classes, the nurse builds on their knowledge during labor.

Relaxation

Promoting relaxation underlies all other methods, both nonpharmacologic and pharmacologic. The nurse should adjust the woman's environment and help her with hygienic measures as discussed in Chapter 6. Water in a tub or shower helps to refresh her and promotes relaxation.

To reduce anxiety and fear, the woman is taught about the labor area, any procedures that are done, and what is happening in her body. The nursing focus should be on the normality of birth. For example, calling the woman by her first name, if that is her preference, promotes an atmosphere of wellness. A partnership style of nurse–client–labor partner relationship is usual in maternity settings.

Looking for signs of muscle tension and teaching her partner to do so help the woman who is not aware of becoming tense. She can change position or guide her partner to massage the area where muscle tension is noted. The laboring woman is guided to release the tension specifically, one muscle group at a time, for example, by saying, "Let your arm relax; let the tension out of your neck . . . your shoulders. . . ." Specific instructions are repeated until she relaxes each body part.

Skin Stimulation

Several variations of massage are often used during labor. Most can be taught to the woman and partner who did not attend prepared childbirth classes. Massage tends to become less effective unless varied periodically.

Effleurage. The woman strokes her abdomen in a circular movement during contractions (Fig. 7–4). If fetal monitor belts are on her abdomen, she can massage between them or on her thigh, or she can trace circles or a figure-8 on the bed. She can use one hand when on her side. Effleurage stimulates the large-diameter nerve fibers that inhibit painful stimuli traveling through the small-diameter fibers. The woman should change methods at intervals because constant use of a single technique reduces its effectiveness (habituation).

Sacral Pressure. Firm pressure against the lower back helps relieve some of the pain of back labor. The woman should tell her partner where to apply the pressure and how much pressure is helpful.

Thermal Stimulation. Heat can be applied with a warm blanket or glove filled with warm water. Warmth can also be applied in the form of a shower if there is no contraindication against doing so. Most women appreciate a cool cloth on the face. Two or three moistened washcloths are kept at hand and changed as they become warm. Do not apply heat or cold to anesthetized areas because the

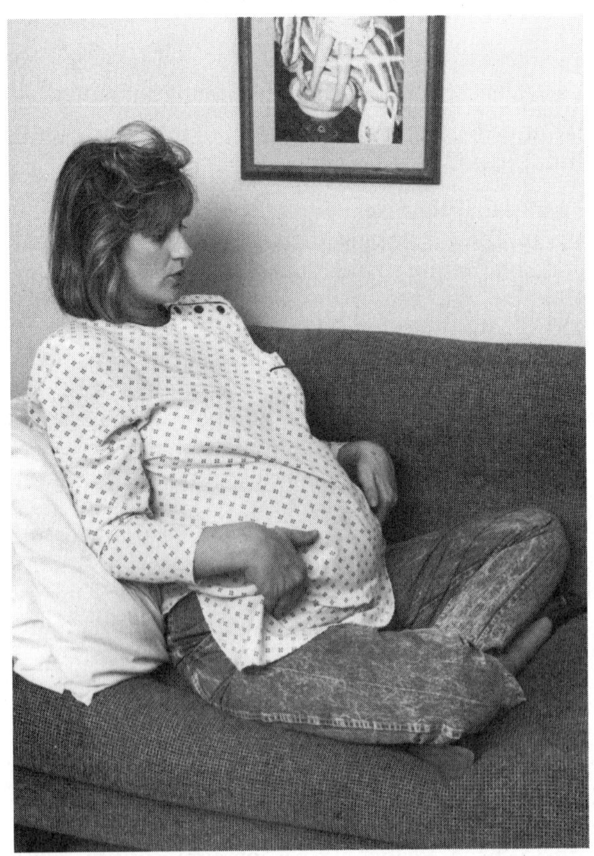

Figure 7–4. • This woman is practicing effleurage, a technique for stimulating the large-diameter nerve fibers, thus interfering with pain transmission. Fingertip pressure should be firm enough to avoid a tickling sensation. (From Gorrie, T.M., McKinney, E.S., & Murray, S.S. [1994]. *Foundations of maternal newborn nursing*. Philadelphia: Saunders.)

woman will not be able to feel tissue injury that might occur.

Positioning

Various positions were described in Chapter 6. Changing position every 30 to 60 minutes relieves muscle fatigue and strain and decreases constant pressure on one area of the body. In addition, position changes promote normal mechanisms of labor. When the woman changes position, she may be more uncomfortable at first but is often more comfortable after a few contractions in that position.

Mental Stimulation

Several methods may be used to stimulate the woman's brain, thus limiting her ability to perceive sensations as painful. All methods direct her mind away from the pain.

Focal Point. The woman fixes her eyes on a picture, an object, or simply a particular spot in the room. Some women prefer to close their eyes during contractions and focus on an internal focal point.

Imagery. The woman learns to create a tranquil mental environment by imagining that she is in a place of relaxation and peace. Preferred mental scenes often involve warmth and sunlight, although some women imagine themselves in a cool environment. During labor, the woman can imagine her cervix opening and allowing the baby to come out, as a flower opens from bud to full bloom. The nurse can help to create a tranquil mental image, even in the unprepared woman.

Music. Favorite music or relaxation recordings divert the woman's attention from pain. Sounds of rainfall, wind, or the ocean contribute to relaxation and block disturbing sounds. Headphones help the woman to concentrate and minimizes external sounds.

Television. Especially during early labor, women often enjoy the diversion of television. The woman may not watch the program, but it provides background noise that reduces intrusive sounds. Some labor rooms have videotape players, and the woman can bring her own tapes to watch during and after birth.

Breathing

Like other techniques, breathing techniques are most effective if practiced before labor. The woman should not use them until she needs them, generally when she can no longer walk or talk through a contraction. She may become tired if she uses them too early or if she moves to a more advanced technique sooner than she must. If the woman has not had prepared childbirth classes, each technique is taught as she needs it.

Each breathing pattern begins and ends with a *cleansing breath,* which is a deep inspiration and expiration, similar to a deep sigh. The cleansing breaths help the woman to relax and focus on relaxing.

First-Stage Breathing

Slow-Paced Breathing. The woman begins with a technique of slow-paced breathing. She starts the pattern with a cleansing breath, then breathes slowly, as during sleep (Fig. 7–5A). A cleansing breath ends the contraction. An exact rate is not important, but about six to nine breaths a minute is average. The rate should be at least half her usual rate to ensure adequate fetal oxygenation.

Modified Paced Breathing. This pattern begins and ends with a cleansing breath. During the contraction, the woman breathes more rapidly and shallowly (Figs. 7–5 B and C). The rate should be no more than twice her usual rate. She may combine slow-paced with modified paced breathing. In this variation, she begins with a cleansing breath and breathes slowly until the peak of the contraction, when she begins rapid, shallow breathing. As the contraction abates, she resumes slow, deep breathing and ends with a cleansing breath.

Hyperventilation is sometimes a problem when the woman is breathing rapidly. She may complain of dizziness, tingling, and numbness around her mouth and may have spasms of her fingers and feet. See Box 7–3 for measures to combat hyperventilation.

Patterned Paced Breathing. Patterned paced breathing is more difficult to teach the unprepared laboring woman because it requires her to focus on the pattern of her breathing. It begins with a cleansing breath, which is followed by rapid breaths punctuated with an intermittent slight blow (Fig. 7–5D), often called pant-blow, or "hee hoo" breathing. The woman may maintain a constant number of breaths before the blow or may vary the number in a specific pattern:

- Constant pattern: pant-pant-pant-BLOW, pant-pant-pant-BLOW, etc.
- Stairstep pattern: pant-BLOW, pant-pant-BLOW, pant-pant-pant-BLOW, pant-pant-BLOW, pant-BLOW

In another variation, her partner calls out random numbers to indicate the number of pants to take before a blow.

If she feels an urge to push before her cervix is fully dilated, the woman is taught to blow in short

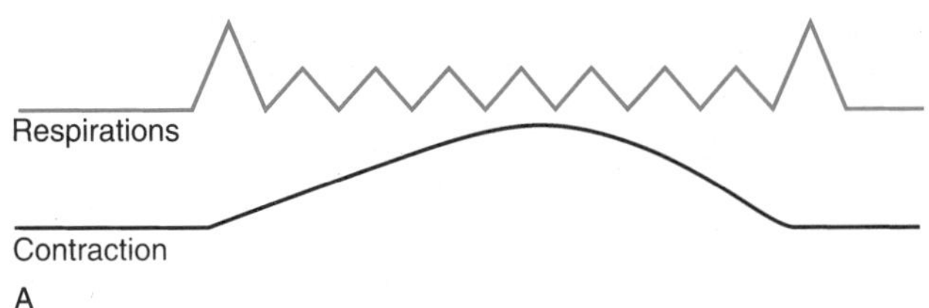

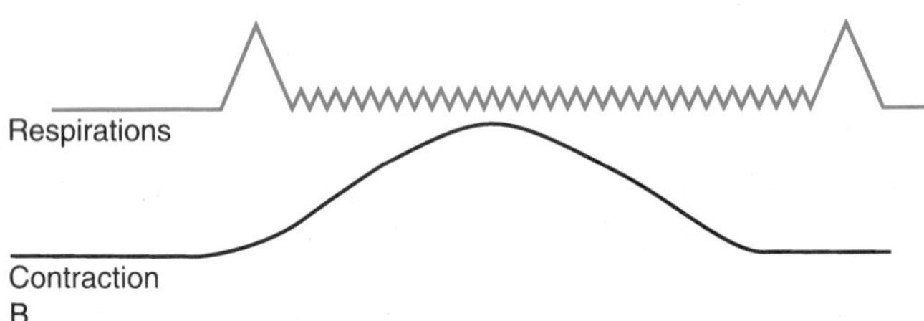

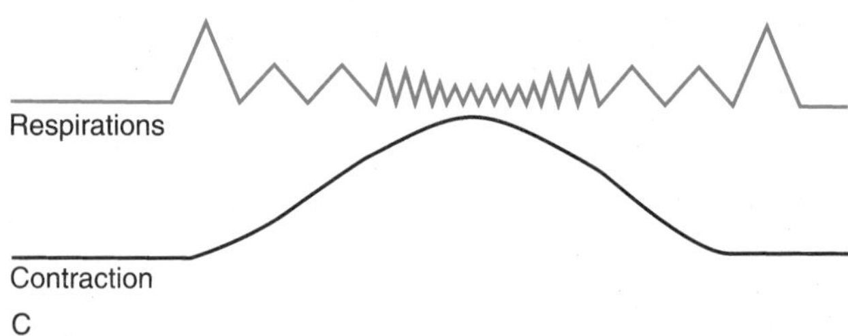

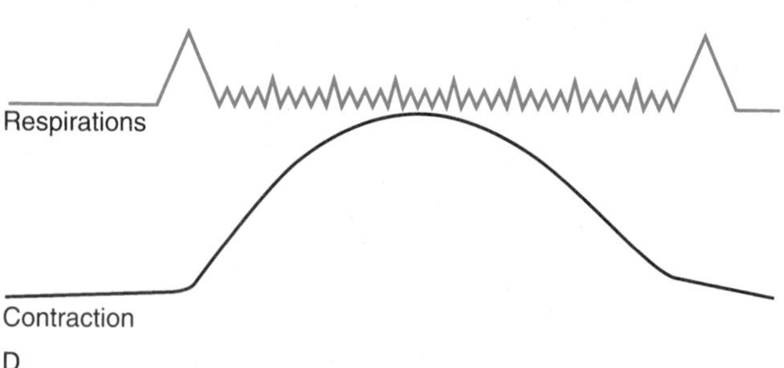

Figure 7–5. • **A,** Slow-paced breathing. The pattern starts with a cleansing breath as the contraction begins. The woman breathes slowly, at about half her usual rate, ending with a second cleansing breath at the end of the contraction. **B,** As labor intensifies, the woman may need to use modified paced breathing. The pattern begins and ends with a cleansing breath. The woman breathes rapidly, no faster than twice her usual respiratory rate, during the peak of the contraction. She ends with another cleansing breath. **C,** In this variation of modified paced breathing, the woman begins with slow paced breathing at the first of the contraction, switching to faster breathing during its peak. A cleansing breath also begins and ends this pattern. **D,** Patterned paced breathing begins and ends with a cleansing breath. During the contraction, the woman emphasizes the exhalation of some breaths. She may use a specific pattern or may randomly emphasize the blow.

breaths to avoid bearing down. Pushing before full cervical dilation may cause cervical edema or lacerations, especially with her first baby, because the cervix is not as stretchable as it is after one or more babies.

Second-Stage Breathing

When it is time for her to push, the woman takes a cleansing breath, then takes another deep breath and pushes down while exhaling to a count of 10. She blows out, takes a deep breath, and pushes again.

There is a difference of opinion among professionals about breath-holding while pushing. Traditional pushing involves sustained breath-holding against a closed glottis (the Valsalva maneuver).

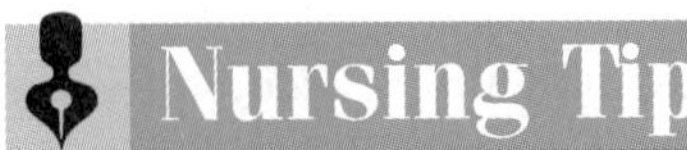

Nursing Tip

If a woman is successfully using a harmless nonpharmacologic pain control technique, do not interfere.

BOX 7–3

HOW TO RECOGNIZE AND CORRECT HYPERVENTILATION

Signs and Symptoms
Dizziness
Tingling of hands and feet
Cramps and muscle spasms of hands
Numbness around nose and mouth
Blurring of vision

Corrective Measures
Breathe slowly, especially in exhalation
Breathe into cupped hands
Breathe into small paper bag
Place a moist washcloth over the mouth and nose while breathing
Hold breath for a few seconds before exhaling

Those who promote this technique believe that the second stage of labor is a dangerous time for the fetus and should be completed quickly.

Others promote a modified pushing technique because they believe it allows better fetal oxygenation. In this form of pushing, the woman pushes with her glottis open. If she holds her breath, it is for no more than 6 seconds.

PHARMACOLOGIC PAIN MANAGEMENT

Pharmacologic pain management methods include analgesics, adjunctive drugs to improve the effectiveness of analgesics or to counteract their side effects, and anesthetics. Analgesics are systemic drugs (affecting the entire body) that reduce pain without loss of consciousness. Anesthetics cause loss of sensation, especially to pain. Regional anesthetics block sensation from a localized area without causing loss of consciousness. General anesthetics are systemic drugs that cause loss of consciousness and sensation to pain. Tables 7–1 and 7–2 summarize intrapartum analgesics, adjunctive drugs, and anesthetic methods.

Anesthetics are administered by various clinicians, depending on the type of drug. Local anesthetics are given by the physician or nurse-midwife at the time of birth. Other anesthetics may be given by the birth attendant or by a specialist in anesthetic administration.

There are two types of anesthesia clinicians: anesthesiologists and certified registered nurse anesthetists (CRNAs). An anesthesiologist is a physician who specializes in giving anesthesia. A CRNA is a registered nurse who has advanced training in anesthetic administration. State licensing laws and individual facility policies affect what anesthetic methods each clinician may administer.

Table 7–1
INTRAPARTUM ANALGESICS AND RELATED DRUGS

Drug/Common Dose/Route of Administration	Nursing Implications
Narcotics to reduce pain	
Meperidine (Demerol), 12.5–50 mg IV every 2–4 hr	Infant's respirations may be depressed; prepare for respiratory support at birth; continue observing newborn's respirations after birth (rate should be 30/min or higher)
Butorphanol (Stadol), 0.5–2.0 mg IV every 3–4 hr	Has mixed narcotic and narcotic-antagonist effects; avoid giving it after a pure narcotic such as meperidine; should not be given to the opiate-dependent (heroin) woman; neonatal effects similar to meperidine
Nalbuphine (Nubain), 10 mg IV every 3–6 hr	Same as butorphanol
Adjunctive drugs to enhance effects of narcotics, reduce nausea and vomiting, and itching from epidural narcotics	
Promethazine (Phenergan), 12.5–25 mg IV every 4–6 hr	Increases risk for infant respiratory depression (see meperidine); action is longer than narcotics
Hydroxyzine (Atarax, Vistaril), 25–100 mg IM Z-track only	Same as promethazine. Hydroxyzine is *not* given intravenously
Diphenhydramine (Benadryl), 10–50 mg IV	Relieves itching from epidural narcotics; dries mouth and mucous membranes; provide fluids, if permitted
Narcotic antagonists to reverse adverse effects of narcotics	
Naloxone (Narcan)	
Adult: 0.4–2 mg IV	Action of naloxone is shorter than most narcotics it reverses; observe for recurrent respiratory depression
For itching from epidural narcotics, 0.04–0.2 mg IV or IV infusion at 5–10 µg/kg/hr	
Neonate: 0.1 mg/kg IV (umbilical vein) or through endotracheal tube during resuscitation	Neonatal resuscitation dose for respiratory depression is higher than when the drug is used in other situations
Naltrexone (Trexan), 3–6 mg PO (1 dose)	Relieves itching from epidural narcotics

Table 7–2
TYPES OF ANESTHESIA FOR CHILDBIRTH

Anesthetic Method	Nursing Implications
Local infiltration. Injection of the perineum with local anesthetic drug just before vaginal birth; administered by nurse-midwife or physician	Injection may burn until area becomes numb; adverse effects are rare; check for allergies to *-caine* drugs or for dental anesthesia allergy
Pudendal block. Injection of the pudendal nerves with local anesthetic just before vaginal birth; local infiltration of the perineum is usually done also; may be used for some forceps births; administered by nurse-midwife or physician	Similar to local infiltration; warn the woman that the long needle is needed to reach the nerve and is shielded by the needle guide or "trumpet", observe for hematoma (collection of blood within tissues), which may become evident during the recovery period and is evidenced by excessive perineal or pelvic pain; pelvic infection sometimes occurs, but is uncommon
Epidural block. Injection of local anesthetic drug into the epidural space, which blocks transmission of pain impulses to brain; epidural narcotics are often added to reduce the amount of anesthetic needed and reduce the adverse effects; used for pain relief during labor and vaginal birth (including forceps-assisted), also for cesarean birth; administered by physician (obstetrician or anesthesiologist) or by nurse-anesthetist	Observe for hypotension and urinary retention; assist woman to maintain position as needed by anesthesia clinician; initially record blood pressure every 5 min after the block is begun and after each reinjection until stable; record fetal heart rates, usually with continuous electronic fetal monitoring; a full bladder may require catheterization if the woman cannot feel the urge to void; ambulate carefully because sensation will be reduced
Subarachnoid (spinal) block. Injection of local anesthetic drug under the dura and arachnoid membranes to block transmission of pain impulses to brain; used primarily for cesarean birth; usually administered by anesthesiologist	Observe for hypotension and urinary retention, as in epidural block—interventions are the same; suspect postspinal headache (usually during postpartum period) if woman complains of a headache that is worse when she is in an upright position; give oral fluids and analgesics as ordered
General anesthesia. Uses a combination of IV and inhalational drugs to produce loss of consciousness; rarely used for vaginal births; used for cesarean birth under some conditions: Woman's refusal of regional block Contraindication for regional block Emergency cesarean when there is not time to establish a regional block	Regurgitation, with aspiration of gastric contents is the primary risk; expect order for an oral antacid, such as sodium citrate with citric acid (Bicitra); IV drugs to reduce gastric acidity or speed up stomach emptying may also be given by the anesthesia clinician; assistant gives cricoid pressure until the woman is intubated to prevent any regurgitated stomach contents from reaching her trachea; anesthesia is light and woman may move on the operating table; postanesthesia recovery care includes observation of level of consciousness, vital signs, oxygen saturation, plus post-cesarean birth care

Advantages of Pharmacologic Methods

Methods that employ drugs are among the most effective for reducing pain during birth and can relieve much of it. Many methods help the woman to be a more active participant in birth. They help her to relax and work with contractions.

Limitations of Pharmacologic Methods

Pharmacologic methods are effective, but they do have limits. One important limitation is that two persons are medicated—the mother and her fetus. Any drug given to the mother can affect the fetus, and the effects may be prolonged in the infant after birth. The drug may directly affect the fetus, or it may indirectly affect the fetus because of effects in the mother (such as hypotension).

Several pharmacologic methods may slow labor's progress if used early in labor. Also, some complications during pregnancy limit the pharmacologic methods that are safe to use. For example, a method that requires infusion of large amounts of intravenous fluids might overload the woman's circulation if she has heart disease. If she takes other medications (legal or illicit), they may interact adversely with drugs used to relieve labor pain.

Analgesics and Adjunctive Drugs

Narcotic (Opioid) Analgesics

Injectable narcotic analgesics are most commonly used during labor. An opioid analgesic is a synthetic drug that is chemically related to opium.

Common analgesics for intrapartum use are butorphanol (Stadol), nalbuphine (Nubain), and meperidine (Demerol).

Butorphanol and nalbuphine have mixed narcotic and narcotic-antagonistic (counteracting) effects. Meperidine is a pure narcotic drug, without mixed effects. It is best to avoid giving butorphanol and nalbuphine after a dose of a pure opioid drug such as meperidine because the effects of the first drug will be partly reversed. They should not be given to the woman who abuses opiate drugs, such as heroin, or they may cause withdrawal effects.

The primary risk of narcotic analgesics is that they cross the placenta and can cause the infant's breathing at birth to be sluggish. This is most likely if the drug reaches its peak effects just as birth occurs. Meperidine has a prolonged action in the newborn and may depress respirations for several hours after birth. Butorphanol and nalbuphine can also cause respiratory depression, but reach a "ceiling," in which further doses do not increase the respiratory depression.

Narcotics are given in small, frequent doses in labor, usually by the intravenous route. This allows the mother to have a rapid and fairly stable level of pain relief and limits the amount of drug the fetus receives.

In general, narcotic analgesics are avoided if birth is expected within an hour. An attempt is made to time administration so the drug does not reach its peak at the time of birth. However, small doses are sometimes given in late labor if the fetus has no problems. The nurse must be prepared to support the respiratory efforts of all infants at birth, regardless of whether the mother received narcotics during labor.

Narcotic Antagonist

Naloxone (Narcan) is used to reverse respiratory depression, usually in the infant, caused by opioid drugs such as meperidine. It is not effective against respiratory depression from other causes, such as intrauterine hypoxia. It can be given by the intravenous route, or it may be given through the endotracheal tube during resuscitation. Intravenous naloxone is given to the neonate immediately after birth via the umbilical cord vein.

Naloxone has a shorter duration of action than most of the narcotics it reverses The nurse should observe for recurrent respiratory depression after each dose of naloxone until the depressant effects of the analgesic cease.

Adjunctive Drugs

Adjunctive drugs enhance the pain-relieving action of analgesics and reduce nausea. They also intensify the tendency of opioid analgesics to cause respiratory depression.

Promethazine (Phenergan) is a common adjunctive drug for labor analgesia. Promethazine remains active longer than most analgesics, and it may not be given with every analgesic dose.

Other adjunctive drugs that may be given include hydroxyzine (Atarax, Vistaril) or diphenhydramine (Benadryl). Hydroxyzine is only given by the intramuscular route using a Z-track technique.

Regional Analgesics and Anesthetics

Regional anesthetics block sensation to varying degrees, depending on the type of regional block used, quantity of medication, and the drugs injected. The woman still feels pressure and may feel some pain. The major advantage of regional anesthetics is that they allow the woman to be awake and participate in birth, yet have satisfactory pain relief.

Local and pudendal blocks are given in the vaginal-perineal area. Epidural and subarachnoid blocks and intrathecal narcotics are given by injecting anesthetic drugs so that they bathe the nerves as they emerge from the spinal cord. The spinal cord and nerves are not directly injected.

Regional blocks use any of several local anesthetic agents. The agents vary in time needed to become effective and in duration of their anesthetic action. The clinician chooses the agent based on the type of regional block and on the desired onset and duration. The names of most agents end in the suffix *-caine.* Common regional agents in obstetrics are bupivicaine, chloroprocaine, lidocaine, and mepivacaine.

Local anesthetic agents for childbirth are related to those for dental work. On admission, the nurse should ask each woman if she is allergic to or if she has had problems with dental anesthesia. If so, her physician or nurse midwife should be alerted to enable her to have the safest pain relief measures.

Local Infiltration

Injection of the perineal area for an episiotomy is done just before birth, when the fetal head is visible (Fig. 7–6). It may also be done after birth to repair a perineal laceration. There is a short delay between injection of the anesthetic agent and loss of pain sensation. The physician or nurse-midwife allows the anesthetic to become effective before beginning the episiotomy. There are virtually no risks if the woman is not allergic to the drug.

Pudendal Block

The pudendal block is used for vaginal births, although its use has become less common as the popularity of the epidural block has increased. It provides adequate anesthesia for an episiotomy and for most low forceps births (see p. 193). It does not block pain from contractions and, like local infiltration, is given just before birth. There is a delay of a few minutes between injection of the drug and onset of numbness.

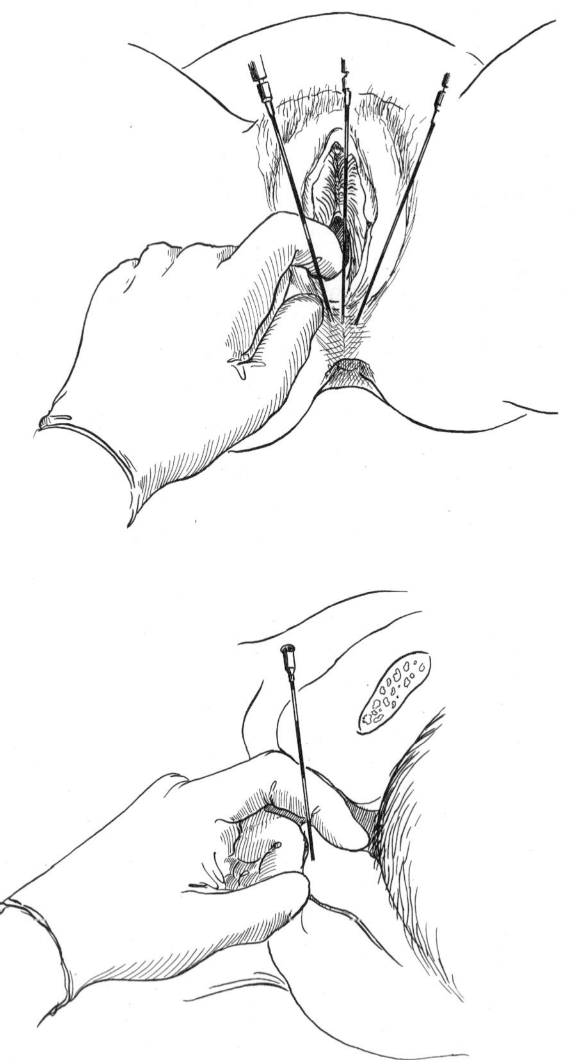

Figure 7–6. • Local infiltration anesthesia. The physician or nurse-midwife injects a local anesthetic agent into the perineal tissues to numb them.

The physician or nurse-midwife injects the pudendal nerves on each side of the mother's pelvis (Fig. 7–7). The nerves may be reached through the vagina or by injection directly through her perineum. A long needle (13–15 cm or 5–6 inches) is needed to reach the pudendal nerves, which are near the mother's ischial spines (see Fig. 7–7). If the injection is done through the vagina, a needle guide ("trumpet") is used to protect the mother's tissues. The needle is only injected about 1.3 cm (0.5 inch) into the woman's tissues. The perineum is also infiltrated because the pudendal block alone does not completely anesthetize the perineum.

Adverse Effects of Pudendal Block. The pudendal block has few adverse effects if the woman is not allergic to the drug. A vaginal hematoma (collection of blood within the tissues) sometimes occurs. An abscess may develop, but this is not common.

Epidural Block

The epidural block, also called a lumbar epidural block, relieves most of pain of labor and birth. It also can be used for cesarean birth and for postdelivery tubal ligation (see p. 195). It is begun after active labor is established (about 4 cm of cervical dilation) or just before a cesarean birth. The woman retains movement and can feel the urge to push if a low concentration of anesthetic agent is used. Higher anesthetic concentrations and a higher level on the woman's body (see Fig. 7–8) are used for cesarean birth or postpartum tubal ligation.

The epidural space is a small space just outside the dura (outermost membrane covering the brain and spinal cord). The woman is in a sitting or side-lying position for the epidural block. Her back is relatively straight, rather than being sharply curved forward, to avoid compressing the tiny epidural space, which is about 1 mm (the thickness of a dime).

The physician or nurse anesthetist penetrates the epidural space with a large needle (16- to 18-gauge). A fine catheter is threaded into the epidural space through the bore of the needle (Fig. 7–9). A test dose (2 to 3 ml) of local anesthetic agent is injected through the catheter. The woman is *not* expected to have effects from the test dose if the catheter is in the right place. Numbness or loss of movement following the small test dose indicates that her dura mater was probably punctured and the drug was injected into the subarachnoid space, as in subarachnoid block, rather than in the epidural space. Numbness around the mouth, ringing in the ears (tinnitus), visual disturbance, or jitteriness are symptoms that suggest injection into a vein. The

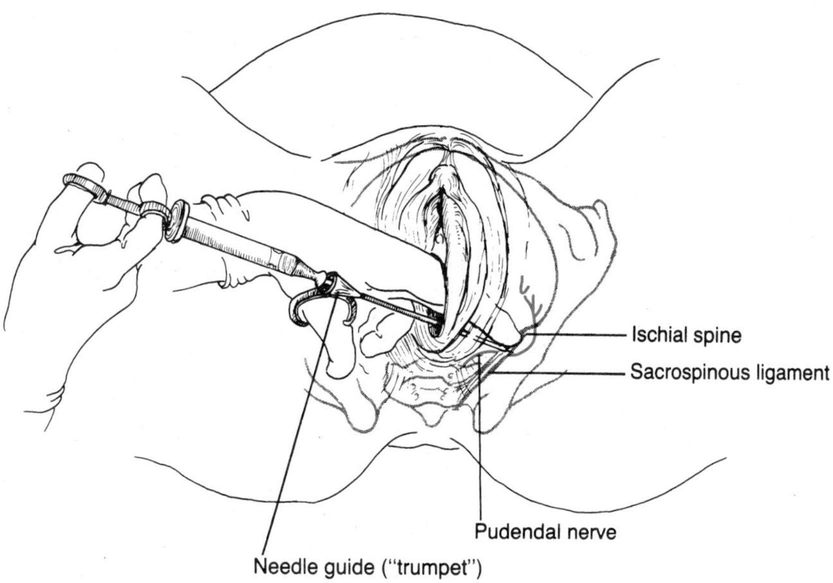

Figure 7–7. • Pudendal block anesthesia. The two pudendal nerves on each side of the pelvis are injected to numb the lower two-thirds of the vagina. In addition, local infiltration of the perineum is usually done, because the pudendal block does not always numb this area fully.

test dose is small enough to avoid long-term adverse effects.

If the test dose is normal (no effects), a larger amount of anesthetic agent is injected to begin the block. A few minutes are needed before the onset of the block. If an epidural block is being used for surgery, such as cesarean delivery or tubal ligation, the anesthesiologist or CRNA will test for the level of numbness before surgery begins.

Local anesthetic drugs are usually combined with a small dose of an opioid analgesic such as fentanyl (Sublimaze). The combination of drugs allows quicker and longer-lasting pain relief with less anesthetic agent and minimal loss of movement. An epidural block for labor is more accurately termed *analgesia* (reducing pain) than *anesthesia* (obliterating all sensation).

The woman can sometimes ambulate when combination-drug epidural is used because the local anesthetic dose is much lower. She can assume any position with this type of block, although any pregnant woman should avoid the supine position.

To maintain pain relief during labor, the anesthetic drug is constantly infused into the catheter.

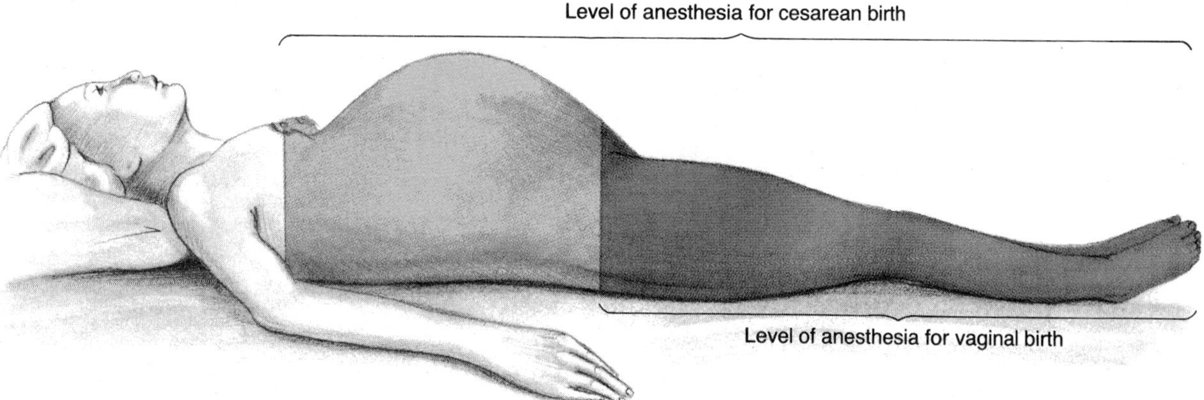

Figure 7–8. • Levels of anesthesia for epidural or subarachnoid blocks. For cesarean birth, numbness reaches the woman's nipple level. For vaginal birth, the level is about at the hips.

Alternatively, repeat intermittent injections of the drug may be given. Patient-controlled analgesia (PCA) epidural infusion is sometimes used.

Long-acting epidural narcotics may be used after cesarean birth to give prolonged postoperative pain relief (up to 24 hours). The woman may need no other analgesia if she receives epidural narcotics, or she may need only oral analgesics for afterpains, such as nonsteroidal antiinflammatory drugs (NSAIDs). Long-acting epidural narcotics can cause respiratory depression that may occur many hours after they are injected. They may also cause intense pruritus (itching), which can be relieved with diphenhydramine (Benadryl) or naltrexone (Trexan).

Dural Puncture. The dura lies just below the tiny epidural space. This membrane is sometimes punctured accidentally ("wet tap") with the epidural needle or the catheter that is inserted through it. If dural puncture occurs, a relatively large amount of spinal fluid leaks from the hole and may result in a headache.

Limitations of Epidural Block. Although it is a popular method of intrapartum pain relief, epidural block is not used if the woman has

- Abnormal blood clotting
- An infection in the area of injection or a systemic infection
- Hypovolemia (inadequate blood volume)

Some women have had back surgery, such as for scoliosis, that make epidural or spinal blocks impossible.

Adverse Effects of Epidural Block. The most common side effects are maternal hypotension, which can compromise fetal oxygenation, and urinary retention. To counteract hypotension, a large quantity (500–1000 ml or more) of warmed intravenous (IV) solution such as Ringer's lactate is infused rapidly before the block is begun. Solutions are warmed because rapid administration of room-temperature intravenous fluids will chill the woman.

The large quantity of intravenous fluids combined with reduced sensation may result in urinary

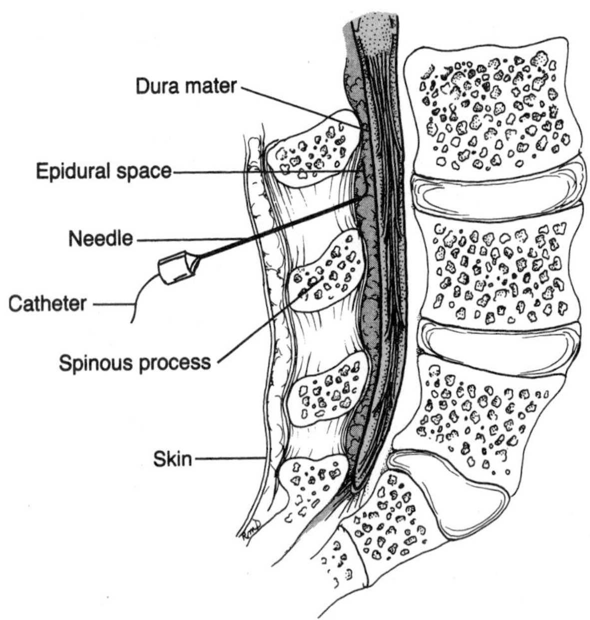

The epidural space is entered with a needle below where the spinal cord ends. A fine catheter is threaded through the needle.

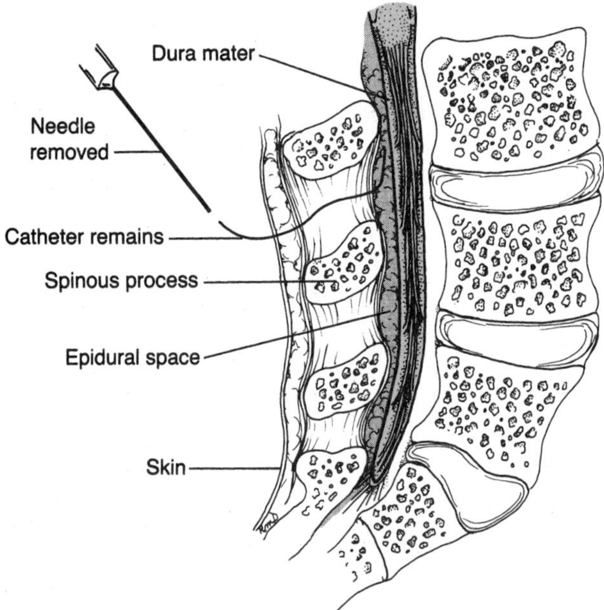

After the catheter is threaded into the epidural space, the needle is removed. Medication can then be injected into the epidural space intermittently or by continuous infusion for pain relief during labor and birth.

Figure 7–9. • Epidural block. A needle is inserted into the epidural space, just outside the dura mater. A small catheter is threaded into the space to allow repeated injections of anesthetic agent. The epidural block can eliminate sensations from both contractions and perineal stretching, and it can be used for cesarean birth or postdelivery sterilization.

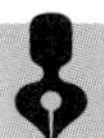

Nursing Tip

Assess the woman for bladder distention regularly if she has epidural or subarachnoid block. A full bladder can delay birth and can cause hemorrhage after birth.

retention. The nurse should palpate the suprapubic area for a full bladder every 2 hours or more often if a large quantity of IV solution was given. If the woman is unable to void, she will need catheterization.

The woman may feel less of an urge to push in the second stage of labor when she has an epidural block, depending on the drugs used for her block. Therefore, this stage may be longer if a woman has an epidural block. There is no arbitrary time limit for the second stage if the maternal and fetal conditions are normal.

Intrathecal Opioid Analgesics

Injection of opioid analgesics into the subarachnoid space (similar to the technique for subarachnoid block) is gaining acceptance. Because the analgesic is so near the nerves that transmit pain to the brain, much smaller doses are needed. The woman feels her contractions, but they are much less painful. Intrathecal analgesics do not produce the anesthesia needed for surgical procedures.

Advantages of intrathecal analgesics include the following:

- Rapid onset of pain relief without sedation
- No loss of movement; the woman may readily change positions or ambulate during labor
- No hypotensive effects

Disadvantages include the following:

- Limited duration of action
- Inadequate pain relief for late labor and the birth itself, requiring added pain-relief measures at that time

Nursing care includes observation for late-occurring respiratory depression. Naloxone should be readily available. Nausea, vomiting, and itching may occur.

Subarachnoid (Spinal) Block

Three membranes cover the brain and spinal cord: the dura mater, arachnoid mater, and pia mater membranes. The dura and arachnoid membranes are so close together that they are like a single membrane. The pia mater is a fragile membrane that tightly covers the nerve tissue. Cerebrospinal fluid circulates between the dura/arachnoid membranes and the pia membrane.

The woman's position for a subarachnoid block is similar to that for the epidural block, except that her back is curled around her uterus in a C-shape. The dura is punctured with a thin (25- to 27-gauge) spinal needle. A few drops of spinal fluid confirms entry into the subarachnoid space (Fig. 7–10). The local anesthetic drug is then injected. A much smaller quantity of drug is needed to achieve anesthesia in the subarachnoid block than in the epidural block. Anesthesia occurs quickly and is more profound than the epidural block; the woman loses movement and sensation below the block.

The subarachnoid block is a "one-shot" block, since it does not involve placing a catheter for reinjection of the drug. It is not often used for vaginal births today, but remains common for cesarean births. Its limitations are essentially the same as those for epidural block.

Adverse Effects of Subarachnoid Block. Hypotension and urinary retention are the main adverse effects of subarachnoid block, as in the epidural block. They are managed as in the epidural block. Hypotension is often more severe.

A postspinal headache sometimes occurs, most likely because of spinal fluid loss. The woman may be advised to remains flat for several hours after the block to decrease the chance of postspinal headache. However, there is no absolute evidence that this precaution is effective (Cunningham et al., 1997).

Postspinal headache is worse when the woman is upright and often disappears entirely when she lies down. Bed rest, analgesics, and oral and intravenous fluids help to relieve the headache. A *blood patch,* done by the nurse-anesthetist or anesthesiologist, may give dramatic relief from postspinal headache. The woman's blood (10–15 ml) is withdrawn from her vein and injected into the epidural space in the area of the subarachnoid puncture (Fig. 7–11). The blood clots and forms a gelatinous seal that stops spinal fluid leakage. The clot later breaks down and is reabsorbed by the body.

General Anesthesia

General anesthesia is rarely used for vaginal births or for most cesarean births. Regional blocks are preferred for cesarean births, if possible. Gen-

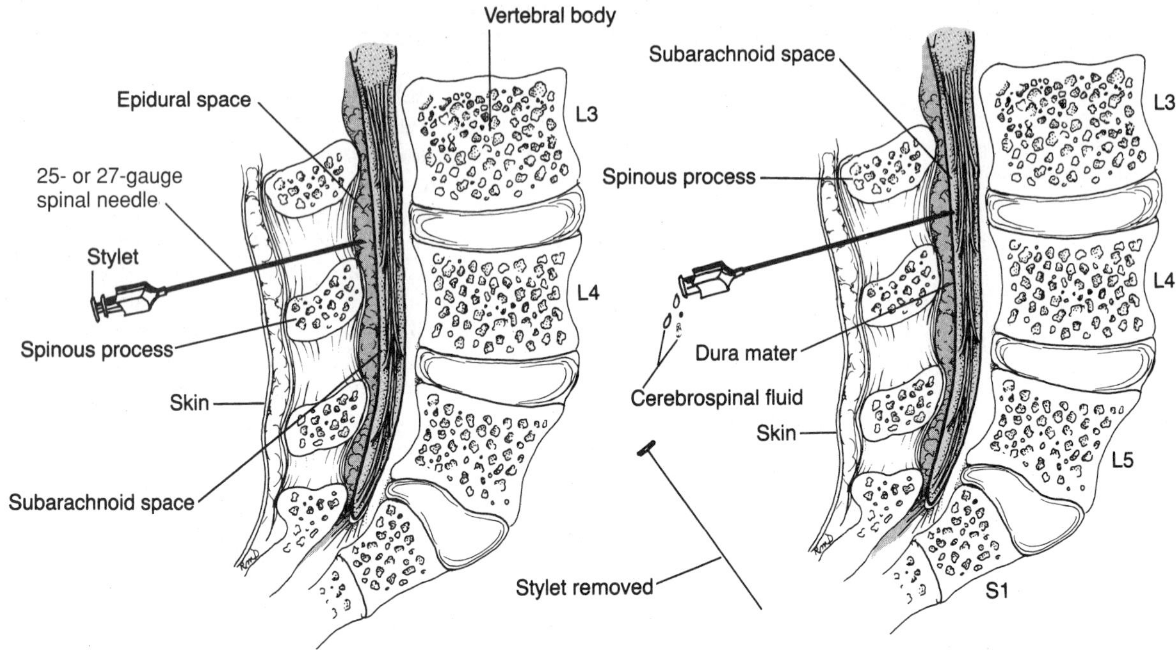

Figure 7–10. • Subarachnoid block. A fine-gauge hollow needle with a stylet to plug it is inserted into the subarachnoid space. The stylet is removed, and a few drops of cerebrospinal fluid confirm that the needle is in the correct space. Local anesthetic agent is injected. Unlike the epidural, repeat injections are not possible with this method.

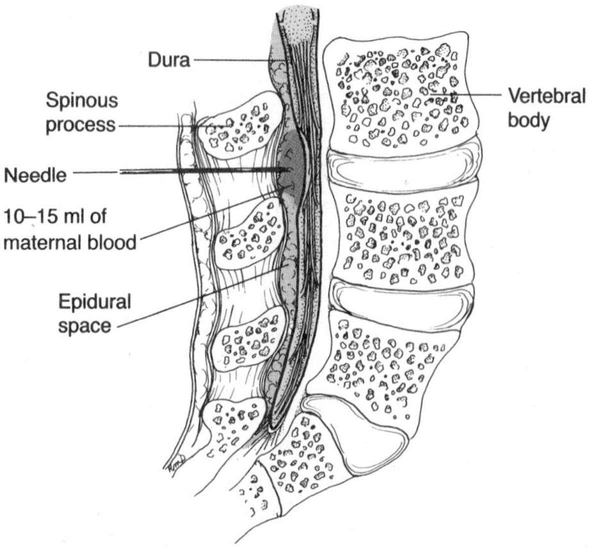

eral anesthesia may be necessary in these circumstances:

- Emergency cesarean birth, when there is not time to establish either an epidural or a subarachnoid block
- Cesarean birth in the woman who refuses or has a contraindication to epidural or subarachnoid block

Combinations of general anesthetic drugs (balanced anesthesia) allow quick onset of anesthesia, minimal fetal effects, and prompt maternal wakening.

Adverse Effects in the Mother

The major adverse effect of general anesthesia is the same during birth as at any other time: regurgitation with aspiration (breathing in) of the acidic stomach contents. This results in a chemical injury to the lungs, *aspiration pneumonitis.* It can be fatal.

Many women begin labor with a full stomach, and their gastric action slows during labor. In addition, the full uterus exerts upward pressure

Figure 7–11. • An epidural blood patch may give dramatic relief from postspinal headache.

against the stomach. For purposes of anesthesia, therefore, every pregnant woman is presumed to have a full stomach.

Several drugs are used to reduce gastric acidity. An oral antacid, such as sodium citrate with citric acid (Bicitra), 15 ml, is commonly given before surgery. Ranitidine (Zantac) or cimetidine (Tagamet) may be given intravenously to reduce gastric acidity or to accelerate emptying of the stomach.

An assistant (often the circulating nurse) gives *cricoid pressure* (Sellick's maneuver) by compressing the esophagus between the rigid trachea and spine. If regurgitation occurs, the gastric contents cannot pass the area of pressure and enter the trachea. After the endotracheal tube is in place and its cuff inflated, stomach contents cannot enter the trachea, and the pressure is released.

General anesthesia can cause the uterus to relax. This is an advantage when uterine inversion occurs (see p. 212), but it may result in hemorrhage after birth (see p. 224 for assessment of the uterine fundus after birth and p. 258 for nursing care in postpartum hemorrhage).

Adverse Effects in the Neonate

Respiratory depression is the main neonatal risk, because drugs given to the mother may cross the placenta. To reduce this risk, the time from induction of anesthesia to clamping of the umbilical cord is kept as short as possible. The woman is prepped and draped for surgery, and all personnel are scrubbed, gowned, and gloved before anesthesia begins. In addition, the anesthesia is kept as light as possible until the cord is clamped. Because the anesthesia is light, the woman may move during surgery, although she does not recall the experience. Respiratory depression can occur in the woman, but this is less common than in the neonate because minimal doses of anesthetic drugs are used.

THE NURSE'S ROLE IN PAIN MANAGEMENT

The nurse has many responsibilities in both nonpharmacologic and pharmacologic pain management during the intrapartum period in addition to those previously discussed under the individual techniques. Nursing care reduces factors that hinder a woman's pain control and enhances factors that benefit it. Nursing Care Plan 7–1 gives examples of nursing measures related to intrapartum comfort.

The Nurse's Role in Nonpharmacologic Techniques

When a woman is admitted, the nurse determines whether she had preparation for childbirth and works with what the woman and her partner learned. The nurse may need to suggest variations in the methods they learned if what they are doing is ineffective. The nurse helps them to identify signs of tension so that the woman can be guided to release it.

If the woman did not have childbirth preparation, the nurse teaches her the simple breathing and relaxation techniques discussed earlier in the chapter. If the woman is extremely anxious and out of control, she will not be able to comprehend verbal instructions. It may be necessary to make close eye contact with her and to breathe with her through each contraction until she can regain control.

The nurse minimizes environmental irritants as much as possible. The lights should be lowered and the woman kept reasonably dry by regularly changing the underpads. The temperature should be adjusted; the nurse provides a warm blanket if that provides the most comfort. See Chapter 6 for other general comfort measures during labor.

The nurse should be cautious not to overestimate or underestimate the amount of pain a woman is having. The quiet, stoic woman may need analgesia, yet be reluctant to ask. A tense body posture or grimacing may indicate she needs additional pain relief measures.

The vocal woman who complains bitterly about her distress in labor is also difficult to assess. It is difficult to evaluate pain relief needs in the woman who moans and cries most of the time. She may need additional pain relief measures, or she may simply be a person who is vocal during labor.

The Nurse's Role in Pharmacologic Techniques

The nurse's responsibility in pharmacologic pain management begins at admission. The woman should be closely questioned about allergy to drugs, including dental anesthetics, to identify pain relief measures that may not be advisable. She should be questioned about her preferences for pain relief. Factors that may impact the choice of pain relief should be noted, such as back surgery, infection in the area where an epidural block would be injected, or blood pressure abnormalities.

The nurse keeps the side rails up if the woman takes pain relief drugs. Narcotics may cause

NURSING CARE PLAN 7–1

Selected Nursing Diagnoses for the Woman Needing Pain Management during Labor

Nursing Diagnosis: Pain related to uterine contractions and descent of fetus in pelvis

Goals	Nursing Interventions	Rationale
The woman will state that her discomfort is manageable during labor using techniques learned in prepared childbirth classes and/or taught by the nurse The woman will have a relaxed facial and body appearance between contractions	1. Assess for presence and character of pain continuously during labor: a. Statement of pain (assess nature of pain, such as location, intensity, whether intermittent or constant) b. Crying, moaning during and/or between contractions c. Tense, guarded body posture or thrashing with contractions d. "Mask of pain" facial expression	1. These are common verbal and nonverbal signs of pain; assessment enables nurse to identify if pain is normal for woman's labor status and to choose the best interventions for pain relief (nonpharmacologic and/or pharmacologic measures); evaluating nonverbal and verbal communication helps nurse to evaluate need for pain relief in women who may not directly communicate their need for pain relief or who do not speak prevailing language
	2. Provide general comfort measures, such as a. Adjust the room temperature and light level for comfort b. Reduce irritants, such as wet underpads c. Provide ice chips, Popsicles, or juices to relieve dry mouth d. Avoid bumping bed	2. These general measures reduce outside irritants that make it harder for woman to use prepared childbirth techniques and are a source of discomfort themselves
	3. Encourage woman to assume positions she finds most comfortable, other than the supine (see Chapter 6 for more information)	3. Position changes promote comfort and help fetus adapt to the size and shape of woman's pelvis; supine position can result in supine hypotensive syndrome, which reduces placental blood flow and fetal oxygenation.
	4. Observe for a full bladder every 1–2 hr or more often if the woman receives large amounts of PO or IV fluids	4. A full bladder is a source of discomfort and can prolong labor by inhibiting fetal descent; it may cause pain that lingers after epidural analgesia is begun
	5. Promote use of prepared childbirth techniques, including labor partner as appropriate: a. Do not stand in front of her focal point b. Offer a back rub or firm sacral pressure; ask her about the best location and amount of pressure; use baby powder to prevent skin irritation c. Encourage woman to switch to more complex patterns only when simpler ones are no longer effective d. Breathe along with woman if she has trouble maintaining patterns; make eye contact	5. These are examples of how to assist woman and her partner in using methods they learned most effectively; use of nonpharmacologic pain relief avoids problems associated with pharmacologic interventions and supplements any drug therapy used; they also give the woman and her partner a sense of control and mastery that enhances perception of birth as a positive experience

Continued on following page

drowsiness or dizziness. Regional anesthetics reduce sensation and movement to varying degrees, so the woman may have less control over her body.

The nurse reinforces explanations given by the anesthesia clinician about procedures and expected effects of the selected pain management method. Women often receive these explanations when they are very uncomfortable and do not remember everything they were told.

The woman is helped to assume and hold the

NURSING CARE PLAN 7–1 *continued*

Selected Nursing Diagnoses for the Woman Needing Pain Management during Labor

Nursing Diagnosis: Pain related to uterine contractions and descent of fetus in pelvis

Goals	Nursing Interventions	Rationale
	6. If woman has signs of hyperventilation (dizziness, numbness or tingling sensations, spasms of the hands and feet), have her breathe into her cupped hands, a small bag, or a washcloth placed over her mouth and nose; or instruct her to hold her breath briefly	6. Hyperventilation often occurs when woman uses rapid breathing patterns because she exhales too much carbon dioxide; these measures help her to conserve carbon dioxide and rebreathe it to correct excess loss
	7. Tell woman and her partner when labor progresses; for example, if she is pushing and her baby's head becomes visible, let her see or feel it	7. Labor does not last forever; knowing that her efforts are having desired results gives her courage to continue and helps her to tolerate pain

Nursing Diagnosis: Knowledge deficit: procedures and expected effects of epidural block

Goals	Nursing Interventions	Rationale
After explanations, the woman will state that she understands what will happen during and after epidural block is begun	1. Explain what to expect as the epidural block is begun (reinforcing explanations of anesthesiologist or nurse-anesthetist): a. An IV will be started and she will receive fluids to offset the tendency of her blood pressure to fall b. Fetus will be monitored by electronic fetal monitoring c. Nurse-anesthetist or anesthesiologist will position her; she should remain still in this position d. A small plastic catheter will be taped to her back to allow constant infusion of medication (or reinjection) e. Her blood pressure will be checked every 5 min when block is first begun	1. This list reflects a common sequence of events for starting an epidural block; anesthesia clinician explains the procedure and expected effects; nurse reinforces explanations as needed because the woman in pain may not be able to concentrate; knowledge reduces anxiety and fear of the unknown; if woman understands that these procedures are a normal part of an epidural block, she is less likely to interpret them as abnormal
	2. If she needs to remain flat briefly to allow the drug to disperse, put a small pillow under her right hip	2. Pillow under hip avoids supine hypotensive syndrome
	3. Explain that she will feel less pain but that she will feel pressure; movement and sensation in her legs and feet will vary	3. Helps woman to understand that epidural block is not expected to abolish pain of labor; leg movement and sensation is affected in varying amounts; if she understands variation in effects, she is less likely to interpret them as abnormal or as evidence that block is not working

Nursing Diagnosis: Risk for injury related to loss of sensation

Goals	Nursing Interventions	Rationale
The woman will not have an injury, such as muscle strain or fall, while her epidural is in effect Fetus will not be born in uncontrolled delivery	1. Check for movement, sensation, and leg strength before ambulating; ambulate cautiously, with an assistant	1. A fall is more likely if she does not have sensation and control over her movements
	2. Observe for signs that birth may be near: a. Increase in bloody show b. Statement of pressure or need to push (may *not* be present, depending on individual response to block) c. Bulging of the perineum or appearance of head	2. Loss of sensation varies among women having epidural block; labor may progress more rapidly than expected; these are signs associated with imminent birth that should be evaluated by the experienced nurse, nurse-midwife, or physician

Nursing Tip

Important admission assessments related to pharmacologic pain management are last oral intake (time and type), adverse reactions to drugs—especially dental anesthetics, and other medications taken.

position for the epidural or subarachnoid block. The nurse tells the anesthesia clinician if the woman has a contraction because it might prevent her from holding still. Also, the anesthetic drug is usually injected between contractions.

The woman is observed for hypotension if an epidural or subarachnoid block is given. Hospital protocols vary, but the blood pressure is usually taken every 5 minutes after the block is begun (and with each reinjection) until her blood pressure is stable. An automatic blood pressure monitor is often used. Some facilities add a pulse-oximeter to monitor oxygen saturation. At the same time, the nurse observes the fetus for signs associated with fetal compromise (see p. 146), as maternal hypotension can reduce placental blood flow.

The epidural block is given during labor and may reduce the mother's sensation of rectal pressure. The nurse coaches her about the right time to start and stop pushing with each contraction if needed. The nurse also observes for signs of imminent birth, such as increased bloody show and perineal bulging, since she may not be able to feel the sensations clearly.

Nursing responsibilities related to general anesthesia include assessment and documentation of oral intake and administration of medications to reduce gastric acidity. The woman should be told that all preparations for surgery will be done *before* she is put to sleep. The nurse reassures her that she will be asleep before any incision is done. Having a familiar nurse in the operating room full of new people is reassuring to the woman before surgery.

The woman who has general anesthesia is usually awake enough to move from the operating table to her bed after surgery. Her respiratory status is observed every 15 minutes for 1 to 2 hours. A pulse oximeter provides constant information about her blood oxygen level. She is given oxygen by face tent or other means until she is fully awake. See a medical-surgical nursing text for more information about postanesthesia nursing care. Her uterine fundus and vaginal bleeding are observed as for any other postpartum woman. Her urine output from the indwelling catheter should be observed for quantity and color.

The nurse should ambulate the woman cautiously and with assistance if she had an epidural or subarachnoid block. She may be able to move her legs yet not be able to feel her feet, which would make her likely to fall.

If the woman receives narcotic drugs, the nurse observes her respiratory rate for depression. Because respiratory depression is more likely to occur in the neonate than in the mother, the neonate is observed after birth. Narcotic effects in the infant may persist longer than in an adult. The nurse has naloxone on hand in case it is needed to reverse respiratory depression in the mother or infant.

The nurse observes the woman for late-appearing respiratory depression and excessive sedation if she had epidural narcotics after cesarean birth. This may be up to 24 hours after administration, depending on the drug given. The woman's respiratory status is monitored with an hourly respiratory rate and sedation assessment, a pulse oximeter, and/or an apnea monitor. Facilities often use a scale to assess for sedation so that all caregivers use the same criteria for assessment and documentation. Additional analgesics are given cautiously and strictly as ordered. If mild analgesics do not relieve the pain, the physician is contacted for additional orders. Analgesics in addition to the epidural narcotic can increase respiratory depression.

KEY POINTS

- Pain during birth is different from other types of pain because it is part of a normal process that results in the birth of a baby. The woman has time to prepare for it, and the pain is self-limiting.
- A woman's pain threshold is fairly constant. Her pain tolerance varies, and nursing actions can increase her ability to tolerate pain. Irritants can reduce her pain tolerance.

- Prepared childbirth classes give the woman and her partner pain management tools they can use during labor. Some tools, such as breathing techniques and effleurage, can be taught to the unprepared woman.
- The nurse should do everything possible to promote relaxation during labor because it enhances the effectiveness of all other pain management methods, nonpharmacologic and pharmacologic.
- Any drug that the expectant mother takes may cross the placenta and affect the fetus. Effects may persist in the baby much longer than in an adult.
- Observe the mother and/or infant for respiratory depression if she received narcotics, including epidural narcotics, during the intrapartum period.
- Regional anesthetics are the most common for birth because they allow the mother to remain awake, including for cesarean birth.
- Closely question the woman about drug allergies when she is admitted. Because drugs used for regional anesthesia are related to those used in dentistry, ask her about reactions to dental anesthesia.
- Observe the mother's blood pressure and the fetal heart rate after epidural or spinal block to identify hypotension or fetal compromise. Urinary retention is also more likely.
- Be prepared to administer a drug to reduce gastric acidity if surgery is anticipated, as general anesthesia may be needed unexpectedly.

MULTIPLE-CHOICE REVIEW QUESTIONS

Choose the most appropriate answer.

1. Specify which of the following situations best describes a woman's use of the gate control theory to manage pain. The woman
   a. breathes slowly at the beginning and end of a contraction but more rapidly at its peak
   b. rubs the palms of her hands on the bed's side rails during each contraction
   c. focuses intently on a photograph that she brought to the birth center
   d. listens to tapes of rain and waterfalls through headphones
2. Which technique is likely to be most effective for "back labor?"
   a. stimulating the abdomen by effleurage
   b. applying firm pressure in the sacral area
   c. blowing out in short breaths during each contraction
   d. rocking side to side at the peak of each contraction
3. What drug should be immediately available when a woman receives narcotics?
   a. fentanyl (Sublimaze)
   b. diphenhydramine (Benadryl)
   c. lidocaine (Xylocaine)
   d. naloxone (Narcan)
4. Choose the most important nursing assessment immediately after a woman has an epidural block.
   a. bladder distention
   b. intravenous site
   c. respiratory rate
   d. blood pressure
5. A woman will have general anesthesia for a repeat cesarean delivery because surgical correction of her scoliosis makes epidural or subarachnoid block impossible. What order related to this anesthetic should the nurse expect?
   a. preoperative antacid
   b. narcotic premedication
   c. 500 ml oral fluids
   d. naloxone (Narcan) injection

BIBLIOGRAPHY AND READER REFERENCE

American Academy of Pediatrics and American College of Obstetricians and Gynecologists. (1997). *Guidelines for perinatal care* (4th ed.). Elk Grove Village, IL: Author.

American College of Obstetricians and Gynecologists. (1996). ACOG technical bulletin number 225: obstetric analgesia and anesthesia. *International Journal of Gynecology and Obstetrics, 54,* 281–292.

Blackburn, S., & Loper, D. (1992). *Maternal, fetal and neonatal physiology: A clinical perspective.* Philadelphia: Saunders.

Boettcher, C. (1997). Reclaiming your spirit in an epidural world. Presentation at AWHONN's Northeast Texas Section Spring Conference, May 2 and 3, 1997, Arlington, TX.

Brucker, M. C., & Zwelling, E. (1997). Pain management during childbirth. In F. H. Nichols & E. Zwelling (Eds.), *Maternal–newborn nursing: Theory and practice* (pp. 823–861). Philadelphia: Saunders.

Creehan, P. A. (1996). Pain relief and comfort measures during labor. In K. R. Simpson & P. A. Creehan (Eds.), *AWHONN's perinatal nursing* (pp. 227–245). Philadelphia: Lippincott.

Cunningham, F. G., MacDonald, P. C., Gant, N. F., Leveno, K. J., Gilstrap, L. C., Hankins, G. D. V., & Clark, S. L. (1997). *William's obstetrics* (20th ed). Stamford, CT: Appleton & Lange.

Dewan, D. M., & Hood, D. D. (1997). *Practical obstetric anesthesia.* Philadelphia: Saunders.

Gorrie, T., McKinney, E., & Murray, S. (1998). *Foundations of maternal–newborn nursing* (2nd ed.). Philadelphia: Saunders.

Kleigman, R. M. (1996). The fetus and the neonatal infant: Delivery room emergencies. In R. E. Behrman, R. M. Kliegman, & A. M. Arvin (Eds.), *Nelson Textbook of Pediatrics* (15th ed., pp. 471–473). Philadelphia: Saunders.

Lowe, N. K. (1996). The pain and discomfort of labor and birth. *Journal of Obstetric, Gynecologic, and Neonatal Nursing, 25*(1), 82–92.

Manning, J. (1996). Intrathecal narcotics: New approach for labor analgesia. *Journal of Obstetric, Gynecologic, and Neonatal Nursing, 25*(3), 221–224.

Simkin, P. (1995). Reducing pain and enhancing progress in labor: A guide to nonpharmacologic methods for maternity caregivers. *Birth, 22*(3), 161–171.

Weber, S. E. (1996). Cultural aspects of pain in childbearing women. *Journal of Obstetric, Gynecologic, and Neonatal Nursing, 25*(1), 67–72.

Youngstrom, P. C., Baker S. W., & Miller, J. L. (1996). Epidurals redefined in analgesia and anesthesia: A distinction with a difference. *Journal of Obstetric, Gynecologic, and Neonatal Nursing, 25*(4), 350–354.

chapter 8

Nursing Care of Women with Complications during Labor and Birth

Outline

OBSTETRIC PROCEDURES
- Amniotomy
- Induction or Augmentation of Labor
- Version
- Episiotomy and Lacerations
- Forceps and Vacuum Extraction Births
- Cesarean Birth

ABNORMAL LABOR
- Problems with the Powers of Labor
- Problems with the Fetus
- Problems with the Pelvis and Soft Tissues
- Psychological Problems
- Abnormal Duration of Labor

PREMATURE RUPTURE OF MEMBRANES

PRETERM LABOR

PROLONGED PREGNANCY

EMERGENCIES DURING CHILDBIRTH
- Prolapsed Umbilical Cord
- Uterine Rupture
- Uterine Inversion
- Amniotic Fluid Embolism
- Trauma

Objectives

On completion and mastery of Chapter 8, the student will be able to

- Define each vocabulary term listed.
- Describe each obstetric procedure discussed in this chapter.
- Explain the nurse's role in each obstetric procedure.
- Describe factors that contribute to an abnormal labor.
- Explain each intrapartum complication discussed in this chapter.
- Explain the nurse's role in caring for women having each intrapartum complication.

Vocabulary

bloodless window
cephalopelvic disproportion
chignon
chorioamnionitis
dystocia
hydramnios
laminaria
macrosomia
shoulder dystocia
tocolytic

Childbirth is a normal, natural event in the life of most women and their families. When the many factors that affect the birth process function in harmony, complications are unlikely. However, some women experience complications during childbirth that threaten their well-being or that of the baby.

OBSTETRIC PROCEDURES

Nurses assist with several obstetric procedures during birth; they also care for women after the procedures. Some, such as amniotomy, are done in uncomplicated births. Other procedures are needed only for women who have complications during birth.

Amniotomy

Amniotomy, abbreviated AROM, is the artificial rupture of the membranes (amniotic sac) by using a sterile sharp instrument. It is performed by a physician or nurse-midwife. Amniotomy is not a nursing function of either the registered or practical nurse. The nurse assists with amniotomy and cares for the woman and fetus afterward.

Amniotomy is done to stimulate contractions. It may provide enough stimulation to start labor before it begins naturally, but it is more often done to enhance contractions that have already begun. It may be done to permit internal fetal monitoring (see p. 146). It also is done just before delivery of the baby through the uterine incision in a planned cesarean birth.

Technique

To determine if amniotomy is safe and indicated, the physician or nurse-midwife does a vaginal examination to assess the cervical effacement and dilation and the station of the fetus. A disposable plastic hook (Amnihook) is passed through the cervix, and the amniotic sac is snagged to create a hole and release the amniotic fluid (Fig. 8–1). Another type of sharp instrument may be used to rupture membranes in a cesarean birth.

Complications

The three complications associated with amniotomy may also occur if a woman's membranes

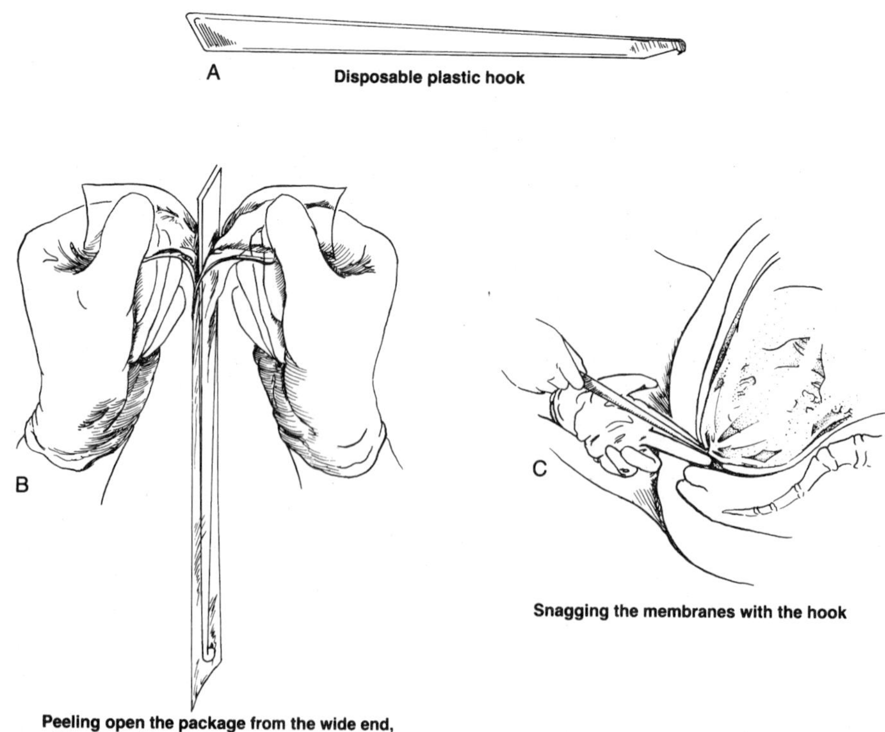

Figure 8–1. • Amniotomy. **A,** The Amnihook disposable plastic hook. **B,** Technique to open the Amnihook package for the physician or nurse-midwife. **C,** Method of rupturing the membranes.

rupture spontaneously (spontaneous rupture of membranes, SROM). These are prolapse of the umbilical cord, infection, and abruptio placentae.

Prolapse of the Umbilical Cord. Prolapse may occur if the cord slips downward with a gush of amniotic fluid (p. 210).

Infection. Infection may occur because the membranes no longer block vaginal organisms from entering the uterus. An amniotomy commits the woman to delivery. The physician or nurse-midwife delays amniotomy until reasonably certain that birth will occur before the risk of infection markedly increases.

Abruptio Placentae. Abruptio placentae (separation of the placenta before birth) is more likely to occur if the uterus is overdistended with amniotic fluid (hydramnios) when the membranes rupture. The uterus becomes smaller with discharge of amniotic fluid, but the placenta stays the same size and no longer fits its implantation site (see p. 91 for more information about abruptio placentae).

Nursing Care

The nursing care after amniotomy is the same as that following spontaneous membrane rupture: identifying complications and promoting the woman's comfort.

Identifying Complications. The fetal heart rate is recorded for at least 1 minute after amniotomy. Rates outside the normal range of 110 to 160 beats per minute (BPM) for a term fetus suggest a prolapsed umbilical cord. A large quantity of fluid increases the risk for prolapsed cord, especially if the fetus is high in the pelvis or is very small.

The color, odor, amount, and character of amniotic fluid are recorded. The fluid should be clear, possibly with flecks of vernix (newborn skin coating) and should not have a bad odor. Cloudy, yellow, or malodorous fluid suggests infection.

The woman's temperature is taken every 2 to 4 hours after her membranes rupture, according to facility policy. A maternal temperature of 38° C (100.4° F) or higher suggests infection. An increase in the fetal heart rate, especially if above 160 BPM, may precede the woman's temperature increase.

Green fluid means that the fetus passed the first stool (meconium) into the fluid before birth.

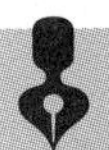

Nursing Tip

Observe for wet underpads and linens after the membranes rupture. Change them as often as needed to keep the woman relatively dry and to reduce the risk for infection.

Meconium-stained amniotic fluid is more common if the gestation is post term (more than 42 weeks) or if the placenta is not functioning well. The fluid may range from barely green-tinged and watery, to thick with meconium and scant ("pea soup"). Meconium-stained amniotic fluid, especially if thick, is associated with fetal compromise during labor and infant respiratory distress after birth (see p. 333).

Promoting Comfort. When amniotomy is anticipated, several disposable underpads are placed under the woman's hips to absorb the fluid, extending from her mid-back to her knees. Amniotic fluid continues to leak from the woman's vagina during labor. Disposable underpads are changed often enough to keep her reasonably dry and to reduce the moist, warm environment that favors growth of microorganisms.

Induction or Augmentation of Labor

Induction of labor the initiation of labor before it begins naturally. *Augmentation* is the stimulation of contractions after they have begun naturally.

Indications

Labor is induced if continuing the pregnancy is more hazardous for the woman and fetus than shortening it by artificial means. Examples of indications are:

- Pregnancy-induced hypertension (see p. 92)
- Ruptured membranes without spontaneous onset of labor
- Infection within the uterus
- Medical problems in the woman that worsen during pregnancy, such as diabetes, kidney disease, or pulmonary disease
- Fetal problems, such as slowed growth, prolonged pregnancy (see p. 210), or incompatibility between fetal and maternal blood types (see p. 99)
- Fetal death

Convenience for the physician or family is not an indication for inducing labor. However, the woman who has a history of rapid labors and lives a long distance from the birth facility may have her labor induced because she has a risk of giving birth en route if she awaits spontaneous labor. Labor may also be induced if a fetal diagnostic procedure has identified a problem that will need treatment at a specialized center or the woman herself may have such a problem. The woman travels to the center and, with equipment and specialists assembled, her labor is induced.

Contraindications

Labor is *not* induced in these conditions:

- Placenta previa (see p. 89)
- Umbilical cord prolapse (see p. 210)
- Abnormal fetal presentation
- High station of the fetus, which suggests a preterm fetus or a small maternal pelvis
- Active herpes infection in the birth canal, which the baby can acquire during birth
- Abnormal size or structure of the mother's pelvis
- Previous classic (vertical) cesarean incision (see p. 196)

The physician may attempt to induce labor in a preterm pregnancy if continuing the pregnancy is more harmful to the woman and/or fetus than the hazards of prematurity would be to the infant.

Technique

Amniotomy may be the only method used to initiate labor, but it is more likely to be used in addition to oxytocin to stimulate contractions. Induction and augmentation of labor may rely on both drug and nondrug methods.

Cervical Ripening. Induction of labor is easier if the woman's cervix is soft, partially effaced, and beginning to dilate. These prelabor cervical changes occur naturally in most women. Methods to hasten the changes, or "ripen" the cervix, ease labor induction if her cervix has not made these changes and is "green."

Prostaglandin in the form of a gel or a commercially prepared vaginal insert softens the cervix when applied before labor induction. It is given in the hospital, and the woman and fetus are observed in the labor area for a short time after application. The woman usually returns home for the night and returns the following morning for induction. Some women who receive cervical ripening products begin labor without additional oxytocin stimulation.

An alternative to prostaglandin for cervical ripening is insertion of one or more laminaria into the cervix. A laminaria is a narrow cone of a substance that absorbs water. The laminaria swells inside the cervix, thus beginning cervical dilation. Oxytocin induction follows, usually on the next day.

Oxytocin Induction and Augmentation of Labor. Initiation or stimulation of contractions with oxytocin (Pitocin) is the most common method of labor induction and augmentation. Oxytocin is administered by registered nurses with additional training in induction of labor and electronic fetal monitoring. Augmentation of labor with oxytocin follows a similar procedure.

Oxytocin for induction or augmentation of labor is diluted in an intravenous solution. The oxytocin solution is a secondary (piggyback) infusion that is inserted into the primary (nonmedicated) intravenous solution line so that it can be stopped quickly while an open intravenous line is maintained.

The infusion of oxytocin solution is regulated with an infusion pump. Administration begins at a very low rate and is adjusted upward or downward according to how the fetus responds to labor and to the woman's contractions. The dose is individualized for every woman. When contractions are well established, it is often possible to reduce the rate of oxytocin. Augmentation of labor usually requires less total oxytocin than induction of labor because the uterus is more sensitive to the drug when labor has already begun.

Continuous electronic fetal monitoring is the usual method to assess and record fetal and maternal responses to oxytocin. Many physicians prefer internal methods of fetal monitoring when oxytocin is used because these techniques are more accurate, especially for contraction intensity.

Nondrug Methods to Stimulate Contractions. The nurse has several nondrug options to help the woman whose contractions have become less effective.

Walking. Many women benefit from a change in activity if their labor slows. Walking stimulates contractions, eases the pressure of the fetus on the mother's back, and adds gravity to the downward force of contractions. If she does not feel like walking, other upright positions often improve the effectiveness of each contraction. She can sit (in a chair, on the side of the bed, or in the bed), squat, kneel while facing the raised head of the bed for support, or maintain other upright positions.

Nipple Stimulation of Labor. Stimulating the nipples causes the woman's posterior pituitary gland to secrete natural oxytocin. This improves the quality of contractions that have slowed or weakened, just as synthetic intravenous oxytocin does. The woman can stimulate her nipples by

- Pulling or rolling them, one at a time
- Gently brushing them with a dry washcloth
- Using water in a whirlpool tub or a shower
- Applying suction with a breast pump

If contractions become too strong with these techniques, the woman simply stops them.

Complications of Oxytocin Induction and Augmentation of Labor

The most common complications, related to overstimulation of contractions, are fetal compromise and uterine rupture. Fetal compromise can occur because blood flow to the placenta is reduced if contractions are excessive. Most placental exchange of oxygen, nutrients, and waste products occurs between contractions. If the contractions are too long, too frequent, or too intense, this exchange is likely to be impaired. See p. 211 for discussion of uterine rupture.

Water intoxication sometimes occurs because oxytocin inhibits the excretion of urine and promotes fluid retention. Water intoxication is not likely with the small amounts of oxytocin and fluids given intravenously during labor, but it is more likely to occur if large doses of oxytocin and fluids are given intravenously after birth.

Oxytocin is discontinued, or its rate reduced, if signs of fetal compromise or excessive uterine contractions occur. Fetal heart rates outside the normal range of 110 to 160 beats/min, late decelerations, and loss of variability (see p. 146) are the most common signs of fetal compromise. Excessive uterine contractions are most often evidenced by contractions closer than every 2 minutes, durations longer than 90 seconds, or resting intervals shorter than 60 seconds. The resting tone of the uterus (muscle tension when it is not contracting) is often higher than normal. Internal uterine activity monitoring allows determination, in millimeters of mercury (mm Hg), of peak uterine pressures and uterine resting tone.

In addition to stopping the oxytocin infusion, the registered nurse chooses one or more of these measures to correct adverse maternal or fetal reactions.

- Increasing the nonmedicated intravenous solution
- Changing the woman's position, avoiding the supine position
- Giving oxygen by face mask

The physician is notified after corrective measures are taken. A tocolytic (drug that reduces uterine contractions) may be ordered if contractions do not quickly decrease after oxytocin is stopped.

Nursing Care

Nursing care in labor induction and augmentation is directed by the registered nurse and by hospital policies. Baseline maternal vital signs are assessed and a fetal monitor tracing is done to identify contraindications to induction or augmentation before the procedure begins.

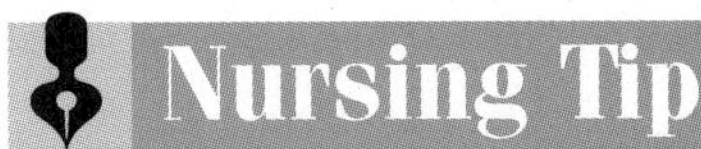

Women who have oxytocin stimulation of labor may find that their contractions are difficult to manage. Help them to stay focused on breathing and relaxation techniques with each contraction.

During induction or augmentation, the principal nursing observations are the fetal heart rate and character of uterine contractions. If abnormalities are noted in either, the nurse stops the oxytocin and begins the measures listed to reduce contractions and increase placental blood flow.

The woman's blood pressure, pulse, and respirations are taken every 30 to 60 minutes. Her temperature is taken every 2 to 4 hours. Recording her intake and output identifies water intoxication.

Version

Version is a method of changing the fetal presentation, usually from breech to cephalic. There are two methods, external and internal. External version is the more common one. A successful version reduces the likelihood that the woman will need cesarean delivery.

Risks and Contraindications

There are few maternal and fetal risks associated with version, especially external version. Version is not indicated if there is any maternal or fetal reason why vaginal birth should not occur, since that is its goal. Examples of maternal or fetal conditions that are contraindications for version are:

- Abnormal uterine or pelvic size or shape
- Previous cesarean birth with a vertical uterine incision
- Disproportion between the mother's pelvis and fetal size
- Multifetal gestation
- Abnormal placental placement
- Active herpesvirus infection
- Inadequate amniotic fluid
- Poor placental function

Version may not be attempted in a woman who has a higher risk for uterine rupture, such as several prior cesarean births or high parity. It is not usually attempted if the fetal presenting part is engaged in the pelvis.

The main risk to the fetus is that it will become entangled in the umbilical cord, thus compressing the cord. This is more likely to happen if there is not adequate room to turn the fetus, such as in multifetal gestation (e.g., twins) or when the amount of amniotic fluid is small. Version is not done if there are signs that the placenta is not functioning normally.

Technique

External version is done after 37 weeks of gestation but before the onset of labor. The procedure begins with a nonstress test or biophysical profile (see Table 5–6, pp. 96–97) to determine if the fetus is in good condition and if there is adequate amniotic fluid to perform the version. The woman receives a tocolytic drug to relax her uterus during the version.

Using ultrasound to guide the procedure, the physician pushes the fetal buttocks upward out of the pelvis while pushing the fetal head downward toward the pelvis in either a clockwise or counterclockwise turn (Fig. 8–2). The fetus is monitored frequently during the procedure.

After the external version is completed (or the effort abandoned), the tocolytic drug is stopped. Rh-negative women receive a dose of Rh immune globulin (RhoGAM).

Internal version is an emergency procedure. The physician performs internal version during vaginal birth of twins to change the fetal presentation of the second twin. An external version may be done for the same purpose.

Nursing Care

Nursing care of the woman having external version includes assisting with the procedure and observing the mother and fetus afterward for 1 to 2 hours. Baseline maternal vital signs and a fetal monitor strip (part of the nonstress test or biophysical profile) are taken before the version. The mother's vital signs and the fetal heart rates are observed to ensure return to normal levels after the version.

Vaginal leaking of amniotic fluid suggests that manipulating the fetus caused a tear in the membranes, and is reported. Uterine contractions usually decrease or stop shortly after the version. The physician is notified if they do not. The nurse reviews signs of labor with the woman because version occurs near term, when spontaneous labor is expected.

Episiotomy and Lacerations

Episiotomy is the surgical enlargement of the vagina during birth. Either the physician or a nurse-midwife performs and repairs an episiotomy.

Lacerations of the perineum and episiotomy incisions are treated similarly. Lacerations are classified according to how far they extend from the vagina toward the anus. First- and second-degree lacerations are usually uncomplicated because they do not affect the rectal sphincter. A third-degree laceration extends into the rectal sphincter; the fourth-degree laceration extends completely through the rectal sphincter. Women with third- and fourth-degree lacerations may have more difficulty if they are constipated after birth.

Indications

Fetal indications are similar to those for forceps or vacuum extraction (see p. 193). Additional maternal indications include the following:

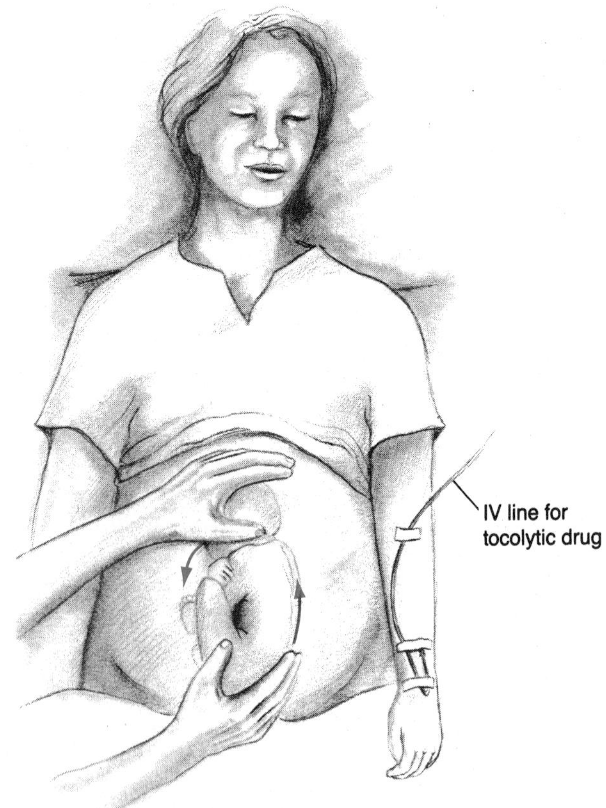

Figure 8–2. • External version. After the uterus is relaxed by a tocolytic drug, the physician pushes the breech of the fetus upward out of the pelvis while at the same time pushing the head downward toward the pelvis.

Nursing Tip

Pay special attention to a woman's diet and fluids if she had a third- or fourth-degree laceration. Roughage in the diet and adequate fluids help to prevent constipation that might result in a break down of the area where the laceration was sutured.

- Better control over where and how much the vaginal opening is enlarged
- An opening with a clean edge, rather than the ragged opening of a tear (controversial)

Routine episiotomy has been challenged by several recent studies that do not support many of its supposed benefits. Nevertheless, it is so common that the nurse is expected to give postpartum care to many women with episiotomies.

Risks

As in other incisions, infection is the primary risk in an episiotomy or laceration. An additional risk is extension of the episiotomy with a laceration into or through the rectal sphincter (third- or fourth-degree).

Technique

The episiotomy is done with blunt-tipped scissors just before birth. One of two directions is chosen (Fig. 8–3):

- *Median (midline),* extending directly from the lower vaginal border toward the anus
- *Mediolateral,* extending from the lower vaginal border toward the mother's right or left

The median episiotomy is easier to repair and heals neatly, but it does not enlarge the opening as much as the mediolateral incision. The mediolateral incision provides more room, but greater scarring during healing may cause painful sexual intercourse. A laceration that extends a median episiotomy is more likely to go into the rectal sphincter than one that extends the mediolateral episiotomy.

Nursing Care

Nursing care for an episiotomy or laceration begins during the fourth stage of labor. Cold packs should be applied for at least the first 12 hours to reduce pain, bruising, and edema. After 12 to 24 hours of cold applications, warmth in the form of heat packs or sitz baths increase blood circulation, enhancing comfort and healing. Mild oral analgesics are usually sufficient for pain management. (See p. 226 for postpartum nursing care of the woman with an episiotomy or laceration.)

Forceps and Vacuum Extraction Births

These two procedures are done by the physician to aid the woman's pushing efforts at the end of labor. Forceps are instruments with curved blades

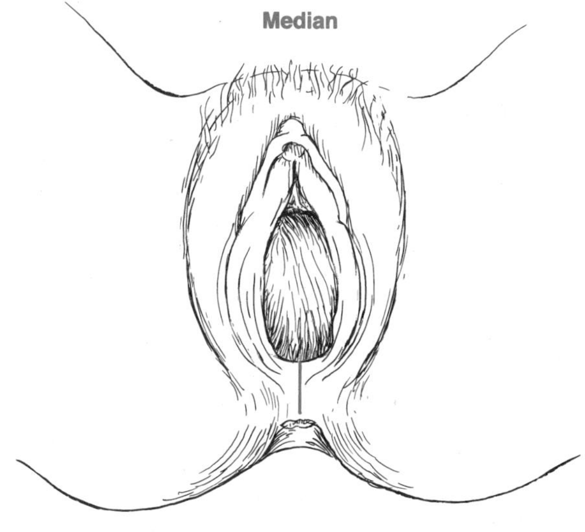

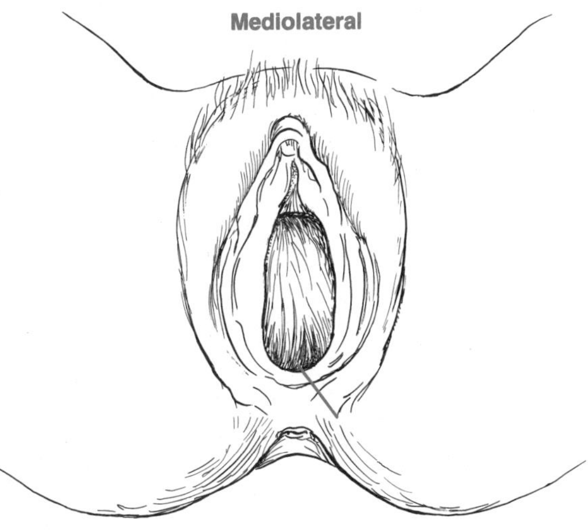

Figure 8–3. • Episiotomies. The median and a left mediolateral episiotomy are shown here.

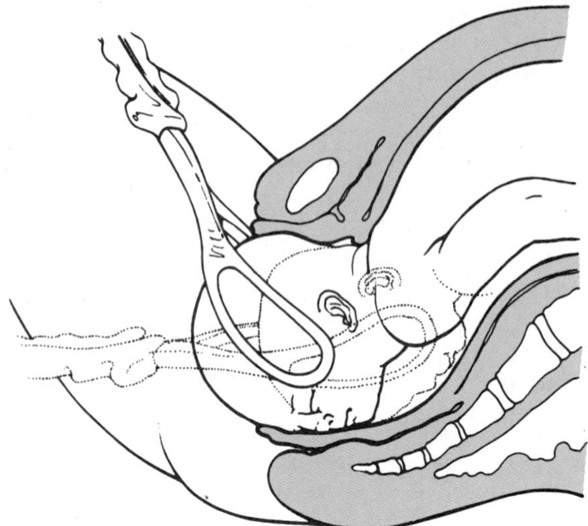

Figure 8–4. • Forceps to assist the birth of the fetal head. After applying the forceps to each side of the fetal head and locking the two blades, the physician pulls, following the pelvic curve.

that fit around the fetal head without unduly compressing it (Fig. 8–4). Several styles are available to assist the birth of the fetal head in a cephalic presentation. Forceps may also help the physician extract the fetal head through the incision during cesarean birth. Piper forceps are a special type used to deliver the head during vaginal birth of the fetus in a breech presentation.

A vacuum extractor uses suction applied to the fetal head so that the physician can assist the mother's expulsive efforts (Fig. 8–5). The vacuum extractor can be used to assist birth of the head during cesarean birth. It cannot be used to deliver the after coming head of a fetus in breech presentation and cannot be used in all variations of the cephalic presentation. One advantage of the vacuum extractor is that it does not take up room in the mother's pelvis, as forceps do.

Indications

Forceps or vacuum extraction may be used to end the second stage of labor if it is in the best interests of the mother and/or fetus. The mother may be exhausted, or she may be unable to push effectively. Women with cardiac or pulmonary disorders often have forceps or vacuum extraction births, because prolonged pushing can worsen these conditions. Fetal indications include conditions in which there is evidence of an increased risk to the fetus near the end of labor. These may include minor degrees of placental disruption or nonreassuring fetal heart rate patterns.

Contraindications

Forceps or vacuum extraction cannot substitute for cesarean birth if the maternal or fetal condition requires a quicker delivery. These techniques are not done if they would be more traumatic than cesarean birth, for example, when the fetus is high in the pelvis or too large for the pelvis.

Risks

Trauma to maternal and/or fetal tissues is the main risk when forceps or vacuum extraction is used. The mother may have a laceration or hematoma (collection of blood in the tissues) in her vagina. The infant may have bruising, facial or scalp lacerations or abrasions, cephalhematoma (see p. 311), or intracranial hemorrhage. The vacuum extractor causes a harmless area of circular edema on the infant's scalp *(chignon)* where it was applied.

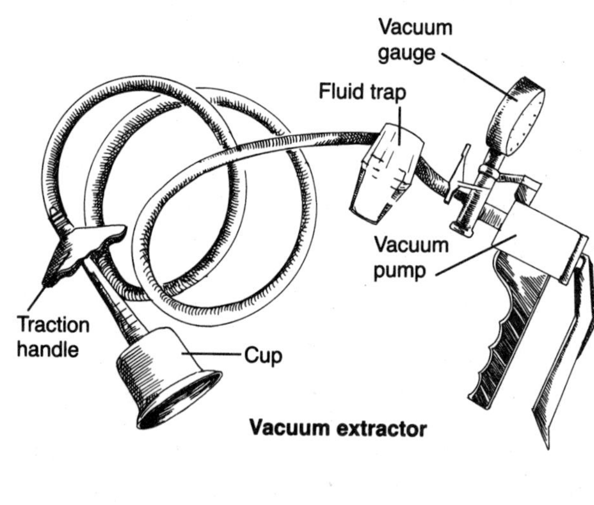

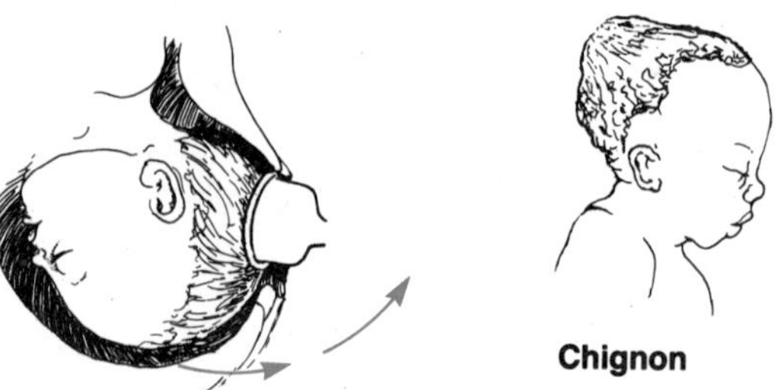

Figure 8–5. • The vacuum extractor cup with its attachments to regulate suction. The chignon is the scalp edema where the cup was applied.

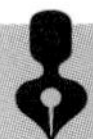

Nursing Tip

Many parents are concerned about the marks made by forceps. Reassure them that they are temporary and usually resolve without treatment.

Technique

If the woman has not urinated recently, the physician catheterizes her to prevent trauma to her bladder and to make more room in her pelvis. After the forceps are applied, the physician pulls in line with the pelvic curve. An episiotomy is usually done. After the fetal head is brought under the mother's symphysis, the rest of the birth occurs in the usual way.

Birth assisted with the vacuum extractor follows a similar sequence. The physician applies the cup over the fetal occiput, and suction is created with a machine to hold it there. Traction is applied by pulling on the handle of the extractor cup.

Nursing Care

If use of forceps or vacuum extraction is anticipated, the nurse places the sterile equipment on the delivery instrument table. A catheter is added to empty the woman's bladder as needed.

After birth, care is similar to that for episiotomy and perineal lacerations. Ice is applied to the perineum to reduce bruising and edema. The physician is notified if the woman has signs of vaginal hematoma, which include severe and poorly relieved pelvic or rectal pain.

The infant's head is examined for lacerations, abrasions, or bruising. Mild facial reddening and molding (alteration in shape) of the head are common and require no treatment. Antibiotic ointment is sometimes ordered for skin breaks. Cold treatments are not used on neonates because they would cause hypothermia.

Pressure from forceps may injure the infant's facial nerve. It is evidenced by facial asymmetry (different appearance of right and left sides), which is most obvious when the infant cries. Facial nerve injury usually resolves without treatment.

Cesarean Birth

Cesarean birth is the surgical delivery of the fetus through incisions in the mother's abdomen and uterus. A goal for the Healthy People 2000 initiative is to reduce the rate of cesarean births to no more than 15%. This goal is not being met at this time. Of all births in the United States, nearly 22% were by cesarean delivery in 1995.

Indications

Several conditions may require cesarean delivery:

- Abnormal labor
- Inability of the fetus to pass through the mother's pelvis (*cephalopelvic disproportion,* also called fetopelvic disproportion)
- Maternal conditions such as pregnancy-induced hypertension or diabetes
- Active maternal herpesvirus, which may cause serious or fatal infant infection
- Previous surgery on the uterus, including some types of previous cesarean incisions
- Fetal compromise, including prolapsed umbilical cord and abnormal presentations
- Placenta previa or abruptio placentae

Contraindications

There are few contraindications to cesarean birth but it is not usually done if the fetus is dead or too premature to survive, or if the mother has abnormal blood clotting.

Risks

Cesarean birth carries risks to both mother and baby. Maternal risks are similar to those of other types of surgery and include the following

- Risks related to anesthesia (see Chapter 7)
- Infection
- Hemorrhage
- Injury to the urinary tract
- Blood clots
- Delayed intestinal peristalsis (paralytic ileus)
- Respiratory complications

Risks to the newborn may include the following

- Inadvertent preterm birth
- Respiratory problems because of delayed absorption of lung fluid
- Injury, such as laceration or bruising

To avoid the unintentional birth of a premature fetus, the physician often performs amniocentesis before a planned cesarean birth to determine if the fetal lungs are mature (see Table 5–6, pp. 96–97).

Technique

Cesarean birth may occur under planned, unplanned, or emergency conditions. Although the sequence is similar for each, preparations are severely abbreviated for cesarean birth under emergency conditions.

Preparations for Cesarean Birth

As in other surgery, several laboratory studies are done to identify anemia or blood clotting abnormalities. Complete blood count, coagulation studies, and blood typing and screening are common. One or more units of blood may be typed and crossmatched if the woman is likely to need a transfusion.

The woman receives a drug to reduce gastric acidity and speed stomach emptying. Most physicians order prophylactic antibiotics to prevent infection. Additional antibiotic doses will be ordered for the woman who has an increased risk for infection (such as prolonged ruptured membranes), displays signs of infection, or is positive for group B streptococcus (GBS).

The woman's abdomen is shaved from just above her umbilicus to her mons pubis, where her thighs come together if a vertical skin incision is expected. If a Pfannenstiel (transverse, or "bikini") skin incision is planned, the upper border of the shave is about 3 inches above her pubic hairline.

An indwelling catheter is inserted to keep the bladder empty during birth and prevent trauma to it. The catheter bag is placed near the head of the operating table so the anesthesiologist can monitor urine output, an important indicator of the woman's circulating blood volume. The circulating nurse will scrub the abdomen by using a circular motion that goes outward from the incisional area.

Types of Incisions

There are two incisions in cesarean birth: a skin incision and a uterine incision. The directions of these incisions are not always the same.

Skin Incisions. The skin incision is done in either a vertical or a transverse direction. The vertical incision allows more room if a large fetus is being delivered, and it is usually needed for an obese woman. In an emergency, the vertical incision can be done more quickly. The transverse, or Pfannenstiel, incision is nearly invisible when healed but cannot always be used in the obese woman or with a large baby.

Uterine Incisions. The more important of the two incisions is the one that cuts into the uterus. There are three types of uterine incisions (Fig. 8–6): low transverse, low vertical, and classic.

Low Transverse. This uterine incision is preferred because it is not likely to rupture during another birth, causes less blood loss, and is easier to repair. It may not be an option if the fetus is large or if there is a placenta previa in the area where the incision would be made. This type of incision makes vaginal birth after cesarean (VBAC) possible for subsequent births.

Low Vertical. This uterine incision produces minimal blood loss and allows delivery of a larger fetus. However, it is more likely to rupture during another birth, although less so than the classic incision.

Classic. This uterine incision is rarely used because it involves more blood loss and is the most likely of the three types to rupture during another pregnancy. However, it may be the only choice if the fetus is in a transverse lie or if there is scarring or a placenta previa in the lower anterior uterus.

Sequence of Events in Cesarean Birth

When the woman is anesthetized, scrubbed, and draped, the physician makes the skin incision. After making the uterine incision, the physician ruptures the membranes (unless they are already ruptured) with a sharp instrument. The amniotic fluid is suctioned from the operative area, and its amount, color, and odor are noted.

The physician reaches into the uterus to lift out the fetal head or buttocks. Forceps or vacuum extraction may be used to assist birth of the head. The infant's mouth and nose are quickly suctioned to remove secretions, and the cord is clamped. The physician hands the infant to the nurse, who receives the infant into sterile blankets or drapes. Care of the infant at birth is essentially the same as that during vaginal birth.

After birth of the baby, the physician scoops out the placenta and examines it for intactness. The uterine cavity is sponged to remove blood clots and other debris. The uterine and skin incisions are then sutured in layers.

Nursing Care

The registered nurse assumes most of the preoperative and postoperative care of the woman. This includes obtaining the required laboratory studies, administering medications, preoperative teaching, and preparing for surgery.

Women who have cesarean birth usually need greater emotional support than those having vaginal births. They are usually happy and excited

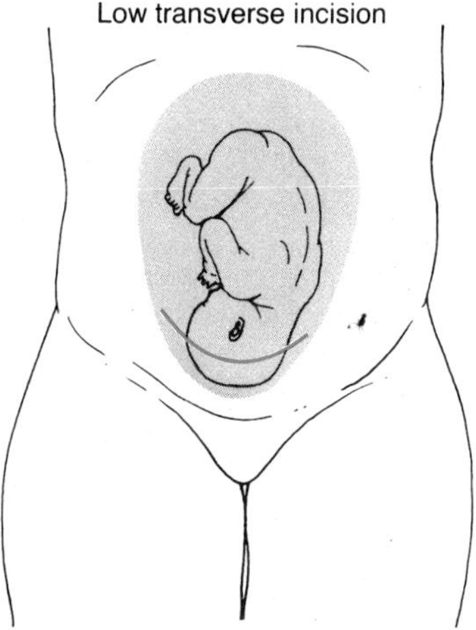

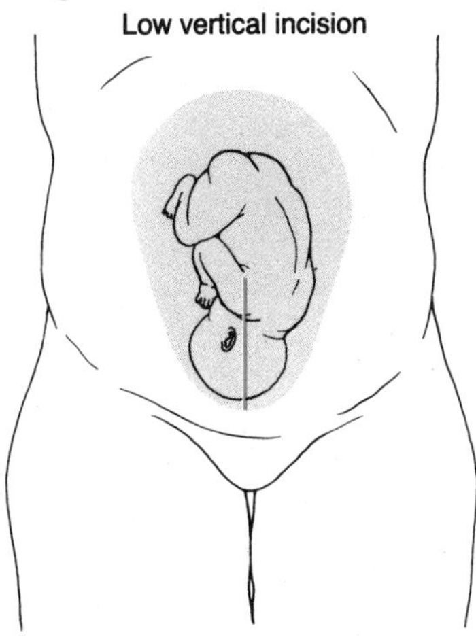

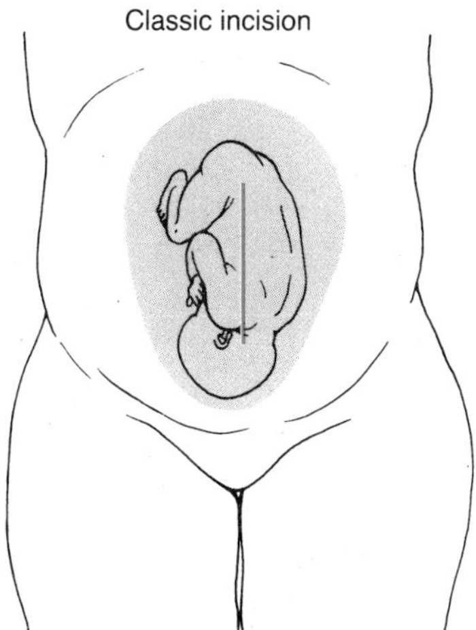

Figure 8–6. • Three types of uterine incisions for cesarean birth. The low transverse uterine incision is preferred, because it is not likely to rupture during a subsequent birth, allowing vaginal birth alter a cesarean birth. The low vertical and classic incisions must occasionally be used. The skin incision and uterine incision do not always match.

about the newborn but may also feel grief, guilt, or anger because the expected course of birth did not occur. These feelings may linger and resurface during another pregnancy.

Women who plan VBAC but need a repeat cesarean delivery often experience diverse feelings. A woman may feel positive in spite of needing another cesarean because she did her best to give vaginal birth a chance. Another woman may have feelings of failure, especially if she strongly wanted a vaginal birth. The nurse should avoid using negative phrases such as "failed VBAC," which a woman may interpret as a personal failure.

Anxiety is normal when confronting a new or unexpected experience. Childbirth, including cesarean childbirth, may be a woman's first hospital experience. Procedures and equipment that are familiar to health care personnel may seem overwhelming at first. Explaining procedures and the role of all persons in the operating room helps to reduce the patient's anxiety. A calm voice and quiet environment promote relaxation.

Emotional care of the partner and family is essential; they are included in explanations of the surgery as much as the woman wishes. The partner may be frightened when an emergency cesarean is needed, but may not express these feelings because the woman needs so much support. The partner may be almost as exhausted as the woman, if cesarean birth is done after hours of labor. The thoughtful nurse includes the partner and promotes his or her emotional and physical well-being.

A support person is present for most cesarean births. The nurse informs the partner of when he or she may enter the operating room, because 1/2 hour or more may be needed to administer a regional anesthesia and for surgical preparations if there is no emergency. During this wait the partner dons surgical attire.

After birth, the mother, infant, and partner are kept together as much as possible, just as in vaginal birth. The woman and her partner are encouraged to talk about the cesarean birth so that they can integrate the experience. The nurse answers questions about events surrounding the birth. The focus is the *birth,* rather than the surgical, aspects of cesarean delivery.

Nursing assessments after cesarean birth are similar to those after vaginal birth, including assessment of the uterine fundus. Assessments are done every 15 minutes for the first 1 or 2 hours, according to hospital policy. Recovery room assessments after cesarean birth include:

- Vital signs to identify hemorrhage or shock; a pulse-oximeter is used to better identify depressed respiratory function

Nursing Tip

Although assessing the uterus after cesarean birth causes discomfort, it is important to do so regularly. The woman can have a relaxed uterus that causes excessive blood loss, regardless of how she delivered her baby.

- Intravenous site and rate of solution flow
- Fundus for firmness, height, and midline position
- Dressing for drainage
- Lochia for quantity, color, and presence of clots
- Urine output from the indwelling catheter

The fundus is checked as gently as possible. The woman flexes her knees slightly and takes slow, deep breaths to minimize the pain of fundal assessments. While supporting the lower uterus with one hand, the fingers of the other hand are gently "walked" from the side of the uterus toward the midline. Massage is not needed if the fundus is already firm.

The woman is told to take deep breaths at each assessment and to cough to move secretions from her airways. A small pillow or folded blanket supports her incision when she coughs or moves, reducing pain. Changing her position every hour or two helps expand her lungs and also makes her more comfortable.

Pain relief after cesarean birth may be by patient-controlled analgesia (PCA) pump or by intermittent injections of narcotic analgesics. Epidural narcotics provide long-lasting pain relief but are associated with delayed respiratory depression and itching (see p. 179), which vary with the drug injected. After about the first 24 hours, the woman is changed to oral analgesics. Nursing Care Plan 8-1 details interventions for selected nursing diagnoses that pertain to the woman with an unplanned cesarean birth.

ABNORMAL LABOR

The "four Ps" of labor (see p. 126) interact constantly throughout the birth. Abnormalities in the powers, passenger, passage, or the psyche may result in a problem labor. In addition, the length of labor may be unusually short or long. Labor abnormalities may require forceps or cesarean delivery, and they are more likely to result in injury to the mother or baby.

Problems with the Powers of Labor

A woman may have contractions that are hypotonic or hypertonic. She may not have adequate pushing efforts to bring about fetal descent.

Hypotonic Labor Dysfunction

A woman has hypotonic labor if her contractions are too weak to be effective. Hypotonic labor usually occurs during active labor. The woman begins labor normally, but contractions diminish during the active phase (after 4 cm of cervical dilation), when the pace of labor is expected to accelerate. Hypotonic labor is more likely to occur if her uterus is overdistended, such as with twins, a large baby, or excess amniotic fluid. Uterine overdistention stretches the muscle fibers and thus reduces their ability to contract effectively. Women who have had many babies (grand multiparas) are more likely to have hypotonic labor, because they have poorer uterine muscle tone.

Medical Treatment. The physician usually does an amniotomy if the membranes are intact. Augmentation of labor with oxytocin or by nipple stimulation increases the strength of contractions. Intravenous or oral fluids may improve the quality of contractions if the woman is dehydrated.

Nursing Care. The woman is reasonably comfortable, but frustrated because her labor is not progressing. In addition to providing care related to amniotomy and labor augmentation, the nurse gives emotional support to the woman and her partner. She is allowed to express her frustrations. The nurse tells her when she makes progress, to encourage continuing her efforts.

Position changes may help to relieve discomfort and enhance progress. Contractions are usually stronger and more effective when the woman assumes an upright position or lies on her side, although they may be less frequent. Walking or nipple stimulation may intensify contractions. Nursing Care Plan 8–2 details interventions for selected nursing diagnoses that pertain to the woman with hypotonic labor dysfunction.

Hypertonic Labor Dysfunction

Hypertonic dysfunction is characterized by contractions that are frequent, cramplike, and poorly coordinated. They are painful but nonproductive.

NURSING CARE PLAN 8–1

Selected Nursing Diagnoses for the Woman with an Unplanned Cesarean Birth*

Nursing Diagnosis: Anxiety related to development of complications

Goals	Interventions	Rationale
The woman and her partner will express decreased anxiety after explanations about the planned surgery	1. Reinforce all explanations given by physician, expressing them in simpler terms, if needed	1. Anxiety tends to narrow attention; although physician may have explained need for surgery, woman and her partner may not have comprehended everything they were told
	2. Encourage woman to continue using breathing and relaxation techniques she learned in prepared childbirth classes; tell her the techniques may help with pain control after birth	2. Learned pain management techniques increase woman's sense of control; control over a situation reduces feelings of helplessness and decreases anxiety
	3. Tell woman what the operating room looks like and who will be present; explain basic equipment, such as catheter, narrow table, monitors for her heart and blood pressure, anesthesia machine, and large overhead lights; explain that personnel will wear protective equipment such as masks, eye protection, gowns, gloves, hats, and shoe covers	3. Commonplace equipment and attire in an operating room can be intimidating for someone who has not seen them before; unfamiliarity increases anxiety; preparation reduces anxiety and fear of the unknown
	4. Describe usual postoperative care—assessment of the vital signs, fundus, vaginal bleeding, dressing, and catheter; tell her she will be asked to take deep breaths and change position regularly	4. If woman understands common postoperative care, she is more likely to cooperate with it, even if assessments are uncomfortable
	5. Encourage her partner to be with her during surgery and do not separate family afterward, if possible	5. Companionship of familiar persons helps to reduce anxiety; keeping new family together promotes attachment to the new baby

Nursing Diagnosis: Pain related to effects of surgery (incisional, slowed gastric peristalsis)

Goals	Interventions	Rationale
The woman will state that pain is manageable with the pharmacologic and nonpharmacologic methods used	1. Assess nature of pain: location, quality, intensity, duration, and factors that increase or decrease it	1. Proper assessment allows nurse to choose most appropriate interventions, such as repositioning or medication
	2. Provide analgesics as ordered, usually intramuscular or patient-controlled analgesia (PCA) pump for the first 24 hr and oral analgesics after this time; do not allow pain to become too intense before medicating woman. See Chapter 7 for information about epidural narcotics	2. Analgesics inhibit brain's ability to interpret pain; early and frequent use of measures to relieve pain allows optimal control and facilitates healing
	3. Assess bowel sounds each shift or more frequently if they are diminished; ask woman to report when she begins passing flatus (gas)	3. Cesarean birth temporarily slows bowel function; accumulation of intestinal gas will cause abdominal distention and cramping; passing flatus indicates return of bowel function
	4. Dangle on side of bed after first 8–12 hr. Ambulate to a chair if woman tolerates dangling Gradually increase ambulation (see Chapter 9)	4. Activity stimulates intestinal peristalsis, which reduces accumulation of gas and limits discomfort from this source
	5. Discourage woman from drinking carbonated drinks or drinking through a straw	5. These tend to increase swallowed gas and can increase gastric discomfort

Continued on following page

NURSING CARE PLAN 8–1 *continued*

Selected Nursing Diagnoses for the Woman with an Unplanned Cesarean Birth*

Nursing Diagnosis: Risk for ineffective airway clearance related to reduced breathing efforts secondary to incisional pain

Goals	Interventions	Rationale
The woman will have a normal respiratory rate of 12–24 breaths/min, clear lung sounds bilaterally	1. Assess vital signs according to length of time since surgery (usually every 15 min during early recovery, increasing to every 4 hr after transfer to postpartum); assess lung sounds each shift	1. Tachypnea or congested lung sounds suggest that woman is not moving secretions from her airways; temperature elevation over 38° C (100.4° F) suggests infection, which could have several sources, including respiratory
	2. Have woman take deep breaths and cough every 2 hr; teach her to press a pillow or folded blanket over her incision area to splint it; teach and verify her use of an incentive spirometer if ordered	2. Deep breathing and coughing help move secretions from airways; splinting incision reduces strain on it and reduces pain so woman can cough more effectively; incentive spirometer provides visual feedback for deep breathing
	3. Encourage changing position every 2 hr before ambulating, turning side to side; encourage oral fluids when allowed	3. Helps to move secretions from airways and prevents congestion, which is a favorable environment for growth of infectious organisms; adequate fluid keeps secretions thinner and easier to move

Nursing Diagnosis: Risk for altered tissue perfusion related to bleeding secondary to uterine atony

Goals	Interventions	Rationale
The woman will have adequate tissue perfusion as evidenced by saturation of no more than one pad per hour during recovery period	1. Assess vital signs every 15 min for first hour, then according to hospital policy	1. Rising pulse and falling blood pressure suggest shock, which is most often due to hemorrhage
	2. Assess uterine fundus for firmness, height, and position (midline or deviated) with vital signs; massage fundus until it is firm if necessary; explain reason for this assessment, and have woman bend her knees and breathe slowly and deeply while you assess fundus; support lower uterus when assessing (see Fig. 9–2)	2. Firm fundus compresses bleeding blood vessels at placenta site; this procedure is often painful if woman had a cesarean birth, especially with a vertical skin incision; if she understands its importance and takes measures to minimize discomfort, she is more likely to accept needed assessment
	3. Assess lochia for amount, color, and odor when uterine fundus is assessed; report over one pad per hour saturated during recovery period or persistent clots	3. Signs of excessive blood loss require prompt medical and nursing intervention to avoid altering tissue perfusion
	4. Assess catheter for patency and for amount of urine output with vital signs and fundal and lochia checks; assess voided output until woman is urinating adequate amounts (at least 100 ml) regularly	4. A full bladder inhibits uterine contraction and can lead to hemorrhage; adequate urine output verifies patency of catheter and reflects an adequate circulating blood volume
	5. Check dressing and incision with each vital sign and fundal check	5. Bloody drainage on dressing suggests breakdown in incision line; gapping of incision (after dressing is removed) suggests infection and can lead to hemorrhage (see Chapter 10 for more information about postpartum infection)

*See also Chapter 9 for postpartum care of the woman having cesarean birth.

NURSING CARE PLAN 8-2

Selected Nursing Diagnoses for the Woman with Hypotonic Labor Dysfunction

Nursing Diagnosis: Risk for infection related to loss of barrier (ruptured membranes)

Goals	Interventions	Rationale
The woman's temperature will remain under 38° C (100.4° F), and the amniotic fluid will remain clear with a mild odor	1. Take woman's temperature every 2–4 hr or more often if elevated; at same time, assess the amniotic fluid drainage for color, clarity, and odor	1. Elevated temperature is a sign of infection; cloudy, yellow, or foul-odored fluid suggests infection; meconium (green) staining suggests fetal compromise but is also seen with prolonged pregnancy
	2. Observe fetal heart rates (see p. 145)	2. Fetal tachycardia (rate >160/min) may be the first sign of infection; poor fetal oxygenation also may occur, especially with abnormal labor
	3. After birth, continue to assess woman's temperature at least every 4 hr; assess the lochia (postbirth vaginal drainage) for a foul odor or brown color	3. Woman may not show these signs of infection until after birth
	4. Observe neonate for a temperature below 36.2° C (97° F) or over 37.8° C (100° F); observe for poor feeding, lethargy, irritability, or "not looking right"	4. Neonate may become infected in utero and display these signs of infection after birth; neonatal sepsis may occur with prolonged rupture of membranes and is a potentially fatal infection

Nursing Diagnosis: Ineffective individual coping related to frustration with slow labor and delayed birth

Goals	Interventions	Rationale
The woman will use breathing and relaxation techniques that she and her partner learned in prepared childbirth class	1. If there is no contraindication, encourage woman to walk or to sit upright in bed or chair; walking may not be wise if membranes are ruptured and fetus is high	1. Upright positions enhance fetal descent; walking strengthens labor contractions; walking when membranes are ruptured and fetal station is high could lead to umbilical cord prolapse
	2. Help woman to use natural methods to stimulate contractions, such as nipple stimulation; encourage a shower or whirlpool if available and not contraindicated	2. Nipple stimulation causes woman's posterior pituitary gland to secrete natural oxytocin, which strengthens contractions; water may help woman relax, which improves labor; all nondrug methods to stimulate labor enhance her sense of control
	3. Assist registered nurse with oxytocin augmentation if it is ordered; observe contractions for excessive frequency (more frequent than every 2 min), duration (over 90 sec), or inadequate rest interval (under 60 sec); observe fetal heart rate for rates outside normal 110–160 beats/min	3. Primary risks of oxytocin augmentation or induction of labor relate to overstimulating the uterus; excessive contractions can reduce fetal oxygen supply; these are signs of potential uterine overstimulation
	4. Explain to woman how each method is expected to help her labor advance; tell her any time she makes progress, either in improved contractions or increasing cervical dilation	4. If woman understands reason for any interventions, she will more likely cooperate with them and feel more in control; knowing that her efforts are having desired effect encourages her to continue with her learned coping methods
	5. Help woman relax and use breathing techniques she learned in prepared childbirth class; praise and support her when she uses them	5. Relaxation promotes normal labor; woman with a long labor may feel that there is no use in continuing relaxation and breathing if she is not making progress; praise encourages her to continue

The uterus is tense, even between contractions, which reduces blood flow to the placenta.

Hypertonic labor dysfunction usually occurs during the latent phase of labor (before 4 cm of cervical dilation). It is less common than hypotonic dysfunction. Box 8–1 summarizes differences between hypotonic and hypertonic labor dysfunction.

Medical Treatment. Medical treatment may include mild sedation to allow the woman to rest. *Tocolytic drugs* (see p. 209), such as terbutaline (Brethine), may be ordered to reduce the high uterine resting tone (resting muscle tension).

Nursing Care. Women with hypertonic dysfunction are uncomfortable and frustrated. Anxiety about the lack of progress and fatigue impair their ability to tolerate pain. They may lose confidence in their ability to give birth.

BOX 8–1

DIFFERENCES BETWEEN HYPOTONIC LABOR AND HYPERTONIC LABOR DYSFUNCTION

Hypotonic Labor

Contractions are weak and ineffective.

It is more common than hypertonic labor dysfunction.

It occurs during active phase, after 4 cm of cervical dilation.

It is more likely if the uterus is overdistended or if woman has had many other births.

Medical management includes amniotomy, oxytocin augmentation, and adequate hydration.

Nondrug stimulation methods include walking, other upright positions, and nipple stimulation.

Other nursing interventions include position changes and encouragement.

Hypertonic Labor

Contractions are poorly coordinated, frequent, and painful.

Uterine resting tone between contractions is tense.

It is less common than hypotonic labor dysfunction.

It is more likely to occur during latent labor, before 4 cm of cervical dilation.

Medical management includes mild sedation and tocolytic drugs.

Nursing interventions include acceptance of the woman's discomfort and frustration and provision of comfort measures.

The nurse should accept the woman's frustration and that of her partner. Both may be exhausted from the near-constant discomfort. It is important not to equate the amount of pain a woman reports with how much she "should" feel at that point in labor. The nurse provides general comfort measures that promote rest and relaxation.

Ineffective Maternal Pushing

The woman may not push effectively during the second stage of labor because she does not understand which techniques to use or she fears tearing her perineal tissues. Epidural or subarachnoid blocks (see pp. 176 and 179) may depress or eliminate the natural urge to push. An exhausted woman may be unable to gather her resources to push out her baby.

Nursing Care. Nursing care focuses on coaching the woman about the most effective techniques for pushing. If she cannot feel her contractions because of a regional block, the nurse tells her when to push, as each contraction reaches its peak.

The exhausted woman may benefit from pushing only when she feels a strong urge or perhaps with every other contraction. The fearful woman may benefit from explanations that sensations of tearing or splitting often accompany fetal descent but that her body is designed to accommodate the baby. Pushing every two or three contractions allows her tissues to gradually adjust to the distention caused by fetal descent.

Problems with the Fetus

Several fetal conditions can contribute to abnormal labor, including fetal size, presentation, or position. Multifetal pregnancies are associated with difficult labor. Some birth defects alter the fetal body in such a way as to impede birth.

Fetal Size

A large fetus *(macrosomia)* is generally considered to be one weighing over 4000 g (8.8 pounds) at birth. The large baby may not fit through the woman's pelvis. A very large fetus also distends the uterus and can contribute to hypotonic labor dysfunction.

Sometimes a single part of the fetus is too large. For example, the fetus may have hydrocephalus, in which there is an abnormal amount of fluid in the head. In that case, the fetal body size and weight may be normal, but the head is too large to fit through the pelvis. These babies are often in an abnormal presentation as well.

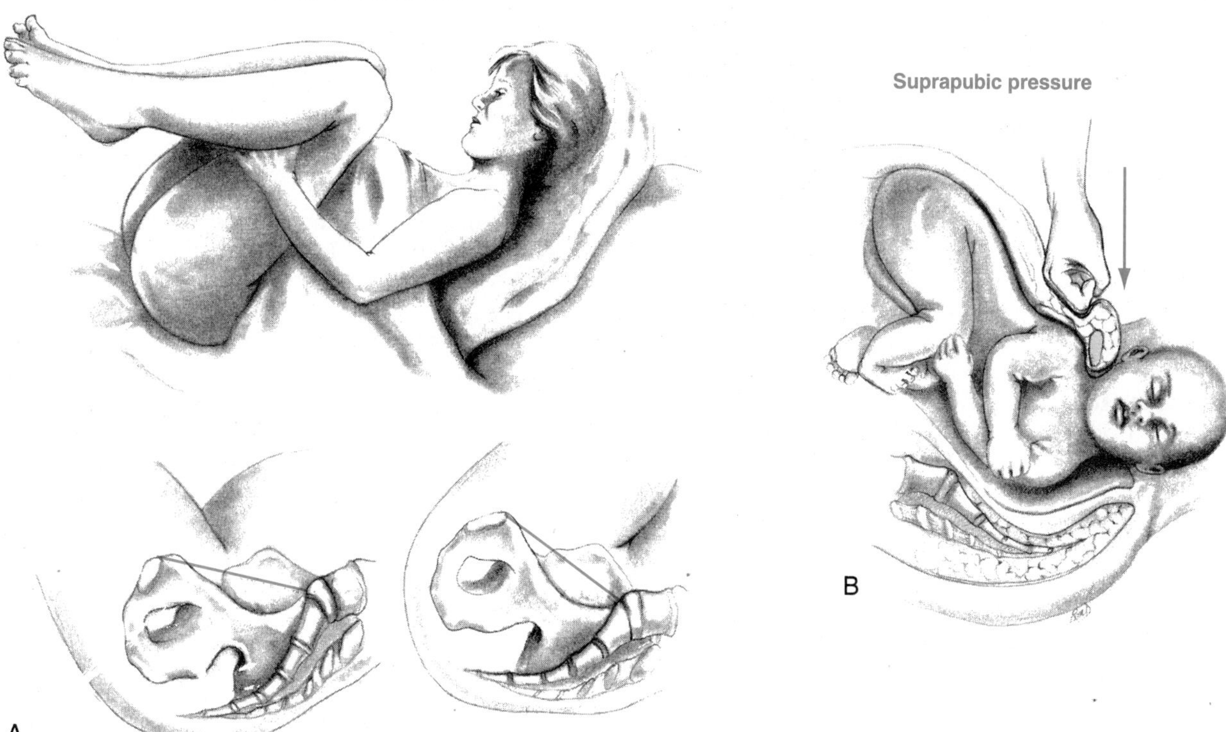

Figure 8–7. • Methods that may be used to relieve shoulder dystocia. **A,** McRobert's maneuver. The woman flexes her thighs sharply against her abdomen, which straightens the pelvic curve somewhat. Squatting has a similar effect and adds gravity to her pushing efforts. **B,** Suprapubic pressure by an assistant pushes the fetal anterior shoulder downward to displace it from above the mother's symphysis. Fundal pressure should not be used, as it will push the anterior shoulder even more firmly against the mother's symphysis. (From Gorrie, T.M., McKinney, E.S., & Murray, S.S. [1994]. *Foundations of maternal newborn nursing.* Philadelphia: Saunders.)

Shoulder dystocia sometimes occurs, usually when the fetus is large. The fetal head is born, but the shoulders become impacted above the mother's symphysis pubis. A shoulder dystocia is an emergency, because the fetus needs to breathe. The head is out, but the chest cannot expand. The cord is compressed between the fetus and the mother's pelvis. The physician may request that the nurse apply firm downward pressure just above the symphysis (suprapubic pressure), to push the shoulders toward the pelvic canal (Fig. 8–7). Squatting or sharp flexion of the thighs against the abdomen may also loosen the shoulders.

Nursing Care. If the woman successfully delivers a large infant, observe mother and child for injuries after birth. The woman may have a large episiotomy or laceration. The large infant is more likely to have a fracture of one or both clavicles (collarbones). The infant's clavicles are felt for crepitus (creaking sensation) or deformity of the bones, and the arms are observed for equal movement. The woman is more at risk for uterine atony and postpartum hemorrhage because her uterus does not contract well after birth to control bleeding at the placental site.

Abnormal Fetal Presentation or Position

Labor is most efficient if the fetus is in a flexed, cephalic presentation and in one of the occiput anterior positions (see p. 133). Abnormalities of fetal presentation and position prevent labor from being most effective.

Abnormal Presentations. The fetus in an abnormal presentation, such as the breech or face presentation, does not pass easily through the woman's pelvis. Abnormal presentations, such as the brow presentation, also increase the relative size of the presenting part (see Fig. 6–6, p. 131). Abnormal presentations prevent smooth dilation of the cervix and interfere with the most efficient mechanisms of labor (p. 135).

In the United States most fetuses in the breech presentation are born by cesarean delivery. During vaginal birth in this presentation the trunk and extremities are born before the head. After the fetal body delivers, the umbilical cord can be compressed between the fetus and the mother's pelvis. The head, which is the single largest part of the fetus, must be quickly delivered so that the infant can breathe. Figure 8–8 illustrates the sequence of delivery for a vaginal breech birth.

Intrapartum nurses must be prepared to assist with a breech birth. Although most breech births are by cesarean, some women will have a planned breech birth. Also, a woman sometimes arrives at the birth facility in advanced labor with her fetus in a breech presentation.

External version is being used to avoid some cesarean deliveries for a breech presentation. However, external version is not always successful, and the fetus sometimes returns to the abnormal presentation.

Abnormal Positions. A common cause of abnormal labor is the fetus's remaining in a persistent occiput posterior position (left [LOP] or right [ROP]). The fetal occiput occupies either the left or right posterior quadrant of the mother's pelvis. In most women, the fetal head rotates in a clockwise or counterclockwise direction until the occiput is in one of the anterior quadrants of the pelvis (left [LOA] or right [ROA]).

Rotation does not occur in every woman. Labor is likely to be longer when the fetus remains in this position. Intense back and leg pain that is poorly relieved characterizes labor when the fetus is in the occiput posterior position. Most women with an average-size pelvis cannot deliver the infants who remain in an occiput posterior position. The physician may use forceps to rotate the fetal head into an occiput anterior position. If forceps rotation is not successful, cesarean delivery is usual.

Nursing Care. During labor the nurse should encourage the woman to assume positions that favor fetal rotation and descent. These positions also reduce some of the back pain. Good positions for back labor include the following:

- Sitting, kneeling, or standing while leaning forward

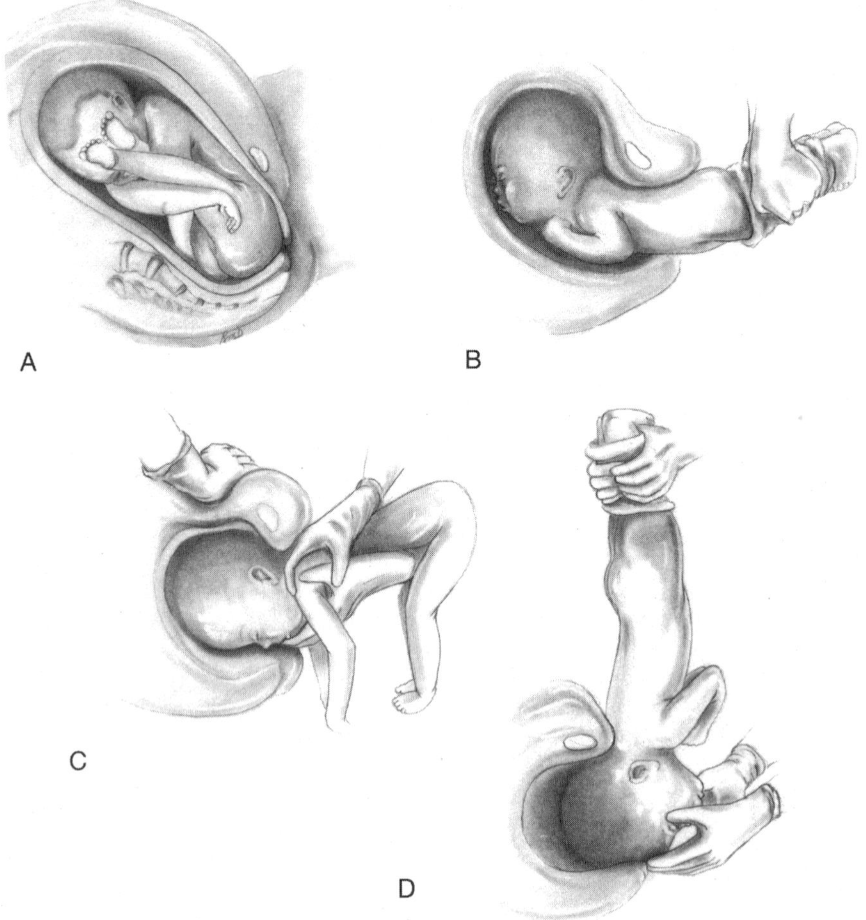

Figure 8–8. • Sequence for vaginal birth in a frank breech presentation. **A,** Descent and internal rotation of the fetal body. **B,** Internal rotation complete; extension of the fetal back as the trunk slips under the symphysis pubis. The birth attendant uses a towel for traction when grasping the wet fetal legs. **C,** After birth of the shoulders, the attendant maintains flexion of the fetal head by using the fingers of the left hand to apply pressure to the lower face; the fetal body straddles the attendant's left arm. An assistant provides suprapubic pressure to keep the fetal head well flexed. **D,** After the fetal head is brought under the symphysis, an assistant grasps the fetal legs with a towel for traction while the attendant delivers the face and head over the mother's perineum. (From Gorrie, T.M., McKinney, E.S., & Murray, S.S. [1994]. *Foundations of maternal newborn nursing.* Philadelphia: Saunders.)

- Hands and knees (Fig. 8–9); rocking the pelvis back and forth encourages rotation
- Side-lying (on the left side for a ROP position, on the right side for a LOP position)
- Squatting (good for second stage labor)
- Lunging by placing one foot in a chair with her foot and knee pointed to that side; she lunges sideways repeatedly during a contraction for 5 seconds at a time (Simkin, 1995)

After birth mother and infant are observed for signs of birth trauma. The mother is more likely to have a hematoma of her vaginal wall (see p. 262) if the fetus remained in the occiput posterior position for a long time. The infant may have excessive molding (alteration in shape) of the head, caput succedaneum (scalp edema), and possibly injury from forceps or the vacuum extractor.

Multifetal Pregnancy

If the woman has more than one fetus, dysfunctional labor is likely for two reasons:

- Uterine overdistention contributes to poor contraction quality.
- Abnormal presentation or position of one or more fetuses interferes with labor mechanisms.

Because of the difficulties inherent in multifetal deliveries, cesarean birth is common. Birth is almost always cesarean if three or more fetuses are involved.

Nursing Care. When the woman has a multifetal pregnancy, each fetus is monitored separately during labor. The woman should avoid lying on her back. An upright or side-lying position with the head slightly elevated aids breathing and is usually most comfortable. Labor care is similar to that for single pregnancies, with observations for hypotonic labor.

The nursery and intrapartum staffs prepare duplicate equipment and medications for every infant expected. An anesthesiologist is often present at birth because of the potential for maternal and/or neonatal problems. One nurse is available for each infant, and one or more pediatricians are usually present. Another nurse focuses on the mother's needs.

Fetal Anomalies

Some birth defects distort the fetal body so that birth is difficult. Hydrocephalus (collection of fluid within the brain) causes the fetal head to be large. The large fetal head usually keeps the fetus from assuming the normal head-down presentation, and it may not fit through the pelvis. Excessive amniotic fluid often occurs with fetal hydrocephalus and may result in uterine overdistention with hypotonic labor. Hydrocephalus is discussed more fully on page 347.

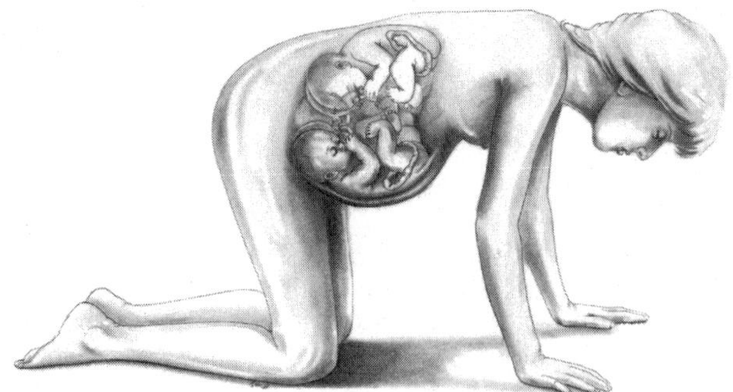

Figure 8–9. • The hands-and-knees position can help the fetus rotate from an occiput posterior to an occiput anterior position. Gravity causes the fetus to float downward toward the pool of amniotic fluid.

Problems with the Pelvis and Soft Tissues

The woman's pelvic size or shape and the characteristics of her soft tissues can either facilitate or impede birth.

Bony Pelvis

Some women have a pelvis that is small or abnormally shaped, thus impeding the normal mechanisms of labor. There are four basic pelvic shapes: gynecoid, which is the most favorable for vaginal birth; anthropoid; android; and platypelloid, which is unfavorable for vaginal birth (see Fig. 2–7). Most women do not have a pure shape, but have a mixture of different pelvic types.

Absolute pelvic measurements are rarely helpful to determine whether a woman's pelvis is adequate for birth. A woman with a "small" pelvis may still deliver vaginally if other factors are favorable. If her fetus is not too large, the head is well flexed, contractions are good, and her soft tissues yield easily to the forces of labor, she often delivers vaginally.

In contrast, some women have vaginally delivered several infants well over 9 pounds but cannot deliver one weighing 10 pounds. Obviously, the pelvis of each was "adequate," or even "large," according to standard measurements. However, the pelvis was not large enough for her largest infant. The ultimate test of a woman's pelvic size is whether her baby fits through it at birth.

Soft-Tissue Obstructions

The most common soft-tissue obstruction during labor is a full bladder. The woman is encouraged to urinate every 1 or 2 hours. Catheterization may be needed if she cannot urinate, especially if regional anesthesia and/or large quantities of intravenous fluids were given, filling her bladder quickly, yet reducing her sensation to void.

Less common soft-tissue obstructions include pelvic tumors, such as benign (noncancerous) fibroids. Some women have a cervix that is scarred from previous infections or surgery. The scar tissue may not readily yield to labor's forces to efface and dilate.

Psychological Problems

Labor is stressful. However, women with adequate social and professional support usually adapt to this stress and can labor and deliver normally. If their stress is too high, however, they perceive more pain and often have inadequate contractions. Their body responds to stress with a "fight-or-flight" reaction that impedes normal labor. For example, the fight-or-flight reaction

- Uses glucose the uterus needs for energy
- Causes secretion of hormones that inhibit uterine contractions
- Diverts blood from the uterus
- Increases tension of pelvic muscles, which impedes fetal descent
- Increases perception of pain, creating greater anxiety and stress and worsening the cycle

Nursing Care. Promoting relaxation and helping the woman to conserve her resources for the work of childbirth are the principal nursing goals. The nurse uses every opportunity to spare her energy and promote her comfort. See Chapter 7 for more information about promoting comfort.

Abnormal Duration of Labor

Labor that is either unusually long or short can cause problems in the mother or in her fetus or infant.

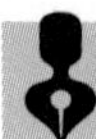

Nursing Tip

In any abnormal labor, observe the fetus for compromised oxygen supply. Observe the woman and newborn for signs of injury or infection after birth.

Prolonged Labor

Any of the previously discussed factors may be associated with a long or difficult labor *(dystocia)*. The average rate of cervical dilation during the active phase of labor is about 1.2 cm/hr for the woman having her first baby and about 1.5 cm/hr if she has had a baby before. Descent is expected to occur at a rate of at least 1.0 cm/hr in a first-time mother and 2.0 cm/hr in a woman who has had a baby before. A *Friedman curve* (Fig. 8–10) is often used to graph the progress of cervical dilation and fetal descent. The graph can help identify normal progress and the type of abnormal labor progress.

Prolonged labor can result in several problems, such as the following:

- Maternal or newborn infection, especially if the membranes have been ruptured for a long time (usually about 24 hours)
- Maternal exhaustion
- Postpartum hemorrhage (see p. 258)
- Greater anxiety and fear in an ensuing pregnancy

In addition, mothers who have difficult and long labors are more likely to be anxious and fearful about their next labor.

Nursing Care. Nursing care focuses on helping the woman to conserve her strength and encouraging her as she copes with the long labor. Observe for signs of infection during and after birth

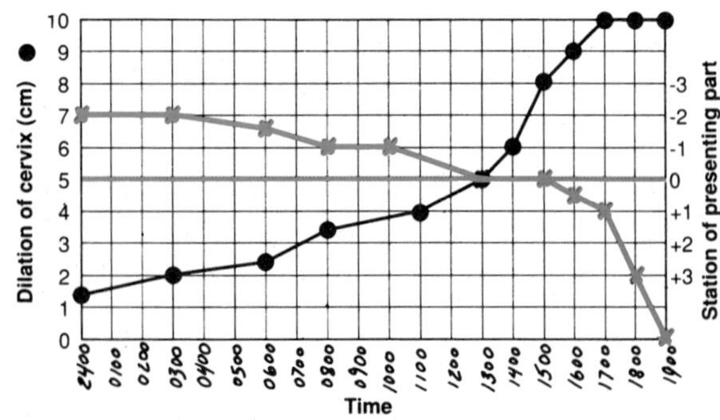

Figure 8–10. • A Friedman graph is a record of the woman's labor progress. Dots indicate cervical dilation; X's indicate fetal station.

in both the mother and newborn, which include the following:

- *Mother.* Temperature 38° C (100.4° F) or higher; foul-smelling cloudy, or yellowish amniotic fluid; foul-odored vaginal drainage after birth
- *Infant.* Axillary temperature under 36.2° C (97.0° F) or over 37.8° C (100° F); lethargy or irritability, poor feeding; not "looking right"

See page 264 for further information about postpartum infection and page 335 for discussion of neonatal infection.

Precipitate Labor

Precipitate labor is completed in less than 3 hours. Labor often begins abruptly and intensifies quickly, rather than having a more subtle onset and gradual progression. Contractions may be frequent and intense, often from the onset.

Precipitate labor is not the same as precipitate birth. A precipitate birth is one that occurs unexpectedly, with no trained birth attendant present. Precipitate birth may occur after a labor of any duration.

If the mother's pelvis is adequate for the size of her baby and her soft tissues yield easily during fetal descent, neither she nor her baby usually has problems. However, if her tissues do not yield easily to the powerful contractions, she may have uterine rupture, cervical lacerations, or hematoma.

Fetal oxygenation can be compromised by intense contractions, because the placenta is resupplied with oxygenated blood between contractions. In precipitate labor, this interval may be very short. Birth injury from rapid passage through the birth canal may become evident in the infant after birth. These injuries can include intracranial hemorrhage or nerve damage.

Nursing Care. Care for the woman in precipitate labor includes methods to promote fetal oxygenation and cope with discomfort. A side-lying position and supplemental oxygen improve fetal oxygenation. A tocolytic drug may be ordered to reduce intense contractions.

Pain control is difficult in precipitate labor. Regional anesthetics may not be effective soon enough to be useful. Narcotics should not be given near the time of birth (usually within 1 hour), to avoid depressing the newborn's respirations. The nurse must rely heavily on the nonpharmacologic techniques discussed in Chapter 7. The nurse stays with the woman and breathes with her to help her focus on coping with each contraction.

After birth the nurse observes the mother and infant for signs of injury. Excessive pain or bruising of the woman's vulva is reported. Cold applications limit pain, bruising, and edema. Abnormal findings on the newborn's assessment (see Chapter 12) are reported to the physician.

Nursing Tip

A woman who had a difficult labor and birth must recover physically before she has much interest in caring for her newborn.

PREMATURE RUPTURE OF MEMBRANES

Premature rupture of the membranes (PROM) is rupture of the membranes at term (38 or more weeks' gestation) before labor contractions begin. A related term, *preterm premature rupture of the membranes* (PPROM), is rupture of the membranes before term (before 38 weeks' gestation), with or without uterine contractions. Medical management of each condition depends on the gestation and whether other complications accompany the ruptured membranes. Infection and umbilical cord compression are the primary complications.

Infection of the amniotic sac, called *chorioamnionitis,* may cause prematurely ruptured membranes; or it may be a consequence of rupture because the barrier to the uterine cavity is broken. After the rupture, the risk for infection increases as time elapses. There is no exact time of infection, but the risk is known to increase after 18 hours.

Group B streptococcus infection is a leading perinatal infection in mothers and infants that is associated with both PROM and PPROM. Most physicians now screen for this organism at 35 to 37 weeks of gestation. Antibiotics are given to those having positive GBS screenings. However, screening cannot identify every woman who carries the organism. Therefore, intrapartum antibiotics are usually given in these other situations:

- Previous infant with GBS infection
- Birth before 37 weeks' gestation (because the woman may not have been screened for GBS)
- Maternal fever during labor
- Membranes ruptured 18 or more hours before birth

See p. 114 for more information about this organism.

Umbilical cord compression may occur because the amniotic fluid cushion is lost. The newborn may have infection, respiratory distress, and other problems of immaturity if born prematurely.

Medical Treatment. Medical therapy depends on the gestation (term or preterm) and on whether there is evidence of or risk for infection, umbilical cord compression, or other complications. PROM at term may simply herald the imminent onset of labor. If the fetus is immature, the physician carefully weighs the benefits of continued maturation against the risk of infection or other complications. If there are no signs of infection, the woman is usually managed at home after a brief hospitalization.

If the fetus is at or near term (about 36 weeks' gestation), the physician usually induces labor with oxytocin if it does not begin spontaneously. Oxytocin induction is rarely successful far from term, because the uterus is not sensitive to the drug.

Nursing Care. Nursing care for the woman who is having labor induced because of PROM has been discussed previously. Intravenous antibiotic therapy is usually added to the protocol in this case. Nursing care for the woman who is not having labor induced right away primarily involves observing for and teaching the woman about complications. Teaching combines information about infection and preterm labor; it includes the following:

- Take the temperature at least four times a day, reporting any that is above 37.8° C (100° F)
- Avoid sexual intercourse or insertion of anything in the vagina, which can increase the risk for infection
- Avoid orgasm, which can stimulate contractions
- Avoid breast stimulation, which can stimulate contractions because of natural oxytocin release
- Maintain any activity restrictions prescribed
- Note any uterine contractions, reduced fetal activity, or other signs of infection (discussed under amniotomy)

See the following discussion of preterm labor for additional care.

PRETERM LABOR

Preterm labor occurs after 20 and before 38 weeks of gestation. The main risks are the problems of immaturity in the newborn.

Just as it is not known exactly why labor begins at term, it is not known why some women begin labor early. However, a large number of factors are associated with preterm labor (Box 8–2).

Early prenatal care can identify many women at risk. One of the Healthy People 2000 goals is that 90% of all pregnant women will have prenatal care starting in the first trimester. The percentage in 1995 was 81% for all women, but was much lower for nonwhite women (National Center for Health Statistics, 1996, 1997). Early prenatal care makes it possible for the woman to reduce or to eliminate some risk factors, including those that contribute to preterm labor. The woman can be taught to observe for signs of preterm labor so that it may be interrupted before a baby is born prematurely.

Preterm labor often has vague symptoms at its onset. Early preterm labor does not usually begin like early labor at term. The symptoms vary considerably, but they include the following:

- Contractions that may be either uncomfortable or painless

BOX 8–2

SOME RISK FACTORS FOR PRETERM LABOR

Exposure to diethylstilbestrol (DES)	Anemia
Underweight	Preterm premature rupture of the membranes
Chronic illness such as diabetes or hypertension	Inadequate prenatal care
Dehydration	Poor nutrition
Preeclampsia	Age under 18 or over 40
Previous preterm labor or birth	Low education level
Previous pregnancy losses	Poverty
Uterine or cervical abnormalities or surgery	Smoking
Uterine distention	Substance abuse
Abdominal surgery during pregnancy	Chronic stress
Infection	Nonwhite

- Feeling that the baby is "balling up" frequently
- Menstrual-like cramps
- Constant low backache
- Pelvic pressure, or a feeling that the baby is pushing down
- A change in the vaginal discharge
- Abdominal cramps, with or without diarrhea
- Pain or discomfort in the vulva or thighs
- "Just feeling bad" or "coming down with something"

Medical Treatment

Medical care involves quickly identifying and halting preterm labor. If birth of an immature infant is likely despite interventions to stop preterm labor, the physician may order drugs to speed maturation of the fetal lungs.

Identifying Preterm Labor Early. A key element of both medical and nursing care is to teach women, especially those at higher risk, about the symptoms of preterm labor. High-risk women have more frequent prenatal visits to identify cervical effacement and dilation that begin before the woman feels anything.

Fetal fibronectin can help the physician decide which women should be treated most aggressively to stop preterm labor. Fetal fibronectin is a protein found in the amniotic fluid and membranes. It is normally present in vaginal secretions up to 22 weeks and reappears near term. If it is found at a time when it should not be present, the fetal membranes may have been weakened by infection or other processes.

The physician may order home uterine activity monitoring for women at risk for preterm labor, although studies of its effectiveness have been mixed. The monitor assesses contractions only; it does not assess fetal heart rates.

Stopping Preterm Labor. The initial measures to stop preterm labor include identifying and treating infection, activity restriction, and hydration. The benefit of hydration is not clear if the woman is not dehydrated, however. Urinary tract infections increase the risk for preterm labor and birth, so urinalysis is done to identify them. GBS infection has already been discussed.

Tocolytic drugs may be given to inhibit uterine contractions and thus delay preterm birth. None of them are likely to be effective if the cervix is more than 3 cm dilated. All of the drugs have significant side effects. Because of the side effects and because complications of prematurity are less severe if a baby is born after 34 weeks' gestation, tocolytics are less likely to be prescribed after that time.

Because of these side effects, other drugs may be given to stop preterm labor. These drugs are well established for other uses, but their use as tocolytics is investigational. They are given for their secondary effect of inhibiting contractions. These drugs include the following:

- Terbutaline (Brethine)
- Magnesium sulfate
- Indomethacin (Indocin)
- Nifedipine Procardia)

Ritodrine (Yutopar) is a drug related to terbutaline. However, it has stronger side effects than terbutaline, and no advantage over terbutaline in stopping preterm labor. A new drug, atosiban, is being investigated as a tocolytic. It appears to have less severe side effects than many other drugs.

Terbutaline is a commonly prescribed tocolytic. Side effects include maternal and fetal tachycardia, hypoglycemia, elevated potassium, and hypotension. The woman on home care may take terbutaline, either orally or by means of a continuous subcutaneous infusion pump. Side effects are most apparent when the drug is given intravenously.

Interventions for magnesium sulfate are the same as those for the drug when given to prevent seizures in pregnancy-induced hypertension (see p. 92). Pulmonary edema and cardiac dysrhythmias may occur because of fluid and electrolyte imbalances.

Speeding Fetal Lung Maturation. If it appears that preterm birth is inevitable, the physician may give the woman steroid drugs to increase fetal lung maturity if the gestation is between 24 and 34 weeks. Dexamethasone and betamethasone are two drugs for this purpose. Steroids may be repeated in 1 week if birth has not occurred.

Activity Restrictions. Bed rest was often prescribed for women at risk for preterm birth. However, the benefits of bed rest are not clear and many adverse maternal effects can occur. Also, physicians cannot predict which women who have preterm labor signs and symptoms will be the ones who actually deliver early. Therefore, total bed rest is prescribed less frequently than in the past. Activity restrictions are often more moderate, such as resting in a semi-Fowler's position or partial bed rest.

Nursing Care

Nurses should be aware of the symptoms of preterm labor because they may occur in any pregnant woman, with or without risk factors. Symptoms are taught and regularly reinforced for women who have risk factors.

If the woman remains at home, the nurse reinforces the exact level of activity the physician prescribed. After a few days, most women begin to think, "It probably won't hurt if I just empty the dishwasher or wash clothes or drive on my carpool day." The nurse should anticipate these temptations and emphasize that maintaining the restrictions is important work that she is doing for her baby right now. If she departs from the physician's recommendations and has recurrent preterm labor, the nurse should not make her feel guiltier about it than she already does.

To reduce boredom the woman can set up two places to rest, such as her living room and bedroom. This provides a change of scenery and helps her to feel more involved in family activities. A telephone should be nearby in both locations. A picnic cooler packed with drinks and snacks limits the need to walk. The nurse helps the woman to identify enjoyable activities that can be done while maintaining activity restrictions. Television, videos, video games, puzzles, reading, letter writing, and hand needlework are some options.

Women with other children have the greatest difficulty in maintaining activity restrictions. The nurse helps them to identify who can assist in child care and transportation to school and other activities.

PROLONGED PREGNANCY

Prolonged pregnancy lasts longer than 42 weeks. Other terms that are often used interchangeably for prolonged pregnancy include *postmature, postdate,* or *postterm.* The term *postmature* most accurately describes the infant that has characteristics consistent with a prolonged gestation (see p. 342) rather than the pregnancy. Many pregnancies seem to be prolonged, yet are really only term, or even preterm. The woman may have had irregular menstrual periods or may have forgotten the date of her last menstrual period. Clarification of an uncertain gestation is much more difficult if the woman has not had regular prenatal care.

Risks. The greatest risks of prolonged pregnancy are to the fetus. As the placenta ages, it delivers oxygen and nutrients to the fetus less efficiently. The fetus may lose weight, and the skin may begin to peel, which are the typical characteristics of postmaturity. Meconium may be expelled into the amniotic fluid, which can cause severe respiratory problems at birth. Low blood sugar is a likely complication after birth.

The fetus with placental insufficiency does not tolerate labor well. Because the fetus has less reserve than needed, the normal interruption in blood flow during contractions may cause excessive stress on the baby.

If the placenta continues functioning well, the fetus continues growing. This can lead to a large fetus and the problems accompanying macrosomia.

There is little physical risk to the mother, other than laboring with a large baby if placental function remains normal. Psychologically, however, she often feels that pregnancy will never end. She becomes more anxious about when labor will begin and when her birth attendant will "do something."

Medical Treatment. The physician or nurse-midwife will evaluate whether pregnancy is truly prolonged or if the gestation has been miscalculated. If she had early and regular prenatal care, ultrasound examinations have usually clarified her true gestation. If the woman's pregnancy has definitely reached 42 weeks, labor is usually induced by oxytocin. Prostaglandin application makes induction more likely to be successful if her cervix is not ripe.

Nursing Care. Nursing care involves careful observation of the fetus during labor to identify signs associated with poor placental blood flow, such as late decelerations (see p. 148). After birth, the newborn is observed for respiratory difficulties and hypoglycemia.

EMERGENCIES DURING CHILDBIRTH

Several intrapartum conditions can endanger the life or well-being of the woman or her fetus. Although these problems do not occur often, they require prompt nursing and medical action to reduce the likelihood of damage. Nursing and medical management often overlap in emergencies.

Prolapsed Umbilical Cord

The umbilical cord prolapses if it slips downward in the pelvis after the membranes rupture. In this position, it can be compressed between the fetal body and the woman's pelvis, interrupting blood supply to and from the placenta. It may slip down immediately after the membranes rupture, or the prolapse may occur later.

A prolapsed cord can be classified in one of three ways (Fig. 8–11):

- *Complete.* The cord is visible at the vaginal opening
- *Palpated.* The cord cannot be seen, but it can be felt as a pulsating structure when a vaginal examination is done
- *Occult.* The prolapse is hidden and cannot be seen

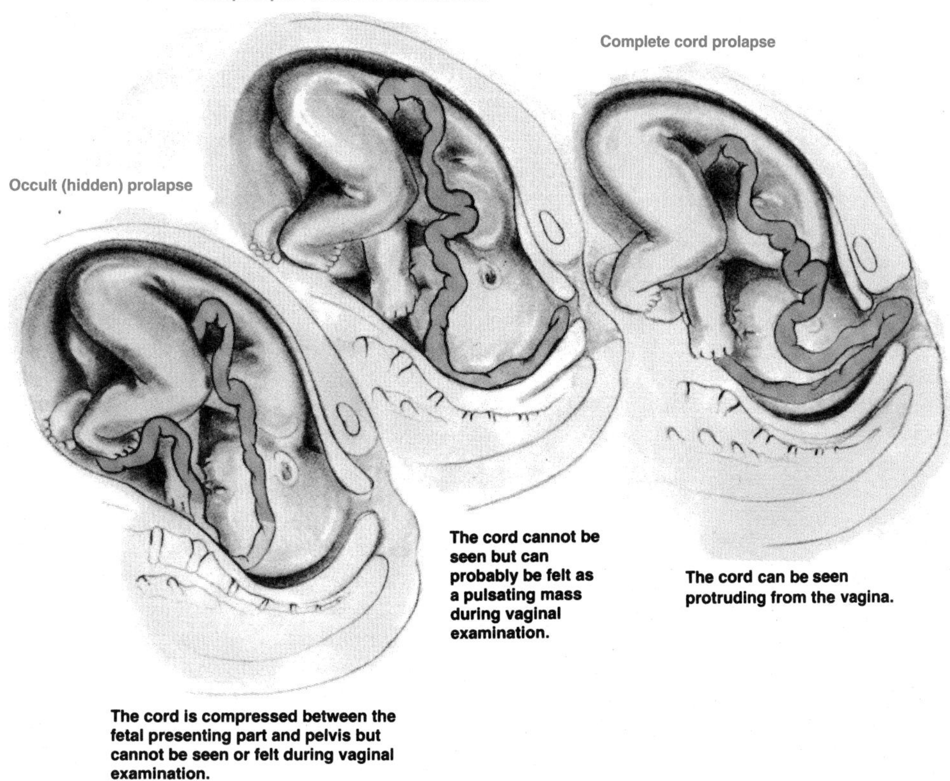

Figure 8–11. • Three different degrees of prolapsed umbilical cord.

or felt; it is suspected on the basis of abnormal fetal heart rates

Risk Factors. Prolapse of the umbilical cord is more likely if the fetus does not completely fill the space in the pelvis or if fluid pressure is great when the membranes rupture. These conditions are more likely in the following situations:

- Fetus high in the pelvis when the membranes rupture
- Very small fetus, as in prematurity
- Abnormal presentations, such as footling breech or transverse lie
- Hydramnios (excess amniotic fluid)

Medical Treatment. The main risk of a prolapsed cord is to the fetus. When prolapsed cord occurs, the first action is to displace the fetus upward to stop compression against the pelvis. Maternal positions such as the knee-chest or Trendelenburg (head-down) accomplish this displacement. Placing the mother in a side-lying position with her hips elevated on pillows also reduces cord pressure. The experienced nurse or physician may push the fetus upward from the vagina. Oxygen and a tocolytic drug, such as terbutaline, may be given. The primary focus is to deliver the fetus by the quickest means possible, usually cesarean delivery.

Nursing Care. In addition to prompt corrective actions and assisting with emergency procedures, the nurse should remain calm to avoid increasing the woman's anxiety. Prolapsed cord is a sudden development; anxiety and fear are inevitable reactions. Calm, quick actions on the part of nurses help the woman and her family to feel that she is in competent hands.

After birth, the nurse helps the woman to understand the experience. She may need several explanations of what happened and why.

Uterine Rupture

A tear in the uterine wall occurs if the muscle cannot withstand the pressure inside the organ (Fig. 8–12). There are three variations of uterine rupture:

- *Complete rupture.* There is a hole through the uterine wall, from the uterine cavity to the abdominal cavity.

- *Incomplete rupture.* The uterus tears into a nearby structure, such as a ligament, but not all the way into the abdominal cavity.
- *Dehiscence.* An old uterine scar, usually from a previous cesarean birth, separates; the separation may be bloodless *(bloodless window).*

Dehiscence is a relatively common occurrence, and the woman may have no signs or symptoms. It may be found during a subsequent cesarean or other abdominal surgery.

Risk Factors. Uterine rupture is more likely if the woman had previous surgery on her uterus, usually a previous cesarean delivery. The low-transverse uterine incision (see p. 196) is least likely to rupture. Because the classic uterine incision is prone to rupture, vaginal birth after this type incision is not recommended.

Uterine rupture may occur in the unscarred uterus if a woman:

- Had many other births (grand multiparity)
- Has intense labor contractions, such as with oxytocin stimulation
- Had blunt abdominal trauma, such as from a vehicle accident or battering

Characteristics. The woman may have no symptoms, or she may have sudden onset of severe signs and symptoms:

- Shock due to bleeding into the abdomen (vaginal bleeding may be minimal)
- Abdominal pain
- Pain in the chest, between the scapulae (shoulder blades), or with inspiration
- Cessation of contractions

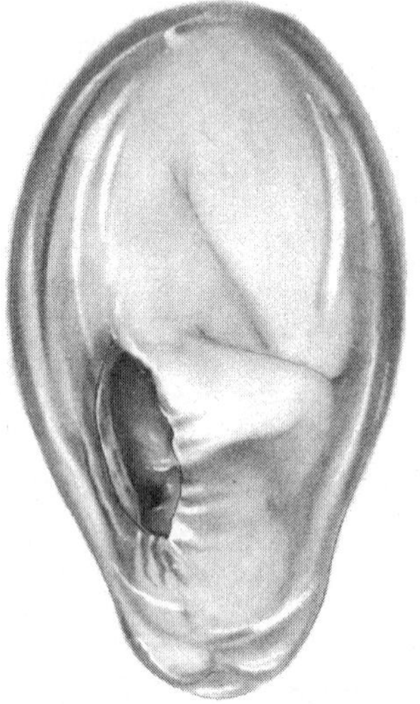

Figure 8–12. • Uterine rupture.

- Abnormal or absent fetal heart rates
- Palpation of the fetus outside the uterus because the fetus is pushed through the torn area

Medical Treatment. If the fetus is living when the rupture is detected and/or if blood loss is excessive, the physician performs surgery to deliver the fetus and stops the bleeding. Hysterectomy (removal of the uterus) is likely for an extensive tear. Smaller tears may be repaired if the woman wants more children.

Nursing Care. Oxytocin is carefully administered during labor, and the woman is observed for excessive contractions. If signs or symptoms of uterine rupture occur, the physician is promptly notified. The nurse incorporates measures to allay the woman's anxiety before and after birth, as discussed with prolapsed umbilical cord.

Uterine rupture is sometimes not discovered until after birth. In these cases, the woman does not have dramatic symptoms of blood loss. However, she may have continuous bleeding that is brighter red than the normal postbirth bleeding. A rising pulse and falling blood pressure are signs of hypovolemic shock, which may occur if blood loss is excessive.

Uterine Inversion

Uterine inversion occurs if the uterus turns inside out after the baby is born. There are varying degrees of uterine inversion. The physician may note a small depression in the top of the uterus or may discover that the uterus is not in the abdomen and protrudes from the vagina with its inner surface showing. Rapid onset of shock is common.

Uterine inversion is more likely to occur if the uterus is not firmly contracted, especially if the birth attendant pulls on the umbilical cord to deliver the placenta. A placenta that adheres to the uterine wall abnormally increases this risk. Inversion can also occur during fundal massage if the uterus is pushed downward toward the pelvis when it is not firm.

Medical Treatment. The physician will try to replace the inverted uterus while the woman is under general anesthesia. The anesthetic agent is chosen to cause uterine relaxation; tocolytic drugs also may be used. After the uterus is replaced, oxytocin is then given to contract the uterus and control bleeding. If replacement of the uterus is not successful, the woman needs a hysterectomy.

Nursing Care. Nursing care during the emergency supplements medical management. Two intravenous lines are usually established to administer fluids and medications and to combat shock.

During the recovery period, the woman's uterus is assessed at least every 15 minutes for firmness, height, and deviation from the midline, supporting the lower uterus at each assessment (see p. 225). Her vital signs and the amount of vaginal bleeding are assessed at the same time. An indwelling catheter may be used to keep her bladder empty so that the uterus can contract well. The catheter is assessed for patency and the output recorded; output may fall below 25 or 30 ml/hr with shock. The patient should take nothing orally until her condition is stable and the physician orders oral intake.

After birth, the nurse provides explanations and emotional support to the woman and her partner. The birth may have been normal until the uterine inversion occurred. Abruptly the woman was surrounded by people who inserted additional intravenous lines in her arm and she was quickly anesthetized. Her partner was probably sent from the room to sit, terrified, in the waiting room. Both will need explanations about what happened and why the actions were taken to correct the problem. The explanations may need to be reinforced several times before they can integrate the experience.

Amniotic Fluid Embolism

This fortunately uncommon embolism occurs when amniotic fluid, with its particles such as vernix, fetal hair, and sometimes meconium, enters the woman's circulation and obstructs small blood vessels in her lungs. It is more likely to occur during a very strong labor because the fluid is "pushed" into small blood vessels that rupture as the cervix dilates.

Amniotic fluid embolism is characterized by abrupt onset of hypotension, respiratory distress, and coagulation abnormalities. However, there is variation among women in the signs and symptoms they present. The woman usually has abrupt and severe respiratory distress and circulatory collapse. Coagulation abnormalities may occur because amniotic fluid is rich in factors that promote blood clotting. These factors cause her normal clotting factors to be consumed and they are then not available to provide normal blood clotting. Immediate cardiac and pulmonary support are begun. Clotting defects are corrected with appropriate blood factors.

The likelihood of death from amniotic fluid embolism is high, especially if meconium was in the fluid. The embolism may occur before or after the infant is born.

Trauma

The pregnant trauma victim may be encountered anywhere, from an accident scene, to the hospital emergency department, to physician's offices and clinics. Battering is a common cause of trauma, and the violence often escalates during pregnancy.

The priority of care is to manage any life-threatening injuries in the woman. Once the woman is stabilized, the fetus can be considered. As the woman's injuries are treated, a small wedge is placed under one hip to displace her uterus from her large blood vessels. This action helps stabilize her blood pressure and improves blood now to the placenta. The staff should remain alert to signs and symptoms that suggest abruptio placentae (see p. 91) and uterine rupture, which are more likely to occur with trauma to the pregnant woman's abdomen. The fetus may also sustain direct injury and should be examined after birth.

KEY POINTS

- The nurse observes the character of the amniotic fluid and the fetal heart rate (FHR) when the membranes are ruptured. Fluid should be clear and mild-odored; the FHR should remain near its baseline level and between 110 and 160 BPM at term.
- The nurse observes the fetal condition and character of contractions if any methods to stimulate labor are used. These methods may include walking, nipple stimulation, amniotomy, or oxytocin infusion.
- After version, the nurse observes for persistent contractions that may indicate labor has begun and leaking amniotic fluid. Before discharge, signs of labor are reviewed with the woman so she will know when to return to the birth center.
- Nursing care after episiotomy or perineal lacerations includes comfort measures, such as cold applications and analgesics.

- Nursing care after cesarean birth is similar to that after vaginal birth with these additions: surgical dressing, indwelling catheter patency, and intravenous flow. The woman and her partner may need extra emotional support after cesarean birth.
- Nursing measures such as encouraging position changes, aiding relaxation, and reminding the woman to empty her bladder can promote a more normal labor.
- Nursing care after births involving instruments (forceps or vacuum extraction) and after abnormal labor and birth includes observations for maternal and newborn injuries or infections.
- Infection is the most common hazard after membranes rupture prematurely, especially if there is a long interval before delivery.
- Nurses should be aware of the subtle symptoms a woman may have at the beginning of preterm labor and encourage her to seek care at the hospital promptly.
- After any kind of emergency, the woman and her family need emotional support, explanations of what happened, and patience with their repeated questions.

MULTIPLE-CHOICE QUESTIONS

Choose the most appropriate answer.

1. Contractions during oxytocin induction of labor are every 2 minutes, they last 95 seconds, and the uterus remains tense between contractions. What action is expected based on these assessments?
   a. no action expected; the contractions are normal
   b. rate of oxytocin will be increased slightly
   c. pain medication or an epidural block will be offered
   d. infusion of oxytocin will be stopped
2. Select the appropriate nursing intervention during the early recovery period to increase the woman's comfort if she had forceps-assisted birth and a median episiotomy.
   a. application of a cold pack to her perineal area
   b. encouragement of perineal stretching exercises
   c. application of warm, moist heat to the perineum
   d. administration of stool softeners as ordered
3. A woman has an emergency cesarean delivery after the umbilical cord was found to be prolapsed. She repeatedly asks similar questions about what happened at birth. The nurse's interpretation of her behavior is that she
   a. cannot accept that she did not have the kind of delivery she planned
   b. is trying to understand her experience and move on with postpartum adaptation
   c. thinks the staff is not telling her the truth about what happened at birth
   d. is confused about events because general anesthesia effects are persisting
4. What nursing intervention during labor can increase space in the woman's pelvis?
   a. promote adequate fluid intake
   b. position on the left side
   c. assist her to take a shower
   d. encourage regular urination
5. A woman is being observed in the hospital because her membranes ruptured at 30 weeks' gestation. While giving morning care, the nursing student notices that the fluid draining has a strong odor. The priority nursing action is to:
   a. caution the woman to remain in bed until her physician visits
   b. ask the woman if she is having any more contractions than usual
   c. take the temperature; report it and the fluid odor to the registered nurse
   d. help to prepare the woman for an immediate cesarean delivery

BIBLIOGRAPHY AND READER REFERENCE

American Academy of Pediatrics & American College of Obstetricians and Gynecologists. (1997). *Guidelines for perinatal care* (4th ed.). Elk Grove Village, IL: Author.

American College of Obstetricians and Gynecologists (ACOG). (1995a). *Technical bulletin no. 196: Operative vaginal delivery.* Washington, DC: Author.

American College of Obstetricians and Gynecologists (ACOG). (1995b). *Technical bulletin no. 218: Dystocia and the augmentation of labor.* Washington, DC: Author.

AWHONN (Association of Women's Health, Obstetric, and Neonatal Nurses). (1993). *Cervical ripening and induction and augmentation of labor.* Washington, DC: Author.

Bachman, J., & Kendrick, J. M. (1996). Childbirth. In K. R. Simpson and P. A. Creehan (Eds.), *AWHONN's perinatal nursing* (pp. 151–186). Philadelphia: J. B. Lippincott.

Bowes, W. A. (1994). Clinical aspects of normal and abnormal labor. In R. K. Creasy & R. Resnick (Eds.), *Maternal–fetal medicine: Principles and practice* (3rd ed., pp. 527–557). Philadelphia: Saunders.

Burke, M. E., & Poole, J. (1996). Common perinatal complications. In K. R. Simpson and P. A Creehan (Eds.), *AWHONN's perinatal nursing* (pp. 109–148). Philadelphia: Saunders.

Creasy, R. K. (1994). Preterm labor and delivery. In R. K. Creasy & R. Resnick (Eds.), *Maternal–fetal medicine: Principles and practice* (3rd ed., pp. 494–523). Philadelphia: Saunders.

Crowther, C. A. (1995). Commentary: Bedrest for women with pregnancy problems. Evidence for efficacy is lacking. *Birth, 22*(1), 13–14.

Cunningham, F. G., MacDonald, P. C., Gant, N. F., Leveno, K. J., Gilstrap, L. C., Hankins, G. D. V., & Clark, S. L. (1997). *Williams' obstetrics* (20th ed.). Norwalk, CT: Appleton & Lange.

Escher-Davis, L. (1996). Fetal fibronectin: A biochemical marker for preterm labor. *AWHONN Voice, 4,*(3), 1, 6–7.

Gardner, M. O., & Goldenberg, R. J. (1995). The clinical use of antenatal corticosteroids. *Clinical Obstetrics and Gynecology, 38*(4), 746–754.

Goodwin, T. M., Valenzuela, G., Silver, H., Hayashi, R., Creasy, G., & Lane, R. (1996). Treatment of preterm labor with the oxytocin antagonist atosiban. *American Journal of Perinatology, 13*(3), 143–146.

Gorrie, T. M., McKinney, E. S., & Murray, S. M. (1998). *Foundations of maternal–newborn nursing* (2nd ed.). Philadelphia: Saunders.

Gupton, A., Heaman, M., & Ashcroft, T. (1997). Bed rest from the perspective of the high-risk pregnant woman. *Journal of Obstetric, Gynecologic, and Neonatal Nursing, 26*(4), 423–430.

Hall, S. P. (1997). The nurse's role in the identification of risks and treatment of shoulder dystocia. *Journal of Obstetric, Gynecologic, and Neonatal Nursing, 26*(1), 25–32.

Mitchell, A. Steffenson, N., Hogan, H., & Brooks, S. (1997a). Group B streptococcus and pregnancy: Update and recommendations. *MCN: American Journal of Maternal/Child Nursing, 22*(5), 242–248.

Mitchell, A., Steffenson, N., Hogan, H., & Brooks, S. (1997b). Neonatal group B streptococcal disease. *MCN: American Journal of Maternal/Child Nursing, 22*(5), 249–253.

National Center for Health Statistics. (1996). *Healthy people 2000 review, 1995–96.* Hyattsville, Md: Author.

National Center for Health Statistics. (1997). *Health, United States, 1996–97, and injury chartbook.* Hyattsville, Md: Author.

Poole, G. V., Martin, J. N., Perry, K. G., Griswold, J. A., Lambert, C. J., & Rhodes, R. S. (1996). Trauma in pregnancy: The role of interpersonal violence. *American Journal of Obstetrics and Gynecology, 174*(6), 1873–1876.

Resnik, R. (1994). Post-term pregnancy. In R. K. Creasy & R. Resnick (Eds.), *Maternal–fetal medicine: Principles and practice* (3rd ed., pp. 521–526). Philadelphia: Saunders.

Simkin, P. (1995). Reducing pain and enhancing progress in labor: A guide to nonpharmacologic methods for maternity caregivers. *Birth, 22*(3), 161–171.

Torgersen, K. (1996). Ask the experts: Please compare prostaglandin E_2 preparation used to ripen the cervix in preparation for induction. *AWHONN Voice, 4*(3), 4.

chapter 9

The Family after Birth

Outline

Objectives

On completion and mastery of Chapter 9, the student will be able to

- Define each vocabulary term listed.
- Describe how to individualize postpartum and newborn nursing care for different clients.
- Describe specific cultural beliefs that the nurse may encounter when providing postpartum and newborn care.
- Explain nursing care of the mother during the fourth stage of labor.
- Describe postpartum changes in maternal systems and the nursing care associated with those changes.
- Modify nursing assessments and interventions for the woman who has a cesarean birth.
- Explain emotional needs of postpartum women and their families.
- Describe nursing care of the normal newborn.
- Describe nursing care to promote optimal infant nutrition.
- Identify signs and symptoms that may indicate a complication in the postpartum mother or infant.
- Plan appropriate discharge teaching for the postpartum woman and her infant.

Vocabulary

acrocyanosis
afterpains
Apgar score
attachment
bonding
colostrum
diastasis recti
fundus
involution
let-down reflex
lochia
postpartum blues
puerperium
suckling

The postpartum period or *puerperium* is the 6 weeks following childbirth. This period is often referred to as the 4th trimester of pregnancy. This chapter addresses the physiological and psychologic changes in the mother and her family and the early care of the newborn.

ADAPTING CARE TO SPECIFIC GROUPS AND CULTURES

The nurse must adapt care to a person's circumstances, such as those of the single or adolescent parent, the poor, families who have a multiple birth, and families from other cultures.

Nursing Considerations for Specific Groups of Clients

Adolescents, particularly younger ones, will need help to learn parenting skills. Their peer group is very important to them, so the nurse must make every effort during both pregnancy and the postpartum period to help them to fit in with their peers. They are often passive in caring for themselves and their infants. They may be single and poor as well. Poor, young adolescent mothers often have several children in a short time, compounding their social problems.

A single woman may have problems making postpartum adaptations if she does not have a strong support system. She often must return to work very soon because she is the sole provider for her family. Some single women are homosexual and want to rear a child with their partner.

Poor families may have difficulty meeting their basic needs before a new infant arrives, and a new family member adds to their strain. Women may have inadequate or sporadic prenatal care, which increases their risk for complications that extend into the puerperium and to their baby. They may need social service referrals to direct them to public assistance programs or other resources.

Families who add twins (or more) face different challenges. The infants are more likely to need intensive care because of preterm birth, delaying the parents' attachment and assumption of newborn care. It is also more difficult for the parents to see the individuality of each infant, rather than attaching to them as a set. The mother is also more likely to have complications during pregnancy and birth, which may further delay her ability to care for her babies. The infants may require care at a distant hospital if their problems are severe. Financial strains mount with each added problem.

Cultural Influences on Postpartum Care

The United States has a diverse population. Special cultural practices are often most evident at significant life events such as birth and even death. The nurse must adapt care to fit the health beliefs, values, and practices of that specific culture to make the birth a meaningful emotional and social event as well as a safe physical event.

Communication

The nurse may need an interpreter to understand and provide optimal care to the woman and her family. If possible, the interpreter should not be a family member if sensitive information is discussed. That person may interpret selectively. The interpreter should not be of a group that is in social or religious conflict with the client and her family, as is the case in many middle Eastern cultures. It is also important to remember that an affirmative nod from the woman may be a sign of courtesy to the nurse rather than a sign of understanding or agreement.

Modesty is important to most women, but especially to Latinas, Middle Eastern, and Asian women. When providing care and teaching, the

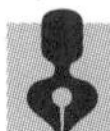

Nursing Tip

To verify that a woman (or family) understands what the nurse has told her, have the woman repeat the teaching in her own words. An affirmative nod may indicate courtesy, not understanding, when the primary languages of the nurse and family are different.

nurse should draw curtains or use a privacy screen in a semi-private room or take the new mother to a separate room.

Some women expect a short period of "small talk" and gracious conversation before approaching the main subject. This may annoy the busy nurse who wants to get to the point of assessments and care. But this short period of courteous talk can smooth client care and increase her receptivity to the nurse's teaching.

Dietary Practices

Some cultures adhere to the "hot" and "cold" theory of diet after childbirth. Temperature has nothing to do with which foods are hot and which are cold, but rather it is the intrinsic property of the food itself that classifies it. For example, many Southeast Asians believe that a woman should eat only "hot" foods after birth, which includes eggs, chicken, and rice. These women may prefer their drinking water hot rather than cool or cold.

Chinese women practice something similar to the hot/cold dietary practice. They believe that a woman's health requires a balance between *yin* foods (such as bean sprouts, broccoli, and carrots) and *yang* foods (such as broiled meat, chicken, soup, and eggs).

Health Beliefs

The nurse should incorporate a family's health beliefs into teaching as much as possible. Examples of the beliefs a nurse may encounter and the groups that hold them include the following:

- *Muslims.* The first sound a child hears should be words of praise and supplication to Allah (God) from the Koran.
- *Southeast Asians.* The spirit resides in the head and patting or rubbing the head should be avoided.
- *Latinas, Southeast Asians.* A postpartum woman should stay warm to avoid upsetting the hot–cold balance. This may include avoiding baths or washing the hair.
- *Southeast Asians.* Colostrum is "unclean" and should be discarded until the milk comes in.

The nurse should accept and support practices that are harmless. If a belief is potentially harmful or a beneficial practice is avoided, such as not feeding the infant the antibody-rich colostrum, the nurse should talk with the family to determine if a compromise can be worked out.

IMMEDIATE POSTPARTUM PERIOD: THE FOURTH STAGE OF LABOR

The fourth stage of labor is the first 1 to 4 hours after birth of the placenta or until the mother is physiologically stable. Nursing care during the fourth stage of labor includes the following general care:

- Identifying and preventing hemorrhage
- Evaluating and intervening for pain
- Observing bladder function and urinary output
- Evaluating recovery from anesthesia
- Promoting bonding and attachment between the infant and family

In many labor-delivery-recovery rooms, the nurse provides initial assessments and care for the infant. Newborn assessments and care are presented after this section and in Chapter 12.

Facility protocols will vary, but a common schedule for assessing the mother during the fourth stage is every 15 minutes for one hour, every 30 minutes during the second hour, and hourly until transfer to postpartum unit. After transfer to postpartum unit, applicable routine assessments are made every 4 to 8 hours. Assessments that should be made each time during the fourth stage include the following:

- Vital signs (temperature may be taken hourly if normal)
- Skin color
- Location and firmness of the uterine fundus (see pp. 224 and 225)
- Amount and color of lochia (see p. 223)
- Presence and location of pain
- Intravenous infusion and medications
- Fullness of the bladder or urine output from a catheter
- Condition of perineum for vaginal birth
- Condition of dressing for cesarean birth or tubal ligation
- Level of sensation and ability to move lower extremities if an epidural or subarachnoid block was used

POSTPARTUM CHANGES IN THE MOTHER

Box 9–1 summarizes nursing assessments for the postpartum woman. Refer to Nursing Care Plan 9–1 for interventions relating to selected diagnoses in the postpartum woman. See Chapter 10 for addi-

NURSING CARE PLAN 9–1

Selected Nursing Diagnoses for the Woman Following Vaginal Birth

Nursing Diagnosis: Risk for altered tissue perfusion related to poor uterine contraction

Goals	Nursing Interventions	Rationale
The woman will maintain adequate tissue perfusion as evidenced by normal vital signs, firm fundus, and saturation of no more than one pad per hour	1. Assess vital signs according to hospital procedure	1. Rising pulse and falling blood pressure may be signs of shock from excessive bleeding
	2. Assess uterine fundus with vital sign checks by evaluating height, position, and firmness; massage if soft until firm	2. A firm fundus compresses bleeding vessels at placental site
	3. Observe lochia when assessing vital signs and uterus for amount, color, persistent clots, and odor	3. Most postpartum hemorrhage is obvious rather than concealed. Lochia that is heavier than expected, large clots, or a return to rubra after progression are associated with postpartum hemorrhage. Foul-odored lochia may occur with infection, which also increases the risk for hemorrhage
	4. Assess bladder and promote regular emptying	4. A full bladder interferes with uterine contraction and increases blood loss.

Nursing Diagnosis: Altered urinary elimination related to birth trauma and altered sensation

Goals	Nursing Interventions	Rationale
The woman will void a minimum of 150 ml at each urination. Fundus will be firm, midline, and at appropriate level for the time since birth	1. Assess uterine fundus for height and deviation from the midline	1. A full bladder elevates the uterine fundus and usually causes it to deviate to one side
	2. Help woman to ambulate to bathroom if sensation and movement have returned; provide privacy; have her squirt warm water over perineum from the peri bottle; run water faucet	2. These measures promote relaxation and voiding
	3. Encourage adequate fluid intake (at least 8–10 glasses per day)	3. Adequate fluid intake promotes urination and reduces urine stasis, which can lead to infection
	4. Catheterize if other measures fail (physician or CNM order required)	4. Some women cannot void despite measures to help them

Nursing Diagnosis: Impaired tissue integrity related to perineal laceration or episiotomy

Goals	Nursing Interventions	Rationale
The woman will state that discomfort is manageable with nursing measures.	1. Assess perineum using REEDA criteria with each vital sign, fundus, and lochia check. Assess amount of tenderness. Teach woman expected findings and what to report	1. Proper healing is indicated by no separation of the suture line, no discharge, and minimal redness, edema, or ecchymosis. Pain should be minimal and quickly decrease. Short stays after birth mean that the woman must know what is normal and what to report
The woman will demonstrate correct self-care for perineal laceration or episiotomy	2. Teach woman to do perineal care after every voiding or defecation. Observe her technique. a. Fill bottle with warm or cool water b. Squirt the water over the perineum in a front-to-back direction c. Blot perineum dry	2. These techniques cleanse organisms from the vaginal area, reducing the risk that they will cause infection. Use of a front-to-back direction prevents contamination with rectal organisms. Observation is the best way to be certain that the woman correctly understands the teaching
	3. Teach nonpharmacologic comfort measures: a. Ice pack for first 12 to 24 hr b. Warm pack after 24 hr c. Sitz bath (warm or cool water)	3. Cold numbs the area and causes vasoconstriction, which reduces bruising and edema. Heat promotes blood flow to the area to promote healing

Continued on following page

NURSING CARE PLAN 9–1 *(Continued)*

Selected Nursing Diagnoses for the Woman Following Vaginal Birth

Nursing Diagnosis: Impaired tissue integrity related to perineal laceration or episiotomy

Goals	Nursing Interventions	Rationale
	4. Provide and teach use of pharmacologic pain relief: a. Topical measures, such as sprays, foam, or witch-hazel pads b. Analgesics	4. These products numb the area, reduce inflammation, or reduce discomfort from hemorrhoids. Analgesics reduce pain perception
	5. Teach woman to squeeze her buttocks together before sitting, then relax them after she sits. Provide an air-ring (donut) or small eggcrate pad	5. Limits stretching of perineal tissues and softens the impact when sitting
	6. Teach measures to reduce constipation: a. Adequate fluid intake b. High-fiber foods c. Activity d. Use of any prescribed stool softeners or laxatives	6. Constipation increases perineal pain when hard stool is passed. Fluid intake and dietary fiber keep the stool soft, making passage easier. Activity stimulates bowel action. Medications may be necessary to supplement nonpharmacologic methods

tional information about postpartum complications.

Reproductive System

The most dramatic changes after birth are in the woman's reproductive system. Nursing care is discussed for each area, if applicable.

Uterus

Involution refers to changes that the reproductive organs, particularly the uterus, undergo after birth to return them to their prepregnancy size and condition. The uterus undergoes a rapid reduction in size and weight after birth. The uterus should return to the prepregnant size by 5 to 6 weeks.

Uterine Lining. The uterine lining (called the *endometrium* when not pregnant and the *decidua* during pregnancy) is shed when the placenta detaches and in the lochia discharge. A basal layer of the lining remains to generate new endometrium to prepare for future pregnancies. The placental site is fully healed in 6 to 7 weeks (Cunningham, 1997).

Descent of the Uterine Fundus. The uterine fundus descends at a predictable rate as the muscle cells contract to control bleeding at the placental site and the size of each muscle cells decreases (Fig. 9–1). Immediately after the placenta is expelled, the uterine fundus can be felt as a firm mass, about the size of a grapefruit, that is located between the mother's umbilicus and symphysis. Within a few hours the fundus ascends to the level of the umbilicus. After 24 hours, the fundus begins to descend about 1 cm (1 fingerbreadth) each day. By 10 days postpartum, it should not be palpable. Women who have had several infants or whose uterus was overdistended, such as a multifetal pregnancy or a large baby, may have a uterine size that is slightly larger. Their uterus should undergo the same pattern for involution, however, and it should remain firmly contracted. A full bladder interferes with uterine contraction. A full bladder pushes the fundus up and causes it to deviate to one side, usually the right side (Fig. 10–1).

Afterpains. Intermittent uterine contractions may cause the mother to have *afterpains* similar to menstrual cramps. The discomfort is self-limiting and decreases rapidly within 48 hours. Afterpains

Nursing Tip

If the mother's uterus is soft, massage it (supporting the lower segment), then expel clots so it will remain contracted. If her bladder is also full, massage the uterus until firm, then address emptying the bladder. Control bleeding first, then keep it controlled by emptying the bladder.

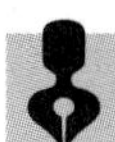

Nursing Tip

The nurse should assess the fundus for descent each shift and teach the mother the expected changes.

NURSING CARE PLAN 9–2

Selected Nursing Diagnoses for the Woman Having a Cesarean Birth

Nursing Diagnosis: Pain related to surgical incision and afterpains

Goals	Nursing Interventions	Rationale
Note: Interventions from Nursing Care Plan 9–1, Selected Nursing Diagnoses for the Woman Following Vaginal Birth, should be incorporated into this care plan as appropriate.		
The woman will state that pain relief is adequate with pharmacologic and nonpharmacologic measures	1. Use a 1 to 10 scale to evaluate pain level before and after interventions	1. Provides a more objective way for the nurse to evaluate the woman's subjective experience of pain. Evaluates adequacy of pain relief
	2. Encourage a woman to change positions regularly, about every 2 hr. Support her body and extremities with pillows	2. Reduces discomfort from constant pressure and having body in one position constantly. Also helps to mobilize respiratory secretions
	3. Teach the woman to use a small pillow pressed to her incision when moving or coughing	3. Supports the incision, reducing pain. Increases the likelihood that she will cough adequately, which expels respiratory secretions
	4. Provide ordered analgesia: a. Patient-controlled anesthesia pump b. Intermittent injections c. Oral analgesia	4. Reduce the perception of pain, which facilitates moving, coughing, and ambulating. Reduces anxiety and fatigue. Promotes mother–infant attachment and breastfeeding

Nursing Diagnosis: Impaired skin integrity related to abdominal incision

Goals	Nursing Interventions	Rationale
The woman will have no excessive redness or tenderness and no separation or discharge from incision. The woman will demonstate knowledge of self-care measures related to her incision by discharge	1. Observe dressing for drainage with each assessment	1. Red drainage indicates bleeding, which should not increase. Foul-odored drainage indicates infection
	2. When dressing is removed, assess incision using REEDA criteria. Assess amount of tenderness	2. Identifies proper healing of incision. A separating suture line, excessive redness or tenderness, or discharge indicates probable infection
	3. Assess temperature every 4 hr	3. A temperature higher than 38°C (100.4°F) after 24 hr is associated with infection
	4. Teach woman self-care measures a. Expected progress of healing and how the incision should look b. How to bathe (plastic over incision, if ordered) c. What to report (signs of bleeding or infection) d. When her staples or sutures should be removed if not done before discharge e. Follow-up appointment	4. Women must assume their own care because of short hospital stays. These guidelines give the woman a framework to know what is normal and what is not and how to care for herself to prevent infection. Follow-up appointments allow her physician to assess how healing is progressing and to identify complications early

occur more often in multiparas or women whose uterus was overdistended. Breastfeeding mothers may have more afterpains because infant suckling causes their posterior pituitary to release oxytocin, a hormone that contracts the uterus.

Lochia. Vaginal discharge after delivery is called *lochia*. It is composed of endometrial tissue, blood, and lymph. Lochia gradually changes characteristics during the early postpartum period:

- *Lochia rubra* is red because it is composed mostly of blood; it lasts for about 3 days after birth.
- *Lochia serosa* is pinkish because of its blood and mucus content. It lasts from about the 3rd through the 10th day after birth.
- *Lochia alba* is mostly mucus and is clear and colorless or white. It lasts from the 10th through the 14th day after birth, although a longer duration of lochia alba discharge is common.

Lochia has a characteristic fleshy or menstrual odor, but should not have a foul odor.

The nurse assesses lochia for quantity, type, and characteristics. A guideline to estimate and chart the amount of flow on the menstrual pad in 1 hour is as follows:

- Scant: Less than a 1-inch (2.5-cm) stain
- Light: Less than a 4-inch (10-cm) stain
- Moderate: Less than a 6-inch (15-cm) stain
- Large or heavy: Larger than a 6-inch stain or one pad saturated within 2 hours
- Excessive: Saturation of a perineal pad within 15 minutes

Many facilities use perineal pads that have cold or warm packs in them. These pads absorb less lochia, so that fact must be considered when estimating the amount. If a mother has excessive lochia, apply a clean pad and check it within 15 minutes. Count the number of peripads applied during a given time period or weigh them to help determine the amount of vaginal discharge. One gram of weight equals about 1 ml of blood. Check her fundus for firmness because an uncontracted

BOX 9–1

SUMMARY OF NURSING ASSESSMENTS OF THE POSTPARTUM WOMAN

After transfer to routine postpartum care, assessments are usually done every 4 to 8 hours unless high-risk factors exist or an abnormality is identified.

General appearance. Observe patient from head to toe (color and warmth of skin, respiratory status, fatigue); assess the responsiveness of patient (level of consciousness or sensation in lower extremities); question about dizziness.

Pulse, respirations, and blood pressure. Assess vital signs according to facility protocol during 4th stage, typically every 15 minutes for 1 hour, every 30 minutes for 1 hour, and hourly until released to routine postpartum care. Assess every 4 to 8 hours thereafter.

Temperature. Assess at beginning of 4th stage, then hourly until released to routine postpartum care. Assess every 4 to 8 hours thereafter. Report a temperature of 38°C (100.4°F) or higher, especially after the first 24 hours.

Fundus. Evaluate the consistency, location, and height of the fundus.

Lochia. Determine the character, color, and amount of lochia, including odor and presence of clots.

Perineum. Observe perineum for edema, bruising, or hematoma.

Episiotomy or perineal laceration. Observe episiotomy site for redness, edema, ecchymosis, discharge, edges well approximated (REEDA); assess degree of tenderness.

Hemorrhoids. Note presence, size, and degree of discomfort.

Bladder. Assess for deviation of uterine fundus; assess quantity of first 2 to 3 voidings; question about unusual frequency, pain, burning on urination.

Cesarean or tubal ligation incision. Assess dressing for drainage. When dressing is removed, assess incision using REEDA criteria.

Breasts. Assess the general appearance, pain, engorgement, nipple condition for tenderness or trauma, onset of lactation. Identify conditions such as flat or inverted nipples or breast engorgement that may interfere with breastfeeding. Assess the mother's perception of how breastfeeding is proceeding.

Extremities. Assess for signs of thrombophlebitis: redness or pallor, pain, tenderness, pain when walking. A positive Homan's sign is not always valuable in the postpartum period.

Pain. Assess location, character, and severity of pain. Determine adequacy of pain relief measures (cold or warm packs, analgesia, use of a donut, splinting an abdominal incision).

Bowels. Determine last defecation. Assess for passage of flatus, bowel sounds, and abdominal distention on a woman who has a cesarean birth.

Hydration. Assess intake and output. For the woman with a vaginal birth, the approximate number of glasses of fluid taken and number of voidings suffices. For the woman with a cesarean birth or other complications, tally the intake (oral and intravenous) and output (urine).

Emotional state. Evaluate for presence of weepiness, depression; evaluate family support and interaction with family members.

Attachment. Observe for attachment behaviors (interest in the newborn; attention to the baby's signals; eye contact; touch and holding). Observe for behaviors that suggest poor attachment (indifference to the newborn; nonresponsiveness to infant signals; limited eye contact; little holding or touching).

Cultural variations. Assess for important cultural beliefs and identify how the staff can incorporate them into care.

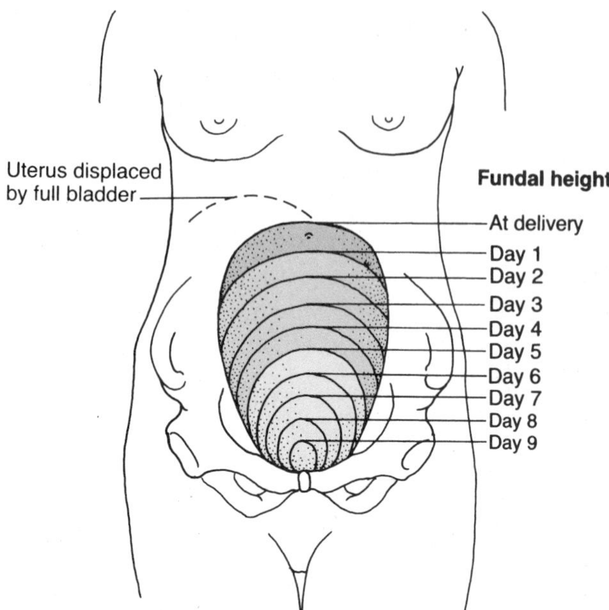

Figure 9–1. • Changes in the height of the uterine fundus each day as involution progresses.

uterus allows blood to flow freely from vessels at the placenta site.

Lochia is briefly heavier when the mother ambulates as lochia pooled in her vagina is discharged when she assumes an upright position. A few small clots may be seen at this time, but large clots should not be present. Lochia may briefly increase when the mother breastfeeds because suckling causes uterine contraction. Lochia increases with exercise. Women who had a cesarean birth have less lochia during the first 24 hours because the uterine cavity was sponged at delivery. Absence of lochia is not normal and may be associated with blood clots retained within the uterus or with infection.

Nursing Care. Assess the fundus for firmness, location, and position in relation to the midline (see procedure for assessing and massaging the uterine fundus and for giving perineal care) at routine intervals. Women who have a higher risk for postpartum hemorrhage (see Chapter 10) should be assessed more often. While doing early assessments, explain the reason they are done and teach the woman how to assess her fundus. If her uterus stops descending she should report that to her birth attendant.

A poorly contracted (soft, or boggy) uterus should be massaged until firm to prevent hemorrhage (Fig. 9–2). Lochia may increase briefly as the uterus contracts and expels it. It is essential *not* to push down on an uncontracted uterus to avoid inverting it (see p. 210). If a full bladder contributes to poor uterine contraction, assist the mother to void in the bathroom or on a bedpan if she cannot ambulate. Catheterization may be necessary if she cannot void.

Medications that may be given to stimulate uterine contraction include:

- Oxytocin (Pitocin), often routinely given in an intravenous infusion after birth
- Methylergonovine (Methergine), given IM or PO.

Infant suckling at the breast has a similar effect because natural oxytocin release stimulates contractions.

Procedure for Assessing and Massaging the Uterine Fundus and for Giving Perineal Care

Materials

Unsterile gloves
Peri bottle filled with warm water
Perineal pad

Method

1. Identify the need for fundal massage. The uterus will be soft and usually higher than the umbilicus. A firm fundus does not need massage.
2. Place the woman in a supine position with the knees slightly flexed. Lower the perineal pad to observe lochia as the fundus is palpated.
3. Place the outer edge of nondominant hand just above the symphysis pubis, and press downward slightly to anchor the lower uterus.
4. Locate and massage the uterine fundus with the flat portion of the fingers of the dominant hand in a firm circular motion.
5. When the uterus is firm, gently push downward on the fundus, toward the vaginal outlet, to expel blood and clots that have accumulated inside the uterus. *Keep the other hand on the lower uterus to avoid inverting it.*
6. If a full bladder contributes to uterine relaxation, have the mother void. Catheterize her (with a doctor's order) if she cannot void.
7. Document the consistency and location of the fundus before and after massage.
8. Give any medications, such as oxytocin, to maintain uterine contraction. Have the mother nurse her baby if she is breastfeeding to stimulate the secretion of natural oxytocin.
9. Report a fundus that does not stay firm.

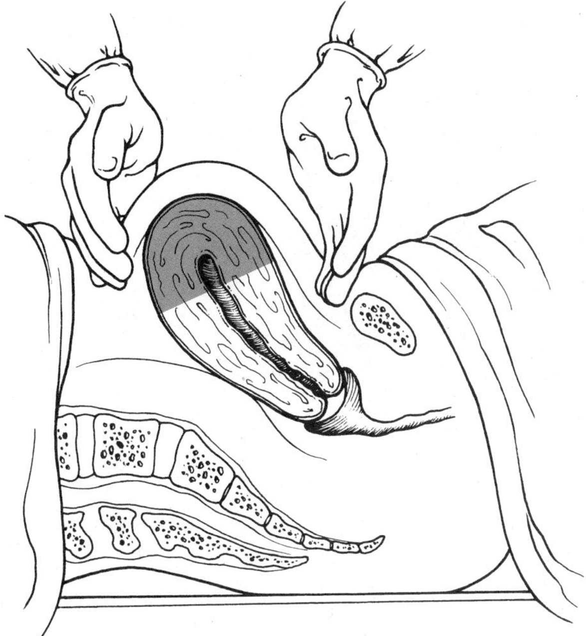

Figure 9–2. • When assessing or massaging the fundus, the nurse keeps one hand firmly on the lower uterus, just above the symphysis pubis. The uterus is massaged in a firm, circular motion. After the uterus becomes firm, the nurse pushes toward the vagina to expel accumulated blood. A firm fundus does not need massage.

Mild analgesics relieve afterpains adequately for most women. The breastfeeding mother will get maximum pain relief if she takes an analgesic 30 minutes before she expects to nurse. Some women find that lying prone with a small pillow against their lower abdomen reduces afterpains. Afterpains persisting longer than the expected time should be reported.

Teach the woman the expected sequence for lochia changes and the amount she should expect. The woman should report any of the following abnormal characteristics:

- Foul-smelling lochia, with or without fever
- Lochia rubra that persists beyond the third day
- Unusually heavy lochia
- Lochia that returns to a bright red color after it has progressed to serosa or alba

Cervix

The cervix regains its muscle tone but never closes as tightly as during the prepregnant state. Some edema persists for a few weeks after delivery. A constant trickle of brighter red lochia is associated with bleeding from lacerations of the cervix or vagina, particularly if the fundus remains firm.

Vagina

The vagina undergoes a great deal of stretching during childbirth. The *rugae,* or vaginal folds, disappear, and the walls of the vagina become smooth and spacious. The rugae reappear 3 weeks postpartum. Within 6 weeks the vagina has regained most of its prepregnancy form, but it never returns to the size it was before pregnancy. Breastfeeding mothers may experience vaginal dryness and discomfort during intercourse. A water-soluble vaginal lubricant such as KY jelly, Lubrin, or Replens makes intercourse more comfortable.

Perineum

The perineum is often edematous, tender, and bruised. An *episiotomy* (incision to enlarge the vaginal opening) may have been done or a perineal laceration may have occurred. Women with hemorrhoids often find that these have temporarily worsened during the pressure of birth.

Perineal lacerations and often episiotomies are described by the amount of tissue involved:

- *First degree.* Involves the superficial vaginal mucosa or perineal skin
- *Second degree.* Involves the vaginal mucosa, perineal skin, and deeper tissues of the perineum
- *Third degree.* Same as second degree, plus involves the anal sphincter
- *Fourth degree.* Extends through the anal sphincter into the rectal mucosa

Some women have a *periurethral laceration* near their urethra. They may require an indwelling catheter for a day or two.

The perineum should be assessed for normal healing and signs of complications. The REEDA acronym helps the nurse remember the five signs to assess:

- ***R**edness.* Redness without excessive tenderness is probably the normal inflammation associated with healing, but pain with the redness is more likely to be infection.
- ***E**dema.* Mild edema is common, but severe edema interferes with healing.
- ***E**cchymosis* (bruising). A few small superficial bruises are common. Larger bruises interfere with normal healing.

- *Discharge.* No discharge from the perineal suture line should be present.
- *Approximation* (intactness of the suture line). The suture line should not be separated. If intact, it is almost impossible to distinguish the laceration or episiotomy from surrounding skin folds.

The REEDA acronym is also useful when assessing a cesarean incision for healing.

Nursing Care. Comfort and hygienic measures are the focus of nursing care and client teaching. Apply an ice pack or chemical cold pack for the first 12 to 24 hours to reduce edema and bruising and numb the perineal area. A disposable rubber glove filled with ice chips and taped at the wrist can also be used. The cold pack should be covered with a paper cover or a washcloth. When the ice melts, leave the cold pack off for 10 minutes before applying another for maximum effect. Asian women who believe that heat has healing properties may resist the use of an ice pack (Schneiderman, 1996).

After 24 hours, heat in the form of a chemical warm pack or a sitz bath increases circulation and promotes healing. The sitz bath (Fig. 9–3) may circulate either cool or warm water over the perineum to cleanse the area and to increase comfort. Sitting in 4 to 5 inches of water in a bathtub has a similar effect.

Teach the woman to do perineal care after each voiding or bowel movement to cleanse the area without trauma. A plastic bottle is filled with warm water and the water is squirted over the perineum in a front-to-back direction. The perineum is blotted dry. Perineal pads should be applied and removed in the same front-to-back direction to prevent fecal contamination of the perineum and vagina.

Topical and systemic medications may be used to relieve perineal pain. Topical perineal medications reduce inflammation or numb the perineum. Commonly prescribed ones include:

- Hydrocortisone and pramoxine (Epifoam)
- Benzocaine (Americaine or Dermoplast)

In addition to these topical medications, witch hazel pads (Tucks) and sitz baths reduce the discomfort of hemorrhoids. Commonly prescribed oral analgesics for postpartum pain, including perineal pain, are listed in Table 9–1.

To reduce pain when sitting, have the mother squeeze her buttocks together as she lowers herself to a sitting position, then relax her buttocks. An air ring, or "donut," takes pressure off the perineal area when sitting. Have the mother inflate the ring about halfway. If it is inflated fully, she tends to topple off when she sits on it. A small eggcrate pad is an alternative to the air ring.

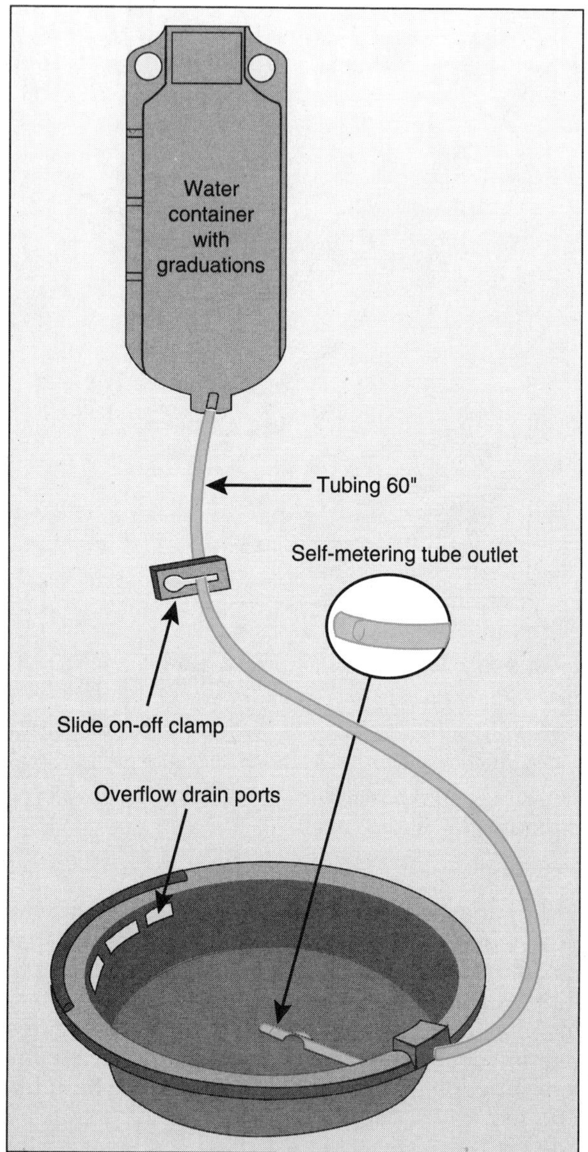

Figure 9–3. • The sitz bath is a plastic basin for individual use that fits on the toilet seat. Cool or warm swirling water cleanses and promotes healing of the perineum. (Courtesy of Baxter Health Care Corporation, McGaw Park, IL. Redrawn with permission.)

Return of Ovulation and Menstruation. The production of placental estrogen and progesterone stops when the placenta is delivered, causing a rise in the production of follicle-stimulating hormone and the return of ovulation and menstruation. Menstrual cycles resume in about 6 to 8 weeks if the woman is not breastfeeding. Nursing mothers show a wide variation in return of menses, from 2 to 18 months. The early menstrual periods may or may not be preceded by ovulation. Return of ovulation is delayed longer in the breastfeeding mother. However, *ovulation may occur at any time after birth, with or without menstrual bleeding, and pregnancy is possible.*

Breasts

Both nursing and nonnursing mothers will experience breast changes after birth. Assessments for each mother are similar, but nursing care differs.

Changes in the Breasts. For the first 2 or 3 days, the breasts are full, but soft. By the 3rd day, the breasts become firm and lumpy as blood flow increases and milk production begins. Breast engorgement may occur in both nursing and nonnursing mothers. The engorged breast is hard, erect, and very uncomfortable. The nipple may be so hard that the infant cannot easily grasp it. The breasts of the nonnursing mother return to their normal size in 1 to 2 weeks.

Nursing Care. Nursing care related to breastfeeding techniques is presented later in this chapter. At each assessment, the nurse checks the woman's breasts for consistency, size, shape, and symmetry. The nipples are inspected for redness and cracking, which makes breastfeeding more painful and is a port for entry of microorganisms. Flat or inverted nipples make it more difficult for the infant to grasp the nipple and suckle.

Both nursing and nonnursing mothers should

Table 9–1
COMMONLY USED DRUGS DURING THE POSTPARTUM PERIOD

Indications	Usual Dosage	Nursing Considerations
Methylergonovine maleate (Methergine)		
Prevention and treatment of hemorrhage due to uterine atony	0.2 mg IM or PO q 6–12 hr	Monitor and record blood pressure, pulse rate, and uterine response; report any sudden change in vital signs, continued uterine relaxation, or excessive lochia
Oxytocin (Pitocin, Syntocinon)		
Reduction of bleeding after expulsion of the placenta	10–40 units in 1000 ml of 5% dextrose in normal saline solution IV at a rate to control bleeding (usually 20 to 40 mU/minute), or 10 units IM	Administer by infusion, not by bolus (a concentrated mass); monitor and record uterine contraction, heart rate, and blood pressure every 15 min; assess and record amount of lochia
Simethecone (Mylicon)		
Flatulence, abdominal distention	Chewable tablets 40–80 mg after each meal and at bedtime	Assess for bowel activity, relief of distention
Ibuprofen (Motrin, Advil)		
Mild to moderate pain	400 mg PO q 4–6 hr	Assess for nausea, vomiting, diarrhea
Acetaminophen (Tylenol, Panadol)		
Mild to moderate pain	325–650 mg PO q 4–6 hr	Side effects rare; assess for allergic reaction, such as skin rash
Percocet (325 mg acetaminophen and 5 mg oxycodone)		
Moderate pain	1–2 tablets PO q 4 hr	Determine sensitivity to acetaminophen or oxycodone; observe for signs of respiratory depression; do not administer with sedatives
Empirin No. 3 (325 mg of aspirin with 30 mg codeine)		
Moderate pain	1–2 tablets q 4 hr	Assess for sensitivity to aspirin or codeine; administer with food to prevent gastric upset
Rh_0 (D) Immune Globulin (RhoGAM, Gamulin Rh, HypRho-D)		
Prevention of sensitization to Rh factor in Rh-negative mothers who gave birth to Rh-positive infants	One vial IM within 72 hr following childbirth	Confirm that administration is necessary; check with second licensed personnel that medication is cross-matched for the specific woman
Rubella virus vaccine, live (Meruvax II)		
To stimulate active immunity against rubella virus	Single-dose vial; administer SC in outer aspect of upper arm	Advise the mother to avoid pregnancy for 3 months; signed informed consent usually required; do not administer if mother is sensitive to neomycin or if she has had a transfusion within the last 3 months

Abbreviations: q, every; PO, orally (per os); IM, intramuscularly; IV, intravenously; mU, milliunit; SC, subcutaneously.
From Gorrie, T. M., McKinney, E. S., & Murray, S. S. (1998). *Foundations of maternal-newborn nursing*, 2nd ed. Philadelphia: Saunders.

wear a bra to support the heavier breasts. The bra should firmly support the nursing mother's breasts but not be so tight that it impedes circulation. The nonnursing mother may also wear an elastic binder to suppress lactation. This binder may be one made specifically for lactation suppression or simply a 6-inch elastic bandage wrapped over the breasts.

The nonnursing mother should avoid stimulating her nipples, which would stimulate lactation. She should wear a bra at all times to avoid having her clothing brush back and forth over her breasts and should stand facing away from the water spray in the shower.

The nipples should be washed with plain water to avoid the drying effects of soap, which can lead to cracking. The nonnursing woman should minimize stimulation when washing her breasts.

Cardiovascular System

Cardiac Output and Blood Volume

Because of a 50% increase in blood volume during pregnancy, the woman tolerates normal blood loss at delivery:

- 500 ml in vaginal birth
- 1000 ml in cesarean birth.

Despite the blood loss, there is a temporary increase in blood volume and cardiac output because blood that was contained in the uterus and in the placenta returns to the main circulation. Added fluid also moves from the tissues into the circulation, further adding to her blood volume. The heart pumps more blood with each contraction (increased stroke volume), leading to bradycardia. After the initial post-birth excitement wanes, the pulse rate may be as low as 50 to 60 beats per minute for about 48 hours after birth.

To reestablish normal fluid balance, the body rids itself of excess fluid in two ways:

- Diuresis (increased excretion of urine), which may reach 3000 ml per day
- Diaphoresis (profuse perspiration)

Coagulation

Blood clotting factors are higher during pregnancy and the puerperium, yet the woman's ability to lyse (break down and eliminate) clots is not increased. Therefore she is prone to blood clot formation, especially if there is stasis of blood in the venous system. This situation is more likely to occur if the woman has varicose veins, a cesarean birth, or must delay ambulation.

Blood Values

The massive fluid shifts just described affect blood values such as hemoglobin and hematocrit, making them difficult to interpret during the early puerperium. Fluid that shifts into the blood stream dilutes the blood cells, causing the hematocrit count to be lower. As the fluid balance returns to normal, the values are more accurately interpreted.

White blood cells (leukocytes) may increase as high as 20,000 to 30,000/mm^3, a level that would ordinarily suggest infection. The increase is in response to inflammation, pain, and stress, and it protects the mother from infection as her tissues heal.

Chills

Many mothers have a chill immediately after birth. They may visibly shake and tremble uncontrollably. Postpartum chills usually decrease within 20 minutes. They are believed to be caused by a nervous response or vasomotor changes in the body. Chills accompanied by fever after the first 24 hours suggest infection.

Orthostatic Hypotension

After the baby's birth, resistance to blood flow in the vessels of the pelvis drops. As a result, the woman's blood pressure falls when she sits or stands, and she may feel dizzy, lightheaded, or even faint.

Nursing Care

After the fourth stage vital signs are taken every 4 hours for the first 24 hours. The temperature, pulse, respirations, and blood pressure help the nurse to identify if assessments are normal. The temperature may rise to 38°C (100.4°F) in the first 24 hours. A higher temperature, or persistence of the elevation later than 24 hours suggests infection.

The pulse rate helps to interpret temperature and blood pressure values. Because of the normal postpartum bradycardia, expand assessments if the pulse rate during the first two days is in the upper range of normal. A high pulse rate often accompanies infection or hypovolemia, usually due to blood loss. The respiratory rate is usually higher as well.

If diaphoresis bothers the woman, remind her that it is temporary. Help her shower or take a sponge bath and provide dry clothes and bedding.

Nursing Tip

The woman who voids frequent, small amounts of urine may have residual urine because her bladder does not fully empty. Residual urine in the bladder may cause hemorrhage from bladder distention and promotes growth of microorganisms.

Check for the presence of edema in the lower extremities, the hands, and the face. Edema in the lower extremities is common, as it is during pregnancy. Edema above the waist is more likely to be associated with pregnancy-induced hypertension, which sometimes first becomes evident during the early postpartum period.

The woman's legs should be checked for evidence of thrombosis at each assessment: a reddened, tender area (superficial vein) or edema, pain, and sometimes pallor (deep vein). Homan's sign (calf pain when the foot is dorsiflexed) is of limited value in identifying thrombosis (Cunningham, 1997).

Early and regular ambulation reduces venous stasis that promotes blood clots. If she cannot ambulate, have her do leg exercises in bed to increase blood flow. TED hose are often ordered for women who have a higher risk for thrombosis.

A warm blanket and drink help to make the chilled woman more comfortable. A portable radiant warmer placed over the woman and her baby warms both while promoting bonding. Reassure the woman that the chill will subside within a few minutes.

To prevent injury from orthostatic hypotension, assist the woman when she is ambulating until she is steady on her feet. Have her sit on the side of the bed and move her legs back and forth before rising to a standing position and ambulating. If she becomes pale, dizzy, or faint, help her to lie down where she is, even if it is on the floor.

Urinary System

Intravenous fluids given in labor and birth plus diuresis cause the woman's bladder to fill quickly. However, decreased bladder muscle tone, trauma to the area during birth, and the effects of some anesthetics may reduce her sensation to urinate. Failure to empty her bladder can lead to postpartum hemorrhage or urinary tract infection.

Nursing Care

Regularly assess the woman's bladder for distention. The bladder may not feel full to her, yet the uterus is high and deviated to one side. If she can ambulate, have her go to the bathroom and urinate. Measure the first 2 to 3 voidings after birth or after a catheter is removed. Women who receive intravenous infusions or have an indwelling catheter continue to have their urine output measured until the infusion and/or catheter are discontinued.

The following measures may help a woman to urinate:

- Provide as much privacy as possible.
- Remain near the woman, but do not rush her by constantly asking her if she has urinated.
- Run water in the sink.
- Have the woman place her hands in warm water.
- Have the woman use the peri bottle to squirt warm water over her perineal area to relax the urethral sphincter. Be sure to measure the amount of water in the peri bottle when it is filled so the amount used can be deducted from the amount of urine voided.

Catheterization may be necessary if other measures fail. Because the perineum may be swollen, it is often difficult to visualize the urinary meatus. Care must be taken not to invade the vagina to avoid introducing more organisms into the uterus.

Some discomfort with early urination is expected because of the edema and trauma in the area. However, continued burning or urgency of urination suggest bladder infection. High fever and chills may occur with kidney infection.

Gastrointestinal System

The gastrointestinal system resumes normal activity shortly after birth. The mother is usually hungry after the hard work and food deprivation of labor. Many women are more thirsty than hungry at first because of the work of labor, breathing techniques that emphasize mouth breathing, diaphoresis, and minimal oral fluid intake. Their appetite quickly returns. Expect to feed and water a new mother often!

Constipation may occur during the postpartum period for the following reasons:

- The relaxing effects of progesterone from the placenta persist for a short while after birth.
- Medications may slow peristalsis.
- Abdominal muscles are stretched, making it more

difficult for the woman to bear down to expel stool. A cesarean incision adds to this difficulty.

- Soreness and swelling of the perineum or hemorrhoids may make the woman fear her first bowel movement.
- Slight dehydration and little food intake during labor make the feces harder.

Encourage the mother to drink lots of fluids, to add fiber to her diet, and to ambulate. A stool softener is usually ordered. These measures are generally sufficient to correct the problem. Because constipation is a common problem during pregnancy, discuss any measures she used to relieve it at that time and build on her knowledge.

The mother who has a cesarean birth usually has intravenous fluids for about the first 24 hours. The nurse should check for bowel sounds and for presence of distention at each assessment. Bowel sounds usually return within 24 hours after birth. The woman is given ice chips at first, progressing to clear liquids and then to a soft diet as her bowel activity returns. She will need adequate oral fluids and ambulation just as the woman who gives birth vaginally to prevent constipation. Foods with dietary fiber should be encouraged as soon as she is on a diet that allows them.

Medications are often ordered to relieve flatus, soften the stool, or as a laxative. Simethecone (Mylicon), 40 to 80 mg after each meal and at bedtime, decreases flatulence and abdominal distention. Stool softeners such as docusate calcium (Surfak) or docusate sodium (Colace) make the stool easier to pass. A common laxative is bisacodyl (Dulcolax), given orally or as a suppository.

Integumentary System

Hyperpigmentation of the skin ("mask of pregnancy," or chloasma, and the linea nigra) disappear as hormone levels decrease. Striae ("stretch marks") do not disappear, but fade from reddish-purple to silver.

Musculoskeletal System

The abdominal wall has been greatly stretched during pregnancy. It may now have a "doughy" appearance. Many women are dismayed to discover that they still look pregnant after they give birth. Reassure them that time and exercise can tighten their lax muscles. It often helps to remind them that it took 9 months to stretch the muscles and that they will not instantly return to their taut state. Also, some women have *diastasis recti*, in which the longitudinal abdominal muscles that extend from the chest to the symphysis pubis are separated. Abdominal wall weakness may remain for 6 to 8 weeks and may contribute to constipation.

A woman can usually begin light exercises as soon as the first day after vaginal birth. Women having a cesarean birth must wait longer. The woman should consult her health care provider for specific instructions about exercise. Common postpartum exercises include the following:

- *Abdominal tightening.* While in the supine or erect position the woman inhales slowly and then exhales slowly while contracting her abdominal muscles. After a count of 10, she relaxes the muscles. She should begin with three repetitions, and increase the number to five, then ten. This may be done three times and then five times daily, up to 10 times each day.
- *Head lift.* The woman lies flat on her bed with her knees bent and inhales. While exhaling, she lifts her head, chin to chest, and looks at her thighs. She holds this position to a count of three, then relaxes. This is repeated several times. After the 3rd week, or when the physician permits, the head lift may progress to include the head and shoulders. This may be done five to 10 times daily.
- *Pelvic tilt.* While lying supine with her knees bent and feet flat, the woman inhales and exhales, flattening her lower back to the bed or exercise surface and contracting her abdominal muscles. She holds the position to a count of three. She begins with five repetitions and works up to 10 repetitions daily.
- *Kegel exercises.* Perineal exercises may be resumed immediately after birth to promote circulation and healing. The mother tightens the muscles of the perineal area, as if to stop the flow of urine, and then relaxes them. She should inhale, tighten for a count of 10, exhale, and relax. She may do the exercise five times each hour for the first few days. Then she may increase the number of repetitions. She should not actually stop her urine flow when urinating, however, because this could lead to urine stasis and urinary tract infection.

Immune System

Prevention of blood incompatibility and of infection are done in the postpartum period according to each woman's specific needs.

Rh Immune Globulin

The woman's blood type and Rh factor and antibody status are determined on an early prenatal visit or on admission if she did not have prenatal care. The Rh-negative woman has antibody titers repeated at intervals during pregnancy. She will receive Rh immune globulin (RhoGAM) at 28 weeks if she is not sensitized to the Rh factor. The newborn of a woman who had RhoGAM during pregnancy often has a positive Coombs test at birth. See p. 364 for further discussion of the Rh factor during pregnancy.

Within 72 hours after the birth of an Rh-positive baby, the Rh-negative mother should receive another dose of Rh immune globulin to prevent sensitization to Rh-positive erythrocytes that may have entered her bloodstream when the infant was born. The drug is crossmatched to the woman and a second licensed person confirms identification and need for administration. *RhoGAM is given to the mother, not the infant* by intramuscular injection into the deltoid muscle. The woman receives an identification card stating that she is Rh-negative and has received RhoGAM on that date.

Rubella (German Measles) Immunization

Rubella titers are done early in pregnancy to determine if a woman is immune to rubella. A titer of 1:8 or greater indicates immunity to the rubella virus. The mother who is not immune is given the vaccine in the immediate postpartum period. The vaccine prevents infection with the rubella virus during subsequent pregnancies, which could cause birth defects. A signed informed consent is usually required to administer the rubella vaccine.

The rubella vaccine is given subcutaneously in the upper arm. The woman may experience mild symptoms of rubella, such as rash, malaise, sore throat, headache, joint pain, and slight fever. The woman should not get pregnant for the next 3 months. Do not administer the vaccine if she is sensitive to Neomycin or if she has had a transfusion within the last 3 months.

Changes after Cesarean Birth

The woman who has a cesarean birth has had surgery as well as given birth. Many of her reactions to the surgical birth depend on whether she expected it. The woman who had an unexpected emergency cesarean will often have many questions about what happened to her and why because there was no time to answer these questions at the time of birth. Also, her anxiety may have limited her ability to comprehend any explanations given. Occasionally a woman may feel that she failed if she was unable to give birth after laboring. Terms such as *failed induction* and *failure to progress* imply that the woman herself was not competent in some way.

Adapting Nursing Care after Cesarean Birth

Some variations of normal postpartum care are needed for the woman who has a cesarean birth.

Uterus. The nurse should check the woman's fundus as on any new mother; it descends at a similar rate. Checking her fundus when she has a transverse skin incision is not much different from checking the woman having vaginal birth. If she has a vertical skin incision, gently "walk" the fingers toward the fundus from the side of her abdominal midline. If the fundus is firm and at its expected level, no massage is necessary. The abdominal dressing is usually light enough to feel the fundus.

Lochia. Lochia is checked at routine assessment intervals, which vary with the time since birth. The quantity of lochia is generally less after cesarean birth.

Dressing. The dressing should be checked for drainage as in any surgical client. When the dressing is removed, the incision is assessed for signs of infection. The wound should be clean and dry and the staples should be intact. The REEDA acronym, previously described, is a good way to remember key items to check on an incision: *r*edness, *e*dema, *e*cchymosis, *d*rainage, *a*pproximation. Staples are usually removed shortly before hospital discharge on the 3rd day. If a woman leaves earlier, the staples may be removed in her physician's office.

The woman can shower as soon as she can ambulate reliably. A shower chair reduces the risk for fainting. The dressing or incision can be covered with a plastic bag, securing the edges with tape. Tell the woman to position herself with her back to the water stream. Change a wet dressing after the woman finishes her bath. A similar technique can be used to cover an intravenous infusion site. A glove can cover the infusion site if it is in her hand.

Urinary Catheter. An indwelling urinary catheter is generally removed within 24 hours. Urine is observed for blood, which may indicate trauma to the bladder during labor or surgery. The blood should quickly clear from the urine as diuresis occurs. Intake and output are measured until both the intravenous infusion and catheter are discontinued. Measure the first 2 to 3 voidings, or until the woman urinates at least 150 ml. Observe and teach the woman to observe for signs of urinary tract infection because the catheter's use increases this risk:

- Fever (low in a bladder infection; high in a kidney infection)
- Burning pain on urination
- Urgency of urination

Frequency of urination is hard to assess in any postpartum client because of normal diuresis. However, frequent voidings of small quantities of urine, especially if associated with the described signs and symptoms, suggest a urinary tract infection in any postpartum client.

Respiratory Care. Lung sounds should be assessed each shift for clarity. Diminished breath sounds, crackles, or wheezes indicate that lung secretions are being retained. When she is confined to bed, have the woman take deep breaths and turn from side to side every 2 hours. Encourage her to cough to move secretions out of her lungs. To reduce incisional pain from coughing or other movement, have her hold a small pillow or folded blanket firmly against her incision. An incentive spirometer may be used to give the woman a "target" for deep breaths. Ambulate the woman as early as possible to mobilize lung secretions.

Preventing Thrombophlebitis. The cesarean birth mother has a greater risk for thrombophlebitis. Have her do simple leg exercises such as alternately flexing and extending her feet or moving her legs from a flexed to an extended position when turning her. Assess for signs of thrombosis as previously described. Early and frequent ambulation also reduces the risk for thrombophlebitis.

Pain Management. Pain control is essential to reduce the woman's distress and facilitate movement that can prevent several complications. Assess the severity, frequency, character, and location of discomfort. Using a 1-to-10 scale helps to quantify the subjective experience of pain better. One would be no pain at all, and 10 would be the worst pain ever. The scale helps the nurse to choose the most appropriate relief methods and provides a method to evaluate the amount of relief the woman receives from the pain interventions.

Some women receive epidural narcotics for long-lasting pain relief. These drugs can cause respiratory depression many hours after they are given, sometimes up to 24 hours. Therefore, hourly respiratory monitoring and a pulse oximeter are usual until the drug's effects have worn off. Naloxone (Narcan) should be readily available to reverse the respiratory depression. If the woman has pain that is not controlled by the epidural narcotic, the anesthesia clinician must be consulted for specific orders.

Many women have a patient-controlled analgesia (PCA) pump to provide them with analgesia. The pump has a syringe of a narcotic analgesic inside. It is programmed to deliver a specific dose of the drug when the woman pushes a button. To prevent overdose, there is a lockout interval, in which pushing the button will have no effect. The drug inside is counted at shift change as any narcotic is, and the facility's protocol for record-keeping is followed to account for all doses of the drug that the woman receives, those remaining, and those wasted when the PCA drug is discontinued.

Most women change to one of the oral analgesics on the day after surgery. Instruct the woman to call for pain medication when she first becomes uncomfortable. Pain is much harder to relieve if it becomes severe.

Reassure the breastfeeding mother that the short-term use of postpartum analgesia does not have harmful effects on her baby. Explain that adequate pain control helps her to relax so she can breastfeed better and have the energy to become acquainted with her baby.

Emotional Care

The birth of a baby brings about physical changes in the mother, but also causes many emotional and relationship changes in all family members.

Mothers. The transition to motherhood brings many hormonal changes, changes in body image, and intrapsychic reorganization. Rubin has described three phases of postpartum change that have been a framework for nursing care for 35 years (Box 9–2). More recent studies have found that women progress through the same three phases, although at a more rapid pace than originally described. The nurse can refer to the three phases when providing postpartum care.

New mothers often experience conflicting feelings of joy and emotional letdown during the first few weeks after birth, often called the *postpartum blues,* or baby blues. The mother experiences periods of weepiness, mood instability, and anxiety. She is often confused about her distress and may not be able to tell anyone why she is upset. She may feel let down, but overall she finds pleasure in life. The cause is unknown, but is thought to relate to the wide hormonal swings she experiences after birth. The symptoms are self-limiting. When providing discharge teaching, the nurse should prepare the woman for these feelings and reassure her that they are normal and temporary.

Postpartum depression is a persistent mood of unhappiness and is discussed on page 271. When teaching about the postpartum blues, explain that

BOX 9–2
RUBIN'S PSYCHOLOGICAL CHANGES OF THE PUERPERIUM

Phase 1: Taking in. Mother is passive and willing to let others do for her. Conversation centers on her birth experience. Great interest in her baby, but willing to let others handle the care; little interest in learning. Primary focus is on recovery from birth and her need for food, fluids, and deep restorative sleep.

Phase 2: Taking hold. Mother begins to initiate action and becomes interested in caring for baby. Becomes critical of her "performance." Increased concern about her body's functions; assumes responsibility for self-care needs. This phase is ideal for teaching.

Phase 3: Letting go. Mothers, and often fathers, work through giving up their previous lifestyle and family arrangements to incorporate the new infant. Many mothers must give up their ideal of their birth experience and reconcile it with what really occurred. They give up the fantasy child so they can accept the real child.

persistent depression is *not* expected and should be reported to her health care provider.

Fathers. New fathers typically display intense interest in their new baby *(engrossment).* Their behaviors with their infant parallel those of the new mother. A man's relationship with his own parents, previous experiences with children, and his relationship to the mother are also important influences on how he will relate to his new baby.

Include fathers when giving instructions about infant care and handling (Fig. 9–4). Many men feel that their only role in childbearing and childrearing is to support the mother. The nurse must be tactful and supportive of a new father who is trying to assume his role as a full parent.

Siblings. The influence of a new baby's birth on siblings depends on their age and developmental level. Toddlers may respond by regression and anger when the mother's attention turns to the infant. Preschool children typically look at and discuss the new baby, but may hesitate to actively touch or hold the infant. Older children often enjoy helping with care of the new baby and are very curious about the newcomer.

Grandparents. The grandparents' involvement with a new baby is often dictated by how near they live to the younger family. Grandparents who live a long distance from them cannot have the close, regular contact that they may desire.

Grandparents also differ in what they expect their role to be. Some feel that their childrearing days are over and want minimal day-to-day involvement in raising the children. Others expect regular involvement in the grandchild's life, second only to the parents (Fig. 9–5). If parents and grandparents agree on their role, little conflict is likely.

Grieving Parents. The postpartum area is usually a happy area, but nurses will occasionally care for grieving parents. For most of these parents, the nurse should simply listen to them and support them. Therapeutic communication techniques such as open-ended questions or reflecting feelings help the parents to express their grief, an early step in resolving it.

It seems strange to talk of grief when a healthy baby is born, but even a healthy baby may be much

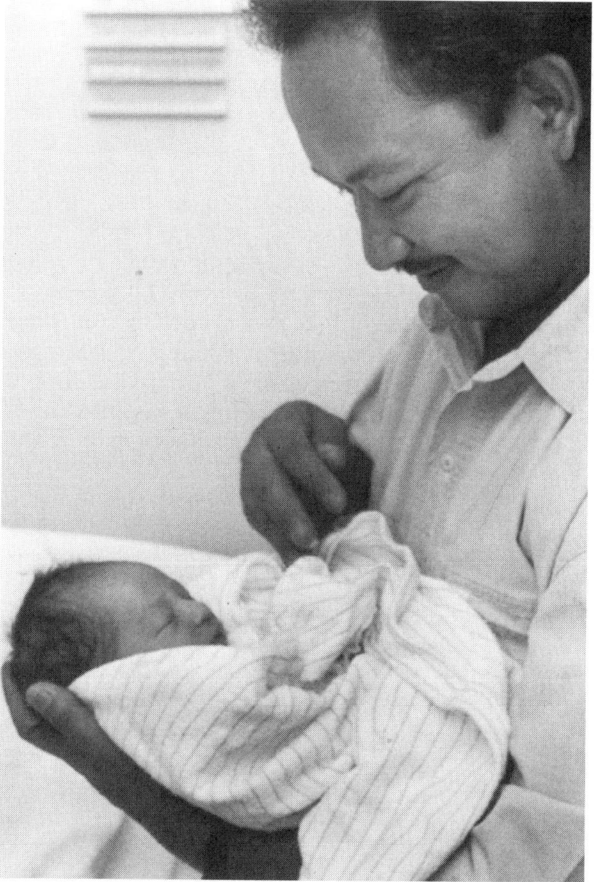

Figure 9–4. • Fathers' reactions to their baby parallels the mother's. The intense fascination is called *engrossment.* (From Gorrie, T. M., McKinney, E. S., & Murray, S. S. [1994]. *Foundations of maternal newborn nursing.* Philadelphia: Saunders.)

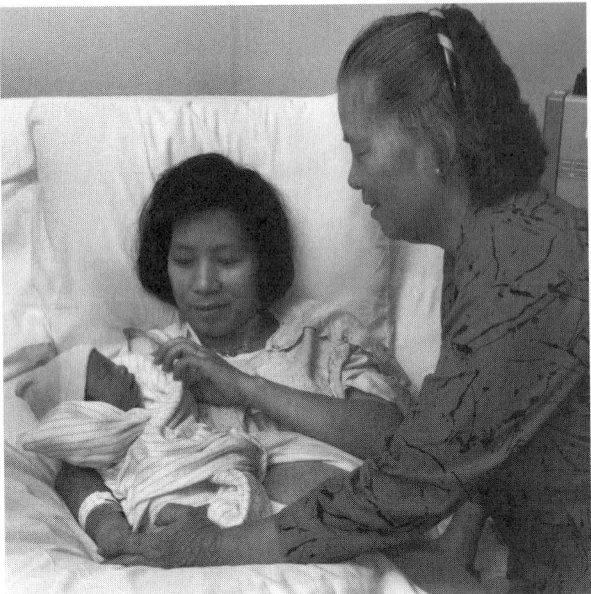

Figure 9–5. • The grandmother can ease adaptation of the young family to their new role as parents. She can reinforce cultural customs, help with infant care, and assist with household tasks. (From Gorrie, T. M., McKinney, E. S., & Murray, S. S. [1994]. *Foundations of maternal newborn nursing.* Philadelphia: Saunders.)

different in size, sex, or appearance from what parents expected. Most parents eventually come to accept their unique infant and his or her characteristics. Their feelings about their baby are not right or wrong—feelings simply exist. The nurse should accept and encourage their expressions of grief to allow them to move forward and accept the baby they have.

A woman who has a spontaneous or induced abortion may experience regret, remorse, and sorrow. This can be one of the most difficult kinds of grief. The woman may question what she could have done differently to prevent the abortion. Anniversaries of these events are painful, and these feelings often last for many years, if not forever. The birth of a new child may awaken grief that parents thought they had resolved ("We have one child, but we almost had two").

If the condition of a newborn is poor, the parents may wish to have a baptism performed. The minister or priest is notified. In an emergency, the nurse may perform the baptism by pouring water on the baby's forehead while saying, "I baptize you in the name of the Father, and of the Son, and of the Holy Spirit." If there is any doubt as to whether the baby is alive, the baptism is given conditionally: "If you are capable of receiving baptism, I baptize you in the name of the Father, and of the Son, and of the Holy Spirit."

If the infant dies, is stillborn, or has a birth defect, the parents' reactions depend on whether the event was expected. If they have known for some time that the fetus is not living, they may have already begun the grief process and will not display all the typical behaviors. If the death was not expected, the nurse is likely to encounter reactions typical of any grieving:

- Shock and disbelief
- Anger, often directed at the physician or staff, but rarely at the infant
- Guilt about what they could have done differently
- Sadness and depression
- Gradual resolution of the sadness

The nurse may encounter grieving families at any point in their grieving process and in many settings. Grieving is often chronic if the infant has a birth defect because of constant reminders of what might have been.

If a newborn dies or is stillborn, nursing units have a protocol to help parents to accept and resolve the event. Allow the parents to progress at their individual pace about when they want to see and hold the baby. Prepare the parents for the baby's appearance. For instance, a stillborn baby may have blue skin that is often peeling. Try to keep the baby warm so it feels more natural to the parents. If this is not possible, prepare them for the coolness of the baby's skin and the limp body. Wrap the baby in a blanket and let them unwrap the baby when and if they want to do so. If an anomaly is present, try to wrap the baby so the most normal part is showing.

Most nursing units make a memory packet containing items such as a lock of hair, footprints on a hospital birth certificate, identification band, a photograph, and clothing or blankets. Some kind of code, such as a flower or ribbon on the mother's door, alerts personnel from other departments that a grieving family is inside. This reduces the chance of well-intentioned, but painful, remarks or questions, such as "What did you have, a boy or girl?"

Parenthood

Whether the parents have one or several children, becoming a parent requires learning new roles and making adjustments. Parents having their first child find themselves in a triangular relationship (the "we" has become an "us"). Many parents say that parenthood, not marriage, made the greatest change in their lives. Adjustments are even greater for women who have professions or who are in the work force, because the changes are more extensive.

The demands of parenthood affect communication between the partners, and there is little doubt that children detract from the relationship at times. It is not unusual for one member to feel left out. The division of responsibility can be a source of conflict, particularly when both parents work. Parents often feel inept, which may cause lower self-esteem, depression, and anger. These feelings can be overwhelming.

Fatigue triggers irritability. Even in the ideal situation, waking up two or three times every night is wearing on anyone. For the new mother, physiologic changes continue to play a part in her emotional lability (instability). Both parents are concerned with increased economic responsibilities. Loss of freedom and a decrease in socialization may give the couple a sense of loneliness.

Preparing parents for the lifestyle changes that occur with a new baby ideally begins before conception. Parenting courses, group discussions, and support from relatives or friends can be explored. Social service agencies, public health nurses, and other professional resources should be suggested, as appropriate. Encouraging parents to share their concerns and worries with one another and to keep communication lines open is foremost. Reestablishing a relationship into which the newborn fits with a minimum of disruption can be accomplished when the parents identify their own needs, set priorities, maintain their sense of humor, and relax their standards.

These tools can make the transition to parenthood, although sometimes difficult, a rewarding experience—one in which the stable family can grow and become stronger. Parents who find themselves at an impasse should seek early intervention with a professional counselor.

CARE OF THE NEWBORN

This chapter will present the early care of the newborn. Newborn assessments and ongoing care are presented in Chapter 12. Care of the preterm and post-term infant is presented in Chapter 13.

Care in the Birthing Room

Initial care of the infant includes the following:

- Maintaining cardiorespiratory function
- Supporting thermoregulation
- Observing for urination
- Identification
- Brief assessment for gestational age and birth injuries or anomalies

The infant will be covered with blood and amniotic fluid at birth. *All caregivers should wear gloves when handling the infant until the first bath.*

Cardiorespiratory Function

Assessment. Breathing should begin within a few seconds after birth. If it does not, resuscitation measures are begun (see discussion under Apgar score). The infant will have a blue color (cyanosis) at birth, but the color should quickly become pink (often except for the hands and feet) as the baby cries. Observe for and report signs of respiratory distress:

- Cyanosis, other than of the hands and feet; cyanosis of the hands and feet *(acrocyanosis)* is due to sluggish peripheral circulation and is normal in the newborn
- Grunting respirations, which may be audible only with a stethoscope
- Retractions of the abdomen under the ribs
- Flaring of the nostrils
- Sustained respiratory rate higher than 60 breaths/min

Oxygen by face mask or placed near the nostrils ("blow by") is often given until the infant is crying vigorously and without cyanosis.

Removing Secretions. Infants expel most respiratory secretions during the first few hours after birth. Fluid and mucus are wiped from the infant's face and the mouth and nose are suctioned by the birth attendant as soon as the head is born. A bulb syringe is usually used for suction, although a catheter with a trap for meconium may be used if the amniotic fluid was meconium stained. After the infant emerges, the birth attendant holds him or her in a head-dependent position or places the baby on the mother's abdomen while suctioning additional secretions with the bulb syringe.

After the cord is cut and the parents see their baby, the infant is handed to the nurse, along with the bulb syringe. The infant is placed in a flat position under a radiant warmer while the nurse dries the skin well. The infant should not remain in a head-dependent position for a prolonged time because this position reduces lung expansion. However, briefly holding the infant in the head-dependent position while large amounts of secretions are cleared may be necessary. When the infant has minimal secretions and a strong cry, tilt the

Table 9–2
APGAR SCORING SYSTEM

Sign	0	1	2
Heart rate	Absent	Below 100 beats/min	100 beats/min or higher
Respiratory effort	No spontaneous respirations	Slow; weak cry	Spontaneous, with a strong lusty cry
Muscle tone	Limp	Minimal flexion of extremities; sluggish movement	Active spontaneous motion; flexed body posture
Reflex irritability	No response to suction or gentle slap on soles	Minimal response (grimace) to stimulation	Prompt response to suction with a gentle slap to sole of foot with cry or active movement
Color	Blue or pale	Body pink, extremities blue	Completely pink (light skin) or absence of cyanosis (dark skin)

Note: The nurse evaluates each sign in the Apgar and totals the score to determine what the infant needs. A score of 8 to 10 requires no action other than continued observation and support of the infant's adaptation. A score from 4 to 7 means the baby needs gentle stimulation such as rubbing the back; the possibility of narcotic-induced respiratory depression should also be considered. Scores of 3 or lower mean that the infant needs active resuscitation.

baby to one side to allow drainage, with the bed position in a flat or slightly elevated position.

When suctioning with a bulb syringe, you should depress the bulb with your thumb, then insert the bulb into the side of the baby's mouth to avoid triggering the gag reflex. The thumb is released to create suction and aspirate secretions into the bulb. The mouth is suctioned before the nose to avoid causing the infant to gasp and aspirate secretions into the lungs.

Teach parents to use the bulb syringe as soon as possible. Keep a bulb syringe with the infant at all times so it is handy for suctioning. Remind parents to carry the bulb syringe with them if they carry the infant away from the crib.

Apgar Scoring. Dr. Virginia Apgar devised a system for evaluating the infant's need for resuscitation at birth (Table 9–2). Five factors are evaluated at 1 minute and 5 minutes after birth and are ranked in order of importance:

- Heart rate
- Respiratory effort
- Muscle tone
- Reflex response to suction or a gentle slap on the soles
- Skin color

The Apgar score is not a predictor of future intelligence or abilities/disabilities. It was meant to identify only the need for neonatal resuscitation measures.

The need for resuscitation can often be anticipated by the history of the mother's pregnancy, complications of pregnancy or labor, size and gestational age of the newborn, and difficulty of delivery. Equipment, medications, and personnel must be readily available for resuscitation at any birth, however, because the need cannot always be anticipated.

Resuscitation methods are directed toward clearing the airway, inflating the lungs, and maintaining circulation. Drugs such as sodium bicarbonate, epinephrine, or blood volume expanders may be needed. Naloxone (Narcan) is used to reverse narcotic-induced respiratory depression.

Tests on a blood sample from the umbilical cord are often done to evaluate and document the infant's respiratory and acid–base status at birth. These tests identify the duration of any hypoxia and help to direct treatment.

Supporting Thermoregulation

Maintenance of body temperature is very important to the newborn infant, who has a less efficient means of generating heat than an older infant. Hypothermia (low body temperature) can cause other problems:

- Hypoglycemia (low blood sugar) as the infant uses glucose to generate heat
- Respiratory distress, because the higher metabolic rate consumes more oxygen, sometimes beyond the baby's ability to supply it

Hypoglycemia can be the cause as well as the result of hypothermia, so the nurse must evaluate both factors. Respiratory distress can also require more glucose for the increased work of breathing, causing hypoglycemia.

Heat is lost by any of four means:

- *Evaporation* of liquids from the skin
- *Conduction,* caused by direct skin contact with a cold surface

- *Convection* of heat away from the body by drafts
- *Radiation,* caused by being near a cold surface, although not in direct contact with it

Conduction, convection, and radiation can also be used to add heat to the body.

Newborns lose heat quickly after birth because amniotic fluid evaporates from their body, drafts move heat away, and they may contact cold surfaces (Table 9–3). The following nursing measures help the baby to conserve heat:

- Preheat the radiant warming unit before the baby is born.
- Dry the infant thoroughly, including the hair immediately after birth. Dry quickly after baths. Remove any wet linens or clothes promptly.
- Place the unclothed infant in the warmer. A skin probe is placed over the infant's liver or spleen area (right or left upper abdomen) to act as a thermostat, increasing or decreasing heat output from the radiant heat unit (Fig. 9–6).
- Do not come between the radiant warmer's heat source and the infant.
- Place the infant in skin-to-skin contact with a parent. A radiant warmer over both mother and infant helps to keep the baby warm and reduces the chill that mothers often experience.
- When not under the radiant warmer, place a hat on the baby's dry head. Placing a hat on wet hair only delays its drying.
- Use warmed blankets to wrap the baby until the temperature is stable.
- Change wet clothing or linens promptly.
- Place the warmer (or bassinet) away from drafts or air conditioner currents.

Observing Urinary Function

Newborns may not urinate for as long as 24 hours and an occasional infant may not void for 48 hours. If an infant urinates in the birthing or operating room, tell the staff nurse and document on the delivery record. If a long period of time elapses before the second voiding, it will have been established that the urinary tract is open.

Identifying the Infant

Bands having preprinted numbers on them are placed on mother, infant, and often the father or other support person in the birthing room as the primary means to identify the infant. Check to be sure that all numbers in the set are identical. Complete other identifying information such as mother's name, birth attendant's name, date and time of birth, sex of the baby, and usually the mother's hospital identification number. The bands are applied relatively snugly on the infant and have only

Table 9–3
NURSING INTERVENTIONS FOR HEAT LOSS IN NEWBORNS

Mechanism of Heat Loss	Conditions Contributing to Heat Loss	Nursing Interventions
Evaporation: drying of wet surface dissipates heat	Wet skin from amniotic fluid, bath water Insensible loss from skin and respiratory tract	Dry baby quickly after birth, including the head (25% of body surface area in the newborn) Wash a small area at a time, then dry it If a hat is used, thoroughly dry head before putting it on
Conduction: direct contact of a cooler surface with the skin	Surfaces such as beds, blankets, scales are cool Cold hands Cold stethoscopes	Prewarm radiant warmer before birth; prewarm stethoscopes or other instruments Use a scale paper when weighing; warm blanket on circumcision restraint Warm blankets and clothing until temperature is stable
Convection: transfer of heat to the air	Drafts from air conditioner vents, open doors Air movement from movement of people Nonwarmed oxygen	Place crib away from drafts Avoid excess movement around babies that have a high risk for heat loss (preterm infants)
Radiation: transfer of heat to cooler objects that are not in direct contact	Placing infant near cold surfaces such as windows or outside walls in winter	Avoid placement of crib near cold windows, walls, or other surfaces Add clothing if cool objects must be nearby

Adapted from Moore, M. L. (1981). *Newborn and family nursing* (2nd ed.). Philadelphia: Saunders.

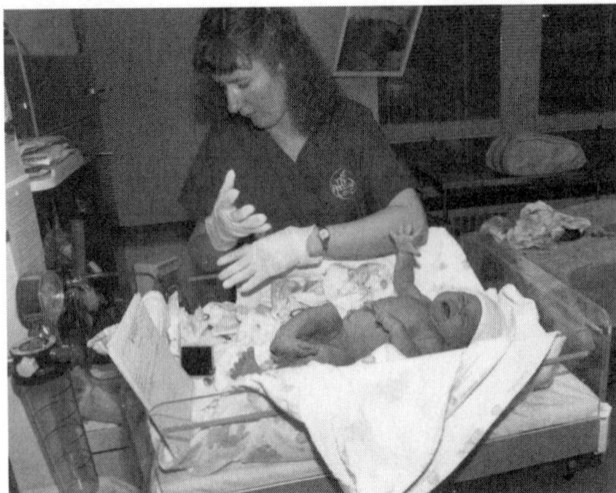

Figure 9–6. • A radiant warmer provides supplemental heat while allowing free access to the baby for care. Note this infant's excellent muscle tone as the nurse prepares to take footprints. The nurse wears gloves until after the infant's first bath.

a fingerwidth of slack because infants lose weight after birth.

Every time the infant returns to the mother after a separation or a mother goes to the nursery to retrieve her baby, check the preprinted band numbers to see that they match. The nurse should either look at the numbers to see that they are identical or have the mother read her band number while looking at the infant's band (Fig. 9–7).

Footprints of the infant and one or both index fingerprints of the mother are usually taken. These are primarily for a keepsake rather than for identification, however. Many birth facilities take a photograph of the infant in the birthing room or very soon after admission and record birthmarks or unique features. This is primarily to identify the infant in the event of an abduction.

Assessment for Gestational Age and Birth Injuries or Anomalies

Gestational Age Evaluation. A thorough gestational age assessment is done using a scale such as the new Ballard or Dubowitz form (see Chapter 13).

Nursing Tip

Do not check bands in this manner: "Is your band number [state number]?" The mother who is sleepy, sedated, or simply distracted may answer affirmatively and receive the wrong baby.

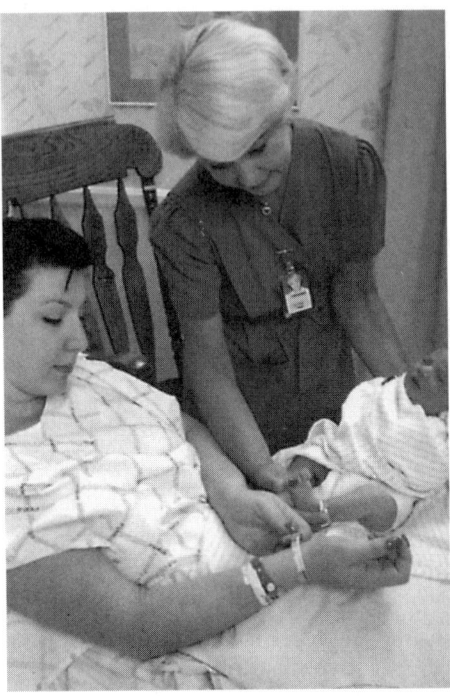

Figure 9–7. • The nurse verifies that she is giving the right infant to the right mother by comparing the identical preprinted numbers on their identification bands. (From Gorrie, T. M., McKinney, E. S., & Murray, S. S. [1998]. *Foundations of maternal-newborn nursing,* 2nd ed. Philadelphia: Saunders.)

However, the birthing room nurse does a quick assessment to evaluate whether the infant seems to be of the appropriate gestational age. The infant who seems to be preterm may be admitted to the nursery sooner than one who is of the expected term gestation. Characteristics to assess include the following:

- *Skin.* Is the skin thin and somewhat transparent (preterm) or peeling (postterm, or possible intrauterine growth retardation [IUGR])?
- *Vernix.* Is this cheesy substance covering most of the skin surface (preterm), or is it only present in creases (term), or is it absent (postterm)? Greenish vernix indicates that meconium was passed before birth, which may indicate that the baby is postterm or had poor placental support.
- *Hair.* Is the skin heavily covered with fine lanugo hair (preterm), or is hair only in a few places (term)? Dark-skinned infants often have more lanugo than light-skinned ones.
- *Ears.* When folded toward the lobe, do the ears spring back slowly (preterm) or quickly (term or postterm)? Abundant vernix can stick the ear in

place, so consider that possibility if the ear does not quickly return to its erect position.

- *Breast tissue.* Is there no or minimal breast tissue under the nipple (preterm), or is there a palpable mass of tissue 5 mm or more (term)? A millimeter is about the thickness of a dime.
- *Genitalia.* For males, is the scrotum smooth and small (preterm) or pendulous and covered with rugae or ridges (term)? For females, are the labia majora and labia minora of near-equal size (preterm) or do the labia majora cover the labia minora (term)?
- *Sole creases.* Are the sole creases on the anterior one-third of the foot only (preterm), the anterior two-thirds (term), or full foot (term or postterm)? Peeling skin may be obvious on the feet in postterm or IUGR babies.

Assessment for Injuries or Anomalies

While performing other assessments and care, the nurse notes signs of injury or anomalies. The infant's movements and facial expression during crying are observed for symmetry and equality of movement. The head and face should be assessed for trauma, especially if forceps were used. A small puncture wound is usually apparent on the scalp if an internal spiral electrode was used for fetal monitoring (see Chapter 6). If the baby was born vaginally in a breech presentation, the buttocks may be bruised.

Many anomalies, such as spina bifida (open spine) or a cleft lip, are immediately obvious. Count the fingers and toes to identify abnormal numbers or webbing. Look at the feet for straightness or determine if deviated feet can be returned to the straight position. Check length equality of arms and legs. Note urination or meconium passage, which confirm patency.

Admission Care of the Newborn

If the infant has adequate cardiorespiratory and heat-regulating functions, he or she usually remains undisturbed while parents and child become acquainted. The nurse can usually assess temperature, heart rate, and respirations while the parents continue to hold their baby. Within an hour, the admitting nurse does a complete physical and gestational age assessment of the baby and gives prophylactic medications. Refer to Chapter 12 for expected characteristics, deviations, and related nursing care of the normal newborn.

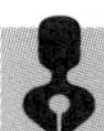

Nursing Tip

If a pacifier is used to provide extra sucking, teach parents to use a one-piece type to prevent choking. They should use a clip to secure the pacifier to the baby's clothing, not place it on a string around the infant's neck, which can cause an active infant to hang himself.

Vital Signs

Vital signs begin while parents and infant are bonding. They are taken at 15- to 30-minute intervals at first, then hourly, and every 4 to 8 hours after the infant is stable.

Respiratory Rate. For best accuracy, assess the respiratory and heart rates before disturbing the infant. Count the respirations for one full minute. Newborn respirations are difficult to count because they are shallow and irregular. The rate can be auscultated by listening with a stethoscope. Placing a hand lightly over the abdomen or watching the cord rise and fall also helps to identify each breath. If the infant is crying, a pacifier or gloved finger to suck may quiet him or her. However, continue to count during crying because the infant breathes at this time, too. Count respirations for one full minute. The normal rate is 30 to 60 breaths per minute, although it may be higher during intense crying.

Heart Rate. The newborn's heart rate is assessed apically. Use a small pediatric head on the stethoscope if possible to limit extraneous noise. Count for one minute. The rate is 120 to 160 beats per minute. It may be slightly slower during sleep or slightly higher if the infant has been crying.

Temperature. Some facilities require an initial rectal temperature for newborns, although many have discontinued this practice. To avoid perforating the rectum, insert the lubricated thermometer

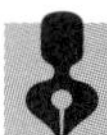

Nursing Tip

In the past newborns were placed in a prone position to facilitate the drainage of mucus. Because the prone position has been associated with sudden infant death syndrome (SIDS) it is now recommended that newborns be placed on their side or back to sleep. Teach all parents this newer information because they may have been taught to keep a previous infant in a prone position.

Nursing Tip

Remember that the artery runs on the *posterior* aspect of the leg when taking a blood pressure in that extremity.

no more than 0.5 inch into the rectum. Hold the thermometer securely near the buttocks while it is in place. *Do not force the thermometer into the rectum because the infant could have an imperforate anus.*

An axillary temperature is most commonly used. Place the thermometer in the axilla, keeping it parallel to the chest wall. Fold the infant's arm firmly against it for the required time.

Tympanic temperatures are less accurate in newborns and not generally used during the neonatal period.

Blood Pressure. A newborn's blood pressure is not routinely taken on a newborn in every facility. It is taken using an electronic instrument. When blood pressure is assessed on a newborn, all four extremities or one arm and one leg are assessed to identify substantial pressure differences between upper and lower extremities, which can be a sign of coarctation of the aorta.

Weighing and Measuring

Weight. The infant is weighed in the birthing room or when admitted to the nursery. Put a disposable paper on the scale and balance it to zero according to the model of the scale. Place the unclothed infant on the scale. The nurse's hand should not touch the baby, but should be kept just above him or her to prevent falls. The weight must be converted to grams for gestational age assessment.

Measuring. Three typical measurements are length, head circumference, and chest circumference. A disposable tape measure is used. Do not slide the tape out from under the baby, to avoid a paper cut. Measures must also be noted in centimeters for gestational age assessment.

Length. There are several ways to measure length. Some facilities have a tape measure applied to the clear wall of a bassinet. The nurse places the infant's head at one end, extends the leg, and notes where the heel ends. Another method is to bring the infant to the bassinet or warmer with the scale paper. Mark the paper at the top of the head, extend the body and leg and mark the paper where the foot is located. Measure between the marks. Still another method is to place the zero end of the tape at the baby's head, extend the body and leg, and stretch the tape to the heel.

Head Circumference. Measure the fullest part of the head just above the infant's eyebrows. Molding of the head may affect the accuracy of the initial measurement.

Chest Circumference. Measure the chest circumference at the nipple line.

Umbilical Cord Care

The birth attendant may leave a long length of umbilical cord. If so, the nurse applies a plastic clamp near the skin and cuts the cord just above the clamp. Take care to clamp only the cord, not the skin.

Assess the cord for the number and type of blood vessels soon after it is cut. The normal umbilical cord has three vessels, two arteries, and one vein. The woman's name "AVA" for "artery-vein-artery" helps the nurse to remember the normal number of vessels. A two-vessel cord is associated with other internal anomalies, often of the genitourinary tract. To distinguish arteries from the vein, look at the freshly-cut end of the cord. The arteries project slightly from the surface and the vein looks like a flattened cylinder that does not project from the cut surface.

Umbilical cord care is aimed at preventing infection. It usually includes an initial application of triple-dye solution or antibiotic ointment. Alcohol applications at each diaper change promote drying of the cord, thus preventing infection. The diaper should be fastened low to allow air circulation to the cord. The cord should become dry and brownish-black in color as it dries. The clamp is removed when the end of the cord is dry and crisp, usually in about 24 hours. Teach the parents to report redness of the area, or a moist, foul-smelling umbilical cord. Tub baths are usually delayed until the cord falls off in about 10 to 14 days.

Bleeding from the cord during the first few hours usually indicates that the cord clamp has become loose. Because of the newborn's small blood volume, even a small amount of bleeding can be a significant percentage of the blood volume. Check the clamp for closure and apply another if needed.

Blood Coagulation

Vitamin K is necessary to form several coagulation factors (VII, IX, X). Newborns have a temporary deficiency of vitamin K because it is manufactured in the intestines by bacteria. The newborn's intestines are sterile until the normal bacterial flora is established. One dose of vitamin K (AquaMephyton), 0.5 to 1 mg, is given in an intramuscular (IM) injection to give the baby the vitamin until their intestinal bacteria produce it.

Intramuscular injections to infants are always given in the anterior thigh. The middle one-third of the anterior lateral thigh (just to the outside of the midline) is preferred. The anterior center of the thigh may be used if necessary.

Preventing Infection

General Measures. Handwashing remains the best way to prevent infection. A 3-minute scrub is commonly required when arriving for work in the newborn nursery. Special clothing is not needed for routine nursery care in terms of preventing infection, although specific clothing may be used as a security measure to help parents to recognize staff. Gloves should be used until after the first bath and for any procedure that involves contact with secretions, including changing diapers.

Eye Care. The infant can acquire infections from an infected mother that can cause blindness, such as gonorrhea and chlamydia. Every state requires eye prophylaxis to prevent these infections. The most common prophylaxis is erythromycin ointment applied as a ribbon to each eye.

To apply erythromycin ointment, first gently wipe any blood and vernix from the eyes with a sterile saline-moistened gauze pad. Place the thumb and forefinger of one hand along the ridges around the eye and open them. Holding the tube horizontally, quickly apply a ribbon of ointment from the inner canthus to the outer canthus without touching the tube end to the eye. Repeat for the other eye. If the skin is slippery, a 2- by 2-inch clean gauze pad under each finger provides traction to open the eye more easily. Excess ointment can be wiped from the eye after one minute. Mild irritation is common for 24 to 48 hours after treatment and requires no treatment.

The infant's vision will be blurred for a short while after the ointment is applied. Therefore, treatment is usually delayed until the parents have had a period of initial bonding.

Hepatitis B Immunization. Many infants are given their first dose of hepatitis B vaccine before discharge home. The parent must sign an informed consent for the infant to receive this drug. The vaccine is given IM in the same manner as vitamin K, but in the opposite leg. The infant should receive subsequent doses at 1 month and 6 months.

Nursing Tip

Advise parents to limit the newborn's exposure to crowds during the early weeks of life, as infants have difficulty forming antibodies against infection until about 2 months of age.

Hypoglycemia

The brain is totally dependent on a steady supply of glucose for its metabolism. Until infants begin regular feedings, they must use the glucose stored in their bodies. A blood glucose level below 40 mg/dl in the term infant indicates hypoglycemia. Screening tests use capillary blood and are less accurate than laboratory tests that use venous blood, so a level of 45 mg/dl is considered hypoglycemic for these tests.

If the screening test indicates hypoglycemia, a venous blood sample is drawn for a more accurate evaluation. The infant is fed formula or is breastfed as soon as the sample is obtained to prevent a further drop in blood glucose.

Some infants have an increased risk for low blood glucose after birth. Infants at higher risk include the following:

- Preterm infants
- Postterm infants
- Infants of diabetic mothers, if maternal glucose is poorly controlled
- Large-for-gestational age infants (LGA)
- Small-for-gestational age infants (SGA)
- Infants with IUGR
- Asphyxiated infants
- Infants that are cold stressed
- Infants whose mother took ritodrine or terbutaline to stop preterm labor

These infants have a blood glucose evaluation shortly after birth and at intervals until their glucose level is stable. They are usually nursed or given formula soon after birth to prevent a fall in their blood glucose.

Although some infants have a higher risk to develop hypoglycemia, any infant can have a fall in blood glucose. Signs of hypoglycemia in the newborn include the following:

- Jitteriness
- Poor muscle tone
- Sweating
- Respiratory difficulty
- Low temperature (which can also cause hypoglycemia)
- Poor suck

- High-pitched cry
- Lethargy
- Seizures

A heel stick is done when obtaining capillary blood for the glucose screening test. The heel stick should avoid the center of the heel where the bone, nerves, and blood vessels are near the surface.

Periods of Reactivity

During adaptation to extrauterine life, the newborn goes through two periods of reactivity separated by a period of sleep. The first period of reactivity begins at birth. The infant is awake, alert, and seems to enjoy gazing at the surroundings. This is an excellent time to promote parent–infant bonding. The first sleep ends the first period of reactivity.

After a deep sleep of 2 to 4 hours, the infant is again awake and alert. At this time, the baby is more interested in feeding and may pass the first meconium stool. Mucus secretions increase and the infant may gag or regurgitate. The second period of reactivity lasts from 4 to 6 hours. After that time, the infant is usually stable.

Screening Tests

Several tests are done to screen for abnormalities that can cause physical or mental disability. The mandatory tests vary according to the state. Most of the disorders have therapy that can prevent many, if not all, of the disabilities that would result if untreated. A test for phenylketonuria (PKU) is mandatory in all states. If the infant has this disorder, a special formula begun in the first 2 months of life can reduce disability and prevent severe mental retardation in most cases. The PKU test is done on the day of discharge for better accuracy and is repeated during early clinic visits. Other tests that are may be done include those for hypothyroidism, galactosemia, sickle cell disease, thalassemia, maple syrup urine disease, and homocystinuria.

Security

The possibility of abduction must be addressed in any facility that cares for infants and children. In the maternal-newborn setting, security begins with identification bands that the nurse matches every time the infant is reunited with the parent.

Recognition of Employees. Parents should be able to recognize employees who are authorized to take the baby from the mother's room. Employees wear photo identification badges and maternal-newborn nurses may have an additional badge. They may wear distinctive uniforms. Some units use a code word that changes on a regular basis. Teach the family very early how to recognize an employee who is allowed to take the baby and to refuse to release their infant to any other person. Reinforce security measures when providing later care.

Teach the mother to keep the baby away from the door to the room. In a semiprivate room, the two bassinets are often placed between the mothers. The mother should not leave her infant alone in the room for any reason. If she is alone in her room have her leave the bathroom door ajar while she toilets, or return the infant to the nursery if she showers or naps. These measures also reduce the risk that the infant would aspirate mucus because no one was present for suctioning.

Observe for suspicious behaviors. Infant abductors are usually female and are often overly curious about routine procedures on the maternal-newborn unit. They may be unable to have a baby or may hope that a child will cement a precarious relationship with their partner. Question anyone holding a package or bundle that might contain a baby. Keep doors locked or alarms set as appropriate for the facility.

Bonding and Attachment

Bonding and *attachment* are terms often used interchangeably, although they differ slightly. *Bonding* refers to a strong emotional tie that forms soon after birth between parents and the newborn. *Attachment* is an affectional tie that occurs over time as infant and caregivers interact. It is important for nurses to promote these processes to help parents to claim their baby as their own. Bonding actually begins during pregnancy as the baby moves and shows individual characteristics. Both fathers and mothers enjoy seeing their baby on a sonogram and usually show these early "baby pictures" and videos to anyone who will watch. Through these pregnancy experiences, they form a "fantasy child" image in their minds.

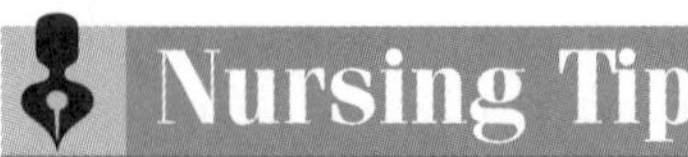

Observe the interaction between parents and infant to evaluate the attachment process.

Both partners should view, hold, and most important, *touch* the baby. They must do this to reconcile the fantasy child of pregnancy with the real child they now have. Many parents are not surprised to know the sex of their baby at birth if the sonogram revealed it earlier. However, some do not want to know the infant's sex before birth and some are surprised when the predicted sex differs from the real sex. Most parents count all fingers and toes.

To prevent infant hypothermia, keep the unclothed infant near the parent's skin. A radiant warmer over both mother and newborn allows the parents to unwrap and thoroughly examine their baby without risk for hypothermia for the baby. Parents soon identify individual characteristics, such as a nose that looks like grandpa's or long fingers like the father or crying just like an older sibling. All of these parental behaviors help to identify the infant as a separate individual.

For some, parental feelings do not come naturally. Assure these parents that with time and caring for the newborn, parental behavior can be learned and acquired. When there is difficulty in bonding or when rejection or indifference is seen in one or both parents, record this observation and consider a referral to social services. Mothers who have little social support may have difficulty forming attachments with their newborn.

Nursing Care to Promote Bonding and Attachment

The nurse observes parenting behaviors, such as amount of affection and interest shown to the baby. The amount of physical contact, stimulation, eye-to-eye contact (*en face* position, see Fig. 9–8), and time spent interacting with the baby are significant. Adults tend to talk with infants in high-pitched voices. The extent to which the parents encourage involvement of siblings and grandparents with the newborn should be noted. This information provides a basis for nursing interventions that may encourage bonding and foster positive family relationships.

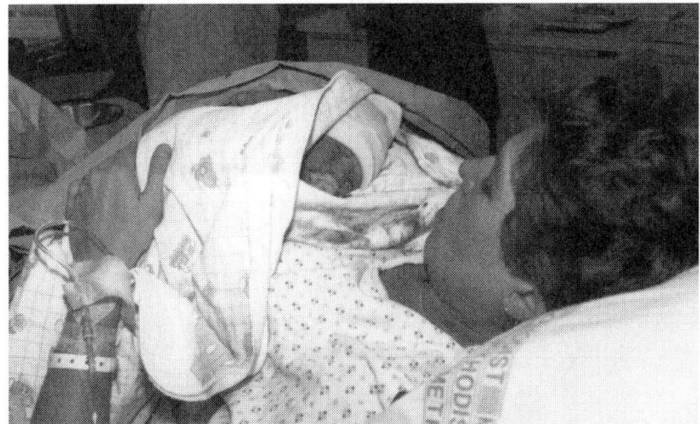

Figure 9–8. • This mother is bonding with her baby shortly after birth. Warm blankets and a cap help keep the infant warm. Note the eye contact the mother and infant make.

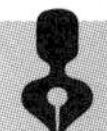

Nursing Tip

On return from the hospital, if siblings are waiting, it is helpful if the father arrives carrying the baby. This leaves the mother's arms free for hugs before turning attention to the new baby.

Parents must learn what their infant's communication cues mean. Soon after birth, most parents begin to recognize when an infant is signaling discomfort from hunger as opposed to discomfort from other causes, such as a wet diaper or boredom. Also, the parents should quickly be able to distinguish their baby's cry from those of other infants. Although this process is just beginning when the mother and baby leave the birth facility, the nurse should note its early signs.

The nurse should observe for parent–infant interactions that dictate a need for additional interventions. Some of these include indifference to infant signals of hunger or discomfort, failure to identify their infant's communication, avoidance of eye contact with the infant, or discussing the infant in negative terms. However, the family's culture should also be considered. In some cultures, the maternal grandmother provides most newborn care during the early weeks, so the nurse should look for signs of attachment between this person and the infant.

Nursing interventions to facilitate parent–infant attachment vary. Calling the baby by name, holding the baby en face, and talking in gentle, high-pitched tones help the nurse to role-model appropriate behavior for the parent. Role modeling is especially important to adolescent mothers who may feel self-conscious when interacting with their baby. Discuss expected infant behaviors and point out unique characteristics to help to enhance the bonding process. This is especially important if the parents' "fantasy child" differs from the "real" child in sex, physical attributes, or health.

Daily Care

A newborn infant stays in the mother's room most of the time unless either mother or infant has a problem that requires separation or when the mother needs to rest. Routine assessments and care provide an opportunity for the nurse to teach the parents normal newborn characteristics, signs of problems that should be reported, and how to provide care for the infant. Involving the parents in care of their infant helps them to learn most successfully. First-time parents may be sensitive to critical remarks, so the nurse should praise their efforts while tactfully giving suggestions for needed improvement.

The infant's heart rate, respiratory rate, heart and breath sounds, and axillary temperature are assessed every 4 to 8 hours after the infant is stable. Skin color is assessed for abnormalities such as cyanosis, pallor, or jaundice. The infant's activity level is assessed for problems such as lethargy or irritability.

Feeding and elimination patterns are assessed by discussing them with the mother as well as observing at diaper changes. Ask the mother how many wet and soiled diapers the baby has had since the last assessment. Voidings are usually totaled for the shift. Stools are also tallied and are described. Meconium stools are expected during the birth facility stay, although they may change to transitional stools before discharge.

If the infant is breastfed, discuss with the mother how well the infant is nursing, the frequency and duration of nursing sessions, and any difficulty she is having. Check her breasts for engorgement and nipples for flatness, inversion, trauma, or tenderness because these problems can impede successful breastfeeding. If the infant is fed formula, ask the mother how many ounces the infant has taken since the previous assessment. This is also a good time to remind the mother that bacteria multiply rapidly in formula, so she should discard any leftovers.

The infant's skin should be observed for jaundice at each assessment. Infants have a large number of erythrocytes because they live in a low-oxygen environment in utero. After birth, the excess erythrocytes are broken down, releasing bilirubin into the bloodstream. High levels of bilirubin cause yellow skin color, starting at the head and progressing downward on the body. Extremely high levels of bilirubin can cause bilirubin encephalopathy (see p. 367).

The infant needs only a shirt and diaper for clothing. A light receiving blanket is used to swaddle the baby and another receiving blanket is placed over the infant. A cap is used for the first few hours and longer for infants at risk for low temperature, such as small or preterm infants. Parents should be cautioned not to overdress the infant. They should be cautioned about placing the infant in drafts or near cold outside windows and walls. A good rule of thumb is to dress the baby in one more layer than would be comfortable for the parent.

Teaching is an important part of mother–baby care. Parent teaching of infant care includes:

- Maintenance of an open airway by positioning and use of the bulb syringe
- Temperature maintenance and assessment after discharge
- Expected increase in the number of voidings
- Changes in the stools
- Feeding
- Signs of illness to report
- Follow-up appointments for well baby care

BREASTFEEDING

Nutrition is especially important in the first few months of life because the brain grows rapidly. Energy use is high because of the newborn's rapid growth. A more in-depth discussion of the nutritional needs of the infant is found in Chapter 15. The mother may choose to nurse her baby or bottle feed. The nurse should support the mother in either decision.

Choosing Whether to Breastfeed

Breastfeeding has many advantages for the newborn:

- Breast milk contains a full range of nutrients that the infant needs and in the right proportions. No commercial formula has the exact nutritional composition of breast milk.
- The composition of breast milk changes to meet the infant's changing needs.
- Breast milk is easily digested by the baby's maturing digestive system.
- Breast milk does not cause infant allergies.
- Breastfeeding provides natural immunity because the mother transfers antibodies through the milk. Colostrum is particularly high in antibodies.
- Breast milk promotes elimination of meconium. Breastfed infants are rarely constipated.
- Suckling at the breast promotes mouth development.
- Breastfeeding is convenient and economical.
- Breastfeeding eliminates risks of a contaminated water supply or improper dilution.
- Infant suckling promotes return of the uterus to its prepregnant state.

- Breast milk production utilizes maternal fat stores, facilitating weight loss.
- Breastfeeding enhances a close mother–child relationship.

There are also some disadvantages and contraindications to breastfeeding:

- There is a potential for most maternal medications to enter breast milk.
- One type of neonatal jaundice occasionally occurs (breast milk jaundice).
- Working mothers may have more difficulty continuing to nurse after they return to work.
- Women who have active tuberculosis, hepatitis B or C, or infection with the human immunodeficiency virus should not breastfeed. Cancer may become worse with the hormonal changes of lactation.
- Women who abuse drugs or alcohol should not breastfeed.

Physiology of Lactation

To better support the nursing mother the nurse needs to understand how breast milk production occurs and how the milk changes over time.

Hormonal Stimulation

Two hormones have a major role in the production and expulsion of breast milk:

- *Prolactin* from the anterior pituitary gland, which causes the manufacture of breast milk
- *Oxytocin* from the posterior pituitary gland, which causes the milk to be delivered from the alveoli (milk-producing sacs) through the duct system, to the nipple (*milk ejection,* or *let-down reflex*); the mother will usually feel a tingling in her breasts and sometimes abdominal cramping as her uterus contracts

During pregnancy, the glandular tissue of the breasts grows under the influence of several hormones. The woman also secretes high levels of prolactin, the hormone that causes milk production. However, other hormones from the placenta inhibit the breasts' response to prolactin. The influence of prolactin is unopposed after birth and the expulsion of the placenta and milk production begins. If milk is not removed from the breast, prolactin secretion abates and the breasts return to their prepregnant state.

Infant suckling at the breast stimulates release of oxytocin so that milk is delivered to the nipple where it is ingested. Prolactin secretion increases as milk is removed from the breasts, thus stimulating further milk production. Therefore, feedings that are infrequent or too short can reduce the amount of milk produced. The opposite is also true, explaining why a mother can produce enough milk for twins.

Very little milk is stored between feedings. Most is manufactured as the baby nurses. The composition of milk changes slightly from the beginning of a feeding until the end of that feeding.

- *Foremilk* is the first milk the infant obtains. It is more watery and quenches the infant's thirst.
- *Hindmilk* is the later milk that has a higher fat content that helps satisfy the infant's hunger. Feedings that are too short do not allow the infant to obtain the hunger-satisfying hindmilk.

Phases of Milk Production

Milk production changes in three phases after birth:

- Colostrum
- Transitional milk
- Mature milk

Late in pregnancy and for the first few days after birth, *colostrum* is secreted by the breasts. This yellowish fluid is rich in protective antibodies. It provides protein, vitamins A and E, and essential minerals, but is lower in calories than milk. It has a laxative effect, which aids in eliminating meconium.

About 7 to 10 days after birth the *transitional milk* emerges, as the breasts gradually shift from production of colostrum to mature milk. Transitional milk has less immunoglobulins and proteins, but lactose (milk sugar), fat, and calorie content increases.

Mature milk is secreted by 14 days after birth. Mature human breast milk has a bluish color, leading women to think that it is not "rich" enough to nourish the infant. The nurse should explain that the apparent "thinness" of the milk is normal but that the milk has 20 kcal/ounce and all the nutrients the infant needs.

Nursing Tip

Anticipatory guidance concerning possible problems associated with breastfeeding helps the mother to see them as common occurrences and not as complications.

Table 9–4
TEACHING THE NEW MOTHER HOW TO BREASTFEED

Instruction	Rationale
Wash hands before feeding; wash nipples with warm water, no soap	Prevents infection of the newborn and breast; use of plain water avoids nipple cracking and irritation
Position	Side-lying position reduces fatigue and pressure on abdominal incision
Comfortably seated in chair or raised bed with back and arm support; hold baby with cradle hold or football hold, supported by pillows	Pillow support of mother's back and arm and the infant's body in any position reduces fatigue; infant is more likely to remain in correct position for nursing
Side-lying with pillow beneath head, arm above head; support baby in side-lying position	Alternating positions facilitates breast emptying and reduces nipple trauma
Turn body of infant to face mother's breast	Prevents pulling on nipple or poor position of mouth on nipple
Stroke baby's cheek with nipple	Elicits rooting reflex to cause baby to turn toward nipple and open mouth wide
Baby's mouth should cover entire areola	Compresses ducts, lessens tension on nipples; suction is more even
Avoid strict time limits for nursing. Nurse at least 10 minutes before changing to other breast, or longer if infant is nursing vigorously; use safety pin as reminder about which breast to start with the next feeding	Let down reflex may take 5 minutes; a too-short feeding will give infant foremilk only, not the hunger-satisfying hindmilk Strict time limits do not prevent sore nipples Alternating breasts increases milk production
Lift baby or breast slightly if breast tissue blocks nose	Provides a small breathing space
Break suction by placing finger in corner of baby's mouth or indenting breast tissue	Removing baby in this way prevents nipple trauma
Nurse baby after birth and every 2–3 hr thereafter	Early suckling stimulates oxytocin from mother's pituitary to contract her uterus and control bleeding Breast milk is quickly digested Early, regular, and frequent nursing reduces breast engorgement
Burp baby halfway through and following feeding	Rids stomach of air bubbles, reduces regurgitation

Assisting the Mother to Breastfeed

Ideally the infant is nursed soon after birth. Although the infant may obtain little colostrum, this first nursing session has other advantages:

- Promotes mother–infant bonding
- Maintains infant temperature
- Infant suckling stimulates oxytocin release to contract the mother's uterus and control bleeding

If the mother is too tired or uncomfortable to nurse at this time or if the infant seems disinterested, reassure her that she can still breastfeed successfully. Table 9–4 reviews techniques the nurse can teach a new mother who wants to breastfeed.

Positions for Nursing

Any of several positions may be used for nursing. The mother may sit in bed or in a chair and hold the baby in a cradle hold, with the head in her antecubital area (Fig. 9–9). To prevent arm fatigue, support the infant's body with pillows or folded blankets. She may prefer the football hold (Fig. 9–10), supporting the infant's head with her hand while the infant's body rests on pillows alongside her hip. The football hold is good for mothers who have a cesarean incision.

She may prefer to lie on her side with the baby's body parallel to hers. Use pillows or folded blankets to support the infant in the proper position. Mothers often use the side-lying position when feeding the infant during the night. It is also good for mothers who have a cesarean birth.

Feeding Technique

Teach the mother to wash her hands before each nursing session. She should wash her breasts gently with plain water.

Have the mother urinate and provide analgesia if she needs relief from perineal or surgical pain before she begins. The mother and infant must be positioned correctly for optimal breastfeeding. Use pillows to support mother and infant to reduce fatigue. If the mother who has a cesarean incision will use the cradle hold, place a small pillow over her incision. Provide privacy and minimize interruptions.

Position of the Mother's Hands. The mother should hold her breast in a C position, with the thumb above the nipple and the fingers below it. The thumb and fingers should be well back from the nipple and the nipple should not tip upward. She can also use the scissors hold to grasp the breast between her index and middle fingers, but her fingers are more likely to slip downward over the nipple. Most infants will not need to have the breast indented for breathing room. The mother can lift the infant's hips higher if her breasts are very large or if the baby buries the nose in her breast.

Latch-on. Teach the mother to allow the infant to become alert and hungry, but not frantic. To elicit latch-on, the mother should hold her breast so the nipple brushes against the infant's lower lip. A hungry infant will usually open the mouth wide

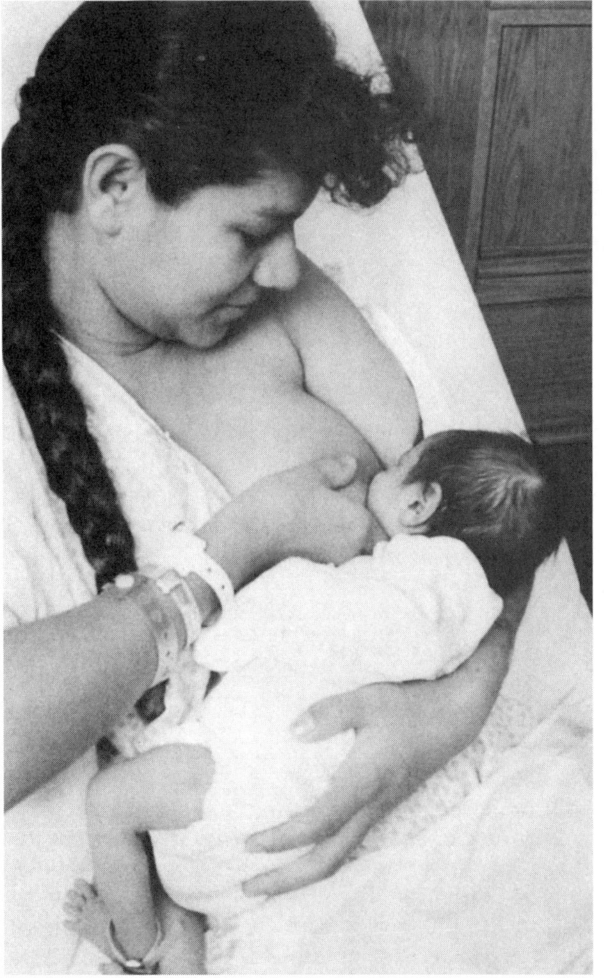

Figure 9–9. • For the cradle hold, the mother positions the baby's head near her antecubital space and level with her nipple with her arms and pillows supporting the infant's body. Her other hand is holding her breast in the C position to guide it to the infant's mouth. (From Gorrie, T. M., McKinney, E. S., & Murray, S. S. [1994]. *Foundations of maternal newborn nursing.* Philadelphia: Saunders.)

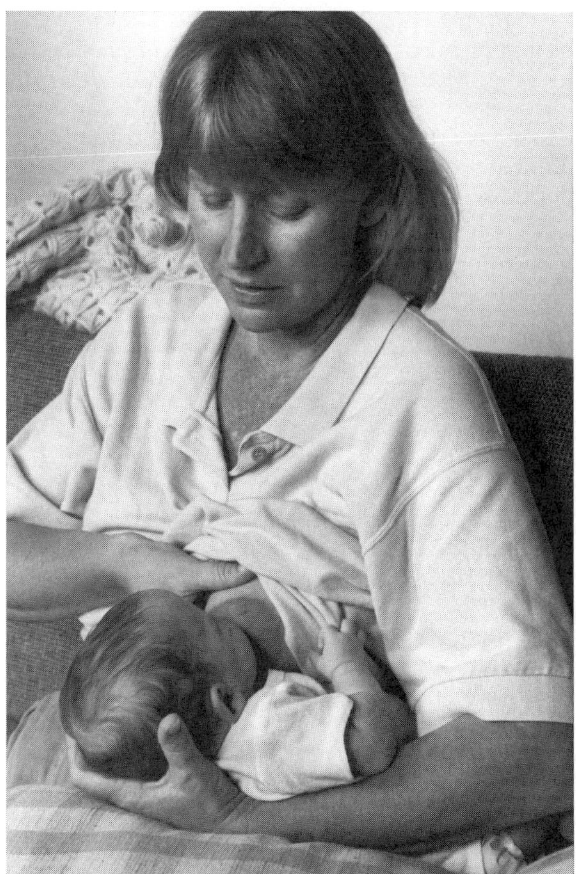

Figure 9–10. • For the football hold, the mother supports the baby's head with her hand. The baby's body is supported alongside her hip with pillows. The football hold helps to avoid pressure on a cesarean incision. (From Gorrie, T. M., McKinney, E. S., & Murray, S. S. [1994]. *Foundations of maternal newborn nursing.* Philadelphia: Saunders.)

with this stimulation. As soon as the infant's mouth opens wide, the mother should bring the infant close to her breast so that her areola is well into the mouth. The lips should flare outward. The infant's tongue position can be checked to be sure it is under the nipple by gently pulling down on the lower lip.

Suckling Patterns. *Suckling* is the term that specifically relates to giving or taking nourishment at the breast. Infants have different suckling patterns when they breastfeed. Some suck several times before swallowing, and others swallow with each suck. A soft "ka" or "ah" sound indicates that the infant is swallowing colostrum or milk (nutritive sucking). Noisy sucking or smacking sounds or dimpling of the cheeks usually indicate improper mouth position. "Fluttering" sucking motions indicate nonnutritive suckling.

Removing the Infant from the Breast. When the infant needs to be repositioned or changed to the other breast, the mother should break the suction and remove the infant quickly. She can break the suction by inserting a finger in the corner of the infant's mouth or indenting her breast near the mouth.

Preventing Problems

Teaching can help new mothers to prevent many problems with breastfeeding. If the mother can avoid problems, she is less likely to become discouraged and stop nursing early. Lactation consultants are available in many birth settings to help with breastfeeding problems. La Leche League chapters may be available to the mother for ongoing support after discharge. Most birth centers have "warm lines" to help with breastfeeding or other problems that occur in mothers and infants after birth.

Frequency and Duration of Feedings. Breastfed infants usually nurse every 2 to 3 hours during the early weeks because their stomach capacity is small and because breast milk is easily digested. Some infants cluster several feedings at frequent intervals and then wait a longer time before nursing again. It is best to maintain flexibility during the early weeks. However, if the infant has not nursed for 3 hours, tell the mother to gently waken the baby and try to nurse.

If feedings are too short, the infant may get little milk, or only the foremilk. It may take as long as 5 minutes for the let-down reflex to occur. The infant will soon be hungry again if he does not receive the richer hindmilk. This can frustrate the mother because her baby wants to "eat all the time." Engorgement will occur if milk is not removed from the breasts, and milk production will decrease or stop.

The infant should nurse at least 10 minutes on the first breast, or longer if still nursing vigorously. The mother should then remove the infant from the first breast and nurse at the second breast until the infant is satisfied. The total duration of early feedings should be at least 15 minutes. The mother should not switch back and forth between breasts several times.

Infants who breastfeed usually do not swallow much air. To burp the baby, the mother can hold the infant in a sitting position in her lap and pat or rub the back to assist a burp (Fig. 9–11). Alternately, the infant can be placed against the mother's shoulder for burping. A soft cloth protects the adult's clothing from spitups.

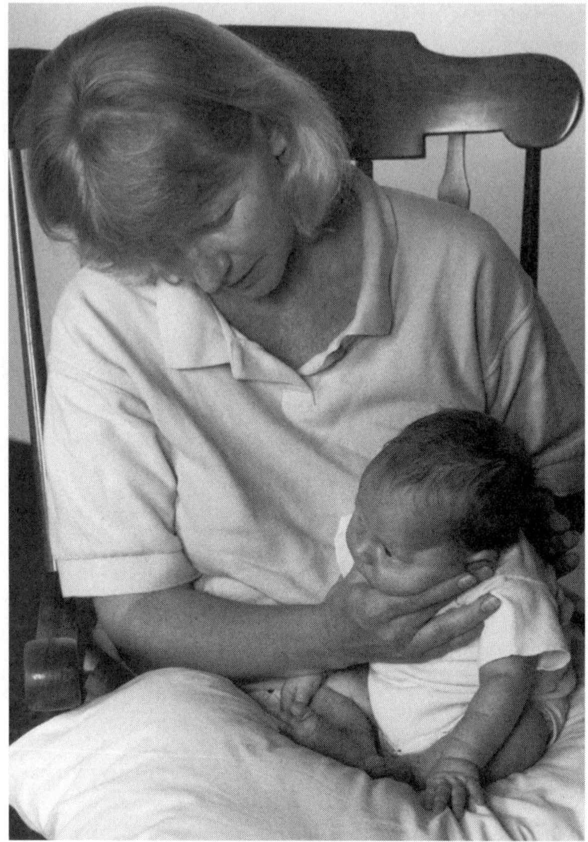

Figure 9–11. • The mother can burp the baby by sitting the baby on her lap while gently patting or rubbing the back. She can easily see the baby's face in case of spitups. (From Gorrie, T. M., McKinney, E. S., & Murray, S. S. [1994]. *Foundations of maternal newborn nursing.* Philadelphia: Saunders.)

The mother should begin the next nursing session using the breast that was used last in the previous session. A safety pin attached to her bra helps her to remember which breast to use each time.

Flat or Inverted Nipples. To help the nipples become erect for feedings, the mother can gently roll them between her thumb and forefinger.

Nipple Confusion. Infants who receive both formula feedings and are breastfed may develop nipple confusion because the sucking action required for the breast and the bottle are different. Milk is easier to obtain from the bottle. Also, formula takes longer to digest, and the infant may not awaken for another feeding for 4 or more hours. This will reduce the amount of breast milk removed from the breast and ultimately reduce the supply. For this reason, nurses should discourage breastfeeding mothers from using formula supplements, particularly during the first 3 to 4 weeks, when milk production is being established. Use of pacifiers can also cause nipple confusion.

Breast Engorgement. Early, regular, and frequent nursing helps to prevent breast engorgement. If engorgement does occur and the breast and areola are very tense and distended, the mother can pump her breasts to get the milk flow started and soften the areola. She may use a breast pump or manual expression of milk. Cold applications between feedings and heat just before feedings may help to reduce discomfort and engorgement.

Manual massage of all segments of the breasts helps to soften them and express milk downward in the duct system. The mother cups her hands around the breast near the chest wall and firmly slides her fingers forward toward the nipple. She rotates her hands to massage all areas of the breast.

Nipple Trauma. Cracks, blisters, redness, and bleeding may occur. Correct positioning of the infant is the best preventive measure, although some minor nipple trauma is common. Feeding formula at this time can worsen the trauma and pain because it is likely to cause engorgement as less milk is removed. Warm water compresses or warm, wet tea bags applied to the breasts offer some relief. Rubbing a small amount of breast milk into the nipples may aid healing. Ointments are not effective; if used, they should be removed before nursing.

Hygiene

The mother should not use soap on her breasts. She should wear a supportive bra 24 hours a day that is not excessively tight.

Special Breastfeeding Situations

Multiple Births. Twins can be fed one at a time or simultaneously. The mother's body adjusts the milk supply to the greater demand. Occasional formula feedings let the father participate more actively.

The mother may want to use the criss-cross hold when nursing simultaneously. She will need help to position two infants at the breast in a cradle hold in each arm. She positions the first infant in a cradle hold, then her helper positions the second infant at the other breast in the crook of her arm. Their bodies cross over each other. Support the infants and the mother's arm with pillows.

Premature Birth. Breastfeeding is especially good for a preterm baby because of its immunological advantages. If the infant cannot nurse, the mother can pump her breasts and freeze the milk for gavage (tube) feedings. See Chapter 13 for further information on the preterm infant.

When nursing the preterm or small infant, the mother may prefer the cross cradle hold. She holds the infant's head with the hand opposite the breast that she will use to nurse. She uses the same arm to support the infant's body. The hand on the same side as the nursing breast is used to guide the breast toward the baby's mouth.

Maternal Nutrition

To maintain her own nutrient stores while providing for the infant, the mother needs 500 additional calories each day over her nonpregnant diet. She should choose foods from each of these groups in the food guide pyramid:

- Meat, fish, poultry, eggs, beans, and nuts
- Milk and other dairy products
- Vegetables
- Fruits
- Breads, cereals, and grains

She needs to drink fluids to satisfy her thirst, about 8 to 10 glasses per day, excluding those containing caffeine. Women with lactose intolerance may use such substitutes as tofu, soy milk, and canned salmon with bones as a substitute for milk products. A calcium supplement will probably be needed to prevent loss from the bones. The birth attendant usually recommends that the nursing mother continue prenatal vitamins during lactation, although routine supplementation has been shown to be unnecessary for the well-nourished mother.

Some foods the mother eats may change the taste of the milk or cause the baby to have gas. Foods that often cause problems are chocolate, cabbage, beans, and broccoli. If the mother suspects that a particular food is causing fussiness or gas, she can eliminate it from her diet for a few days to determine if the infant has fewer problems. These problems do not indicate an allergy to breast milk, only irritation with some food by-product that is contained in the milk.

Excess caffeine in the diet can cause infant irritability. Caffeine intake should be restricted to two caffeinated drinks per day.

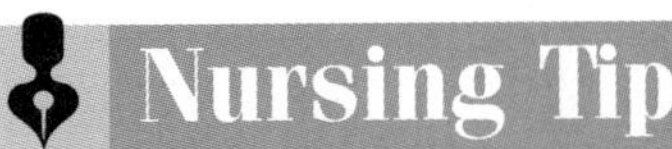

Lactation uses fat stores from pregnancy to produce milk, assisting weight loss.

Other Concerns

Alcohol can interfere with the let-down reflex and may be harmful to the infant. The nursing mother should not take more than an occasional single glass of an alcoholic beverage.

Cigarette smoking exposes the infant to nicotine and may reduce milk production.

Many medications taken by the mother are secreted in breast milk, but in varying concentrations depending on the drug. In general, if a medication can be taken by a newborn, it is safe to be taken by a lactating woman. Timing the drug dose so that it passes its peak of action before the infant's nursing sessions can reduce the amount delivered to the baby.

Weaning

Gradual weaning is preferred to abrupt weaning. Abrupt weaning can cause engorgement and lead to mastitis; it can be upsetting to the infant.

There is no one best time to wean. Even a short period of breastfeeding provides the infant with many immunologic and digestive advantages. As the infant matures, he or she will gradually become less interested in the breast, especially when solid foods are added to the diet around 6 months.

The nurse can teach mothers the following tips when she wants to wean her baby:

- Eliminate one feeding at a time. Wait several days and eliminate another one. The young infant will need formula from a bottle; the older infant may be weaned from the breast to a cup.
- Omit daytime feedings first, starting with the one the baby is least interested in.
- Eliminate the baby's favorite feeding last. This will often be the early morning or bedtime feeding.
- Expect the infant to need "comfort nursing" if tired, ill, or uncomfortable.

If the mother must wean abruptly for some reason she should wear a firm support bra and bind her breasts with a breast binder or a 6-inch elastic bandage. She should avoid nipple stimulation as discussed in the postpartum care section. Lactation-suppressing drugs are not advised.

FORMULA FEEDING

Women choose to formula feed for many reasons.. Some are embarrassed by breastfeeding or are very modest. They may have little social support because family and friends had poor experiences with breastfeeding. Others are uncomfortable when they cannot see the amount of milk the infant takes each feeding. Women who have many other commitments and cannot maintain the flexibility needed when lactation is established may find that formula feeding is the only realistic choice. A few women must take medications or have other illnesses that make breastfeeding unwise. Regardless of the mother's reason for choosing to formula feed her baby, the nurse should fully support the mother and reassure her that her baby can receive good nutrition and emotional closeness.

Some nursing mothers want to feed an occasional bottle of formula while they work or go out. They are advised to wait until lactation is well established (3 to 4 weeks) before offering the baby a bottle.

Types of Formulas

Most formulas are modifications of cow's milk. Examples of *cow's milk formulas* are Similac and Enfamil. Infants who do not tolerate cow's milk formulas or who come from a family with many allergies may be given soy or protein hydrolysate formulas. *Soy formulas* include ProSobee and Isomil; Nutramigen is a *protein hydrolysate* formula. Other formulas are available to meet special needs, such as those of the preterm infant or the infant with PKU.

Common formulas come in three forms:

- Ready-to-feed, either in cans or in glass bottles
- Concentrated liquid
- Powdered

Preparation

The parent should wash the hands before preparing formula and feeding the baby. Bottles and nipples can be washed in hot soapy water and rinsed well. Bottles can be washed in a dishwasher, but nipples should be washed by hand to slow deterioration. Bottles of formula can be prepared

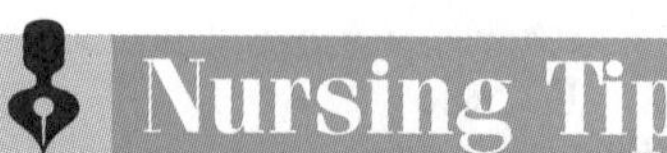

Over- or underdilution of concentrated liquid or powdered formulas can result in serious illness.

one at a time or a 24-hour supply can be prepared. Refrigerate formula promptly and keep refrigerated until ready to use.

Ready-to-feed formulas require no dilution. Diluting them with water reduces the amount of nutrients the infant receives and can be dangerous. Ready-to-feed formula for home use comes in cans. The mother should wash the can's lid and open it with a freshly washed can opener. She then pours the approximate amount the infant will take at a feeding into a bottle and caps the bottle.

Concentrated liquid formula also comes in a can. After washing the can and opening it, the mother pours recommended proportions of concentrated liquid formula and tap water into the bottles and caps them. The usual proportions are one part concentrated liquid formula plus one part tap water. Water for formula dilution does not need to be boiled unless its safety is questionable.

Powdered formula is a popular choice for nursing mothers who want to feed their baby an occasional bottle of formula. The parent measures the amount of tap water into the bottle and adds the number of scoops recommended for that quantity.

Sterilization is not required unless the quality of the water is in doubt. To sterilize formula, either of two methods are safe:

- *Aseptic method:* All equipment (bottles, nipples, caps, tongs) are boiled for 5 minutes. Water for dilution is boiled separately. The bottles are filled with formula, capped, and refrigerated until used.
- *Terminal method:* Bottles are filled with formula and loosely capped. The bottles are then placed in a sterilizer or pan of water where they are boiled for 25 minutes. They are allowed to cool, the lids are tightened, and they are refrigerated until used.

Feeding the Infant

Formula is digested more slowly than breast milk. Most formula-fed infants feed about every 3 to 4 hours at first. The formula feeding mother should also be encouraged to avoid rigid scheduling.

Many mothers prefer to warm the formula somewhat, although warming is not needed. Placing the bottle in a container of hot water takes the chill off the milk. Microwave heating of infant formula is *not* recommended. The center of the formula becomes very hot in a microwave although the outside feels cool. If formula is heated, it should always be tested

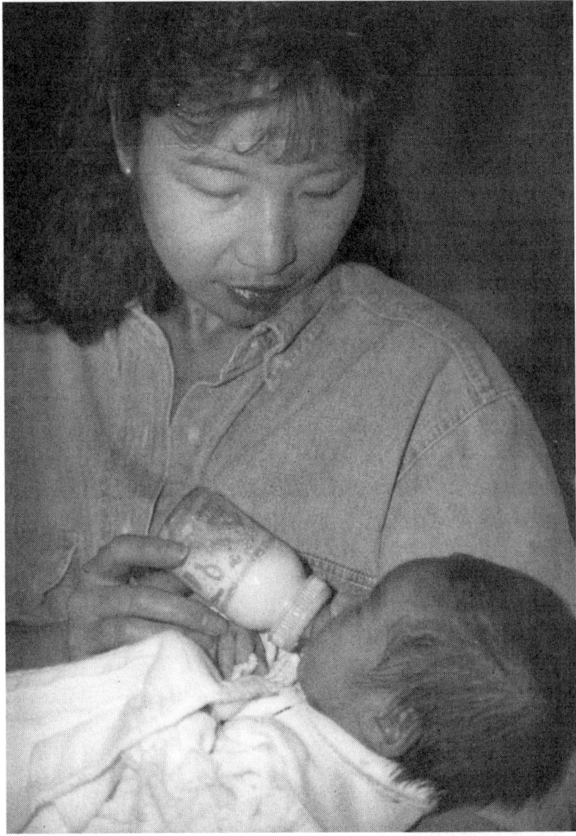

Figure 9–12. • Bottle feeding can be a time of closeness with the baby as breastfeeding is. The mother positions the bottle so the nipple remains filled with milk to prevent the baby from swallowing air. (From Gorrie, T. M., McKinney, E. S., & Murray, S. S. [1994]. *Foundations of maternal newborn nursing.* Philadelphia: Saunders.)

before giving it to the baby by sprinkling a few drops on the inside of the wrist.

The mother should hold the baby in a semi-upright position in a cradle hold. The nipple should be kept full of formula to reduce the amount of air the baby swallows (Fig. 9–12). The baby is burped about every ½ to 1 ounce at first, gradually increasing the amount between burps as the stomach capacity enlarges. The baby is also burped at the end of a feeding. Slightly elevating the upper body at the end of the feeding reduces regurgitation.

If milk is running out of the baby's mouth during sucking, the nipple holes may be too large. The nipple should be discarded and replaced with a new one. The baby should not be coaxed to finish the bottle. Leftover formula should be discarded as microorganisms from the mouth grow rapidly in warm formula.

The nurse should caution parents not to prop the bottle, even when the baby is older. Propping the bottle may cause the infant to aspirate formula and is associated with dental caries (cavities) and ear infections.

Fathers or significant others are encouraged to assist with feedings. Some families choose formula feeding for this very reason: to involve the father in the infant's care. When teaching new parents about infant care, involve the father or other support person. This will aid his or her involvement and attachment to the infant and enhance support for the mother as well.

DISCHARGE PLANNING

Discharge planning begins on admission or even earlier, when parents attend childbirth classes. Because mothers and babies are discharged quickly after birth, often after 24 hours, teaching self-care and infant care must often begin before the mother is psychologically ready to learn. Some birth facilities use *clinical pathways,* also called care maps, care paths, or multidisciplinary action plans (MAPs), to ensure that important care and teaching is not overlooked. These plans guide the nurse to identify areas of special need that require referral as well as a means to keep up with the many facets of routine care needed after birth. The nurse must take every opportunity to teach during the short birth facility stay. Ample written materials for both new mother and infant care should be provided to refresh the memory of parents who may be tired and uncomfortable when teaching must occur.

Postpartum Self-Care Teaching

The nurse teaches the new mothers how to best care for themselves to reduce their risk for complications. The birth attendant may give more specific instructions in some areas.

Follow-Up Appointments

Most physicians and nurse-midwives want to see postpartum women at 2 weeks and 6 weeks after birth. The nurse should emphasize the importance of these follow-up appointments to verify that *involution* is proceeding normally and to identify any complications as soon as possible. Signs of problems the woman should report have been discussed in previous sections.

At the 2-week appointment, the healing of the mother's perineum or cesarean incision is assessed. She is questioned about signs of complications. Problems that she may be having, such as constipation or breastfeeding difficulties, are addressed. Postpartum blues may have occurred, and the woman should be reassured about their temporary nature.

At the 6-week appointment, the mother's general health and recuperation from birth are assessed. The physician or nurse-midwife does a vaginal exam to check the uterus to ensure that involution is complete. Any incision is assessed for healing. The breasts are carefully examined for any signs of problems. Occasionally a complete blood count is done, and vitamins or iron supplements, or both, are ordered if anemia is present.

The woman has the opportunity to discuss any problems she may be having, whether physical or psychological. The physician and the nurse usually inquire about how she is adapting to motherhood. Is she getting enough rest? How is breastfeeding coming along? Does she have help at home? How is the father adapting to his new role?

Rest

The mother should avoid strenuous activity and do no heavy lifting. Napping when the baby is napping is recommended. Women, particularly those having cesarean birth, are advised to pick up nothing heavier than their baby until after their checkup.

Hygiene

A daily shower or bath is refreshing and cleanses the skin of perspiration that may be more profuse in the first days after birth. Perineal care should be continued until the lochia stops. Douches and tampons should not be used for sanitary protection until after the 6-week checkup.

Sexual Intercourse

Coitus should be avoided until the episiotomy is fully healed and the lochia flow has stopped. Having sexual relations earlier can lead to infection and trauma. A water-soluble lubricant makes intercourse more comfortable. The woman or partner can feel the perineum for areas of tenderness as part of foreplay.

Ovulation, and therefore pregnancy, can occur before the 6-week checkup. The birth attendant usually discusses contraception with the woman, but the nurse must often clarify or reinforce any explanations. It is important to emphasize that breastfeeding is not a reliable contraceptive.

Diet

A well-balanced diet promotes healing and recovery from birth. Because constipation may be a problem, teach the mother about high-fiber foods (such as whole-grain fruits and vegetables with the skins). Breastfeeding mothers should not try to lose weight while nursing. The formula-feeding mother should delay a strict reducing diet until released by her physician to do so. Most birth attendants recommend that new mothers continue any prenatal vitamins that were prescribed until after the 6-weeks checkup.

Danger Signs

By teaching the mother changes to expect as she returns to the prepregnant state, the nurse gives her a framework to recognize when something is not progressing normally. Hemorrhage, infection, and thrombosis are the most common complications. The mother should therefore report:

- Fever higher than 38°C (100.4°F)
- Persistent lochia rubra or lochia that has a foul odor
- Bright red bleeding, particularly if the lochia has changed to serosa or alba
- Prolonged afterpains, pelvic or abdominal pain, or a constant backache
- Signs of a urinary tract infection, previously described
- Pain, redness, or tenderness of the calf
- Localized breast tenderness or redness
- Discharge, pain, redness, or separation of any suture line (cesarean, perineal laceration, or episiotomy)
- Prolonged and pervasive feelings of depression or being let down; generally not enjoying life

Newborn Discharge Care

Discharge planning for the infant begins at birth. Because of short stays after birth, the nurse must teach the parents how to care for their newborn at every opportunity. Discharge teaching will then be more of a summary than an attempt to crowd all teaching into a short time.

Infants who are discharged sooner than 48 hours after birth should have a check by a health care professional within 48 hours of discharge. The infant is assessed at this early check for jaundice, feeding adequacy, urine and stool output, and behavior. The assessment focuses on identifying jaundice, inadequate feeding or other feeding problems, and infection.

Infants are usually seen again at 6 to 8 weeks after birth to begin well-baby care. When providing discharge teaching, the nurse should emphasize the value of these visits. Explain that immunizations can be given to prevent many illnesses. The physician or nurse-practitioner assesses the baby for growth and development, nutrition, and any problems the parents or infant are having. Teaching to prepare them for the baby's upcoming needs (anticipatory guidance) helps them to plan ahead to prevent injuries.

The nurse should teach parents the importance of using infant car safety seats (Fig. 9–13), and the correct use of them. The newborn should be placed in semi-reclining position in the car's back seat (never in the front), facing the rear until 1 year *and* 20 pounds (see Fig. 17–10). The seat's harness is snugly fastened and the seat is secured to the automobile seat with the seat belt. Parents should consult their car's instruction manual for specific instructions on securing safety seats. The National Highway Traffic Safety Administration also has a toll-free number to help parents to solve problems when using car safety seats: 800-424-9393.

It is especially important to make parents aware of the dangers of air bags to infants or small children. Air bags can prevent serious injuries to older children and adults. However in a crash, the

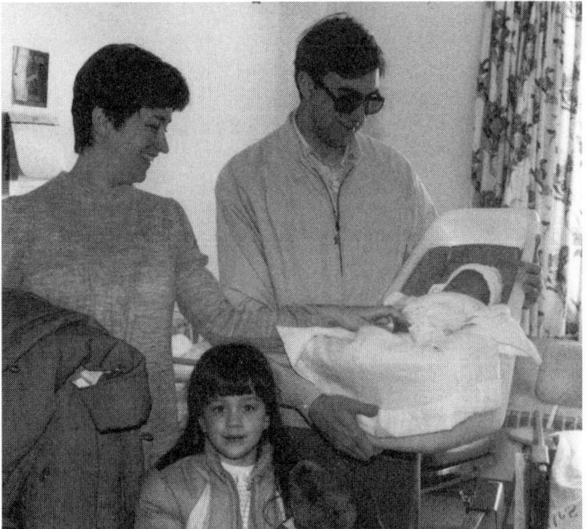

Figure 9–13. • A new family prepares to leave the birth facility. The infant is secured in a car safety seat that will be held by the car's seat belt for the ride home. (Courtesy of St. Joseph Hospital, Nasuau, NH.)

air bag thrusts an infant toward the rear, causing a whip-like motion that can seriously injure the neck or head (see Fig. 17–10).

Because of the well-publicized dangers of air bags to youngsters and what seems like a great deal of trouble to use a car seat, some parents are tempted to hold the baby in their arms, especially for short trips. Emphasize to the parent that even in a low-impact accident, their baby will probably be thrust from their arms and become a missile in the car or even be ejected from the car. Death is a likely result.

New parents are often overwhelmed at the volume of information given in such a short time. Reassure them that the birth facility staff is available 24 hours a day to help them to care for their baby and to refresh their memory if they forget what they have been told.

KEY POINTS

- It is essential to consider each client individually to better incorporate their special needs into the plan of care.
- The major risk for the fourth stage of labor is hemorrhage, usually from a poorly contracted uterus. Regular assessment of the fundus, lochia, and vital signs helps to identify hemorrhage quickly for prompt intervention.
- From its level at the umbilicus, the uterus should descend about one fingerbreadth per day. It should no longer be palpable at 10 days postpartum. Women who have had several babies or whose uterus was overdistended may have a slightly larger uterine size at any stage postpartum.
- A slow pulse is common in the early postpartum period. A pulse rate that would be high normal at other times may indicate hemorrhage or infection.
- A full bladder interferes with uterine contraction, which can lead to hemorrhage.
- Measures to prevent constipation should be emphasized at each assessment: fluid intake, a high-fiber diet, and activity.
- RhoGAM is given within 72 hours to the Rh-negative mother who delivers a Rh-positive infant.
- Early care of the newborn focuses on maintaining adequate cardiorespiratory function, normal temperature regulation, and adequate glucose levels.
- Screening tests such as PKU identify disorders that can be treated to reduce or prevent disability.
- The nurse must always keep the possibility of infant abductions in mind when providing care. The facility's specific protocol should be maintained during care. Most persons will not be offended by precautions, but will be grateful for the security.
- Bonding and attachment require contact between parents and infant. The nurse should promote this contact by every possible means.
- More breast milk removed equals more milk produced. Early, regular, and frequent nursing promotes milk production and lessens engorgement.
- Duration of nursing on the first breast should be at least 10 minutes to stimulate milk production.
- The nursing mother needs 500 extra calories each day plus enough fluid to relieve thirst (about 8 to 10 glasses).
- Weaning from the breast should be gradual, starting with the feeding the baby is least interested in and ending with the one in which he or she has most interest.
- The three major formula types are modified cow's milk, soy protein, or protein hydrolysate. They are available in ready-to-feed, concentrated liquid, or powdered form. Dilution, if required, must be followed exactly according to instructions.
- Discharge planning should take place with every instance of mother or newborn nursing care as the nurse teaches the mother normal findings, significance, and what to report. Written materials should augment all teaching.

MULTIPLE-CHOICE REVIEW QUESTIONS

Choose the most appropriate answer.

1. Which of these assessments is expected 24 hours after birth?
   a. Scant amount of lochia alba on the perineal pad
   b. Fundus firm and in the midline of the abdomen
   c. Breasts distended and hard with flat nipples
   d. Slight separation of a perineal laceration
2. Nursing the infant promotes uterine involution because it
   a. uses maternal fat stores accumulated during pregnancy.
   b. stimulates additional secretion of colostrum.
   c. causes the pituitary to secrete oxytocin to contract the uterus.
   d. promotes maternal formation of antibodies.
3. The best way to maintain the newborn's temperature immediately after birth is to
   a. dry the baby thoroughly, including the hair.
   b. give the baby a bath using warm water.
   c. feed 1 to 2 ounces of warmed formula.
   d. limit the length of time parents hold the baby.
4. When teaching new parents to use the bulb syringe, the nurse should tell them to
   a. insert the tip of the bulb syringe into the center of the mouth.
   b. compress the bulb after the tip is inserted into the mouth.
   c. suction the mouth before suctioning the nose.
   d. place the baby in a prone position after suctioning is completed.
5. A new mother asks how often she should nurse her baby. The nurse should tell her to feed the baby
   a. on a regular schedule, every 2 hours.
   b. on demand, about every 2 to 3 hours.
   c. at least every 4 hours during the day.
   d. whenever the baby is interested.

BIBLIOGRAPHY AND READER REFERENCE

American Academy of Pediatrics (AAP) & American College of Obstetricians and Gynecologists (ACOG). (1997). *Guidelines for perinatal care* (4th ed.). Elk Grove Village, IL, and Washington, DC: Authors.

Ashwill, J. A., & Droske, S. C. (1997). *Nursing care of children: Principles and practice.* Philadelphia: Saunders.

Blackburn, S. T., & Loper, D. L. (1992). *Maternal, fetal, and neonatal physiology: A clinical perspective.* Philadelphia: Saunders.

Cunningham, F. G., MacDonald, P. C., Gant, N. F., et al. (1997). *Williams Obstetrics,* 20th ed. Stamford, CT: Appleton & Lange.

Ferguson, S. L., & Engelhard, C. L. (1997). Short stay: The art of legislating quality and economy. *Lifelines, 1*(1), 17–23.

Gorrie, T. M., McKinney, E. S., & Murray, S. S. (1998). *Foundations of maternal-newborn nursing* (2nd ed.). Philadelphia: Saunders.

Grohar, J. (1996). Postpartum care. In K. R. Simpson & P. A. Creehan (Eds.), *AWHONN's perinatal nursing* (pp. 249–270). Philadelphia: Lippincott.

Johnson & Johnson Consumer Products, Inc., & Association of Women's Health Obstetric, and Neonatal Nurses. (1996). *Compendium of postpartum care.* Skillman, NJ: Authors.

Kowalski, K. (1996). Loss and bereavement: Psychological, sociological, spiritual, and ontological perspectives. In K. R. Simpson & P. A. Creehan (Eds.), *AWHONN's perinatal nursing* (pp. 271–286). Philadelphia: Lippincott.

Miklos, A. B., & Creehan, P. A. (1996). Newborn physical assessment. In K. R. Simpson & P. A. Creehan (Eds.), *AWHONN's perinatal nursing* (pp. 307–336). Philadelphia: Lippincott.

Moore, K., & Chute, G. (1996). Newborn nutrition. In K. R. Simpson & P. A. Creehan (Eds.), *AWHONN's perinatal nursing* (pp. 337–354). Philadelphia: Lippincott.

Moran, C. F., Holt, V. L., & Martin, D. P. (1997). What do women want to know after childbirth? *Birth, 24*(1), 27–34.

Penny-MacGillivray, T. (1996). A newborn's first bath: When? *Journal of Obstetric, Gynecologic, and Neonatal Nursing, 25*(6), 481–487.

Reimann, D., & Coughlin, M. (1996). Newborn adaptation to extrauterine life. In K. R. Simpson & P. A. Creehan (Eds.), *AWHONN's perinatal nursing* (pp. 289–306). Philadelphia: Lippincott.

Schneiderman, J. U. (1996). Postpartum nursing for Korean mothers. *MCN: American Journal of Maternal-Child Nursing, 21*(3), 155–158.

U.S. Public Health Service. (1995). Put prevention into practice: Newborn screening. *Journal of the American Academy of Nurse Practitioners, 7*(10), 513–517.

chapter 10

Nursing Care of Women with Complications Following Birth

Outline

Objectives

On completion and mastery of Chapter 10, the student will be able to

- Define each vocabulary term listed.
- Describe signs and symptoms for each postpartum complication.
- Identify factors that increase a woman's risk for developing each complication.
- Explain nursing measures that reduce a woman's risk for developing specific postpartum complications.
- Describe additional problems that may result from the original postpartum complication.
- Describe medical management of postpartum complications.
- Explain general and specific nursing care for each complication.

Vocabulary

atony
curettage
hematoma
hypovolemic shock
involution
mania
mastitis
metritis
mood
psychosis

Most women who have a baby recover from pregnancy and childbirth uneventfully. However, some have complications after birth that slow their recovery. Most childbearing women fully recover from these complications, but the problems interfere with their ability to assume their new role.

A woman can have any medical problem after a birth, but most complications fall into one of five categories:

- Hemorrhage
- Thromboembolic disorders
- Infections
- Subinvolution of the uterus
- Mood disorders

Of these classifications, hemorrhage and infection are the two most commonly encountered. Thromboembolic disorders may occur either during pregnancy or after birth.

Each type of complication has specific risk factors, although a woman who has no identified risk factor may also have complications. If a woman has any risk factors for a complication, the nurse should be especially alert for its development.

HEMORRHAGE

Postpartum hemorrhage is traditionally defined as blood loss greater than 500 ml after vaginal birth, or 1000 ml after cesarean birth. Postpartum blood losses that exceed 500 ml are fairly common, but losses exceeding 1000 ml are unusual. Because the average-size woman has 1 to 2 liters of added blood volume from pregnancy, she can tolerate this amount blood loss better than would otherwise be expected.

Most cases of hemorrhage occur immediately after birth, but some are delayed up to several weeks.

- Early postpartum hemorrhage occurs within 24 hours of birth
- Late postpartum hemorrhage occurs after 24 hours until 6 weeks after birth

Overview

The major risk of hemorrhage is *hypovolemic* (low-volume) *shock,* which interrupts blood flow to body cells. This prevents normal oxygenation, nutrient delivery, and waste removal at the cell level. Although a less dramatic problem, anemia is likely to occur after hemorrhage.

Hypovolemic Shock

Hypovolemic shock occurs when the volume of blood is depleted and cannot fill the circulatory system. The woman will die if blood loss does not stop and if the blood volume is not corrected.

Body Response to Hypovolemia. The body initially responds to reduced blood volume with increased heart and respiratory rates. These reactions increase the oxygen content of each erythrocyte (red blood cell) and more quickly circulate the remaining blood. *Tachycardia (rapid heart rate) is usually the first sign of inadequate blood volume (hypovolemia).* The first blood pressure change is a narrow pulse pressure (a falling systolic pressure and rising diastolic pressure). The blood pressure continues falling, and eventually cannot be detected.

Blood flow to nonessential organs gradually stops to make more available for vital organs, specifically the heart and brain. This change causes the woman's skin and mucous membranes to become pale, cold, and clammy (moist). As blood loss continues, flow to the brain falls, resulting in mental changes, such as anxiety, confusion, restlessness, and lethargy. As blood flow to the kidneys decreases, they respond by conserving fluid. Urine output decreases and eventually stops.

Medical Management. Medical management of hypovolemic shock resulting from hemorrhage may include any of the following actions:

- Stopping the blood loss
- Giving intravenous fluids to maintain circulating volume and to replace fluids
- Giving blood transfusions to replace lost erythrocytes
- Giving oxygen to increase saturation of remaining blood cells; a pulse oximeter is used to assess oxygen saturation of the blood
- Placing an indwelling (Foley) catheter to assess urine output, which reflects kidney circulation

Intensive care may be required to allow invasive hemodynamic monitoring of the woman's circulatory status. Nursing Care Plan 10–1 specifies interventions for the woman at high risk for altered tissue perfusion related to hemorrhage.

Anemia. Anemia occurs after hemorrhage because of the lost erythrocytes. Anemia resulting from blood loss occurs suddenly, and the woman may be dizzy or lightheaded and is likely to faint. These symptoms are more likely to occur if she changes position quickly, particularly from a lying position to an upright one.

Until her hemoglobin and hematocrit counts return to near-normal values, she will probably be exhausted and have difficulty meeting her needs and those of her infant. She is more likely to develop an infection while her body defenses are down.

Iron supplements are prescribed to provide adequate amounts of this mineral for manufacture of more erythrocytes. Many physicians and nurse-midwives have the woman continue taking the remainder of her prenatal vitamins, which provide enough iron to correct mild anemia.

Early Postpartum Hemorrhage

Early postpartum hemorrhage is due to one of three causes:

- Uterine atony
- Lacerations (tears) of the reproductive tract
- Hematomas in the reproductive tract

Of these three, uterine atony is the most common. Table 10–1 summarizes care for these causes of hemorrhage.

Uterine Atony

Atony describes a lack of normal muscle tone. The uterus is a large, hollow organ that has three layers of muscle. The middle layer has interlacing "figure-eight" fibers. The uterine blood supply must pass through this network of muscle fibers to supply the placenta. Contraction of the uterine muscle after birth is essential to limit blood loss after the placenta is expelled from its site.

Blood clotting is not adequate to control blood loss after the birth of the placenta; blood flows from open uterine vessels too rapidly to allow clotting. After the placenta detaches, the uterus contracts and the muscle fibers compress bleeding vessels. If the uterus is atonic, these muscle fibers are flaccid and do not compress the vessels. Uterine atony allows the blood vessels at the placenta site to bleed freely and usually massively.

Normal Postpartum Changes. After birth, the uterus should easily be felt through the abdominal wall as a firm mass about the size of a grapefruit. Immediately after the placenta is expelled, the fundus (top) is about halfway between the umbilicus and symphysis (see Chapter 9). Within a few hours, the fundus rises to about the umbilicus level and then begins descending at a rate of about 1 fingerbreadth (1 cm) each day.

Lochia rubra should be dark red. The amount of lochia during the first few hours should be no more than one saturated perineal pad within 1 hour. (Perineal pads containing cold packs absorb less than regular perineal pads.) A few small clots may appear in the drainage, but large clots are not normal.

Characteristics of Uterine Atony. When uterine atony occurs, the woman's uterus is difficult to feel, and when found, it is boggy (soft). The fundal height is high, often above the umbilicus. If the bladder is full, the uterus is higher and pushed to one side rather than being in the midline of the abdomen (Fig. 10–1). The uterus may or may not be soft if the bladder is full. However, a full bladder interferes with the ability of the uterus to contract and if not corrected, eventually leads to uterine atony.

Lochia is increased, and may contain large clots. The bleeding may be dramatic, but it also may be just above normal for a long time. Some lochia will be retained in the relaxed uterus because the cavity is enlarged. Thus, the true amount of blood loss may not be immediately apparent. Collection of blood within the uterus further interferes with contraction and worsens uterine atony and postpartum hemorrhage.

Risk Factors. Uterine atony can occur in women who have no added risk factors, but it should be anticipated in some women. Uterine atony is more common in many situations, explaining why it is the most common cause of early postpartum hemorrhage. Some of the these risk factors include the following:

- Urinary bladder distention
- Abnormal labor (see p. 198)
- Uterine overdistention from any cause, such as a multifetal pregnancy, large infant, or excessive amniotic fluid (hydramnios)
- Multiparity, especially over five births
- Stimulation of labor with oxytocin
- Abnormal labor pattern such as prolonged or precipitate
- Placental abnormalities
    - Previa (low implantation)
    - Accreta (abnormally adherent)
    - Retention of a large piece

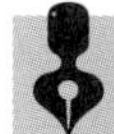

Nursing Tip

To determine blood loss most accurately, weigh perineal pads before and after applying them. One gram of weight equals about 1 ml of blood lost.

NURSING CARE PLAN 10–1

Selected Nursing Diagnoses for the Woman with Postpartum Hemorrhage

Nursing Diagnosis: Risk for altered tissue perfusion related to excessive blood loss secondary to uterine atony or birth injury

Goals	Intervention	Rationale
The woman's blood pressure and pulse will be within 10% of her values when she was admitted. The woman will not have signs or symptoms of hypovolemic shock	1. Identify whether woman has added risk factors for postpartum hemorrhage	1. Women who have risk factors should be assessed more frequently than those who do not
	2. Assess woman's a. Fundus for height, firmness, and position b. Lochia for color, quantity, and clots; count pads and degree of saturation (weigh pads for greater accuracy); check blood pressure, pulse and respiratory rates	2. The fundus must be firm to compress bleeding vessels at the placenta site; bladder distention interferes with uterine contraction and causes the fundus to be high and displaced to one side; a rising pulse rate is often first sign of inadequate blood volume; a rising pulse and falling blood pressure also occur; most blood lost after birth is visible rather than concealed, observing lochia provides an estimate of actual blood loss
	3. Observe for less obvious signs of bleeding: a. Constant trickle of brighter red blood with a firm fundus b. Severe, poorly relieved pain, especially if accompanied by changes in the vital signs or shock signs and symptoms	3. Most postpartum hemorrhage is caused by uterine atony, which often produces dramatic dramatic blood loss, however, blood loss from a laceration or hematoma can be significant, even though it is less obvious
	4. Observe for other signs and symptoms of hypovolemic shock	4. Excessive blood loss can result in hypovolemic shock
	5. If signs of hemorrhage are noted, take appropriate actions, according to probable cause for hemorrhage: a. Uterine atony: massage uterus until firm—do not overmassage; expel blood from uterine cavity when uterus is firm; have breastfeeding woman nurse baby; notify registered nurse and/or physician or nurse-midwife for orders and medication if uterus does not become firm and stay firm b. Lacerations: notify registered nurse and/or physician or nurse-midwife to examine woman c. Hematomas on the vulva: place cold pack on the area	5. Hemorrhage can cause death of a new mother if not promptly corrected; most minor episodes of uterine atony are easily corrected with fundal massage and infant suckling; if the uterus does not remain firm, physician or nurse-midwife examines woman to identify and correct cause of bleeding; oxytocin (Pitocin) infusions are often ordered to contract the uterus. Other drugs, such as methylergonovine (Methergine) or prostaglandin, may be needed; overmassage of uterus can tire it, possibly resulting in inability to contract. Trauma such as laceration or hematoma may require repair by physician or nurse-midwife; small hematomas on vulva can be limited by cold applications because they reduce blood flow to area; cold applications also numb area and make woman more comfortable

Nursing Diagnosis: Risk for injury (falls) related to anemia secondary to blood loss

Goals	Intervention	Rationale
The woman will not fall or have other injury while in birth facility	1. Caution woman not to get out of bed without help until her condition has stabilized	1. While lying in bed, woman may not realize that she is likely to be dizzy or lightheaded when she ambulates

Continued on following page

NURSING CARE PLAN 10–1 *(Continued)*

Selected Nursing Diagnoses for the Woman with Postpartum Hemorrhage

Nursing Diagnosis: Risk for injury (falls) related to anemia secondary to blood loss *(Continued)*

Goals	Intervention	Rationale
	2. When helping woman out of bed, partially elevate head of bed, then help to rise slowly to a sitting position on the side of the bed	2. Blood loss reduces amount of circulating blood volume; woman may not have enough volume to maintain circulation to all parts of her body if she changes position quickly
	3. Before she stands or walks, have her sit on side of bed for a few minutes; have her rotate her feet and ankles and move her legs as she sits on bed	3. Gradual changes of position reduce risk that she will fall because her circulatory system adapts to the change; moving her feet and legs prevents blood from pooling in her lower extremities
	4. Remain with woman when she walks; after she is stable and has been up several times, a family member can walk with her	4. Someone accompanying woman can prevent her from falling if she becomes dizzy or faint
	5. If woman feels faint, have her sit down immediately; if she faints, gently lower her to floor	5. Prevents injury due to a fall if woman does faint

- Medications that relax the uterus, such as magnesium sulfate, tocolytic drugs (see p. 209), some general anesthetics
- Operative birth (cesarean, forceps- or vacuum extractor-assisted)
- Clotting abnormalities worsen hemorrhage

A woman who has risk factors should have more frequent postpartum assessments of the uterus and lochia.

Medical and Nursing Treatment. Care of the woman with uterine atony combines nursing and medical measures. When the uterus is boggy, it should be massaged until firm (see Procedure p. 224). One nurse institutes emergency measures, such as fundal massage, while another notifies the physician or nurse-midwife if blood loss is severe.

The uterus should not be overmassaged. Because it is a muscle, excessive stimulation to contract the uterus will tire it and can actually worsen uterine

Table 10–1
TYPES OF EARLY POSTPARTUM HEMORRHAGE

	Uterine Atony	Lacerations	Hematoma
Characteristics	Soft, high uterine fundus that is difficult to feel through the woman's abdominal wall Heavy lochia, often with large clots or sometimes a persistent moderate flow Bladder distention that causes uterus to be high and usually displaces it to one side Possible signs of hypovolemic shock	Continuous trickle of blood that is brighter than normal lochia Fundus is usually firm Onset of hypovolemic shock that may be gradual and easily overlooked	If visible, blue or purplish mass on the vulva Severe and poorly relieved pain and/or pressure in vulva, pelvis, or rectum Large amount of blood lost into tissues, which causes signs and symptoms of hypovolemic shock Lochia that is normal in amount and color
Contributing factors	Bladder distention Abnormal or prolonged labor Overdistended uterus Multiparity (>5 births) Use of oxytocin during labor Medications that relax uterus Placental abnormalities Operative birth	Rapid labor Use of instruments, such as forceps or vacuum extractor, during birth	Prolonged or rapid labor Large infant Use of forceps or vacuum extractor

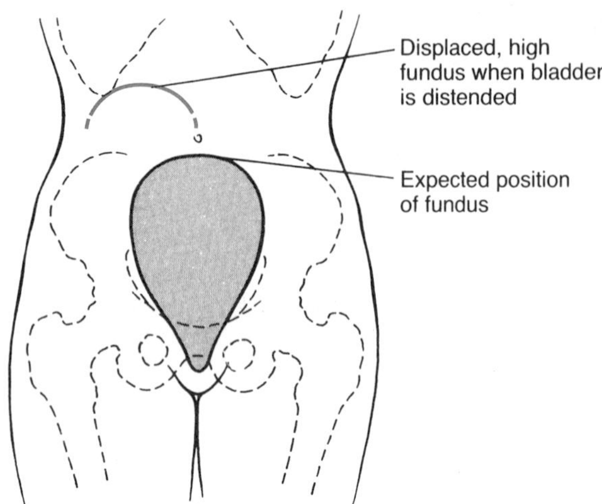

Figure 10–1. • A distended bladder pushes the uterus upward and usually to one side of the abdomen. The fundus may be boggy or firm. If not emptied, a distended bladder can result in uterine atony and hemorrhage because it interferes with normal contraction of the uterus.

atony. If the uterus is firmly contracted, leave it alone.

Bladder distention is an easily corrected cause of uterine atony. If the woman cannot urinate in the bathroom or on a bedpan, the nurse should catheterize her. Any clots or blood pooled in the vagina should be expelled by pressing toward the vagina *after the uterus is firm.* Most physicians and nurse-midwives include an order for catheterization to avoid delaying this corrective measure. First, massage the uterus to firmness, then empty the bladder to keep the uterus firm.

Infant suckling at the breast stimulates the woman's posterior pituitary gland to secrete oxytocin, which causes uterine contraction. Dilute oxytocin (Pitocin) infusion is the most common drug ordered to control uterine atony. Other drugs to increase uterine tone include methylergonovine (Methergine) or prostaglandin $F_{2\alpha}$. Methylergonovine increases blood pressure and should not be given to a woman with hypertension.

The physician may examine the woman in the delivery or operating room to determine the source of her bleeding and correct it. The physician may perform bimanual compression, a technique to compress the uterus between one hand in her vagina and the other on her abdomen. Rarely, hysterectomy is needed to remove the bleeding uterus that does not respond to other measures. The woman should have nothing by mouth until her bleeding is controlled.

Lacerations of the Reproductive Tract

Lacerations of the perineum, vagina, cervix, or area around the urethra (periurethral lacerations) can cause postpartum bleeding. They are more likely to occur if the woman has a rapid labor or if forceps or a vacuum extractor were used. Blood lost in lacerations is usually a brighter red than lochia and flows in a continuous trickle. Typically, the uterus is firm.

Treatment. If the woman has signs of a laceration, bleeding with a firmly contracted uterus, the physician or nurse-midwife should be notified. The injury is usually sutured in the delivery or operating room.

Nursing Care. Report signs and symptoms of a bleeding laceration. *A continuous trickle of blood can result in as much or more blood loss than the dramatic bleeding associated with uterine atony.* Keep the woman NPO until further orders are received because she may need a general anesthetic for repair of the laceration.

Hematomas

A *hematoma* is a collection of blood within the tissues. Hematomas resulting from birth trauma are usually on the vulva or inside the vagina. They may be easily seen as a bulging, bluish, or purplish mass (Fig. 10–2). Hematomas deep within the vagina are not visible from the outside.

Discomfort after childbirth is normally minimal and easily relieved with mild analgesics. The woman with a hematoma usually has severe, unrelenting pain that analgesics do not relieve. Depending on the amount of blood in the tissues, she also may describe pressure in the vulva, pelvis, or rectum. She may be unable to urinate because of the pressure.

The woman does not have unusual amounts of lochia, but she may develop signs of concealed blood loss if the hematoma is large. Her pulse and respiratory rates rise, and her blood pressure falls. She may develop other signs of hypovolemic shock if blood loss into the tissues is substantial.

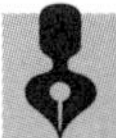

Nursing Tip

The woman who develops a hemorrhagic complication should be kept NPO until the physician or nurse-midwife evaluates her in case she needs general anesthesia to correct the problem.

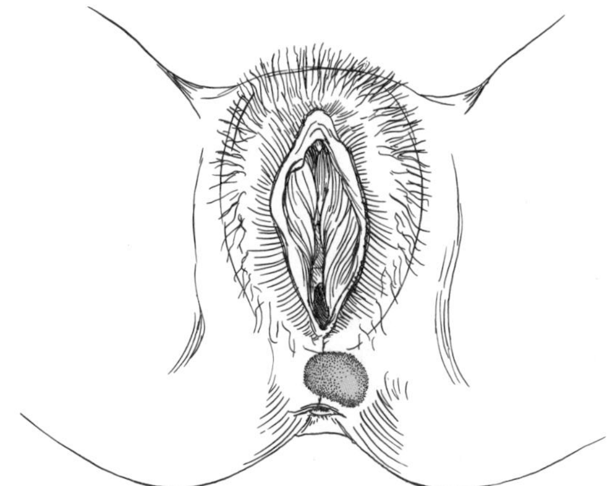

Figure 10–2. • A hematoma on the vulva is a collection of blood within the soft tissues. It is a blue or purple mass. Cold applications may limit the hematoma.

Risk factors for development of a hematoma include:

- Prolonged or rapid labor
- Large baby
- Use of forceps or vacuum extractor

Treatment. Small hematomas usually resolve without treatment. Larger ones may require incision and drainage of the clots. The bleeding vessel is ligated or the area packed with a hemostatic material to stop bleeding.

Nursing Care. An ice pack to the perineum is sufficient for most small hematomas and requires no order. Observe and report for the classic symptom: excessive, poorly relieved pain. Report signs of concealed blood loss accompanied by maternal complaints of severe pain, perineal or vaginal pressure, or the inability to void. Notify the physician promptly if the woman has symptoms of a hematoma, even if none can be seen on the outside. Keep her NPO until the physician examines her and other orders are received.

Late Postpartum Hemorrhage

Late postpartum hemorrhage (after 24 hours to 6 weeks after birth) is usually due to

- Retention of placental fragments
- Subinvolution of the uterus (discussed on p. 271)

Late postpartum hemorrhage usually occurs after discharge. It begins without warning and may be profuse.

Placental fragments are more likely to be retained if the placenta does not separate cleanly from its implantation site after birth. Clots form around these retained fragments and slough several days later, sometimes carrying the retained fragments with them. Retained placental fragments are more likely to occur if the placenta is manually removed (removed by hand, rather than being pushed away from the uterine wall spontaneously as the uterus contracts). It is also more likely to occur if the placenta grows more deeply into the uterine muscle than is normal.

Treatment. Treatment consists of drugs, such as oxytocin, methylergonovine, or prostaglandins, to contract the uterus. Firm uterine contraction often sweeps the retained fragments out and no other treatment will be needed. Ultrasonography may be used to identify remaining fragments. If bleeding continues, *curettage* (scraping or vacuuming the inner surface of the uterus) is done to remove small blood clots and placental fragments. Antibiotics are prescribed if infection is suspected.

Nursing Care. The nurse should teach each postpartum woman what to expect about changes in the lochia (see p. 222). Teach her to report signs of late postpartum hemorrhage to her physician or nurse-midwife:

- Persistent red bleeding
- Return of red bleeding after it has changed to pinkish or white

If a late postpartum hemorrhage occurs, the nurse assists in implementing drug and surgical treatment.

THROMBOEMBOLIC DISORDERS

Venous thrombosis is more likely to occur when three conditions exist:

- Presence of increased clotting factors
- Venous stasis
- Injury to the inner surface (intima) of the vein

In normal pregnancy, two of these conditions exist: increased clotting factors and venous stasis caused by pressure of the growing uterus on veins that return blood to the heart. Injury to the inner vein surface is unlikely to occur unless the woman has a pelvic infection or cesarean delivery.

Risk Factors. Some women have added risk factors for thrombus formation. These may include the following:

- Varicose veins
- Obesity
- Smoking
- Age over 35 years
- Cesarean birth
- Over three pregnancies

Manifestations. Signs and symptoms depend on whether the disorder is a superficial vein thrombosis or deep vein thrombosis.

- *Superficial vein thrombosis* is characterized by a painful, hard, reddened, warm vein that is easily seen.
- *Deep vein thrombosis* is characterized by pain, calf tenderness, leg edema, color changes, pain when walking, and sometimes a positive Homan's sign (pain when the foot is dorsiflexed), although the Homan's sign is not reliable during the postpartum period.

The greatest risk of deep vein thrombosis is that a clot will break off (embolize) and lodge in the blood vessels of the lungs (pulmonary embolism).

Pulmonary embolism may have dramatic signs and symptoms, such as sudden chest pain, cough, dyspnea (difficulty breathing), depressed consciousness, and signs of heart failure. A small pulmonary embolism may have nonspecific signs and symptoms, such as shortness of breath, palpitations, hemoptysis (bloody sputum), faintness, and low-grade fever. Table 10–2 compares the manifestations and likelihood of pulmonary embolism of superficial vein thrombosis with those of deep vein thrombosis.

Table 10–2
ASSESSMENT OF VENOUS THROMBOSIS

Location	Manifestations	Pulmonary Embolism
Superficial vein thrombosis	Tender, painful hard, reddened area along warm vein; easily visible	Rare
Deep vein thrombosis	Increased pain and calf tenderness; leg edema, color and temperature changes; positive Homan's sign may be present but is unreliable during the postpartum; occasional fever rarely over 101°F (38.3°C)	Possible

Treatment. Superficial vein thrombosis is treated with analgesics, local application of heat, and elevation of the legs to promote venous drainage. Deep vein thrombosis is treated similarly, with the addition of heparin anticoagulation. Anticoagulant therapy is continued with heparin or warfarin (Coumadin) for 6 weeks after birth to minimize the risk of embolism. Antibiotics are prescribed if infection is a factor. See a medical-surgical nursing text for treatment and nursing care of pulmonary embolism.

Nursing Care. Observe for signs and symptoms that suggest venous thrombosis before and after birth. Dyspnea, coughing, and chest pain suggest pulmonary embolism and must be reported immediately.

Pregnant women should not cross their legs, which impedes venous blood flow. When the legs are elevated, there should not be sharp flexion at the groin or pressure in the popliteal space behind the knee, which would restrict venous flow. Measures to promote venous flow should be continued during and after birth, because levels of clotting factors remain high for several weeks.

Teach the woman who will be on anticoagulant therapy at home to give herself the drug and about signs of excess anticoagulation (prolonged bleeding from minor injuries, bleeding gums, nosebleeds, unexplained bruising). Teach her to use a soft toothbrush and to avoid minor trauma that can cause prolonged bleeding or a large hematoma. Home nursing visits are often prescribed to obtain blood for laboratory clotting studies and to help the woman to cope with therapy.

INFECTION

New mothers may acquire a variety of infections after birth. Many of these have their origins during pregnancy or labor but may not become apparent until after birth. The most likely sites for postpartum infection are

- Wounds such as from an episiotomy, laceration, or surgical incision
- Uterus
- Urinary tract
- Breast

Table 10–3 lists characteristics, medical treatment, and nursing care for these infections.

Table 10–3
POSTPARTUM INFECTIONS

	Wound Infections	Endometritis (Uterus)	Urinary Tract	Mastitis (Breast)
Characteristics	Signs of inflammation (redness, edema, heat, pain) Separation of suture line Purulent drainage	Tender, enlarged uterus Prolonged, severe cramping Foul-smelling lochia Fever and other systemic signs of infection Signs of uterine subinvolution	Cystitis (bladder) Low temperature Burning, urgency, and frequency of urination Pyelonephritis (kidneys) High fever with a pattern of spikes Chills Pain in the costovertebral angle or flank Nausea and vomiting	Reddened, tender, hot area of the breast Edema and a feeling of heaviness in the breast Purulent drainage may occur if an abscess forms
Medical treatment	Culture and sensitivity of wound exudate Antibiotics	Culture and sensitivity of uterine cavity Antibiotics by IV route initially	Clean-catch or catheterized urine specimen for culture and sensitivity testing Antibiotics (initially by IV route for pyelonephritis)	Antibiotics (usually oral, although may be IV initially if woman has an abscess) Incision and drainage of abscess
Nursing care	Aseptic/sterile technique for all wound care, as indicated Teach proper perineal hygiene to reduce fecal contamination Sitz baths for perineal wound infections	Teach woman usual progression of lochia, since infection often occurs after discharge Fowler's position to facilitate drainage of infected lochia Analgesics Observation for absent bowel sounds, abdominal distention, and nausea or vomiting, which suggest spread of infection	Teach perineal hygiene Encouraging fluid intake of 3 l/day Teaching which foods increase acidity of urine, such as apricots, cranberry juice, plums, and prunes	Teach effective breastfeeding techniques Moist heat applications with a warm pack Warm shower before nursing to start milk flow Massage of affected area to reduce congestion and start milk flow Regular and frequent nursing or pumping to keep breasts empty

Overview

Regardless of their location or the causative organism, postpartum infections have several common features.

Manifestations. Puerperal (postpartum) morbidity (illness) is defined as a temperature of 38°C (100.4°F) or higher after the first 24 hours and occurring on at least 2 days during the first 10 days after birth. Slight temperature elevations, with no other signs of infection, often occur during the first 24 hours because of dehydration. The nurse should look for other signs of infection if the woman's temperature is elevated, regardless of the time since birth. A pulse that is higher than expected plus an elevated temperature are often found if the woman has an infection.

Nursing Tip

Because postpartum women often have a slow pulse, suspect hypovolemic shock or infection if the pulse rate is higher than 100 beats/min.

Other signs and symptoms of infection may be localized (in a small area of the body) or systemic (throughout the body). Redness, edema, and pain are examples of localized signs and symptoms. Fever, malaise, achiness, and loss of appetite are examples of systemic signs and symptoms of infection.

White blood cells (leukocytes) are normally elevated during the early postpartum period to about 20,000 to 30,000/dl, which limits the usefulness of the blood count to identify infection. Leukocyte counts in the upper limits are more likely to be associated with infection than lower counts, however.

Risk Factors. Birth involves some amount of trauma, providing a portal of entry for microorgan-

NURSING CARE PLAN 10-2

Selected Nursing Diagnosis for the Woman with Postpartum Infection

Nursing Diagnosis: Risk for infection related to loss of skin integrity (cesarean incision) and increased risk factors (prolonged labor)

Goals	Interventions	Rationale
The woman will not have signs of infection, as evidenced by oral temperature below 38°C (100.4°F) and normal progression of lochia that does not have a foul odor	1. Use handwashing when providing care; teach woman personal hygiene measures, such as handwashing, perineal care, regular changes of perineal pads	1. Limits transfer of infectious organisms between clients and from one area of the body to another; regular pad changes also reduce amount of time organisms have to multiply in its warm, dark, and moist environment
	2. Assess vital signs every 4 hr or more frequently if signs of infection are present	2. An elevated temperature and rising pulse are signs of infection; if they occur, woman should be assessed for other signs and symptoms of infection
	3. Assess lochia for amount, color, and odor with vital signs	3. Endometritis is more common if a woman has a cesarean birth and is evidenced by foul-smelling lochia that may be increased or decreased; it is sometimes brown
	4. Assess uterus for height, firmness, and descent	4. Metritis is characterized by an enlarged, tender uterus
	5. Assess for cramping or other pain	5. Prolonged cramping may occur with metritis; a wound infection may be painful
	6. Assess the wound each shift for redness, edema, discharge, and intactness	6. A wound infection is characterized by signs of inflammation; the suture line may separate if there is infection in the area
	7. Assess for signs and symptoms of urinary tract infection (see p. 269). Encourage high fluid intake (3 liters/day)	7. Identifies possible presence of urinary tract infection so that it can be reported to the physician; high fluid intake regularly flushes microorganisms from bladder and reduces chance that they will infect the urinary tract

Continued on following page

isms that naturally inhabit the vaginal and rectal area. Breastfeeding can result in small cracks in the nipples. The warm, dark, moist environment of the uterus provides a good growth medium for bacteria. Additionally, the vagina is less acidic after birth, which fosters the growth of microorganisms.

The organs of the reproductive tract are especially vulnerable to infection because they are interconnected. During pregnancy and for a time after birth, the reproductive organs are richly supplied with blood. These two characteristics make it easy for an infection in one organ to spread to another or to enter the circulation and infect a distant part of the body.

Some women have added risk for infection. Conditions that increase a woman's risk for developing infection include the following:

- Cesarean birth
- Use of forceps or vacuum extractor
- Long labor
- Prolonged rupture of membranes, especially for longer than 24 hours
- Urinary catheterization
- Repeated vaginal examinations during labor
- Retained fragments of placenta
- Hemorrhage or anemia

Nursing Tip

Proper handwashing is the primary method to avoid spread of infectious organisms. Gloves should be worn when contacting any body secretion.

NURSING CARE PLAN 10–2 *(Continued)*

Selected Nursing Diagnosis for the Woman with Postpartum Infection

Nursing Diagnosis: Risk for altered nutrition, less than body requirements, related to increased demand for nutrients

Goals	Interventions	Rationale
After teaching, the woman will verbalize foods that provide nutrients she needs for healing	1. Determine foods woman usually eats	1. Identifies her preferences and areas of nutrient adequacy or inadequacy; nurse can build on her preferences and dislikes
	2. Teach sources of foods high in protein, vitamin C, and iron: a. *Protein:* eggs, meats, cheeses, milk, legumes, combinations of grain foods b. *Vitamin C:* citrus fruits and juices, strawberries, cantaloupe, tomatoes, broccoli, peppers, cabbage c. *Iron:* meats, enriched cereals and breads, dark-green leafy vegetables, dried beans and fruits	2. Protein and vitamin C are necessary for healing; anemia, which is usually related to iron deficiency, can be corrected by high-iron foods; vitamin C may improve body's ability to use iron
	3. Reinforce physician's orders about vitamin supplements	3. Many physicians have woman take remainder of her prenatal vitamins to be certain she has adequate nutrients
	4. If woman is breastfeeding, incorporate diet recommendations for nursing mother into teaching (see p. 253)	4. Nursing mother requires added nutrients to meet her own needs for healing and restoration, plus enough to make breast milk
	5. Have woman restate appropriate foods to meet her nutritional needs	5. Evaluates what she learned and identifies need for further teaching
	6. Refer to social services for financial assistance, such as the Women, Infants, and Children (WIC) program for food supplementation	6. Helps to overcome financial barriers to obtaining adequate food

- Poor nutritional state
- Medical conditions such as diabetes mellitus

These risk factors are often linked to one another. For example, the woman who has a long labor often has prolonged ruptured membranes, many vaginal examinations, and a forceps or cesarean birth.

General Medical Treatment. The goals of medical treatment are to

- Limit the spread of infection to other organs
- Eliminate the infection

A culture and sensitivity of the site of the suspected infection is done to determine what antibiotics are effective. A culture and sensitivity requires 2 or 3 days to complete. In the meantime, antibiotics that are effective against typical organisms that cause the infection are given to limit the spread of infection to nearby structures.

General Nursing Care. Nursing care objectives focus on preventing infection and if one occurs, on facilitating medical treatment. To achieve these goals, the nurse should

- Use and teach hygienic measures to reduce the number of organisms that can cause infection, such as handwashing and perineal care
- Promote adequate rest and nutrition for healing
- Observe for signs of infection
- Teach signs of infection that the woman should report after she is discharged
- Teach the woman to take all of the antibiotics prescribed rather than stopping them after her symptoms go away

Women should be taught to wash their hands before and after doing self-care that may involve contact with secretions. The nurse should explore ways to help the woman get enough rest. Nursing Care Plan 10–2 details interventions for the woman at high risk for infection.

Ultimately, a woman's own body must overcome infection and heal any wound. Nutrition is an essential component of her body defenses. The nurse, and sometimes a dietitian, teaches her about foods that are high in protein (meats, cheese, milk, legumes) and vitamin C (citrus fruits and juices, strawberries, cantaloupe) because these nutrients are especially important for healing. Foods high in iron to correct anemia include meats, enriched cereals and breads, and dark-green, leafy vegetables.

Wound Infection

Wound infections can occur in a surgical incision, episiotomy, or lacerations. The REEDA criteria discussed in Chapter 9 are good to assess any type of wound for healing or presence of infection. The signs and symptoms are typical of localized infection anywhere in the body:

- Redness
- Warmth
- Edema
- Pain and localized tenderness
- Purulent (pus-containing) drainage which may have a foul odor
- Separation of suture line

The woman also may experience systemic signs and symptoms, such as fever and malaise. Septic pelvic thrombophlebitis occasionally occurs as the infection spreads along the venous system and thrombophlebitis develops.

Medical Treatment. The physician or nurse-midwife usually obtains a sample of the wound's exudate for a culture and sensitivity. Antibiotics are prescribed, usually by the oral route unless the infection is severe. The wound may be opened to allow drainage of the purulent exudate. Analgesics are usually prescribed.

Nursing Care. Nursing care begins with regular assessment of wounds for the signs of infection and teaching the woman what to observe. If they are found, they should be reported to the physician. Teach the woman signs to report because facility stays after birth are very short and most local infections will not be identified before discharge.

Cleanliness is promoted by using and teaching a good handwashing technique. Teach the woman to do perineal care following each urination or a bowel movement. To reduce the risk of carrying fecal organisms from the rectum to the vagina, teach her to use a front-to-back motion when she

- Performs perineal care
- Applies a perineal pad
- Wipes the perineal area after toileting

Teach the woman who has a cesarean birth to keep her incision clean and dry.

Observe for signs of infection and teach the woman to report fever or increasing pain from any wound to her physician or nurse-midwife. Normally, pain after birth decreases steadily. Persistent or increasing pain is often associated with infection. Any drainage should be reported as well.

Sitz baths several times each day may increase comfort and speed healing of infections located in the perineal area (see p. 226). The woman should use the sitz bath about 20 minutes at a time. Staying longer in the sitz bath will not harm her, but it has no added benefit. Warm compresses have a similar effect.

Uterine Infection

Metritis, also called *endometritis,* is an infection of the uterine lining, often at the site of the placenta. The woman has most systemic signs and symptoms of infection and looks sick. Specific signs and symptoms of metritis include

- Uterine tenderness
- Enlarged uterus
- Prolonged and severe cramping
- Foul-smelling lochia that may be increased or decreased in amount

Complications. The organisms causing metritis may spread to nearby organs or enter the circulation (Fig. 10–3). Infection from the uterus may spread to the

- Fallopian tubes (salpingitis)
- Ovaries (oophoritis)
- Connective tissues and ligaments (parametritis)
- Lining of the abdomen and pelvis (peritonitis)

Medical Treatment. Therapy includes culture and sensitivity studies, followed by immediate initiation of antibiotic treatment. Common antibiotics are ampicillin, cephalosporins, clindamycin, and gentamicin. The antibiotics are usually begun by the intravenous route and may be continued by the oral route after the acute phase of the infection. Two antibiotics may be combined. Analgesics for pain are ordered, and antipyretics are given to lower fever.

The breastfeeding mother may have to stop nursing to conserve her energy for healing if she is quite ill. A few antibiotics cannot be taken during breast feeding. If the mother wants to resume nursing

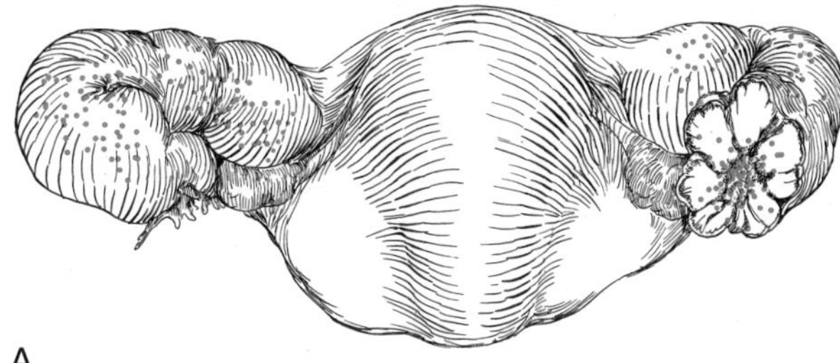

A

Salpingitis: Infection in fallopian tubes causes them to become enlarged, hyperemic, and tender

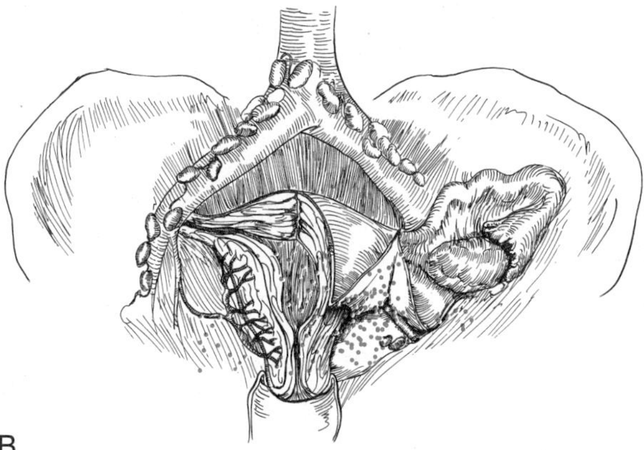

B

Parametritis: Infection spreads via lymphatics through uterine wall to connective tissue of broad ligament or entire pelvis

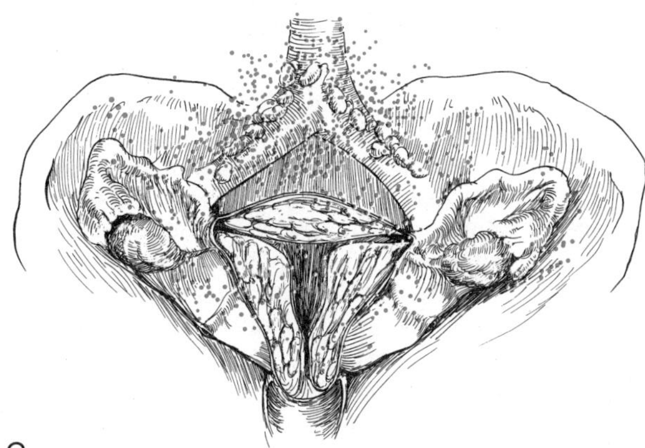

C

Peritonitis: Infection spreads via lymphatics to peritoneum: formation of a pelvic abscess may occur

Figure 10–3. • **A–C.** Metritis can spread to nearby organs if it is not eradicated promptly.

after the infection, she may pump her breasts to maintain lactation.

Nursing Care. Place the woman in a Fowler's (semi-sitting) position to promote drainage of the infected lochia. Regular perineal care and pad changes make the woman more comfortable. Perineal hygiene reduces the number of infectious organisms that may spread to the reproductive organs, an episiotomy incision or laceration, or the urinary tract. Give antibiotics and analgesics ordered. Comfort measures include warm blankets, cool compresses, sponge baths, perineal care, cold or warm drinks, or use of a heating pad.

Observe for signs of improvement or worsening of her condition. Her fever and discomfort should decline. Persistent or worsening discomfort, absence of bowel sounds, abdominal distention, or nausea and vomiting suggest that the infection has spread beyond the uterus.

Urinary Tract Infection

Infections of the bladder or kidneys are common after birth. Trauma during birth and incomplete emptying of the bladder increase the risk for infection. Many women are catheterized during labor, sometimes several times, which can carry organisms from the lower urethra into the bladder.

Infection may occur in the bladder (cystitis) or the kidneys (pyelonephritis). Cystitis is characterized by

- Low fever
- Burning pain during urination
- Urgency to urinate
- Increased frequency of urination, with small amounts voided each time

Pyelonephritis has more severe signs and symptoms:

- High fever with a spiking (abrupt up-and-down) pattern
- Chills
- Pain in the back, about the waistline, when the area is tapped (costovertebral angle [CVA] tenderness)
- Flank pain
- Nausea and vomiting

Medical Treatment. Oral antibiotics, such as ampicillin, are prescribed for cystitis. Intravenous antibiotics and supplemental fluids are ordered for pyelonephritis.

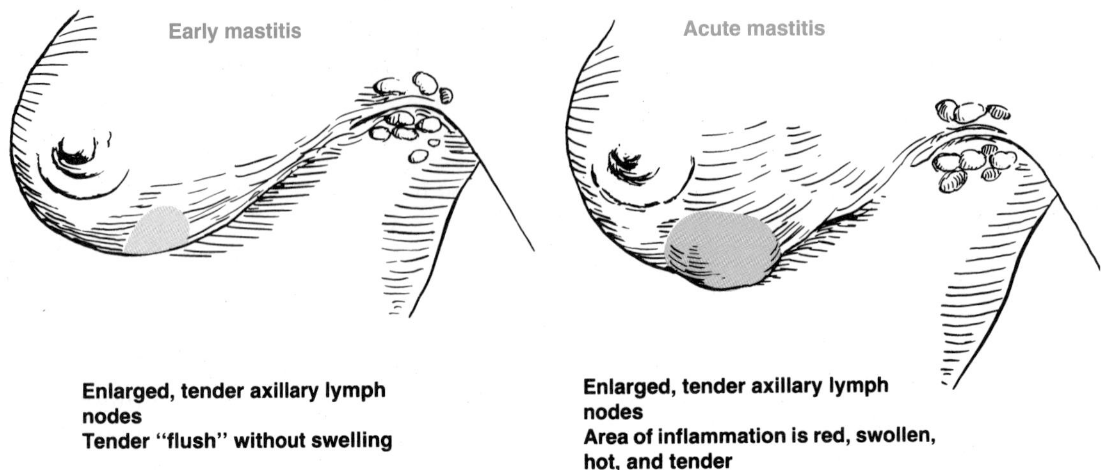

Figure 10–4. • Mastitis typically occurs several weeks after birth in the woman who is breastfeeding. Bacteria usually enter the breast through small cracks in the nipples. Breast engorgement and milk stasis increase the risk for mastitis.

Nursing Care. Maintain the prescribed antibiotic therapy to help eliminate the infection. Teach the woman how to take the prescribed drug because it is usually continued after discharge.

Most microorganisms in the urinary tract are flushed out with each voiding. The woman should drink large quantities (about 3 liters) of liquid each day to promote the self-cleaning action of the urinary tract. Acidic urine inhibits growth of infectious organisms. Foods that increase urine acidity include apricots, cranberry juice, plums, and prunes.

Many women are prone to recurrent episodes of urinary tract infection, usually cystitis. The postpartum period is a good time to teach preventive measures, such as adequate fluid intake and foods to acidify the urine. Urination immediately after sexual intercourse flushes out organisms that may have entered the urethra.

Breast Infection

Mastitis is an infection of the breast. It usually occurs about 2 or 3 weeks after birth (Fig. 10–4). Mastitis occurs when organisms from the skin or the infant's mouth enter small cracks in the nipples or areola. These cracks may be microscopic. Breast engorgement and inadequate emptying of milk are associated with mastitis.

Signs and symptoms of mastitis include:

- Redness and heat in the breast
- Tenderness
- Edema and a heaviness in the breast
- Purulent drainage (may or may not be present)

The woman usually has fever, chills, and other systemic signs and symptoms. If not treated, the infected area becomes walled off, and an abscess forms. The infection is usually outside the ducts of the breast, and the milk is not contaminated. However, if an abscess develops, it may rupture into the ducts and contaminate the milk.

Medical Treatment. Antibiotics and continued removal of milk from the breast are the primary treatment for mastitis. Mild analgesics make the woman more comfortable. The woman may need an incision and drainage of the infected area if an abscess forms. Intravenous antibiotics are needed to treat breast abscess.

The mother can usually continue to breastfeed unless an abscess forms. If she should not nurse for any reason, she should pump her breasts and discard the milk. She should not wean her baby when she has mastitis, because weaning leads to engorgement and stasis of milk, which worsens the mastitis.

Nursing Care. Teach nursing mothers proper breastfeeding techniques to reduce their risk for mastitis (see Chapter 9). Nursing care for mastitis centers on relieving pain and on maintaining lactation. Heat promotes blood flow to the area, comfort, and complete emptying of the breast. Moist heat can be applied with chemical packs. An inexpensive warm pack can be made by wetting a disposable diaper with hot water and applying it to the breasts. A warm shower provides warmth, cleanliness, and stimulates the flow of milk if done just before nursing.

Both breasts should be emptied regularly (every 1½ to 2 hours) to reduce milk stasis, which increases the risk for abscess formation. If the affected breast is too painful for the mother to breastfeed she can use a pump to empty it. She can massage the area of inflammation to improve milk flow and reduce stasis. Nursing first on the unaffected side starts the milk flow in both breasts and can improve emptying with less pain.

Other nursing measures include

- Encouraging fluid intake, about 3 liters a day
- Wearing a good support bra to support the breasts and limit movement of the painful breast; the bra should not be too tight or it will actually cause milk stasis
- Supporting the woman emotionally and reassuring her that she can continue to breastfeed

SUBINVOLUTION OF THE UTERUS

Involution is the return of the uterus to its nonpregnant condition after birth. *Subinvolution* is a slower-than-expected return of the uterus to its nonpregnant condition. Infection and retained fragments of the placenta are the most common causes of uterine subinvolution.

The expected changes in the uterine size and progression of lochia (see Chapter 9) do not occur at the normal pace in subinvolution of the uterus. Two typical signs of subinvolution are:

- Fundal height greater than expected for the amount of time since birth
- Persistence of lochia rubra or a slowed progression through the three phases

Other signs and symptoms are similar to those of endometritis, and the two conditions often occur together. The other signs and symptoms are:

- Pelvic and back pain
- Tenderness of the uterus
- Fatigue and general malaise

The woman often has fever and other signs that accompany infection.

Medical Treatment. Medical treatment is selected to correct the cause of the subinvolution. It may include any or all of these measures:

- Methylergonovine (Methergine) to maintain firm uterine contraction
- Antibiotics for infection
- Dilation of the cervix and curettage to remove fragments of the placenta from the uterine wall.

Nursing Care. The mother has almost always been discharged when subinvolution of the uterus occurs. Teach all new mothers about the normal changes to expect so that they can recognize a departure from the normal pattern. Women should report fever, persistent pain, persistent red lochia (or return of bleeding after it has changed), or foul-smelling vaginal discharge.

The woman may be admitted to the hospital on the gynecology unit. Nursing care involves assisting with medical therapy and providing analgesics and other comfort measures. Specific nursing care depends on whether the subinvolution is due to infection or another cause.

DISORDERS OF MOOD

"Postpartum blues," or "baby blues," are common after birth. The woman has periods when she feels let down, but overall she finds pleasure in life and in her new role as mother. Her roller-coaster emotions are self-limiting as she adapts to the changes in her life.

A *mood* is a pervasive and sustained emotion that can color one's view of life. A *psychosis* involves serious impairment of one's perception of reality. Postpartum depression and postpartum psychosis are disorders of mood. They are more serious than postpartum blues.

Postpartum Depression

The woman with persistent postpartum depression (2 weeks or longer) exhibits characteristics such as these:

- Lack of enjoyment in life
- Disinterest in others; loss of normal give-and-take in relationships
- Intense feelings of inadequacy, unworthiness, guilt; inability to cope
- Loss of mental concentration
- Disturbed sleep

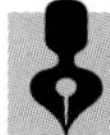

Nursing Tip

If a postpartum woman seems depressed, the nurse should not assume that she has the common "baby blues" or that she will "snap out of it." Explore her feelings to determine if they are persistent and pervasive.

- Constant fatigue and feelings of ill health
- Sleep disturbances
- Panic attacks
- Obsessive thinking

The woman who has postpartum depression has impaired function because she is listless and withdrawn most of the time. However, she remains in touch with reality. Nevertheless, postpartum depression can seriously disrupt her life and that of her family. It may persist for months before it finally lifts.

Depressed women are more tense and feel less competent as mothers. They interact with their babies less and are slower to respond to their infant's cues. Their babies are often more fussy.

No specific cause of postpartum depression is identified. Factors associated with the disorder include:

- Anger at the pregnancy
- Complications of pregnancy or birth
- Complications in the newborn
- History of depression, mental illness, or alcoholism in the woman or in her family
- Immature personality
- Low self-esteem
- Isolation from sources of support
- Poor relationship with her partner
- Financial worries
- Rapid changes in hormone levels after birth

As in many other complications, one of these factors often leads to another. For example, complications during pregnancy may result in the birth of an infant who is ill.

Treatment. Treatment of postpartum depression includes psychotherapy, increased social support, and antidepressant medications. The woman's family is included in her care.

Nursing Care. The nurse is more likely to encounter the woman with postpartum depression in the physician's office or a pediatric clinic. The nurse may help the mother by being a sympathetic listener. Women may be reluctant to express dissatisfaction with their new role, especially if they have waited a long time for a baby.

The nurse should elicit the new mother's feelings about motherhood and her infant. Observe for complaints of sleeplessness or chronic fatigue. Pursue the mother's expressions of feeling to help her to better express them. Help her to see that there is hope for her problem, but do not minimize her feelings by saying things like, "You'll get over it."

Isolation can be both a cause and a result of depression. Help the new mother identify sources of emotional support among her family and friends. Many of her friends may have stopped including her because she has withdrawn from them. She may not have the emotional energy to reach out to them again.

The woman who is physically depleted often has an exaggerated feeling of let-down and depression. Determine whether she is getting enough exercise, sleep, and proper nutrition to improve her physical health and sense of well-being. Help her to identify ways to meet her own needs and reassure her that she is not being selfish.

A new mother may feel guilty because she is not happy all the time. Explain that feelings are not right or wrong—feelings simply exist. Refer her to support groups if these are available. Discussing her feelings with others who have similar difficulties can help her to realize that she is not alone.

Postpartum Psychosis

Women having a postpartum psychosis have an impaired sense of reality. Psychosis is much less common than postpartum depression. A woman may have any psychiatric disorder, but those more often encountered are:

- *Bipolar disorder.* A disorder characterized by episodes of *mania* (hyperactivity, excitability, euphoria, and a feeling of being invulnerable) and depression
- *Major depression.* A disorder characterized by deep feelings of worthlessness, guilt, serious sleep and appetite disturbance, and sometimes delusions about the infant's being dead

Postpartum psychosis can be fatal for both mother and infant. The mother may endanger herself and her baby during manic episodes because she uses poor judgment and has a sense of being invulnerable. Suicide and infanticide are possible, especially during depressive episodes.

Care of the woman with postpartum psychosis requires psychiatric professionals and is beyond the scope of maternity nursing. The patient is usually treated in the same way as other people with similar disorders. Hospitalization is usually needed.

KEY POINTS

- The nurse must be aware of women who are at higher risk for postpartum hemorrhage and assess them more often.
- A constant small trickle of blood can result in significant blood loss, as can a larger one-time hemorrhage.
- Persistent and more severe pain than expected is characteristic of a hematoma in the reproductive tract.
- It is essential to identify and limit an infection before it spreads to adjacent organs or through the blood stream to a distant site.
- The nurse should teach new mothers about normal postpartum changes and indications of problems they should report.
- Careful listening and observation can help the nurse to identify a new mother who is suffering from postpartum depression.
- Postpartum psychoses are serious disorders that are potentially life-threatening to the woman and others, including her infant.

MULTIPLE-CHOICE REVIEW QUESTIONS

Choose the most appropriate answer.

1. The earliest finding in hypovolemic shock is usually
   a. low blood pressure.
   b. rapid pulse.
   c. pale skin color.
   d. soft uterus.
2. A bleeding laceration typically exhibits
   a. a soft uterus that is difficult to locate.
   b. low pulse and blood pressure.
   c. bright red bleeding and a firm uterus.
   d. profuse dark red bleeding and large clots.
3. The white blood cell (leukocyte) count is normally ____________ during the postpartum period.
   a. Higher
   b. Lower
   c. Unchanged
4. How does high fluid intake help to resolve urinary tract infection?
   a. Reduces fever.
   b. Decreases bladder muscle tone.
   c. Increases urine acidity.
   d. Removes microorganisms.
5. A woman is having her checkup with her nurse-midwife 6 weeks after birth. She seems disinterested in others, including her baby. She tells the nurse she does not think she is a very good mother. The nurse should
   a. reassure her that almost all new mothers feel let down after birth.
   b. ask her how her partner feels about the new baby.
   c. explore her feelings with sensitive questioning.
   d. refer her to a psychiatrist.

BIBLIOGRAPHY AND READER REFERENCE

Beck, C. T. (1995). Perceptions of nurses' caring by mothers experiencing postpartum depression. *Journal of Obstetric, Gynecologic, and Neonatal Nursing, 24*(9), 819–825.

Clark, R. A. (1995). Infections during the postpartum period. *Journal of Obstetric, Gynecologic, and Neonatal Nursing, 24*(6), 542–548.

Cunningham, F. G., MacDonald, P. C., Gant, N. F., Leveno, K. J., Gilstrap, L. C., Hankins, G. D. V., & Clark, S. L. (1997). *Williams Obstetrics* (20th ed.). Norwalk, CT: Appleton & Lange.

Ely, J. W., Rijhsinghani, A., Bowdler, N. C., & Dawson, J. D. (1995). The association between manual removal of the placenta and postpartum endometritis following vaginal delivery. *Obstetrics and Gynecology, 86*(6), 1002–06.

Gorrie, T. M., McKinney, E. S., & Murray, S. M. (1998). *Foundations of maternal-newborn nursing* (2nd ed.). Philadelphia: Saunders.

Grohar, J. (1996). Postpartum care. In K. R. Simpson and P. A. Creehan (Eds.), *AWHONN's perinatal nursing*. Philadelphia: Lippincott.

chapter 11

The Nurse's Role in Women's Health Care

Outline

PREVENTIVE HEALTH CARE FOR WOMEN
- Breast Care
- Vulvar Self-Examination
- Pelvic Examination

MENSTRUAL DISORDERS
- Amenorrhea
- Abnormal Uterine Bleeding
- Menstrual Cycle Pain
- Endometriosis
- Premenstrual Syndrome

INDUCED ABORTION
- Treatment
- Nursing Care

GYNECOLOGIC INFECTIONS
- Toxic Shock Syndrome
- Sexually Transmissible Diseases
- Pelvic Inflammatory Disease

FAMILY PLANNING
- Abstinence
- Hormonal Contraceptives
- Intrauterine Device
- Barrier Methods
- Natural Family Planning
- Sterilization
- Unreliable Contraceptive Methods

INFERTILITY CARE
- Social and Psychological Implications
- Factors Affecting Infertility
- Evaluation of Infertility
- Therapy for Infertility
- Outcomes of Infertility Therapy
- Nursing Care Related to Infertility Treatment

MENOPAUSE
- Physical Changes
- Psychological and Cultural Variations
- Hormone Replacement Therapy
- Therapy for Osteoporosis
- Nursing Care of the Menopausal Woman

PELVIC FLOOR DYSFUNCTION
- Vaginal Wall Prolapse
- Uterine Prolapse

OTHER FEMALE REPRODUCTIVE TRACT DISORDERS
- Cervical Polyps
- Uterine Leiomyomas
- Ovarian Cysts

Objectives

On completion and mastery of Chapter 11, the student will be able to

- Define each vocabulary term listed.
- Explain aspects of preventive health care for women.
- Describe each menstrual disorder and its care.
- Describe care related to induced abortion.
- Explain each gynecologic infection in terms of cause, transmission, treatment, and care.
- Describe the various methods of birth control, including side effects and contraindications of each method.
- Describe how to use natural family planning methods for contraception or infertility management.

(Continued)

Objectives (Continued)

- Describe possible causes and treatment of infertility.
- Explain the changes that occur during the perimenopausal period and after menopause.
- Explain medical and nursing care of women who are nearing or have completed menopause.
- Discuss medical and nursing care of women with pelvic floor dysfunction or problems related to benign growths in the reproductive tract.

Vocabulary

amenorrhea	menorrhagia
climacteric	metrorrhagia
coitus interruptus	mittelschmerz
dysmenorrhea	myoma
dyspareunia	osteoporosis
endometriosis	retrograde ejaculation
hypospadias	spermicide
laminaria	spinnbarkeit
leiomyoma	stress incontinence

The nurse plays an important role in many aspects of women's health care. The nurse will encounter women seeking preventive health care, help controlling their fertility, or treatment for gynecologic disorders in many settings; such as clinics, outpatient surgery centers, acute care hospitals, and the community.

PREVENTIVE HEALTH CARE FOR WOMEN

The goal of preventive health care, or health maintenance, is the prevention or early identification of disease. The value of preventive health care is that some disabling conditions can be avoided or their severity lessened by specific measures, such as altering the diet or detecting the disorder early, at a more treatable stage. Preventive care for women may include disorders that are:

- Exclusive to women, such as cervical cancer
- Dominant in women, such as breast cancer or osteoporosis
- Prevalent in the general population, such as hypertension or colorectal cancers

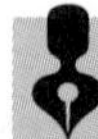

Nursing Tip

Encouraging women to practice preventive health care can help to avoid some disorders or to identify them when they are the most treatable.

This discussion will focus on those disorders that are exclusive or dominant in women.

Much of preventive health care involves screening tests. These tests are not diagnostic, but can identify whether additional testing is needed. Examples of screening tests that are common in women's health care include mammography to identify breast cancer and Papanicolaou (Pap) tests for cervical cancer.

Breast Care

Three approaches are needed for early detection of breast cancer:

- Monthly breast self-examination
- Professional breast examination
- Mammography as appropriate

The nurse's role is to educate women about the benefit of all three examinations and of self-examination. See a medical-surgical text for additional information about diagnosis and treatment of breast cancer.

Breast Self-Examination

Breast self-examination (BSE) should be performed by all women after age 20 at about the same time each month. The best time for BSE is 1 week after the beginning of the menstrual period. If she is not menstruating, the woman may choose any day that is easy for her to remember, such as the first day of each month. Box 11–1 describes how to teach a woman BSE.

The chief value of BSE is that a woman learns how her own breasts feel. This is particularly valuable if she has fibrocystic breast changes, in which there are often many lumps that may change with hormonal fluctuations. The woman is more likely to know when something is different about *her* breasts.

BOX 11–1

TEACHING WOMEN TO PERFORM BREAST SELF-EXAMINATION

Perform breast self-examination monthly. If you are menstruating, do the examination 1 week after the beginning of your period because your breasts are less tender then. If you are not menstruating, choose any day that you can easily remember, such as the first day of each month. Examine your breasts 3 ways: before a mirror, lying down, and in the shower.

Before a Mirror

Inspect your breasts in 4 steps: (1) arms at your sides; (2) arms over your head; (3) with your hands on your hips, pressing them firmly to flex your chest muscles; (4) and bending forward. At each step, note any change in the shape or appearance of your breasts. Note skin or nipple changes such as dimpling of the skin. Squeeze each nipple gently to identify any discharge.

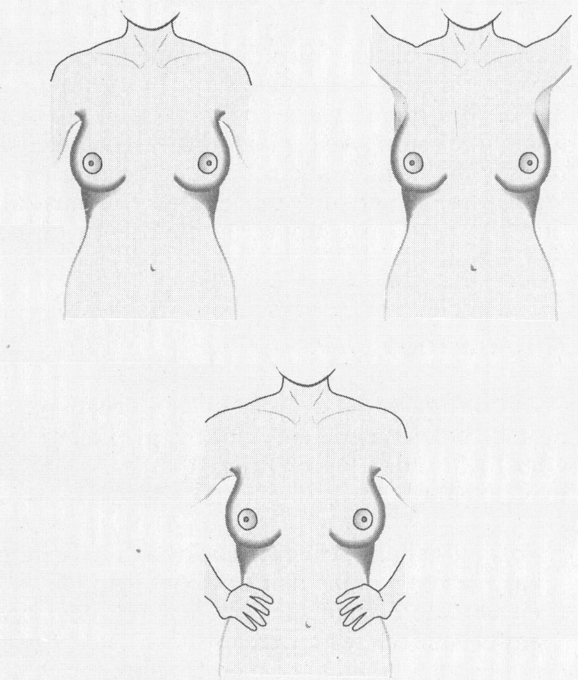

Lying Down

Place a small pillow under your right shoulder and put your right hand under your head while you examine your right breast with your left hand. Use the sensitive pads of your fingers to press gently into the breast tissue. Use a systematic pattern to check the entire breast. One pattern is to feel the tissue in a circular pattern, spiraling inward toward the nipple. Another method is to use an up-and-down pattern. Use the same systematic pattern to examine the underarm area because breast tissue is also present here. Repeat for the other breast.

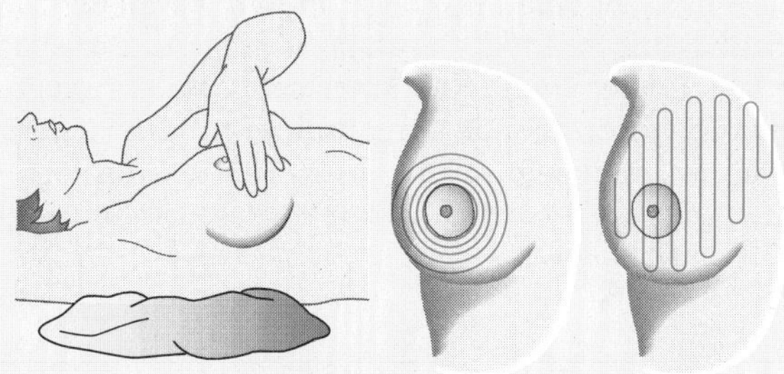

In the Shower

Raise your right arm. Use your soapy fingers to feel the breast tissue in the same systematic pattern described under Lying Down.

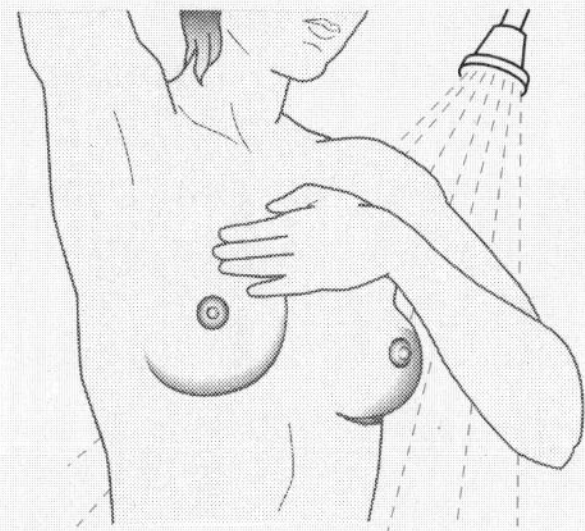

For Additional Information

Contact the American Cancer Society at 1-800-ACS-2345 or visit their website at http://www.tx.cancer.org

Professional Breast Examination

Breast self-examination is a supplement to, rather than a substitute for, regular professional examinations. Although the woman who does regular BSE knows what is usual for her own breasts, professionals have the training and experience to identify suspicious breast masses. It is part of every annual gynecologic examination and is done more frequently for women who have a high risk for breast cancer. It is recommended at yearly intervals for all

Nursing Tip

Preventive care for breast health involves self-examination, professional examinations, and mammography at the appropriate ages.

women over age 20. The professional examination is similar to that for BSE.

Mammography

Mammography uses very-low-dose x-rays to visualize the breast tissue. It can detect breast tumors very early, long before the woman or a professional can feel them. The breast is compressed firmly between two plates, which is briefly uncomfortable. Scheduling the mammogram following a menstrual period reduces the discomfort because the breasts are less tender then. The American Cancer Society currently recommends a mammogram every year for all women age 40 or over (1997). Women at higher risk for breast cancer may begin mammography earlier.

Vulvar Self-Examination

Women over age 18 (or younger, if sexually active) should perform a monthly examination of the external genitalia to identify lesions or masses that may indicate infection or malignancy. The woman should use a hand mirror in a good light to systematically inspect her vulva for any new growths of any kind, any painful or inflamed areas, ulcers, sores, or changes in skin color. She should palpate these tissues to identify any masses.

Pelvic Examination

The pelvic examination should be scheduled between menstrual periods, and the woman should not douche or have sexual intercourse for at least 48 hours before the examination to avoid altering the Pap test. The purpose of the pelvic examination is to identify conditions such as tumors, abnormal discharge, infections, or unusual pain.

The examiner first checks the external organs to identify signs of problems similar to those noted in vulvar self-examination. Next, a speculum is inserted to visualize the woman's cervix and vagina for inflammation, discharge, or lesions. The speculum is warmed and lubricated with warm water only. A Pap test is obtained to screen for changes in the tissues that may be precancerous.

The current American Cancer Society recommendations (1996) for the Pap test are:

- Yearly for all women age 18 or older
- After three or more normal exams, the Pap test may be performed less frequently at the health care provider's discretion.

After the Pap test is obtained, the examiner will perform an internal, or bimanual, examination to evaluate the internal organs. The index and middle fingers of one hand are inserted into the vagina and the other is placed on the abdomen to permit palpation of the cervix, uterus, and ovaries between the fingers.

After the internal examination, a single lubricated finger is inserted into the rectum to identify hemorrhoids or other lesions. A test for fecal occult blood may be done at this time (see a medical-surgical text for details).

MENSTRUAL DISORDERS

Menstrual cycle disorders can cause many women distress. The nursing role in each depends on the disorder's cause and treatment. Common nursing roles involve explaining any recommended treatments, such as medications, and caring for the woman before and after procedures. The nurse also provides emotional support to the client who may be frustrated.

Amenorrhea

Amenorrhea is the absence of menstruation. It is normal before menarche, during pregnancy, and after menopause. Amenorrhea that is not normal may be either:

- *Primary.* Failure to menstruate by age 16 if the girl has breast or pubic hair development; failure to menstruate by age 14 if she has not developed any secondary sex characteristics
- *Secondary.* Cessation of menstruation for at least 3 cycles or 6 months in a woman who previously had an established pattern of menstruation

Treatment of amenorrhea begins with a thorough history, physical exam, and laboratory examinations to identify the cause. Pregnancy testing will be done for any sexually active woman.

The specific treatment depends on the cause that

is identified. For example, women who are very thin or have a low percentage of body fat may have amenorrhea because fat is necessary for estrogen production. These women may include athletes, but may also include clients who have eating disorders such as anorexia or bulimia. Therapy for their eating disorder may allow resumption of normal periods. Other treatments are aimed at correcting the cause, which may be an endocrine imbalance.

Abnormal Uterine Bleeding

Abnormal uterine bleeding is (1) too frequent, (2) too long in duration, or (3) excessive in amount. *Metrorrhagia* is uterine bleeding that is usually normal in amount, but that occurs at irregular intervals. *Menorrhagia* refers to menstrual bleeding that is excessive in amount. Common causes for any type of abnormal bleeding include the following:

- Pregnancy complications, such as an unidentified pregnancy that is ending in spontaneous abortion
- Lesions of the vagina, cervix, or uterus (benign or malignant)
- Break-through bleeding (BTB) that may occur in the woman taking oral contraceptives
- Endocrine disorders such as hypothyroidism
- Failure to ovulate or respond appropriately to hormones secreted with ovulation (dysfunctional uterine bleeding)

Treatment of abnormal uterine bleeding depends on the identified cause. Pregnancy complications are treated appropriately, as are any benign or malignant lesions identified. Break-through bleeding may be relieved by a change in the oral contraceptive used. Abnormal hormone secretion will be treated with the appropriate medications. Surgical dilation and curettage (D&C) may remove intrauterine growths or aid in diagnosis. Hysterectomy may be done for some disorders if the woman does not want other children. A newer technique, *laser ablation,* can permanently remove the abnormally bleeding uterine lining without a hysterectomy.

Menstrual Cycle Pain

Mittelschmerz

Mittelschmerz ("middle pain") is pain that many women experience around ovulation, near the middle of their menstrual cycle. Mild analgesics are usually sufficient to relieve this discomfort. The nurse can teach the woman that this discomfort, while annoying, is harmless.

Dysmenorrhea

Dysmenorrhea, or "cramps," affects many women. It occurs soon after the onset of menses, and is spasmodic in nature. Discomfort is in the lower abdomen and may radiate to the lower back or down the legs. Some women also have diarrhea, nausea, and vomiting. It is most common in young women who have not been pregnant (nulliparas).

Prostaglandins from the endometrium (uterine lining) play an important role in dysmenorrhea. Some women produce excessive amounts of prostaglandins from the endometrium, and these substances are potent stimulants of painful uterine contractions. Three treatments may give relief:

- Prostaglandin inhibitor drugs, such as ibuprofen (Motrin, Advil) or naproxen (Naprosyn, Anaprox). Prostaglandin inhibitors are most effective if taken before the onset of menstruation and cramps.
- Heat application to the lower abdomen or back.
- Oral contraceptives, which reduce the amount of endometrium built up each month, and therefore reduce prostaglandin secretion.

Endometriosis

Endometriosis is the presence of tissue that resembles endometrium outside the uterus. This tissue responds to hormonal stimulation just as the uterine lining does. As the lesions build up and slough during menstrual cycles, they may cause pain, pressure, and inflammation to adjacent organs.

Endometriosis causes pain in many women that is either sharp or dull. It is more constant than the spasmodic pain of dysmenorrhea. *Dyspareunia* (painful sexual intercourse) may be present. Endometriosis appears to cause infertility in some women. Some women with endometriosis have few symptoms and no problems conceiving, however.

Treatment of endometriosis may be either medical or surgical. Medications such as danazol and analogues of gonadotropin releasing hormone (GnRH) may be given to reduce the buildup of tissue by inducing an artificial menopause. The woman may have hot flashes and vaginal dryness, similar to symptoms occurring at natural menopause. She is also at increased risk for other problems that occur after menopause, such as osteoporosis and serum lipid changes.

Surgical treatment includes the following:

- Hysterectomy with removal of the ovaries and all lesions if the woman does not want another pregnancy
- Laser ablation (destruction) of the lesions if she wants to maintain fertility

Premenstrual Syndrome

Premenstrual syndrome (PMS) involves both physical and behavioral symptoms that occur regularly in the last half of each menstrual cycle. It can be most distressing for women and their families. Its cause is unknown, adding to their frustration and making treatment difficult. The manifestations a woman experiences may be physical, behavioral, or both (see Box 11–2).

Many women experience some type of physical and emotional changes during their menstrual cycles. The following criteria are used to diagnose true PMS:

- The signs and symptoms must occur during the last half of each menstrual cycle.
- The woman should be symptom free before ovulation; there must be at least 7 symptom-free days during each cycle.
- Symptoms must be severe enough to impact work, lifestyle, and relationships.
- Diagnosis must be based on symptoms charted by the woman as they occur, rather than by her recall of past problems. PMS diaries are available for this purpose.

BOX 11–2

SIGNS AND SYMPTOMS OF PREMENSTRUAL SYNDROME (PMS)

Physical Manifestations	Behavioral Manifestations
Edema	Anxiety
Weight gain	Depression
Abdominal bloating	Irritability
Constipation	Mood swings
Hot flashes	Aggressive behavior
Breast pain	Increase appetite
Headache	Food cravings
Acne	Fatigue
Rhinitis	Inability to concentrate
Heart palpitations	Insomnia

BOX 11–3

TEACHING RELIEF MEASURES FOR PREMENSTRUAL SYNDROME

In addition to medications your health care provider may order, some women have found these measures to improve the discomforts of premenstrual syndrome.

Diet

Reduce intake of caffeine, including coffee, tea, colas, and chocolate. Read labels to determine what foods and medicines contain caffeine.

Avoid simple sugars such as those found in candy, cookies, and cake.

Reduce intake of salty foods such as chips, pickles, and many fast-food items.

Drink at least 2 quarts of *water* each day. Do not include other beverages in this total.

Eat six small meals each day to keep your blood sugar more stable.

Avoid alcohol.

Exercise

Increase exercise to relieve tension. Do aerobic exercise such as walking or jogging several times each week.

Stress Management

Note the time when your PMS symptoms are more severe. Try to arrange your schedule to minimize the amount of stress in your life at these times.

Guided imagery, conscious relaxation techniques, warm baths, and massage may help to reduce stress.

Sleep and Rest

Maintain a regular schedule for sleep.

Drink a glass of milk just before bedtime.

Schedule exercise in the early morning or early afternoon.

Do activities that are relaxing for you just before bedtime.

Treatment depends on the signs and symptoms each woman experiences. They may include mild diuretics, vitamin B_6, progesterone, antianxiety medications, and various stress-reduction measures. Box 11–3 describes measures the nurse can teach the woman about reducing the symptoms of PMS.

INDUCED ABORTION

Induced abortion is an issue heavily laden with legal, social, moral, and ethical conflicts. Women end a pregnancy for a variety of reasons, such as preservation of their health, prevention of the birth of an abnormal infant, social or economic factors, or prevention of birth in cases of rape or incest. For this discussion, a *therapeutic abortion* is one that is done to preserve the woman's health, and an *elective abortion* is one that the woman requests but that does not involve preservation of health. Laws may vary from state to state concerning parental consent when a minor is involved; for counseling or a required waiting period after decision to have an elective abortion; and the timing of the elective abortion related to the probable viability of the fetus. These issues remain controversial and laws often change.

Although abortion is currently legal in the United States, there are circumstances in which it is not legal. If the abortion is performed in an inappropriate facility and/or by an unqualified person, it is illegal, just as any other medical procedure performed under these conditions would be. Women who cannot afford a legal abortion and cannot get public funding for one may resort to illegal abortionists. They are more likely to suffer life-threatening hemorrhage or infection (septic abortion).

Treatment

The physician chooses the most appropriate method to end the pregnancy. The choice depends on gestational age and the woman's physical condition. A vacuum aspiration or D&C (see Table 5–1, p. 84) is most often used to end a pregnancy during the first trimester. Methods used to end a second-trimester pregnancy include:

- Dilation and evacuation (D & E), a procedure that is similar to D&C but that requires greater cervical dilation
- Induction of labor with prostaglandins. *Laminaria* (cones of a water-absorbing material) are often inserted into the cervix to begin the dilation process as they swell and enlarge.
- Injection of hypertonic saline or hypertonic urea into the uterus (uncommon in the United States).

Oxytocin can hasten labor that has already begun, but it cannot be used alone to induce labor during the second trimester as it can during late pregnancy.

Possible new options for induced abortion include FDA approval of the medication mifepristone (RU 486) that has been used in other countries, methotrexate (a chemotherapeutic drug not currently approved for induced abortion), or misoprostol. These drugs interfere with embryonic growth or stimulate uterine contractions to expel the products of conception.

Nursing Care

Physical Care

Nursing care of the woman depends on the method of induced abortion. Care after the procedure is similar to that following spontaneous abortion (see p. 83). Rh immune globulin should be administered to the Rh-negative woman.

Recognizing Personal Beliefs and Values

The nurse who cares for women having an induced abortion must examine personal beliefs and biases so that they do not interfere with the woman's care. The woman needs nonjudgmental, compassionate care. The nurse who has ethical or moral objections to caring for a woman undergoing induced abortion must make this fact known before being employed in an agency that provides these services. It is unethical to wait until being assigned to care for a client who is having any procedure that violates the nurse's moral, ethical, or religious beliefs, and then refuse to care for that client if the situation could have been foreseen.

GYNECOLOGIC INFECTIONS

Three classes of gynecologic infections will be covered in this section:

- Toxic shock syndrome
- Sexually transmissible diseases
- Pelvic inflammatory disease

Toxic Shock Syndrome

Toxic shock syndrome (TSS) is a rare disorder that is potentially fatal. It is caused by strains of *Staphylococcus aureus* that produce toxins that can cause shock, coagulation defects, and tissue damage if they enter the bloodstream. Toxic shock syndrome is associated with trapping of the bacteria within the reproductive tract for a prolonged time. Factors that increase the risk of TSS include use of high-absorbency tampons and use of a diaphragm or cervical cap for contraception.

Signs and symptoms of TSS include the following:

- Sudden spiking fever
- Flulike symptoms
- Hypotension
- Generalized rash that resembles sunburn
- Skin peeling from the palms and soles 1 to 2 weeks after the illness

The incidence of TSS has decreased, but the nurse continues to play a role in prevention. The nurse's role is primarily one of education. The following should be included:

Tampon Use

- Wash hands before and after inserting a tampon
- Change tampons at least every 4 hours
- Do not use superabsorbent tampons
- Use pads rather than tampons when sleeping because tampons will likely remain in the vagina longer than 4 hours

Diaphragm or Cervical Cap Use

- Wash hands before and after inserting the diaphragm or cervical cap.
- Do not use a diaphragm or cervical cap during the menstrual period.
- Remove the diaphragm or cervical cap at the time recommended by the health care provider.

Sexually Transmissible Diseases

Sexually transmissible diseases (STDs) are those that can be spread by sexual contact, although several of these have other modes of transmission as well. It is important that all sexual contacts, even those who are asymptomatic, be completely treated to eradicate the infection. Refer to Table 11–1 for specific information about STDs that the nurse may encounter.

Nursing care related to STDs primarily focuses on client education to prevent spread of these infections. Nurses may do the following:

- Teach signs and symptoms that should be reported
- Explain diagnostic tests
- Teach measures to prevent spread of infection, such as use of a condom
- Explain treatment measures
- Emphasize the importance of completing treatment and follow-up and of treating all partners to eliminate the spread of infection

> **Nursing Tip**
>
> To prevent toxic shock syndrome, the woman should be taught to wash her hands well when using tampons or a diaphragm. The diaphragm should not be used during menstruation. Tampons should be changed every 4 hours and not used during sleep, which usually lasts longer than 4 hours.

Pelvic Inflammatory Disease

Pelvic inflammatory disease (PID) is an infection of the upper reproductive tract. Asymptomatic, STDs are a common cause of PID. The cervix, uterine cavity, fallopian tubes, and pelvic cavity are often involved. Infertility may be the result.

The woman's symptoms vary according to the area affected. Fever, pelvic pain, abnormal vaginal discharge, nausea and anorexia, and irregular vaginal bleeding are common. When examined, the abdomen and pelvic organs are often very tender. Laboratory tests identify common general signs of infection, such as elevated leukocytes and an elevated sedimentation rate. Cultures of the cervical canal will be done to identify the infecting organism. Urinalysis is usually done to identify infection of the urinary tract.

Treatment may be administered on an inpatient or outpatient basis, depending on the severity of the infection. Antibiotics are begun promptly to treat the infection. The antibiotic(s) will be changed if culture and sensitivity testing indicates that another one would be more effective.

FAMILY PLANNING

Family planning (birth control) may be part of the nurse's work in family-planning clinics, physician or nurse-midwife practices, or on the postpartum or gynecology units of an acute-care hospital. Also, family members and friends may turn to the nurse as a resource person who can answer their ques-

Table 11–1
SEXUALLY TRANSMISSIBLE DISEASES

Infection and Causative Organism	Signs and Symptoms	Diagnosis	Treatment	Comments
Candidiasis (yeast) *(Candida albicans)*	Itching and burning on urination, inflammation of vulva and vagina, "cottage cheese" appearance to discharge	Signs and symptoms; identification of the spores of the causative fungus	Miconazole nitrate (Monistat), clotrimazole (Gyne-Lotrimin), nystatin (Mycostatin), fluconazole (Diflucan)	Medications are available over the counter (OTC), but the woman should seek medical attention to diagnose her first infection or if she has persistent or recurrent infections
Trichomoniasis *(Trichomonas vaginalis)*	Thin, foul-odored, greenish-yellow vaginal discharge, vulvar itching, edema, redness	Identification of the organism under microscope in a wet-mount preparation	Metronidazole (Flagyl) if not pregnant during the first trimester; clotrimazole (Gyne-Lotrimin) for symptomatic relief during the first trimester	Organism thrives in an alkaline environment. Most infections are thought to be transmitted by sexual contact
Bacterial vaginosis *(Gardnerella vaginalis)*	Thin, grayish-white discharge that has a fishy odor	Microscopic evidence of clue cells (epithelial cells with bacteria clinging to their surface)	Bacteria is normal inhabitant of the vagina but overgrows. Treatment is aimed at restoring the normal balance of vaginal bacterial flora. Metronidazole (Flagyl) may relieve symptoms	Avoid alcohol during treatment with metronidazole and for 24 hours after
Chlamydia *(Chlamydia trachomatis)*	Symptoms similar to gonorrhea, such as yellowish discharge and painful urination. Often asymptomatic in women, which delays treatment	Culture to identify the organism is best. Rapid detection tests, such as enzyme-linked immunosorbent assay (ELISA) and monoclonal antibody tests are used but are often nonspecific	Azithromycin, doxycycline, tetracycline	Untreated chlamydial infection can ascend into the fallopian tubes where it causes scarring. Infertility or ectopic pregnancy may result. Can be spread to the neonate's eyes by contact with infected vaginal secretions
Gonorrhea *(Neisseria gonorrhoeae)*	Purulent discharge, painful urination, dyspareunia	Culture of organism	Cephtriaxone plus doxycycline, azithromycin	Can result in pelvic inflammatory disease with tubal scarring

Table continued on following page

tions about contraception. The nurse's role in family planning includes the following:

- Answering general questions about contraceptive methods
- Explaining different methods that are available, including accurate information about their advantages and disadvantages
- Teaching the correct use of the method or methods of contraception that the client chooses

Factors that influence one's choice of a contraceptive include the following:

- Age
- Health status, including risk for STD
- Religion
- Culture
- Impact of an unplanned pregnancy on the woman or family
- Desire for future children
- Frequency of intercourse

Table 11–1
SEXUALLY TRANSMISSIBLE DISEASES *(Continued)*

Infection and Causative Organism	Signs and Symptoms	Diagnosis	Treatment	Comments
Syphilis *(Treponema pallidum)*	3 stages: *Primary.* Painless chancre on the genitalia, anus, or lips *Secondary.* Two months after primary syphilis; enlargement of spleen and liver, headache, anorexia, generalized skin rash, wartlike growths on the vulva *Tertiary.* May occur many years after secondary syphilis and cause heart, blood vessel, nervous system damage	*Primary.* Examining material scraped from the chancre with darkfield microscopy to identify the spirochete organism; serologic tests are not positive this early *Secondary or tertiary.* Serologic tests (VDRL (less specific), RPR, and FTA-ABS (more specific)	Penicillin; doxycycline, tetracycline, or erythromycin if allergic. Tetracycline is not recommended during pregnancy; desensitization of the woman is recommended	Primary and secondary stages are the most contagious. Spread is through sexual contact, by inoculation (sharing needles), or through the placenta from an infected mother
Herpes genitalis (herpes simplex virus [HSV], types I and II)	Clusters of painful vesicles (blisters) on the vulva, perineum, and anal areas. Vesicles rupture in 1–7 days and heal in 12 days	By signs and symptoms; confirmed by viral culture	No cure exists; acyclovir (Zovirax) reduces symptoms	HSV II usually causes genital lesions. The first episode is usually most uncomfortable. The virus "hides" in the nerve cells and can reemerge in later outbreaks that are as contagious as the first
Condylomata acuminata (human papilloma virus [HPV])	Dry, wartlike growths on the vagina, labia, cervix, and perineum	By typical appearance and location	Removal with cryotherapy (cold), electrocautery, or laser Podophyllin applications are an alternative	Also known as venereal or genital warts; associated with higher rates of cervical cancer; women should have more frequent Pap tests
Acquired immunodeficiency syndrome (AIDS) (human immunodeficiency virus [HIV])	Initially, no symptoms; later symptoms include weight loss, night sweats, fever and chills, fatigue, enlarged lymph nodes, skin rashes, diarrhea. Late symptoms include immune suppression, opportunistic infections, and malignancies	Serology tests: positive ELISA, followed by positive Western blot test	No cure available yet; zidovudine (AZT, Retrovir) and didanosine (Videx) may slow progression. Research is ongoing into new drugs	Transmitted through contact of nonintact skin or mucous membranes with infectious secretions, exposure to blood, and transmission from mother to fetus. Standard precautions reduce risk for caregivers. Condom use reduces risk for sexual transmission

- Convenience and degree of spontaneity that is important to the couple
- Expense
- Degree of comfort the partners have with touching their bodies
- Number of sexual partners

A couple's choice of contraception often changes as needs change.

Contraception does not always prevent pregnancy. An important consideration for clients is how likely the method is to fail. Other than abstinence, which has no failure rate, each method has two failure rates:

- The *theoretic* (ideal, or perfect) failure rate refers to a problem with the method itself rather than the client's use of the method. This would mean, for example, that the woman takes her oral contraceptive *every* day, at the same time every day, and that she never misses a dose.
- The *typical* (actual, or user) failure rate is most relevant to real people. It refers to how likely pregnancy is to occur if its use is occasionally imperfect. Failures are often due to inconsistent or incorrect use, rather than to a problem with the method itself.

Two Healthy People 2000 goals are relevant to provision of family planning services:

- Reduce the percentage of unintended pregnancies to no more than 30%
- Reduce the percentage of women who have an unintended pregnancy despite the use of a contraceptive method to no more than 7%.

The nurse can play a part in helping couples to choose and to use contraceptive methods that enable them to have children that are both wanted and well timed.

Abstinence

Abstinence is 100% effective in preventing pregnancy and STDs, including infection with the human immunodeficiency virus (HIV). However, most couples believe that their sexual relationship adds to the quality of life. Therefore, abstinence is rarely an option the couple will consider. Most religious groups support abstinence among unmarried people and adolescents.

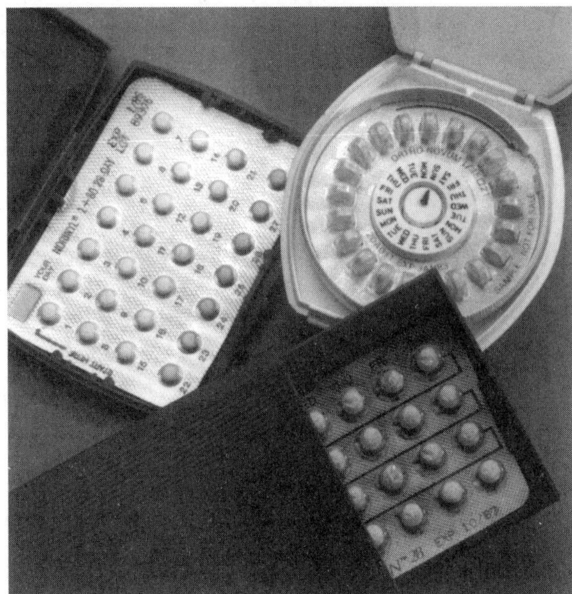

Figure 11–1. • Oral contraceptives. (Courtesy of Planned Parenthood Federation of America, Inc., New York, NY.)

Hormonal Contraceptives

Hormonal contraceptives have one or more of the following contraceptive effects:

- Prevent ovulation
- Make the cervical mucus thick and resistant to sperm penetration
- Make the uterine endometrium less hospitable if a fertilized ovum does arrive

Hormonal contraceptives do not protect either partner from STDs, including HIV infection.

Oral Contraceptives ("The Pill")

Oral contraceptives (OCs) are a popular, highly effective, and reversible method of birth control (Fig. 11–1). They contain either combined hormones (estrogen and progestin) or progesterone alone ("minipill"). Combination OCs are highly effective in preventing ovulation. Minipills are slightly less

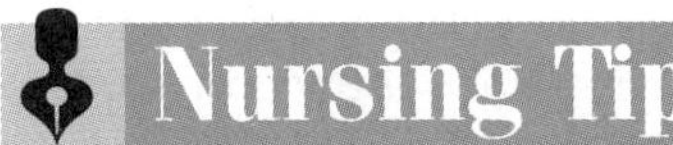

Smoking increases the chance of experiencing complications related to oral contraceptives, particularly in women over 35.

Nursing Tip

The more birth control pills a woman misses, the greater her risk for a pregnancy occurring.

effective in preventing ovulation; their main contraceptive effect is to thicken the cervical mucus and make the endometrium unfavorable for implantation. Minipills are useful for the woman who cannot take estrogen.

Oral contraceptives require a prescription. The woman's history will be taken and she will have a physical examination, including breast and pelvic examinations and Pap test. She should have a yearly physical examination, Pap test, breast examination, and blood pressure check.

Dosing Regimens. Combination OCs are available in 21- or 28-pill packs. If the woman has a 21-pill pack, she takes a pill each day at the same time for 21 days then stops for 7 days. The woman who has a 28-day pack takes a pill each day; the last 7 pills of the pack are inert but maintain the habit of taking the pill each day. Menstruation occurs during the 7-day period during which no pills or inert pills are ingested.

Some pills are multiphasic, in that their estrogen and progesterone content changes during the cycle to mimic natural hormonal activity. If the woman takes multiphasic pills, it is very important that she take each pill in order. Taking the pills at the same time each day is important to maintain a stable blood level of the hormones, regardless of the type of OC the woman is prescribed.

Oral contraceptives are occasionally prescribed as a "morning-after pill" to reduce the risk of pregnancy after unprotected intercourse. The woman takes a larger-than-usual dose of the pills within 72 hours of intercourse and another dose 12 hours after the first. This use is ineffective if pregnancy has already occurred. Nausea and vomiting are common with the high dose of hormones.

Benefits. Oral contraceptives have a failure rate of 0.1% for combined pills and 0.5% for minipills. They reduce the risk for ovarian and endometrial cancer. Their effect on the risk for breast and cervical cancer risks is not yet clear. Women tend to have less cramping, and lighter periods (and therefore less anemia) when taking oral contraceptives. Oral contraceptives may improve PMS symptoms for some women.

Side Effects and Contraindications. Common side effects of oral contraceptives include nausea, headache, breast tenderness, weight gain, and spotting between periods or amenorrhea. These effects generally decrease within a few months and are less frequently seen when low-dose OCs are taken.

Some women should not take OCs or should take them with caution. These women include those who have:

- Thromboembolic disorders (blood clots)
- Cerebrovascular accident or heart disease
- Estrogen-dependent cancer or breast cancer
- A smoking pattern of more than 15 cigarettes a day for women older than 35 (the pill is safe for women over 35 if they do not smoke)
- Impaired liver function
- A confirmed pregnancy or who may be pregnant
- Undiagnosed vaginal bleeding

Combination OCs decrease milk supply and should be given postpartum only after lactation is well established; the minipill does not have this drawback. Women should be taught to inform the health care provider of any preexisting health condition or any change in their condition that may affect their use of OCs. The ACHES acronym can help a woman recall warning signs to report:

- *Abdominal pain* (severe)
- *Chest pain,* dyspnea, bloody sputum
- *Headache* (severe), weakness or numbness of the extremities
- *Eye problems* (blurring, double vision, vision loss)
- *Severe leg pain* or swelling; speech disturbance

Some medications decrease the effectiveness of OCs. These include:

- Some antibiotics, such as ampicillin and tetracycline
- Anticonvulsants

Nursing Care. The woman needs thorough teaching if the pill is to be a satisfactory contraceptive for her. Teaching should be done in her own language, supplemented by generous written materials if she can read. Teaching points should include:

- How to take the specific drug
- What to do if a dose is missed or if she decides to stop using it and does not want to become pregnant
- Common side effects and signs and symptoms that should be promptly reported
- Backup contraceptive methods, such as barrier methods discussed later in this chapter

- Supplemental barrier methods of contraception to use in addition to OCs to reduce the risk of STDs, including HIV infection

Hormone Implants (Norplant)

Hormone implants involve the placement of six matchstick-size capsules that release progestin under the skin of the upper arm (Fig. 11–2). Progestin, is released slowly and in small amounts to provide contraception for 5 years. Like the minipill, the hormone implant inhibits ovulation, development of the endometrium, and causes the cervical mucus to impede sperm passage. Its effectiveness is almost 100%. Its advantages are that it does not need to be taken daily and is unrelated to intercourse. It can be removed at any time with prompt return of fertility. The initial cost of hormone implants is high, but if the woman keeps them for 5 years, they cost about the same as 5 years of OCs.

Side Effects and Contraindications. The benefits, side effects, and contraindications of the hormone implant are essentially the same as for OCs. A common side effect of the hormone implant is menstrual irregularity. Other side effects include headaches, weight gain, acne, dizziness, and mood changes. Infection may occasionally occur.

Nursing Care. The woman should be taught about side effects of hormone implants. Menstruation is likely to be very irregular or absent when the implants are first inserted. This makes many women anxious because they associate a missed period with pregnancy.

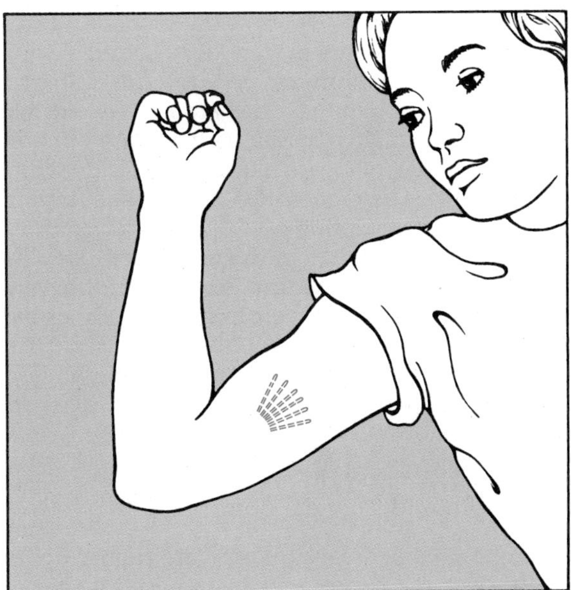

Figure 11–2. • The Norplant contraceptive system.

Hormonal Injection (Depo-Provera)

Depo-Provera is an injectable form of slow-release progestin. Its contraceptive action is similar to that of the minipill and hormone implant. It provides 3 months of highly effective contraception. Fertility returns in about 4 to 9 months. The injection is given deep IM within 5 days of the menstrual period. If it is given later than 5 days after the menstrual period, the woman should use another form of contraception because ovulation may have already occurred. The breastfeeding woman usually starts hormone injections 6 weeks after birth to allow lactation to be well established.

Side Effects and Contraindications. Side effects and contraindications are similar to those of OCs and hormone implants. Menstrual irregularities, breakthrough bleeding, or amenorrhea are common complaints and often the reason why women stop taking the drug.

Nursing Care. Teach the woman about the side effects and problems to report. Emphasize that she should return every 3 months for another injection if she wants to maintain a constant level of hormone and thus prevent pregnancy. Teach a backup contraceptive method if she decides to stop the injections or is delayed in returning for subsequent injections.

Intrauterine Device

Intrauterine devices (IUDs) are a reversible prescription method of birth control. Two types are currently approved for use in the United States: ParaGard and Progestasert (Fig. 11–3). The ParaGard is a small T-shaped plastic device containing copper that is effective for 10 years. Progestasert is also T-shaped and contains progesterone in the stem. The Progestasert must be replaced yearly as its progesterone is depleted.

The exact mechanism by which IUDs prevent pregnancy is not known, but may include the following factors:

- Immobilization of sperm
- Speeding transport of the ovum through the fallopian tube
- A sterile inflammation of the endometrium that prevents implantation

The IUDs are effective (98% effectiveness or greater), reversible, and unrelated to intercourse. Their initial cost is high, but their cost is similar to that of OCs over the long term.

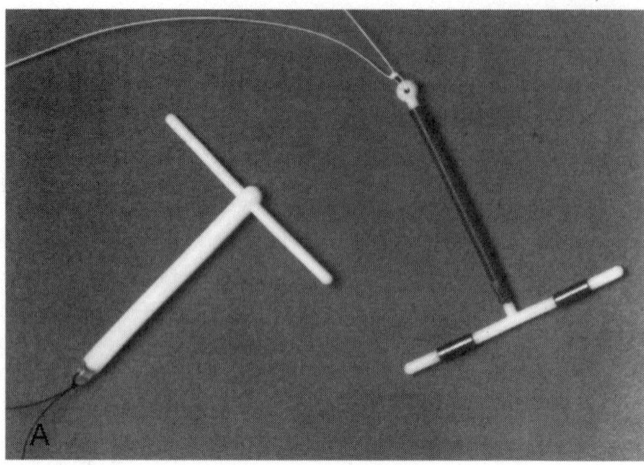

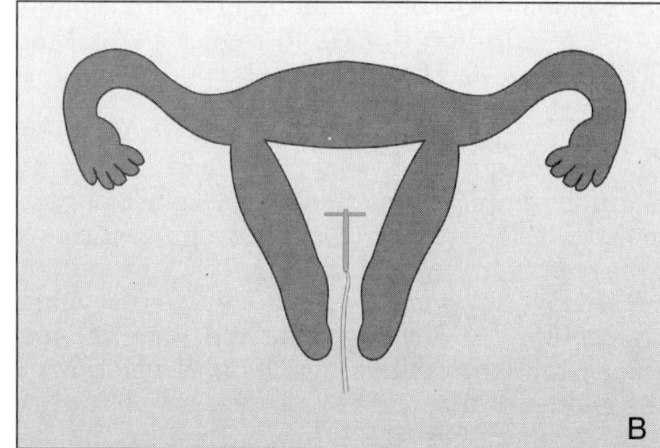

Figure 11–3. • **A** and **B.** The intrauterine device. (From *A.* Courtesy of Planned Parenthood Federation of America, Inc., New York, NY.)

The initial history and examination before insertion of an IUD are similar to those for hormonal contraceptives. The woman is reevaluated in 1 year. She is evaluated for the presence of STDs or other pelvic infection because the IUD can increase the risk of the spread of infection. The IUD should be used only for women who are in mutually monogamous relationships and at low risk for contracting STDs.

Side Effects and Contraindications. Cramping and bleeding are likely to occur with insertion. Increased menstruation and dysmenorrhea may occur and are common reasons a woman decides to have the IUD removed. The woman who has heavier periods may need iron supplementation.

Possible complications besides infection include expulsion of the IUD or perforation of the uterus. If the woman becomes pregnant with an IUD in place, she is more likely to have a spontaneous abortion, ectopic pregnancy, or a preterm baby.

Nursing Care. Teach the woman about side effects and how to take iron supplements if they are prescribed. The woman will need to feel for the fine plastic strings (tail) that are connected to the IUD to verify that it is in place. She should check the tail weekly for the first 4 weeks after insertion, then monthly. Teach her to report if she cannot feel the tail or if it is longer or shorter than previously. Teach her signs of infection (fever, pain, change in vaginal discharge) and signs of ectopic pregnancy (see p. 85) that should be promptly reported.

Nursing Tip

The intrauterine device should be used only by women who have no current pelvic infection and are in a mutually monogamous relationship.

Barrier Methods

Barrier methods work by blocking the entrance of semen into the woman's cervix. Spermicides (sperm-killing chemicals) are part of some of these methods. They avoid use of systemic hormones. Some barrier methods provide some protection against STDs by providing a barrier to contact.

Some barrier methods must be used just before intercourse (condoms, spermicidal foams, and suppositories), while others can be inserted several hours earlier (diaphragm, cervical cap). Spermicidal foams and suppositories are messy and may drip from the vagina. These methods are not suitable for people who are uncomfortable touching their bodies. They are often used as a backup method of contraception.

Barrier methods are inexpensive per use. The diaphragm and cervical cap require a fitting and prescription, adding to their initial cost. Other barrier methods are over-the-counter purchases. These methods are often chosen as backup methods or when the woman is lactating or if she does not tolerate OCs or an IUD.

Diaphragm and Cervical Cap

Diaphragms and cervical caps are rubber domes that fit over the cervix and are used with spermicides that kill sperm that pass the mechanical bar-

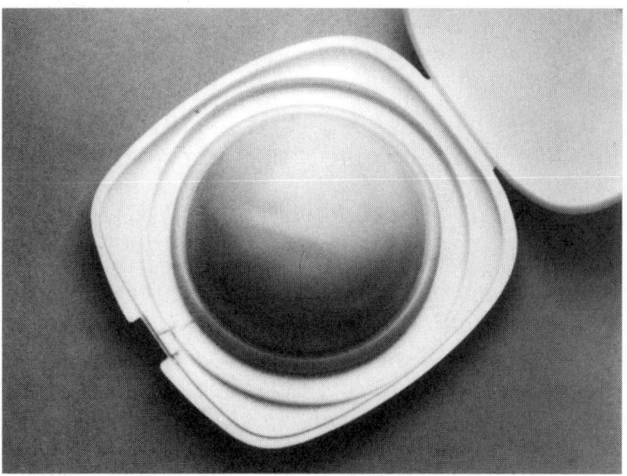

Figure 11–4. • The diaphragm. (Courtesy of Planned Parenthood Federation of America, Inc., New York, NY.)

rier (Figs. 11–4 and 11–5). The cervical cap is much smaller than the diaphragm. Cervical caps do not come in as many sizes as diaphragms, but women who cannot be fitted with a diaphragm may be able to use the cervical cap.

The diaphragm and cervical cap are fitted by a nurse-practitioner, nurse-midwife, or physician. The woman must learn how to insert and remove the diaphragm or cervical cap and to verify proper placement. User misplacement, especially of the small cervical cap, is a common reason for unintended pregnancy.

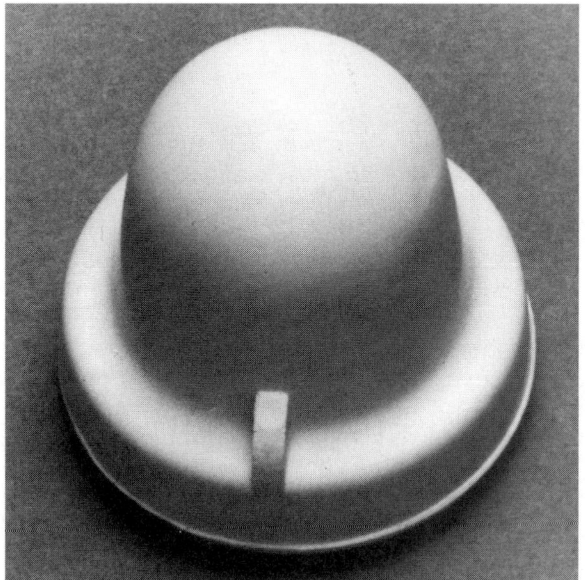

Figure 11–5. • The cervical cap. (Courtesy of Planned Parenthood Federation of America, Inc., New York, NY.)

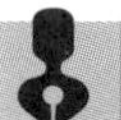

Nursing Tip

Adolescents must be educated about contraception, reproductive health, and the dangers of unprotected sex.

The woman should check either device for weak spots or pinholes before insertion by holding it up to the light. Spermicidal jelly or cream is applied to the ring and center of the diaphragm before inserting and positioning it over the cervix. It may be inserted several hours before intercourse and should remain in place for at least 6 hours after intercourse. Leaving the diaphragm or cervical cap in longer than necessary increases the risk for toxic shock syndrome. More spermicidal jelly or cream must be inserted into the vagina if the couple repeats coitus within 6 hours.

Use of the cervical cap is similar to that of the diaphragm except that it may remain in place for up to 48 hours. Spermicide is applied to the center of the cap. Use of added spermicide for repeat episodes of intercourse is optional.

The diaphragm must be refitted after each birth or a weight change of 10 pounds or more. The cap must be refitted yearly and after birth, abortion, or surgery.

Side Effects and Contraindications. Women who have an allergy to rubber or spermicides are not good candidates for the diaphragm or cervical cap. These devices are not recommended for women who have a history of toxic shock syndrome because the diaphragm or cap must remain in the body for several hours. Some women who have uterine anomalies or birth injuries cannot be fitted. Pressure from the diaphragm on the urethra may interfere with complete emptying of the bladder, increasing the woman's risk for bladder infections. They should not be worn during menstruation or in cases of vaginal bleeding because of the risk for infection.

Nursing Care. The health care provider who fits the device will provide much of the teaching on insertion, verification of placement, and removal. The nurse often reinforces the teaching, especially about the use and reapplication of spermicide for repeat intercourse. The nurse should teach the woman about signs of uterine infection (pain, foul-odored drainage, or fever) and of sensitivity to the product (irritation or itching). The woman also should be taught to report signs and symptoms of urinary tract infection: fever, pain or burning with urination, urgency, or urinary frequency.

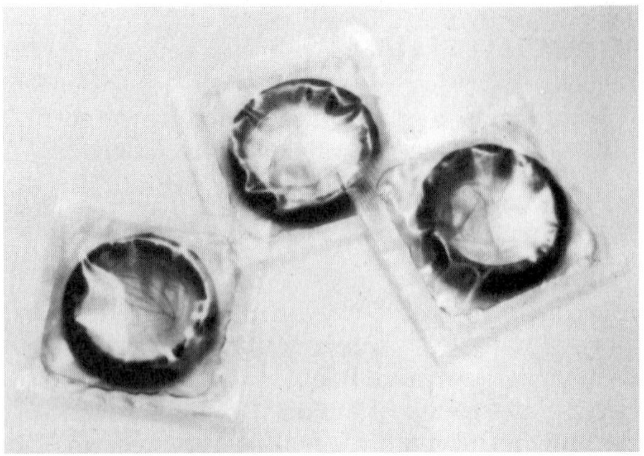

Figure 11–6. • The male condom. (Courtesy of Planned Parenthood Federation of America, Inc., New York, NY.)

Male Condom

Male condoms are sheaths of thin latex, polyurethane, or natural membrane ("skins") worn on the penis during intercourse (Fig. 11–6). Condoms collect semen before, during, and after ejaculation. They come in various styles, such as ribbed, lubricated, and colored, and with or without spermicide. They are single-use, low-cost items that are widely available from vending machines, drugstores, and family planning clinics. Latex condoms provide some protection from STDs, including HIV. Natural membrane condoms do not prevent the passage of viruses, including HIV. See Box 11–4 for correct use of the condom.

Water-soluble lubricants should be used if the condom or vagina is dry to avoid breakage. These lubricants do not damage the latex or cause breakage as petroleum jelly or other oil-based lubricants may. The penis should be withdrawn immediately if the man feels that the condom is breaking or becoming dislodged. The condom is removed and replaced.

Condoms are not reused, because even a pinhole can lead to pregnancy or permit the entry of viruses, including HIV. The condom package should be checked for expiration date.

Side Effects and Contraindications. Side effects and contraindications are rare. Either of the partners may be allergic to latex. The polyurethane condom can often be used successfully for those who are sensitive to latex.

Female Condom

Female condoms are essentially used for the same purpose as male condoms, to prevent pregnancy and to protect the woman from HIV and other STDs (Fig. 11–7). There are currently two styles of female condoms:

- Two flexible rings, one that fits into the vagina and one that remains outside, connected by a polyurethane sheath
- A bikini-panty style that has a pouch that fits inside the vagina

Female condoms are prelubricated, single-use items that are available over the counter.

The female condom is less effective than a latex condom at preventing infections. However, it gives the woman control over her exposure to infections without having to rely on the cooperation of her partner. Its failure rate in pregnancy prevention is 21%. Many women find it unattractive.

Side Effects and Contraindications. There are few problems with use of the female condom. Few people are sensitive to polyurethane.

Nursing Care Related to Male and Female Condom Use. The nurse should emphasize that condoms are single-use items that can deteriorate with age. Water-soluble lubricants should be used to avoid breakage, which would defeat their contraceptive and infection-prevention purposes. Condoms containing spermicides are more effective in preventing pregnancy and also provide lubrication, which can prevent breakage. A condom must be in place before *any* penile contact with the vagina because sperm are contained in the preejaculation secretions from the penis. The condom should be removed so as to avoid spillage of semen before the penis becomes soft.

Spermicides

Spermicidal foam, cream, jelly, film, and suppository capsules are over-the-counter contraceptives. They are inserted into the vagina before intercourse. They neutralize vaginal secretions, destroy sperm, and block entrance to the uterus. Each product has specific directions for use. Vaginal films and suppositories must melt before they are effective, which takes about 15 minutes. Most spermicides are effective for no more than 1 hour. Reapplication is needed for repeated coitus. The woman should not douche for at least 6 to 8 hours after intercourse.

Adolescents often choose this type of contraception because it is inexpensive and easy to obtain. Teenagers should be taught that products labeled "for personal hygiene use" do not have contraceptive action. Spermicides have an actual failure rate of 21%. The use of a condom with the spermicide increases the contraceptive effectiveness.

The drawbacks of spermicides used alone as a contraceptive method include their relatively high failure rate. Many couples also consider them messy or complain that they interfere with lovemaking. Dissatisfaction with their use often means that couples will take risks and not use the spermicide, with pregnancy as a possible outcome.

Side Effects and Contraindications. Spermicides can cause local irritation in the vagina or on the penis. The irritation can cause tiny cracks

BOX 11–4

TEACHING USE OF THE MALE CONDOM

Use a new condom each time. Check the expiration date on packages, as condoms deteriorate over time.

Apply the condom before you have any contact with the woman's vagina because there are sperm in the secretions before you ejaculate.

1. Squeeze the air from the tip when placing the condom over the end of your penis. Leave a half inch of space at the tip to allow sperm to collect and to prevent breakage.

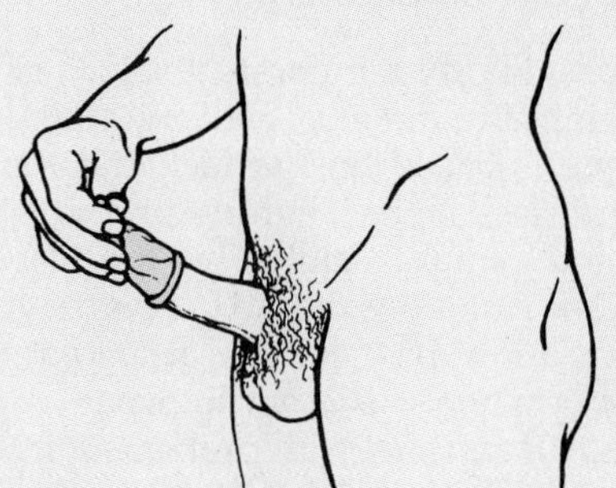

2. Hold the tip while you unroll the condom over the erect penis.

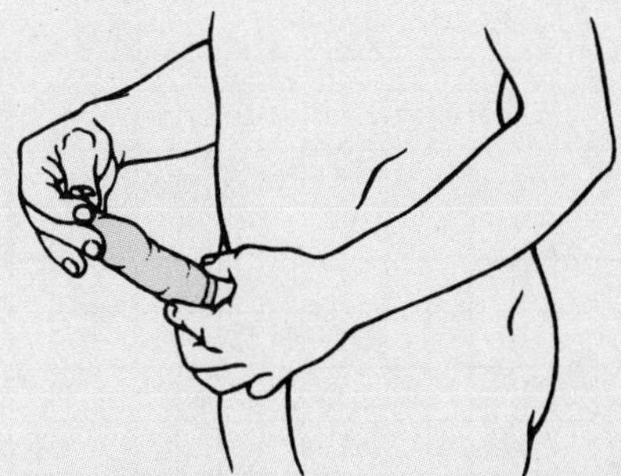

3. Do not use petroleum jelly, grease, or oil as lubricants because they can cause the condom to burst. Instead, use a water-soluble lubricant such as K-Y Jelly.

4. Hold on to the condom at the base of the penis to prevent spillage as you withdraw from the vagina.

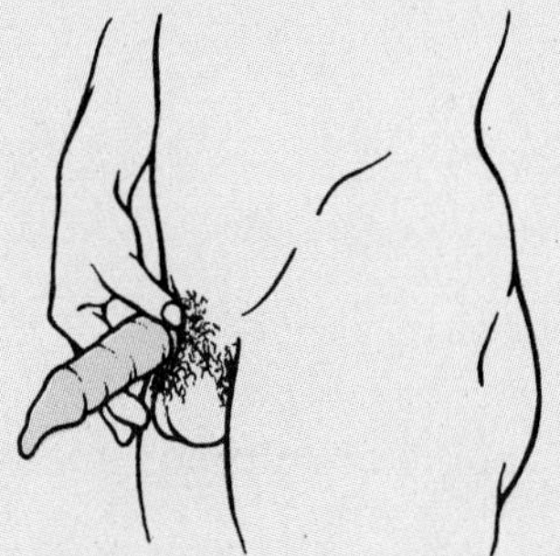

5. Remove the condom carefully to be sure that no semen spills from it.

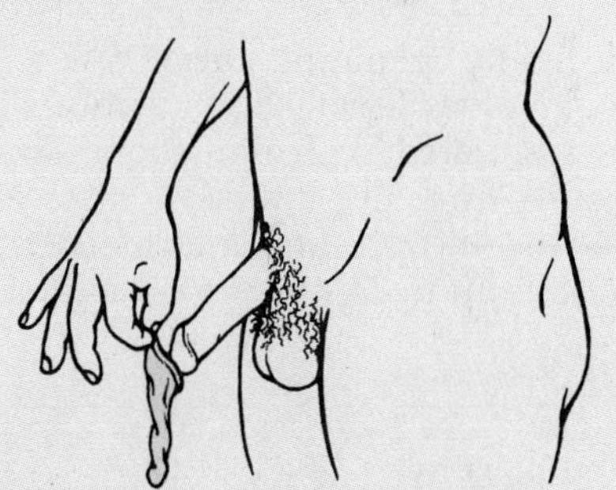

6. Place the condom in the trash or in some safe disposal.

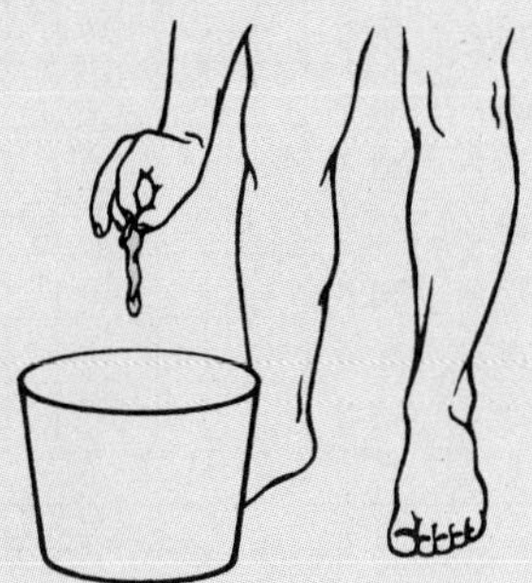

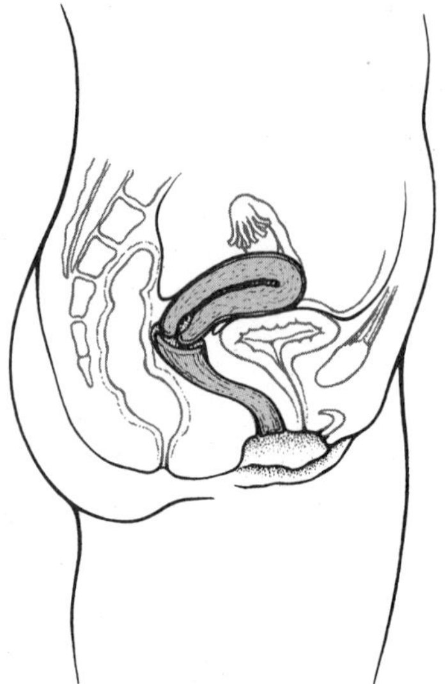

Figure 11–7. • The female condom can protect the woman from sexually transmitted disease and offer her a sense of control over her own body.

that provide a portal of entry for infection, including HIV.

Natural Family Planning

Natural family planning, also called fertility awareness, involves learning to identify signs and symptoms associated with ovulation. The couple either abstains from intercourse or uses a barrier method during the presumed fertile period. The ovum is viable up to 24 hours after ovulation and sperm are viable for up to 72 hours, although most die within 24 hours.

Natural family planning methods are acceptable to most religions. They require no systemic hormones or insertion of devices. They are not only reversible, but also can actually be used to increase the odds of achieving pregnancy when the couple desires a child.

Natural family planning requires extensive assessment and charting of all the changes in the menstrual cycle. The woman must be highly motivated to track the many factors that identify ovulation. Both partners must be willing to abstain from intercourse for much of the woman's cycle if the method is used to avoid pregnancy. They must also be willing to accept the high failure rate of 20%. There are three ways for a woman to predict when she is fertile. A woman may select only one method, but most women use a combination of the three to increase the predictive value of the methods.

Basal Body Temperature

The basal body temperature (BBT) is taken upon awakening before any activity (Fig. 11–8). This technique is based on the fact that the basal temperature rises very slightly at ovulation (about 0.4°F) and remains higher in the last half of the cycle. Unfortunately, the BBT is better at identifying that ovulation has *already* occurred rather than predicting when it is *about* to occur.

A *basal thermometer* is calibrated in tenths of a degree or is an electronic digital one to detect these tiny changes. The woman charts each day's temperature to identify her temperature pattern. A rise in the BBT for the last 14 days of the cycle means

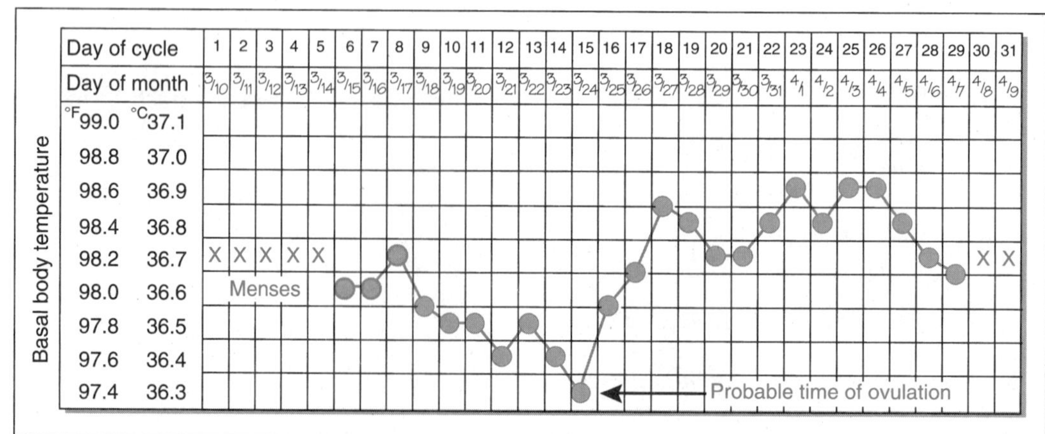

Figure 11–8. • Basal body temperature chart. By taking and recording her temperature, the woman can determine the probable time of ovulation.

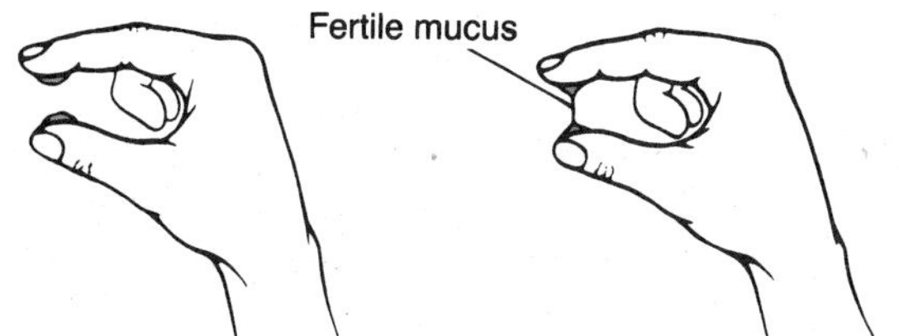

Figure 11–9. • Spinnbarkeit. The woman tests the ability of her cervical mucus to stretch. This helps to determine the time of ovulation.

that ovulation has probably occurred. Some electronic models have a memory to retain each day's temperature and display the pattern on a small screen.

Many factors can interfere with the accuracy of the BBT in predicting ovulation. Poor sleep, illness, jet lag, sleeping late, alcohol intake the evening before, or sleeping under an electric blanket or on a heated water bed can make the BBT unreliable.

Cervical Mucus

This method is also called the Billings method to predict ovulation. The character of cervical mucus changes during the menstrual cycle as estrogen and progesterone influence the mucus-secreting glands of the cervix. Immediately after menstruation, the cervical mucus is sticky, thick, and white. As ovulation nears, the mucus becomes thin, slippery, and clear to aid the passage of sperm into the cervix. The slippery mucus can be stretched 6 cm or more and has the consistency of egg white (Fig. 11–9). The stretching of the mucus is called *spinnbarkeit.* After ovulation, the mucus again becomes thicker. Factors that interfere with the accuracy of cervical mucus assessment include use of antihistamines, vaginal infections, contraceptive foams or jellies, sexual arousal, and recent coitus.

Calendar, or Rhythm, Method

The woman charts her menstrual cycles on a calendar for several months. If they are regular, she may be able to predict ovulation. The rhythm method is based on the fact that ovulation usually occurs about 14 days *before* the next menstrual period. This would be about halfway through a 28-day cycle, but would be on day 16 of a 30-day cycle.

Sterilization

Sterilization is a permanent method of birth control that is almost 100% effective in preventing pregnancy. Although the procedure may be reversed in some cases, it is expensive and not always successful. Therefore, clients should carefully think about this decision and consider it permanent.

Advantages

The advantages to sterilization is that the person can consider their risk of pregnancy to be near zero. Minimal anxiety about becoming pregnant may help them to enjoy their sexual relationship more.

Disadvantages

A major disadvantage of sterilization is the same as its primary advantage: permanence. Divorce, marriage, death of a child, or a change in attitude toward having children may make the person regret his or her decision. The procedures require surgery, and although the risks are small, they are the same as for other surgical procedures: hemorrhage, infection, injury to other organs, and anesthesia complications.

Male Sterilization

Male sterilization, or *vasectomy,* is performed by making a cut in each side of the scrotum and cutting each vas deferens, the tube through which the sperm travel (Fig. 11–10). Because sperm are already in the system distal to the area of ligation,

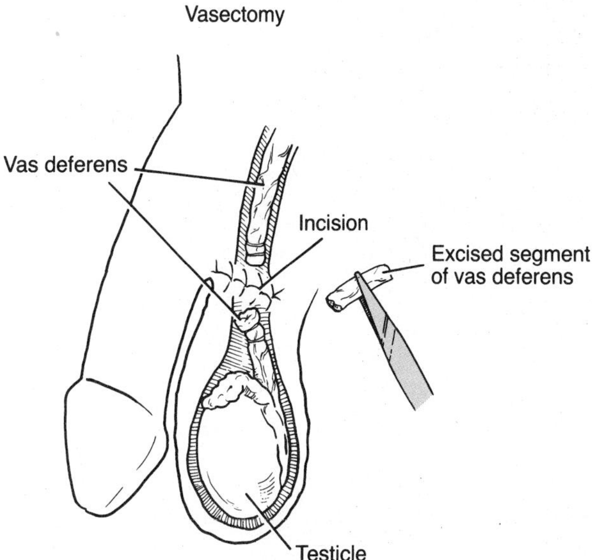

Figure 11–10. • Vasectomy. (From Black, J. M., & Matassarin-Jacobs, E. [1993]. *Luckmann and Sorensen's medical-surgical nursing: A psychophysiologic approach* [4th ed.]. Philadelphia: Saunders.)

Nursing Tip

When discussing sexual issues with a couple, the nurse should use the word *partner* until the couple indicates a preference for an alternative term.

sterility is not immediate. Another method of birth control must be used until all sperm have left the system, usually about 1 month. The man should return to his physician for analysis of his semen to verify that it no longer contains sperm. Men need information about the anatomy and physiology of their sex organs. They need reassurance that they will still have erections and ejaculations and that intercourse will remain pleasurable.

The surgery takes about 20 minutes and is performed on an outpatient basis under local anesthesia. There is some pain, bruising, and swelling after the surgery. Rest, a mild analgesic, and the application of an ice pack are comfort measures. As in other surgeries, the man should report:

- Bleeding or substantial bruising
- Separation of the suture line, drainage, or increasing pain

Female Sterilization

Female sterilization, called *tubal ligation,* involves blocking or ligating the fallopian tubes. It can be accomplished by using electrocautery or clips. Tubal ligation is easy to perform during the immediate postpartum period because the fundus, to which the tubes are attached, is large and near the surface. Any of three methods may be used:

- A *minilaparotomy,* nicknamed "Band-Aid surgery," uses an incision near the umbilicus in the immediate postpartum period or just above the symphysis at other times. The surgeon makes a tiny incision, brings each tube through it, and ligates and cuts the tube.
- *Laparoscopic surgery* is similar, but the tubes are identified and ligated through a lighted tube called a laparoscope (Fig. 11–11).
- Traditional approach during other abdominal surgery, usually a cesarean birth.

The discomfort following the minilaparotomy or laparoscopy is usually easily relieved with oral analgesia. Some women experience nausea from the anesthesia. Even though this is not considered major surgery, the woman requires 1 or 2 days to recuperate. She should report signs of bleeding or infection, as in the male vasectomy.

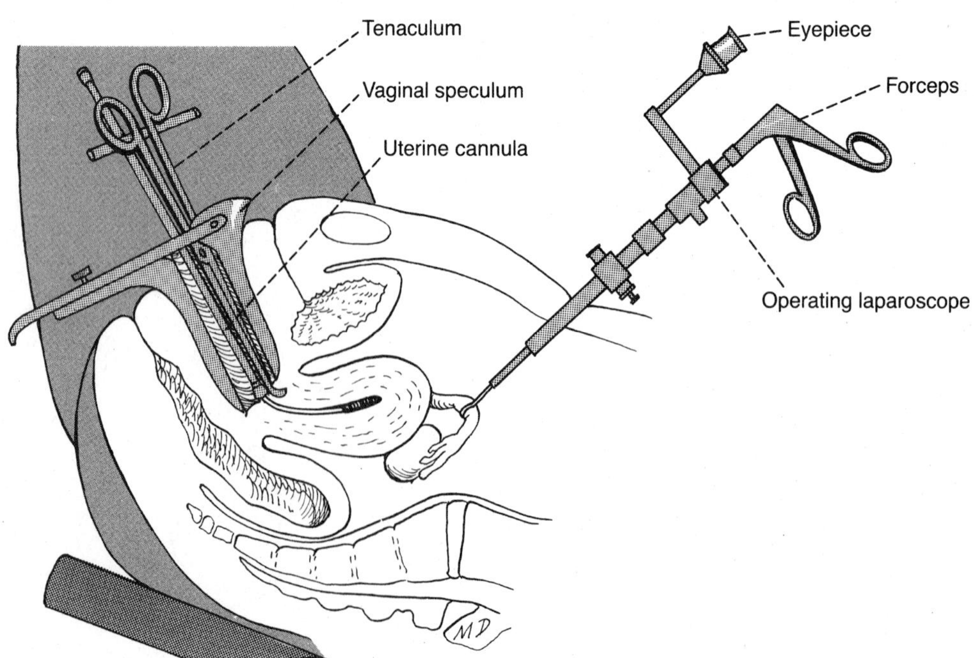

Figure 11–11. • Laparoscopy for tubal ligation. (From Black, J. M., & Matassarin-Jacobs, E. [1993]. *Luckmann and Sorensen's medical-surgical nursing: A psychophysiologic approach* [4th ed.]. Philadelphia: Saunders.)

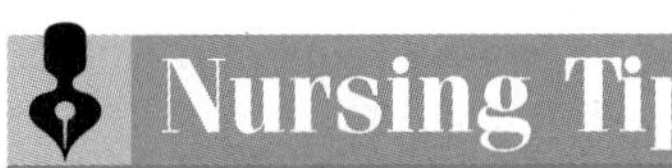

A woman can become pregnant while breastfeeding.

Unreliable Contraceptive Methods

Withdrawal

Withdrawal, or *coitus interruptus,* is withdrawal of the penis before ejaculation. It demands more self-control than most men can achieve. Preejaculatory secretions often contain sperm which can fertilize an ovum.

Douching

Douching after intercourse is not a form of birth control and may actually transport sperm farther into the birth canal.

Breastfeeding

Breastfeeding inhibits ovulation in many women as long as the infant receives at least 10 feedings in 24 hours. The prolactin secreted to stimulate milk production also inhibits ovulation. If the woman supplements with formula or when the infant begins taking solids, milk intake, and thus prolactin secretion, falls. Ovulation is then likely. Remember that ovulation *precedes* menstruation—pregnancy can occur before the first menstrual period after birth.

INFERTILITY CARE

Infertility is the inability to conceive when desired. The strict definition of infertility is that a couple who has regular, unprotected sexual intercourse for 1 year cannot conceive. Infertility is *primary* if conception has never occurred and *secondary* when there have been one or more pregnancies before the infertility. The definition is usually expanded to couples who conceive but repeatedly lose a pregnancy.

About 15% of U.S. couples cannot achieve pregnancy when they desire (Edwards & Brody, 1995). More couples are seeking help for infertility for many reasons, including the following:

- Delaying childbearing until the mid to late 30s when a natural decline in fertility occurs
- New treatments that may cause couples to reconsider their acceptance of childlessness and initiate or resume infertility therapy

Social and Psychological Implications

Becoming a parent is a role that most people expect to assume at some time. Because parenting is such an expected and necessary part of society, infertility has implications that go far beyond its physical implications.

Assumption of Fertility

Most couples assume that they are fertile and work hard to avoid pregnancy as they pursue educational or career goals. They expect to conceive in a few months at the most when they do decide to have a baby. They enjoy being with parents and expectant parents because they foresee joining their ranks shortly. They often begin making preparations for living space and supplies that a baby will need.

As the months pass and the woman's period comes each month, they become less certain that they will join the ranks of other parents. Once-joyful occasions, such as baby showers, become melancholy or anxiety-provoking events. The potential grandparents may think their children are waiting too long to start a family or even believe they are selfish if they do not realize that the younger couple is trying to conceive.

If the couple considers whether to seek help for infertility, they must discuss several factors:

- How important is a baby in their lives? Conflicts may occur if one member of the couple is more eager to get help and start treatment than the other one.
- Are they willing to share intimate information? Infertility specialists will ask for no more information than is required, but still a great deal of intimate information about their sexual relationship and function will have to be shared.

Nursing Tip

Avoid using the word *fault* when discussing which member of the infertile couple has the identified problem. Although a problem may be identified in only one person, many unknown factors impact fertility.

- What are their ages? The woman who is 40 years old has less time to pursue pregnancy than the woman who is 30.
- Can they afford infertility therapy? Some diagnostic tests and therapies are relatively inexpensive, whereas others are very expensive. The newest techniques are usually experimental and not covered by health insurance. A couple must often reevaluate financial commitments at decision points along the way.
- Can they commit the time and energy necessary for treatment? Some tests and treatments are simple, but others are difficult and time-consuming. Couples may be involved in treatment for a decade or more. The woman is most often the one who must chart her menstrual periods, take medications, have studies on a daily basis near ovulation, and take medications. She may feel that having a baby is her new job; many women do stop or decrease their work commitments to undergo infertility therapy.
- What is the probability of success of treatment? This is a recurring decision for couples whose tests and treatments become progressively more difficult.

The couple must often reevaluate their commitment to treatment at decision points along the way.

Psychological Reactions

Shock is often a couple's first reaction to infertility. Their reactions vary on how easily the infertility is alleviated, their personality and self-images, and their relationship.

Guilt. The partner who has the identified problem may feel guilty because he or she is depriving the other one of children. Either partner may regret past choices that now affect their fertility, such as sexual practices that resulted in infections that scarred the fallopian tubes.

Isolation. Infertile couples often feel different from those who have no problem conceiving. They may isolate themselves from these people to avoid emotional pain. In doing so, they may also isolate themselves from sources of support.

Depression. Infertility challenges one's sense of control and self-image. The couple may experience a roller-coaster of hope alternating with despair as the woman has her period each month. They may become judgmental and angry at others.

Stress on the Relationship. Either or both partners may feel unlovable because their self-esteem has been shaken by the problem. A man often finds it difficult to perform sexually "on demand" for semen specimens or at specific times each month. Their sexual relationship may take on a clinical air rather than one of love and support.

Cultural and Religious Considerations

In many cultures, fertility, or lack thereof, is considered strictly a female problem. It may be closely linked to the woman's social status. The stigma of infertility can lead to divorce and rejection from family and society. To choose treatment for infertility may go against the couple's societal norms, particularly if the male must be treated to achieve pregnancy.

Religious norms influence what tests and treatments a couple is willing to pursue. Surrogate parenting, in vitro fertilization, or other techniques may not be acceptable in terms of the couple's personal or religious beliefs. Conflict can arise if a potentially successful therapy is acceptable to one member of the couple, but not to the other.

Factors Affecting Infertility

Many factors that cause infertility are unknown. Some couples may have a problem that makes it unlikely that they would conceive, yet they have several children. Others have no identified problem, but still cannot conceive.

Male Factors

To achieve pregnancy, the man must deposit a sufficient number of normal sperm near the cervix, and the sperm must be protected from the acidic vaginal secretions until they enter the cervix. The sperm must be able to swim purposefully to the waiting ovum. Male factors in infertility can be divided into abnormalities of the sperm, erections, ejaculation, or seminal fluid.

Abnormal Sperm. A man may have a sperm count that is too low to achieve fertilization. He may have a sufficient number of sperm, but too many of these are dead or abnormally formed. Sperm are continuously formed, and many factors can affect their formation. Some factors that can interfere with normal sperm formation and function include:

- High scrotal temperature from hot tubs, saunas, or fever
- Abnormal hormone stimulation
- Infections
- Anatomic abnormalities such as a varicocele (enlarged veins in the testicles)
- Medications, illicit drugs, excessive alcohol intake
- Exposure to toxins

Abnormal Erections. Anything that impairs nervous system function or blood flow to the penis can interfere with erections. Some drugs, notably antihypertensives, reduce or shorten erections.

Abnormal Ejaculation. Some drugs and nervous system disorders may cause *retrograde ejaculation,* in which semen is released into the bladder rather than from the penis. *Hypospadias* (urethral opening on the underside of the penis rather than the tip) causes semen to be deposited closer to the vaginal outlet rather than near the cervix.

Abnormal Seminal Fluid. Seminal fluid carries the sperm into the vagina, but only sperm enter the cervix to fertilize the ovum. Semen coagulates immediately after ejaculation, then liquifies within 30 minutes to allow sperm to swim toward the cervix. Sperm will be trapped or will not survive if the seminal fluid remains thick or if its composition does not protect the sperm from the vaginal secretions.

Female Factors

A woman's fertility depends on regular production of normal ova, having an open path from the ovary to the uterus, and having a uterine endometrium that supports the pregnancy.

Disorders of Ovulation. Normal ovulation depends on a balanced and precisely timed interaction between the hypothalamus, pituitary, and ovary (see Chapter 2). If the hypothalamus and/or pituitary do not properly stimulate the ovary, ovulation will not occur. Conversely, the ovary may not respond despite normal hormonal stimulation. Chemotherapeutic drugs for cancer, excessive alcohol intake, and smoking can interfere with ovulation. Sometimes ovulation does not occur because the woman is entering the climacteric early.

Abnormalities of the Fallopian Tubes. Infections such as chlamydia and gonorrhea can cause scarring and adhesions of the fallopian tubes that block them. Adhesions may also occur because of endometriosis, pelvic surgery, appendicitis, peritonitis, or ovarian cysts. If the tubal obstruction allows the smaller sperm to pass but is too narrow for the resulting fertilized ovum, ectopic tubal pregnancy may occur (see p. 85). The same conditions may cause abnormal transport of the ovum through the tube.

Abnormalities of the Uterus, Cervix, or Ovaries. Congenital abnormalities of the reproductive tract or uterine *myomas* (benign uterine muscle tumors) may interfere with normal implantation of the ovum or may result in repeated spontaneous abortion or early preterm labor. Women with polycystic ovaries have abnormalities of ovulation and menstruation that accompany the hormonal dysfunction associated with this disorder.

Hormone Abnormalities. In addition to interfering with ovulation, abnormal hormone stimulation can interfere with proper development of the uterine lining, resulting in an inability to conceive or in repeated spontaneous abortions. Abnormalities in amount or timing of any hormone necessary for endometrial buildup, ovum development and release, or support of the conceptus can result in infertility.

Evaluation of Infertility

Both members of a couple are evaluated for infertility. The evaluation begins with a thorough history and physical examination to identify evidence of other conditions that may also be affecting their fertility. Information that directly relates to fertility will be collected:

- The woman's menstrual pattern
- Any pregnancies and their outcomes, including pregnancies with the same partner and those with any other partner(s)
- Pattern of intercourse in relation to the woman's menstrual cycles
- Length of time the couple has had unprotected intercourse
- Any home tests or techniques (such as basal body temperature) the couple has already used

Diagnostic Tests

Testing proceeds from the simple to the complex. However, testing may be accelerated if the woman is older because of her natural decline in fertility with age.

Male Testing. A semen analysis is the first male test performed. Semen is best collected by masturbation, although it can be collected in a condom if this is unacceptable. Endocrine tests identify the hormonal stimulation that is necessary for sperm formation. Ultrasonography can identify anatomical abnormalities. Testicular biopsy is an invasive test to obtain a sample of testicular tissue for analysis.

Female Testing. The methods for predicting ovulation discussed in natural family planning can also be used to evaluate infertility. Ultrasonography is used to assess the structure of reproductive organs, to identify maturation and release of the ovum, and to ensure proper timing for other tests, such as the postcoital test. Ultrasonography is also used to identify multifetal pregnancies. The postcoital test is done 6 to 12 hours after intercourse to evaluate the action of sperm within the woman's cervical mucus at the time of ovulation. Endocrine tests evaluate hormone stimulation of ovulation and buildup of the uterine lining to prepare for pregnancy.

More invasive tests are sometimes required. The hysterosalpingogram is an X-ray using contrast medium to evaluate the structure of the reproductive organs. An endometrial biopsy is done to obtain a sample of uterine lining to assess its response to hormones. Hysteroscopy and laparoscopy use an endoscope (instrument that allows visual inspection of internal organs) to examine the uterine interior and the pelvic organs.

Therapy for Infertility

The specific therapy depends on what cause, if any, was identified by testing. Possible therapies are discussed here.

Medications

Medications may be given to either the man or woman to improve semen quality, induce ovulation, prepare the uterine endometrium for pregnancy, or support the pregnancy once it is established. Several of the drugs are given with another drug to mimic natural function. Some of the drugs that may be prescribed include the following:

- Bromocriptine (Parlodel). Corrects excess prolactin secretion by the pituitary, which would interfere with implantation of the fertilized ovum
- Clomiphene (Clomid). Induces ovulation. It may also increase sperm production although this is an unlabeled use
- Gonadotropin-releasing hormone (GnRH, Lutrepulse). Stimulates production of other hormones that, in turn, stimulate ovulation in the female and production of testosterone and sperm in the male
- Leuprolide (Lupron). Reduces endometriosis
- Menotropins (Pergonal). Stimulates ovulation and sperm production
- Nafarelin (Synarel). Reduces endometriosis
- Progesterone. Promotes implantation of the fertilized ovum
- Urofollitropin (Metrodin). Stimulates ovulation.

Medications given to induce ovulation also increase the risk of multifetal gestations. Although most of these multiple gestations are twins, higher multiples present a much higher risk for maternal, fetal, and neonatal complications. The parents of high multiples may have to make a decision about which, if any, of their fetuses to abort so that the others have a better chance of achieving maturity. This situation, although uncommon, presents a difficult ethical situation for both parents and professionals.

Surgical Procedures

Surgery may be used to correct anatomic abnormalities such as varicocele, adhesions, or tubal obstruction.

Therapeutic Insemination

Once called "artificial insemination," therapeutic insemination may use the male partner's sperm or sperm from an anonymous donor. Therapeutic insemination may be used by a woman who wants a biological child without a relationship with a man. If sperm are placed directly in the uterus, they are washed and concentrated to improve their chances of fertilizing an ovum. Donors are screened for genetic defects, infections, and high-risk behaviors. Donor sperm is held frozen for 6 months to reduce the risk of transmitting a disease that was not apparent at the initial screening. Reputable centers limit the number of times a man may donate his sperm to reduce the chance of inadvertent consanguinity (blood relationship) between his offspring when they grow up.

Surrogate Parenting

A surrogate mother may donate the use of her uterus only, with the sperm and ovum coming from the infertile couple who has a problem carrying a pregnancy. Or she may be inseminated with the male partner's sperm, thus supplying both her genetic and her gestational components. Surrogate mothering cannot be anonymous and the birth mother inevitably forms bonds with the baby during the months of pregnancy.

Advanced Reproductive Techniques

The field of advanced reproductive technologies (ARTs) gives new hope to couples who may have once considered their infertility to be irreversible (Table 11–2). However, some of the newest techniques are still considered experimental and are thus not covered by insurance.

Bypassing Obstacles to Conception. These techniques place intact sperm and ova together to allow fertilization. Each begins with ovulation induction by medications to obtain several ova and thus improve the likelihood of a successful pregnancy.

- *In vitro fertilization (IVF).* Several ova are obtained and mixed with the partner's or a donor's semen. Up to four resulting embryos are then returned to the uterus two days later.
- *Gamete intrafallopian transfer (GIFT).* Ova are obtained and mixed with sperm. The gametes are placed in the fallopian tubes where fertilization and entry into the uterus occur normally.
- *Tubal embryo transfer (TET),* also called zygote intrafallopian transfer (ZIFT). The ova are fertilized outside the woman's body and returned to the fallopian tube at an earlier stage than with IVF.

In general, GIFT and TET have a higher pregnancy rate than IVF. These techniques can result in a multifetal pregnancy. It is rare that all ova or embryos returned to the uterus actually implant.

Microsurgical Techniques. In these techniques, the surgeon "operates" on the ovum itself to inject a sperm into it. The fertilized ovum is placed into the uterus, as with IVF.

Outcomes of Infertility Therapy

Three outcomes are possible after infertility therapy:

- Achievement of a "take home" baby
- Unsuccessful therapy resulting in a decision about adoption
- Pregnancy loss after treatment

Becoming pregnant changes the couple's anxiety, but does not eliminate it. Because of past disappointments, they may be reluctant to invest emotionally in the pregnancy. They may delay preparations for birth because they expect to be disappointed again or fear that something will go wrong at the last minute. Even when their baby is born, they may have unrealistic expectations of themselves as parents after all their hard work in achieving pregnancy.

Couples who decide to pursue adoption must consider their preferences and the realities of the adoption "market." Most couples prefer to adopt an infant of the same race, but that child may not be available. Some couples fear that they will have a biological child after adoption and wonder if they can love the two children equally. When a pregnancy is lost after treatment, the couple may feel optimism mixed with sadness. On one hand, they proved that they could conceive. On the other hand, they did not get a baby.

Nursing Care Related to Infertility Treatment

Much of the nursing role involves supporting the couple as they undergo diagnosis and treatment. The nurse must use tactful therapeutic communication to help each member of the couple to discuss their feelings. Encourage partners to accept their feelings. Reinforce the normality of feelings that seem out of place (such as ambivalence about a pregnancy after working so hard to achieve it). Help the couple to identify ways to communicate with each other.

Table 11–2
SUMMARY OF ASSISTED REPRODUCTIVE THERAPIES (ARTS)

Therapy	Description
Therapeutic insemination	Donor sperm are placed in the uterus or fallopian tube; sperm may be the partner's or a donor's
In vitro fertilization (IVF)	After inducing ovulation, ova are recovered by laparoscopy or transvaginal aspiration under sonography; they are then fertilized with sperm from the partner or a donor in the laboratory and transferred to her uterus two days later
Gamete intrafallopian transfer (GIFT)	Oocytes are retrieved into a catheter that contains prepared sperm; up to two ova are injected into each fallopian tube, where fertilization occurs. The woman must have at least one open tube
Tubal embryo transfer (TET), also called zygote intrafallopian transfer (ZIFT)	Ova are fertilized as in IVF, but are transferred to the fallopian tube as soon as fertilization occurs. The resulting embryos enter the uterus normally for implantation
Donor oocyte	Multiple ova are retrieved from a woman. They are fertilized and placed in the prepared uterus of the infertile woman
Surrogate mother	A woman allows her ova to be inseminated by the partner or another donor. She then carries the fetus and agrees to relinquish the infant after birth
Gestational surrogate	The infertile couple undergoes IVF, but the resulting embryos are placed in the prepared uterus of a woman who has agreed to carry the fetus for them. The woman does not donate any of her genetic components.

Increase the couple's sense of control as much as possible. Reinforce their positive coping skills and explore more constructive alternatives to poor coping. They may benefit from relaxation techniques, support groups, and other stress-management methods. Support groups can also reduce their sense of isolation. Help the couple explore their options at each decision point. Only the person(s) involved can make the decision, but the nurse can help them to explore their feelings.

MENOPAUSE

Strictly speaking, *menopause* occurs when a woman's menstrual periods have ceased for a period of 1 year. The *climacteric* (or "change of life") is the time in a woman's life surrounding this event, when many physical and psychological changes occur. The early part of the climacteric is also referred to as the *perimenopausal period.* The term *menopause* is often used to describe both the climacteric and the actual cessation of menstruation, however.

Women often live 30 or more years after menopause. Changes of aging that accelerate after menopause, such as bone loss and heart disease, require the woman to make important decisions that may affect her health for many years. She must also evaluate her goals and priorities to deal with the physical, psychological, and social changes of aging.

Physical Changes

The final menstrual period usually occurs at about 51.5 years in natural menopause. The changes that precede cessation of menstruation occur gradually over 3 to 5 years. Any spontaneous bleeding after cessation of menstrual periods should be investigated because it suggests endometrial cancer. Menopause may be induced at any age by hysterectomy, pelvic irradiation, or extreme stress.

Perimenopausal symptoms are due to a decrease in ovarian function and changes in hormone production. There is an increase in follicle-stimulating hormone (FSH) to stimulate the maturation and release of an ovum, but the ovaries become more resistant to its effects. Ovarian production of estrogen and progesterone stop as ovulation gradually ceases. As estrogen and progesterone production fall, the woman's menstrual periods become more irregular until they finally cease.

Vasomotor changes often accompany these fluctuations. "Hot flashes" are a well-known phenomenon. The woman suddenly feels a burning or hot sensation of her skin followed by perspiration. Hot flashes often occur during the night, and some women have several sleep interruptions because of them. They are more likely to occur when menopause is artificial, such as through oophorectomy (removal of the ovaries), rather than when it occurs naturally. The woman may also notice chills, palpitations, dizziness, and tingling of the skin as part of the vasomotor instability.

The reproductive organs are estrogen-dependent, leading to changes as the estrogen level declines. The uterus shrinks and the ovaries atrophy. The sacral ligaments relax and pelvic muscles weaken, which can result in pelvic floor dysfunction. The cervix becomes pale and shrinks. The vagina becomes shorter, narrower, and less elastic. There is less lubrication. Some women notice a change in *libido* (sexual desire) at this time. Coitus may be uncomfortable because of vaginal dryness. Urinary incontinence may be a problem as the muscles controlling urine flow atrophy. The breasts atrophy.

Loss of estrogen secretion also means an end to its protective effect on the woman's cardiovascular and skeletal systems. Estrogen increases the amount of high-density lipoproteins, which carry cholesterol from body cells to the liver for excretion. The incidence of heart disease rises dramatically after menopause because low-density lipoproteins, which carry cholesterol into body cells (including blood vessels), increase.

Estrogen assists the deposition of calcium in the bones to strengthen them. Loss of bone mass accelerates as estrogen levels fall, resulting in *osteoporosis.* Osteoporosis is a leading cause of vertebral, hip, and other fractures in postmenopausal women because the bones become very fragile. Both males and females lose bone mass as they age. Females, who have a lower bone mass to begin with because they are smaller, lose more in proportion to the total amount as they age. Also, they live longer than males, so the loss continues longer. Therefore, problems such as hip fractures related to age affect many more women than men. The bones may be so fragile that a fracture occurs and causes a fall, rather than the fracture being the result of a fall.

Psychological and Cultural Variations

Women from different cultures have different experiences of menopause. How the society views aging, the role of the female, and femininity itself has a bearing. In countries in which age is revered, menopause is practically a "non-event." In the

United States, with its emphasis on youth, sex appeal, and physical beauty, menopause can threaten the woman's feelings of health and self-worth. A positive aspect of menopause is that it is a time of liberation from monthly periods, cramps, and the fear of unwanted pregnancy. It can be the beginning of a satisfying postreproductive life.

Hormone Replacement Therapy

Hormone replacement therapy (HRT) may be prescribed to relieve many of the uncomfortable symptoms of menopause. Additionally, HRT prolongs the protective effects of estrogen on the woman's cardiovascular and skeletal systems. Estrogen cannot prevent osteoporosis, but it can slow bone loss if the woman also takes in adequate calcium.

Estrogen may be administered in various forms depending on the woman's needs. Estrogen comes in tablets, transdermal skin patches, vaginal creams, injections, and pellets. The goal of therapy has a bearing on the dosage and form prescribed (e.g., whether for temporary relief of hot flashes or for osteoporosis). Vaginal changes can be treated locally with vaginal creams or systemically, or both ways. However, vaginal creams have no effect on osteoporosis.

Any of three regimens for HRT are used, depending on the woman's needs and whether she has a uterus.

- *Cyclic regimen.* Estrogen is given for a specific period, often 25 days, with progestin added for part of the month. The woman will have withdrawal bleeding during the interval when she does not take hormones.
- *Combined regimen.* Estrogen and progestin are given continuously. The woman will not have withdrawal bleeding with this treatment plan, although she may have some irregular bleeding for up to 6 months.
- *Estrogen only.* Estrogen is given for 25 days of each month or daily, with no medication-free interval. This regimen is used only for women who have had a hysterectomy because they have no risk for overstimulating the endometrium.

Side Effects and Contraindications. Side and adverse effects of estrogen include nausea, vomiting, headache, dizziness, intolerance to contact lenses, jaundice, and breast tenderness. The most common side effect of progesterone is irregular bleeding when therapy begins. The less frequent side effects of progesterone include symptoms similar to those of premenstrual syndrome, fluid retention, and depression. Both drugs are contraindicated for the woman who has thromboembolic disease. The fluid retention associated with progesterone therapy may complicate other conditions, such as asthma, heart disease, or renal disorders.

Therapy for Osteoporosis

Osteoporosis occurs when loss of calcium from the bones is faster than its deposition in the bones. Estrogen replacement can slow bone loss if the woman's calcium intake is adequate, particularly if given in the first few years after menopause. Additional therapies for osteoporosis include adequate intake of calcium, alternate medications for some women, and exercise.

Calcium Intake. Prevention of osteoporosis begins during youth, when calcium is deposited in growing bones. Adults and young women should have at least 1200 mg/day. Postmenopausal women need 1500 mg/day. Vitamin D is needed for calcium to be absorbed from the intestine, so 400 to 800 units is often recommended. Food sources for calcium include dairy products, leafy dark-green vegetables, soybeans, and wheat bread.

A woman should consult her medical care provider about her need for and recommended dose of calcium supplements because preparations vary and may differ in absorption. A high calcium intake does not substitute for HRT but complements it.

Alternatives to HRT. Some women cannot take estrogen, such as many breast cancer survivors. Several medications have been introduced that not only slow bone loss, but also can actually increase the woman's bone density. All must be taken with an adequate calcium intake to achieve the desired results. These medications and their chief nursing implications include the following:

- Calcitonin (Calcimar, Miacalcin) nasal spray or injection. Nasal irritation is the chief side effect of the spray.
- Alendronate (Fosamax). Esophageal irritation or gastric discomfort are chief side effects. The woman should take the drug with plain water upon arising and wait at least 30 minutes before taking any other food, beverage, or medication. She should not lie down for at least 30 minutes after taking the drug to reduce esophageal irritation.

Exercise. Weight-bearing exercise can increase bone density in the lumbar vertebrae. Walking, hiking, stair climbing, and dancing are good weight-bearing exercises. High-impact exercises should be avoided, as should those which have a high risk of causing a fall.

Nursing Care of the Menopausal Woman

Refer to Nursing Care Plan 11–1 for nursing interventions in addition to those discussed here. Assess the woman's knowledge of the changes surrounding menopause. Identify any symptoms that she is having if she is near the age for the climacteric to begin. Clarify any treatments or tests that the woman will have, such as bone density studies. Determine the woman's understanding of the risks and benefits of HRT when helping her to decide about the therapy. Provide written information to reinforce verbal teaching.

Teach the woman what signs and symptoms she should report, such as vaginal bleeding that recurs after cessation of menstrual periods. She should also report signs of vaginal irritation or signs of urinary tract infection because these are more common with atrophy of vaginal tissues.

Teach the woman how to take prescribed medications properly. For example, teach her that calcium is best utilized if she also takes Vitamin D. Taking foods or other medications before allowing at least 30 minutes (preferably 1 hour) for alendronate to be absorbed will negate the benefit of that dose. Lying down after taking alendronate can cause severe esophageal irritation.

Teach the woman medication-related side effects that should be reported. She should contact her health care provider if she has headaches, visual disturbances, signs of thrombophlebitis, heaviness in her legs, chest pain, or breast lumps because these symptoms may indicate adverse side effects associated with HRT. She should contact her health care provider for the best plan if she decides to stop HRT to reduce the distress associated with abrupt cessation of therapy.

Teach the woman about the value of weight-bearing exercise in slowing bone loss. Help her identify suitable exercises that she enjoys and caution her about the high-impact ones that she should avoid. Because even "minor" falls can result in disabling fractures in women who have osteoporosis, teach the woman ways to make her environment safer. Safety needs may be as simple as making sure there are adequate lights with handy switches and that loose cords and obstructions are secured outside of walking paths. Non-skid bath and shower floors and convenient grab bars reduce the risk of falls when bathing.

PELVIC FLOOR DYSFUNCTION

Pelvic floor dysfunction occurs when the muscles, ligaments, and fascia that support the pelvic organs are damaged or weakened. The dysfunction may occur as a result of childbirth injury, but often does not become obvious until the perimenopausal period. There are two classifications of pelvic floor dysfunction, and they often occur together:

- Vaginal wall prolapse, which includes cystocele, enterocele, and rectocele
- Uterine prolapse

Vaginal Wall Prolapse

The vaginal wall may prolapse in either the anterior or posterior wall or in both walls.

Cystocele

A *cystocele* occurs when the upper vaginal wall becomes too weak to support the bladder that contains urine. *Stress incontinence* may result when the woman loses urine with a sudden increase in intraabdominal pressure, such as with laughing, coughing, or sneezing.

Enterocele

An *enterocele* occurs when the upper posterior vagina is weakened, allowing a loop of bowel to herniate downward between the rectum and uterus.

Rectocele

A *rectocele* occurs when the posterior vaginal wall becomes weakened. When the woman strains to defecate, feces are pushed against the weakened wall rather than being directed toward the rectal sphincter for elimination. The woman may use digital pressure against her posterior vaginal wall to facilitate defecation.

Uterine Prolapse

A *uterine prolapse* occurs when the ligaments that support the uterus and vagina are weakened. The uterus sags downward in the vagina. It is more likely to occur in the woman who has had several vaginal births or one who had large infants. Symptoms of uterine prolapse include pelvic fullness, a dragging sensation, pelvic pressure, fatigue, and a low backache. The woman will often have symptoms characteristic of vaginal wall prolapse as well.

NURSING CARE PLAN 11–1

Selected Nursing Diagnoses: The Woman Experiencing Perimenopausal Symptoms

Nursing Diagnosis: Altered comfort related to vasomotor symptoms (hot flashes)

Goals	Nursing Interventions	Rationales
The woman will verbalize measures to increase her comfort during vasomotor symptoms	1. Suggest that she wear layered cotton clothes	1. This allows the woman to take off or put on clothes during hot flashes or chills; cotton allows easier passage of air than synthetic fabric
	2. Advise her to avoid caffeine (coffee, tea, colas, chocolate)	2. Hot flashes often occur at night; caffeine is a stimulant and will contribute to insomnia and perspiration
	3. Explain that stress exacerbates the condition; explore activities that she finds relaxing	3. Stress affects virtually every system of the body, including endocrine and cardiovascular systems, worsening the hot flashes
	4. Suggest she discuss hormone replacement therapy (HRT) with her physician	4. HRT is effective at relieving vasomotor symptoms, but its benefits and risks must be evaluated by the individual client
	5. Vitamin E, ginseng, and other herbs may reduce vasomotor symptoms	5. Some women should not take or choose not to take HRT, and these measures provide an alternative

Nursing Diagnosis: Altered sexuality patterns related to painful intercourse

Goals	Nursing Interventions	Rationales
The woman will state measures to reduce vaginal dryness The woman will express no discomfort with coitus	1. Teach woman to use water-soluble lubricant before intercourse	1. Thinning of vaginal walls and drying of secretions can lead to discomfort during intercourse unless additional lubrication is used; oil-based lubricants can promote bacterial growth
	2. Teach that products, such as Replens and Lubrin, are available without a prescription to provide relief of vaginal dryness for several days	2. These products lubricate vagina for a longer period of time, reducing tissue trauma
	3. If estrogen vaginal cream is prescribed, teach that it should be inserted at bedtime	3. Topical applications of estrogen reduce vaginal atrophy; applying at bedtime reduces loss and increases absorption

Nursing Diagnosis: Risk for urinary incontinence and infection related to genital atrophy

Goals	Nursing Interventions	Rationales
The woman will restate measures to promote urinary tract health	1. Teach Kegel exercises: Contract muscles as if to stop urine flow. Repeat 10 times. Do the cycle of 10 Kegel exercises 5 times each day. Do not actually stop urine flow while urinating	1. Kegel exercises increase muscle tone around the urinary meatus and the vagina. Repeatedly stopping the stream of urine could cause retention that could lead to infection
	2. Drink at least 8 glasses of water each day. Caffeine-containing drinks should not be included in the target amount of fluid	2. Adequate intake of liquid dilutes urine and promotes regular emptying, both of which discourage bacterial growth. Caffeine acts as diuretic, which reverses some of the benefits of the fluid taken in
	3. Urinate regularly; do not allow the bladder to become overdistended	3. Prevents stasis of urine, which promotes growth of bacteria
	4. Wipe from front to back after toileting	4. Avoids bringing anal organisms to the urinary meatus or vagina, where they could cause infection

Management of Pelvic Floor Dysfunction

Medical management of pelvic floor dysfunction depends on several factors, such as age, physical condition, sexual activity, and extent of the problem. Surgical correction gives the most definitive relief. The vaginal wall(s) may be repaired and a vaginal hysterectomy is often done for uterine prolapse. The two surgeries are often combined. If the woman cannot have surgery, a *pessary,* which is a device to support the pelvic structures, may be inserted into her vagina.

Nursing Care of the Woman with Pelvic Floor Dysfunction

Kegel exercises can help to strengthen the pubococcygeal muscle, a major support for the urethra, vagina, and rectum. The woman should contract her muscles as if stopping the flow of urine. She should not actually do the exercise while urinating. She should repeat the contraction 10 times and perform this cycle 5 times each day. The woman should continue Kegel exercises for the rest of her life to maintain pelvic muscle tone.

To reduce some of the low back and pelvic discomforts associated with pelvic relaxation, the woman can be taught to lie down with her feet elevated. Assuming the knee-chest position for a few minutes may also help. Measures to prevent constipation, such as adequate fluid and fiber intake, reduce hard feces that would put further pressure on a rectocele.

OTHER FEMALE REPRODUCTIVE TRACT DISORDERS

A woman may have other reproductive tract disorders during her life. An overview of some common benign ones will be presented here. For more information about these and information about malignant female reproductive tract disorders, consult a medical-surgical nursing text.

Cervical Polyps

Polyps are very small tumors that generally grow on a stemlike structure called a pedicle. They may cause erratic vaginal bleeding. Polyps are usually surgically removed in an outpatient setting. Any growth removed is sent for a pathological examination to rule out cancer.

Uterine Leiomyomas

Most women know of these growths by the name *fibroids.* Uterine fibroids are benign growths of uterine muscle cells and are a very common gynecologic condition. They grow under the influence of estrogen and are thus most prominent during the childbearing years and often atrophy after menopause. The growths may be within the uterine muscle mass, near the inside or outside uterine surface, or on a pedicle. They may be evident in the pregnant woman as a knotty growth felt on her uterus.

Many women have no problems with fibroids, but they sometimes cause irregular bleeding, pressure on the bladder, or pelvic pressure. If they are not troubling the woman, they are only observed and reevaluated periodically. If the woman is symptomatic, surgical treatments may include hysterectomy if the woman is finished with childbearing or a myomectomy (excision of the muscle tumor only) if she wants to preserve her uterus. Hormone treatment with GnRH may also shrink the tumors.

Ovarian Cysts

A follicular ovarian cyst may develop if the follicle fails to rupture and release its ovum during the menstrual cycle. This type of cyst usually regresses with the next menstrual cycle. A lutein cyst may occur when the corpus luteum that develops after ovulation fails to regress. The lutein cyst is more likely to cause pain. An ovarian cyst that ruptures or becomes twisted and infarcted as its blood supply is cut off can cause pelvic pain and tenderness.

Diagnosis is by transvaginal ultrasound examination. A laparoscopy may aid in diagnosing and differentiating the ovarian cyst pain from that caused by endometriosis. Laparotomy may be required to remove the cyst.

KEY POINTS

- Preventive care is cost-effective and reduces distress.
- Teaching a woman breast care can reduce her risk of death from breast cancer.
- Although the exact cause of premenstrual syndrome is unknown, several self-help measures can relieve some of its symptoms.
- Prevention of toxic shock syndrome involves not allowing microorganisms the time to grow in the woman's reproductive tract.
- Sexually transmissible diseases must be adequately treated in all sexual contacts to stop the transmission and to avoid resistance to antibiotics.
- Contraception is an individual choice. The nurse must avoid incorporating personal preferences when educating clients about contraceptive methods.
- Fertility awareness methods can be used both to avoid pregnancy and to increase the chance of achieving it.
- Except for abstinence, condoms (male and female) offer the best protection from sexually transmissible diseases, including the human immunodeficiency virus.
- Nursing care of infertile couples includes helping them to evaluate their options at different phases during evaluation and treatment.
- Common menopausal symptoms, such as "hot flashes" and vaginal dryness, stem from the cessation of ovulation and decrease in hormonal activity, particularly that of estrogen and progesterone.
- Prevention of disabling osteoporosis begins with adequate calcium and vitamin D intake during youth to achieve maximum bone mass. Reducing osteoporosis after menopause is best accomplished by adequate calcium and vitamin D coupled with supplemental estrogen. Alternative drugs are available for women who can not take estrogen.

MULTIPLE-CHOICE REVIEW QUESTIONS

Choose the most appropriate answer.

1. Choose the correct teaching for breast self-examination (BSE).
   a. Monthly BSE eliminates the need for a professional examination until after age 40.
   b. BSE should be done one week after the beginning of each menstrual period.
   c. Dry fingers make it easier to feel very small lumps that are just under the skin.
   d. Look at each breast from the side in a mirror.
2. The women's health nurse practitioner recommends ibuprofen to relieve Jenny's menstrual "cramps." The nurse should teach her to take the drug
   a. with a full glass of water and wait 30 minutes before taking any food.
   b. on a full stomach, but only if her cramps seem to be getting more severe.
   c. three times per day for one week before she expects her period to begin.
   d. with food, just before her period begins or soon after it begins.
3. Choose the sexually transmissible disease that may cause infertility.
   a. *Chlamydia*
   b. Syphilis
   c. Herpes genitalis
   d. *Candida*
4. To reduce the risks of complications from an IUD, the woman should
   a. avoid aspirin or nonsteroidal antiinflammatory drugs.
   b. be in a mutually monogamous relationship with her partner.
   c. avoid crossing her legs or standing for prolonged periods.
   d. limit her intake of caffeine and chocolate.
5. Nursing teaching to prevent osteoporosis in the menopausal woman should include
   a. limiting total calcium intake to 1000 mg per day.
   b. using pillows to maintain good body alignment when sleeping.
   c. taking alendronate (Fosamax) with the evening meal.
   d. doing low-impact weight-bearing exercise several times each week.

BIBLIOGRAPHY AND READER REFERENCE

American Cancer Society. (1996). *Cancer facts for women.* Author.

American Cancer Society. (1997). *Learn to give yourself breast examinations.* Author.

Chez, R. A., & Chapin, J. (1997). Emergency contraception: The pill's little-known secret goes public. *Lifelines, 1*(5), 28–31.

Creehan, P. A. (1995). Toxic shock syndrome: An opportunity for nursing intervention. *Journal of Obstetric, Gynecologic, and Neonatal Nursing, 24*(6), 557–561.

Cunningham, F. G., MacDonald, P. C., Gant, N. F., Leveno, K. J., Gilstrap, L. C., Hankins, G. D. V., & Clark, S. L. (1997). *Williams Obstetrics* (20th ed.). Stamford, CT: Appleton & Lange.

Cutter, V. T. (1997). Hormonic convergence: Finding balance through hormone replacement therapy. *Lifelines, 1*(1), 37–42.

Edwards, R. G., & Brody, S. A. (1995). *Principles and practices of assisted human reproduction.* Philadelphia: Saunders.

Ferreira, N. (1996). Sexually transmitted *Chlamydia trachomatis. Nurse Practitioner Forum, 7*(1), 40–46.

Gallo, A. M. (1996). Building strong bones in childhood and adolescence: Reducing the risk of fractures in later life. *Pediatric Nursing, 22*(5), 369–422.

Galsworthy, T. D., & Wilson, P. L. (1996). Osteoporosis: It steals more than bone. *American Journal of Nursing, 96*(6), 27–33.

Kinzy, J. (1996). Sexually transmitted diseases. In R. E. Rakel (Ed.), *Saunders manual of medical practice* (pp. 442–444). Philadelphia: Saunders.

LeBoeuf, F. J., and Carter, S. G. (1996). Discomforts of the perimenopause. *Journal of Obstetric, Gynecologic, and Neonatal Nursing, 25*(2), 173–180.

Mahan, L. K., & Escott-Stump, S. (1996). *Krause's food, nutrition, & diet therapy* (9th ed.). Philadelphia: Saunders.

McHugh, D. R. (1996). Syphilis: An old disease with modern health concerns. *Nurse Practitioner Forum, 7*(1), 34–39.

Moore, A. A., & Noonan, M. D. (1996). A nurse's guide to hormone replacement therapy. *Journal of Obstetric, Gynecologic, and Neonatal Nursing, 25*(1), 24–31.

National Center for Health Statistics. (1996). *Healthy people 2000 review, 1995–96.* Hyatsville, MD: Public Health Service.

O'Connell, M. L. (1996). The effect of birth control methods on sexually transmitted disease/HIV risk. *Journal of Obstetric, Gynecologic, and Neonatal Nursing, 25*(6), 476–480.

Selleck, C. S. (1997). Identifying and treating bacterial vaginosis. *American Journal of Nursing, 97*(9), 16AAA–16DDD.

Wasaha, S., & Angelopoulos, F. M. (1996). What every woman should know about menopause. *American Journal of Nursing, 96*(1), 24–32.

Youngkin, E. Q. (1995). Sexually transmitted diseases: Current and emerging concerns. *Journal of Obstetric, Gynecologic, and Neonatal Nursing, 24*(8), 743–758.

chapter 12

The Term Newborn

Outline

ADJUSTMENT TO EXTRAUTERINE LIFE

PHYSICAL CHARACTERISTICS AND NURSING ASSESSMENT
- Nervous System
- Respiratory System
- Circulatory System
- Musculoskeletal System
- Genitourinary System
- Integumentary System
- Gastrointestinal System

PREVENTING INFECTION

DISCHARGE PLANNING

HOME CARE
- Furnishings
- Clothing

Objectives

On completion and mastery of Chapter 12, the student will be able to

- Define each vocabulary term listed.
- Briefly describe three normal reflexes of the neonate, including the approximate age of their disappearance.
- State four methods of maintaining the body temperature of a newborn.
- State the cause and appearance of physiologic jaundice in the newborn.
- Define the following skin manifestations in the newborn: lanugo, vernix caseosa, mongolian spots, milia, acrocyanosis, desquamation.
- State the methods of preventing infection in newborns.

Vocabulary

acrocyanosis
caput succedaneum
cephalohematoma
circumcision
dancing reflex
Epsteins pearls
fontanel
icterus neonatorum
lanugo
meconium
milia
molding
mongolian spots
Moro reflex
rooting reflex
scarf sign
tonic neck reflex
vernix caseosa

The arrival of the newborn, or *neonate,* begins a highly vulnerable period during which many psychological and physiologic adjustments to life outside the uterus must be made. The fetus that remains in the uterus until maturity has reached a major goal. The baby's genetic background, the health of the recent uterine environment, a safe delivery, and the care during the 1st month of life contribute to this adjustment.

The *infant mortality rate* is the ratio between the number of deaths of infants younger than 1 year of age during any given year and the number of live births occurring in the same year. The rate is usually expressed as the number of deaths per thousand live births. The infant death rate is highest in the first month and is referred to as the *neonatal mortality rate.* The first 24 hours of life are the most dangerous ones. The infant mortality rate is considered to be one of the best means of determining the health of a country. To obtain accurate figures, all births and deaths must be registered. In the United States, this registration is required by law. Each birth certificate is permanently filed with the state Bureau of Vital Statistics.

In the United States, the current neonatal death rate is 5 deaths per 1000 live births and the infant death rate is approximately 8 deaths per 1000 live births. Most of the causes of death are related to perinatal problems (Wong, 1997).

Morbidity (*morbidus,* "sick") refers to the state of being diseased or sick. Morbidity rates show the incidence of disease in a specific population during a certain time frame. *Perinatology* is the study and support of the fetus and neonate. The term *perinatal mortality* designates fetal and neonatal deaths related to prenatal conditions and delivery circumstances.

Low-birth-weight newborns and limited access to health care are major causes of infant morbidity. Reducing infant morbidity rates can reduce the resulting disability that can impact the growth and development of children. The nurse can play a vital role in educating new parents about health care and the developmental needs of their new baby.

ADJUSTMENT TO EXTRAUTERINE LIFE

When a baby is born, an orderly, continuous adaptation from fetal life to extrauterine life takes place. All the body systems undergo some change. Respirations are stimulated by chemical changes within the blood and by chilling. Sensory and physical stimuli also appear to play a role in respiratory function. The first breath opens the alveoli. The baby then enters the world of air exchange, at which time an independent existence begins. This process also instigates cardiopulmonary interdependence. The newborn's ability to metabolize food is hampered by the immaturity of the digestive system, particularly deficiencies in enzymes from the pancreas and liver. The kidneys are structurally developed but their ability to concentrate urine and maintain fluid balance is limited because of a decreased rate of glomerular flow and limited renal tubular reabsorption. Most neurologic functions are primitive (see discussion of the individual body systems in this chapter).

PHYSICAL CHARACTERISTICS AND NURSING ASSESSMENT

This discussion covers the physical characteristics and nursing assessment of the newborn, by body system. Refer to Chapter 9 for immediate postpartum care of the newborn.

Nervous System

Reflexes. The nervous system directs most of the body's activity. Newborns can move their arms and legs vigorously but cannot control them. The reflexes full-term babies are born with, such as blinking, sneezing, gagging, sucking, and grasping (Fig. 12–1), help to keep them alive. They can cry, swallow, and lift their heads slightly when lying on their

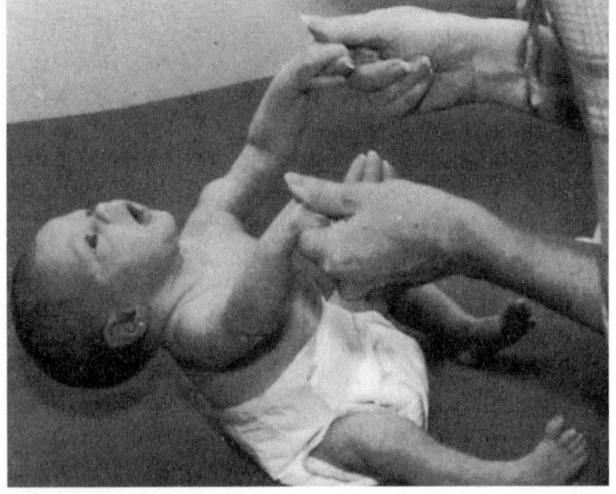

Figure 12–1. • Grasp reflex and head lag help to determine the maturity of the newborn. (From Marlow, D. R., & Redding, B. A. [1988]. *Textbook of pediatric nursing* [6th ed., p. 369]. Philadelphia: Saunders.)

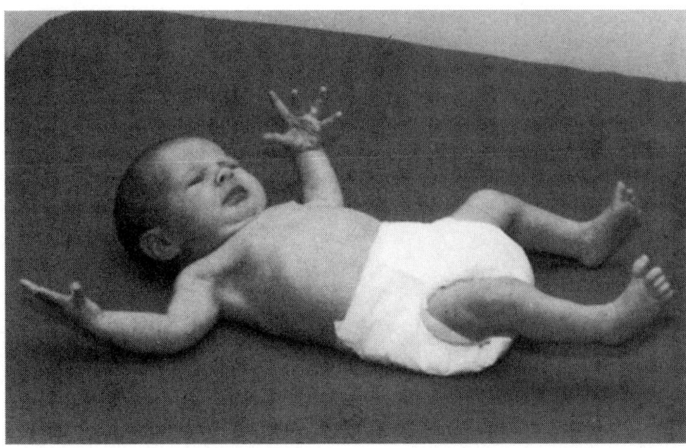

Figure 12–2. • Moro reflex. Sudden jarring causes extension and abduction of the extremities and spreading of the fingers. (From Marlow, D. R., & Redding, B. A. [1988]. *Textbook of pediatric nursing.* [6th ed., p. 369]. Philadelphia: Saunders.)

stomach. If the crib is jarred, they draw their legs up and the arms fan out and then come toward midline in an embrace position. This is normal and is called the *Moro reflex* (Fig. 12–2). Its absence may indicate abnormalities of the nervous system. The *rooting reflex* causes the infant's head to turn in the direction of anything that touches the cheek, in anticipation of food. The nurse utilizes this when helping a mother to breastfeed her infant. A breast touching the cheek causes the infant to turn toward it to find the nipple.

The *tonic neck reflex* is a postural reflex that is sometimes assumed by sleeping babies. The head is turned to one side, and the arm and leg are extended on the same side, while the opposite arm and leg are flexed in a "fencing" position. This reflex disappears about the 20th week of life (Fig. 12–3). Prancing movements of the legs, seen when a baby is held upright on the examining table, are termed the *dancing reflex.* Table 12–1 lists ages at which the neurologic signs of infancy appear and disappear.

Head. The newborn's head is large in comparison with the rest of the body, for the brain grows rapidly before birth. The normal limits of head circumference range from 13.2 to 14.8 inches (Fig. 12–4A). The head may be out of shape from *molding* (the shaping of the fetal head to conform to the size and shape of the birth canal) (Fig. 12–4B). There may also be swelling of the soft tissues of the scalp, which is termed *caput succedaneum* (Fig. 12–4C). It gradually subsides without treatment. Occasionally, a *cephalohematoma* (*cephal,* "head," *hemato,* "blood," *toma,* "tumor") protrudes from beneath the scalp (Fig. 12–4D). This condition is caused by a collection of blood beneath the periosteum of the cranial bone. It may be seen on one or both sides of the head but *does not cross the suture line.* This condition usually recedes within a few weeks. Some newborns have much hair, which eventually is replaced by new hair. When the hair is washed, the nurse holds the newborn in a football hold (see Fig. 22–4).

The *fontanels* are unossified spaces or soft spots on the cranium of a young infant. They protect the head during delivery by the process of molding and allow for further brain growth during the next 1½ years. The *anterior fontanel* is diamond-shaped and

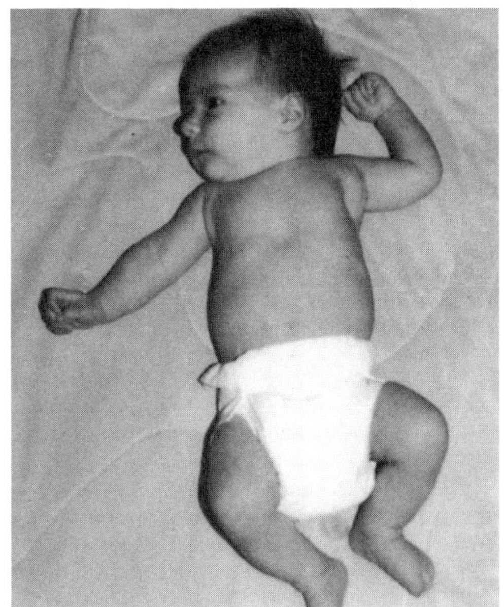

Figure 12–3. • Spontaneous tonic neck reflex. (From Marlow, D. R., & Redding, B. A. [1988]. *Textbook of pediatric nursing* [6th ed., p. 369]. Philadelphia: Saunders.)

Table 12–1
AGES OF APPEARANCE AND DISAPPEARANCE OF NEUROLOGIC SIGNS PECULIAR TO INFANCY

Response	Age at Time of Appearance	Age at Time of Disappearance
Reflexes of position and movement		
Moro reflex	Birth	1–3 mo
Tonic neck reflex (unsustained)*	Birth	5–6 mo (partial up to 2–4 yr)
Palmar grasp reflex	Birth	4 mo
Babinski reflex	Birth	Variable†
Responses to sound		
Blinking response	Birth	
Turning response	Birth	
Reflexes of vision		
Blinking to threat	6–7 mo	
Horizontal following	4–6 wk	
Vertical following	2–3 mo	
Postrotational nystagmus	Birth	
Food reflexes		
Rooting response awake	Birth	3–4 mo
Rooting response asleep	Birth	7–8 mo
Sucking response	Birth	12 mo
Other signs		
Handedness	2–3 yr	
Spontaneous stepping	Birth	
Straight line walking	5–6 yr	

*Arm and leg posturing can be broken by child despite continued neck stimulus.
†Usually of no diagnostic significance until after age 2 yr.
Adapted from Ross Laboratories. (1986). *Children are different.* Columbus, OH: Author. Copyright 1986.

located at the junction of the two parietal and two frontal bones. It usually closes by 12 to 18 months of age. The *posterior fontanel* is triangular and located between the occipital and parietal bones. It is smaller than the anterior fontanel and is usually ossified by the end of the 2nd month. These areas are covered by a tough membrane, and there is little chance of their being injured during ordinary care. The features of the newborn's face are small. The mouth and lips are well developed, as they are necessary to obtain food. The newborn can both taste and smell. In fact, the newborn can recognize the scent of the mother's breast pad.

Visual Stimuli and Sensory Overload. The healthy newborn can see and can fixate on points of contrast. The newborn shows preference for observing a human face and follows moving objects. Visual stimulation is thus an important ingredient in newborn care. Toys that make sounds and have contrasting colors attract the newborn. Tears will be absent in the newborn and may first appear when the infant cries after he is 2 to 3 weeks old. Sensory overload can occur if there is too much detrimental stimulation. This overload can happen in the hospital environment, where lights are bright and voices carry. The nurse can help to modify this situation by responding quickly to alarms and by speaking quietly when working near the baby.

Hearing. The ears are well developed at birth but are small. The hearing ability of the newborn is well developed at birth, but the sick or premature newborn may not respond to sounds that are heard. The presence of amniotic fluid in the ear canal can diminish hearing, but normal drainage and sneezing that occurs shortly after birth help clear the ear canal. The newborn will react to sudden sound by an increase in pulse and respiration or a display of the startle reflex. Newborn infants who do not respond should be referred for a hearing test. Increased responses to vocal stimulation, particularly higher-pitched female voices, have been documented. The ability to discriminate between the mother's voice and others' may occur as early as 3 days of age. Hearing is important to the development of normal speech. The nurse observes and records how the newborn reacts to sound, such as a rattle or the voice of the caretaker. The infant will respond to voices by decreasing motor activity and sucking activity and turning the head toward the sound. One test used to measure infant hearing is a Crib-O-Gram. It analyzes hearing by comparing the movement of the newborn before and after a sound. The sensor is placed beneath the mattress, and a readout is generated by a microprocessor (Wong, 1997).

The ears and nose need no special attention, except for cleansing with a soft cloth during the bath. Occasionally, they may be *externally* cleansed with a cotton ball moistened slightly with water. The bony canal of the external ear is not well developed and the tympanic membrane is vulnerable to injury. Do *not* insert applicators. They may cause serious injury to the tympanic membrane if inserted too far into the ear canals or if the baby moves suddenly.

Sleep. The baby sleeps approximately 15 to 20 hours a day. There is a gradual change in the quantity and quality of sleep as the newborn matures. At birth the newborn passes through phases of sleep–wake states as part of its adjustment to life outside of the uterus.

- *First reactive phase.* During the first 30 minutes of life the newborn is alert and this is the best time to initiate bonding between the parent and the newborn.
- *Sleep phase.* During the next few hours of life the infant gradually becomes more sleepy and less responsive.
- *Second reactive phase.* After a deep sleep the infant again becomes responsive and alert.
- *Stability phase.* After 24 hours of age the sleep–

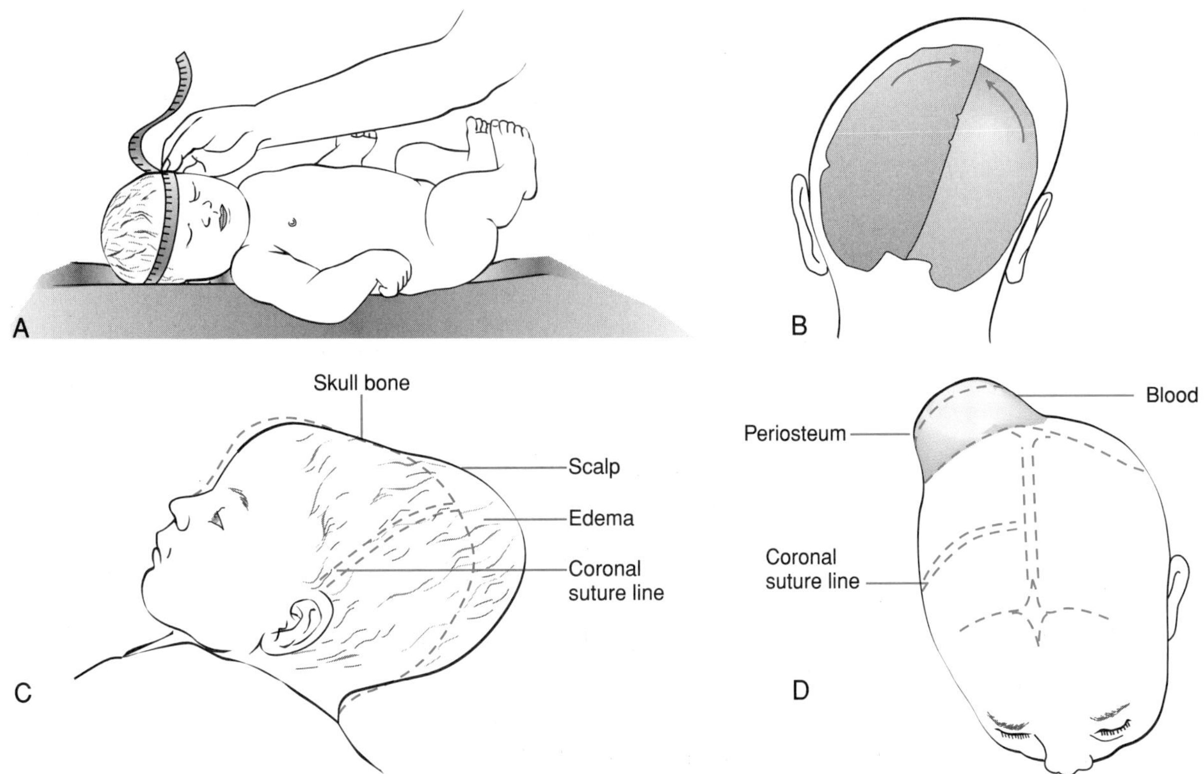

Figure 12–4. • **A,** The circumference of the head is measured from top of the eyebrow to the widest part of the occiput. **B,** Molding of the head occurs as a result of overriding of the parietal bones as the head passes through the birth canal. The head appears to be longer than normal. This condition disappears without treatment within a few weeks. **C,** Caput succedaneum is a collection of fluid under the scalp. **D,** Cephalohematoma. Blood vessels rupture, and blood collects between the surface of the cranial bone and the periosteal membrane.

wake pattern becomes more stabilized. The pattern of sleep gradually develops into one in which the newborn is awake during the day and asleep during the night.

The environment plays a large role in the infant's sleep behavior. The nurse can help the parent to understand that normal conversational tones can quiet a newborn, whereas high noise levels can cause increased crying. Wrapping an infant snugly can maintain temperature and promote sleep, as can gentle *horizontal* rocking. An infant held upright on the shoulder and rocked in a *vertical* fashion is likely to maintain an alert state. Newborns exhibit a specific *pattern of reactivity* that can influence the response to stimuli and bonding:

- *Quiet sleep.* Infant sleeps, does not move.
- *REM sleep.* During rapid eye movement respirations are more irregular. Eye movements are evident beneath the eyelid and movement of limbs and mouth may be seen.
- *Active alert.* The infant displays diffuse motor activity.
- *Quiet alert.* The infant is awake, relaxed, and quiet. In this state the infant is most responsive to testing and to bonding efforts.
- *Crying.* The infant's cry is accompanied by vigorous motor activity of extremities.
- *Transitional.* The infant is moving between one of the above states. The infant may be quiet and relaxed but not very responsive to the environment.

Pain. In the past, it was believed that newborns did not experience pain because of immaturity of

Nursing Tip

Advise parents that even the youngest of babies can roll off a changing table or bed when left unattended.

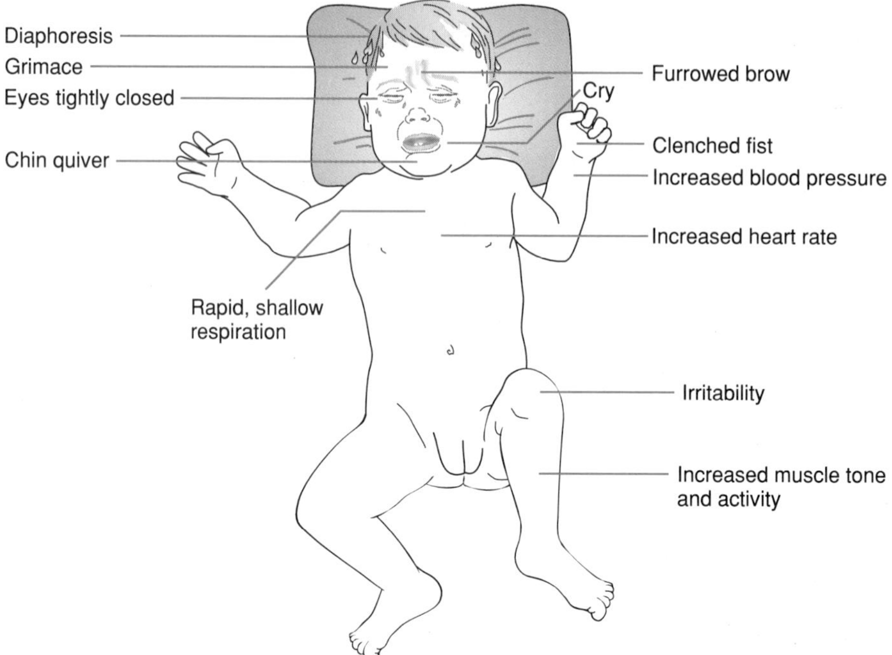

Figure 12–5. • Observing signs of pain in the neonate.

the nerve pathways to the brain. It is now thought that fibers that conduct pain stimuli to the spinal cord are in place early in fetal life. These are called *nociceptors* (*noci,* "pain," *ceptus,* "to receive"). The newborn also produces catecholamines and cortisol in response to stress. Heart rate and respiratory rates change. Blood pressure increases and blood glucose levels rise. Newborns should be medicated for pain when discomfort is anticipated.

Adequate pain relief in newborns who undergo painful procedures (such as circumcision) can reduce postoperative morbidity. Evaluation of pain in the neonate can be based on changes in vital signs and behavior of the infant and decreased oxygen saturation rates (Fig. 12–5). Swaddling, cuddling, rocking, nonnutritive sucking, and a quiet environment are noninvasive methods of pain relief for newborn infants. Morphine, Fentanyl, and topical anesthetics can be safely used for pain in neonates. The nurse must be aware of safe dose ranges and observe infants closely for side effects or signs of withdrawal when the medication is gradually decreased and then discontinued.

Conditioned Responses. A conditioned response or reflex is one that is learned over time. It is an unconscious response to an external stimulus. An example is the hungry baby who stops crying merely at the sound of the caregiver's footsteps, even though food is not yet available. Emotions are particularly subject to this type of conditioning. As an infant matures, the mere sight of an object that once caused pain can precipitate fear.

Neonatal Behavioral Assessment Scale. The Neonatal Behavioral Assessment Scale, developed by T. B. Brazelton, has increased our understanding of the newborn's capabilities. Among other areas of assessment, the scale measures the inherent neurologic capacities of the newborn and responses to selected stimuli. Areas tested include alertness, response to visual and auditory stimuli, motor coordination, level of excitement, and organizational process in response to stress.

Respiratory System

The unborn fetus is completely dependent on the mother for all vital functions. The fetus needs oxygen and nourishment to grow. These nutrients are supplied through the blood stream of the pregnant woman by way of the placenta and umbilical cord. The fetus is relieved of the waste products of metabolism by the same route. The lungs are not inflated and are almost completely inactive. The circulatory system is adapted only to life within the uterus. Little blood flows through the pulmonary artery because of natural openings within the heart and vessels that close at birth or shortly thereafter. When the umbilical cord is clamped and cut, the

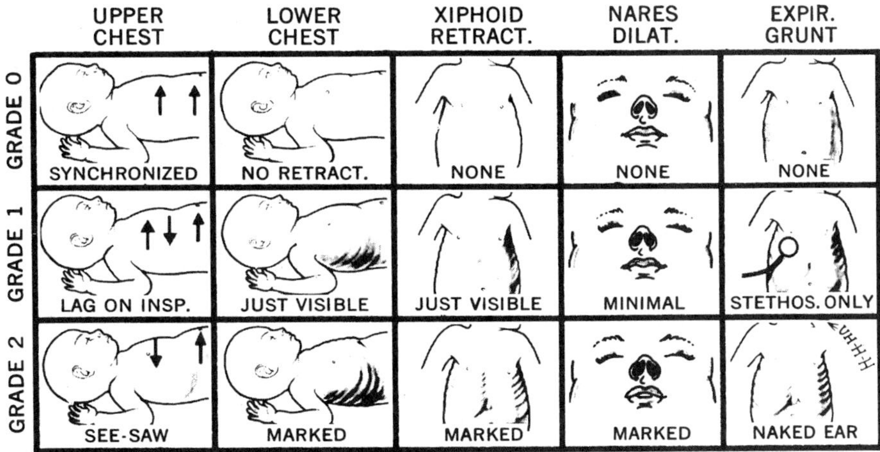

Figure 12–6. • Criteria of respiratory distress. Grade 0 for each criterion indicates no respiratory distress; grade 2 for each criterion indicates severe distress. (dilat., dilation; expir., expiratory; insp., inspiration; retract., retraction; stethos., stethoscope.) (Courtesy of Mead Johnson, Evansville, IN. Modified from Silverman, W., & Andersen, D. [1956]. Controlled clinical trial of effects of water mist on obstructive respiratory signs, death rate, and necropsy findings among premature babies. Reproduced by permission of *Pediatrics, 17*(1), copyright 1956.)

lungs take on the function of breathing oxygen and removing carbon dioxide. The first breath helps to expand the collapsed lungs, although full expansion does not take place for several days. The physician assists the first respiration by holding the newborn's head down and removing mucus from the passages to the lungs. The baby's cry should be strong and healthy. The most critical period for the newborn is the 1st hour of life, when the drastic change from life within the uterus to life outside the uterus takes place.

The nurse can assist the newborn to maintain a patent airway by positioning him or her on his or her back or side and dressing him or her in clothing to maintain warmth while allowing full expansion of the lungs. The nurse should record vital signs and suction mucous as needed, first from the mouth and throat and then the nose.

Apgar Score. The Apgar score is a standardized method of evaluating the newborn's condition immediately after delivery. Five objective signs are measured: heart rate, respiration, muscle tone, reflexes, and color. The score is obtained at 1 and 5 minutes (see Table 9–2 in Chapter 9). On admission of the newborn to the nursery, the Apgar score is reviewed to determine any particular difficulties encountered during the birth process. The physician's orders are noted. The nurse must observe the newborn *very closely.* Respiratory distress may be evidenced by the rate and character of respirations (Fig. 12–6), color (watch for cyanosis), and general behavior. Sternal retractions are reported immediately (Fig. 12–7). Mucus may be seen draining from the nose or mouth. It is wiped away with a sterile gauze square. Gently clearing mucus with a bulb syringe may also be indicated. The bulb is depressed, and then the tip is inserted into the nose or mouth. The depression is slowly released, creating the necessary suction (Fig. 12–8). When this procedure is done orally, the tip is inserted into the side

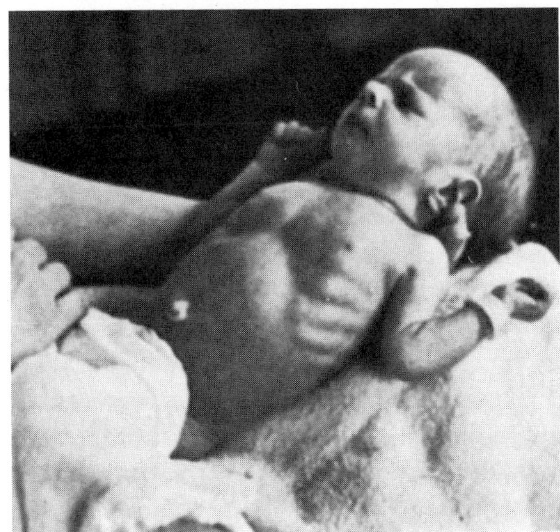

Figure 12–7. • Sternal retractions. Note the triangular indentation over the area of the chest, which indicates marked retraction during inspiration. Intercostal retractions are also evident. The infant is inactive. All of his energy is being used to breathe. (From Kalafatich, A. [1966]. *Pediatric nursing.* New York: Putnam's. Copyright 1966, The Putnam Publishing Group.)

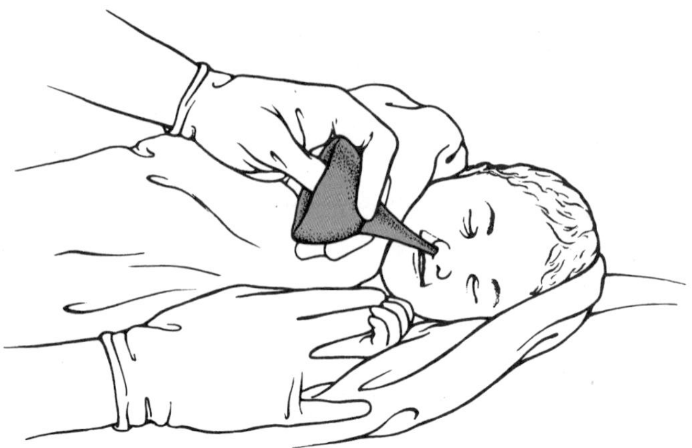

Figure 12–8. • Nasal and oral suctioning. The bulb is compressed before it is inserted into the nose or mouth; then the bulb is released. If the bulb is depressed after being inserted mucus will be forced farther into the respiratory passages.

of the mouth to avoid stimulating the gag reflex. Parents are taught how to use the bulb syringe and instructed to keep one next to the newborn during the early weeks.

Circulatory System

The mother's blood has brought essential oxygen to each cell of the fetus in the uterus. The obstetrician cuts off this supply by severing the umbilical cord. Thereafter, the newborn depends on his own systemic circulation and pulmonary circulation.

The circulation of the fetus differs from that of the newborn in that most of the fetal blood bypasses the lungs (Fig. 3–5). Some of the blood goes from the right atrium to the left atrium of the heart through an opening (the foramen ovale) in the septum. Some goes from the pulmonary artery to the thoracic aorta by way of the ductus arteriosus. These normal openings close soon after birth. If they fail to close or if there are congenitally abnormal openings, the baby may be cyanotic because part of the blood continues to bypass the lungs and does not pick up oxygen.

Nursing Tip

The nurse must adhere to universal precautions while working in the delivery room and/or nursery. These guidelines are of particular importance during the initial care of the newborn, when exposure to secretions, blood, and amniotic fluid is high.

Murmurs are caused by blood leaking through openings that have not yet closed. Murmurs may be thought of as functional (innocent) or organic (due to improper heart formation). Functional murmurs are due to the sound of blood passing through normal valves. Organic murmurs are due to blood passing through abnormal openings or normal openings that have not yet closed. The majority of heart murmurs are not serious. However, they should be checked periodically to rule out other possibilities. The newborn has approximately 300 cc of circulatory blood volume.

Providing Warmth. The newborn has an unstable heat-regulating system. Body temperature falls immediately after birth to about 96°F. Within a few hours, it climbs slowly to a range of 98 to 99°F (36.6 to 37.2°C). The body temperature is influenced by that of the room and the number of blankets covering the baby. The temperature of the nursery, or of the mother's room in the case of rooming-in, is kept at 68 to 75°F. The humidity should be 45% to 55%. The air in the room must be fresh, but there should be no drafts. The hands and feet are not

Nursing Tip

Changing Lab Values

	Newborn	7 days	3 mo
Hgb (g/100 mm)	19	17	11.3
Hct	61	56	33
WBC	18,000	12,000	12,000
Bilirubin	6 mg/Dcl	12 mg/Dcl	1 mg/Dcl

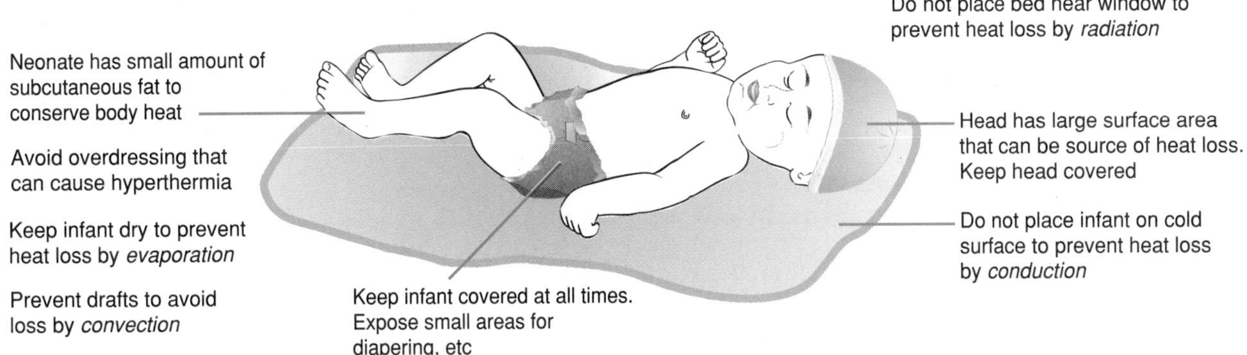

Figure 12–9. • Maintaining body temperature of the newborn. Chilling causes increased metabolism and oxygen consumption in the neonate because the infant cannot shiver, as the adult can, to raise body temperature.

used as a guide to determine warmth because the baby's extremities are cooler than the rest of the body. *Acrocyanosis* (*acro,* "extremity," and *cyanosis,* "blue color") is also evident. The newborn cannot adapt to changes in temperature. The nurse wraps the baby in a blanket whenever the baby leaves the nursery. Because the baby's heat perception is poor, the nurse must be careful when applying any form of external heat.

Since the sweat glands do not function effectively during the neonatal period, the newborn infant is at risk for developing an elevated temperature if overdressed or placed in an overheated environment. A red skin rash may develop in response to overheating. Maintaining body temperature in the newborn is discussed in Chapter 9 and summarized in Fig. 12–9.

Obtaining Temperature, Pulse, and Respirations. Some birth facilities recommend that the initial temperature of the newborn be taken by rectum to determine that it is patent. When the temperature is taken rectally, the nurse must be gentle to avoid injuring the rectal mucosa. Daily routine temperatures are taken by axilla. To obtain the axillary temperature, the thermometer is held firmly in the center of the axilla for 5 minutes. During this time, the arm is held against the baby's side. Digital thermometers are read when the indicator sounds.

The newborn's pulse and respirations are counted before the temperature is taken because the baby is apt to cry when disturbed. Figure 12–10 illustrates the apical pulse being obtained from a newborn infant. The newborn's pulse is irregular and rapid, varying from 110 to 160 beats/min. Blood pressure is low and may vary with the size of the cuff used. The average blood pressure at birth is 80/46. The respirations are approximately 35 to 50 breaths/min. The nurse always reports the following changes:

- Temperature elevated to 100°F or below 97°F
- Pulse elevated above 160 beats/min or below 110 beats/min
- Respirations elevated above 60 breaths/min or below 30 breaths/min
- Noisy respirations
- Nasal flaring or chest retraction

Musculoskeletal System

Movements, Eye Coordination, and Tremors. The bones of the newborn are soft because they are chiefly made up of cartilage, in which there is only a small amount of calcium. The skeleton is flexible. The joints are elastic to accommodate the passage through the birth canal. Because the bones of the child are easily molded by pressure, position must

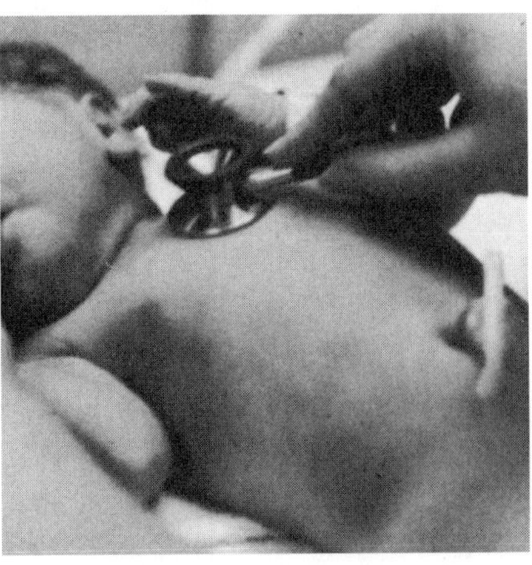

Figure 12–10. • Assessing an apical pulse.

be changed frequently. If the baby lies constantly in one position, the bones of the head can become flattened.

The movements of the newborn are random and uncoordinated. The newborn lacks the muscular control to hold the head steady. The development of muscular control proceeds from head to foot and from the center of the body to the periphery (see discussion of cephalocaudal and proximodistal control, p. 378 and Fig. 15–1). Therefore, the baby holds the head up before sitting erect. In fact, the head and neck muscles are the first ones under control. The legs are small and short and may appear bowed. There should be no limitation of movement. Fingers clenched in a fist should be separated and observed.

An examination of the newborn for maturity includes checking for the *Scarf sign* (see pp. 331–332). This refers to the full-term infant's resistance to attempts to bring one elbow farther than the midline of the chest. No resistance would be observed in the preterm infant.

Most newborns appear cross-eyed because their eye muscle coordination is not fully developed. At first, the eyes appear to be blue or gray; however, the permanent coloring becomes fixed between 6 and 12 months. The eyelids are closed most of the time. Tears do not appear until approximately 1 to 3 months because of the immaturity of the lacrimal gland ducts.

The baby needs freedom of movement. The infant stretches, sucks, and makes faces and vigorously moves the whole body when crying. Tremors of the lips and extremities during crying are normal. Constant tremors during sleep may be pathologic. These are often accompanied by eye movements and are not related to particular stimuli. The morning bath provides excellent opportunities for the newborn to exercise and the nurse to inspect and assess the baby's condition. When handled, the infant should not feel limp. General body proportions are noted. Bathing is also an excellent means of stimulation for the newborn.

Length and Weight. The length of the average newborn is 19 to 21½ inches (46 to 56 cm). The weight varies from 6 to 9 pounds (2700 to 4000 g) (Fig. 12–11). Girls generally weigh a little less than boys. African-American, Asian-American, and Native-American babies may be somewhat smaller. *In the first 3 to 4 days after birth, the baby loses about 5% to 10% of the birthweight.* The loss may be as high as 15% for preterm infants. This may be due to withdrawal from maternal hormones, fluid shifts, and the loss of feces and urine. Mothers should be prepared for this and reassured that weight will normalize after 3 or 4 days and the infant will regain birthweight by 10 days of age. Newborns are weighed at the same time each day, when morning care is given. (Instructions for measuring and weighing the baby are provided in Figs. 12–11 and 15–2.)

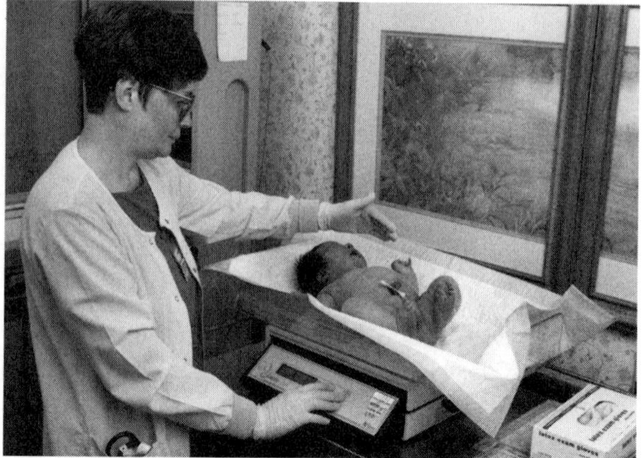

Figure 12–11. • **Weighing the infant.** Note the barrier placed under the infant and the nurse's hand held above the infant for safety and protection. The scale used may be a balance scale or a digital scale that locks-in and displays the weight in pounds and/or kilograms. The newborn weighs 2700 to 4000 g (6 to 9 pounds). Weight loss of about 10% occurs within the first 2 days because of fluid shifts. (From Gorrie, T. M., McKinney, E. S., & Murray, S. S. [1994]. *Foundations of maternal newborn nursing*. Philadelphia: Saunders.)

Genitourinary System

The kidneys function normally at birth but are not fully developed. The glomeruli are small. Renal blood flow is only about one-third that of the adult. The ability to handle a water load is reduced, as is the excretion of drugs. The renal tubules are short and have a limited capacity for reabsorbing important substances such as glucose, amino acids, phosphate, and bicarbonate. There is a decrease in the ability to concentrate urine and to cope with fluid imbalances. It is important to note the first voiding of the newborn. This may occur in the delivery room or may not occur for several hours. *If voiding does not occur within the first 8 hours, the physician is notified.* The nurse must keep an accurate record of the frequency of urination. Anuria, changes in color, and any unusual findings are brought to the attention of the physician. The newborn should have about 6 wet diapers per day.

Male Genitalia. The genitals of the male are developed at birth, although their maturation varies. The testes of the male descend into the scrotum before birth. Occasionally, they remain in the abdomen or inguinal canal. This condition is called *cryptorchidism,* or undescended testes, and is described on pages 763–765. With proper surgical treatment, the prognosis is good. The location of the urethral opening should be at the tip of the penis in newborn boys. A white cheesy substance called *smegma* is found under the foreskin.

Routine retraction of the foreskin of the newborn for cleansing is no longer recommended. Behrman, Kleigman, and Arvin (1996) states that nonretractability is normal in newborns. The foreskin and glans penis gradually separate, beginning in the prenatal period. This process is generally completed between 3 and 5 years. Parents are instructed to test occasionally for retraction during the daily bath. If it has occurred, gentle washing of the glans is begun. The foreskin is then returned to its unretracted position.

Circumcision. Circumcision is the surgical removal of the foreskin on the penis. Circumcision has both advantages and disadvantages. The disadvantages include infection and hemorrhage. Infants with congenital anomalies of the penis, such as hypospadias (the opening of the urethra on the undersurface of the penis), should not be circumcised because the skin may be needed for surgery. Benefits of circumcision include possible prevention of cancer, less urinary tract infections and less occurrence of sexually transmitted diseases such as HIV later in life. A discussion of the pros and cons of this procedure is included as part of prenatal and postpartum education. Regardless of whether the male is circumcised, at an appropriate age he is taught daily hygiene of the genitals. This includes special attention to skin folds, retraction and replacement of the foreskin, cleansing of the penis, and examination for lumps or swelling.

The baby should be at least 12 hours old before circumcision. This allows a period of time for the newborn to become stabilized. This stress should be avoided immediately following delivery, when it may also interfere with bonding. The newborn is restrained on a circumcision board (Fig. 12–12). The Gomco clamp and the Plastibell clamp are two devices commonly used for performing circumcisions. If the Gomco clamp is used, a thin layer of petroleum jelly (Vaseline) or petroleum jelly–impregnated gauze may be applied to the end of the penis to protect it from moisture and from sticking to the diaper. The area is observed for bleeding, infection, and irritation. Voidings are recorded.

When a Plastibell is used, the foreskin is tied over a fitted plastic ring and the excess prepuce cut away. The rim usually drops off 5–8 days after circumcision. Parents are instructed not to remove it prematurely. No special dressing is required, and the baby is bathed and diapered as usual. A dark brown or black ring encircling the plastic rim is natural. This disappears when the rim drops off. Parents are instructed to consult their physician if there are any questions, if there is increased swelling, if the ring has not fallen off within 8 days, or immediately if the ring has slipped onto the shaft of the penis. The Jewish religious custom of circumcision, comparable to baptism in the Christian faith, is performed on the 8th day after birth if the newborn's condition permits. The baby receives his Hebrew name at that time.

The nurse's role in circumcision includes assessing parental knowledge, checking to see that the surgical consent has been signed and preparing the newborn. The baby is not fed for 1 to 2 hours prior to the procedure to prevent possible vomiting and aspiration. A bulb syringe is kept handy in case suctioning is required. A light blanket is placed under the infant on the "circ" board, and the diaper is removed. A heat lamp is positioned to avoid cold stress. The physician may administer a local anesthetic to minimize pain during the procedure and to prevent irritability and sleep disturbances following it. Additional comfort measures include holding and soothing the baby and using a pacifier. If bleeding occurs, gentle pressure is applied to the site with a sterile gauze pad and the physician is notified. The amount and characteristics of the urinary stream are recorded, as edema could cause an obstruction.

Female Genitalia. The female genitals may be slightly swollen. A thin white or blood-tinged mucus (pseudo-menstruation) may be discharged from the vagina. This discharge is due to hormonal withdrawal from the mother at birth. The nurse cleanses the vulva *from the urethra to the anus,* using a clean cotton ball or different sections of a wash cloth for each stroke to prevent fecal matter from infecting the urinary tract. The importance of this is stressed to parents.

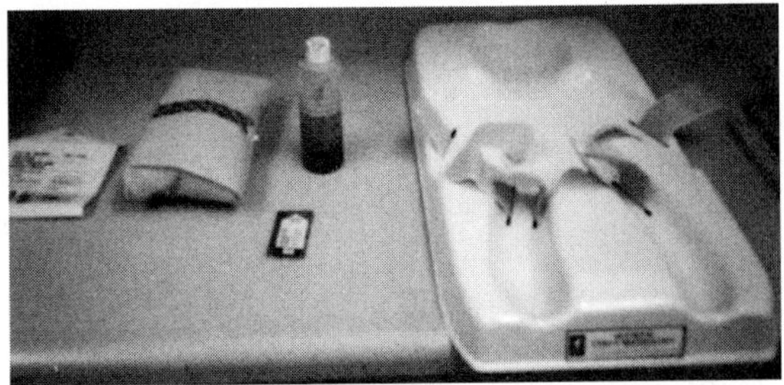

Figure 12–12. • Circumcision board, sterile instruments, surgical blade, antiseptic, and gloves. (Courtesy of Columbia/HCA Portsmouth Regional Hospital, Portsmouth, NH).

Integumentary System

Skin. The skin of newborn Caucasian babies is red to dark pink. The skin of African-American babies is reddish-brown. Infants of Latin descent may appear to have an olive or yellowish tint. The body is usually covered with fine hair called *lanugo,* which tends to disappear during the 1st week of life. This is more evident in premature infants. *Vernix caseosa,* a cheeselike substance that covers the skin of the newborn, is made of cells and glandular secretions; it is thought to protect the skin from irritation and the effects of a watery environment in utero. White pinpoint pimples caused by obstruction of sebaceous glands may be seen on the nose and chin. These are called *milia* and disappear within a few weeks. Milia type lesions on the midline of the hard palate are called *Epsteins pearls. Stork bites* (telangiectatic nail nevi) are flat, red areas seen on the nape of the neck and on the eyelids. They result from the dilation of small vessels (see Color Figure 1).

Mongolian spots, bluish discolorations of the skin, are common in babies of African-American parents, Native-American parents, and parents of Mediterranean races. They are usually found over the sacral and gluteal areas (see Color Figure 2). They disappear spontaneously during the early years of life. *Acrocyanosis,* or peripheral blueness of the hands and feet, is normal, and is due to poor peripheral circulation. The hands or feet should not be used to determine general body warmth in the newborn. Central body areas are not cyanotic in normal newborns. Pallor is not normal and should be reported because it may indicate neonatal anemia or another more serious condition.

Tissue turgor refers to the hydration or dehydration of the skin. To test tissue turgor (elasticity), the nurse gently grasps and releases the skin. It should spring back to place immediately. When the skin remains distorted, tissue turgor is considered poor. Figure 12–13 illustrates the method of testing tissue turgor.

Desquamation, or peeling of the skin, occurs during the early weeks of life. Skin in areas such as the nose, knees, elbows, and toes may break down because of friction from rubbing against the sheets. The involved area is kept dry, and the baby's position is changed frequently. The buttocks need special attention. A wet diaper should be changed immediately to prevent chafing. The buttocks are washed and dried well.

Physiologic jaundice, also called *icterus neonatorum,* is characterized by a yellow tinge of the skin. It is caused by the rapid destruction of excess red blood cells, which the baby does not need now, being in an atmosphere that contains more oxygen than was available during prenatal life. Plasma levels of bilirubin rise from a normal 1 mg/dl to an average of 5 to 6 mg/dl between the 2nd and 4th days. Physiologic jaundice becomes evident between the 2nd and the 3rd days of life and lasts for about 1 week. This is a normal process and is not harmful to the baby. However, genetic and ethnic factors may affect its severity, resulting in pathologic hyperbilirubinemia. Blanch the skin over the nose or chest to evaluate for presence of jaundice. Evidence of jaundice is reported and charted, and the newborn is frequently evaluated to ensure safety.

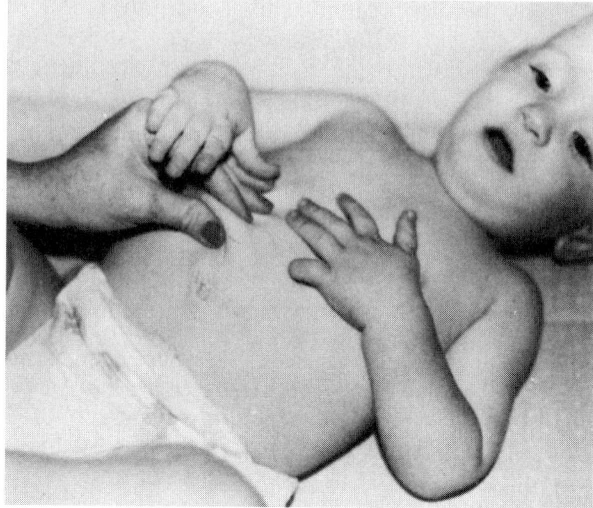

Figure 12–13. • Testing tissue turgor. *Turgor* refers to the elasticity of the skin, which is affected by the extent of hydration. The nurse tests turgor by gently grasping the skin. When the skin is released it should instantly spring back into place; if it does not, tissue turgor is considered poor. (From Thompson, E. D., & Ashwill, J. W. [1992]. *Pediatric nursing: An introductory text* [6th ed., p. 92]. Philadelphia: Saunders.)

Table 12–2 discusses nursing interventions for common skin manifestations of the newborn infant.

Bathing the Baby. The bath is an excellent time to observe the naked newborn for behavior, muscle activity, and general well-being, as well as providing basic hygiene. Special attention must be given to areas of the skin that come in contact with each other because chafing may occur there. These areas

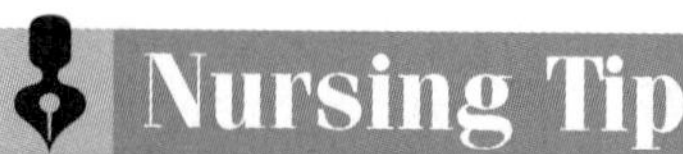

Jaundice that appears in the first day of life is not normal and should be recorded and reported.

Table 12–2
COMMON SKIN MANIFESTATIONS IN THE NEWBORN

	Appearance	Intervention
Acrocyanosis	Cyanoses of the hands and feet in the first week of life is caused by a combination of a high hemoglobin level and vasomotor instability	Parent education concerning this normal phenomenon is helpful
Cutis marmorata	A lacelike red or blue pattern on the skin surface of a newborn's body	A normal vasomotor response to low environmental temperature. Wrap infant warmly. Intense or persistent appearance should be reported
Desquamation	Peeling of the skin at birth may indicate postmaturity. Early removal of vernix can be followed by desquamation in term newborns	Instruct parents to avoid harsh soaps. Some hospitals do not vigorously remove vernix from skin of newborn
Epsteins pearls	Pearly white pinpoint papules in midline of upper palate	Distinguish from thrush lesion (see p. 741)
Erythema toxicum	Splotchy erythema with firm yellow-white papules that have red base.	Can occur at 2 days of age. No intervention is required as erythema will spontaneously clear
Forcep marks	A bruised area on skin following the shape of forcep or pattern of vacuum extractor	The bruising and swelling fades within a few days and does not require intervention other than parental support and teaching
Harlequin color change	An imbalance of autonomic vascular regulatory mechanism. Deep red color over half of body, pallor on the longitudinal half of body. Usually occurs with preterm infants who are placed on their side	The phenomenon disappears with muscular activity. Changing position of infant is helpful. Condition is temporary and does not usually indicate a problem
Milia	Pearly white pinpoint papules on face and nose of newborn	No treatment. Will spontaneously disappear. Educate parents not to attempt to "squeeze out" the white material as infection can occur
Mongolian spots	Dark blue or slate grey discolorations most commonly found in lumbar-sacral area. The intensity and hue of color remain until fading occurs	These lesions are due to melanin deposits in dark-skinned persons and will gradually disappear in a few years. The nurse needs to distinguish these lesions from hematoma of child abuse
Nevi	Known as *stork bites.* These are pink, easily blanched patches that can appear on eyelids, nose, lips, and nape of the neck	These marks gradually fade and are of no clinical significance
Portwine stain	Known as *nevus flammeus.* Is a collection of capillaries in the skin. It is a flat, red-purple lesion that does not blanch on pressure	This is a permanent skin marking that darkens with age and can become elevated and vulnerable to injury. If a large area of face or neck is involved, laser surgery may be indicated to preserve the child's self-image. Can be associated with genetic disorders

are found in the neck, behind the ears, in the axillae, and in the groin. They should be dried well. Powder is seldom used in the hospital because it can irritate the respiratory tract. Parents are educated about this fact. The use of lotions and oil and the type of soap vary with each institution. The baby is bathed when his or her temperature is stable; the first bath removes blood and excess vernix. The nurse adheres to universal precautions during the procedure.

The temperature of the bath water should be approximately 100 to 105°F in a warm 75 to 80°F room environment. Special care should be taken to keep the infant covered to prevent chilling. Items such as cotton swabs should *not* be inserted into the nose or ears. Sponge baths, using plain tap water should be given to newborns until the cord is well-healed. A mild soap can be used for heavily soiled areas. Alkaline soaps and oils and lotions alter the pH of the skin and should be avoided. Parents should be taught to start bathing the face and then proceed in a cephalocaudal direction, turning the surface of the wash cloth as the bath progresses. The eyes should be cleansed with a moist cottonball from the inner canthus to the outer, using a clean cotton ball for each eye. The genitals should be cleansed with a front to back motion to prevent urinary tract infection. The nurse may use a football hold to shampoo the hair. Figure 22–4 depicts the football hold as a safe method for holding a baby. The shampoo is given last because the large surface area of the head predisposes infant to heat loss. The general principles of the baby bath should be explained to parents to foster good techniques at home. Cord care is discussed on p. 240.

Gastrointestinal System

Stools. The intestinal tract functions as an outlet for amniotic fluid as early as the 5th month of fetal life. The normal functions of the gastrointestinal tract begin after birth: Food is prepared for absorption into the blood and is absorbed and waste products are eliminated.

Meconium, the first stool, is a mixture of amniotic fluid and secretions of the intestinal glands. It is dark greenish-black, thick, and sticky and is passed 8 to 24 hours following birth. The stools gradually change during the 1st week. They become loose and are greenish-yellow with mucus. These are called *transitional* stools (see Color Figures following page 328).

The stools of a breastfed baby are *bright yellow, soft, and pasty.* There may be three to six stools a day. With age the number of stools decreases. *The bowel movements of a bottle-fed baby are more solid than those of the breastfed baby.* They vary from yellow to brown and are generally fewer in number. There may be one to four a day at first, but this gradually decreases to one or two a day. The stools are darker when a baby is receiving oral iron supplements and green when a baby is under the phototherapy lamp. Small, puttylike stools or diarrhea and bloody stools are abnormal. When there is a question, the nurse saves the stool specimen for the physician to observe. The nursery nurse keeps an accurate record of the number and character of stools each newborn passes daily.

Constipation. Constipation refers to the passage of hard dry stools. Newborns differ in regularity. Some pass a soft stool every other day. This is not constipation. The nurse explains to parents that straining in the newborn period is due to undeveloped abdominal musculature. This is normal and no treatment is required. In the first month of life, a breastfed infant will pass at least four stools a day. After the second month of life, the infant will increase stool volume and decrease stool frequency. Even if 5 to 6 days pass without a stool, it is not considered constipation if the stool passed is large in volume and soft or pasty in character. As the baby grows older and if a formula change is made, constipation is sometimes seen. Increasing water intake may be all that is necessary to remedy this constipation. If the baby is on solid foods, an increase in intake of fruits, vegetables, and whole-grain cereals is usually sufficient. The nurse encourages mothers to telephone their physician's office when questions arise and ask to speak to the nurse. This is particularly emphasized to new mothers, who may be afraid of appearing "ignorant." Very often a simple solution can relieve hours of anxiety.

Hiccups. Hiccups appear frequently in newborns and are normal. Most disappear spontaneously. Burping the baby and offering warm water may help.

Digestion. Breastfeeding is discussed in Chapter 9. Breastfed babies may be put to the breast while the mother is on the delivery table to help to stimulate milk production and for psychological benefits. Bottle feedings are begun in about 5 hours. A baby's hunger is evidenced by crying, restlessness, fist sucking, and the rooting reflex. The capacity of the stomach is about 90 ml. Emptying time is 2 to 3 hours, and peristalsis is rapid. Feeding the newborn often stimulates the *gastrocolic reflex,* which results in the infant passing a stool. The immature cardiac sphincter of the stomach causes the young infant to be prone to regurgitation. For this reason parents should be educated to avoid overfeeding their infant and to position the infant on the right side after feeding. Deficiency of pancreatic enzymes such as lipase limits fat absorption. Breast milk contains some lipase enzyme that aids infant digestion. Whole cow's milk does not contain this enzyme and therefore should not be fed undiluted to newborns or young infants.

The salivary glands do not secrete saliva until the infant is 2 to 3 months of age. Drooling in the newborn is considered a sign of pathology and should be reported. The liver is immature, especially in its ability to conjugate bilirubin, regulate blood sugar, and coagulate blood.

Vitamins. Babies need extra vitamins C and D. Breast milk contains sufficient vitamin C if the mother's diet is rich in citrus fruits and certain vegetables. Vitamin D may be added to commercial milk, labeled "vitamin D milk." Commercial concentrated vitamin preparations may also be prescribed. The fluid is drawn up in the dropper to the prescribed amount (0.3 or 0.6 ml) and is placed directly in the baby's mouth. This is done each morning at approximately the same time to avoid forgetting the vitamins. Bonding and attachment are discussed in Chapter 9.

PREVENTING INFECTION

Infections that are relatively harmless to an adult may be fatal to the newborn. The newborn's response to inflammation and infection is slow because of the immaturity of the immune system.

- IgG is an immunoglobin that crosses the placenta and provides the newborn with passive immunity to infections the mother was immune to. This type of immunity rarely lasts longer than 3 months.
- IgM is an immunoglobin produced by the newborn, and an elevated level suggests serious infection.
- IgA is an immunoglobin produced after the neonatal period (about one month of age) that is contained in breast milk and provides some resistance to respiratory and gastrointestinal infections. Before one month of age, infants are at risk for such infections.

Every newborn has an immature immune system and an open wound (the umbilical cord) that can be a portal of entry for infection. Measures to prevent infections in the newborn nursery includes *universal precautions, handwashing, cleansing, and replacement of equipment*, and *proper disposal of diapers and linen.*

Nursery standards are developed and enforced by various professional agencies, such as the American Academy of Pediatrics, hospital accreditation boards, and local health agencies. The infection control nurse in each hospital also provides education and surveillance. Provisions governing space, control of temperature and humidity, lighting, and safety from fire and other hazards are considered. Each newborn has an individual crib, bath equipment, and linen supply. Any communal equipment is sterilized following each use.

Protective precautions may be employed for patients in pediatric units, especially preterm babies, newborns, and infants. The meaning of protective precautions is implied by the name; they protect the patient from microorganisms. Children with burns or leukemia and persons receiving certain therapeutic regimens, such as body irradiation or steroids, may also be on protective precautions. *Handwashing is the most reliable precaution available.* The nursery nurse washes her hands between handling different babies. The nurse stresses to parents the need for proper handwashing in the home.

In many hospitals, nursery personnel wear clean scrub gowns while in the nursery for the purpose of infection control and/or security. Physicians, technicians, and other nonnursery personnel wear a cover gown when on duty in the nursery. Universal precautions are adhered to to protect personnel.

Health examination of personnel before employment minimizes the spread of infection by unhealthy persons. The nurse who has signs of a cold earache, skin infection, or intestinal upset should not work in the nursery or care for ill children. Visitors are instructed not to come to the hospital or be around hospital patients if they are not feeling well.

DISCHARGE PLANNING

Discharge teaching ideally begins with the admission of the woman to the hospital or birthing center. Many hospitals have flowsheets, which are helpful in ensuring that all topics have been addressed and that patients understand what has been explained to them. Areas of concern include:

1. Basic care of the baby, including bathing, cord care, feeding, and elimination
2. Safety measures
3. Immunizations
4. Support groups, such as La Leche League
5. Return appointments for well-baby care
6. Telephone number of Nursery (note 24-hour availability)
7. Signs and symptoms of problems and who to contact; for example, temperature above 38°C (100.4°F) by axilla, refusal of two feedings in a row, two green watery stools, frequent or forceful vomiting, lack of voiding or stooling

The nurse should guide the parents in assessing, bathing and feeding the newborn so that questions can be answered early and parents can demonstrate understanding of skills and behaviors. The following critical pathway for the newborn specifies nursing interventions for assisting the mother, parents, or other caregivers in caring for the infant during and after discharge from the hospital.

HOME CARE

Furnishings

It helps if the newborn has a separate room or a separate area within a room. Simple, durable, easy-to-clean furnishings are necessary. A crib with a firm mattress is a suitable place for the infant to sleep for several years. Crib slats should adhere to safety standards. Mattress covers of thin rubber that are large enough to tuck in at the sides may be used. *Plastic bags are never used for this purpose.* Sheeting that has a flannelette backing on both sides stays in place. Contour sheets are convenient. Blankets of lightweight cotton are warm and easy to launder. A knitted shawl stays tucked in and is also a nice wraparound for going places. The newborn does not require a pillow.

Pictures are attached securely to the wall with wall tapes. Thumbtacks may be swallowed by the

(Text continued on p. 326)

Clinical Pathway 12–1

CLINICAL PATH DAY		EXPECTED PATIENT/ FAMILY OUTCOMES	MULTIDISCIPLINARY ASSESSMENT	TESTS	CONSULT
Immediate Newborn Care	Date & Time	☐ Apgar score >7 at 5 min. [4] ☐ Maintains axillary temp of 36.5C to 37.2C while in radiant warmer or in double blankets [1] ☐ Physiologic parameters WNL [4} ☐ Demonstrates proper latch when breastfeeding [2]	☐ Apgar score 1 & 5 min. ☐ Transitional newborn assessment q 30 min. ☐ Suck reflex	☐ Hypoglycemia protocol when indicated	☐ ________
Newborn Admission	Date & Time	☐ Maintains axillary temp of 36.5C to 37.2C while in radiant warmer or in double blankets [1] ☐ Physiologic parameters WNL [4] ☐ Tolerates initial feeding [2] ☐ Mother's blood type O/Rh- ☐ ________	☐ Weight ☐ V/S q 30 min x 4 ☐ Multisystem admission assessment ☐ Suck reflex ☐ ________	☐ Hypoglycemia protocol when indicated ☐ ________	☐ ________ ☐ ________
Day of Birth	Date	N D E ☐☐☐ Maintains axillary temp of 36.5C to 37.2C independent of external heat source [1] ☐☐☐ Parents/family verbalize understanding of safety & security measures [6] ☐☐☐ Physiologic parameters WNL [4] ☐☐☐ Parent(s)/family & infant demonstrate attachment behaviors [3] ☐☐☐ Feeding [2] ☐☐☐ Latch score is 7 or greater for breastfed newborn [2] ☐☐☐ No jaundice [4] ☐☐☐ Infant seen by physician within 12 hours [6]	N D E ☐☐☐ Temp, apical pulse, neuro, cardiac, resp., GI, GU, integ. q shift ☐☐☐ Parent/infant attachment ☐☐☐ Positioning and LATCH score of breastfed newborn ☐☐☐ Freq. and amount of bottlefeeding ☐☐☐ ________	N D E ☐☐☐ Hypoglycemia protocol when indicated ☐☐☐ ________	N D E ☐☐☐ ________ ☐ Social service consult if indicated

NAME	INITIALS	NAME	INITIALS

8035 (4/96)

An example of a clinical pathway for a newborn from birth to discharge on the second day. This is used by all caregivers to plan and document care. (Courtesy of Women's and Children's Services of the York Health System. York, PA. Modified with permission.)

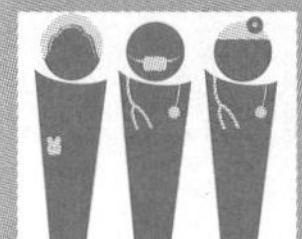

Clinical Pathway 12–1 *(Continued)*

DOCUMENTATION CODES
Initial = Meets Standard
★ = Exception on pathway identified
C = Chronic problems
N/A = Not applicable

PATIENT/FAMILY PROBLEMS
1. Thermoregulation
2. Nutrition
3. Parent-Infant attachment
4. Potential alteration in newborn metabolism
5. Risk for infection
6. Infant safety
7. ____________________
8. ____________________

TREATMENTS	MEDS	NUTR.	EDUC & DC PLANNING
☐ Clamp cord ☐ Dry newborn ☐ Radiant warmer or double blanket while being held until temp stable ☐ ID bands	☐ Neonatal eye prophylaxis & Aquamephyton ☐ HBIG if indicated	☐ Determine if bottlefeeding or breastfeeding ☐ Assist with initial breastfeeding	☐ Initiate safety & security measures with parents/ family ☐ Teach breastfeeding mother proper latch
☐ Cord care ☐ Admission bath	☐ ____________	Initial feeding: ☐ ____________	
N D E ☐☐☐ Cord care ☐☐☐ Circumcision care when indicated ☐☐☐ ____________	N D E ☐☐☐ ____________	N D E ☐☐☐ Breast/bottle feed on demand (breast: q 2–3 hrs, bottle: q 3–4 hrs)	N D E ☐☐☐ Reinforce safety and security measures w/ parents/family ☐☐☐ Observe & reinforce proper latch and instruct breastfeeding mother/family in alternative positioning ☐☐☐ Give and review new pamphlets: -Message to mothers -Newborn screening -Car seat -Health insurance for newborns -Preparing formula -Breastfeeding, A Guide for Success

NAME	INITIALS	NAME	INITIALS

(Continued)

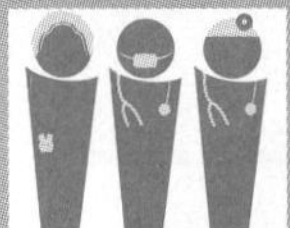

Clinical Pathway 12–1 *(Continued)*

CLINICAL PATH DAY		EXPECTED PATIENT/ FAMILY OUTCOMES	MULTIDISCIPLINARY ASSESSMENT	TESTS	CONSULT
Day 1	Date	N D E ☐☐☐ Maintains axillary temp of 36.5C to 37.2C independent of external heat source [1] ☐☐☐ Parent(s)/family & newborn demonstrate attachment behaviors [3] ☐☐☐ Physiologic parameters WNL [4] ☐☐☐ Feeding [2] ☐☐☐ LATCH score 7 or greater for breastfed newborn [2] ☐☐☐ No jaundice [4] ☐☐☐ No signs of infection [5] ☐☐☐ ________	N D E ☐☐☐ Temp, apical pulse, cardiac, resp., neuro, GI, GU, integ. q 8 hr. ☐ N/A N/A Weight ☐☐☐ Parent(s)/family & infant attachment behaviors ☐☐☐ LATCH score of breastfed newborn ☐☐☐ Frequency & amt. of bottle feeding ☐☐☐ ________	N D E ☐☐☐ ________	N D E ☐☐☐ Referral made to lactation consultant for LATCH score <7 ☐☐☐ ________
Day 2	Date	☐☐☐ Maintains axillary temp of 36.5C to 37.2C independent of external heat source [1] ☐☐☐ Parent(s)/family & newborn demonstrate attachment behaviors [3] ☐☐☐ Physiologic parameters WNL [4] ☐☐☐ Feeding [2] ☐☐☐ LATCH score 7 or greater for breastfed newborn [2] ☐☐☐ No jaundice [4] ☐☐☐ No signs of infection [5] ☐☐☐ ________	☐☐☐ Temp, apical pulse, cardiac, resp., neuro, GI, GU, integ. q 8 hr. ☐ N/A N/A Weight ☐☐☐ Parent(s)/family & infant attachment behaviors ☐☐☐ LATCH score of breastfed newborn ☐☐☐ Frequency & amt. of bottle feeding ☐☐☐ ________	☐☐☐ ________	☐☐☐ Referral made to lactation consultant for LATCH score <7 ☐☐☐ ________
Discharge	Date	☐ Maintains axillary temp of 36.5C to 37.2C independent of external heat source [1] ☐ Parent(s)/family & newborn demonstrate attachment behaviors and appropriate care of newborn [3] ☐ Physiologic parameters WNL [4] ☐ Circumcision w/o bleeding [5] ☐ Voided at least x 1 [4] ☐ Stooled at least x 1 [4] ☐ Feeding [2] ☐ LATCH score 7 or greater for breastfed newborn [2] ☐ Parent(s)/family verbalize newborn D/C instruction [6] ☐ No jaundice [4] ☐ Physician aware of Coombs results ☐ Discharge Day 2 ☐ No signs of infection	☐ Temp, apical pulse, cardiac, resp., neuro, GI, GU, integ. q 8 hr. ☐ Discharge weight ☐ Parent(s)/family & infant attachment behaviors ☐ LATCH score of breastfed newborn ☐ Frequency & amt. of bottle feeding ☐ ________	☐ Newborn screening tests prior to D/C ☐ ________	☐ Referral made to lactation consultant for LATCH score <7 ☐ ________

NAME	INITIALS	NAME	INITIALS

NOTE: EACH PATIENT REQUIRES AN INDIVIDUAL ASSESSMENT & TREATMENT PLAN. THIS CLINICAL PATH IS A RECOMMENDATION FOR THE AVERAGE PATIENT WHICH REQUIRES MODIFICATION WHEN NECESSARY BY THE PROFESSIONAL STAFF.

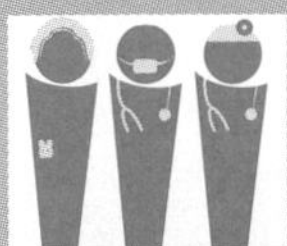

Clinical Pathway 12–1 *(Continued)*

TREATMENTS	MEDS	NUTR.	EDUC & DC PLANNING
N D E N/A N/A Cord care Circumcision care when indicated __________	N D E __________	N D E Breast/bottle feed on demand (breast: q 2–3 hrs, bottle: q 3–4 hrs)	N D E Observe return demonst. of breast-feeding mother's use of -alternative positioning -infant's suck, swallow Observe parent(s) providing appropriate newborn care; reinforce. __________
N/A N/A Cord care Circumcision care when indicated __________	__________	Breast/bottle feed on demand (breast: q 2–3 hrs, bottle: q 3–4 hrs)	Observe return demonst. of breast-feeding mother's use of -alternative positioning -infant's suck, swallow Observe parent(s) providing appropriate newborn care; reinforce. __________
☐ Cord care ☐ Circumcision care when indicated ☐ Cord clamp removed prior to D/C ☐ __________	☐ Hepatitis B vaccine per order ☐ __________	☐ NPO for circumcision when indicated ☐ Breast/bottle feed on demand (breast: q 2–3 hrs, bottle: q 3–4 hrs)	☐ Review D/C instructions with parent(s)/family ☐ Discuss plan for follow-up care ☐ D/C to mother's care

NAME	INITIALS	NAME	INITIALS

growing child. A chest of drawers for clothing, an adult chair (preferably a rocker), and a flat-topped table for changing clothes are necessary. The baby needs a separate bathtub, which may be merely a plastic basin. A tray containing frequently used articles saves time and energy. These might include a thermometer, hairbrush and comb, baby wipes, and baby oil or lotion. A diaper pail may also be necessary.

Clothing

Clothing must be soft, washable, of the proper size, and easy to put on and take off. Instruct parents to launder new clothing and sheets before using them to prevent skin irritation. Nightgowns with drawstring necks are avoided because they may lead to strangulation. Buttons need to be sewed on tightly. Snaps or Velcro fasteners are safer. If the mother does not have a clothes dryer, she needs a clothes rack to dry the infant's garments when the weather is inclement.

Disposable diapers are commonly used in hospitals and homes. They have an outer waterproof layer. Diapers are made of gauze, knitted cotton, or bird's-eye or cotton flannel. Contoured and prefolded types are available and are convenient if a diaper service is used. However, they take longer to dry when laundered at home and are more costly. *Diaper liners* are specially treated tissues placed within the diaper. When diapers are soiled, the stool is rinsed into the toilet. The diapers are soaked in cold water, washed with a mild soap, rinsed thoroughly, and dried by clothes dryer or outdoors in the sun. Diapers that have been improperly washed and rinsed may aggravate rashes.

Waterproof pants should be loose and cut so that air can circulate through them. They are not used when the skin is irritated. If a rash is present, the buttocks are kept exposed to the air as often as possible. Diapers are changed as soon as they are wet. Disposable diapers are avoided when a diaper rash is present because the plastic covering prevents evaporation. If a rash becomes increasingly worse, the physician is consulted.

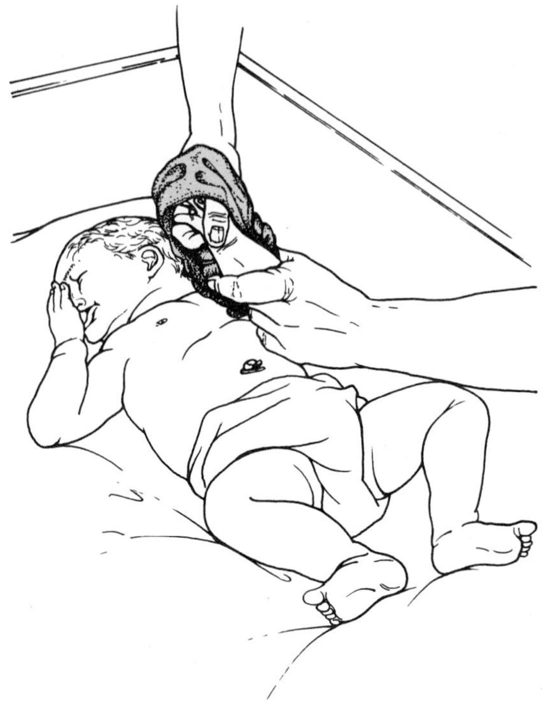

Figure 12–14. • The simplest way to dress the newborn is to put your hand through the sleeve, grasp the baby's hand, and gently pull it through.

The quantity of items that the mother needs is determined by her washing facilities and the climate of the area in which she lives. It is wise to obtain sufficient amounts of the few articles that have to be changed often, for example, three or four dozen diapers, six shirts and blankets, six nightgowns, and two or three sweater sets. Figure 12–14 illustrates the simplest way to dress the newborn.

KEY POINTS

- Assessment of the newborn includes gestational age, weight and measurement, reflexes, system assessment, and bonding with parents.
- Heat loss occurs in the newborn via conduction, convection, evaporation, and radiation.
- The newborn is born with certain reflexes. Three of these are the Moro reflex, the rooting reflex, and the tonic neck reflex.
- The Apgar score is a standardized method of evaluating the newborn's condition immediately following delivery. Five objective signs are measured. These include heart rate, respiration, muscle tone, reflexes, and color.

- The most critical period for the newborn is the 1st hour of life, when drastic change from life within the uterus to life outside it takes place.
- Physiologic jaundice becomes evident between the 2nd and 3rd day of life and lasts for about 1 week.
- The newborn has an unstable heat-regulating system and must be kept warm.
- Although the kidneys function at birth, they are not fully developed. Likewise, the immune system is not fully activated.
- Vernix caseosa is a cheeselike substance that covers the skin of the newborn at birth.
- Meconium, the first stool of the newborn, is a mixture of amniotic fluid and secretions of the intestinal glands. They change in color from tarry greenish-black, to greenish-yellow (transitional stools), to yellow-gold (milk stools).
- Proper handwashing is essential in prevention of infection in newborn infants.
- Nursery standards are developed and enforced by various professional agencies.
- The nutritional status of newborns can be evaluated by determining the number and consistency of stools, frequency of voiding, appearance of sunken fontanels, and status of tissue turgor.
- The normal newborn infant will lose about 10% of the birth weight in the first few days of life but will regain the birth weight by 10 days of age.
- Discharge teaching begins before birth and continues to discharge date. It includes infant care, follow-up visits, evaluation of support systems, and use of car safety seats.
- The fontanels are spaces between the skull bones of the newborn that allows for molding and provides space for the brain to grow. They are known as "soft spots" on the infant's head.
- Caput succedaneum is edema of the infant's scalp that occurs during the birth process.
- Cephalohematoma is a collection of blood under the periosteum of a cranial bone. The swelling does *not* cross the suture line of the skull bone.

MULTIPLE-CHOICE REVIEW QUESTIONS

Choose the most appropriate answer.

1. The mother of a newborn reports to the nurse that her infant has had a black tarry stool. The nurse would tell the mother that
   a. this is most likely caused from blood the infant may have swallowed during the birth process.
   b. the doctor will be promptly notified.
   c. the infant want will be placed on Nothing by Mouth (NPO) until a stool culture is taken.
   d. this is a normal stool in newborn infants.
2. The soft spots on a newborn's head are termed
   a. hematomas.
   b. fontanels.
   c. sutures.
   d. petechiae.
3. Infections in the newborn require prompt intervention because
   a. they spread more quickly.
   b. infections that are relatively harmless to an adult can be fatal to the newborn.
   c. the portals of entry and exit are more numerous.
   d. the newborn has no defenses against infection.
4. White pinpoint pimples caused by obstruction of sebaceous glands seen on the nose and chin of the newborn are termed
   a. vernix caseosa.
   b. acrocyanosis.
   c. milia.
   d. mongolian spots.
5. The normal respiratory rate of a newborn is
   a. 12 to 16 breaths/min
   b. 16 to 20 breaths/min
   c. 20 to 30 breaths/min
   d. 30 to 60 breaths/min

BIBLIOGRAPHY AND READER REFERENCE

American Nursing Association. (1995). *ANA Position statement on home care for mother, infant and family following birth.* Washington, DC: Author.

Arnand, M. (1996). Early assessment of the breastfeeding infant. *Contemporary Pediatrics, 13*(10), 142.

Association of Woman's Health. Obstetric and Neonatal Nurses (AWHONN). (1994). *Didactic content and clinical skills verification for professional nurse providers of perinatal home care.* Washington, DC.: Author.

Behrman, R., Kleigman, R., & Arvin, A. (1996). *Nelson's textbook of pediatrics* (15th ed.). Philadelphia: Saunders.

Betz, C., Hunsberger, M., Wright, S. (1994). *Family centered nursing care of children* (2nd ed.). Philadelphia: Saunders.

Beyea, S. (1996). *Critical pathways for collaborative nursing care.* Reading, MA: Addison-Wesley.

Braveman, P., et al. (1995). Early discharge of newborns and mothers: A critical review of literature. *Pediatrics, 96*(4), 716–726.

Brazelton, T. B. (1973). *The neonatal behavioral assessment scale.* Philadelphia: Lippincott.

Britton, J., Britton, H., & Beebe, S. (1994). Early discharge of the term newborn: A continued dilemma. *Pediatrics, 94,* 3.

Bruno, J. B. (1995). "Systemic neonatal assessment and intervention." *MCN.* 20(1):21–24.

Cookfair, J. (1996). *Nursing care in the community.* St. Louis, MO: Mosby.

Fanaroff, A. A., & Martin, R. J. (1995). *Neonatal and perinatal medicine: Diseases of fetus and infant.* (6th ed.) St. Louis, MO: Mosby.

Garner, J. (1996). Hospital Infection Control Practices Advisory Committee. Guidelines for isolation precautions in hospitals. *Infection Control Hospital Epidemiol, 17,* 53–80.

Gorrie, T., McKinney, E., & Murray, S. (1997). *Foundations of maternal-newborn nursing.* Philadelphia: Saunders.

Rabinowitz, R., & Hulbert, W. C. (1995). Newborn circumcision should not be performed without anesthesia. *Birth, 22*(1): 45–46.

Short, J. D. (1994). Interdependence needs and nursing care of the new family. *Issues in Comprehensive Pediatric Nursing, 17,* 1–14.

U.S. Department of Health and Human Services. (1991). *Healthy People 2000.* National Health Promotion and Disease Prevention Objectives. DHHS Publication No. 9150212. Washington, DC: U.S. Government Printing Office.

U.S. Department of Health and Human Services. (1992). Acute pain management in infants, children and adolescents: Operative and medical procedures. (AHCPR920020). Washington, DC: U.S. Government Printing Office.

Weiss, M. E., & Richards, M. T. (1994). Accuracy of electronic axillary temperature measurement in term and preterm neonates. *Neonatal Network, 13*(8), 35–40.

Wong, D. (1997). *Whaley & Wong's:* Essentials of pediatric nursing (5th ed.). St. Louis, MO: Mosby.

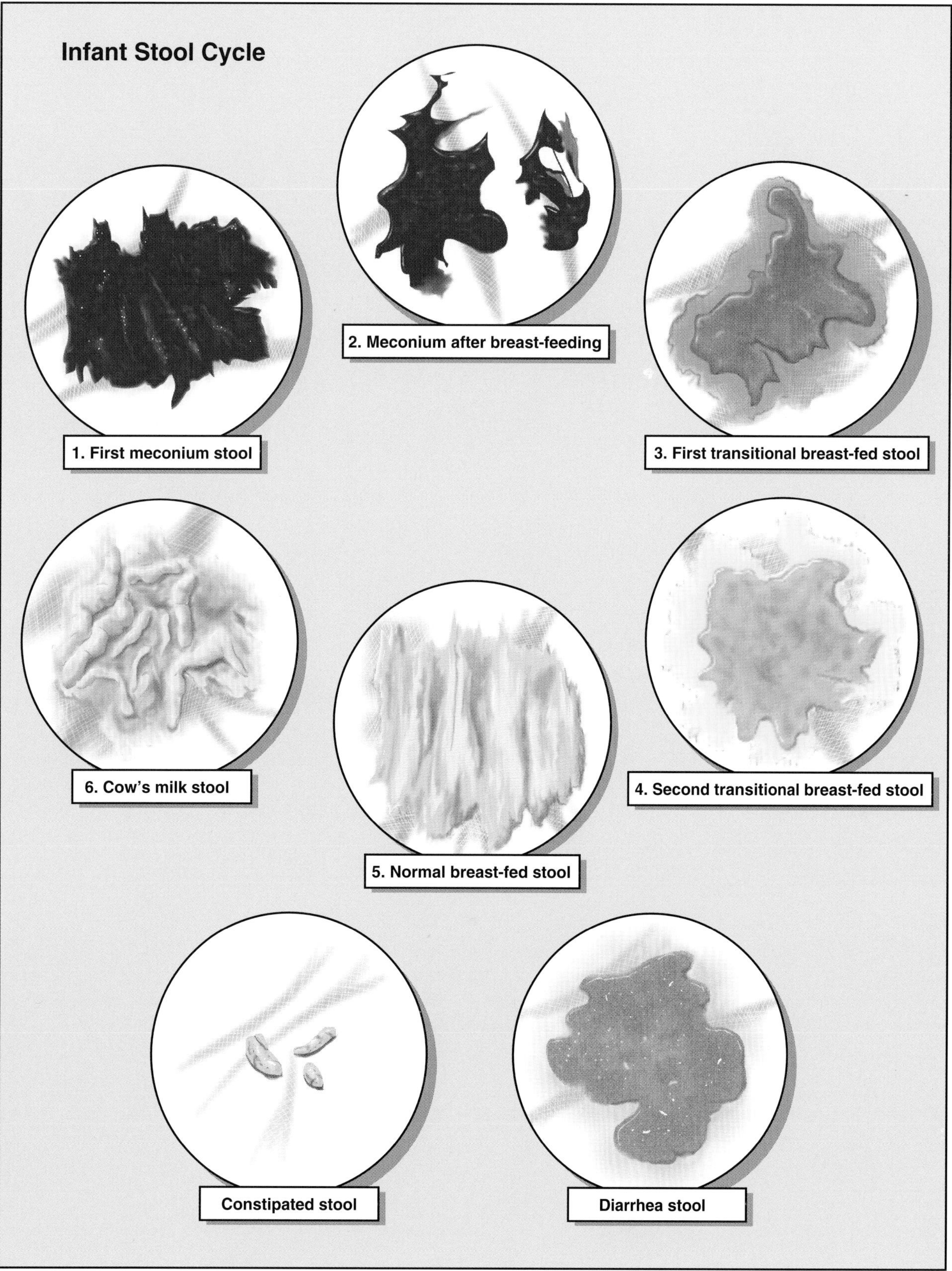

The Infant Stool Cycle. (Redrawn from *Clinical Education Aid #3*. Courtesy of Ross Labs, 1978)

chapter 13

Preterm and Postterm Newborns

Outline

Objectives

On completion and mastery of Chapter 13, the student will be able to

- Define each vocabulary term listed.
- Differentiate between the preterm and the low-birth-weight newborn.
- List three causes of preterm birth.
- Describe selected handicaps of preterm birth and the nursing goals associated with each handicap.
- Contrast the techniques for feeding preterm and full-term newborns.
- Describe the symptoms of cold stress and methods of maintaining thermoregulation.
- Discuss two ways to help to facilitate maternal–infant bonding for a preterm newborn.
- Describe the family reaction to preterm infants and nursing interventions.
- List three characteristics of the postterm baby.

Vocabulary

apnea
bradycardia
bronchopulmonary dysplasia
cold stress
Dubowitz score
gestational age
high risk
hyperbilirubinemia
hypocalcemia
hypoglycemia
icterus
Kangaroo care
lanugo
necrotizing enterocolitis
postterm
preterm
previability
pulse oximeter
respiratory distress syndrome
retinopathy of prematurity
sepsis
surfactant
thermoregulation
total parenteral nutrition

THE PRETERM NEWBORN

The preterm (also known as premature) newborn is the most common admission to the intensive care nursery. With increased specialization and sophisticated monitoring techniques, many babies who in the past would have died are now surviving. The nurse's role has become more and more complex, with greater emphasis placed on subtle clinical observations and technology. This chapter acquaints the student with the preterm baby to encourage an appreciation of this baby's struggle for survival and the intense responsibility placed on those entrusted with this care. The words *preterm* and *premature* are used synonymously, although the former is now considered more accurate.

Any newborn whose life or quality of existence is threatened is considered to be in a high-risk category and requires close supervision by professionals. Preterm newborns constitute a majority of these patients and account for the largest number of admissions to the neonatal intensive care unit. Premature birth is responsible for more deaths during the 1st year of life than any other single factor. Preterm babies also have a higher percentage of birth defects. Prematurity and low birth weight are often concomitant, and both factors are associated with increased neonatal morbidity and mortality. The less a baby weighs at birth, the greater the risks to life during delivery and immediately thereafter.

In the past, a newborn was classified solely by birth weight (Fig. 13–1). Emphasis is now placed on gestational age and level of maturation. Current data also indicate that intrauterine growth rates are not the same for all babies and that individual factors must be considered. *Gestational age* refers to the actual time, from conception to birth, that the fetus remains in the uterus. For the *preterm* this is less than 38 weeks, for the *term* baby it is 38 to 42 weeks, and for the *postterm* baby it is beyond 42 weeks. One standardized method used to estimate gestational age is the *Ballard scoring system,* based on the baby's external characteristics and neurologic development (Figs. 13–2 and 13–3).

Level of maturation refers to how well developed the baby is at birth and the ability of the organs to function outside the uterus. The physician can de-

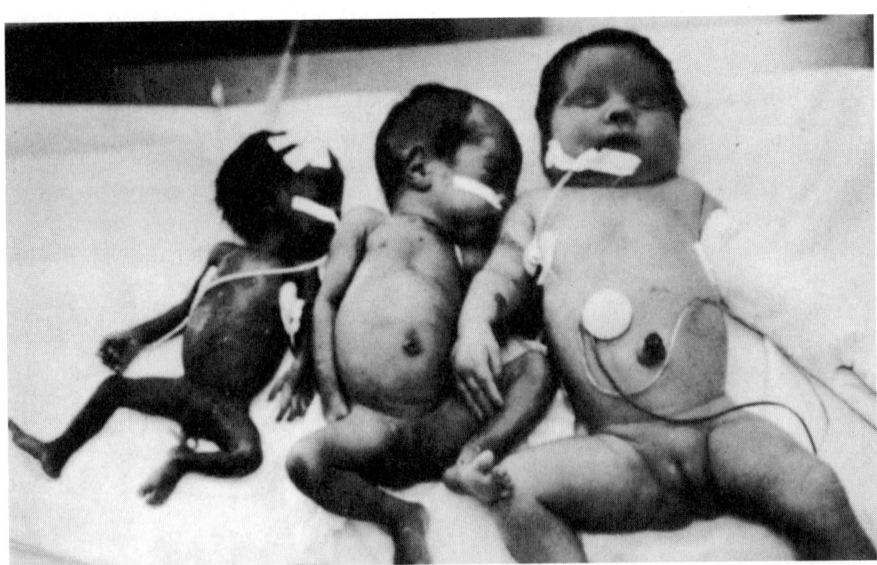

Figure 13–1. • Three babies of the same gestational age (32 weeks) weighing 600, 1400, and 2750 g, respectively, from left to right. (From Korones, S. B. [1986]. *High risk newborn infants: The basis of intensive nursing care* [4th ed.]. St. Louis, MO: Mosby.)

MATURATIONAL ASSESSMENT OF GESTATIONAL AGE (New Ballard Score)

A

NEUROMUSCULAR MATURITY

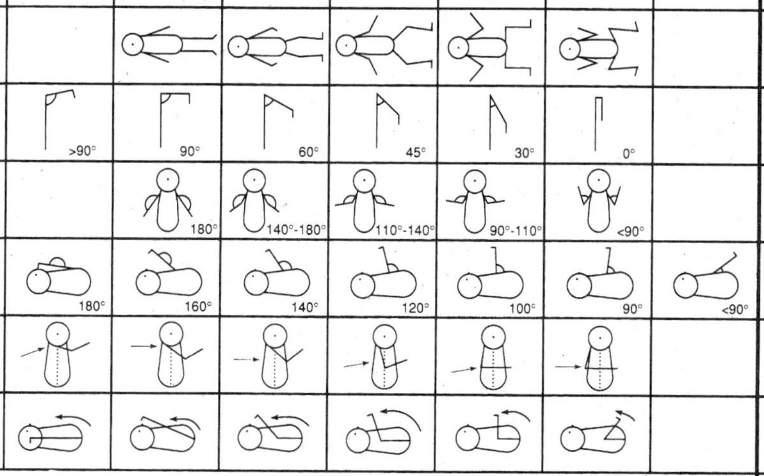

NEUROMUSCULAR MATURITY SIGN	SCORE -1	0	1	2	3	4	5	RECORD SCORE HERE
POSTURE								
SQUARE WINDOW (Wrist)	>90°	90°	60°	45°	30°	0°		
ARM RECOIL		180°	140°-180°	110°-140°	90°-110°	<90°		
POPLITEAL ANGLE	180°	160°	140°	120°	100°	90°	<90°	
SCARF SIGN								
HEEL TO EAR								
							TOTAL NEUROMUSCULAR MATURITY SCORE	

B

PHYSICAL MATURITY

PHYSICAL MATURITY SIGN	SCORE -1	0	1	2	3	4	5	RECORD SCORE HERE
SKIN	sticky friable transparent	gelatinous red translucent	smooth pink visible veins	superficial peeling &/or rash, few veins	cracking pale areas rare veins	parchment deep cracking no vessels	leathery cracked wrinkled	
LANUGO	none	sparse	abundant	thinning	bald areas	mostly bald		
PLANTAR SURFACE	heel-toe 40-50 mm:-1 <40 mm:-2	>50 mm no crease	faint red marks	anterior transverse crease only	creases ant. 2/3	creases over entire sole		
BREAST	imperceptible	barely perceptible	flat areola no bud	stippled areola 1-2 mm bud	raised areola 3-4 mm bud	full areola 5-10 mm bud		
EYE/EAR	lids fused loosely: -1 tightly: -2	lids open pinna flat stays folded	sl. curved pinna; soft; slow recoil	well-curved pinna; soft but ready recoil	formed & firm instant recoil	thick cartilage ear stiff		
GENITALS (Male)	scrotum flat, smooth	scrotum empty faint rugae	testes in upper canal rare rugae	testes descending few rugae	testes down good rugae	testes pendulous deep rugae		
GENITALS (Female)	clitoris prominent & labia flat	prominent clitoris & small labia minora	prominent clitoris & enlarging minora	majora & minora equally prominent	majora large minora small	majora cover clitoris & minora		
							TOTAL PHYSICAL MATURITY SCORE	

Reference
Ballard JL, Khoury JC, Wedig K, et al: New Ballard Score, expanded to include extremely premature infants. *J Pediatr* 1991; 119:417-423. Reprinted by permission of Dr Ballard and Mosby-Year Book, Inc.

SCORE

Neuromuscular________

Physical________

Total________

MATURITY RATING

score	weeks
-10	20
-5	22
0	24
5	26
10	28
15	30
20	32
25	34
30	36
35	38
40	40
45	42
50	44

C

GESTATIONAL AGE (weeks)

By dates________

By ultrasound________

By exam________

Figure 13–2. • The new Ballard scale estimates gestational age based on the neonate's neuromuscular (A) and physical maturity (B). A newborn will score 45 for a 42-week gestation, or only 20 for a 32-week gestation (C). (From Ballard, J.L., Khoury, J., Wedig, K., et al. New Ballard score expanded to include extremely premature infants. *Journal of Pediatrics*, 1991, 119:417–423. St Louis: Mosby Yearbook.)

termine much about the maturity of the newborn by careful physical examination, observation of behavior, and family history. A baby who is born at 34 weeks' gestation, weighs 3½ pounds at birth, has not been damaged by multifactorial birth defects, and has had a good placenta may be healthier than a full-term, "small for date" baby whose placenta was insufficient for any of a number of reasons. It is also probably in better condition than the heavy, but immature, baby of a diabetic mother. Each child has different, distinct needs.

Causes

The predisposing causes of prematurity are numerous; in many instances the cause is unknown. Prematurity may be caused by multiple births, illness of the mother (e.g., malnutrition, heart disease, diabetes mellitus, or infectious conditions), or the hazards of pregnancy itself, such as pregnancy-induced hypertension, placental abnormalities that may result in premature rupture of the membranes, placenta previa (the placenta lies over the cervix

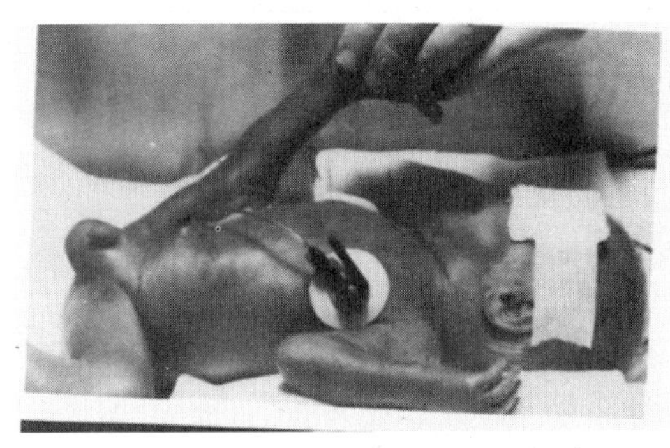

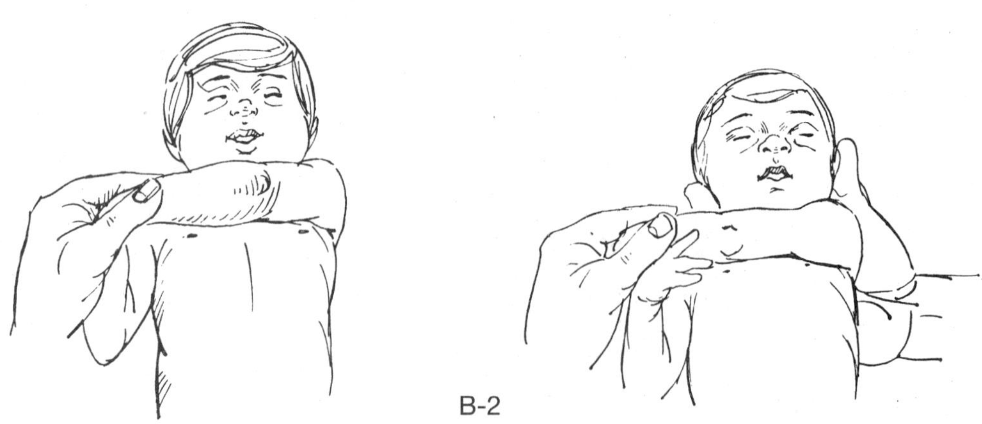

Figure 13–3. • **A,** The Dubowitz or new Ballard assessment of the newborn. The popliteal angle of this newborn is 180 degrees, rating a score of 0. (From Moore, M. L. [1982]. *Family, newborn, and nurse.* Philadelphia: Saunders.) **B-1,** In the full-term infant, when the arm is pulled across the chest, the elbow will go only as far as the chin in the midline. This is called the *scarf sign.* **B-2,** In the premature infant, when the arm is pulled across the chest, it can be pulled into a straight line, the elbow passing the chin at the midline. (From Leifer, G. [1982]. *Principles and techniques in pediatric nursing.* Philadelphia: Saunders.)

instead of higher in the uterus), and premature separation of the placenta.

Studies also indicate relationships between prematurity and poverty, smoking, alcohol consumption, and cocaine and other drug abuses. Adequate prenatal care to prevent preterm birth is extremely important. Following delivery, early parental interaction with the baby is recognized as essential to the bonding (attachment) process. The presence of parents in special care nurseries is commonplace. Some preterm babies are born into families with numerous other problems. The parents may not be prepared to handle the additional financial and emotional strain imposed by a preterm infant. Multidisciplinary care including parent aides and other types of home support and assistance are vital particularly because current studies indicate a correlation between high-risk births and child abuse and neglect.

Physical Characteristics

Preterm birth deprives the newborn of the complete benefits of intrauterine life. The baby whom the nurse sees in the incubator may resemble a fetus of 7 months' gestation. The skin is transparent and loose. Superficial veins may be seen beneath the abdomen and scalp. There is a lack of subcutaneous fat, and fine hair *(lanugo)* covers the forehead, shoulders, and arms. The cheeselike vernix caseosa is abundant. The extremities appear short. The soles of the feet have few creases, and the abdomen protrudes. The nails are short. The genitals are small. In girls, the labia majora may be open.

Related Handicaps

Inadequate Respiratory Function. Important structural changes occur in fetal lungs during the second half of the pregnancy. The alveoli, or air sacs, enlarge, which brings them closer to the capillaries in the lungs. The failure of this phenomenon leads to many deaths attributed to previability (*pre,* "before," and *vita,* "life"). In addition, the muscles that move the chest are not fully developed; the abdomen is distended, causing pressure on the diaphragm; the stimulation of the respiratory center in the brain is immature; and the gag and cough reflexes are weak because of inadequate nerve supply.

Respiratory Distress Syndrome. Respiratory distress syndrome (RDS), also called hyaline membrane disease, is a result of immaturity of the lungs, which leads to decreased gas exchange. An estimated 30% of all neonatal deaths result from RDS or its complications (Behrman, Kleigman, & Arvin, 1996). In this disease, there is a deficient synthesis or release of *surfactant,* a chemical in the lungs. Surfactant is high in lecithin, a fatty protein necessary for absorption of oxygen by the lungs. A test to determine the amount of surfactant in amniotic fluid is the lecithin/sphingomyelin (L/S) ratio. Areas of *atelectasis,* or collapse, also occur, and the functional residual capacity (FRC) of the lungs fails to develop.

Manifestations. The symptoms of respiratory distress are generally apparent after delivery, although they may not be manifested for several hours (Fig. 13–4). Respirations increase to 60 or more breaths/min. Rapid respirations (tachypnea) are accompanied by gruntlike sounds, nasal flaring, cyanosis, and intercostal and sternal retractions. As the condition becomes more severe, edema, lassitude, and apnea occur. Mechanical ventilation may be necessary. The treatment of these babies is ideally carried out in the neonatal intensive care unit.

Treatment. Surfactant is produced by the infant's alveoli at 22 weeks' gestation and is at an adequate level to enable the infant to breathe adequately at birth by 34 weeks' gestation. If insufficient amounts of surfactant are detected through amniocentesis, it is possible to increase its production by giving the mother injections of corticosteroids, such as betamethasone. Administration 1 or 2 days before delivery may reduce the chances of RDS. In preterm infants, surfactant can be administered via endotracheal (ET) tube at birth or when symptoms of respiratory distress syndrome occur, with improvement of lung function seen within 72 hours. Surfactant production is altered during cold stress, hypoxia, and poor tissue perfusion, conditions often present in the premature infant.

Vital signs are monitored closely, arterial blood gas analyzed, and the infant is placed in a warm incubator with gentle and minimal handling to conserve energy. Intravenous fluids are prescribed and the nurse observes for signs of overhydration or dehydration. Oxygen therapy may be given via hood (Fig. 13–5) or ventilator in concentrations necessary to maintain adequate tissue perfusion. Oxygen toxicity is a high risk for infants receiving prolonged treatment with high concentrations of oxygen. *Bronchopulmonary dysplasia* is the toxic response of the lung to oxygen therapy. Atelectasis, edema, and thickening of the membranes of the lung interferes with ventilation. This often results in prolonged dependence on oxygen and ventilators that have long-term complications.

Apnea. *Apnea* is defined as the cessation of breathing for 20 seconds or longer. It is not uncommon in the preterm newborn. An apneic episode

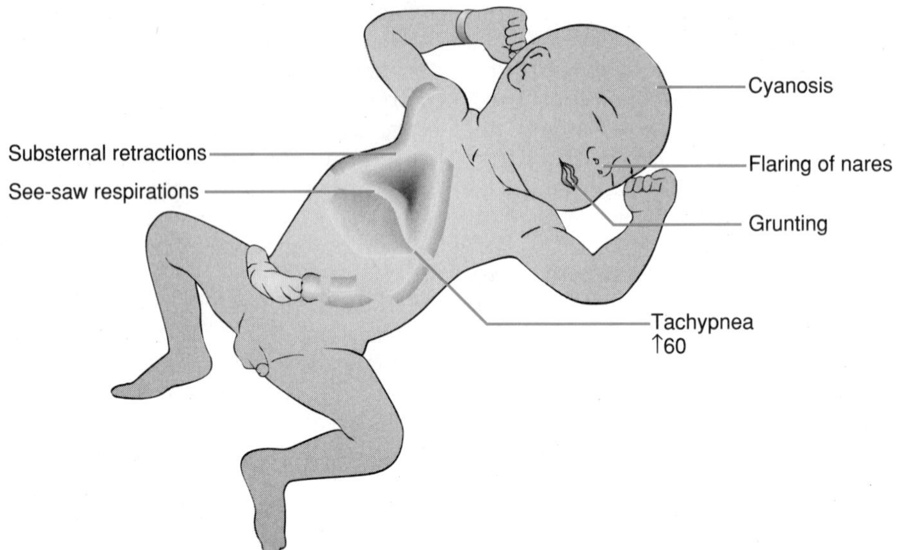

Figure 13–4. • Signs of respiratory distress in premature infant.

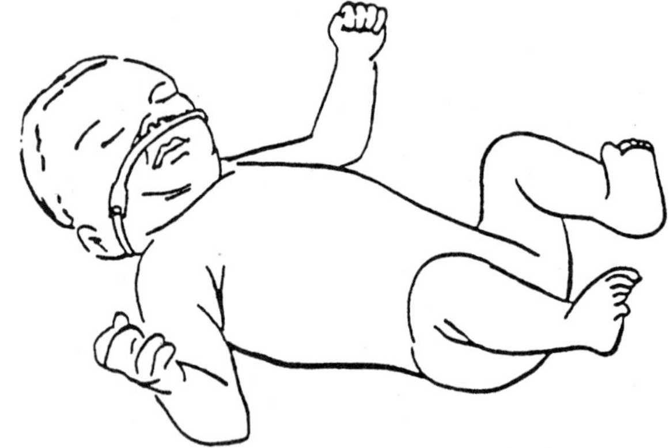

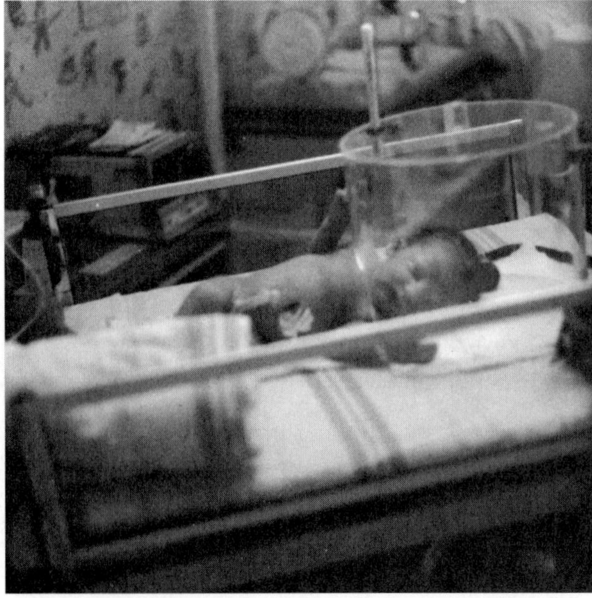

Figure 13–5. • **A,** O_2 via nasal cannula. **B,** Oxygen is administered by means of a plastic hood.

may be accompanied by *bradycardia* (fewer than 100 beats/min) and cyanosis. Apnea monitors alert nurses to this complication. Gentle rubbing of the baby's feet, ankles, and back may stimulate breathing following this occurrence. When these measures fail, suctioning of the nose and mouth and raising of the baby's head usually facilitates breathing. If breathing does not begin, an Ambu bag is utilized. Apnea is believed to be related to immaturity of the nervous system.

Sepsis. Sepsis is a generalized infection of the bloodstream. Preterm newborns are at risk for developing this complication because of the immaturity of many body systems. The liver of the premature infant is immature and forms antibodies poorly. Body enzymes are inefficient. There is little or no immunity received from the mother, and stores of nutrients, vitamins, and iron are insufficient. There may be no local signs of infection, which also hinders diagnosis. Some signs of sepsis include a low temperature, lethargy or irritability, poor feeding, and respiratory distress. Maternal infection and complications during labor can also predispose the preterm infant to sepsis.

Treatment involves administration of intravenous antibiotics, maintenance of warmth and nutrition, and close monitoring of vital signs, including blood pressure. Organization of care will conserve energy. An incubator separates the infant from other infants in the unit and facilitates close observation. Maintenance of strict (standard) universal precautions is essential.

Poor Control of Body Temperature. Keeping the preterm infant warm is a nursing challenge. Heat loss in the preterm is due to several factors:

- The preterm infant has a lack of fat, which is the body's insulation.
- There is excessive heat loss by radiation from a surface area that is large in proportion to body weight. The large surface area of the head predisposes the infant to heat loss.
- The heat-regulating center of the brain is immature.
- The sweat glands are not functioning to capacity.
- The premature infant is inactive, the muscles are weak and less resistant to cold, and the baby cannot shiver.
- The posture of the preterm infant's extremities is one of leg extension. This increases the surface area exposed to the environment and increases heat loss.
- Metabolism is high, and the preterm infant is prone to low blood glucose (hypoglycemia).

These and other factors make the preterm newborn vulnerable to *cold stress,* which causes an increased need for oxygen and glucose. Early detection can prevent complications.

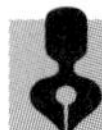

Nursing Tip

Signs and symptoms of cold stress include:
- Decreased skin temperature
- Increased respiratory rate with periods of apnea
- Bradycardia
- Mottling of skin
- Lethargy

Nursing Care. The infant's skin temperature will fall before the core temperature falls. A skin probe is used to monitor the temperature of preterm infants. The skin probe is placed in the right upper quadrant of the abdomen. Care should be taken to ensure the probe is not directly over a bony prominence, in the line of cool oxygen input, or under a diaper.

The infant is placed under a radiant warmer or in an incubator to maintain a warm environment. The temperature of the incubator is adjusted so that the infant's body temperature is at an optimal level (97–98°F).

Hypoglycemia and Hypocalcemia. Hypoglycemia (*hypo,* "below," and *glycemia,* "sugar in the blood") is common among preterm babies. They have not remained in the uterus long enough to acquire sufficient stores of glycogen and fat. This condition is aggravated by the need for increased glycogen in the brain, heart, and other tissues as a result of asphyxia, sepsis, RDS, unstable body temperature, and the like. Any condition that increases energy requirements places more stress on these already deficient stores. Plasma glucose levels of less than 40 mg/dl are indicative of hypoglycemia.

The brain needs a steady supply of glucose and hypoglycemia must be anticipated and treated promptly. Any condition that increases metabolism increases glucose needs. The preterm infant may be too weak to suck and swallow formula and often requires gavage or parenteral feedings to supply their 120 to 150-Kcal/Kg/day needs.

Nursing Tip

Signs of hypoglycemia in the preterm infant include:
- Tremors
- Weak cry
- Lethargy
- Convulsions
- Plasma glucose lower than 40 mg/dl

Nursing Tip

When an infant is given IV calcium gluconate the nurse should monitor the heart rate closely and report bradycardia.

Hypocalcemia (*hypo,* "below," and *calcemia,* "calcium in the blood") is also seen in preterm and sick newborns. Calcium is transported across the placenta throughout pregnancy, but particularly during the 3rd trimester. Early birth can result in babies with lower serum calcium levels.

In early hypocalcemia, the parathyroid fails to respond to low calcium levels in the preterm infant. Infants stressed by hypoxia, birth trauma, or receiving sodium bicarbonate are at high risk. Infants born to mothers who are diabetic or who have had low vitamin D intake are also at risk for developing early hypocalcemia.

Late hypocalcemia usually occurs about 1 week of age in newborn or preterm infants who are fed cow's milk. Cow's milk increases serum phosphate levels, which cause calcium levels to fall.

Hypocalcemia is treated by administering IV calcium gluconate. During intravenous therapy the nurse should monitor the infant for bradycardia. Adding calcium lactate powder to the formula also lowers phosphate levels. (Calcium lactate tablets are insoluble in milk and must not be used.) When calcium lactate powder is slowly discontinued from the formula, the nurse should again monitor the infant for signs of neonatal tetany.

Increased Tendency to Bleed. Premature babies are more prone to bleeding than full-term babies because their blood is deficient in prothrombin, a factor of the clotting mechanism. Fragile capillaries of the head are particularly susceptible to injury during delivery, causing intracranial hemorrhage. Ultrasonography is helpful in detecting this problem. The nurse should monitor the neurological status of the infant and report bulging fontanels, lethargy, poor feeding, and seizures. The bed should be in a slight Fowler's position, and unnecessary stimulation that can cause increased intercerebral pressure should be avoided.

Retinopathy of Prematurity. Retinopathy of prematurity (ROP) is a condition in which there is separation and fibrosis of the retina, which can lead to blindness. Damage to immature blood vessels is thought to be caused by high oxygen levels of arterial blood. The condition was formerly termed *retrolental fibroplasia,* but the term ROP is currently used because it is more precise. It is the leading cause of blindness in newborns weighing less than 1500 g. It was believed at first to be caused by oxygen toxicity alone, but now many other factors have been discovered, some of which are not fully understood. The disorder is classified into several stages, and preterm babies who have milder forms of the disorder may have no residual effects or visual disabilities (Behrman et al., 1996). Prevention of preterm births and the problems that beset preterm infants are the key to resolving ROP. Careful monitoring of arterial blood gases in high-risk infants with a *pulse oximeter* continues to be a priority in the nursery (Fig. 13–6). Gorrie, McKinney, and Murray (1997) clarify further that it is the level of oxygen in the blood, rather than the amount of oxygen received, that is of importance. Maintaining a sufficient level of vitamin E and avoiding excessively high concentrations of oxygen may help to prevent this condition. Cryosurgery may reduce long-term complications of ROP. Consultation with an experienced ophthalmologist is necessary when pathologic signs appear.

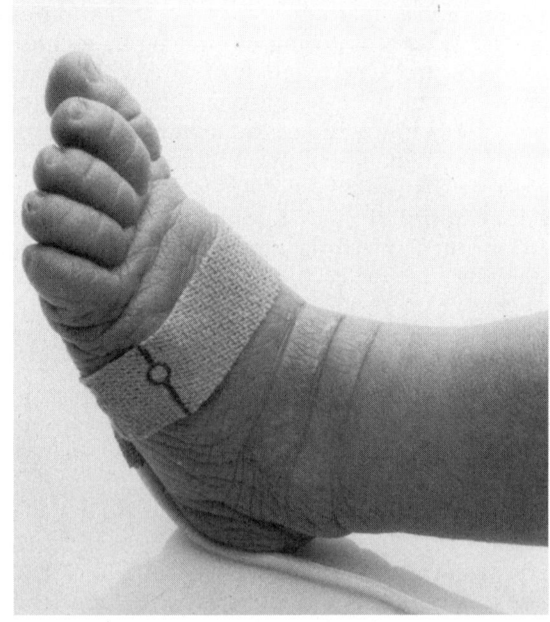

Figure 13–6. • Pulse oximeter. A lead with two sensors opposite each other is placed on the toe or foot of the newborn. A red light passes from one sensor, through the vascular bed of the toe and registers on the sensor on the opposite toe. The determination of oxygen saturation in the blood is shown on the monitor, which displays the heart rate as well as the oxygen saturation level. The foot sensor above is in place. The circle indicates location of the sensor on the footband. (From Mini-Ox® V pulse oximeter. MSA Patient Monitoring Products brochure.)

Poor Nutrition. The stomach capacity of the premature baby is small. The sphincter muscles at both ends of the stomach are immature, contributing to regurgitation and vomiting, particularly after overfeeding. Sucking and swallowing reflexes are immature. The baby's ability to absorb fats is poor (this includes fat-soluble vitamins). The inadequate store of nutrients in the preterm infant and the need for glucose and nutrients to promote growth and prevent brain damage contribute to the nutritional problems of the preterm infant. Parenteral or gavage feedings are usually required until the infant is strong enough to tolerate bottle feedings without compromising cardiorespiratory status.

Necrotizing Enterocolitis. *Necrotizing enterocolitis* (NEC) is an acute inflammation of the bowel that leads to bowel *necrosis.* Preterm newborns are particularly susceptible to NEC. Factors implicated include diminished blood supply to the lining of the bowel wall due to hypoxia or sepsis that causes a decrease in protective mucus and results in bacterial invasion of the delicate tissues. When the infant is fed a milk formula or hypertonic gavage feeding a source for bacterial growth occurs.

Signs include abdominal distention, bloody stools, diarrhea, and bilious vomitus. Specific nursing responsibilities include observing vital signs, maintaining infection control techniques, and carefully resuming oral fluids as ordered. Measuring the abdomen and listening for bowel sounds are also important. Treatment includes antibiotics and the use of parenteral nutrition to rest the bowels. Surgical removal of the necrosed bowel may be indicated.

Immature Kidneys and Skin. Improper elimination of body wastes contributes to electrolyte imbalance and disturbed acid–base relationships. Dehydration occurs easily. Tolerance to salt is limited, and susceptibility to edema is increased.

The nurse should document the intake and output for all preterm infants. The nurse should weigh the dry diaper and subtract its weight from the infant's wet diaper to determine the urine output. The urine output should be between 1 and 3 ml/kg/hr. The infant should be observed closely for signs of dehydration or overhydration. The nurse should document the status of the fontanels, tissue turgor, weight, and urine output.

Jaundice (Hyperbilirubinemia). The liver of the newborn is immature, which contributes to a condition called *icterus* or jaundice (Table 13–1). Jaundice causes the skin and whites of the eyes to assume a yellow-orange cast. The liver is unable to clear the blood of bile pigments that result from the normal postnatal destruction of red blood cells. The amount of bile pigment in the blood serum is expressed as milligrams of bilirubin per deciliter. The higher the bilirubin level, the deeper the jaundice and the greater the risk. An increase of more than 5 mg/dl in 24 hours requires careful investigation. Physiologic jaundice is normal and is discussed on page 318. Pathologic jaundice is more serious. It occurs within 24 hours of birth and is secondary to an abnormal condition such as ABO-Rh incompatibility (see p. 364). In preterm infants the normal rise in bilirubin levels (icterus neonatorum) is slower than in full-term infants and lasts longer, which predisposes the infant to *hyperbilirubinemia* (*hyper* "excessive," *bilirubin* "bile," and *emia* "blood"), excessive bilirubin levels in the blood.

Table 13–1
NEONATAL JAUNDICE

Type	Appears	Peak Bilirubin Concentration	Duration
Physiologic			
Full-term	2–3 days	10–12 mg/dl	4–5 days
Preterm	3–4 days	15 mg/dl	7–9 days
Pathologic	1st day	Unlimited	Varies
Breast milk	4–7 days	15–20 mg/dl	10 weeks

There is more evidence of jaundice in babies who are breastfed. Breast milk jaundice begins to be seen about the 4th day, when the mother's milk supply develops. The newborn usually does well but is carefully monitored to rule out problems. Supplemental feedings of 5% dextrose or water to breastfeeding infants can increase bilirubin levels and should be discouraged. Occasionally breastfeeding may be temporarily discontinued for 1 or 2 days and formula prescribed.

The aims of treatment for hyperbilirubinemia are to prevent *kernicterus,* a serious neurologic complication that can cause brain damage, and to reverse the hemolytic process that causes the bilirubin level to rise. The nursing care and treatment for hyperbilirubinemia consists of observing the infant's skin, sclera, and mucous membranes for jaundice. (Blanching the skin over bony prominences enhances evaluation for jaundice.) Monitoring and reporting bilirubin lab values and response phototherapy should be documented.

Special Needs

The doctor appraises the physical status of the preterm newborn at delivery. The immediate needs are to clear the baby's airway and to provide warmth. The baby is given care for the umbilical

BOX 13–1

NURSING GOALS FOR THE PRETERM NEWBORN

The nursing goals in caring for the preterm newborn are to

- Improve respiration
- Maintain body heat (keep the "premie" warm)
- Conserve energy
- Prevent infection
- Provide proper nutrition and hydration
- Give good skin care
- Observe the baby carefully and record observations
- Support and encourage the parents

cord and eye care and is then properly identified. Weighing is sometimes omitted until later if the baby's condition is poor. The baby is placed naked in an incubator and taken to the nursery. The nurse in charge is given a report on the general condition of the newborn, the type of delivery, and any complications that have occurred. Many hospitals transfer their preterm infants to special centers geared to care for them. The transport team is briefed by the neonatologist and is dispatched to the referring hospital. A life-support infant-transport incubator that can be carried by ambulance, and sometimes helicopter, is utilized. Box 13–1 lists some nursing goals for care of the preterm newborn.

Thermoregulation (Warmth)

Thermoregulation (*thermo* "heat" and *regulation* "maintenance of") involves maintaining a stable body temperature and preventing hypothermia (low temperature) and hyperthermia (high temperature). A stable body temperature is essential in the survival and management of preterm infants.

The Incubator. The preterm newborn is placed in an incubator to maintain environmental conditions similar to those of the uterus. The incubator is designed to provide proper heat, humidity, oxygen and mist; isolation; and protection from infection. The top of the incubator is transparent to enable personnel to view the newborn clearly at all times. Models include alarms to indicate overheating or lack of circulating air, facilities for positioning, and a scale to weigh the baby without removal from the warm environment. Nurses must understand how to use the incubators available in the nurseries to which they are assigned (Fig. 13–7A). They should request assistance if needed. The temperature of the incubator is adjusted to a level that will maintain an optimal body temperature in the infant. Smaller infants may require higher incubator temperatures. The nurse records the temperature of the infant and the incubator every 2 hours. The temperature of the baby is monitored with a heat-sensitive probe, which is taped to the abdomen. Axillary temperatures may also be taken. A relative humidity of 60% or higher is desirable. Overheating should be avoided because it increases the baby's oxygen and caloric requirements.

Radiant Heat. Radiant heat cribs that supply overhead heat have the advantage of providing easier access to the patient while maintaining a neutral environment (Fig. 13–7B). Refer to Nursing Care Plan 13–1 to find nursing interventions for selected nursing diagnoses pertinent to care of the preterm newborn.

Kangaroo Care. *Kangaroo care* is a method of care for preterm infants that uses skin-to-skin contact. This method of holding the baby is similar to the way a kangaroo keeps its offspring warm in its pouch (Fig. 13–8). The practice began in 1979 in Bogota, Colombia, in response to a shortage of incubators and staff and is currently a popular practice in the United States. The baby, wearing only a diaper and small cap, rests at the mother or father's naked breast. The skin warms and calms the child and promotes bonding.

Nutrition. Feeding of the preterm newborn varies with gestational age and health status. There is currently controversy about the type and timing of feedings. One reason for this controversy is that the optimal growth rate is unclear. In the past, the preterm newborn was given nothing by mouth for the first 24 to 72 hours. Today, early feedings and intravenous glucose solutions are given to prevent dehydration, hyperbilirubinemia, and hypoglycemia (low blood sugar). The preterm newborn is at risk because early birth has denied the baby time to store needed nutrients, such as glycogen and fat. In addition, water and caloric requirements are higher.

Human milk is ideal because its fat is absorbed readily. The use of milk obtained from milk banks or donors is no longer popular because of many factors, including the risk of human immunodeficiency virus and cytomegalovirus infections. A number of commercial formulas for the preterm infant are available.

The preterm may be fed orally, by gavage (tube feeding), or parenterally. Oral feedings are ordered in milliliters; as little as 2 to 4 ml may initially be given. Special nipples that are small and soft are used. Often the infant is fed while still in the incubator or warming bed. Fluids may be administered intravenously. Again, only very small amounts of fluid are given, sometimes as little as 5 ml/hr. Because the preterm infant's suckling may be weak and swallowing reflexes are immature, gavage feedings may be necessary. Supplemental vitamins (C, D, and E) may be prescribed.

The technique of formula feeding is similar to that for the term newborn, with adjustments for the preterm infant's smaller stomach capacity, lower gastric acidity, and poor absorption of fats. The feeding should take no longer than 15 to 20 minutes to avoid the expenditure of excessive calories. Overfeeding is dangerous. The hazards of aspiration are increased because the gag and cough reflexes are weak, which makes airway clearance more difficult. Careful burping is necessary. Following the feeding, the preterm is placed on the right side with the head slightly raised unless the position is contraindicated by other conditions.

The nurse reports the number of voidings and color of the infant's urine and watches for signs of edema. The hydration needs of the infant are reviewed daily on the basis of intake, output, weight, blood chemistries, and general appearance. *Hyperalimentation,* that is, *total parenteral nutrition,* provides fluid, calories, electrolytes, and vitamins to sustain growth. It may be lifesaving for an infant whose birth weight is very low.

Close Observation. The doctor examines the preterm newborn and writes specific orders for treatment and nursing care. When the doctor leaves

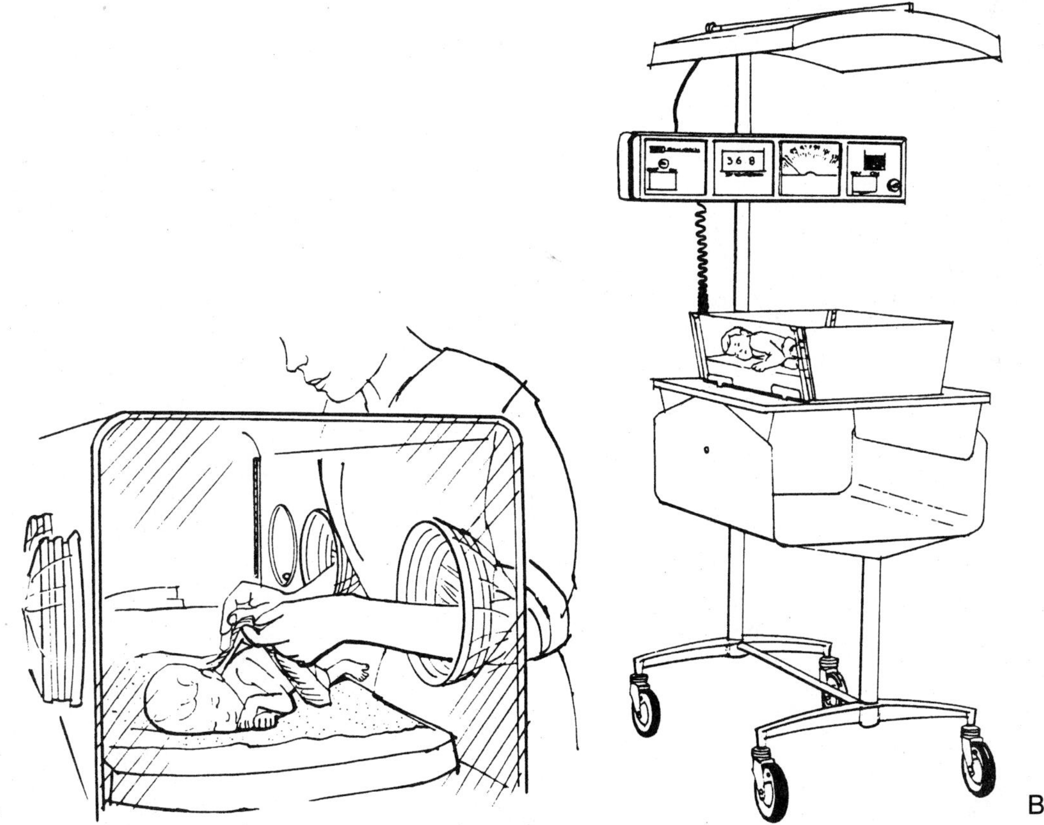

Figure 13–7. • **A,** The incubator. The infant is dressed only in a diaper. Portholes facilitate routine infant care without disturbing the atmospheric conditions in the incubator. The infant can be assessed through plexiglass windows. Levers under the mattress can place the bed in Fowler's or Trendelenburg position. Openings at the head and foot of the incubator can be used to remove soiled linen, using principles of aseptic technique. The door of the incubator can be lowered to form a platform that makes the bed accessible for special treatments or tests. The nurse must make sure the door is *locked* in the closed position when the incubator is in use. To promote circadian rhythms, a blanket may be placed over the top of the incubator to shield infant from environmental lights. **B,** The radiant warmer conserves the infant's body heat. The nurse must be sure there is no obstruction between the overhead heat implement and the infant. (From Leifer, G. [1982]. Principles and techniques in pediatric nursing [4th ed.]. Philadelphia: Saunders.)

NURSING CARE PLAN 13–1

Selected Nursing Diagnoses for the Preterm Newborn

Nursing Diagnosis: High risk for hypothermia related to decreased subcutaneous tissue, immature body temperature control

Goals	Nursing Interventions	Rationale
Baby's temperature will remain at 97.6°F with Servocontrol	1. Monitor temperature with skin probe or by axillary method	1. These methods provide best indication of infant's core temperature and are less invasive
	2. Adjust incubator or radiant warmer to maintain skin temperature	2. A neutral thermal environment permits baby to maintain a normal core temperature with minimum oxygen consumption and caloric expenditure
	3. Observe for signs of cold stress, such as decreased temperature, pallor, and lethargy	3. Preterm babies have little or no muscular activity; they remain in an extended posture because of lack of muscle tone; they cannot shiver
	4. Use discretion in bathing	4. The temperature of a wet baby drops quickly as a result of evaporation
	5. Avoid cold surfaces	5. Conductive heat loss occurs when a baby is weighed on a cold scale; prewarm surfaces or use receiving blanket for protection

Nursing Diagnosis: High risk for impaired skin integrity related to immature skin, poor nutrition, and immobility

Goals	Nursing Interventions	Rationale
Skin will remain intact	1. Change position regularly	1. This prevents pressure sores and aids respiration and circulation
	2. Be gentle when removing dressings, tape, and electrodes	2. The preterm's skin is fragile and bruises easily; use as little tape as possible
	3. Cleanse skin with clear water or approved cleansers	3. Avoid hexachlorophene cleaners because of their toxic effect; all products need to be carefully assessed before use because permeability of perterm's skin fosters absorption of ingredients
	4. Observe skin for signs of infection while recognizing that there may be no local inflammatory response, only vague signs and symptoms	4. Heel pricks and other invasive procedures are often necessary; preterm baby's immune system is immature and healing becomes difficult

the nursery, the nurse is responsible for reporting any significant changes in the baby's condition. The experienced nurse in the preterm nursery observes and charts care and treatment in great detail. Table 13–2 lists *general* observations to guide care of the preterm newborn. Sudden changes are immediately reported.

Positioning and Skin Care. The preterm newborn is positioned on the back with the head of the mattress slightly elevated unless contraindicated. In this position the abdominal contents do not press against the diaphragm and impede breathing.

Positioning the preterm infant should be compatible with drainage of secretions and prevention of aspiration. Propping the infant on the side or placing the infant prone can decrease respiratory effort and improve oxygenation. An enclosed space, or *nesting,* can provide a calming, supportive environment for the preterm infant (Fig. 13–9). The baby should not be left in one position for long periods because it is uncomfortable and may harm the lungs. Changing the position also prevents breakdown from pressure on the infant's delicate skin. If such a breakdown should occur, the area is exposed to the air, and a suitable ointment is applied as prescribed by the doctor (see Table 12–2 and pp. 773–774 for a more extended discussion on the skin of the newborn).

Prognosis

In the absence of severe birth defects and complications, the growth rate of the preterm newborn nears that of the term baby by about the 2nd year. Very-low-birth-weight infants may not catch up, especially if there has been chronic illness, insuffi-

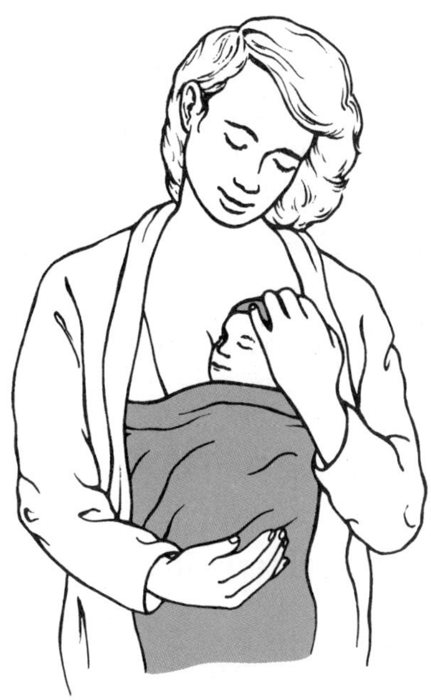

Figure 13–8. • Kangaroo care (nature's incubator).

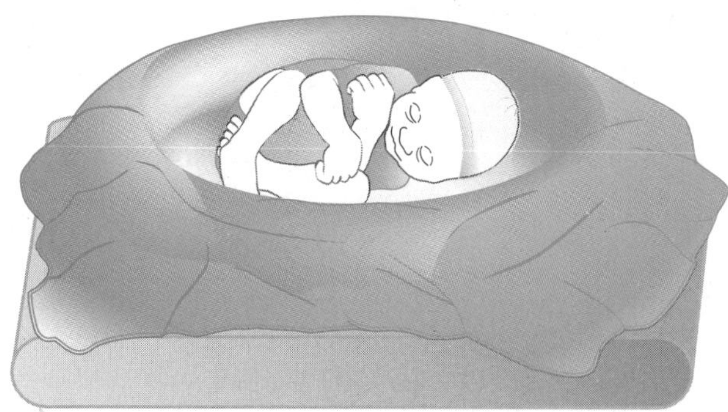

Figure 13–9. • Infant nesting. Providing an enclosed space, bounded by small blanket rolls encircling the preterm infant provides a calming supportive environment.

cient nutritional intake, or inadequate caretaking (Behrman, et al., 1996). Additional studies are needed to determine the effects of these factors at various age levels. Parents need to be prepared for relatives' comments on the baby's small size and slower development. In general, growth and development of the preterm infant are based on current age minus the number of weeks before term the infant was born; for example, if born at 36 weeks' gestation, a 1-month-old infant would be at a newborn's achievement level. This calculation ensures that no one has unrealistic expectations for the infant.

Table 13–2
NURSING OBSERVATIONS IN CARE OF THE PRETERM BABY

Observation	Signs to Look For
Color	Paleness, cyanosis, jaundice
Respirations	Regularity, apnea, sternal retractions, labored breathing
Pulse	Rate and regularity
Abdomen	Distention
Stools	Frequency, color, consistency
Skin	Rashes, irritations, pustules, edema
Cord	Discharge
Eyes	Discharge
Feeding	Sucking ability, vomiting or regurgitation, degree of satisfaction
Mucous membranes	Dryness of lips and mouth, signs of thrush
Voiding	Initial, frequency
Fontanels	Sunken, flat, or bulging
General activity	Increase or decrease in movements, lethargy, twitching, frequency and quality of cry, hyperactivity

Encourage parents to talk about their feelings and fears concerning the preterm baby. Answer questions about home care.

Family Reaction

Nursing care of the preterm infant includes measures to provide short periods of stimulation during the alert phase of activity. The parents can be taught to provide stimulation by using a black-and-white mobile, stroking gently, talking to the infant, rocking, or providing range-of-motion activity. During gavage feeding a pacifier should be used to provide nonnutritive sucking. Care should be taken not to overstimulate or tire the infant. The nurse should assist the parents to cope with their responses to having a small, preterm infant.

Parents need guidance throughout the infant's hospitalization to help to prepare them for this new experience. They may be disheartened by the unattractive appearance of the preterm newborn. They may believe that they are to blame for the baby's condition. They may fear that the baby will die but may be unable to express their feelings. They need time to look at and touch the baby and to begin to see the child as uniquely their own. This touch and immediate human contact are vital for the infant as well. The mother is usually concerned with her ability to care for such a small and helpless creature. When she feels ready, she may assist the nurse in diapering, bathing, feeding, and so on. During these times, other aspects of baby care are also stressed.

The nurse should collaborate with pediatricians, social workers, nutritionists, psychologists, and staff from other disciplines to plan and coordinate

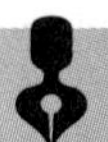

Nursing Tip

Encourage parents to talk about their feelings and fears concerning the preterm baby. Answer questions about home care.

follow-up care of the preterm infant after discharge. Often a mother is discharged without her baby. This is difficult for the entire family and makes attachment and bonding more complicated. The nurse encourages the family to keep in touch by telephone and by visits. Parents can help siblings to accept the infant by addressing the child by name, sharing news of progress, taking pictures of the infant, and encouraging communication by drawings and cards. Listening to what siblings are saying provides information for discussion.

Discharge planning begins at birth. The parents will need to demonstrate and practice in routine and/or specialized care. Visits by the nurse to assess home care and provide additional support are valuable. Continued medical supervision is important. The nurse stresses the importance of well-baby examinations, immunizations, and prevention of infection. Good prenatal care for subsequent pregnancies is emphasized because the mother is at high risk for future preterm births.

THE POSTTERM NEWBORN

The newborn is considered *postterm* if a pregnancy goes beyond 42 weeks. *Postmaturity* refers to the infant's showing characteristics of the postmature syndrome. Identification of babies who are not tolerating the extra time in the uterus is the major goal of treatment. Death is uncommon today because of early detection and intervention. What causes postmaturity is not yet clear; however, it is known that the placenta does not function adequately as it ages, which could result in fetal distress. The mortality rate of late babies is higher than that of newborns delivered at term. Morbidity rates are also higher. Once the baby makes it through delivery, the risks are fewer.

The late birth is a psychological strain on the mother, father, and other members of the family, who are eagerly awaiting the arrival of the baby. The nurse encourages parents to verbalize their feelings and concerns about the delay. Very large newborns, such as those of diabetic mothers, are not necessarily postmature but are larger than normal because of rapid abnormal growth before delivery.

The following problems are associated with postmaturity:

- Asphyxia due to chronic hypoxia while in the uterus due to a deteriorated placenta
- Meconium aspiration; hypoxia and distress may cause relaxation of the anal sphincter; meconium can be aspirated into the fetal lungs
- Poor nutritional status; depleted glycogen reserves cause hypoglycemia
- Increase in red blood cell production (polycythemia) due to hypoxia
- Difficult delivery due to increased size of baby
- Birth defects
- Seizures as a result of the hypoxic state

Physical Characteristics and Care

The postterm infant is long and thin and looks as though weight has been lost. The skin is loose, especially about the thighs and buttocks. There is little lanugo (downy hair) or vernix caseosa. Loss of the cheeselike vernix caseosa leaves the skin dry; it cracks, peels, and is almost like parchment in texture. The nails are long and may be stained with meconium. The baby has a thick head of hair and looks alert. Many postterm babies suffer few adverse effects from the delay, but they still require careful observation in the nursery.

Cesarean deliveries are commonly performed if the pregnancy is determined, by testing, to be past 42 weeks or if there are signs of fetal distress or maternal risk. Nursing care involves observing for respiratory distress (usually due to aspiration of meconium-stained amniotic fluid), hypoglycemia (due to depleted glycogen stores), and hyperbilirubinemia (due to polycythemia). The infant may be placed in an incubator because fat stores have been used in utero for nourishment and the infant is vulnerable to cold stress.

TRANSPORTING THE HIGH-RISK NEWBORN

Transportation of the high-risk newborn to a regional neonatal center requires the organization and the expertise of a special team. A nurse and sometimes a doctor accompany the baby unless specialists (e.g., life-flight helicopter personnel) are part of the transport team. Stabilization of the baby before discharge is important. Baseline data, such as vital signs and blood work (blood gases and glucose levels), are obtained. The baby is weighed if this is not contraindicated. Copies of all records are made, including the baby's record, the mother's prenatal history and delivery, and pertinent admission data. A transport incubator is provided for warmth. Batteries are kept fully charged.

The nurse is responsible to place an identification band on the infant before transport and verify the identification name and number with the mother's identification band. The mother should be reassured the identification will stay with the baby. The parents should be given the name and location of the hospital the infant is transported to and the name and telephone number of a doctor to contact for follow-up information and visits.

The mother is shown the newborn before departure. If the mother is unable to hold the baby because of its condition, the incubator is wheeled to the bedside for her observation. A picture is taken and given to the parents. On occasion, a mother is unable to see her baby because of her own unstable condition. Such situations require special empathy from nursing personnel. Once the baby has safely reached its destination, the parents are contacted by telephone. It is also thoughtful if the receiving hospital personnel provide feedback to the transport team so that they may enjoy the results of their efforts.

KEY POINTS

- Early identification of the high-risk fetus facilitates treatment and nursing care.
- Studies indicate that there is a relationship between prematurity and poverty, smoking, alcohol consumption, narcotics use, and lack of prenatal care.
- Preterm infants have poor muscle tone and less subcutaneous fat, but more vernix and lanugo than full-term infants.
- Observe the preterm infant for jaundice, low oxygen saturation levels, and unstable vital signs. Monitor intake and output on all preterm infants.
- Organize care of preterm infants to minimize handling and stimulation.
- Use blanket rolls to provide an enclosed space for preterm infants.
- Support parents and encourage participation in care.
- The postterm newborn has little lanugo and vernix and the skin is dry and peeling.
- Respiratory distress syndrome has a high mortality rate, and it may precipitate long-term effects.
- Problems associated with prematurity include asphyxia, meconium aspiration, hypoglycemia, hypocalcemia, hemorrhage from fragile vessels, poor resistance to infection, and inadequate nutrition.
- Heat or thermoregulation is essential for the preterm newborn's survival. Cold stress is to be avoided.
- Nursing goals in caring for the preterm newborn are to improve respirations, maintain body heat, conserve baby's energy, prevent infection, provide nutrition and hydration, give good skin care, and support and encourage the parents.
- Oxygen is administered very carefully to preterm newborns to help to prevent eye complications, such as retinopathy of prematurity.
- The postterm newborn is born after 42 weeks of gestation and shows certain characteristics that place the baby at risk, such as hypoxia, poor nutritional stores and polycythemia.

MULTIPLE-CHOICE REVIEW QUESTIONS

Choose the most appropriate answer.

1. A standardized method of determining gestational age based on appearance and neuromuscular criteria is the
   a. Gesell graph.
   b. Dubowitz score.
   c. Washington guide.
   d. Friedman curve.
2. Some preterm babies are fed by gavage because of
   a. poor digestion.
   b. overdeveloped gag and cough reflexes.
   c. refusal of formula.
   d. weak sucking and swallowing reflexes.
3. A characteristic sign of necrotizing enterocolitis (NEC) in the newborn is
   a. bloody diarrhea.
   b. necrosis of the abdomen.
   c. projectile vomiting.
   d. high fever.
4. The actual time that the fetus remains in the uterus is termed
   a. gestational age.
   b. intrauterine growth rate.
   c. neurologic age.
   d. level of maturation.
5. Providing high oxygen concentrations to a preterm newborn may cause
   a. hyaline membrane disease.
   b. cyanosis.
   c. retinopathy of prematurity.
   d. primary atelectasis.

BIBLIOGRAPHY AND READER REFERENCE

Affonso, D., Bosque, E., Wahlberg, V., & Brady, J. P. (1993). Reconciliation and healing for mothers through skin to skin contact provided in an American tertiary level intensive care nursery. *Neonatal Network, 12,* 25–32.

American Academy of Pediatrics Committee on Injury and Poison Prevention and Committee on Newborn. (1996). Safe transportation of premature and LBW infants. *Pediatrics, 97*(5), 758–760.

Ashwill, J., & Droske, S. (1997). *Nursing care of children: Principle and practice.* Philadelphia: Saunders.

Behrman, R., Kleigman, R., Arvin, A. (1996). *Nelson's textbook of pediatrics* (15th ed.). Philadelphia: Saunders.

Betz, C., Hunsberger, M., & Wright, S. (1994). *Family-centered nursing care of children.* Philadelphia: Saunders.

Blackburn, S., & Loper, D. (1992). *Maternal, fetal, and neo-natal physiology.* Philadelphia: Saunders.

Creasy, R., & Resnik, R. (1992). *Maternal-fetal medicine.* Philadelphia: Saunders.

Gale, G., Franch, L., & Lund, C. (1993). Skin to Skin (Kangaroo holding of the intubated premature infant). *Neonatal Network, 12*(6), 49–57.

Gorrie, T., McKinney, E., & Murray, S. (1998). *Foundations of maternal newborn nursing.* Philadelphia: Saunders.

Klaus, M. H., & Fanaroff, A. A. (1993). *Care of the high-risk neonate* (4th ed.). Philadelphia: Saunders.

Ludington-Hoe, S. M., et al. (1994). Kangaroo care research results and practice implications and guidelines. *Neonatal Network, 13*(1), 19–27.

Wong, L. (1997). *Whaley and Wong's essentials of pediatric nursing* (4th ed.). St. Louis, MO: Mosby.

chapter 14

The Newborn with a Congenital Malformation

Outline

Objectives

On completion and mastery of Chapter 14, the student will be able to

- Define each vocabulary term listed.
- List and define the more common disorders of the newborn.
- Describe classifications of birth defects.
- Outline the nursing care for the infant with hydrocephalus.
- Discuss the prevention of neural tube anomalies.
- Outline the preoperative and postoperative nursing care of a newborn with spina bifida cystica.
- Discuss the dietary needs of an infant with phenylketonuria.
- Describe the symptoms of increased intracranial pressure.
- Differentiate between cleft lip and cleft palate.
- Discuss the early signs of dislocation of the hip.
- Discuss the care of the newborn with Down syndrome.
- Outline the causes and treatment of hemolytic disease of the newborn (erythroblastosis fetalis).
- Devise a plan of care for an infant receiving phototherapy.
- Describe home phototherapy.

Vocabulary

birth defect
cheiloplasty
clubfoot
congenital malformation
erythroblastosis
habilitation
hydrocephalus
hyperbilirubinemia
macrosomia
meningocele
meningomyelocele
myelodysplasia
Ortolani's sign
Pavlik harness
phototherapy
RhoGAM
shunt
spica cast
spina bifida
transillumination

Congenital defects that are apparent at birth occur in 3% to 4% of all live births, affecting millions of families. The rate is even higher if the defects that become evident later in life are counted. An abnormality of structure, function, or metabolism may result in a physical or mental handicap, may shorten life, or may be fatal. Box 14–1 shows the system of classification of birth defects. Because these disorders include so many conditions, it has been necessary to limit the number discussed in this chapter and to place others in relevant areas of the text (see Index for specific conditions). Fetal alcohol syndrome and environmental influences on fetal growth is discussed in Chapter 5. Congenital heart is discussed in Chapter 25.

Defects present at birth often involve the skeletal system; limbs may be missing, malformed or duplicated. Some abnormalities, such as congenital hip dysplasia, are more subtle, and the nurse must be alert to detect them. *Inborn errors of metabolism* include a number of inherited diseases that affect body chemistry. There may be an absence or a deficiency of a substance necessary for cell metabolism. The deficient substance is usually an enzyme. Almost any organ of the body may be damaged. Examples of inborn errors of metabolism include cystic fibrosis and phenylketonuria (PKU). In *disorders of the blood,* there is a reduced or missing blood component or an inability of a component to function adequately. Sickle cell anemia, thalassemia, and hemophilia fall into this category. *Chromosomal abnormalities* number in the hundreds. Most involve some type of mental retardation, and some are incompatible with life. The newborn with Turner's syndrome or Klinefelter's syndrome may be retarded in physical growth and sexual development.

BOX 14–1

CLASSIFICATION OF BIRTH DEFECTS

Malformations Present at Birth
Structural defects, such as hydrocephalus,* spina bifida,* congenital heart malformations, cleft lip and palate,* clubfoot,* and developmental hip dysplasia*

Metabolic Defects (Body Chemistry)
Cystic fibrosis, phenylketonuria,* Tay-Sachs disease, family hypercholesterolemia or high cholesterol that often causes early heart attack, and others

Blood Disorders
Sickle cell anemia, hemophilia, thalassemia, defects of white blood cells and immune defense, and others

Chromosomal Abnormalities
Down syndrome,* Klinefelter's syndrome, Turner's syndrome, Trisomies 13 and 18, and many others; most involve some combination of mental retardation and physical malformations ranging from mild to fatal

Perinatal Damage
Infections, drugs, maternal disorders, abnormalities unique to pregnancy (Rh disease,* difficult labor or delivery, premature birth)

*Topics discussed in this chapter.

Perinatal damage has many causes and is seen in a variety of forms, the most common of which is premature birth.

As the March of Dimes Birth Defect Foundation (1992) points out, "Few birth defects can be attributed to a single cause. The majority are thought to result from an interplay between environment and heredity, depending on inherited susceptibility, stage of pregnancy, and degree of environmental hazard." Newborns with birth defects may have to remain in the neonatal unit for an extended period.

MALFORMATIONS PRESENT AT BIRTH

This discussion covers *congenital malformations,* or those present at birth, according to body systems.

Nervous System

Hydrocephalus

Description. *Hydrocephalus* (*hydro,* "water," and *cephalo,* "head") is a condition characterized by an increase of cerebrospinal fluid (CSF) in the ventricles of the brain, which causes pressure changes in the brain and an increase in head size. It results from an imbalance between production and absorption of CSF. Hydrocephalus may be congenital or acquired. It is most commonly caused by an obstruction, such as a tumor, or by improper formation of the ventricles. It may occur with a meningomyelocele or as a sequella of infections (encephalitis, or meningitis) or perinatal hemorrhage. The symptoms depend on the site of obstruction and the age at which it develops.

Hydrocephalus is classified as noncommunicating (obstructive) or communicating. *Noncommunicating hydrocephalus* results from obstruction of CSF flow from the ventricles of the brain to the subarachnoid space. *Communicating hydrocephalus* results when CSF now is not obstructed in the ventricles but is inadequately reabsorbed in the subarachnoid space (Fig. 14–1).

Manifestations. The signs and symptoms of hydrocephalus depend on the time of onset and the severity of the imbalance. The classic sign is an increase in head size. If hydrocephalus occurs in utero, the enlarged head will require caesarean section delivery. At birth, the *head enlarges rapidly* and the fontanels bulge. The *cranial sutures separate* to accommodate the enlarging mass. The scalp is shiny, and the veins are dilated. In advanced cases, the pupil of the eyes may appear to be looking downward, while the sclera may be seen above the pupil, much like the look of a *setting sun* (Fig. 14–2). A foreshortened occiput suggests pathology of the 4th ventricle with the brain stem protruding through the cervical canal. This is called the *chiarri* type malformation (Behrman, Kleigman, & Arvin, 1996). When the enlarged head involves a prominent occiput, the pathology usually involves an atresia of the foramen of Lushka and Magendie and is known as the *Dandy-Walker syndrome.* In the older child, headache is the prominent symptom with cognitive slowing, personality changes, spasticity,

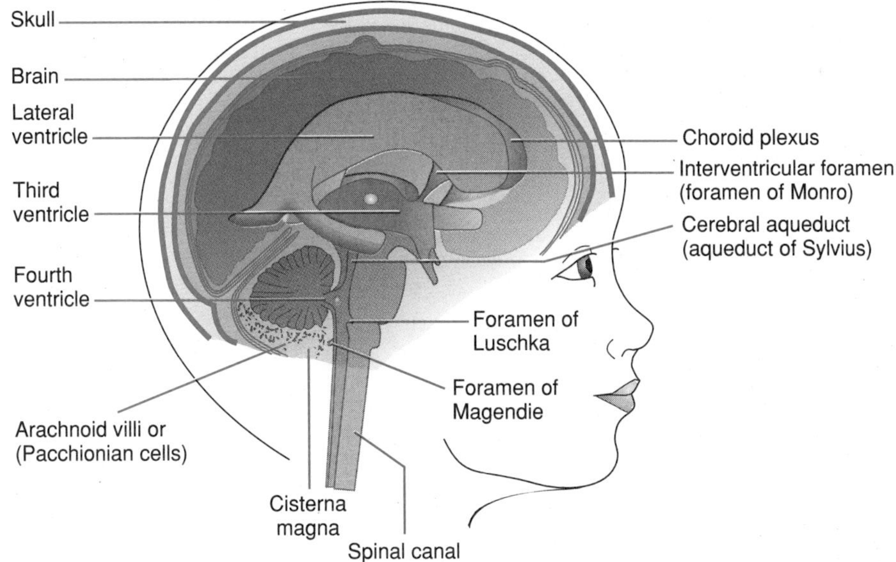

Figure 14–1. • Cerebrospinal fluid circulation. Cerebrospinal fluid is formed in the choroid plexus. The total volume of CSF is approximately 50 cc in the infant and 150 cc in the adult. It flows from the lateral ventricles through the foramen of Monro to the 3rd ventricle. From the 3rd ventricle, the CSF fluid flows through the aqueduct of sylvius to the 4th ventricle and then through the foramen of Luschka and the foramen of Magendie into the cisterns at the base of the brain. Flow continues to the spinal canal. Then the CSF is absorbed by the arachnoid villi (which are also known as Pacchionian cells). When the arachnoid villi are malformed or malfunction, communicating or nonobstructive hydrocephalus will occur. When the tiny aqueducts of sylvius is obstructed within the ventricles, noncommunicating or obstructive hydrocephalus results. When hydrocephalus occurs, excessive CSF causes the ventricles to enlarge and press the brain tissue against the bony skull.

and other neurologic signs. The infant is helpless and lethargic. The body becomes thin, and the muscle tone of the extremities is often poor. The cry is shrill and high-pitched. Irritability, vomiting, and anorexia are present, and convulsions may occur.

Diagnosis. Transillumination (*trans,* "across," and *illuminare,* "to enlighten"), the inspection of a cavity or organ by passing a light through its walls, is a simple diagnostic procedure useful in visualizing fluid. A flashlight with a sponge-rubber collar is held tightly against the infant's head in a dark room. The examiner observes for areas of increased luminosity. A small ring of light is normal, a large halo effect is not (Fig. 14–3). The child's head is measured daily. Echoencephalograph, computed tomography (CT) scan, and magnetic resonance imaging (MRI) are used to visualize the enlarged ventricles and to identify the area of obstruction. A ventricular tap or puncture may be performed in the treatment room using sterile technique. The equipment needed is the same as for a lumbar puncture. A specimen is labeled and sent to the laboratory for analysis.

Treatment. After careful evaluation of preoperative test results, the decision of whether to operate is made. The surgeon attempts to bypass, or *shunt,* the point of obstruction. The CSF may thus be carried to another area of the body, where it is absorbed and finally excreted. This is accomplished by inserting special tubing, which is replaced at intervals as the child grows. The procedure, known as a *ventriculoperitoneal shunt* (Fig. 14–4), allows the excess fluid to drain into the peritoneal cavity where it is absorbed.

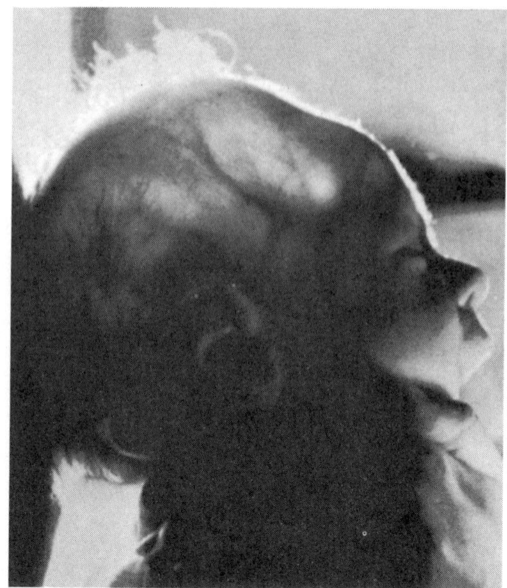

Figure 14–3. • A halo of light through the skull indicates a loss or thinning of cerebral cortex. (From Jarvis, C. [1992]. *Physical examination and health assessment.* Philadelphia: Saunders.)

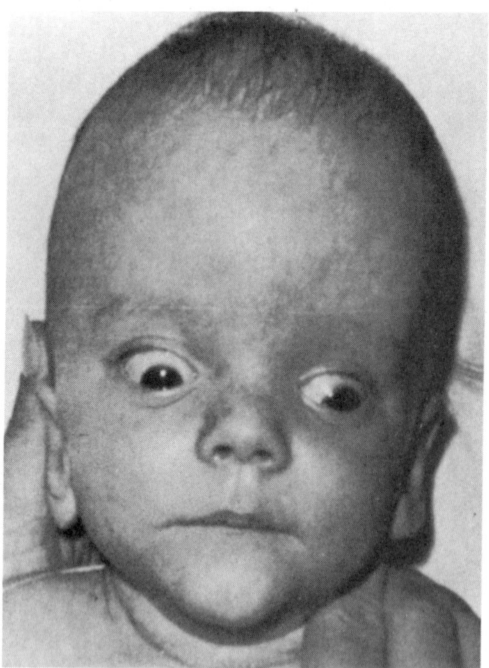

Figure 14–2. • Marked hydrocephalus with "setting sun" sign and divergence of the eyes. (From Youmans, J. R. [1982]. *Neurological surgery* [2nd ed.]. Philadelphia: Saunders.)

The prognosis for the child with this condition has improved with modern drugs and surgical techniques. If the brain is not seriously damaged before the operation, mental function may be preserved. Motor development is sometimes slower if the child cannot lift the head normally. Complications of shunts are usually mechanical (kinking or plugging of tubing) or infection. The shunt acts as a focal spot for infection and may need to be removed if infection persists.

Preoperative Nursing Care. The general nursing care of an infant with hydrocephalus who has not undergone surgery presents several challenges. The child may be barely able to raise the head. Mental development is delayed. Lack of appetite, a tendency to vomit easily, and poor resistance to infections present challenging problems.

The position of the patient must be changed frequently to prevent hypostatic pneumonia and pressure sores. Hypostatic pneunonia occurs when the circulation of the blood in the lungs is poor and the infant remains in one position too long. It is particularly prevalent in infants who are poorly nourished or weak or who have a debilitating disease. When the nurse turns a patient who has hydrocephalus, the head must always be supported. To turn the infant in bed, the weight of the head is borne in the palm of one hand, and the head and body are rotated together to prevent a strain on the neck. When the infant is lifted from the crib, the head must be supported by the nurse's arm and chest.

Pressure sores may occur if the infant's position is not changed at least every 2 hours. The tissues of the head and ears as well as the bony prominences have a tendency to break down. A pad of lamb's wool or sponge rubber placed under the head may help to prevent these lesions. If the skin becomes broken, it is given immediate attention to prevent infection. The infant must be kept dry, especially around the creases of the neck, where perspiration may collect.

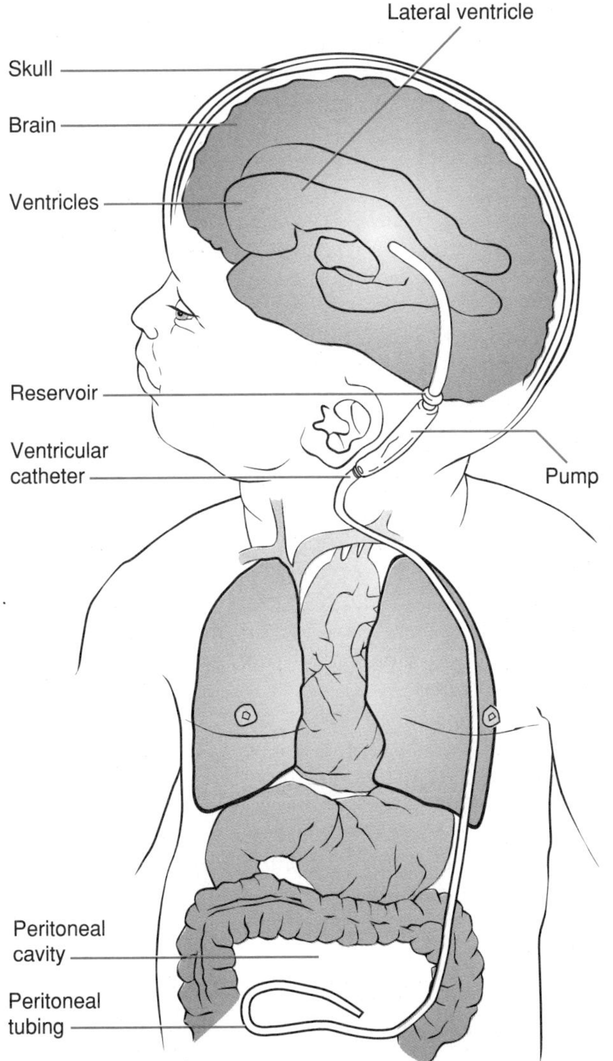

Figure 14–4. • Shunting procedure for hydrocephalus, in which a catheter drains the ventricular system into the peritoneal cavity. Note the pump behind the ear that can be depressed intermittently to clear mucus plugs.

In most cases the nurse may hold the infant for feedings. The nurse sits with the arm supported because the baby's head is heavy. A calm, unhurried manner is necessary. The room should be as quiet as possible. After the feeding, the infant is placed on the side. The patient is not disturbed once settled since vomiting occurs easily. The nurse must organize daily care so that it does not interfere with meals.

Observations to be made include type and amounts of food taken, vomiting, condition of skin, motor abilities, restlessness, irritability, and changes in vital signs. Fontanels are inspected for size and signs of bulging. Head circumference is measured around the occipito-frontal area and recorded on the chart. Symptoms of increased pressure within the head are an increase in blood pressure and a decrease in pulse and respiration. Signs of a cold or other infection are immediately reported to the nurse in charge and are recorded.

Postoperative Nursing Care. In addition to routine postoperative care and observations, the nurse observes the patient for signs of increased intracranial pressure (ICP) and of infection at the operative site or along the shunt line.

Bacterial infection is a life-threatening complication that sometimes necessitates removing the shunt. Signs of infection include an increase in vital signs, poor feeding, vomiting, pupil dilation, decreased levels of consciousness, and seizures. The operative area is observed for signs of inflammation. An internal flushing device may be used to ensure patency of the shunt tube when increased ICP is suspected. The physician may order the pump to be routinely depressed a certain number of times each day to facilitate drainage. This is accomplished by compressing the antechamber or reservoir that is under the skin behind the ear (Fig. 14–4).

Positioning of the patient depends on several factors and may vary with the patient's progress. If the fontanels are sunken, the infant is kept flat because too rapid a reduction of fluid may lead to seizures or cortical bleeding. If the fontanels are bulging, the patient is usually placed in the semi-Fowler's position to promote drainage of the ventricles through the shunt. The patient is always positioned so as to avoid pressure on the operative site. The surgeon leaves orders for the patient's position and activity. Assessment of skin remains a priority. Head and chest measurements are recorded. In patients with peritoneal shunts, the abdomen is measured or observed to detect malabsorption of fluid.

The infant should be observed for signs of increased ICP. The development of a high-pitched cry, unequal pupil size or response to light, bulging fontanels, irritability or lethargy, poor feeding or abnormal vital signs should be reported and recorded. The need for pain control should be assessed and medications given as needed. A careful intake and output is recorded and the infant observed closely for signs of fluid overload. The infant is usually fed after active bowel sounds are heard The surgical suture lines should be kept clean and dry and the infant's diaper kept well below the abdominal suture line to prevent contamination. Parent education, support, and guidance are essential. Parents are taught signs indicating shunt malfunction, how and when to "pump" the shunt by pressing against the valve behind the ear, and the need for multidisciplinary follow-up care. Community resources, such as the National Hydrocephalus Foundation, and information concerning special car seats for children with special needs, should be made known to the parents. There is approximately an 80% survival rate for infants treated early, and approximately one third of the cases result in normal physical and neurological functioning. Other survivors may have varying degrees of developmental disabilities.

Myelodysplasia and Spina Bifida

Myelodysplasia refers to a group of central nervous system disorders characterized by malformation of the spinal cord, one of which is spina bifida.

Description. Spina bifida (divided spine) is a congenital embryonic neural tube defect in which there is an imperfect closure of the spinal vertebrae. There are two forms, occulta (hidden) and cystica (sac or cyst) (Fig. 14–5).

Spina bifida occulta is a relatively minor variation of the disorder in which the opening is small and there is no associated protrusion of structures. It is often undetected and occurs most commonly at L5 and S1 levels. There may be a tuft of hair, a dimple, a lipoma, or a port-wine birthmark at the site. Generally, treatment is not necessary unless neuromuscular symptoms appear. These symptoms consist of progressive disturbances of gait, footdrop, or disturbances of bowel and bladder sphincter function.

Spina bifida cystica consists of the development of a cystic mass in the midline of the spine (Fig. 14–6). Meningocele and meningomyelocele are two types of spina bifida cystica. A *meningocele* (*meningo*, "membrane," and *cele*, "tumor") contains portions of the membranes and CSF. The size varies from that of a walnut to that of a newborn's head.

More serious is a protrusion of the membranes and spinal cord through this opening, or a *meningomyelocele.* Although it resembles a meningocele, there may be associated paralysis of the legs and poor control of bowel and bladder functions (Fig. 14–7). Hydrocephalus is common. Prenatal detection is possible by ultrasonography and by testing for increased alpha$_1$-fetoprotein (AFP) in the amniotic fluid of the mother.

Prevention. The specific cause of meningomyelocele is unknown but a genetic predisposition may exist. The use of drugs during early pregnancy such as Valproic acid may contribute to the development of a neural tube defect. The American Academy of Pediatrics recommends that all women of childbearing age take a daily multivitamin that contains 0.4 mg of folic acid and that they continue the intake of folic acid until the 12th week of pregnancy when the basic neural tube development is completed. Studies have shown that the intake of folic acid before conception dramatically decreases the occurrence of neural tube defects such as spina bifida.

Treatment. The treatment for spina bifida is surgical closure. The prognosis for patients with these conditions depends on the extent of involvement. In a meningocele patient with no weakness of the legs or sphincter involvement, surgical correction is performed with excellent results. Surgery is also indicated in a meningomyelocele patient for cosmetic purposes and to help to prevent infection. A multidisciplinary approach is necessary because depending on the extent of the defect the child may have difficulties associated with hydrocephalus, orthopedic problems, and problems relating to urinary function.

Habilitation is necessary after the operation because the legs remain paralyzed and the patient is incontinent of urine and feces. Habilitation, rather than rehabilitation, is the term used to describe this treatment because the patient is handicapped from birth and therefore is learning, not relearning. The aim of habilitation is to minimize the child's dis-

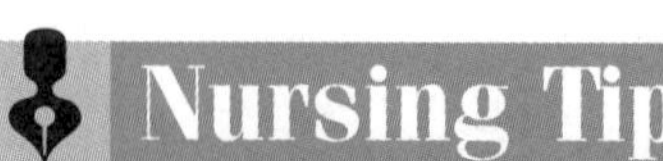

The intake of a daily multivitamin containing 0.4 mg of folic acid before conception can reduce the risk of neural tube defects such as spina bifida.

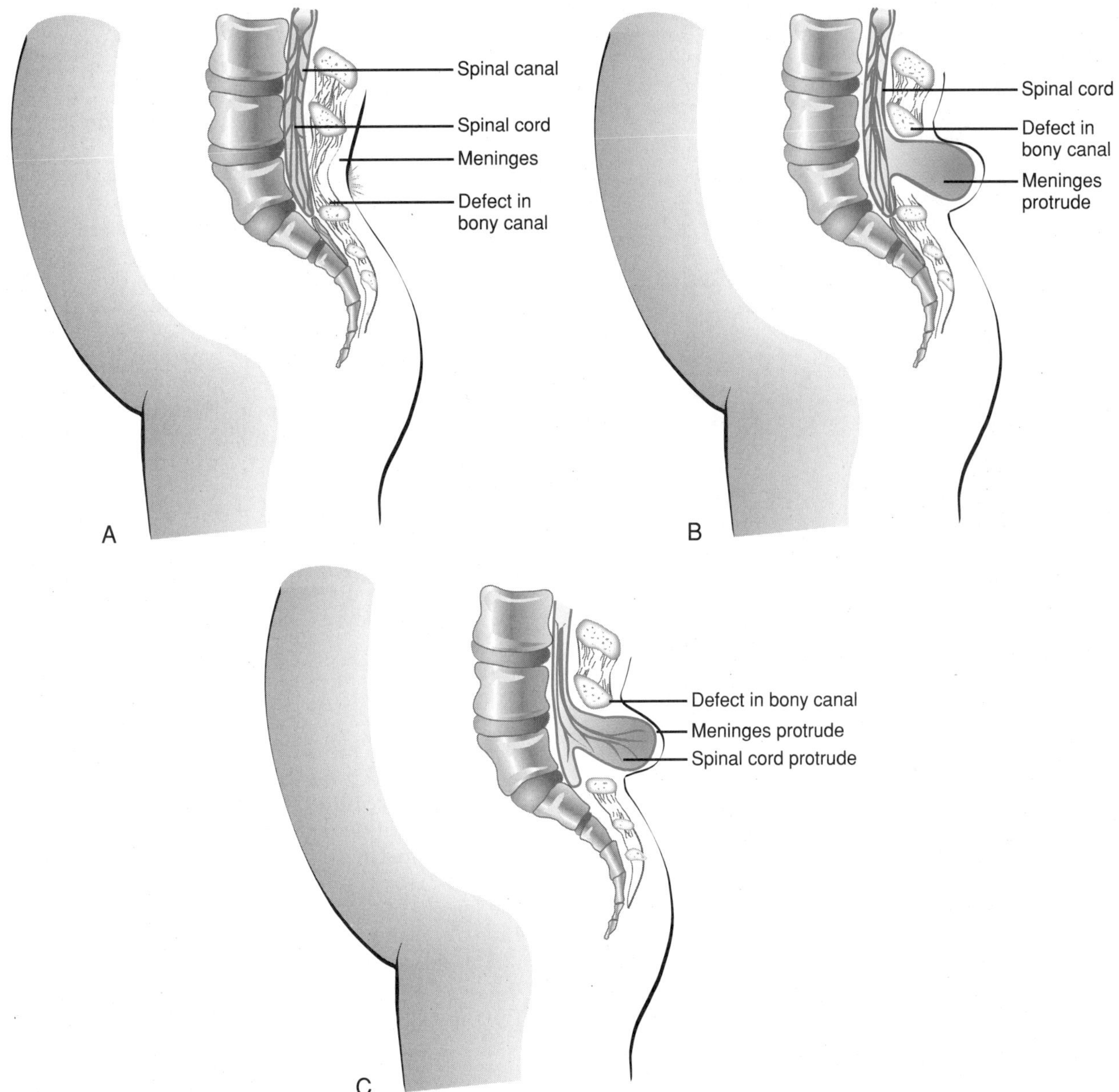

Figure 14–5. • Types of spina bifida. **A,** *Spina bifida occulta.* There is a defect in the bony canal. The meninges and spinal cord are normal. **B,** *Spina bifida cystica* **meningocele.** There is a defect in the bony canal. The meninges protrude through the defect. The spinal cord is normal. **C,** *Spina bifida cystica* **meningomyelocele.** There is a defect in the bony canal. The meninges protrude and the spinal cord protrudes through the defect.

ability and put to constructive use the unaffected parts of the body. Every effort is made to help the child to develop a healthy personality so that a happy and useful life may be experienced. Eventually, the child can be taught to use a wheelchair and possibly to walk with braces and crutches. The implantation of an artificial urinary sphincter in early childhood can help some children to become continent and prevent the complications associated with constant urinary dribble. Medications are available to increase bladder storage, such as Ditropan (oxybutynin chloride). Children can also be "bowel trained" with the use of suppositories that promote timed bowel movements and avoid the social rejection that can be caused by bowel incontinence.

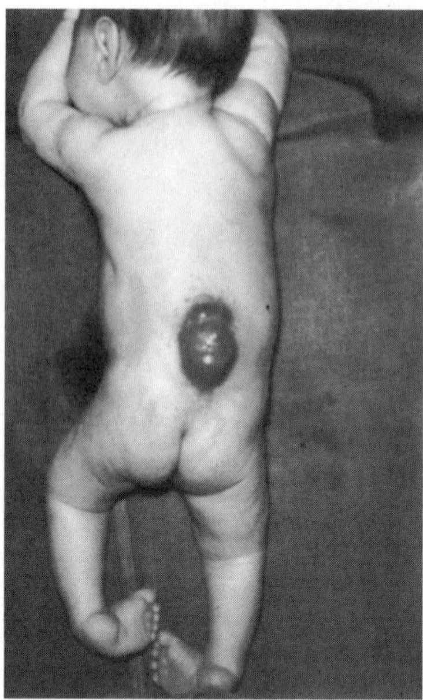

Figure 14–6. • Newborn with spina bifida and bilateral clubfoot. (From Moore, K. L., & Persaud, T. V. N. [1993]. *The developing human: Clinically oriented embryology* [5th ed., p. 377]. Philadelphia: Saunders.)

Nursing Care. The main objectives of the nursing care include prevention of infection of or injury to the sac; correct position to prevent pressure on the sac and deformities; good skin care, particularly if the baby is incontinent of urine and feces; adequate nutrition; tender, loving care; accurate observations and charting; education of the parents; continued medical supervision; and habilitation.

- Immediate care of the sac is essentially the same regardless of whether the cord is involved. On delivery the newborn is placed in an incubator. Moist, sterile dressings of saline or an antibiotic solution may be ordered to prevent drying of the sac. Some method of protecting the mass is necessary if surgery is to be delayed. Protection from injury and maintenance of a sterile environment for the open lesion is essential.
- Pertinent nursing observations must be made:
  - The newborn is assessed.
  - The size and area of the sac are checked for any tears or leakage.
  - The extremities are observed for deformities and movement. There may be spasticity or paralysis of the limbs, or they may be normal, depending on the type and location of the cyst.
  - The head is measured to determine the possibility of associated hydrocephalus.
  - Fontanels are observed to provide baseline data.
  - The lack of anal sphincter control and dribbling of urine are significant in the differential diagnosis (see Fig. 14–7). In general, the higher the defect is on the spine, the greater the neurologic deficit.

Data are recorded along with the routine observations made for every newborn.

- Positioning of the infant is of importance. The goal is to avoid pressure on the sac and to prevent postural deformities. When positioning infants with multiple deformities, the nurse must try to guard against aggravating existing problems. The infant is usually placed prone with a pad between the legs to maintain abduction and to counteract hip subluxation. A small roll is placed under the ankles to maintain foot position. Some infants may be supported in a side-lying posture to provide periods of relief. The disadvantage of

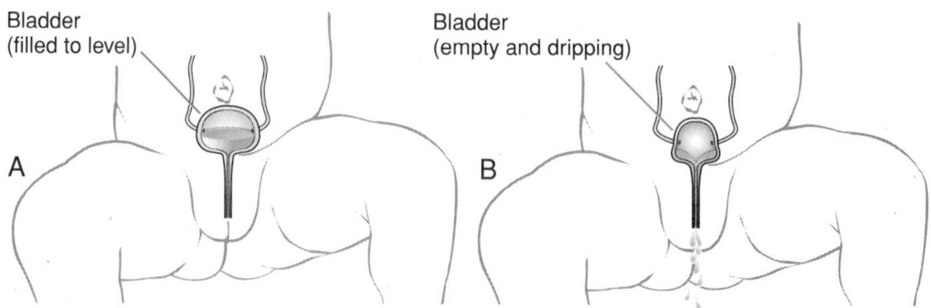

Figure 14–7. • Incontinence in the newborn. **A,** Normally, when the bladder fills to a certain level, a sensor stimulates contraction of the bladder and expulsion of a volume of urine into the diaper occurs. A normal newborn has about 6 wet diapers a day. **B,** A newborn is considered *incontinent* when the sensor does not function and the bladder does not fill to its capacity before emptying. There is a constant dribble of urine into the diaper. The diaper is *always* wet.

this position is that it reduces movement of the arms and flexes the hips. The physical therapy staff may provide a helpful consultation. Fortunately, surgery is generally done early.

- Postoperative nursing care involves neurologic assessment and prevention of infection. The status of the fontanels and any signs of increased ICP, such as irritability or vomiting, are significant. Sometimes a shunt is performed shortly after closure of the spine, if hydrocephalus is present. Complications that can be life-threatening include meningitis, pneumonia, and urinary tract infection.
- Urologic monitoring is essential, since many of these infants have urinary incontinence (Fig. 14–7). Medication to prevent urinary tract infections is routinely given. In infants, the Credé method of bladder emptying may be employed. Older children may be taught intermittent, clean self-catheterization. This technique can be performed by parents and learned by children.
- Skin care is a challenge. Diapering is generally contraindicated. Constant dribbling of feces and urine irritates the perineal area and can infect the sac or the incision. Meticulous cleanliness is necessary. Bedding must be dry and wrinkle-free. Frequent cleansing, application of a prescribed ointment or lotion, and light massage help to maintain skin integrity. If range-of-motion exercises are ordered they are performed gently.
- Feeding of the patient is facilitated by early closure of the defect. In delayed cases, gavage may be used. These patients need cuddling and sensory stimulation. An infant that cannot be held can be soothed by touch. The nurse talks to the baby and, when possible, provides face-to-face (en-face) communication. Mobiles are placed appropriately. Periodically moving the incubator or crib provides diversity of view. Soft music is also soothing.
- Many infants with spina bifida develop a latex allergy. A latex-free environment should be initiated whenever possible. Parents should be educated that latex products such as balloons, kooshballs, tennis balls, and adhesive strips can cause allergic reactions that may include rashes and wheezing. In some cases, antihistamines and steroids may be prescribed before and after surgery or contact with latex gloves that may be used for specific procedures.
- Special consideration must be given to the establishment of parent–infant relationships. This problem is complicated if the infant is transferred to a large medical center. Understanding and support are given to the parents, who may be overwhelmed. It is not unusual for them to be repulsed by the cyst. Most experience a sense of loss for what was to have been their "perfect baby." Steps of the grieving process may be recognized by the astute nurse. If the malformation is complex and incompatible with life, a decision must be made about the feasibility of surgical intervention. This is a crisis situation for the most mature of people and an area in which guidelines are not clearly defined. Information and education about this disorder can be obtained from the Spina Bifida Association of America.

Gastrointestinal System

Cleft Lip (Harelip)

Description. A *cleft lip* is characterized by a fissure or opening in the upper lip (Fig. 14–8). It is a result of the failure of the maxillary and median nasal processes to unite during embryonic development, usually between the 7th and 8th week of gestation. In many cases, it seems to be caused by hereditary predisposition but occasionally can be caused by environmental influences during the stage of oral development. This disorder appears more frequently in boys than in girls and may occur on one or both sides of the lip. The extent of the defect may vary from slight to severe. Sometimes it is accompanied by a *cleft palate,* a fissure in the midline of the roof of the mouth. Cleft lip and palate are common congenital anomalies, occurring

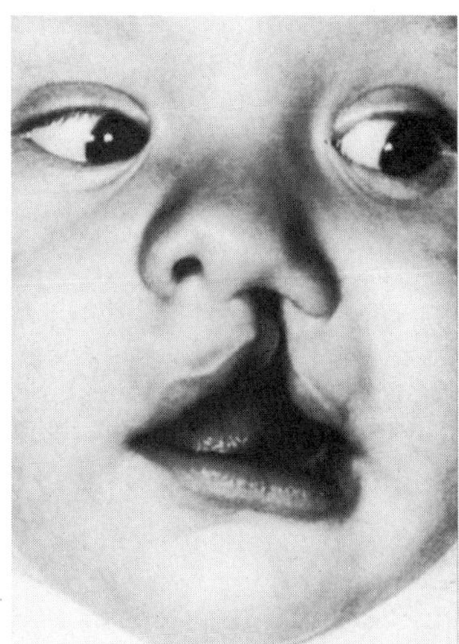

Figure 14–8. • Cleft lip. (From Behrman, R. E., & Kliegman, R. M. [1996]. *Nelson textbook of pediatrics* [15th ed.]. Philadelphia: Saunders.)

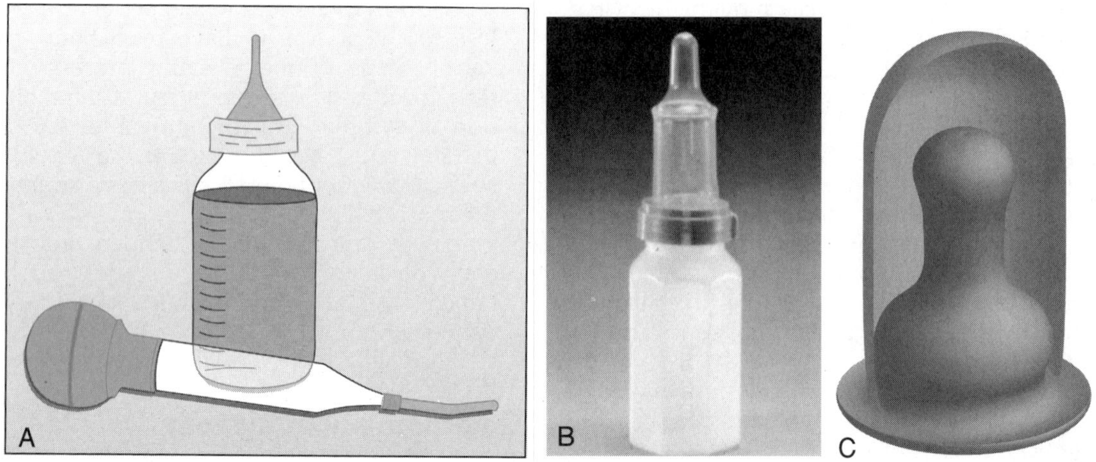

Figure 14–9. • Equipment to feed the infant with a cleft lip or palate. **A,** Gravity feeder, cleft-lip nipple. **B,** shows the Haberman feeder. (B, Courtesy of Medela, Inc., McHenry, IL.) **C,** Cleft palate obturator. The rubber phalange over the top of the nipple adheres to the upper palate over the deformity, allowing the infant to suck on the nipple.

in about 1 in 600 to 1250 births. Transculturally, they occur more often in Asian Americans and Native Americans and less commonly in African Americans (Behrman et al., 1996).

Treatment and Nursing Care. The initial treatment for cleft lip is surgical repair known as *cheiloplasty.* The cleft lip is repaired by 2 months of age when weight gain is established and the infant is free of infection. Surgery not only improves the infant's sucking but also greatly improves appearance. Indirectly, this influences bonding and the amount of affection the baby receives, because some refrain from cuddling a baby who is obviously disfigured.

Before surgery, a complete physical examination is done and routine blood tests are ordered. Photographs may also be taken. Any signs of oral respiratory or systemic infection are reported to the nurse manager. The doctor may order elbow restraints to prevent the patient from scratching the lip and to acquaint the baby with them because they are necessary postoperatively. An Asepto syringe with a rubber tip, a Haberman feeder, or a medicine dropper are used to feed the baby before and after surgery, since sucking motions must be avoided to decrease tension on the suture line (Fig. 14–9).

Postoperative Nursing Care. Postoperative nursing goals for this patient include:

- Preventing the baby from sucking and crying, which could cause tension on the suture line.
- Careful positioning (never on the abdomen) to avoid injury to the operative site.
- Prevention of infection and scarring by gentle cleansing of the suture line to prevent crusts from forming.
- Prevention of injury to the operative site by using elbow restraints. A Logan bow, which is a device used to immobilize the upper lip may be applied for a short time postoperatively.
- Providing for the infant's emotional needs by cuddling and other forms of affection. This is of particular importance because the baby cannot obtain the usual satisfactions from sucking.
- Providing appropriate pain relief and sedation that may be required for active infants.

Feeding. The infant receives feedings by dropper until the wound is completely healed (1–2 weeks). The infant is usually fed as soon as clear liquids are tolerated postoperatively. Care should be taken to avoid touching the suture line when inserting the medicine dropper or breck feeder. Sucking is avoided until the suture line is healed. Placing a small amount of formula into the infant's mouth and allowing time for swallowing will prevent aspiration. Offering small amounts of sterile water will cleanse the mouth following feeding. Formula or drainage is gently cleaned from the suture line with saline and an ointment may be applied to the skin as prescribed. Holding the infant during feedings, burping frequently and placing the infant in an infant seat after feeding or on the right side propped with a rolled blanket will aid in a positive outcome for this infant. The mother who has fed her baby preoperatively and has been allowed to assist with feedings during hospitalization will feel more confident after discharge. The immediate improvement as a result of surgery is encouraging to the parents, particularly if the child must have further surgery for cleft palate repair.

Cleft Palate

Description. A cleft palate is a failure of the hard palate to fuse at the midline during the 7th to 12th week of gestation. The separation forms a passageway between the nasopharynx and the nose, which not only complicates feeding but also easily leads to infections of the respiratory tract and middle ear. It is generally responsible for the speech difficulties that occur in later life. The cleft may not be readily apparent at birth and is the reason careful examination of the oral cavity and upper palate at birth is essential. Feeding is a problem because the cleft prevents negative pressure from being formed within the mouth that is necessary for successful sucking.

Treatment. The best time for surgery is a subject of controversy, although some surgeons prefer to operate before 18 months of age if at all possible, so that speech patterns are minimally affected. To facilitate communication, a dental speech appliance may be used if surgery has been deferred or has been contraindicated because of extensive malformation. This appliance must be changed periodically as the child grows.

Treatment of the child with a cleft lip and palate requires multidisciplinary teamwork with a psychologist, speech therapist, pediatric dentist, orthodontist, social worker, and pediatrician. The Public Health nurse should be responsible for coordinating parental counseling and referral as needed. Emotional problems that sometimes occur with this condition require more extensive attention than does the repair itself. A child born with a facial deformity encounters many problems. Feedings are difficult and are not relaxed in the initial period. As the child grows, irregular tooth eruptions, drooling, delayed speech, and the need for intermittent hospitalization and frequent clinic appointments can be frustrating. It is difficult not to be attractive when society places such emphasis on good looks.

Psychosocial Adjustment of the Family. A mother's first reaction to a disfigured newborn is one of shock, hurt, disappointment and guilt. Some parents regard the deformity as a result of their inadequacies. They may desire to hide the child from relatives and friends. The developing child senses the parents' feelings and acquires either a positive or a negative self-image. The patient and family need understanding, a concrete basis for hope, and practical advice.

Follow-Up Care, Home Care. In large cities, special cleft palate clinics are available in which several specialists can work together in convenient consultation. The parents are instructed about the resources available in the state in which they live. The American Cleft Palate Association, the Cleft Palate Foundation, the March of Dimes Birth Defect Foundation, and state programs for children with special needs are examples of community referrals that should be offered to parents.

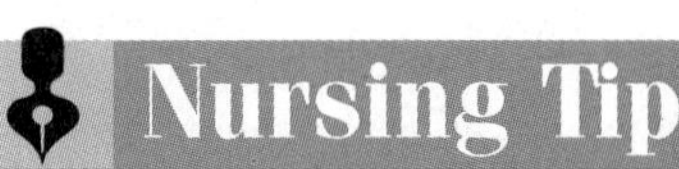

Suctioning the mouth should be avoided in infants who have a cleft palate repair.

Postoperative Treatment and Nursing Care

Nutrition. Fluids are taken by a cup, although a gravity feeder may be desirable in some cases. The method varies with the plastic surgeon. The diet is progressive. At first it consists of clear fluids and then full fluids. By the time of discharge, a soft diet can generally be taken. Hot foods and liquids are avoided to prevent injury to the operative site. The patient must not suck on a straw. When feeding with a spoon, place only its side into the mouth. The spoon must not touch the roof of the mouth. The nurse teaches parents that objects such as the child's thumb, tongue blades, toast, cookies, forks, and pacifiers are to be kept out of the mouth. The child is prevented from placing fingers or objects in the mouth by the use of elbow restraints. The diet is advanced only on consultation with the physician.

Oral Hygiene. The mouth is kept clean at all times. Feedings are followed by a little water. The doctor may prescribe a mild antiseptic mouthwash.

Restraints. Elbow restraints are generally sufficient. They are removed one at a time and periodically, to prevent constriction of circulation and to allow normal movement. In the home, they may be made of rolled cardboard tied with string.

Speech. It is helpful to speak slowly and distinctly to the child. The child is encouraged to pronounce words correctly. Children who have had extensive repairs or have associated deafness need the help of a speech therapist. The speech therapist evaluates the child and assists the parents in specific activities that will facilitate speech development.

Diversion. Crying is to be avoided as much as possible. Play should be quiet, particularly in the immediate postoperative period. The nurse reads, draws, or colors with the child.

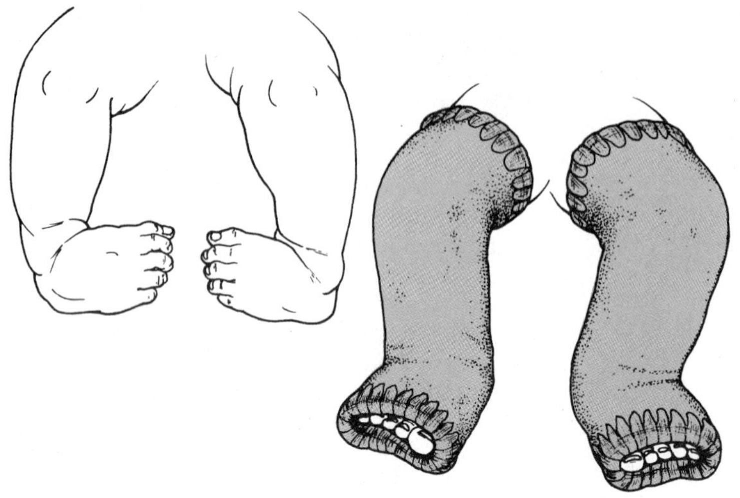

Figure 14–10. • Bilateral talipes equinovarus (clubfoot) before and after application of plaster casts. Adhesive "petals" have been placed around the ends of the casts to prevent plaster from irritating the skin.

Complications. Earaches and dental decay may accompany this condition. Parents are instructed to take the child to the doctor at the first signs of earache. Regular visits to the dentist are scheduled. Throughout the long term care, a stable goal in the care of this infant is to promote optimum growth and development and to establish a positive self-esteem.

Musculoskeletal System

Clubfoot

Description. Clubfoot, one of the most common deformities of the skeletal system, is a congenital anomaly characterized by a foot that has been twisted inward or outward. The incidence is about 1 in 1000 live births. Many mild forms are due to improper position in the uterus, and these clear up with little or no treatment when the extremity is allowed unrestricted activity. In contrast, true clubfoot does not respond to simple exercise. Several types are recognized. Talipes (*talus,* "heel," and *pes,* "foot") equinovarus (*equinus,* "extension," and *varus,* "bent inward") is seen in 95% of patients. The feet are turned inward, and the child walks on the toes and the outer borders of the feet. It generally involves both feet. Boys are affected twice as often as girls.

Treatment and Nursing Care. The treatment of clubfoot is started as early as possible, otherwise the bones and muscles continue to develop abnormally. During infancy, conservative treatment, consisting of manipulation and casting to hold the foot in the right position, is carried out (Fig. 14–10). A Denis Browne splint may also be used, usually for children under 1 year of age. It is made of two footplates attached to a crossbar. When it is fitted to the shoes, the feet may be put in various positions of angulation by sets of screws. When the infant kicks, the feet are automatically forced into the correct position. Passive stretching exercises may also be recommended. If these methods are not effective, surgery is indicated. The infant with a clubfoot is under medical supervision for a long time. Parents need to be instructed in developmental behaviors of the infant as well as the clinical aspects of care. Ongoing support is paramount.

Cast Care. Casts are made of plaster or synthetic materials such as fiberglass or polyurethane. The plaster cast consists of crinoline that has powdered plaster in its meshwork. It is placed in warm water before being applied over cotton wadding or a stockinette. The wet plaster of Paris hardens as it dries. This type of cast dries from the inside out and takes 24 to 48 hours to dry.

If the patient returns to the unit before the cast is dry, the cast must be left uncovered and protected from pressures that could cause a depression in it. If the doctor orders that the leg and foot be elevated on pillows to prevent swelling, the nurse who assists must use the palms of the hands, not the fingers, to hold the cast. Indentations made in a wet

Nursing Tip

In the long-term care of orthopedic patients, educating the parents about orthopedic devices, cast care, exercise, hygiene, and treatment goals is necessary. The nurse explains the importance of frequent clinic visits, reinforces doctors' information, and clarifies directions as necessary.

cast by fingers can press on the underlying skin and cause damage. This precaution is also explained to parents. Lighter synthetic casts dry in less than 30 minutes; however, they are less strong and more expensive.

The toes are left exposed for observation. The nurse checks them for capillary refill and signs of poor circulation, pallor, cyanosis, swelling, coldness, numbness, pain, or burning. If circulation is impaired the doctor may split the cast in order to relieve the pressure, or the cast may need to be removed and reapplied. The nurse also reports irritation of the skin around the edges of the cast and lack of movement of the toes. Adhesive petals may be placed around the edges of the cast to prevent skin irritation.

It is difficult to keep a child's cast free of food particles, which cause skin irritation. Careful supervision during mealtime is necessary in order to prevent the child from placing bits of food under the edges of the cast. Powder and oil are not used following the bath because they may cause irritation.

The cast may need to remain in place for weeks or months. Since the infant grows rapidly, the parent should be taught how to check for impairment of circulation that could be caused by a tight cast. The cast may need to be changed periodically.

If surgery on tendons and bones has been performed the nurse also observes the cast for evidence of bleeding. If a discolored area appears on the cast, it is circled and the time is recorded. Further bleeding can then be estimated If bleeding is noted, the patient's vital signs are also checked and compared with preoperative readings. After surgery, the cast is changed about every 3 weeks to bring the foot gradually into position. When the cast is removed for the final time, exercise and special shoes may be indicated.

Emotional Support. The nurse is an important figure in the care of the long-term patient with clubfoot. Nurses review the normal growth and development of children in the patient's age range to anticipate problems and to educate caretakers in parenting.

Children in a cast may be slow in developing certain motor abilities, and many regress to more babyish behavior. This is particularly true of bowel and bladder control. The nurse does not shame a child if an "accident" occurs. The parents can give much helpful information about their child. The nurse must be a good listener. Parents are encouraged to participate in the care of their child because it brings them satisfaction and a sense of control and reassures the child. Parents play a key role in the long-term care of the infant. Education concerning the therapy and referral for follow-up care is an important nursing responsibility. The financial burdens of hospitalization, surgery, special shoes, and continued medical supervision pose a serious problem. If the nurse suspects that the parents need financial help, a social-service referral is made.

Developmental Hip Dysplasia

Description. Developmental hip dysplasia, formerly known as congenital hip dysplasia, is a common orthopedic deformity. The incidence is about 1 in 1000 births. The term *hip dysplasia* is a broad description applied to various degrees of deformity: subluxation or dislocation, either partial or complete. The head of the femur is partly or completely displaced from a shallow hip socket (acetabulum). Hereditary and environmental factors appear to be causal factors. Hip malformation, joint laxity, breech position, and maternal hormones may all contribute. Developmental hip dysplasia is seven times more common in girls than in boys. Newborn infants seldom have complete dislocation. However, the baby beginning to walk exerts pressure on the hip, which can cause complete dislocation. Therefore, early detection and treatment are of particular importance.

In cultures where the newborn is wrapped snugly with the hips in adduction and extension there is a high risk for developmental hip dysplasia. In cultures where the infant is carried straddled on the mother's waist with the infant's hips flexed and widely abducted there is a low risk for developmental hip dysplasia.

Manifestations. A dislocation of the hip is commonly discovered at the periodic health examination of the baby during the 1st or 2nd month of life. One of the most reliable signs is a limited abduction of the leg on the affected side. When the infant is placed on the back with knees and hips flexed, the doctor can press the thigh of the normal hip backward until it almost touches the examining table. This can be accomplished only partially on the affected side. The knee on the side of the dislocation is lower, and the skin folds of the thigh are deeper and often asymmetric (Fig. 14–11). When the infant is prone, one buttock appears higher than the other.

Barlow's test is a test performed by a doctor to detect a dislocation of the hip. The doctor adducts and extends hips while stabilizing the pelvis and may "feel" the dislocation occur as the femur leaves the acetabulum.

In some infants with developmental dislocation of the hip, the doctor can actually feel and hear the femoral head slip back into the acetabulum under

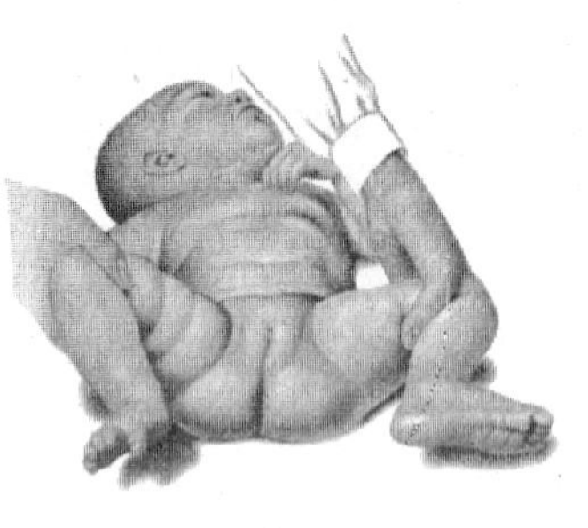

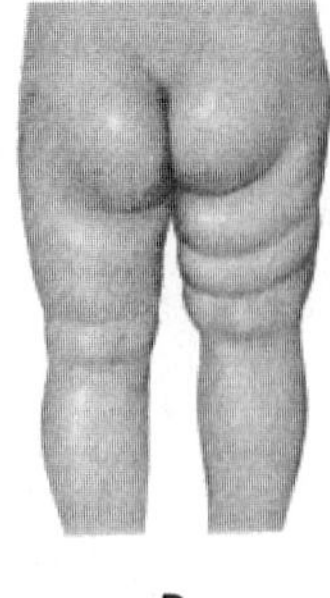

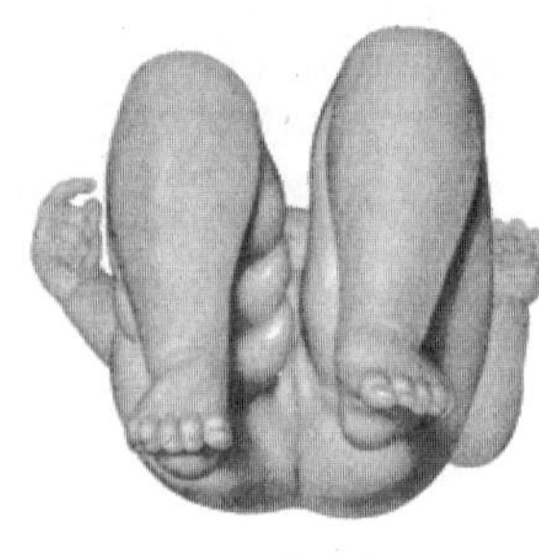

Figure 14–11. • Early signs of dislocation of right hip. **A,** Limitation of abduction. **B,** Asymmetry of skin folds. **C,** Shortening of femur. (From Ross Laboratories. [1986]. *Clinical education aid no. 15.* Columbus, OH: Author. Reproduced with permission of Ross Laboratories.)

gentle pressure. This is called *Ortolani's sign* or Ortolani's click and is also considered diagnostic of the disorder. The child who is walking and has had no treatment displays a characteristic limp. Bilateral (*bi,* "two," and *latus,* "side") dislocation may occur; however, unilateral (*uni,* "one," and *latus,* "side") dislocation is more common. X-ray studies confirm the diagnosis.

Treatment. Treatment begins immediately on detection of the dislocation. The hips are maintained in constant flexion and abduction for 4 to 8 weeks to keep the head of the femur within the hip socket. This constant pressure enlarges and deepens the acetabulum; thus, it corrects the dislocation.

There is some controversy over the exact course of treatment; however, some device to maintain abduction of the hips is used. A triple thick diaper may be used in the newborn to maintain a "froglike" abduction of the legs, and a *Pavlick harness* may be required for infants 1 to 6 months of age (Fig. 14–12). If the dislocation is severe or is not detected until the child begins to walk, it may be necessary to use traction. This pulls the head of the femur down to the correct position opposite the acetabulum and helps to overcome muscle spasm. Casting in a froglike position is then done. This type of cast, known as a *body spica cast,* is shown in Figure 14–13.

The length of time spent in a cast varies according to the patient's progress and growth and the condition of the cast; however, it is usually 5 to 9 months. During this time, the cast may be changed about every 6 weeks. In infants over 18 months of age, surgery may be required. If so, open reduction of the dislocation or repair of the shelf of the hip bone are done. After surgery, a cast is applied to keep the femur in the correct position.

Nursing Care. The nursery nurse carefully observes each infant during the morning bath to detect signs of a hip dysplasia.

- When the baby is prone, the nurse observes the buttocks for variation in size.
- The legs of the infant should be equal in length.
- The infant should be kicking both legs, not just one leg.
- The depth of the skin folds of the baby's upper thighs should be symmetrical.
- In the well-baby clinic, the nurse notes the posture and gait of older children and records observations.

Infants who progress well with the Pavlik harness (Fig. 14–12) or Frejka splint, or a similar brace, remain at home. The mother and baby visit the doctor regularly. The parents need assurance that the baby may be held and may sit in a chair. They should be encouraged to ask questions of the clinic nurse and doctor.

The child who is admitted to the hospital with a diagnosis of a developmental hip dysplasia is given as much personal attention as possible. The first admission sets the pattern for future hospitalization; therefore, the child must make a satisfactory adjustment. The nurse becomes familiar with the child's habit and care sheet. Every effort is made to provide a homelike environment for children who are hospitalized for many weeks.

The Spica Cast. The body spica cast encircles the waist and extends to the ankles or toes. Neurovascular assessment, discussed on page 625, should be reviewed at this point. Nursing Care Plan 14–1 gives selected nursing diagnoses and interventions for the patient with a spica cast.

Firm, plastic-covered pillows are required. These are placed beneath the curvatures of the cast for support. Older children may benefit from an overhead bar and trapeze. The room should be adequately ventilated. A fracture pan should be available at the bedside.

The head of the patient's bed is slightly elevated so that urine or feces drain away from the body of the cast. One should not elevate the head or shoulders of a child in a body cast by means of pillows, as this thrusts the patient's chest against the cast and causes discomfort or respiratory difficulty. The child who is not toilet-trained may be placed on a Bradford frame to facilitate nursing care. Frequent change of position is important; bed patients need to be turned often. Infants may be held in the nurse's lap after the cast has dried. A ride on a stretcher to the playroom or around the hospital provides changes of position and scenery.

Technique for Turning the Child in a Body Cast

Two people, one on each side of the bed, are needed to turn a child in a body cast.

- Move the child to the edge of the bed as far as possible, so that the nurse who receives the child is farther away from him or her.
- The nurse nearer to the child places one hand under the head and back and one hand under the leg part of the cast and turns the child to the midway point on the side.
- The nurse farther away then accepts the support of the child and cast as the child is turned completely on to the abdomen.

The supporting bar between the legs should not be used as a lever when turning the child. All body curvatures are supported with pillows or sheet rolls. Whenever possible, the older child should be on the abdomen during mealtime to facilitate swallowing and self-feeding. When placing a child in a body cast on a fracture pan, support the upper back and legs with pillows so that body alignment is maintained.

Itching is a problem for the patient in a body cast. If at all possible, before applying the cast, a strip of gauze is placed beneath the cast, extending through the opened area required for toilet needs. It is

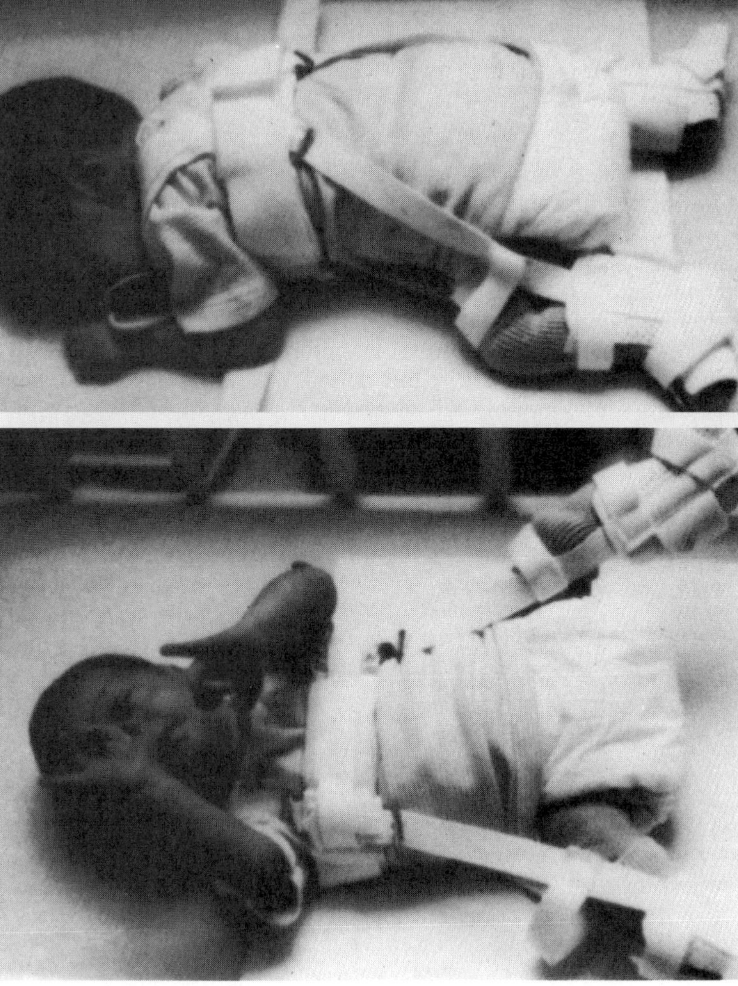

Figure 14–12. • The Pavlik harness maintains abduction of the hips. (From Behrman R. E., & Kliegman, R. [1992]. *Nelson textbook of pediatrics* [14th ed.]. Philadelphia: Saunders.)

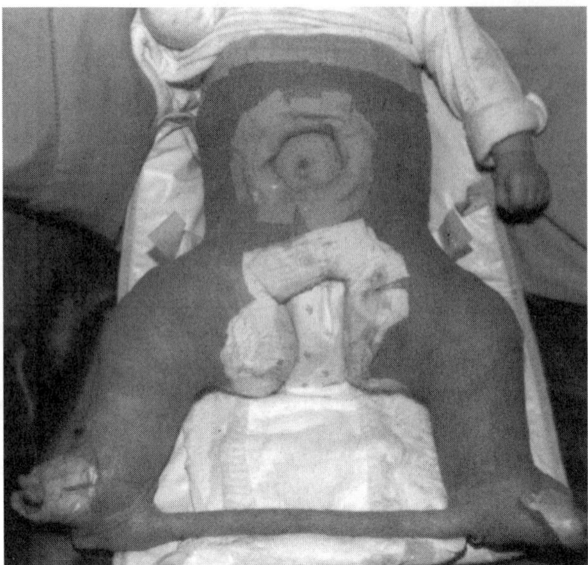

Figure 14–13. • A spica body cast. This cast maintains the legs in a froglike position and is used to treat congenital dislocations of the hip. Note that the infant is able to move her toes freely. The opening in the center allows for auscultation of bowel sounds.

gently moved back and forth to relieve itching. When the strip becomes soiled, a clean one is tied to one end of the soiled gauze and pulled through the cast; this soiled portion is removed. Other methods that might cause injury to the skin beneath the cast are discouraged because any break in the skin under a cast is difficult to heal.

The child with this long-term disability needs help in meeting everyday needs. This child is growing and developing rapidly. Therefore, frequent adjustments in home and clinic care are necessary. Dressing and clothing are a problem. The child cannot fit into regular furniture and much of the play equipment enjoyed by other children. Transportation is difficult. A special wagon built up with pillows may be used during hospitalization. A referral for home health care should be made upon discharge.

METABOLIC DEFECTS

The infant with an inborn error of metabolism has a genetic defect that is not apparent before birth. As the infant adjusts to the birth process and begins to ingest nourishment, symptoms can rapidly emerge that quickly become life- threatening. Symptoms such as lethargy, poor feeding, hypotonia, a unique odor to the body or urine, tachypnea and vomiting must be reported by the nurse in the newborn nursery to avoid long-term or life-threatening sequellae. The nurse must also be prepared to offer psychological support and help parents to deal with the impact of having an infant with a genetic problem.

Phenylketonuria

Description. Classic phenylketonuria (PKU) is a genetic disorder caused by the faulty metabolism of phenylalanine, an amino acid essential to life and found in all protein foods. The hepatic enzyme phenylalanine hydrolase, normally needed to convert phenylalanine into tyrosine, is missing. When the baby is fed milk, phenylalanine begins to accumulate in the blood. It can rise to as high as 20 times the normal amount. Its by-product, phenylpyruvic acid, appears in the urine within the first weeks of life. This inborn error of metabolism, which is transmitted by an autosomal recessive gene, is termed *classic PKU* and is associated with blood phenylalanine levels above 20 mg/dl. It results in severe retardation that is evidenced in infancy. Early detection and treatment are paramount. By the time the urine test is positive, brain damage has already occurred. The baby appears normal at birth but begins to show delayed development at about 4 to 6 months of age. The child may show evidence of failure to thrive, have eczema or other skin conditions, have a peculiar musty odor, or have personality disorders. About one-third of the children have seizures. PKU occurs mainly in children who are blond and blue-eyed; these features are due to a lack of tyrosine, a necessary component of the pigment melanin. Less severe forms of the disorder are now recognized. They are designated as "atypical PKU" and "mild hyperphenylalaninemia."

Diagnosis. The *Guthrie blood test* is widely used and is currently considered the most reliable test. Blood is obtained from a simple heel prick. A few drops of capillary blood are placed on a filter paper and mailed to the laboratory for screening. It is recommended that the blood be obtained after 48 to 72 hours of life, preferably after ingestion of proteins, to reduce the possibility of false-negative results. Many states require that the test be done on all newborns before they leave the nursery, but because of early discharge the test may be repeated within 3 weeks. The infant can be tested at home by a public health nurse or at the clinic or physician's office. Confirmation of the diagnosis requires quantitative elevations of phenylalanine compound in both blood and urine (Behrman et al., 1996). Screening programs for pregnant women have also been advocated to detect elevated phenylalanine levels that could have an effect on the newborn.

NURSING CARE PLAN 14-1

Selected Nursing Diagnoses for the Infant/Child with a Spica Cast

Nursing Diagnosis: High risk for altered tissue perfusion due to cast constriction

Goals	Nursing Interventions	Rationale
Tissues and circulation appear adequate as evidenced by pink, warm skin, good capillary refill, and lack of numbness or swelling Parents understand signs of inadequate circulation and explain the importance of seeking immediate assistance if these signs appear	1. Observe exposed extremities and skin distal to the cast every 30 min for the first few hours of a new cast and every 1 to 4 hr thereafter; watch for signs of pallor, cyanosis, swelling, coldness, numbness, pain, or burning	1. Circulation can be impaired, leading to ischemia. Peripheral nerves in contrast to muscles do not degenerate with disuse, but loss of *innervation* can take place if nerves are damaged by pressure or if the blood supply is disrupted
	2. Circle any drainage on cast with date and time; monitor and record findings	2. An increase in size of circle indicates further bleeding or possibly a draining infection
	3. Observe nonverbal communication for signs of pain; ask older child if pain is experienced	3. Unrelieved pain, especially after a few days, may indicate *compartment syndrome;* compartment syndrome appears in a group of muscles and fascia where an increase in pressure within this closed space may disrupt circulation within the space
	4. Educate parents and patient, if old enough, in all of above	4. Education reduces stress of parents and patient
	5. Written instructions are provided	5. Written instructions provide reinforcement and help to ensure the success of other interventions

Nursing Diagnosis: High risk for injury related to awkwardness and weight of cast

Goals	Nursing Interventions	Rationale
Patient will remain safe and as independent as possible	1. Restrain patient adequately when on Bradford frame with vests and belts	1. These restraints prevent falls; active children may turn without assistance or move suddenly
	2. Inform older child when turning as to how and when you are going to proceed (e.g., "ready, set, go")	2. Involving child in procedure as age-appropriate gives patient a sense of control; procedure will go more smoothly
	3. Leave articles and toys within reach	3. Child will not need to strain or move awkwardly to reach articles; patient will feel greater mastery if articles can be obtained independently
	4. Some car seats are adapted to accommodate a small child in a spica cast	4. These children need protection in a car

Treatment and Nursing Care. Treatment consists of close dietary management and frequent evaluation of blood phenylalanine levels. Because phenylalanine is found in all natural protein foods, a synthetic food providing enough protein for growth and tissue repair but little phenylalanine must be substituted. The most commonly used formulas are *Lofenalac* for infants, Phenyl-Free for children and Phenex-2 for adolescents. The goals of the diet are to provide enough essential proteins to support growth and development while maintaining phenylalanine blood levels between 2 and 10 mg/dl. A phenylalanine level below 2 mg/dl may result in growth retardation and above 10 mg/dl can result in significant brain damage.

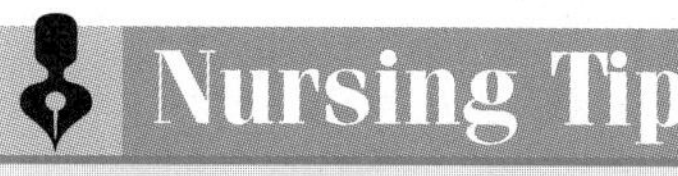

Children with PKU need to avoid the sweetener aspartame (NutraSweet) because it is converted to phenylalanine in the body.

There is a low phenylalanine content in breast milk and infants can be partially breastfed and supplemented with Lofenalac while monitoring phenylalanine blood levels. Solid foods that are low in phenylalanine are added at the same age as are solid foods for infants without PKU. Phenyl-Free is introduced between the ages of 3 and 8 years. Cookbooks and family recipes provide variety. Eventually the child learns to assume full management of the diet.

A dietician may be consulted concerning parental guidance and support in maintaining the dietary regime, especially for the school-age child and adolescent. Many foods that contain a high level of phenylalanine are clearly labeled and provide easier choices for parents at the supermarket. A single 12 oz. can of diet cola containing NutraSweet or Equal (aspartame) will not significantly raise blood levels of phenylalanine, but the intake of most meat, dairy products, and diet drinks need to be restricted. An exchange list for food selection can aid the child in participating in and monitoring his progress. Flavoring the milk substitute with a fruit-flavored powder or a chocolate such as "Quick" can increase compliance by the child.

Genetic counseling is important for the affected child for future family planning. Women of childbearing age who have PKU must be on a low phenylalanine diet before conception to avoid brain damage of the fetus during development.

Maple Syrup Urine Disease

Description. Maple syrup urine disease is caused by a defect in the metabolism of the branched-chain amino acids. It causes marked serum elevations of leucine, isoleucine, and valine. This results in acidosis, cerebral degeneration, and death within two weeks if left untreated.

Manifestations. The infant appears healthy at birth but soon develops feeding difficulties, loss of Moro reflex, hypotonia, irregular respirations, and convulsions. The urine, sweat, and cerumen (ear wax) have a characteristic sweet or maple syrup odor. This is due to ketoacidosis, a process similar to that which may occur in diabetic children, and causes a fruity odor of the breath. However, the condition does not resolve with correction of blood glucose levels. The urine contains high levels of leucine, isoleucine, and valine. Diagnosis is confirmed by a blood and urine test.

Treatment and Nursing Care. Early detection in the newborn period is extremely important. The nursery nurse should report any newborn whose urine has a sweet aroma. Initial treatment consists of removing these amino acids and their metabolites from the tissues of the body. This is accomplished by hydration and peritoneal dialysis to decrease serum levels. The patient is placed on a lifelong diet low in the amino acids leucine, isoleucine, and valine. Several formulas specifically for this disease are available. Exacerbations are most often related to the degree of abnormality of the leucine level. These exacerbations are frequently related to infection and can be life-threatening. The nurse must frequently assess the patient and instruct parents about the need to prevent infections.

Galactosemia

Description. In galactosemia the body is unable to use the carbohydrates galactose and lactose. In the healthy person the liver converts galactose to glucose. In the galactosemia patient, because an enzyme is defective or missing, there is a disturbance in a normally occurring chemical reaction. The result is an increase in the amount of galactose in the blood (galactosemia) and in the urine (galactosuria). This can cause cirrhosis of the liver, cataracts, and mental retardation if left untreated. Because galactose is present in milk sugar, early diagnosis is necessary so that a milk substitute can be used.

Manifestations. The symptoms begin abruptly and worsen gradually. Early signs of galactosemia consist of lethargy, vomiting, hypotonia, diarrhea, and failure to thrive. These commence as the newborn begins breastfeeding or ingesting formula. Jaundice may be present. Diagnosis is made by observing galactosuria, galactosemia, and evidence of decreased enzyme activity in the red blood cells. Screening tests are available.

Treatment and Nursing Care. Milk and lactose-containing products are eliminated from the diet of the patient with galactosemia. The nursing mother must discontinue breastfeeding. Lactose-free formulas and those with a soy-protein base are frequently substituted. The nurse must realize the frustration and anxiety that this diagnosis creates. Parents experience periods of feeling overwhelmed and inadequate. They can also become totally absorbed in the dietary program. When a disease is rare, it creates feelings of isolation and uncertainty. Because surveillance is ongoing, some of the emotional characteristics of the family with a child who has a chronic disease are pertinent.

CHROMOSOMAL ABNORMALITIES

Down Syndrome

Description. Down syndrome is one of the most common chromosomal abnormalities. Its incidence

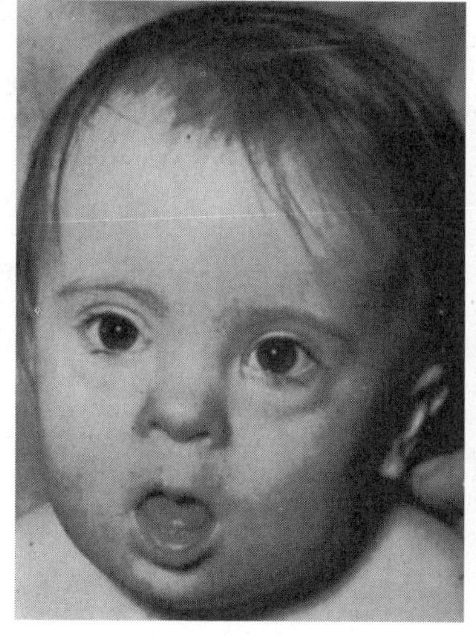

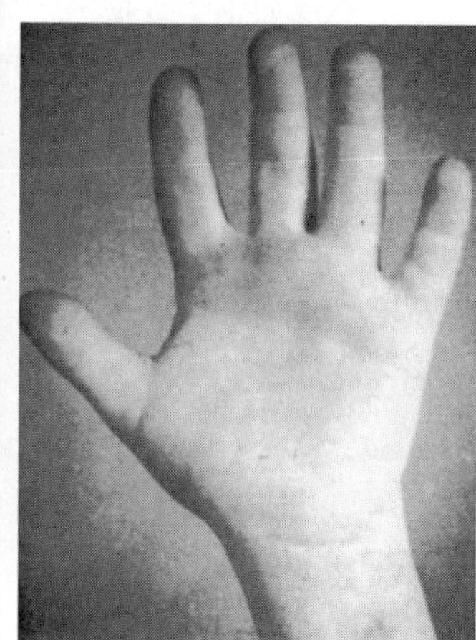

A B

Figure 14–14. • **A,** Typical facial appearance of an infant with Down syndrome. (From Smith, D. W. [1982]. *Recognizable patterns of human malformation* [3rd ed.]. Philadelphia: Saunders.) **B,** Typical broad, spade-like hand of a 12-year-old boy with Down syndrome. Note the shortness of all fingers. (From Vaughan, V. C., et al. [1979]. *Nelson textbook of pediatrics* [11th ed.]. Philadelphia: Saunders.)

is approximately 1 in 600 to 800 live births. It is higher among children of mothers 35 years or older. Paternal age is also a factor, particularly when the father is 55 or over. Sometimes, the first baby of a young mother has Down syndrome; however, subsequent children are usually born free of the defect. Children born with this birth defect have mild to severe mental retardation and generally some physical abnormalities. In the past, children with this condition were called "mongoloid" because of the Oriental ("Mongolian") appearance of their faces, but this term is now considered inappropriate.

Three phenotypes (genetic makeups) of Down syndrome are seen. These are: (1) trisomy 21; (2) mosaicism; and (3) translocation of a chromosome.

The most common type, trisomy 21 syndrome, accounts for 95% of patients. In this instance there are three number 21 chromosomes, rather than the normal two. It is a result of *nondisjunction,* the failure of a chromosome to follow the normal separation process into daughter cells. The earlier in the embryo's development this occurs, the greater is the number of cells affected.

When nondisjunction occurs late in development, both normal and abnormal cells are present in the newborn. This condition is *mosaicism.* Patients with this condition tend to be less severely affected in physical appearance and intelligence. The third condition is *translocation.* In translocation, a piece of chromosome in pair 21 breaks away and attaches itself to another chromosome.

What causes these disruptions is unknown. Current information points to multiple causes. Down syndrome has been reported to occur in all races.

Manifestations. Down syndrome can be diagnosed by the clinical manifestations, but a chromosomal analysis will confirm the specific type. The signs of Down syndrome, which are apparent at birth, are close-set and upward-slanting eyes, small head round face, flat nose, protruding tongue that interferes with sucking, and mouth breathing (Fig. 14–14A). The hands of the baby are short and thick, and the little finger is curved (Fig. 14–14B). There is a deep straight line across the palm, which is called the *Simian crease.* There is also a wide space between the first and the second toes. The undeveloped muscles and loose joints enable the child to assume unusual positions. Physical growth and development may be slower than normal (Tables 14–1 and 14–2). The child is limited intellectually. Some children have been found to have IQs in the borderline to low-average range. Congenital heart deformities are also associated with this condition.

These children are very lovable. They may be restless and somewhat more difficult to train than the normal youngster. Their resistance to infection is poor, and they are prone to respiratory and ear infections. They are also prone to speech and hearing problems. The life spans of children with Down syndrome has been increased with the widespread use of antibiotics. The incidence of acute leukemia is higher in these children than in the normal population and Alzheimer's disease is common to those who reach middle-adult life.

The limp, flaccid posture of the infant, due to hypotonicity of the muscles, make positioning and holding more difficult and contributes to heat loss from the exposed surface areas. The infant should be warmly wrapped to prevent chilling. The hypo-

Table 14–1

TIME OF OCCURRENCE OF DEVELOPMENTAL MILESTONES IN NORMAL CHILDREN AND THOSE WITH DOWN SYNDROME (IN MONTHS)

	Children with Down Syndrome		Normal Children	
Milestone	Average	Range	Average	Range
Smiling	2	1.5–4	1	0.5–3
Rolling over	8	4–22	5	2–10
Sitting alone	10	6–28	7	5–9
Crawling	12	7–21	8	6–11
Creeping	15	9–27	10	7–13
Standing	20	11–42	11	8–16
Walking	24	12–65	13	8–18
Talking, words	16	9–31	10	6–14
Talking, sentences	28	18–96	21	14–32

From Levine, M. D., Carey, W. B., & Crocker, A. C. (1992). *Developmental-behavioral pediatrics* (2nd ed.). Philadelphia: Saunders.

tonicity of muscles also causes respiratory problems and excess mucus accumulation. Bulb suctioning may be necessary prior to feedings. Hypotonicity of muscles also contributes to the development of constipation which can be controlled by dietary intervention.

Nursing Responsibilities

Counseling Parents. The counseling of families of Down syndrome children is ongoing. It takes exceptional strength and time to accept this diagnosis. Maternity nurses need to be aware of their own feelings before they can effectively support parents. They, too, will feel saddened at the birth of an imperfect child. They may identify with the parents. It is appropriate to express one's feelings of initial helplessness, and it may encourage the parents to verbalize their concerns. The nurse must listen and provide honest, tactful, and compassionate support.

Sometimes parents cannot accept the fact that their baby is retarded and are ashamed to tell anyone of the baby's condition. The nurse can support and encourage the parents' need to cry. Empathy from the nurse is particularly important. Involving parents in the care and planning for the infant from the start facilitates bonding. The need for the staff's warm concern cannot be overestimated. Pampering the baby by putting a little curl in the hair, for example, shows that others care even though the baby is different.

Counseling Family. Siblings of the patient need to be informed and included in discussions about the new baby. Even very young children are aware of parental distress, and their imaginations can be more frightening than the reality. Open communications early on will prevent isolation, avoid misconceptions, and promote an easier transition period. The nurse should connect the family with a Down syndrome support group in their area if there is one. Other parents with a Down syndrome child are an important resource. The National Association for Down Syndrome is one organization that provides education and support to families. (For further discussion of nursing care of the mentally retarded child, see Chapter 23.)

Table 14–2

TIME OF OCCURRENCE OF SELF-HELP SKILLS IN NORMAL CHILDREN AND THOSE WITH DOWN SYNDROME (IN MONTHS)

	Children with Down Syndrome		Normal Children	
Milestone	Average	Range	Average	Range
Eating				
Finger feeding	12	8–28	8	6–16
Using spoon and fork	20	12–40	13	8–20
Toilet training				
Bladder	48	20–95	32	18–60
Bowel	42	28–90	29	16–48
Dressing				
Undressing	40	29–72	32	22–42
Putting clothes on	58	38–98	47	34–58

From Levine, M. D., Carey, W. B., & Crocker, A. C. (1992). *Developmental-behavioral pediatrics* (2nd ed.). Philadelphia: Saunders.

PERINATAL DAMAGE

Hemolytic Disease of the Newborn: Erythroblastosis Fetalis

Description. Erythroblastosis fetalis (*erythro*, "red," and *blast*, "a formative cell," and *osis*, "disease condition") is a disorder that becomes apparent in fetal life or soon after birth. It is one of many congenital hemolytic diseases found in the newborn. There is an excessive destruction of the red blood cells of the baby due to maternal antibodies that pass through the placenta. The terms *isoimmunization* and *sensitization* refer to this process (see Box 14–2). The incidence of erythroblastosis fetalis has greatly decreased as a result of the protective administration of an Rh vaccine (RhoGAM) to women at risk. Incompatibility of ABO factors is

BOX 14–2

TERMS HELPFUL IN UNDERSTANDING RH SENSITIZATION

Antigen (*anti,* "against," and *gen,* "to produce"): A substance that induces the formation of antibodies; the antigen–antibody reaction is the basis of immunity

Coombs test: *Indirectly* measures Rh-positive antibodies in *mother's* blood; *directly* measures antibody-coated Rh-positive red blood cells in *baby's* blood

Erythroblastosis fetalis: The severe form of this disease produces anemia in the *fetus* as a result of the incompatibility of the red blood cells of the mother and those of the fetus

Rh_0(D) immune globulin (RhoGAM): Immunoglobulin given after delivery of an Rh-positive fetus to an Rh-negative mother, to prevent the maternal Rh immune response

Sensitization (isoimmunization): The phenomenon in which the Rh-negative mother develops antibodies against the Rh-positive fetus

now more common and generally less severe than Rh incompatibility (Box 14–3).

The process of maternal sensitization is depicted in Figures 14–15 and 14–16. The mother accumulates antibodies with each pregnancy; therefore, the chance that complications may occur increases with each gestation. If large numbers of antibodies are present, the baby may be severely anemic. In the gravest form, *hydrops fetalis,* the progressive hemolysis causes fetal *hypoxia, anasarca* (generalized edema), and heart failure. This is rare today because of early detection methods.

Diagnosis and Prevention. An extensive history is obtained. Of particular interest are previous sensitizations, an ectopic pregnancy, abortion, blood transfusions, or children who developed jaundice or anemia during the neonatal period. The mother's blood titer is carefully monitored. An *indirect Combs test* on the mother's blood will indicate previous exposure to Rh-positive antigens. Not every Rh-negative woman has erythroblastosis babies. Some women never become sensitized even though they bear several Rh-positive children.

Diagnosis of the disease in the prenatal period is confirmed by amniocentesis and monitoring of bilirubin levels in the amniotic fluid. Information gained from these tests helps to determine early interventions such as induction of labor or intrauterine exchange transfusion. In the latter procedure, a needle is inserted into the abdomen of the fetus. The position of the needle is guided and verified by ultrasonography, and a transfusion is given. Repeated transfusions may be required. Intravascular transfusions are now being performed in utero (Behrman et al., 1996). These procedures are hazardous; therefore, they are done only in carefully selected cases, and the parents are informed of possible complications. Improved intrauterine diagnosis has led to fewer fetal deaths.

Prevention of erythroblastosis by the use of Rh_0 (D) immune globulin (RhoGAM) is now routine. An intramuscular injection is given to the mother within 72 hours of delivery of an Rh-positive infant, provided she has not previously been sensitized (Fig. 14–16). RhoGAM may also be given to the pregnant woman at 28 weeks' gestation. This is important in a primigravida who may have unknowingly miscarried or in a multigravida who may not have received her postpartum RhoGAM. It is also administered, when appropriate, following a spontaneous or therapeutic abortion, following amniocentesis, and to women who have bleeding during pregnancy, because fetal blood may leak into

BOX 14–3

ABO INCOMPATIBILITY

Hemolytic disease with symptoms similar to those of erythroblastosis can occur with ABO incompatibility. A mother who has an "O" blood type gives birth to an infant with an A or B blood group is the most commonly seen ABO incompatibility. Treatment and Nursing care are the same as for erythroblastosis.

Nursing Tip

RhoGAM is administered to Rh-negative mothers by the intramuscular route after normal delivery, after an ectopic pregnancy, or after an abortion to prevent the development of Rh-positive antibodies. RhoGAM has no effect on existing Rh-positive antibodies.

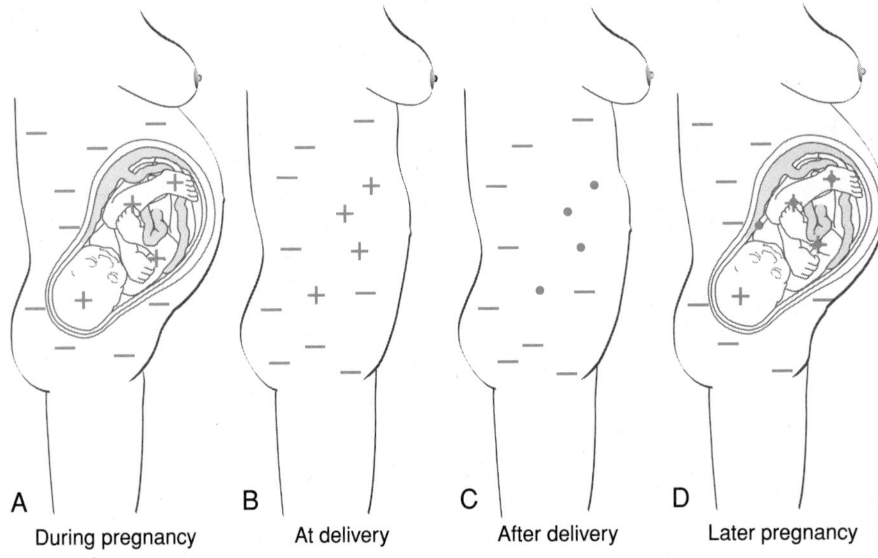

Figure 14–15. • Maternal sensitization producing erythroblastosis in newborn. **A,** An Rh-negative mother is carrying an Rh-positive baby. **B,** Some of the baby's Rh-positive blood enters the mother's body. **C,** Her body produces antibodies against this factor. **D,** When she carries a subsequent Rh-positive baby, the antibodies cross the placenta and attack the baby's red blood cells.

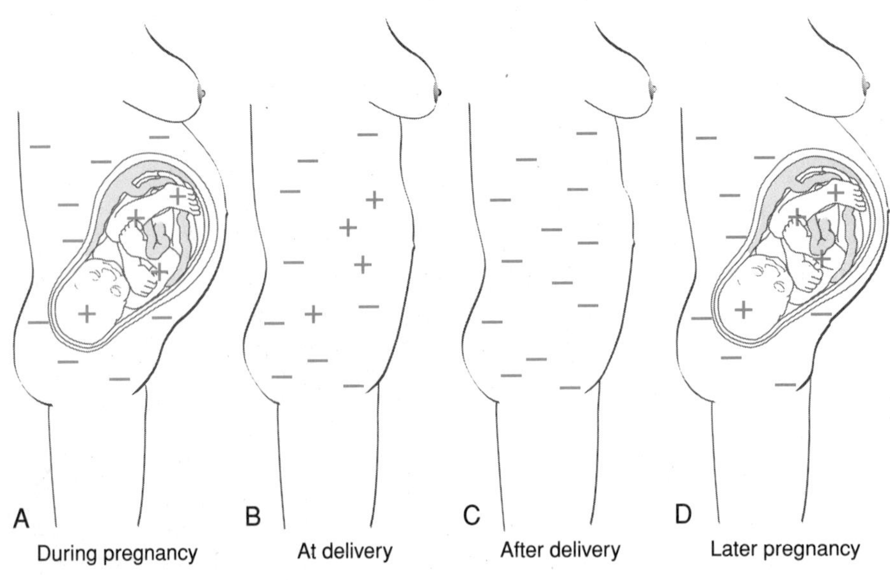

Figure 14–16. • The effect of RhoGAM on maternal sensitization. **A,** After birth, the baby's blood is tested. **B,** If the blood is Rh-positive, RhoGAM is given to the Rh-negative mother within 72 hours after delivery. **C,** It prevents formation of Rh antibodies. **D,** The next Rh-positive fetus is protected. The procedure is repeated with each pregnancy or miscarriage.

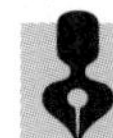

Nursing Tip

Jaundice occurring on the first day of life is always pathological and requires prompt intervention.

Nursing Tip

An infant born with cardiac failure and edema as a result of hemolytic disease is a candidate for immediate exchange transfusion with fresh whole blood.

the mother's circulation at these times. Mothers who deliver at home and are potential candidates for sensitization must not be overlooked.

Manifestations. At the time of delivery, a sample of the baby's cord blood is sent to the laboratory. The *direct Combs test* detects damaging antibodies. The symptoms of erythroblastosis fetalis vary with the intensity of the disease. Anemia and jaundice are present. The anemia is due to hemolysis of large numbers of erythrocytes. This *pathologic jaundice* differs from *physiologic jaundice* in that it becomes evident within 24 hours following delivery. The liver is unable to handle the massive hemolysis, and bilirubin levels rise rapidly, causing *hyperbilirubinemia* (*hyper,* "excess," *bilis,* "bile," *rubor,* "red," and *emia,* "blood"). Early jaundice is immediately reported to the physician.

Enlargement of the liver and spleen and extensive edema may develop. The circulating blood usually contains an excess of immature nucleated red blood cells (erythroblasts) caused by the baby's attempts to compensate for the destruction of cells. The oxygen-carrying power of the blood is diminished as is the blood volume, so shock or heart failure may result. Severe jaundice may cause *kernicterus* (accumulation of bilirubin in the brain tissues). This may cause serious brain damage, may leave the newborn mentally retarded and frequently results in death.

Treatment and Nursing Care. Treatment includes prompt identification, laboratory tests, drug therapy, phototherapy, and exchange transfusion if indicated. Phototherapy may be utilized to reduce serum bilirubin levels. It may be used alone or in conjunction with an exchange transfusion. It may decrease the need for an exchange transfusion or the number required. The newborn is placed in an incubator under a bank of fluorescent lights (Fig. 14–17). The eyes and gonads are protected from the lights and specific protocols are carried out. Although this procedure may prevent the rise of bilirubin, it has no effect on the underlying cause of jaundice. The nursing care of the infant receiving phototherapy is presented in Nursing Care Plan 14–2.

During an exchange transfusion, a plastic catheter is inserted into the umbilical vein of the newborn, small amounts of blood (10–20 ml) are withdrawn, and equal amounts of Rh-negative blood are injected. The amount of donor blood used is about twice the infant blood volume to a limit of 500 cc. In this way, healthy cells are added to the infant's blood and antibodies are removed. Additional small transfusions may be necessary later. After a second exchange transfusion approximately 85% of the baby's blood will have been replaced. Antibiotics may be given to prevent infection. The nurse is usually responsible for the following: observing the newborn's color and reporting any evidence of jaundice during the 1st and 2nd day; applying wet, sterile compresses to the umbilicus if ordered, until an exchange transfusion is completed; stressing to mothers the importance of good prenatal care for subsequent pregnancies; helping to interpret the treatment to parents by giving reassurance as needed; observing and assisting the physician with the exchange transfusion.

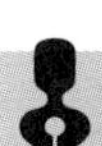

Nursing Tip

Assessing jaundice:

- The skin and the whites of the eyes assume a yellow-orange cast.
- Blanching the skin over the bony prominences enhances evaluation of jaundice.

Home Phototherapy

Home phototherapy programs are being utilized for newborns with mild to moderate physiologic (normal) jaundice. These programs are advocated because bilirubin levels generally begin to rise on the 2nd or 3rd day after birth, when the mother and newborn are discharged. Currently, many women are leaving the hospital within 12 to 24 hours of birth, and a rise in bilirubin levels necessitates the newborn's return to the hospital and possible separation of mother and baby. Home therapy is less costly. Referral for home care is made by the baby's pediatrician on the basis of the

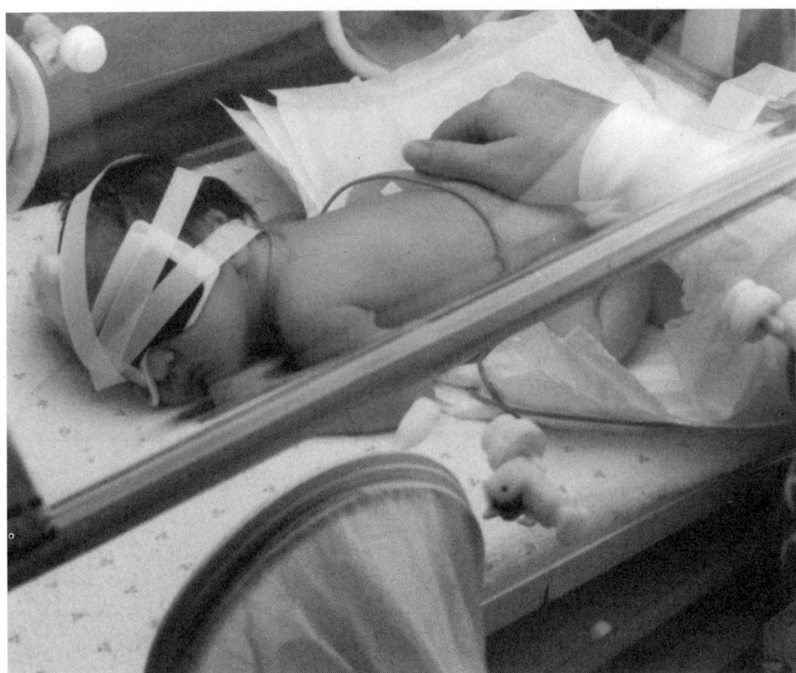

Figure 14–17. • Incubator with phototherapy lights. When an infant receives phototherapy in an incubator, the eyes are protected from the fluorescent lights.

newborn's health, bilirubin levels (generally between 10 and 14 mg/dl), evidence of jaundice, and suitability of the family for complying with the home program.

Lights may be rented from vendors of medical supplies. Fiberoptic phototherapy blankets or pads (Fig. 14–18) are also being utilized. They allow for holding the baby and decrease the risk of eye damage. Written instructions are given to the parents. Parents keep a daily record of their baby's temperature, weight, intake and output, stools, and feedings. (See Nursing Care Plan for the baby receiving phototherapy.) Phototherapy tips are listed in Box 14–4.

Intracranial Hemorrhage

Description. Intracranial hemorrhage, the most common type of birth injury, may result from trauma or anoxia. It occurs more frequently in the preterm infant, whose blood vessels are fragile. Blood vessels within the skull are broken, and bleeding into the brain occurs. When the diagnosis is made, the specific location of the hemorrhage may be noted, that is, subdural, subarachnoid or intraventricular. This injury may also occur during precipitate delivery or prolonged labor or when the newborn's head is large in comparison with the mother's pelvis.

Manifestations. The symptoms of intracranial hemorrhage may occur suddenly or gradually. Some or all symptoms are present, depending on the severity of the hemorrhage. They include poor muscle tone, lethargy, poor sucking reflex, respiratory distress, cyanosis, twitching, forceful vomiting, a high-pitched shrill cry, and convulsions. Opisthotonic posturing may be observed (see p. 599, Fig. 23–9). The fontanel may be tense and under pres-

BOX 14–4

PHOTOTHERAPY TIPS

If infant is in an incubator:

- Eyes must be covered while the infant is under lights.
- A small diaper should cover the gonad area.
- Turn the infant frequently to expose all skin surfaces.
- The infant should be in an incubator to prevent chilling.
- Loose greenish stools caused by photodegradation products must be distinguished from true diarrhea.

Lay the covered light pad on the mattress or other flat surface with the white, illuminating side facing up. Place the infant's back or chest directly on the white side of the pad with the tip of the pad at the baby's shoulders and the pad's cable at the infant's feet.

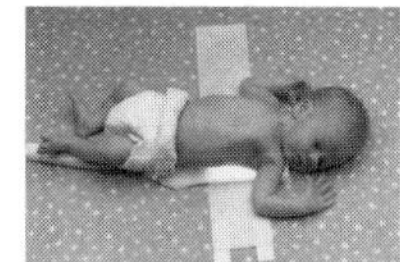

Ensure that:

- as much of the infant's skin is in direct contact with the lighted section of the pad as is possible (diapers may be worn).
- there is nothing between the infant's skin and the light pad other than the disposable cover (clothing may be worn over the pad).
- the baby's eyes are not directly exposed to the covered light pad.

The baby may be clothed or bundled in a blanket and will continue to receive effective phototherapy treatment as long as the lighted section of the pad remains in contact with the skin. It is possible to hold and nurse the infant while continuing treatment.

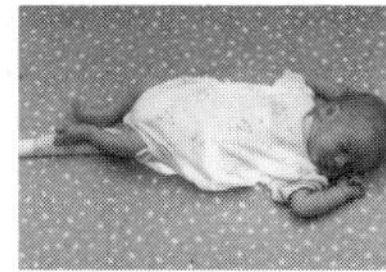

Figure 14–18. • Phototherapy pad or blanket. A phototherapy blanket is a fiberoptic blanket or pad wrapped around the baby. Light generated by the blanket/pad reduces bilirubin levels. The infant can be held during the treatment and eye shields are not necessary. The phototherapy blanket/pad is ideal for home phototherapy. (Courtesy of Ohmeda Inc.)

sure, rather than soft and compressible. The pupil of one eye is likely to be small and the other large. If the symptoms are mild most patients have a good chance of complete recovery. Death results if there is a massive hemorrhage. The infant who survives an extensive hemorrhage may suffer residual defects, such as mental retardation or cerebral palsy. The diagnosis is established by the history of the delivery, computed tomography (CT) scan, magnetic resonance imaging (MRI), evidence of an increase in pressure of the cerebrospinal fluid, and the symptoms and course of the disease.

Treatment and Nursing Care. The newborn is placed in an incubator, which allows proper temperature control, ease in administering oxygen, and continuous observation (p. 339). The baby is handled gently and as little as possible. The head is elevated. The doctor may prescribe vitamin K to control bleeding and phenobarbital if twitching or convulsions are apparent. Prophylactic antibiotics as well as vitamins may be used. The baby is fed carefully because the sucking reflex may be affected. The infant vomits easily. The nurse observes the baby for signs of increased intracranial pressure (see p. 350) and convulsions and assists the doctor with such procedures as lumbar punctures and aspiration of subdural hemorrhage. Performing neurochecks, monitoring vital signs and head circumference, and palpating fontanels are essential.

If a convulsion occurs, observation of its character aids the doctor in diagnosing the exact location of the bleeding. The following are of particular importance: Were the arms, legs, or face involved? Was the right or left side of the body involved? Was the convulsion mild or severe? How long did it last? What was the condition of the infant before and after the seizure? The nurse records observations in the nurses' notes.

INFANT OF A DIABETIC MOTHER

Diabetes in the mother presents various problems for the newborn infant. These are determined by the severity and duration of the disease in the mother, the degree of control of her condition, and the gestational age of the baby. Diabetes in pregnancy is discussed on page 103. When diabetes of the mother is under good control from conception

NURSING CARE PLAN 14–2

Selected Nursing Diagnoses for the Baby Receiving Phototherapy

Nursing Diagnosis: High risk for injury to eyes and gonads related to phototherapy

Goals	Nursing Interventions	Rationale
Baby does not have eye drainage or irritation Genitals are protected	1. Apply eye patches over infant's closed eyes before placing infant under lights 2. Remove patches at least once per shift to assess eyes for conjunctivitis 3. Remove patches to allow eye contact during feeding 4. Cover ovaries or testes with diaper	1. Closing eyes prevents corneal abrasion, and protects retina from damage by high-intensity light 2. Facilitates early detection of inflammation and jaundice (sclera may yellow) 3. Provides for visual stimulation and bonding 4. Protects gonads from damage by heat

Nursing Diagnosis: Altered skin integrity related to immature structure and function, immobility

Goals	Nursing Interventions	Rationale
Skin remains intact as evidenced by absence of skin rash, excoriation, or redness	1. Observe for maculopapular rash 2. Cleanse rectal area gently, as stools are often green and liquid 3. Reposition at least every 2 hr 4. Assess for jaundice or bronzing (note: serum bilirubin may be high, even though baby may not appear jaundiced under lights) 5. Observe for pressure areas	1. Rashes and burns have been known to occur as a result of phototherapy 2. Frequent stools may cause breakdown of skin; loose stools are result of increased bilirubin excretion 3. Repositioning provides exposure of all skin areas 4. Observation of jaundice may be initial sign of hyperbilirubinemia Bronze baby syndrome appears in preterms who do not excrete the photooxidation products adequately 5. Early intervention prevents skin breakdown

Nursing Diagnosis: High risk for fluid volume deficit related to increased water loss through skin and loose stools

Goals	Nursing Interventions	Rationale
Baby does not become dehydrated, as evidenced by good skin turgor, normal fontanels, and moist tongue and mucous membranes Weight maintenance, urine output satisfactory	1. Monitor intravenous fluids 2. Check skin turgor 3. Observe for depressed fontanel 4. Anticipate the need for additional water between feedings 5. Daily weights unless contraindicated	1. IV fluids are sometimes used to prevent dehydration or in anticipation of exchange transfusion 2. Helps to determine extent of dehydration 3. Sign of dehydration 4. Adequate hydration facilitates elimination and excretion of bilirubin 5. Assess progress; helps to determine extent of dehydration

Nursing Diagnosis: High risk for hyperthermia or hypothermia

Goals	Nursing Interventions	Rationale
Baby does not become overheated or chilled; temperature will be maintained between 36.3 and 37.4°C (97.4 and 99.4°F)	1. Monitor baby's temperature 2. Adjust incubator to maintain neutral thermal environment	1. Hyperthermia and hypothermia are common complications of phototherapy 2. Avoid overheating incubator or warming unit

and throughout pregnancy, the adverse effects on the newborn infant are minimal.

Many newborn infants of diabetic mothers have serious complications. When the mother is hyperglycemic, large amounts of glucose are transferred to the fetus. This makes the fetus hyperglycemic. In response, the fetal pancreas (islet cells) produces large amounts of fetal insulin. Hyperinsulinism, along with excess production of protein and fatty acids, often results in a newborn infant who weighs over 9 pounds. Such a baby is designated large for gestational age (LGA). The condition is termed

NURSING CARE PLAN 14–2 *continued*

Selected Nursing Diagnoses for the Baby Receiving Phototherapy

Nursing Diagnosis: High risk for neurologic injury related to nature of hyperbilirubinemia

Goals	Nursing Interventions	Rationale
Baby will show no signs of neurologic involvement (lethargy, twitching)	1. Anticipate daily bilirubin blood levels	1. Phototherapy success determined by frequently measuring serum bilirubin levels
	2. Turn off phototherapy lights when blood is being drawn to avoid false readings	2. Promotes accuracy of blood test
	3. Observe parameters for neurologic deficit (e.g., twitching, lethargy)	3. Kernicterus (brain damage) is rare but is evidenced by neurologic sequella, such as hypotonia, diminished reflexes, twitching, lethargy

Nursing Diagnosis: Nutrition alterations: less than body requirements

Goals	Nursing Interventions	Rationale
Baby receives adequate nutrients as evidenced by stabilization of weight, laboratory reports	1. Provide feedings as ordered	1. Early feedings within 4 to 6 hr following delivery tend to decrease high bilirubin levels as well as to provide nourishment
	2. Assist mother to reestablish breastfeeding if temporarily halted	2. Encourages mother, helps her to feel more in control, promotes bonding; opinions of physicians vary as to discontinuance of breastfeeding, as the cause of breast milk jaundice is not known

Nursing Diagnosis: High risk for injury related to immobility, electrical apparatus

Goals	Nursing Interventions	Rationale
Baby will show no signs of burns or other breaks in skin integrity	1. Ascertain that all electrical outlets are grounded	1–3. Safety is an important consideration in all procedures involving patients and equipment
	2. Record number of hours lights have been in use, change as necessary	
	3. Use plexiglass cover or shield to protect baby in case of lamp breakage	

Nursing Diagnosis: Parental anxiety related to knowledge deficit, crisis of having a baby with jaundice

Goals	Nursing Interventions	Rationale
Parents express fears concerning baby's welfare	1. Explain procedures and treatment	1. Information decreases parental stress
	2. Provide reassurance	2. Parents are in need of support persons
	3. Provide follow-up	3. Follow-up care is reassuring to parents and medical personnel that family is progressing nicely without complications

macrosomia (*macro* "large," *soma* "body"). This infant is prone to injuries at birth because of its size. Following delivery, it often has *low blood sugar* levels because of the abrupt loss of maternal glucose and hypertrophy of the pancreatic islet cells that result in a temporary overproduction of insulin.

Hypoglycemia in the first days of life is defined as a blood sugar that falls below 40 mg/dl. The babies have a characteristic *cushingoid* appearance owing to increased subcutaneous fat. The face is round and appears puffy; the babies appear lethargic. The size of these newborn infants makes them appear healthy, but this is deceptive as they often have developmental deficits and may suffer complications of respiratory distress syndrome (RDS) or congenital anomalies. In contrast, an infant born to a mother with severe diabetes may be small for gestational age (SGA) because of poor placental perfusion. These babies suffer from hypoglycemia, hypocalcemia, and hyperbilirubinemia. The nursing care of the infant of a diabetic mother includes close monitoring of vital signs, early feeding, and frequent blood glucose levels for the first two days of life. Hypoglycemia can result in rapid and permanent brain damage. The infant should be closely watched for signs of irritability, tremors, and respiratory distress.

KEY POINTS

- The nurse manages communication between parents and the multidisciplinary health care team to meet the needs of the newborn with congenital problems and of their families.
- Measuring the size of the infant's head is important in babies with hydrocephalus.
- Spina bifida is a congenital embryonic neural tube defect in which there is an imperfect closure of the spinal vertebrae.
- Folic acid supplementation during the early weeks of pregnancy can prevent neural tube anomalies.
- Postoperative nursing care of the baby with a cleft lip includes preventing the baby from sucking and crying, which could impair the suture line.
- Newborns feel pain and adequate pain control following invasive procedures and surgery is essential.
- The body spica cast encircles the waist and extends to the ankles or toes. It is used to treat congenital dislocations of the hip.
- A positive Barlow's test and Ortolani sign are indicative of developmental hip dysplasia.
- Newborn infants are routinely screened for phenylketonuria.
- Lofenalac is a formula used for infants with phenylketonuria.
- RhoGAM is given after delivery of an Rh-positive fetus to an Rh-negative mother to prevent the maternal Rh sensitization.
- Hyperbilirubinemia results from rapid destruction of red blood cells.
- Pathological jaundice occurs in the first 24 hours of life.
- Distinguishing pathological jaundice from physiological jaundice can facilitate early intervention and prevention of serious complications.
- Macrosomia is a condition where the infant is large for gestational age (LGA) and usually occurs in infants of diabetic mothers.
- In intracranial hemorrhage, blood vessels within the skull are broken and bleeding into the brain occurs.

MULTIPLE-CHOICE REVIEW QUESTIONS

Choose the most appropriate answer.

1. The inspection of a cavity by passing a light through its wall to visualize fluid is called
   a. transillumination.
   b. phototherapy.
   c. hydrotherapy.
   d. photosynthesis.
2. A congenital defect that results in enlargement of the patient's head and pressure changes within the brain is
   a. hydrocephalus.
   b. microcephalus.
   c. hydrocele.
   d. anencephaly.
3. Meningomyelocele is
   a. a protrusion of the meninges through an opening in the spine.
   b. primarily a disorder of the muscular tissue of the body.
   c. a protrusion of the membranes and cord through an opening in the spine.
   d. a tumor in the meningele space.
4. A Pavlik harness is sometimes used to correct
   a. clubfoot.
   b. juvenile arthritis.
   c. developmental hip dysplasia.
   d. fractured femur.
5. When bathing an infant, the nurse observes the hips for dislocation. Which of the following observations may indicate developmental hip dysplasia?
   a. Toes turned inward.
   b. Limitation of abduction of legs.
   c. Asymmetry of epicanthal folds.
   d. Shortening of patella.

BIBLIOGRAPHY AND READER REFERENCE

Ahlfors, C. E. (1994). Criteria for exchange transfusions for newborns. *Pediatrics, 93*(3), 488–494.

Behrman, R. E., Kleigman, R., & Arvin, A. (1996). *Nelson's textbook of pediatrics* (15th ed.). Philadelphia: Saunders.

Bell, R., & McGrath, J. (1996, June). Implementing a research-based Kangaroo Care program in the NICU. *Nursing Clinics of North America, 31*(2), 387.

Blackburn, S. (1995). Hyperbilirubinemia and neonatal jaundice. *Neonatal Network, 14*(7), 15–25.

Bowden, V., Dickey, S., & Greenberg, C. (1998). *Children and their families: A continuum of care.* Philadelphia: Saunders.

Bruno, J. (1995). Systematic neonatal assessment and intervention. *MCN, 20*(1).

Eichner, R. (10/94). Circadian Rhythms. *Sports Medicine, 22*(10), 82.

Elias, E., & Hobbs, N. (1998). Spinabifida: Sorting out the complexities of care. *Contemporary Pediatrics, 15*(4), 156.

George, P., & Lynch, M. (1994). Ohmedi Biliblanket vs. Wallaby Phototherapy System for reduction of bilirubin levels in home care settings. *Clinical Pediatrics, 33,* 178–180.

Hegyi, T., et al. (1994). Blood pressure ranges in premature infants. *Journal of Pediatrics, 124*(4), 627–633.

Hysmith, T., Hysmith, S., et al. (1993). *Comparison of Olympic Fluorescent bank lights and the Ohmeda Biliblanket® for the treatment of unconjugated hyperbilirubinemia of the newborn in a home health care environment.* Paper presented at the 9th National Meeting of Associated Neonatal Nurses, September 8–12.

Klaus, M. H., & Fanaroff, A. A. (1993). *Care of the high-risk neonate* (4th ed.). Philadelphia: Saunders.

Krechel, S. W., & Bildner, J. (1995). Cries: A new neonatal postoperative pain measurement score. *Pediatric Anesthesiology, 5,* 53–61.

Levine, M. D., Carey, W. B., & Crocker, A. C. (1992). *Developmental-behavioral pediatrics* (2nd ed.). Philadelphia: Saunders.

Mainous, R. O. (1995). Research utilization: Pharmacologic management of neonatal pain. *Neonatal Network, 14*(4), 71–74.

March of Dimes Birth Defects Foundation. (1992). *Birth Defects.* White Plains, NY: Author.

Omenaca, F., Paredes, C., et al. (1994). *A multi-center, open label, controlled randomized clinical trial using fiberoptic light for treatment of jaundice in neonates.* Paper presented at the Japanese Society for Newborn Medicine, Tokyo, Japan, October 28–29.

Schuett, V. (1993). *Low protein cookery for phenylketonuria.* Madison: University of Wisconsin Press.

Selekman, J., & Malloy, E. (1995). Difficulties in symptom recognition in infants. *Journal of Pediatric Nursing, 10*(2), 89.

Sinai, L. N., et al. (1995). PKU screening: Effects of early newborn discharge. *Pediatrics, 96*(4), 605–608.

Tan, K. L. (1994). Comparison of efficacy of fiberoptic and conventional phototherapy for neonatal hyperbilirubinemia. *Journal of Pediatrics, 125*(4), 607–612.

Weinbert, S. H. (1995). Shortened stays and PKU testing. *Maternal Child Nursing, 20*(2), 76.

Winter, S. (1993). Diagnosing metabolic disorders: One step at a time. *Contemporary Pediatrics, 10*(10), 35.

Wordinsky, T. D. (1994). Visual clues to diagnosis of birth defects and genetic disease. *Journal of Pediatric Health Care, 8,* 63.

Yule, K. A. (1996). PKU. In P. L. Jackson & J. A. Vessey, Eds., Primary care of a child with a chronic condition (2nd ed.). St. Louis, MO: Mosby.

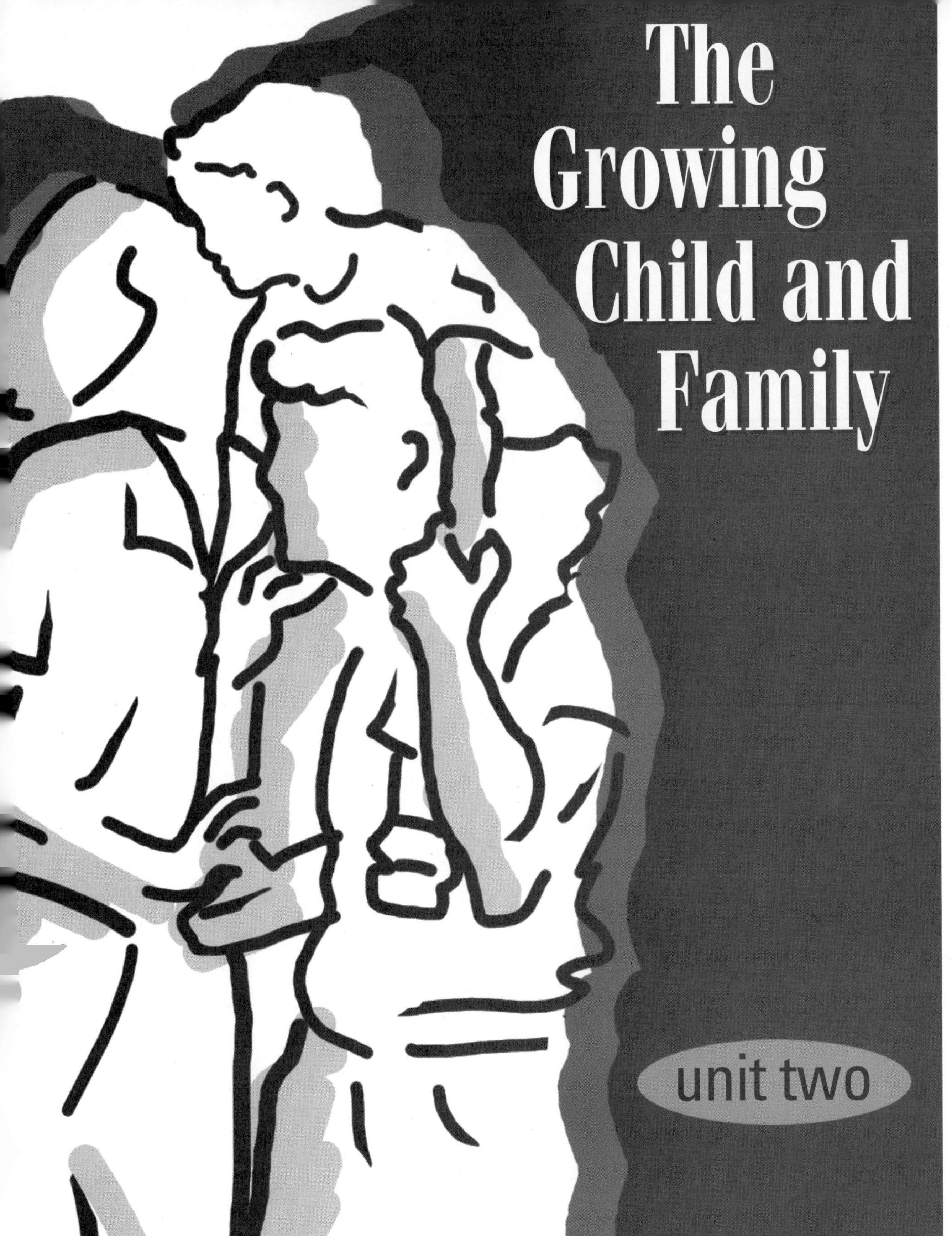
The Growing Child and Family
unit two

chapter 15

An Overview of Growth, Development, and Nutrition

Outline

Objectives

On completion and mastery of Chapter 15, the student will be able to

- Define each vocabulary term listed.
- Explain the differences between growth, development, and maturation.
- Recognize and read a growth chart for children.
- List five factors that influence growth and development.
- Discuss the nursing implications of growth and development.
- Describe three developmental theories and their impact on planning nursing care of children.
- Discuss the nutritional needs of growing children.
- Differentiate between permanent and deciduous teeth and list the times of their eruption.
- Recognize the influence of the family and cultural practices on growth, development, nutrition, and health care.
- Understand the characteristics of play at various age levels.
- Describe the relationship of play to physical cognitive and emotional development.
- Understand the role of computers and computer games in play at various ages.
- Define therapeutic play.
- Understand the use of play as an assessment tool.
- Discuss the importance of family-centered care in pediatrics.

Vocabulary

adolescent	length
cephalocaudal	Maslow
cognition	maturation
community	metabolic rate
competitive play	neonate
cooperative play	nursing caries
deciduous	nuclear family
dysfunctional family	parallel play
Erikson	personality
extended family	Piaget
fluorosis	proximodistal
growth	syndrome
height	therapeutic play
infant	toddler
Kohlberg	

AN OVERVIEW OF GROWTH, DEVELOPMENT, AND MATURATION

The main difference between caring for the adult and caring for the child is that the latter is in a continuous process of growth and development. This process is orderly and proceeds from the simple to the more complex (Box 15–1). Although the process is orderly, it is not steadily paced. Growth spurts are often followed by plateaus. One of the most noticeable growth spurts is at the time of puberty. The rate of growth varies with the individual child. Each baby has an individual timetable that revolves about established norms. Siblings within a family vary in growth rate. Growth is measurable and can be observed and studied. This is done by comparing height, weight, increase in vocabulary, physical skills, and other parameters. There are variations in growth within the systems and subsystems. Not all parts mature at the same time. Skeletal growth approximates whole-body growth, whereas the brain, lymph, and reproductive tissues follow distinct and individual sequences.

The Impact of Growth and Development on Nursing Care

Pediatrics is a subspecialty of medical-surgical nursing. On the adult acute care units in a hospital, there may be a separate neurology unit, a separate cardiac unit, a separate medical unit, and a separate surgical unit. On the pediatric acute care unit in the hospital, all medical-surgical specialties are housed on one unit, caring for clients from newborn to the teenage years age group. The developmental needs of the child impact the response of the child to illness as well as the approach required by the nurse in developing a plan of care. Choosing the right words to explain to a child what will happen to him or her is essential. For example, if the nurse states we will "put you to sleep" before the operation, will the child relate that to a pet at home being "put to sleep" and never heard from again? The fractured jaw of an 8-month-old after a motor vehicle accident may affect his developmental process more seriously than the same injury in a 4-year-old because the 8-month-old is in the oral phase of development.

Since the child differs from the adult both anatomically and physiologically, differences in response to therapy as well as manifestations of illness can be anticipated. The nurse must understand the normal to recognize deviations within any age group and plan care to take into account these developmental differences (Box 15–2).

Terminology

The stages of growth and development that are referred to throughout this text are as follows:

- *Fetus.* Conception to birth
- *Neonate.* Birth to 4 weeks
- *Infant.* 4 weeks to 1 year
- *Toddler.* 1 to 3 years
- *Preschool.* 3 to 6 years
- *School age.* 6 to 12 years
- *Adolescence.* 12 to 18 years

Growth refers to an increase in physical size, measured in inches and pounds. *Development* refers to a progressive increase in the function of the body. The two are inseparable. *Maturation* (*maturus,* "ripe") refers to the total way in which a person grows and develops, as dictated by inheritance (Box 15–3). Although maturation is independent of environment, its timing may be affected by environment.

Directional Patterns. Directional patterns are fundamental to all humans. *Cephalocaudal* development proceeds from head to toe. The infant is able to raise the head before being able to sit, and he or she gains control of the trunk before walking. The second pattern is *proximodistal,* or from midline to the periphery. Development proceeds from the center of the body to the periphery (Fig. 15–1). These patterns occur bilaterally. Development also proceeds from the general to the specific. The infant grasps with the hands before pinching with the fingers.

Height. *Height* refers to standing measurement, whereas *length* refers to measurement while the infant is in a recumbent position. At birth the newborn has an average length of about 20 inches (50 cm). Linear growth is caused mainly by skeletal growth. Growth fluctuates throughout life until maturity is reached. Infancy and puberty are both rapid growth periods. Height is generally a family trait, although there are exceptions. Good nutrition and general good health are instrumental in pro-

BOX 15–1

EMERGING PATTERNS OF BEHAVIOR FROM 1 TO 5 YEARS OF AGE

15 Months

Motor. Walks alone; crawls up stairs.

Adaptive. Makes tower of three cubes; makes a line with crayons; inserts pellet in bottle.

Language. Jargon; follows simple commands; may name a familiar object (ball).

Social. Indicates some desires or needs by pointing; hugs parents.

18 Months

Motor. Runs stiffly; sits on small chair; walks up stairs with one hand held; explores drawers and waste baskets.

Adaptive. Makes a tower of four cubes; imitates scribbling; imitates vertical stroke; dumps pellet from bottle.

Language. 10 words (average); names pictures; identifies one or more parts of body.

Social. Feeds self; seeks help when in trouble; may complain when wet or soiled; kisses parent with pucker.

24 Months

Motor. Runs well; walks up and down stairs, one step at a time; opens doors; climbs on furniture; jumps.

Adaptive. Tower of seven cubes (6 at 21 mo); circular scribbling; imitates horizontal stroke; folds paper once imitatively.

Language. Puts three words together (subject, verb, object).

Social. Handles spoon well; often tells immediate experiences; helps to undress; listens to stories with pictures.

30 Months

Motor. Goes up stairs alternating feet.

Adaptive. Tower of nine cubes; makes vertical and horizontal strokes, but generally will not join them to make a cross; imitates circular stroke, forming closed figure.

Language. Refers to self by pronoun "I"; knows full name.

Social. Helps put things away; pretends in play.

36 Months

Motor. Rides tricycle; stands momentarily on one foot.

Adaptive. Tower of 10 cubes; imitates construction of "bridge" of three cubes; copies a circle; imitates a cross.

Language. Knows age and sex; counts three objects correctly; repeats three numbers or a sentence of six syllables.

Social. Plays simple games (in "parallel" with other children); helps in dressing (unbuttons clothing and puts on shoes); washes hands.

48 Months

Motor. Hops on one foot; throws ball overhand; uses scissors to cut out pictures; climbs well.

Adaptive. Copies bridge from model; imitates construction of "gate" of five cubes; copies cross and square; draws a man with two to four parts besides head; names longer of two lines.

Language. Counts four pennies accurately; tells a story.

Social. Plays with several children with beginning of social interaction and role-playing; goes to toilet alone.

60 Months

Motor. Skips.

Adaptive. Draws triangle from copy; names heavier of two weights.

Language. Names four colors; repeats sentence of 10 syllables; counts 10 pennies correctly.

Social. Dresses and undresses; asks questions about meaning of words; domestic-role playing.

Data are derived from those of Gesell (as revised by Knobloch), Shirley, Provence, Wolf, Bailey, and others. After 5 years the Stanford-Binet, Wechsler-Bellevue, and other scales offer the most precise estimates of developmental level. To have the greatest value, they should be administered only by an experienced and qualified person.

From Behrman, R., Kleigman, R., & Arvin, A. (1996). *Nelson's textbook of pediatric* (15th ed.). Philadelphia: Saunders.

BOX 15–2

THE NURSING PROCESS APPLIED TO GROWTH AND DEVELOPMENT

Assess

Obtain height and weight and plot a standard growth chart.

Record developmental milestones achieved related to age.

Observe infant, interview parents.

Analysis/Nursing Diagnosis

Determine appropriate nursing diagnosis related to parenting, coping skills, and unmet developmental needs.

Planning

Offer guidance and teaching to family, school personnel, and child to meet child's developmental needs. For example, the toddler and preschooler may have specific needs related to safety or the use of age-appropriate toys.

Implementation

Interventions that foster growth and development in the hospital setting can include encouraging age-appropriate self-care. In the home, the school-age diabetic child may be taught to participate in accuchecks and insulin administration. Anticipatory guidance may be given to parents so they will understand changes in behavior, eating habits, and play of the growing child.

Evaluation

Ongoing evaluation of growth and development of the child and follow-up of teaching and anticipatory guidance offered at prior clinic/home visits are essential.

moting linear growth. Height is measured during each well-child conference (Fig. 15–2). The length of the infant usually increases about 1 inch per month for the first 6 months. By one year of age, the birth length increases by 50% (mostly in the trunk area).

Weight. Weight is another good index of health. However the weight of a newborn infant does not always imply gestational maturity. (See assessing gestational maturity Figs. 13–2 and 13–3.) The average full-term newborn weighs 6 to 9 pounds or 2.72 to 4.09 kilograms (kg) with a general average of 7½ pounds. About 5% to 10% of the birth weight is lost

BOX 15–3

KEY TERMS IN CHILD DEVELOPMENT

Growth. An increase in physical size, measured in feet or meters and pounds or kilograms

Development. A progressive increase in the function of the body (e.g., baby's increasing ability to digest solids)

Maturation. The total way in which a person grows and develops, as dictated by inheritance

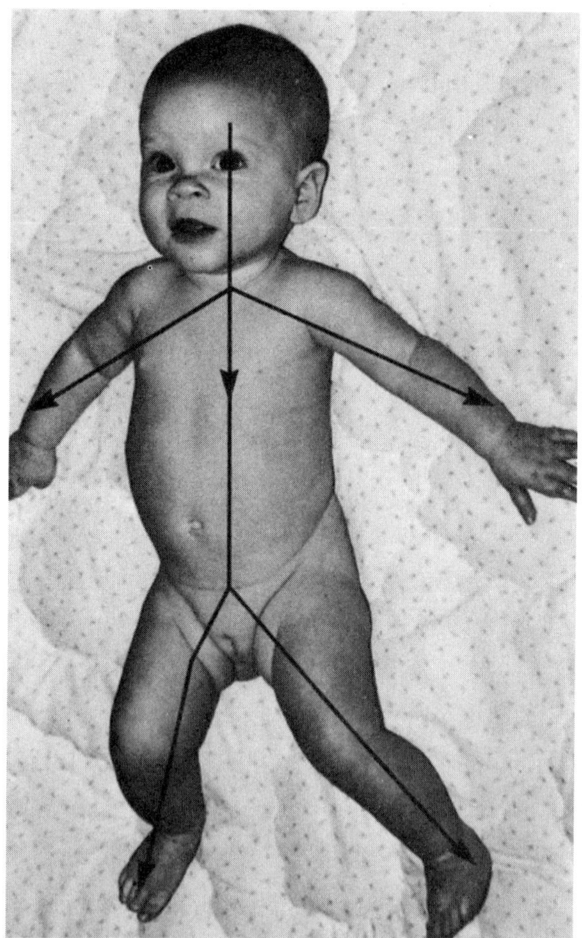

Figure 15–1. • The development of muscular control proceeds from head to foot (cephalocaudally) and from the center of the body to its periphery (proximodistally). (From Betz, C., Hunsberger, M., & Wright, S. [1994]. *Family-centered nursing care of children* [2nd ed.]. Philadelphia: Saunders.)

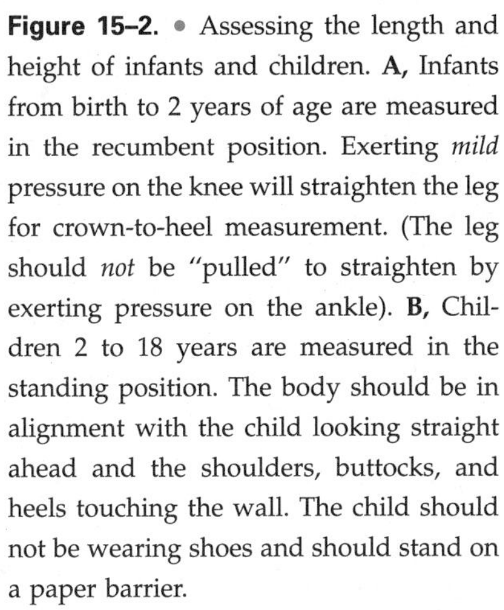

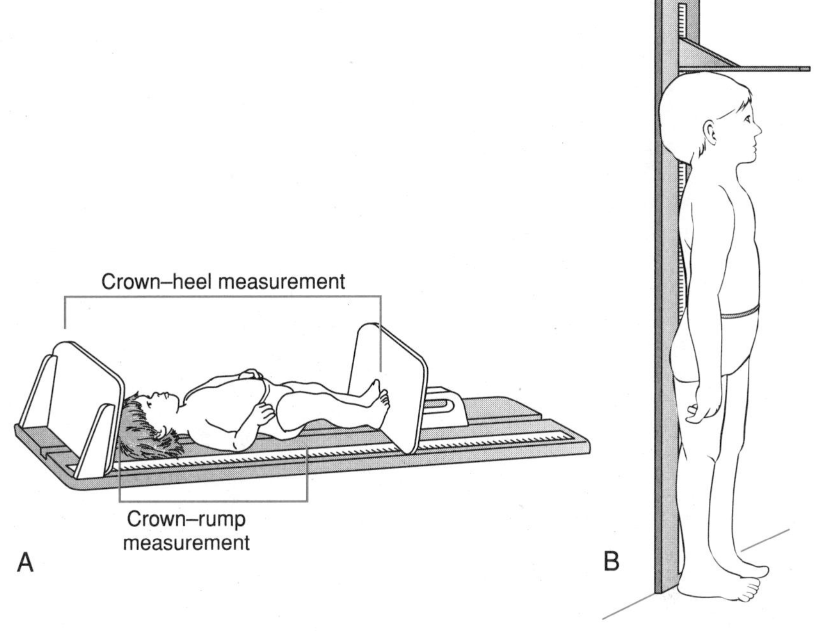

Figure 15–2. • Assessing the length and height of infants and children. **A,** Infants from birth to 2 years of age are measured in the recumbent position. Exerting *mild* pressure on the knee will straighten the leg for crown-to-heel measurement. (The leg should *not* be "pulled" to straighten by exerting pressure on the ankle). **B,** Children 2 to 18 years are measured in the standing position. The body should be in alignment with the child looking straight ahead and the shoulders, buttocks, and heels touching the wall. The child should not be wearing shoes and should stand on a paper barrier.

by 3 or 4 days of age. This is the result of the passage of stools and a limited fluid intake. The infant usually regains his birth weight by 10 to 12 days of age. *Birth weight usually doubles by 5 to 6 months and triples by 1 year of age.* After the 1st year, weight gain levels off to approximately 4 to 6 pounds (1.81 to 2.72 kg) per year until the pubertal growth spurt begins. Weight is determined at each office visit. A marked increase or decrease requires further investigation. The body weight of a newborn is composed of a higher percentage of water than in the adult. This extracellular fluid falls from 40% in the newborn to 20% in the adult. The high proportion of extracellular fluid in the infant can cause a more rapid loss of total body fluid, and therefore every infant needs to be closely monitored for dehydration. (See technique of weighing infants see Chapter 12, p. 316.)

Body Proportions. Body proportions of the child differ greatly from those of the adult (Fig. 15–3). The head is the fastest growing portion of the body during fetal life. During infancy the trunk grows rapidly, and during childhood growth of the legs becomes the predominant feature. At adolescence, characteristic male and female proportions develop as childhood fat disappears. Alterations in proportions in the size of head, trunk, and extremities are characteristic of certain disturbances. Routine measurements of head and chest circumference are important indexes of health.

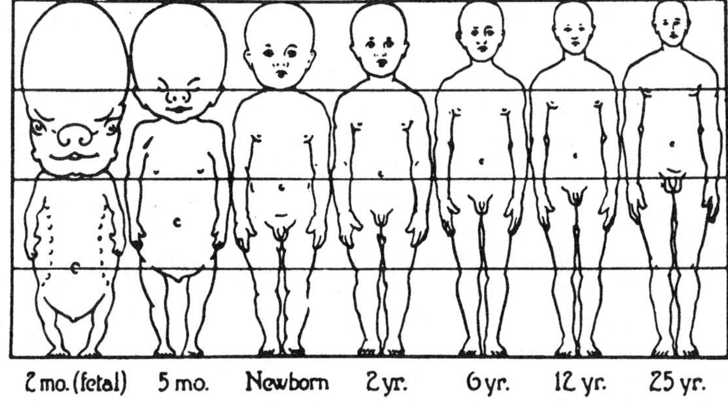

Figure 15–3. • Changes in body proportions. Approximate changes in body proportions from fetal life through adulthood are shown. These changes in body proportions affect body surface areas that are used to determine the percentages of body burns in burn injuries. See "rule of nines" on page 783. (From Robbins, W. J., Brody, S., Hogan, A. G., et al. [1928]. *Growth.* New Haven: Yale University Press. By permission of the Publisher.)

Metabolic Rate. The metabolic rate in children is higher than in adults. Infants require more calories, minerals, vitamins, and fluid in proportion to weight and height than do adults. Higher metabolic rates are accompanied by increased production of heat and waste products. The body surface area of young children is far greater in relation to body weight than that of adults. The young child loses relatively more fluid from the pulmonary and integumentary systems.

Respirations. The respirations of infants are irregular and abdominal. Small airways can become easily blocked with mucus. The short, straight eustachian tube connects with the ear and predisposes the infant to middle-ear infections. The chest wall is thin and muscles are immature, therefore pressure on the chest can interfere with respiratory efforts.

Cardiovascular System. The muscle mass of the right and left ventricles of the heart in neonates is almost equal. An increased need for cardiac output is often met by an increase in *heart rate.* Newborns have a high oxygen consumption and require a high cardiac output in the first few months of life. The presence of fetal (immature) hemoglobin in the first months of life also contributes to the need for a high cardiac output. The disappearance of fetal hemoglobin along with the loss of maternal iron stores contributes to the development of *physiological anemia* in infants between 3 and 4 months of age.

Immunity. The newborn is protected for the first 3 months of life from illnesses the mother was exposed to. The infant gradually produces his or her own immune globins until adult levels are reached by the age of puberty. The infant and child therefore need to be protected from nosocomial infections in the hospital and from unnecessary exposure to pathogens. Immunizations against common childhood communicable diseases is discussed on page 823.

Kidney Function. Kidney function matures by the end of the second year of life. Therefore, drugs that are eliminated from the body via the kidney can accumulate in the body to dangerous levels before 2 years of age. Immature kidney function also predisposes the infant to dehydration. Nursing responsibilities for children under 2 years of age include monitoring for dehydration and observing closely for toxic effects of drug therapy.

Nervous System. Maturation of the brain is evidenced by increase in coordination, skills, and behaviors in the first years of life. Primitive reflexes, such as the grasp reflex, are replaced by purposeful, controlled movement. In the first 6 months of life, the head circumference increases 1.5 cm per month to 43 cm at 6 months of age. During the second 6 months of life, the head circumference increases 0.5 cm per month to approximately 46 cm at 1 year of age. The age-appropriate toy is correlated with nervous system maturation. When selecting play activities, the nurse should consider the diagnosis and the child's developmental level and abilities to be sure the toy is safe.

Sleep Patterns. Sleep patterns vary with age. The neonate will sleep 8 to 9 hours per night and nap an equal amount of time during the day. The 2-year-old may sleep 10 hours during the night and have only one short daytime nap. The 7-year-old usually requires 8 to 8½ hours of sleep and rarely has a daytime nap. These patterns may be altered by cultural practices. For example, Israeli Kibbutzim often have *all* family members nap after work or school and before dinner.

Bone Growth. Bone growth provides one of the best indicators of biologic age. Bone age can be determined by x-ray films. In the fetus, bones begin as connective tissue, which later is converted to cartilage. Through ossification, cartilage is converted to bone. The maturity and rate of bone growth vary within individuals; however, the progression remains the same. Growth of the long bones continues until *epiphyseal* fusion occurs. Bone is constantly synthesized and reabsorbed. In children, bone synthesis is greater than bone destruction. Calcium reserves are stored in the ends of the long bones. Vitamin A, vitamin D, sunlight, and fluorine are necessary for growth and development of skeletal and soft tissue.

Critical Periods. There appear to be certain periods when environmental events or stimuli have their maximum impact on the child's development. The embryo, for example, can be adversely affected during times of rapid cell division. Certain viruses, drugs, and other agents are known to cause congenital anomalies during the first 3 months following conception. It is believed that these sensitive periods also apply to factors such as developing a sense of trust during the 1st year of life (and) learning readiness.

Integration of Skills. As the child learns new skills, they are combined with ones previously mastered. For instance, the child who is learning to walk may sit, pull the body up to a table by grasping it, balance, and take a cautious step. Tomorrow the child may take three steps! Children connect and perfect each skill in preparation for learning a more complex one.

Growth Standards

Growth is measured in dimensions such as height, weight, volume, and thickness of tissues, but measurement alone, without any standard of comparison, limits interpretation of the data. A number of standards have been developed to make it possible (1) to compare the measurement of a child to others of the same age and sex, and ideally race; and (2) to compare that child's present measurements with the former rate of growth and pattern of progress. These standards, available as *growth charts,* are among the tools that have been used to assess the child's overall development (Fig. 15–4).

Length refers to horizontal measurement; it is used before a child can stand, usually between birth to 2 years. Height is measured with the child standing, usually between 2 and 18 years. Some pointers in reading and interpreting growth charts follow:

- Children who are in good health tend to follow a consistent pattern of growth.
- At any age, there are wide individual differences in measured values.
- Percentile charts are customarily divided into seven percentile levels designated by lines. These lines generally are labeled 97th, 90th, 75th, 50th, 25th, 10th, and 3rd, or 95th, 90th, 75th, 50th, 25th, 10th, and 5th.
- The median (middle), or 50th percentile, is designated by a solid black line. Percentile levels show the extent to which a child's measurements

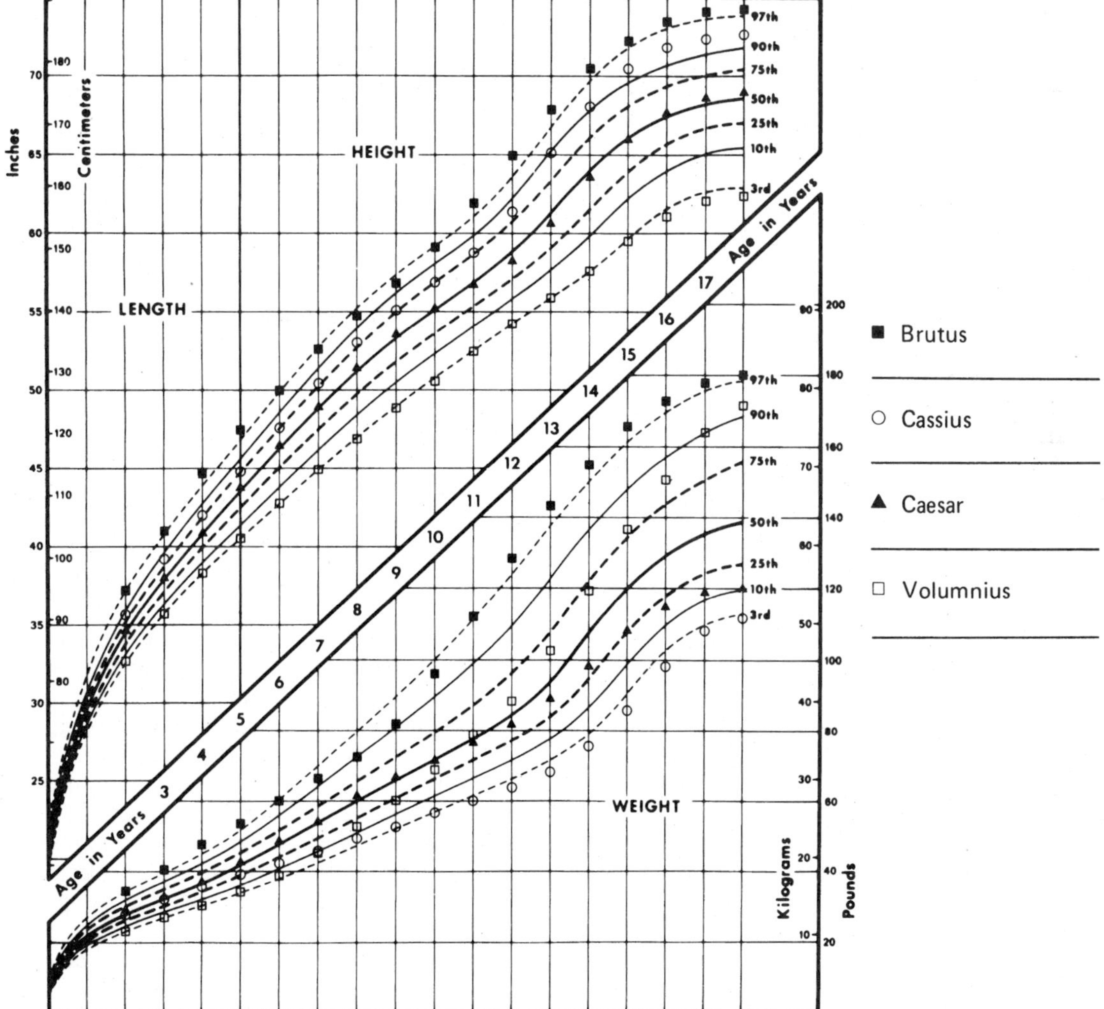

Figure 15–4. • Sample of a complete growth chart. Note the percentile for length, height, and weight for four boys from birth to age 18 years. (From Valadian, I., & Porter, D. [1977]. *Physical growth and development from conception to maturity.* Boston: Little, Brown.)

Nursing Tip

"Catch-up" growth refers to the process by which a child who has been sick or malnourished and whose growth has slowed or stopped experiences a more rapid period of recovery as the body attempts to compensate.

deviate from the 50th percentile or middle measurement. A child whose weight is at the 75th percentile line is *one percentile above* the median. A child whose height is at the 25th percentile is *one percentile below* the median.
- A difference of two or more percentile levels between height and weight may suggest an underweight or overweight condition and prompts further investigation.
- Deviations of two or more percentile levels from an established growth pattern require further evaluation.

Developmental Screening. Developmental screening is a vital component of child health assessment. One widely used tool is the Denver II, a revision of the Denver Developmental Screening test (Fig. 15–5). This tool assesses the developmental status of children during the first 6 years of life in four categories: personal-social, fine motor-adaptive, language, and gross motor. It is *not* an intelligence test. Its purpose is to identify children who are unable to perform at a level comparable to their agemates. A low score merely indicates a need for further evaluation. It is designed for use by both professionals and paraprofessionals. Proper administration and interpretation will aid in developing an individualized plan of care for the child.

Influencing Factors

Growth and development are influenced by many factors, such as heredity, nationality, race, ordinal position in the family, sex, and environment. These factors are closely related and dependent on one another in their effect on growth and development. They make each person unique. If a child is ill, physically or emotionally, the developmental processes may be delayed.

Hereditary Traits. Characteristics derived from our ancestors are determined at the time of conception by countless genes within each chromosome. Each gene is made of a chemical substance called deoxyribonucleic acid (DNA), which plays an important part in determining inherited characteristics. Examples of these inherited traits are the color of eyes and hair and physical resemblances within families.

Nationality and Race. Many physical differences among people of various nationalities and races, who were formerly distinguished with ease, have become less apparent in our age of common environment and customs. For instance, one thinks of a person of Japanese origin as being of short stature. However, Japanese children living in the United States are comparable in height to other children in this country. Nevertheless, ethnic differences extend into many areas, including speech, food preferences, family structure, religious orientation, and code of conduct. The nurse should ascertain cultural beliefs and practices when collecting data for nursing assessment.

Ordinal Position in the Family. Whether the child is the youngest, middle, or oldest in the family has some bearing on growth and development. The youngest and middle children learn from their older sisters and brothers. However, motor development of the youngest may be prolonged if the child is babied by the others in the family. The only child or the oldest child may excel in language development because conversations are mainly with adults. These children are often subject to greater parental expectations.

Sex. The male infant often weighs more and is longer than the female. He grows and develops at a slightly different rate. Parents and relatives may treat boys differently from girls by providing "sex-appropriate" toys and play and by having different expectations of them. Current trends promote unisex activities in play and career development.

Environment. The physical condition of the newborn is influenced by the prenatal environment. The health of the mother at the time of conception and the amount and quality of her diet during pregnancy are important for proper fetal development. Infections or diseases may lead to malformations of the fetus. A healthy and strong newborn can easily adapt to its surroundings.

The home greatly influences the infant's physical and emotional growth and development. If a family is financially strained by an added member and the parents are unable to provide nourishing foods and suitable housing, the infant is directly affected. An uneducated mother may not know how to properly cook foods to preserve their nutritional value. Immunizations and other medical attention may be neglected. The baby senses tension within the family and is affected by it.

In contrast, when the surroundings are secure and stable, and the infant feels secure, wanted, and

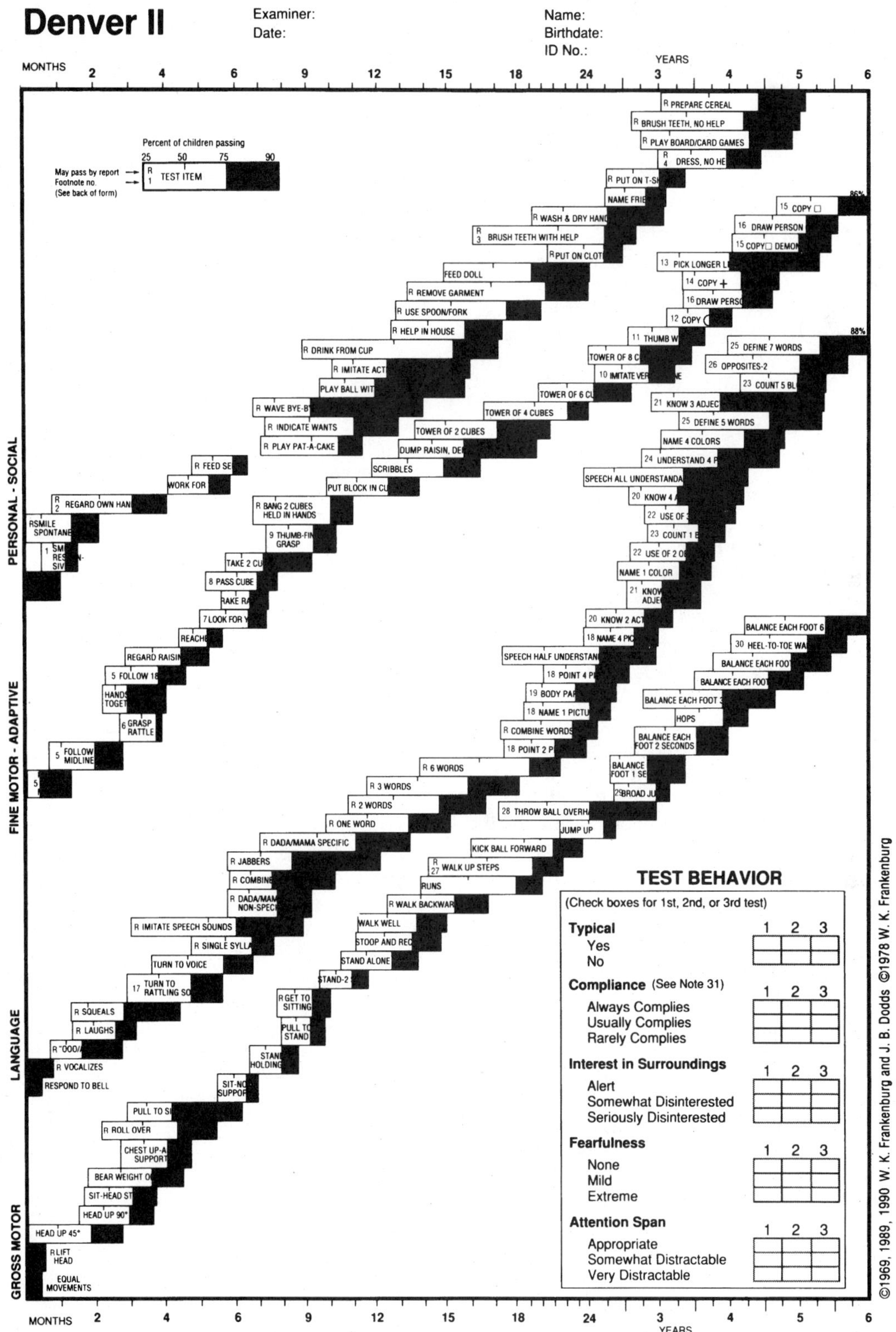

Figure 15–5. • Denver II. Denver Developmental Screening Test-II. (From Frankenburg, W. K., Dodds, J., Archer, P., Shapiro, H., & Bresnick, B. [1992]. The Denver II: A major revision and restandardization of the Denver Developmental Screening Test. *Pediatrics, 89,* 91.) Usually the physician or school nurse initiates the test, which can indicate developmental delays that may require early intervention.

Nursing Tip

"Different" does not mean "inferior."

loved, energies can be directed toward positive development. Most environments are neither completely positive nor completely negative but fall somewhere between the two extremes. Intelligence plays an important role in social and mental development. Potential intelligence is believed to be inherited but greatly affected by the environment.

The Family

The *family* has been defined in many different ways and fulfills many different purposes. Traditionally, the *nuclear,* or biologic, family has been the basic unit of structure in American society (mother, father, siblings). Today, many nuclear families do not share the same household because of single parenthood, divorce, and remarriage. Kinship lines have become blurred and fundamental changes are occurring in the family as it was once perceived. The *extended* family refers to three generations: grandparents, parents, and children. Because of an increasing life span, however, there are a greater number of living grandparents and great-grandparents, and the proportion of them living in the family home may increase. Table 15–1 lists various types of families and a description of each.

Table 15–1
VARIETIES OF FAMILY LIVING

Type of Family*	Comment
Nuclear	Traditional—husband, wife, children (natural or adopted)
Extended	Grandparents, parents, children, relatives
Single parent	Women or men establishing separate households through individual preference, divorce, death, illegitimacy, desertion
Foster parent	Parents who care for children who require parenting because of dysfunctional families, no families, or individual problems
Alternative	Communal family
Dual career	Both parents work because of desire or need
Blended	Remarriage of persons with children
Polygamous	More than one spouse
Homosexual	Two persons of the same sex who have adopted children or who have had children from a previous marriage
Cohabitation	Heterosexual or homosexual couples who live together but remain unmarried

*Not all may be legally sanctioned.

By far, the *interactions* of family unit members is most influential in the growth and development of the child. The nurse must understand the interaction of the family unit to affect a positive change that may be necessary to prevent or treat childhood illnesses. Some families have solid support systems and use available community resources to maintain health. Other families may lack support systems and require closer follow-up care and encouragement by the health team. Parenting is a learned behavior, often modeled by past experience and modified by acceptance of specific roles and responsibilities. A family that does not provide for the optimum physical, psychological, and emotional health of the children is called a *dysfunctional family.* A dysfunctional family does not necessarily imply that its members are not loving and caring. A dysfunctional family does not know how to be successful in their efforts and interactions and requires intervention.

Historically in middle-class families, the father was the breadwinner and the mother managed the home and raised the children. This trend has shifted. Because of changing economic conditions, both parents' earnings may be necessary to maintain the family's standard of living. In dual-career families, a father and mother are often absent for most of the day because of long commutes or the demands of the working environment. Both parents may share child care and domestic chores. The parents may have to transfer to different locations to maintain their careers. This decreases extended family support and makes it necessary for children to change schools frequently.

Divorce, separation, death, and pregnancy outside marriage create many one-parent families. The percentage of children living in single-parent families has more than doubled since the 1970s. Most single-wage families have an economic disadvantage, but families with women as the single wage earner often have considerably lower incomes than those with men. The problem of providing good

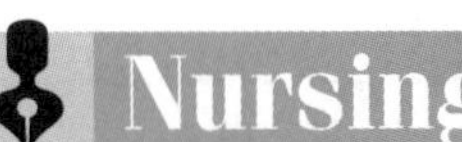

Acceptance of the child's value system and cultural beliefs will assist in positive nurse–child interactions.

Nursing Tip

Special care may be required to assist in the growth and development of infants who are blind or whose parents are chronically depressed.

affordable child care is a serious one for both dual-career families and single parents. Relatives and the noncustodial parent may assist in raising the child. Many single parents remarry, creating the *blended* family. The addition may be merely a stepfather or stepmother, or two families may unite. These family units must make many adjustments. To succeed, parents and children have to learn problem-solving techniques, communication skills, and flexibility.

A *family APGAR* first described by Smilkstein (1984) is a tool that can be used as a guide today to assess family functioning. This assessment is valuable in determining the approach to home care needs:

- **A***daptation.* How the family helps and shares resources
- **P***artnership.* Lines of communication and partnership in the family
- **G***rowth.* How responsibilities for growth and development of child are shared
- **A***ffection.* Overt and covert emotional interactions among family members
- **R***esolve.* How time, money, and space are allocated to prevent and solve problems

Questions concerning each of these areas should be posed and evaluated. The goal in family assessment is to enable the nurse to develop interventions that will aid the family to achieve a healthier adaptation to the child's health needs or problems.

The Family as Part of a Community. The term *community* is defined in many ways, but here it is used to refer to the immediate geographic area in which the family lives and interacts (e.g., "I come from the South Side"). Families are greatly influenced by the communities in which they reside. Nurses must understand the makeup of the community in which they work or to which the patient will return (Table 15–2). Assessment of the community is particularly important in creating discharge plans for families from various cultures. Their lives may be broadened or restricted, depending on the facilities of the community. A few factors to consider are housing, access to public transportation, city services, safety, and health care delivery. The nurse with her immediate access to the patient becomes an important liaison between various agencies addressing specific needs.

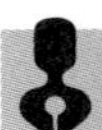

Nursing Tip

An infant hypersensitive to noise or touch needs the parent to understand the need for quiet surroundings. A chronically depressed parent may interpret fussiness or lack of smiling as rejection. Therefore an assessment of parent–child interaction is essential in the home, clinic, or hospital setting.

The Homeless Family. The homeless family with children is a modern-day problem that impacts the growth, development, and health of the child. Often support systems and financial resources are lacking and the school nurse or emergency room (ER) nurse may be the first to identify this family. Community referrals to provide shelter, food, education, and financial aid are primary needs that must be met before health teaching can be effective.

It is imperative that nurses take advantage of the strengths of the family while attending to its weaknesses. Nurses are in an excellent position to help the health professions to move toward truly contemporary models of family-centered care. The nuclear family of the past is no longer dominant. Pediatric nursing research and care must reflect this phenomenon.

Personality Development

Most people tend to equate personality with social attractiveness: "She has a lot of personality, and he has no personality"; or "There's an example of personality plus." The term *personality* is more broadly defined by psychologists. One definition states that personality is a "unique organization of characteristics that determine the individual's typical or recurrent pattern of behavior." No two persons are exactly alike. An individual's personality is the result of interaction between biologic and environmental heritages.

Although no one group of theories can explain all human behavior, each can make a useful contribution to it. Many experts have devoted their lives to understanding why children and families behave as they do. Some, called *systems theorists,* believe that everyone in the family or system is affected by each of its members. This theory focuses on the interre-

Table 15–2
CULTURAL INFLUENCES ON THE FAMILY

Cultural Group	Family and Kinship Structure	Communication	Health Beliefs and Practices	Family and Child Care Practices
Hispanics Mexican American	Family is an extensive network composed of nuclear and extended family members. Father is provider and decision maker; mother is family caretaker. Decisions made by father after discussion with older or extended family members. Divorce is uncommon. Out-of-wedlock relationships are common. Children are center of family life.	Eye contact may be considered rude. Looking at or admiring a baby without touching the child can bring about mal ojo (evil eye).	Health represents an equilibrium between hot and cold, wet and dry. An imbalance in these forces causes disease. Cold remedies used to treat hot diseases, and hot remedies used to treat cold diseases. Balance and harmony are accomplished through avoiding some foods and consuming others. Seek curandero, a folk healer, for treatment remedies and spiritual healing ceremonies. May combine advice from curandero with the antibiotics or other therapies from a physician. Resort to prayer or home remedies (remedias caseras) before seeking help from folk practitioner or physician. Often delay seeking medical attention and obtaining screening examinations and immunizations. Tend to have jobs with no health insurance. Mother unlikely to sign consent for child's health care without discussion with the father.	Delay breast-feeding until milk comes in. Feel stress and anger make milk bad and infant can become ill. Neutralize infant bowel when weaning from breast to bottle by feeding only anise tea for 24 hours. More likely to have children without prenatal or postnatal care. Mal ojo or evil eye is an illness that affects children and occurs when someone with special powers looks at or admires a child but does not touch or hold the child. A curandero can treat the child through massage and prayer. Wearing special amulets or charms can protect child from the evil eye. Practice of binding the umbilicus of the newborn is done to prevent bad air from entering the baby. Parent-child relationship is warm and nurturing. Parents are often quite permissive in respect to their child's behavior.
Puerto Rican	Extended and patriarchial family.	Bilingual—Spanish and English.	Avoid iron supplements because they are considered "hot" medication. Classify foods and medication as hot, cold, and cool. Classify foods as hot and cold.	Children viewed as gift from God. Children taught to obey and respect parents.
Cuban	Strong family ties, which continue as children grow into adulthood.	Bilingual—Spanish and English.	Health promotion important. Belief in biomedical model, although supernatural forces (evil eye) are thought to cause some illnesses that can be cured by ethnic treatments or magic spells. Amulets on a bracelet or necklace may be worn to ward off evil eye. Diet is high in fat, cholesterol, sugar, and fried foods.	Mother primary child caretaker. Plump babies and young children are idealized. School system assumes much of child rearing responsibilities.

Table 15–2
CULTURAL INFLUENCES ON THE FAMILY *(Continued)*

Cultural Group	Family and Kinship Structure	Communication	Health Beliefs and Practices	Family and Child Care Practices
Haitian	Extended family is important as support system. Males are the decision makers and direct caregivers.	Rely on native language.	Believe that God's will must prevail. Rely on folk foods and treatments for illness management. Believe in hot-cold theory. Avoid eggplant, okra, tomatoes, black pepper, cold drinks, milk, rice, bananas, and fish during pregnancy. White foods believed to cause increased vaginal discharge in pregnancy.	Usually breast-feed and believe strong emotions affect quality of milk.
African American	Family of great importance. Many headed by mother in absence of father. In two-parent families egalitarian structure is most prominent. Not uncommon to have extended family living together and older members assisting with child care.		Wife or mother source of advice on medical ailments and when to seek medical treatment. Many believe illness comes from germs. Others believe illness can be due to natural causes (e.g., exposure to wind, rain) or unnatural causes (witchcraft, voodoo, punishment for sin). Poverty and lack of health insurance lead to inadequate health care. Many rely on folk remedies passed on from one generation to next before seeking care from physician. "Granny" or "old lady" is woman in community with knowledge of herbs to treat common illnesses. Spiritualist is someone with special gift from God to heal certain diseases. Prayer is commonly used in response to illness. A diet high in fat and sodium is considered an indication of well-being. Many individuals have lactose intolerance; therefore milk may be inadequate from diets of pregnant women and children.	Begin cereal consumption in infancy at early age. Culture least likely to breast-feed. Strong religious orientation (Baptist predominant). Use belly band or binder to protect newborn's umbilicus from dirt, injury, or hernias. Strict parenting practices are encouraged and meant to develop effective coping abilities in children to prepare them for the presence of racial discrimination they are likely to encounter in society. High respect for authority figures, strong work ethic, and emphasis on achievement. Expression of emotions by males and females is encouraged. Children are expected to use their time wisely, assume responsibilities at an early age, and participate in decision making. Physical forms of discipline often used.

Table continued on following page

latedness of the various persons as opposed to an analysis of an individual in the group. Nurses using systems theory focus on caring for the child by caring for the whole family. They see the family as protector, educator, resource, and health provider for the child. In turn, they see the child's health as having an impact on each member of the family as a whole.

Table 15–2
CULTURAL INFLUENCES ON THE FAMILY *(Continued)*

Cultural Group	Family and Kinship Structure	Communication	Health Beliefs and Practices	Family and Child Care Practices
Asian Vietnamese	Patriarchal in structure. Extended families predominant. Primogeniture (first son inherits family's worth).	Avoid confrontations with health care professionals, perhaps answering questions with what they believe the other person wants to hear. May consider health practitioners to be loud and boisterous. Do not touch children on the head. The head is considered sacred because it is where one's consciousness lies. Eye contact may be considered rude. Beckoning with one's hand or finger is the gesture used to beckon dogs and is considered insulting when used with people.	Forces of yang (light, heat, or dryness) and yin (darkness, cold, and wetness) influence the balance and harmony of person's state of health. Seek shaman, a physician-priest, for treatment remedies and spiritual healing ceremonies. Evil spirits enter the body through open orifices such as ears, nose, and mouth, causing infection. If the opening is covered, the bad spirits cannot enter and the illness is cured. Health represents an equilibrium between hot and cold, wet and dry. An imbalance in these forces causes disease.	May delay breast-feeding for 3 days because colostrum is considered "dirty." Breast-feeding low among immigrant Southeast Asians. Breast-feed boys longer than girls. Delay introduction of solid foods up to 18 months. Diet may consist of breast milk and rice water; diet is low in calcium and iron. Excessive consumption of cow's milk (up to eight bottles a day) in the second year of life is common, as is the continual use of the bottle instead of the cup into the third year of life. Avoid praising an infant for fear that a spirit may overhear the praise and be tempted to steal the baby. Parents have an approach to child rearing that is more controlling, achievement oriented, and more encouraging of independence than that of white parents. Balance and harmony are accomplished.
Chinese	Needs of the family come before the needs of the individual. Children repay their parents' love and care by providing for them in their old age. Extended family important, with elderly respected and cared for in the homes of the adult children. Frown upon interracial marriages.	Silence does not necessarily indicate the end of a conversation; it may mean the speaker wishes the listener to consider the content before the speaker continues.	Forces of yang (light, heat, or dryness) and yin (darkness, cold, and wetness) influence the balance and harmony of person's state of health. Health is a state of physical and spiritual harmony with nature. Prevention is key to healthy living. Traditional Chinese medicine is sought first before Western medical services.	Primary responsibility for child care belongs to mother. Grandparents may be asked to assist in child care. Cultural healing practices can cause visible bruising or injury to child's skin. Important for children to exhibit self-control. Children socialized not to challenge authority. Pregnancy means woman has "happiness in her body."

Many see human development as a composite of various theories. Abraham Maslow's hierarchy of needs is depicted in Figure 15–6, and the developmental theories of Erik Erikson, Sigmund Freud, Lawrence Kohlberg, Harry Stack Sullivan, and Jean Piaget are presented in Table 15–3. Other theorists are briefly contrasted within appropriate chapters devoted to specific age groups. Theories provide a

Table 15–2

CULTURAL INFLUENCES ON THE FAMILY *(Continued)*

Cultural Group	Family and Kinship Structure	Communication	Health Beliefs and Practices	Family and Child Care Practices
Chinese *(Continued)*			Use acupuncture, herbal medicines, massage, cupping, skin scraping, and moxibustion as therapies to restore yin and yang. Avoid eating soy sauce during pregnancy because believed to darken baby's skin, shellfish believed to cause allergies in baby, and iron supplements believed to harden bones and lead to difficult delivery.	Many breast-feed until child is 4 to 5 years old. Jade is often worn in form of a charm to keep the child safe.
Japanese	Value social group harmony over individual needs and autonomy. Extended and patriarchal family structure. Women traditionally passive.	Silence does not necessarily indicate the end of a conversation; it may mean the speaker wishes the listener to consider the content before the speaker continues. Handshakes are acceptable; pat on the back is not acceptable. Direct eye contact considered a lack of respect.	When in pain, patients stoically withstand discomfort. Women labor in silence. After delivery long periods of rest and recuperation are encouraged. Use natural herbs—Kampō medicine. Use both Western and traditional Oriental healing methods.	Mother has primary responsibility for child rearing and assuring their success in school. Mother may sleep with her child. Colostrum not fed to babies. Only half of all breast-fed babies continue after 1 month of age.
Hmong	Extended family structure.	Do not touch children on the head. The head is considered sacred because it is where one's consciousness lies.	Seek shaman, a physician-priest, for treatment remedies and spiritual healing ceremonies.	Avoid praising an infant for fear that a spirit may overhear the praise and be tempted to steal the baby. Babies may wear colorful hats so that they are disguised as "flowers" and the spirits will not notice them.
European American White Protestant	Nuclear family highly valued. Divorce and remarriage common practice. Goal of individual often seen as more important than goal of the family. Success is measured in terms of financial wealth and status in society.	Pat children on head to show affection or approval. Uncomfortable with periods of silence. Expect people to look you in the eye when they are speaking to you. Avoiding eye contact can be considered an indication that a person is lying.	Rely on modern medicine and health care professionals to treat illness.	Authoritative style of parenting. Children encouraged to value individual differences, the future rather than the present, material well-being, and competition and to consider many options when making decisions. Adults readily praise infant's and child's behavior and appearance. Self-reliance is highly valued.

Table continued on following page

framework for the practitioner; however, humans are not a gathering of isolated parts, even though these parts need to be dissected for investigative purposes.

Cognitive Development. *Cognition* (*cognoscere,* "to know") refers to one's intellectual ability. Children are born with inherited potential, but it must be developed. "It requires opportunities for explo-

Table 15–2

CULTURAL INFLUENCES ON THE FAMILY *(Continued)*

Cultural Group	Family and Kinship Structure	Communication	Health Beliefs and Practices	Family and Child Care Practices
Irish American	Strong family bonds. Emphasis placed on well-being of family, not individual member.	May communicate with flowery and sometimes exaggerated words. May be overly verbose in descriptions of their condition.	Health comes when person is goal oriented and nurtures a strong religious faith. Health is maintained with a great deal of sleep combined with fresh air, exercise, and balanced diet. Home remedies or treatments are first resort to treat illness. Medical assistance should be sought only in cases of emergency.	Strict followers of the church typically Protestant or Catholic.
Italian American	Traditional family roles. Father is head of household, and mother is heart of the household, although mother has powerful sway over internal family matters. Children are valued members and are showered with love and affection. Family a source of comfort and pride for individual members. Members maintain close contact or close proximity with nuclear and extended family. Divorce is uncommon in traditional families. Large family size is attributed to adherence to Catholic beliefs and traditions.	Complaining loudly and making demands are often rewarded with attention.	Health is maintained by strong religious influence (Catholic primarily). Faith in God and saints will see them through illness. Beliefs about the cause of illness have been found to include winds and currents that bear diseases, contagion or contamination, heredity, supernatural or human causes, and psychosomatic explanations.	Important to keep child warm in cold weather, stay out of drafts, and not go outside with wet hair. Maintain health with a nutritious diet of fruit, vegetables, pasta, hard cheese, and wine. Children introduced to water-wine mixture at young age.
Native American	Grandparents retain important role in parenting their grandchildren. Extended family network valued. Many Native Americans have married into other tribes and other ethnic groups.	Silence is critical during interactions. Strong need to sit quietly and think before responding to questions. Eye contact may be considered rude. May consider health practitioners to be loud and boisterous.	Wellness exists when there is harmony in body, mind, and spirit. Seek shaman, a physician-priest, for treatment remedies and spiritual healing ceremonies. High incidence of lactose intolerance. Eat nonperishable food items because of lack of refrigeration. Beans main source of protein. Frequent problems with obesity and alcoholism. Often feel that Western medicine places too much emphasis on medications. A holistic approach to healing is valued. Alcoholism is major problem for many families.	High rate of breast-feeding. Mothers retain primary responsibility for child rearing and discipline.

From Bowden, V., Dickey, S., & Greenberg, C. (1998). *Children and their families: The Continuum of care.* Philadelphia: Saunders.

ration that are neither too easy nor too hard" (Levine, Corey, & Crocker, 1992). The development of logical thinking and conceptual understanding is a complex process. One outstanding authority on cognitive development was Piaget, a Swiss psychologist. He proposed that intellectual maturity is attained through four orderly and distinct stages of development, all of which are interrelated. These stages include *sensorimotor* (up to 2 years), *preoperational* (2–7 years), *concrete operations* (7–11 years), and *formal operations* (11–16 years). The ages are approximate, and each stage builds on the preceding one.

Piaget believed that intelligence consists of interaction and coping with the environment. Babies begin their interaction by reflex response. As they grow older, their use of symbolism (particularly language) increases. Gradually they acquire a here-and-now orientation (concrete operations) and finally a fully abstract comprehension of the world (formal operations). In Table 15–4, Piaget's theory is related to feeding and nutrition. It is a good example of how a knowledge of development can help one understand the behavior of a child at a particular time.

Moral Development. Lawrence Kohlberg, a childhood theorist, suggests that moral development in children is sequential. His theories on moral development are based on Piaget's cognitive development investigations. He describes three levels with two stages at each level. The three levels are *preconventional, conventional,* and *postconventional.* In the preconventional stage (4–7 years), children try to be obedient to their parents for fear of punishment. During the conventional phase (7–11 years), children show conformity and loyalty, and they focus on obeying rules. In the postconventional level (12 years and older), *moral values* are developed to solve complex problems. There is an emphasis on the conscience of the individual within the society. Although rules are still important, changing them to meet the needs of a culture is considered.

Nursing Implications

An understanding of growth and development, including its predictable nature and individual variation, has value in the nursing process. Such knowledge is the basis of the nurse's anticipatory guidance of parents. For example, the nurse who knows when the infant is likely to crawl can, at the appropriate age, expand teaching on safety precautions. The nurse also incorporates these precautions into nursing care plans in the hospital. *Age-appropriate care cannot be administered without an understanding of growth and development.*

While explaining various aspects of child care to families, the nurse stresses the importance of individual differences. Parents tend to compare their children's development and behavior with those of other children and with information in popular magazine articles. This may relieve their anxiety or cause them to impose impossible expectations and standards. In addition, many parents had poor role models who influenced their own experiences as children. Lack of knowledge about parenting can be recognized by the nurse and suitable interventions begun.

The nurse who understands that each child is born with an individual temperament and "style of behavior" can help frustrated parents to cope with a newborn who has difficulty settling into the new environment. Specific parameters can be used to

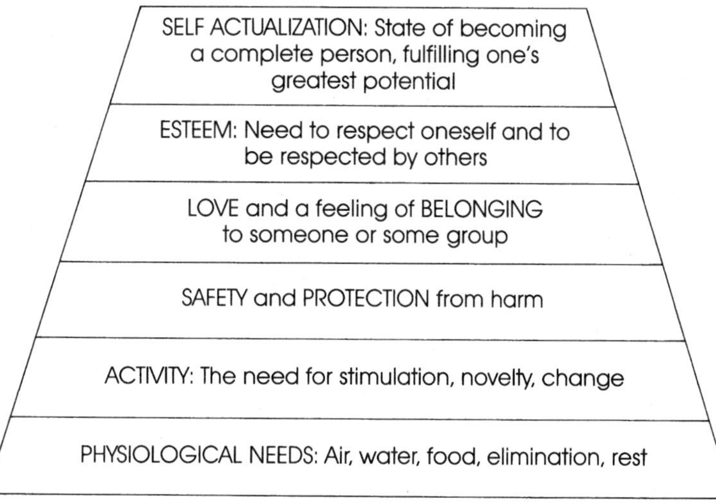

Figure 15–6. • Maslow's hierarchy of basic needs. The needs at the bottom of the pyramid must be met before one can fulfill needs at the next higher level.

Table 15–3
COMPARISON OF THE DEVELOPMENTAL THEORIES OF ERIKSON, FREUD, KOHLBERG, SULLIVAN, AND PIAGET

Developmental Period	Erikson	Freud	Kohlberg	Sullivan	Piaget
Infancy	Trust/mistrust Getting Tolerating frustration in small doses Recognizing mother as distinct from others and self	Orality—understanding the world by exploring with the mouth		Security, patterns of emotional response, organization of sensation	Sensorimotor stage (birth to 2 yr)—At birth, responses limited to reflexes; begins to relate to outside events; concerned by sensations and actions that affect self directly
Early childhood	Autonomy/shame and doubt Trying out own powers of speech Beginning acceptance of reality versus pleasure principle	Anality—learning to give and take		Mastery of space and objects	Preoperational (2–7 yr)—Child is still egocentric; thinks everyone sees world as self does
Late childhood	Initiative/guilt Questioning Exploring own body and environment Differentiation of sexes	Phallic/oedipal phase—Becoming aware of self as sexual being	Preconventional or premoral morality—Rules are absolute; breaking rules results in punishment (4–7 yr)	Speech and conscious need for playmates, interpersonal communication	Perceptual (4–7 yr)—Capable of some reasoning but can concentrate on only one aspect of a situation at a time
School age	Industry/inferiority Learning to win recognition by producing things Exploring, collecting Learning to relate to own sex	Latency—Focusing on peer relations, learning to live in groups and to achieve	Conventional morality—Rules are created for the benefit of all; adhering to rules is the right thing to do (7–11 yr)	Chumship, one-to-one relationship, self-esteem, compassion (homosexuality)	Concrete operations (7–11 yr)—Reasoning is logical but limited to own experience; understands cause and effect
Adolescence	Identity/role diffusion Moving toward heterosexuality Selecting vocation Beginning separation from family Integrating personality (e.g., altruism)	Genitality	Principled morality (autonomous stage) (12 yr on)—Acceptance of right or wrong on basis of own perceptions of world and personal conscience	Capacity to love, empathy, partnership (heterosexuality)	Formal operational stage (11–16 yr)—acquires ability to develop abstract concepts for self; oriented to problem solving

determine whether an infant is merely on an individual timetable or whether the infant varies from normal.

The nurse must also recognize when to intervene to prevent disease and/or accidents. For example, a brief visit with a caretaker may reveal that the child's immunizations are not up-to-date. A review of the characteristics of a 2-year-old with a teenage mother may prevent the ingestion of poisons. Complications of the newborn can be avoided by advising the expectant mother to avoid alcohol and cigarettes. Other threats to health may likewise be anticipated. Knowing that specific diseases are prevalent in certain age groups, the nurse maintains a high level of suspicion when interacting with these patients. This approach, based on developmental knowledge, experience, and effective communication, helps to ensure a higher level of family care. Finally, the nurse must understand how to

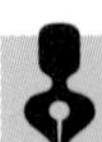

Nursing Tip

The nursing approach should be governed by the developmental level of the child, and family values, offering choices and active participation when appropriate.

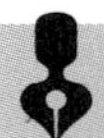

Nursing Tip

Arnold Gesell, founder of the Clinic for Child Development at Yale University, was the first to study children scientifically over a period of time. He coined the term *child development.*

provide nursing care to children of various ages so that their physical, mental, emotional, and spiritual development is enhanced according to their specific needs and comprehension.

The Growth and Development of a Parent

Erikson's stages of child development demonstrate the various tasks that need to be mastered at each age for the child to achieve optimum maturity. Each stage builds on the successful completion of the previous stage. Achievement of the tasks of childhood do not occur in isolation. Parents must *interact* appropriately to assist the child to achieve successfully at his or her developmental level. For example, if the parent constructs a school project for a child, the child will not achieve a sense of industry. If the parent does not accept a positive attitude toward the pregnancy and attempts to abort unsuccessfully, the parent may become overprotective or abusive to the newborn infant and bonding will not occur. Table 15–5 shows the task of the parent that relates to the child's developmental task and some suggestions for nursing interventions that can assist in the growth and development of a parent and a child.

Parents should be guided not to attempt to prevent frustration in the lives of their children. Childhood experiences in dealing with challenges and disappointments prepares the child to function independently in adulthood. Parents should encourage a child to deal with successes and failures, provide socially acceptable outlets, and intervene only if the frustrations become overwhelming. The parent's task is to provide the child with skills and tools appropriate at each age level to deal with events. Current tips concerning parenting skills can be accessed on computer via www.iamyourchild.org.

Table 15–4
PIAGET'S THEORY OF COGNITIVE DEVELOPMENT IN RELATION TO FEEDING AND NUTRITION

Developmental Period	Cognitive Characteristics	Relationships to Feeding and Nutrition
Sensorimotor (Birth–2 yr)	Progression from newborn with automatic reflexes to intentional interaction with the environment and the beginning use of symbols	Progression is made from sucking and rooting reflexes to the acquisition of self-feeding skills Food is used primarily to satisfy hunger, as a medium to explore the environment and to practice fine motor skills
Preoperational (2–7 yr)	Thought processes become internalized; they are unsystematic and intuitive Use of symbols increases Reasoning is based on appearances and happenstance Approach to classification is functional and unsystematic Child's world is viewed egocentrically	Eating becomes less the center of attention than social, language, and cognitive growth Food is described by color, shape, and quantity, but there is limited ability to classify food into "groups" Foods tend to be classed as "like" and "don't like" Child can identify food as "good for you," but reasons are unknown or mistaken
Concrete operations (7–11 yr)	Child can focus on several aspects of a situation simultaneously Cause-effect reasoning becomes more rational and systematic Ability to classify, reclassify, and generalize emerges Decrease in egocentrism permits child to take another's view	Child begins to realize that nutritious food has a positive effect on growth and health but has limited understanding of how or why this occurs Mealtimes take on a social significance Expanding environment increases the opportunities for, and influences on, food selection (peer influence rises)
Formal operations (11–16 yr)	Hypothetic and abstract thought expand Understanding of scientific and theoretic processes deepens	The concept of nutrients from food functioning at physiologic and biochemical levels can be understood Conflicts in making food choices may be realized (knowledge of nutritious food versus preferences and nonnutritive influences)

From Mahan, L. K., & Escott-Stump, S. (1996). *Krause's food, nutrition and diet therapy* (9th ed.). Philadelphia: Saunders.

Table 15–5
THE GROWTH AND DEVELOPMENT OF A PARENT

Stage of Child's Development	Child's Tasks	Parent's Task	Nursing Intervention
First prenatal trimester	Growth	Develop attitude toward new baby: Happy about baby? Parent of one handicapped child? Unwed mother? These factors and others will affect developing attitude of the mother	Develop positive attitude in both parents concerning expected birth of child. Use referrals and agencies as needed
Second prenatal trimester	Growth	Mother focuses on infant because of fetal movements felt. Parents picture what baby will look like and what future it will have, etc.	Parents' focus is on baby care and needs and providing physical environment for expected infant. Therefore, information concerning care of the newborn should be given at this time.
Third prenatal trimester	Growth	Mother feels large. Attention focuses on how fetus is going to get out	Detailed information should be presented at this time concerning the birth processes, preparation for birth, breastfeeding, and care of sibling at home
Birth	Adjust to external environment	Elicit positive responses from child and respond by meeting child's need for food and closeness. If parents receive only negative responses (e.g., sleepy baby, crying baby, difficult feeder, congenital anomaly), then development of the parent will be inhibited	Encourage early touch, feeding, etc. Explain behavior and appearance of newborn to allay fears. Help parents to identify positive responses. (Utilize infant's reflexes, such as grasp reflex, to identify a positive response by placing mother's finger into infant's hand)
Infant	Develop trust	Learn "cues" presented by infant to determine individual needs of infant	Help parents assess and interpret needs of infant (avoid feelings of helplessness or incompetence). Do not let in-laws take over parental tasks. Help parents cope with problems such as colic, etc.
Toddler	Autonomy	Try to accept the pattern of growth and development. Accept some loss of control but maintain some limits for safety	Help parents to cope with transient independence of child, e.g., allow child to go on tricycle but don't yell "don't fall" or anxiety will be radiated
Preschool	Initiative	Learn to separate from child	Help parents show standards but "let go" so child can develop some independence. A preschool experience may be helpful
School age	Industry	Accept importance of child's peers. Parents must learn to accept some rejection from child at times Patience is needed to allow child to do for himself even if it takes longer. Do not ***do*** the school project ***for*** the child. Provide chores for child appropriate to his age level	Help parents to understand that child is developing his or her own limits and self-discipline. Be there to guide child, but don't constantly intrude. Help child get results from his or her own efforts at performance
Teenager	Establish identity Accept pubertal changes Develop abstract reasoning Decide on career Investigate lifestyles Control feelings	Parents must learn to let child live his or her own life and not expect total control over child. Expect, at times, to be discredited by teenager. Expect differences in opinion and respect them. Guide but don't push	Help parents to adjust to changing role and relationship with teenager (e.g., as child develops his or her own identify, he may become a Democrat if parents are Republican). Expose child to varied career fields and life experiences. Help child to understand emerging emotions and feelings brought about by puberty

From Leifer, G. (1982). *Principles and techniques in pediatric nursing* (4th ed.). Philadelphia: Saunders.

NUTRITION

The Child's Nutritional Heritage

Good nutrition begins before conception. Nutritional needs during pregnancy are discussed in Chapter 4. The dependent child is fed for many years by adults whose eating habits may be based on misinformation, income level, folklore, fads, or religious, cultural, and ethnic preferences. Table 15–6 describes some common, selected food patterns of various cultures found in the United States. Many families are poor, others have inadequate knowledge of how to prepare foods, and many rely on convenience foods to save time.

Some families do not consider food a priority in the home. Optimum nutrition is essential for the child to reach his or her growth potential. Lack of adequate nutrition can lead to mental retardation. The obese child may be subject to decreased motor skills and peer rejection, leading to low self-esteem. The nurse is in a position to identify children at risk and to help families to modify eating habits to ensure proper nutrition. *An important resource for the nurse is the nutritionist in the Community or on the staff of the health agency where the nurse is employed.*

Family Nutrition

The U.S. Departments of Agriculture and Health and Human Services' guidelines for good eating are shown in the food pyramid (Chapter 4, p. 65). They are intended to help Americans to make informed decisions about what they eat. *Families who practice such principles are educating their children by good*

Table 15–6
CULTURALLY DIVERSE FOOD PATTERNS OF AMERICANS

Culture	Historical Dietary Pattern*
African American	All meats, fish, and chicken; pork often consumed (spareribs, bacon, and sausage); vegetables cooked in salt pork for long periods of time; grits and cornbread muffins; some lactose intolerance. Popular vegetables include collard greens, beet greens, and sweet potatoes
Chinese American	Rich in vegetables (bean sprouts, broccoli, bamboo shoots, and mushrooms). Vegetables cooked until crisp; meat consumed in small portions with other food. Soy sauce, tofu, peanut butter; limited milk and cheese; fish baked with native spices; soups with egg, meat, and vegetables. Tea is China's national beverage. Rice is staple of diet
Jewish American	Diet varies according to whether family is Orthodox, Reform, or Conservative. For Orthodox family, food must be kosher (clean); meat is soaked in salt water to remove blood; only meat eaten is that of divided hoofed animals that chew a cud; fish without scales (shellfish) and pork are prohibited; milk and meat cannot be combined. Favorites are gefilte fish, lox (smoked salmon), herring, eggs, bagels, cream cheese, and matzo
Laotian American	Numerous varieties of freshwater fish and shellfish (eaten fresh, dried, or salted); pork, beef, chicken, rabbit, often mixed with vegetables and spices; eggs, peanuts, black-eyed peas; vegetables eaten raw, as juice, or cooked with meat or fish and preserved by drying or pickling; sticky rice, rice or bean thread noodles, and legumes often used in desserts; soybean drink, sugar cane drink, tea, and coconut juice. Popular seasonings include padek, chilies, curry, tamarind, and red and black pepper
Italian American	All meats, fish, and chicken, including cold cuts (salami, mortadella) and Italian pork sausage; pasta (staple of diet), breads, olive oil, wine, cheese, and all varieties of fruits and vegetables
Japanese American	Fish and seafood (fresh, smoked, and raw) and beef. Food is cut into small portions. Principal fruit is nasi, which tastes much like a pear. Many vegetables are eaten, such as seaweed, bamboo shoots, onions, beans, and dried mushrooms (shitake); enjoy pickled vegetables. Rice is national staple. Beverages include tea and sake. Little cheese, milk, butter, or cream is consumed. Chief cooking fat is soybean oil or rice oil
Mexican American	Chicken, pork chops, wieners, cold cuts, hamburger, eggs (used frequently), beans (eaten mashed or refried with lard), potatoes (basic item, usually fried), chilies, fresh tomatoes, corn (maize—often used as basic grain), tortillas, packaged cereals; little milk because of lactose intolerance
Native American Indian	Acorn flour, a staple food made into mush or bread; salmon, fresh or dried; other varieties of fish, deer, duck, geese, and other small game; nuts such as buckeye and hazel; wild berries, seeds, and roots
Puerto Rican American	Meat cooked in stews; poultry, pork, fish, dried beans or peas mixed with rice; milk in combination with coffee (cafe con leche), variety of fruits, starchy vegetables (plantains, cassava, sweet potatoes), salad, soft drinks
Vietnamese American	Pork—most common meat; meats cut into small pieces and fried, boiled, or steamed; fish—all types of freshwater and saltwater fish and shellfish, often fried and dipped in fish sauce; eggs, soybeans, legumes, and wide variety of fruits and vegetables; rice often eaten with every meal; seasonings including oyster sauce, soy sauce, monosodium glutamate, ginger, garlic, nuoc mam sauce; tea, coffee, soft drinks, soybean milk

*More diverse eating patterns occur as future generations of a culture become assimilated.
Data from Mahan, L. K., & Escott-Stump, S. (1996). *Krause's food, nutrition and diet therapy* (9th ed.). Philadelphia: Saunders, and other sources.

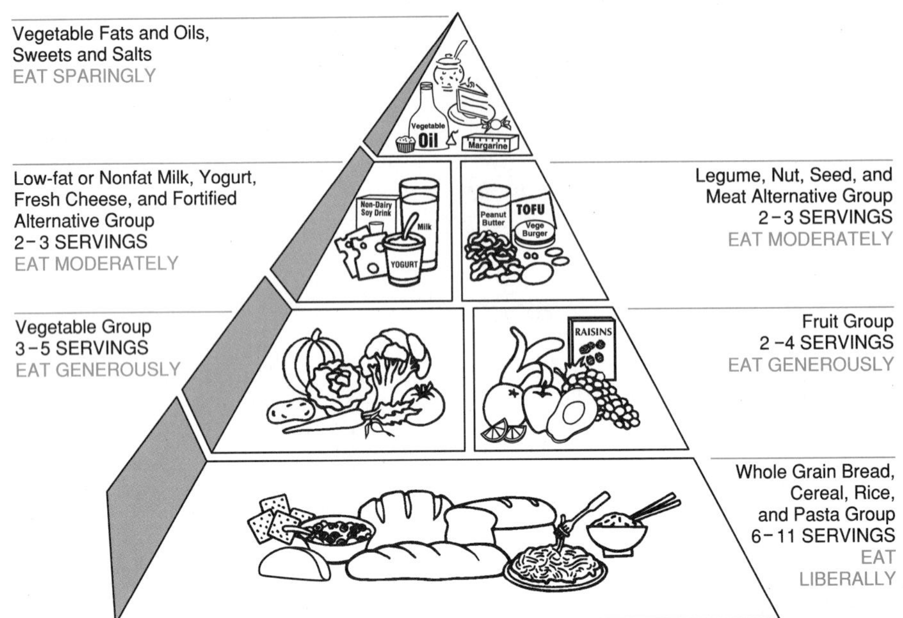

Figure 15–7. • The Vegetarian Food Pyramid. A food pyramid designed for vegetarians will promote compliance when teaching parents and children concerning recommended dietary intakes for a balanced diet that will promote growth and development. (Courtesy of the Health Connection, 55 W Oak Ridge Drive, Hagerstown, MD 21740. Reprinted with permission.)

example. Many families are vegetarian and the use of teaching tools that respect the dietary limitations will encourage compliance. Figure 15–7 demonstrates a modification of the standard food pyramid that is distributed by the U.S. Department of Agriculture and Health and Human Services. This food pyramid is directed to vegetarian families and applies to children as young as 2 years of age. The nurse should assess restricted foods in the vegetarian diet and ensure that the diet is adequate in protein, vitamins, and minerals to promote growth and development in children. Children on vegetarian diets often consume large amounts of high-fiber foods. Foods high in fiber cause increased losses of calcium, zinc, magnesium, and iron in the stool. A diet containing meat, poultry, or fortified foods lessens this nutrient deficiency.

There are different kinds of fiber contained in foods (Box 15–4). The water-soluble fiber found in oats, apples, and citrus fruits delays intestinal transit and decrease serum cholesterol. The water-insoluble fiber found in whole-grain breads, wheat bran, and some cereals accelerate intestinal transit and slow starch digestion.

A well-balanced diet supplies all the essential nutrients in the amounts that we need. Food provides heat and energy, builds and repairs tissues, and regulates body processes. A given food is a mixture of elements, such as minerals (e.g., calcium, phosphorus, sodium, iron), compounds (carbohy-

BOX 15–4

HIGH-FIBER FOODS FOR RELIEF OF MILD CONSTIPATION IN CHILDREN OVER 12 MONTHS OF AGE

Type of Food	Service Size	Example*
Cereals, bread	1 oz	Raisin Bran®, Grapenuts®, Shredded Wheat®, Bran Chex®
	1 slice	Whole-grain bread
	1 med.	Bran muffin
	2½″ square	Corn bread
Fruits	½ cup	Cooked prunes
	½ cup	Spinach
	1 med	Corn-on-the-cob
Meat substitute	½ cup	Beans (baked, black, garbanzo, kidney, lima, pinto, lentil)

*All products indicated are registered trademarks of their respective companies.

Adapted from Baker, S. (1994, Summer). Introduce Fruits, Vegetables, and Grains but Don't Overdo High Fiber Foods. *Pediatric Basics,* #69.

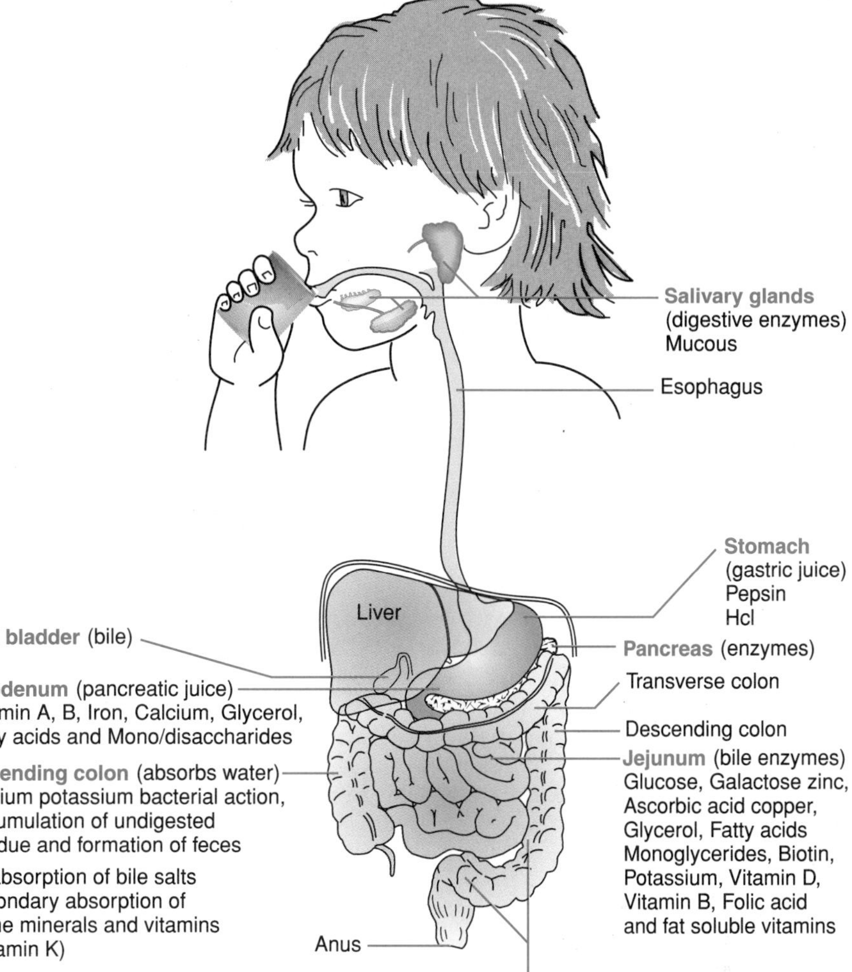

Figure 15–8. • Nutrient digestion. The sites of absorption of major nutrients are shown in this illustration. Most nutrient absorption occurs in the duodenum and jejunum of the small intestine. Most water absorption occurs in the large intestine. Absorption of nutrients depends on adequate secretion of digestive enzymes, normal motility, and normal villi on the mucosal surface of the intestines. Portal circulation, lymphatic circulation, and hormones also play a role in the digestion and absorption of nutrients.

drates, fats, proteins, some vitamins), and water. The body needs approximately 50 nutrients, which it absorbs at various sites (Fig. 15–8). Table 15–7 specifies the recommended dietary allowances for energy and protein for children.

Children are susceptible to nutritional deficiencies because they are growing and developing. Infants require more calories, protein, minerals, and vitamins in proportion to their weight than do adults. Fluid requirements are also higher for infants. Eating a *variety* of foods selected from the

Nursing Tip

The American Academy of Pediatrics recommends 0.5 g of fiber per kg of body weight in childhood, gradually increasing to adult levels of 20 to 35 g per day by the end of adolescence. High-fiber foods can fill the small stomach capacity and provide few of the nutrients and calories needed by the active, growing child.

Table 15–7

DIETARY ALLOWANCES FOR ENERGY AND RECOMMENDED PROTEIN FOR CHILDREN

	Kilocalories		Grams of Protein		
Age	**Daily**	**Per Kilogram (kg)**	**Per Centimeter (cm)**	**Daily**	**Per Kilogram**
1–3	1300	102	14.4	16	1.2
4–6	1800	90	16.0	24	1.1
7–10	2000	70	15.2	28	1.0

Reprinted with permission from *Recommended Dietary Allowances: 10th Edition.* Copyright 1989 by the National Academy of Sciences. Courtesy of the National Academy Press, Washington, D.C.

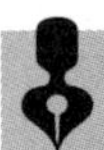

Nursing Tip

Raw fruits that contain seeds, or some raw vegetables and nuts may not be appropriate foods for infants and young children because of the risk of choking. Beans and vegetables should be well cooked.

basic food groups ensures good health for children. The *amount* and *size* of portions are important in maintaining a reasonable weight. *There are no known advantages to consuming excessive amounts of any nutrients, and there are risks for overdoses.*

Nutritional Care Plan

The nutritional care plan can be used in the hospital, home, or outpatient department. Parts of the care plan may already have been collected by other professionals, so the nurse should refer to the patient's chart for pertinent data. The care plan provides information and stores it in one place. It can also be put on a computer for easy retrieval.

Nutrition and Health

Digestion. The digestive system of the newborn is immature and functions minimally during the first 3 months. Saliva is minimal; hydrochloric acid and renin in the stomach and trypsin aid in the digestion of milk. Amylase, a pancreatic enzyme, and lipase are not in adequate quantity before 4 months of age, and so complex carbohydrates and fats cannot be digested effectively. Excess fiber intake in the young infant results in loose bulky stools. The liver's ability to function is limited in the first year of life. The teeth are not present for chewing before 6 to 8 months of age. The physiology of digestion, therefore, is the basis for food introduction in the first year of life. Breast milk or iron-fortified formula are the food of choice for the first 6 months to 1 year of life. Introduction of baby food prior to 5 to 6 months of age is not for the purpose of nutritional gain. Overnutrition and its link to obesity in adults have been explored. The effects of childhood nutrition on adult health and illness patterns, such as heart disease, have been established.

Nutrition and Illness

Therapeutic diets, such as the diabetic diet, are well established in medical care. Some foods can promote dental caries and other contain protective fiber that are known to prevent some diseases. Atherosclerosis can be prevented by starting healthy dietary patterns in childhood. However, restrictive diets are not advised for infants and young children. Fat and cholesterol are needed for calories and the development of the central nervous system. The sodium content of baby foods have been decreased because the average diet contains adequate sodium, and developing a taste for salty foods may predispose to hypertension later in life. Some food additives, such as aspartame, an artificial sweetener, may be harmful to children with phenylketonuria. Food additives that prolong the shelf life of foods and food dyes that make food look more attractive should be minimized in the child's diet. Fast-food chains, often depended on by working parents and preferred by adolescents, make available to the consumer the nutrient content of their foods served. The caloric content of the menu often depends on the foods selected and the toppings added. Therefore, a "salad bar" is not necessarily synonymous with a low-calorie meal.

Height and weight should be plotted on a growth chart at each clinic visit to enable early identification of health problems related to dietary intake. The weight or tricep skinfold thickness greater than the 85th percentile or below the 3rd percentile indicates a need for further evaluation. Often the role of the grandparents in providing a diet that may lead to obesity needs to be addressed because

BOX 15–5

METHODS TO REDUCE CHOLESTEROL IN SCHOOL-AGE CHILDREN

- Exercise more with your children.
- Provide fresh fruit and vegetables rather than empty calories such as found in doughnuts and store-bought pastries.
- Decrease trips to fast-food restaurants.
- Switch to low-fat foods; use vegetable oil cooking sprays in place of butter; bake or broil foods instead of frying.
- If you have a family history of heart disease, have child's as well as adult's levels of cholesterol tested.
- Seek advice of nutritionist.

principles of good nutrition that were adhered to twenty or thirty years ago may not currently be valid. Concern is expressed over the level of cholesterol in children. Methods to reduce cholesterol in families are listed in Box 15–5. The National Cholesterol Education Program's recommendations are cited in Box 15–6.

Dietary supplements, formulas, and nutritional support techniques for preterm babies, children with cancer, and those with long-term disorders, such as cystic fibrosis, have become sophisticated and are successfully utilized. Total parenteral nutrition allows the physician to choose preparations ranging from amino acids and intravenous fats to complete multivitamins. Total parenteral nutrition and enteral feedings allow care of children who need nutritional support to be at home, thus greatly enhancing the quality of life.

In the 1990s, an oral rehydration solution (ORS) used by Third World populations for treating acute diarrhea in children has gained acceptance and is now produced and distributed by the World Health

BOX 15–6

NATIONAL CHOLESTEROL EVALUATION PROGRAM (NCEP) RECOMMENDATIONS FOR DETECTING AND MANAGING HYPERCHOLESTEROLEMIA IN CHILDREN AND ADOLESCENTS

The NCEP made recommendations for managing hypercholesterolemia to be applied to adolescents and children over the age of about 2 years.

For the general population of children and adolescents in the United States, NCEP recommended that eating patterns be adopted to meet the following criteria:

- Nutritionally adequate, varied diet
- Adequate energy intake to support growth and development and maintain appropriate body weight
- Saturated fat—less than 10% of total calories
- Total fat—an average of no more than 30%
- Dietary cholesterol—less than 300 mg/day

To implement these patterns means involving the entire community—parents, in the selection and preparation of food; schools, by modification of school food service; health care clinics, by providing health education; government, by mandating improvement of food labeling; and the food industry, by developing low-saturated-fat, low-fat foods appealing to children.

NCEP also aims to identify and treat individual children and adolescents who have hypercholesterolemia and a family history of premature cardiovascular disease, or whose parents have hypercholesterolemia. For this group, NCEP recommends:

- Blood cholesterol screening of children and adolescents whose parents or grandparents, at 55 yr or younger, were found to have coronary atherosclerosis; suffered myocardial infarction, peripheral vascular disease, cerebrovascular disease, or sudden death; or underwent invasive cardiac therapy (balloon angioplasty or coronary artery bypass surgery)
- Blood cholesterol screening of offspring of a parent with a blood cholesterol of 240 mg/dl or greater
- Appropriate levels for total cholesterol and low-density-lipoprotein (LDL) cholesterol. For children with levels above these, dietary change is recommended:

Category	Total Cholesterol	LDL Cholesterol
Acceptable	<170 mg/dl	<110 mg/dl
Borderline	170–199 mg/dl	110–129 mg/dl
High	≥200 mg/dl	≥130 mg/dl

If after 6 months to 1 year of dietary therapy there is insufficient blood lipid lowering, drug therapy can be considered in children over 10 years of age.

Adapted from Mahan, L. K., & Escott-Stump, S. (1996). *Krause's food, nutrition, and diet therapy* (9th ed.). Philadelphia: Saunders.

Table 15–8
NURSING INTERVENTIONS FOR MEETING THE NUTRITIONAL NEEDS OF CHILDREN

Age	Comment	Nursing Interventions
Newborns and infants	High energy maintenance because of immature systems (e.g., heat loss)	Assist mother with breastfeeding Assist family with bottle feeding Teach formula preparation
	Immature digestive system	Place infant on right side following feeding Burp infant frequently Observe infant for tolerance to formula
	Nutrient requirements related to body size	Consider vitamin C and D supplementation Anticipate iron deficiencies (particularly in preterm newborns)
	Need for additional nutrients, satiety	Introduce solids when age-appropriate, at about six months, starting with rice cereal, which is the least allergenic. Fruits and then vegetables may be added one at a time in one or two week intervals to allow time to observe for adverse responses. (consider variety, portions, texture) Instruct parents not to add salt or sugar to baby foods to avoid high sodium and calorie intake.
	Danger of choking decreases as swallowing matures	Anticipate allergies. As teething progresses, junior or chopped foods can be substituted for strained food. Explain selection and makeup of soy-based formulas if prescribed
	Prevention of dental decay	Encourage use of fluorides (after six mo of age) If fluoride content of community water supply is less than 0.6 ppm Encourage weaning as appropriate to prevent bottle-mouth caries Rinse infant's mouth after feedings
	Continued requirements for basic food groups	Assess educational and financial needs of family Utilize supplemental food programs (e.g., Women, Infants, and Children [WIC] program)
Toddlers and preschoolers	Slower rate of growth; although body needs are still high, energy requirements decrease	Emphasize that from a nutritional viewpoint, child can regulate intake if appropriate foods are offered
	Picky eater	Provide nutritional snacks Respect need for independence; do not force child to eat Use colored straws; offer cheese, yogurt (not fortified with vitamin D) if milk refused; add milk to potatoes Offer meat in bite-sized portions Add fruit to cereal Reduce sweets Invite playmate to lunch Relax at meals Promote harmony
Children of school age	Growth rate that continues to be slow but steady until puberty, some spurts and plateaus	Maintain education in nutrition Introduce new foods when eating out Assist child in preparing nutritious lunches Provide fruits and raw vegetables for snacks when competition exists for meals Encourage parents to include children in meal planning, preparation, and food shopping

Organization. It is composed mainly of electrolytes, glucose, and water. Health workers are able to teach parents how to save the lives of their infants by using this simple solution. Medicine women, the respected leaders of some tribes, are being incorporated into the educational process. One example of a commercial preparation available in the United States is Pedialyte.

A cereal-based oral rehydrating solution can be made by mixing ½ to 1 cup of infant rice cereal, 2 cups water, and ¼ tsp. table salt (Bartholmey, 1994). Often the older child who refuses the oral rehydrating solution can be offered a saltine cracker with half-strength apple juice.

Feeding the Healthy Child

Table 15–8 specifies the nursing interventions that help to meet the nutritional needs of children, from infancy to adolescence.

The Infant. Infants, in proportion to their weight, require more calories, protein, minerals, and vitamins than adults do. Their fluid require-

Table 15–8
NURSING INTERVENTIONS FOR MEETING THE NUTRITIONAL NEEDS OF CHILDREN *(Continued)*

Age	Comment	Nursing Interventions
Adolescent girls	Girls' caloric requirements less than those of boys Concern with body image may lead to anorexia or bulimia	Emphasize that skipping meals can lead to decrease in essential nutrients Encourage physical exercise to maintain body weight Educate as to proper nutrients to maintain body weight (e.g., skim milk, fruits) Avoid high-calorie fast foods Consider emotional components related to foods (difficulty with peers, need for love and approval, and so on)
	Athletic activities	See interventions for adolescent boys
	Oral contraceptives	Explain that oral contraceptives increase requirements for several nutrients (folic acid, vitamin B_6, ascorbic acid)
	Adolescent pregnancy	Educate client concerning increased nutritional needs to complete growth and nourish fetus
Adolescent boys	Concern with body image, bodybuilding	Instruct as to proper nutrition for sports Avoid quack claims Promote proper conditioning, well-balanced diet (increased calories), proper hydration without supplements—salt tablets unnecessary
	Overnutrition	Explain that this can lead to adult obesity Teach clients in order to lose weight: Eat a variety of foods low in calories and high in nutrients Eat less fat and fewer fatty foods Eat less sugar and fewer sweets Drink less alcohol Eat more fruits, vegetables, whole grains Increase physical activity

ments are also high. Breast milk is excellent, and a nursing mother may continue this even when her baby is hospitalized. The nurse stresses that the mother should avoid fatigue because it affects milk production. Breast milk can be manually expressed and refrigerated at the hospital, then given in the mother's absence.

Some babies are unable to tolerate milk because of intestinal bleeding, allergy, or other negative reactions. Many milk substitutes are available for therapeutic use. Among these are soybean mixtures (such as ProSobee and Isomil) for patients with milk-protein sensitivity. Most products come in dry and liquid forms, and parents need to be made aware of what concentrations the doctor intends.

The nurse needs to be aware of the problems of underfeeding and overfeeding infants. Underfeeding is suggested by restlessness, crying, and failure to gain weight. Overfeeding is manifested by such symptoms as regurgitation, mild diarrhea, and too rapid a weight gain. Diets high in fat delay gastric emptying and cause abdominal distention. Diets too high in carbohydrates may cause distention, flatus, and excessive weight gain. Constipation may be the result of too much fat or protein or a deficiency in bulk. Increased amounts of cereals, vegetables, and fruits can often correct this problem.

Most infants naturally adapt to a schedule of three meals a day by the 1st year of life. At this time, the appetite fluctuates as the growth rate slows somewhat. The child may not be interested in eating. Spills are frequent. At 1 year of age, children cannot manipulate a spoon, but hand-to-mouth coordination is good enough that they enjoy holding a piece of toast while the nurse assists. In the hospital, children in highchairs wear jacket restraints. The nurse remains in constant attendance. Developmental advancements that change eating patterns are explained to parents to prevent feeding difficulties.

The Toddler. By the end of the 2nd year, toddlers can feed themselves. This is important to developing a sense of independence. The toddler may be rebellious at times, and food may be pushed away

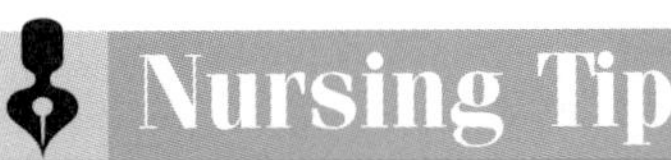

Whole milk should not be introduced before 1 year of age.

or completely refused. Toddlers benefit most from the caretakers' presence at mealtime. Feeding difficulties may result from anxieties of parents and lack of time.

The Preschool Child. Preschoolers and toddlers like finger foods. Dawdling is common in this age group, as is regression. Preschoolers in general are more vulnerable to protein-calorie deficiencies; their younger siblings receive priority at home, and older brothers and sisters receive the benefits of school lunch programs. The nurse recognizes this problem and offers nourishing snacks, such as dry cereal out of the box, graham crackers, fruit juices, milk, and ice cream.

The School-Age Child. School-age children need food from the basic food groups, but in increased quantities to meet energy requirements. Their attitudes toward food are unpredictable. Intake of protein, calcium, vitamin A, and ascorbic acid tends to be low. The intake of sweets decreases the appetite and provides empty calories.

The Adolescent. During the adolescent years, nutrition is particularly important. Teenagers are growing rapidly and expending large amounts of energy. Food needs are great. The nurse attempts to involve the teenager in selecting foods that are nutritious and appetizing. This may be done by reviewing choices made on the daily menu. Sometimes it helps to stress how important good nutrition is to physical appearance and fitness. The need for peer approval is at its height during adolescence, and food fads and skipped meals may result in malnutrition, even in families of means. Fatigue is a common complaint at this age. If it is accompanied by a lack of appetite and irritability, anemia should be suspected.

Table 15–9 reviews some of the community programs available to children.

Feeding the Ill Child

Children in the hospital are in the process of growing. Well-nourished children:

- Nearly always show steady gains in weight and height
- Are alert
- Have shiny hair
- Have no fatigue circles beneath the eyes
- Have a skin color within normal limits
- Have a flat abdomen
- Have an erect posture
- Have well-developed muscles
- Have mouth and gum mucous membranes that are firm and pink, not swollen or bleeding
- Have no mouth or tongue lesions
- Have teeth that are erupting on schedule
- Have a generally good appetite and eliminate regularly
- Sleep well at night, have energy and vitality, and are not irritable

This picture changes somewhat during illness, but the child who is basically well nourished can easily be distinguished from one who is malnourished.

Many hospitalized children have poor appetites. This may be due to age, the nature of the illness, the type of diet, sudden exposure to strange foods and strange environment, reaction to hospitalization, and the degree of satisfaction obtained during mealtimes. The child may also refuse to eat in an attempt to manipulate the parents, particularly if lack of appetite was a concern in the past.

The nurse observes the patient's tray to determine if the food is of the right consistency. Does the child have any teeth? Do lesions in the mouth prevent chewing? Can the child use a knife and fork? Children with bandaged limbs or those receiving intravenous fluids require assistance. The size of servings is important. One should serve less than one hopes will be eaten. A tablespoonful of food (not heaping) for each year of age is a good guide to follow. More is given if the patient appears hungry. One item at a time is placed before small children who feed themselves, so that they will not become overwhelmed. The nurse avoids showing personal dislikes because negative attitudes are easily transmitted. The nurse proceeds slowly with unfamiliar children to determine their level of mastery. Food is served warm, and sufficient time is allotted. Sweet drinks and snacks should not be served just before meals. Treatments such as chest physiotherapy should not be scheduled immediately following a meal.

Infants who are placed on "nothing by mouth" (NPO) should be provided with a pacifier to meet their sucking needs. Some children prefer to use their thumb for non-nutritive sucking (Fig. 15–9).

Food–Drug Interactions

Whenever a child is ill and treated with prescription medications, the nurse is responsible for monitoring drug–drug interactions, drug–food interactions, and drug–environment interactions. Drug–drug interactions involve a knowledge of the side effects of each drug prescribed. Drug–environment interactions involves the effects of a drug on the response of the patient to his or her environment.

Table 15–9
NUTRITION RESOURCES WITHIN THE COMMUNITY

Program	Eligibility	Program Content
Maternal and child health	Pregnant women and children of low-income families	Free or reduced price Improved health care services for mothers and children at a clinic affiliated with a specific hospital Free vitamins, immunizations
Special Supplemental Food Program for Women, Infants, and Children (WIC)	Individuals at nutritional risk: Pregnant women up to 6 mo postpartum Nursing mothers up to 1 yr Infants and children up to age 5 identified as being at nutritional risk: must live in geographically determined low-income area and be eligible for reduced price or free medical care; must be certified by WIC staff member Periodic assessment of risk status	Provision of supplemental foods: >1 yr: iron-fortified formula and infant cereals, fruit juice high in vitamin C Women and children: whole fluid milk or cheese, eggs, iron-fortified hot or cold cereal, fruit or vegetable high in vitamin C Food distribution: directly from participating agency, via voucher system, or home delivery Nutrition education is an integral part of program
Program for Children with Special Health Needs (formerly Crippled Children's Services)	Children with developmental disabilities	Under Title V Free nutrition counseling Funds available for equipment or supplies
Child Care Food Program (CCFP)	Preschool children in nonprofit facilities, Head Start, day care, afterschool facilities	Year-round program Cash in lieu of commodities available
School Breakfast Program	All public and nonprofit private schools Public and licensed nonprofit residential child care institutions For needy children or those who travel great distances to school	As set by U.S. Dept of Agriculture Nonprofit breakfasts meeting nutritional standards Served free or at a reduced price to children from low-income families Costs to schools reimbursed by federal funds
National School Lunch Program	All public and nonprofit private school pupils of high-school grade or under, some residential institutions and temporary shelters	As set by U.S. Dept of Agriculture Nonprofit nutritious lunches offered free or at a reduced price to those who cannot pay Lunch follows specified guidelines and meets one-third or more of daily dietary allowance Schools reimbursed by federal and state funds
Summer Food Service Programs for children	Public agency-sponsored preschool and school-age recreation programs, summer camps	Free lunch to children in summer programs Federal monetary support
Special Milk Program	Schools, child care centers, summer camps	Federal reimbursement for all or part of the milk served
Food Distribution (donated foods)	Supplemental programs for mothers and infants	Distribution of surplus food to eligible persons, schools, institutions
Food Stamps	Eligibility based on total income, expenses, number being fed in household Each applicant is considered on an individual basis	Client should apply at local Food Stamp Office within the community, presenting wage slips, sources of income, rent receipts, utility bills Food Stamps are given free of charge, depending on eligibility needs Used like cash to purchase food at authorized food stores (nonfood items and alcoholic beverages not allowed)

For example, certain antibiotics have photosensitivity as a side effect. Nurses armed with this knowledge advise the patient or parent to avoid prolonged exposure to sunlight. Drug–food interactions are often overlooked, but can impact treatment and/or growth and development of the child. A selected group of interactions is reviewed in Table 15–10 to encourage the nurse to remain alert to food–drug interactions while dealing with the sick child.

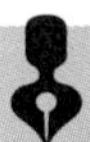

Nursing Tip

Foods containing essential minerals such as iron, zinc, and calcium should be combined with citrus, fish, or poultry to enhance absorption of the minerals. Vitamin D and lactose sugars also enhance mineral absorption in the body.

The Teeth

Deciduous Teeth. The development of the 20 deciduous, or baby, teeth begins at about the 5th month of intrauterine life. The health and diet of the expectant mother affect their soundness. Primary teeth erupt during the first 2½ years of life. It is a normal process and is generally accompanied by little or no discomfort. Wide individual differences in tooth eruption occur in normal, healthy infants. Occasionally a baby is born with teeth, but the neonatal tooth is removed to prevent the possibility of choking if it should fall out. A delay in teething is significant if other forms of immaturity or illness are present. The physician evaluates the process of teething during the baby's regular health checkups.

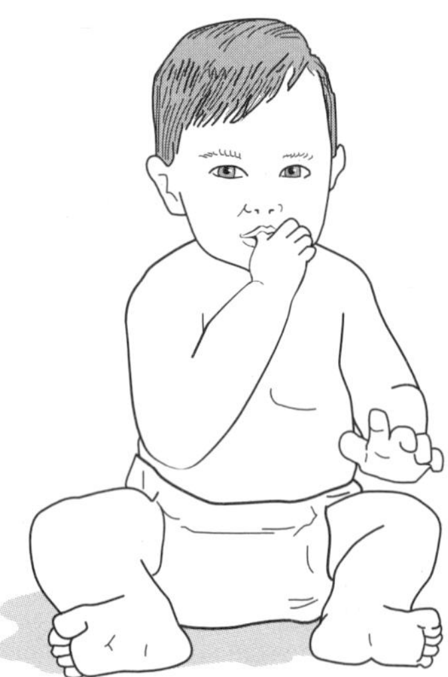

Figure 15–9. • Nonnutritive sucking. Nonnutritive sucking involving the finger or a pacifier is common in infants under one year of age and fulfills the needs of the oral phase of development. Generally, malocclusion from nonnutritive sucking will not be a problem if the habit is discontinued before age 3. *Frequency, duration,* and *intensity* of sucking influence the occurrence of malocclusion associated with finger or pacifier use. Behavior modification can help to decrease thumb sucking (e.g., a dental appliance or substances placed on the finger). The child needs to be physically and emotionally "ready" to discontinue thumbsucking and appropriate rewards should be predetermined.

The first tooth generally appears at about the 6th or 7th month. The 1-year-old has about six teeth, four above and two below. The order in which the teeth appear is almost always the same (Fig. 15–10). They are shed in about the same order in which they appear, that is, lower central incisors first, and so forth. Although the Academy of Pediatric Dentistry recommends that the first dental visit occur by 1 year, the majority of children begin seeing the dentist at about 3 years of age. Tetracycline antibiotics stain developing teeth a yellowish-brown and are to be avoided during pregnancy and in the first 8 years of life.

Parents and nurses must not neglect baby teeth, thinking that they will eventually be lost. A 2-year-old who wants to brush his teeth when Mommy does is encouraged to do so. The deciduous teeth serve not only in the digestive process but also in the development of the jaw. When the deciduous teeth are lost early because of neglect, the permanent teeth become poorly aligned. The nurse checks that all patients 3 years of age and older have toothbrushes. Children sometimes need to be reminded of oral hygiene at bedtime.

Permanent Teeth. The 32 permanent teeth develop just before birth and during the 1st year of life. They do not erupt through the gums, however, until the 6th year. Nutrition and general health during the 1st year of life affect the formation of permanent teeth. This process is not completed until the wisdom teeth appear at about the age of 18 to 23 years. The first permanent teeth do not replace any of the deciduous teeth but appear behind the deciduous molars. They are important teeth because the whole denture develops around them. Cavities in them are frequently neglected because they are mistaken for baby teeth. The most common site of decay in children is the fissures of the molar teeth. These areas can be protected by the professional application of plastic sealants.

Oral Care in Health and Illness. Good dental care begins with proper diet that supplies adequate nutrients while the teeth are developing in the jaws, especially during the prenatal period and the 1st year. The many essential elements found in milk include calcium, phosphorus, vitamins A and B complex, and protein. Vitamin D, the sunshine

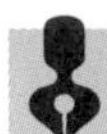

Nursing Tip

To assess the number of teeth a child under 2 years is expected to have, use the formula: Age in Months – 6.

Table 15–10
SELECTED FOOD–DRUG INTERACTIONS

Drug and Nutrient	Interaction	Nursing Intervention
Anticonvulsants and folic acid	Dilantin and mysoline can cause a folic acid deficiency. Folic acid supplements can decrease effectiveness of these drugs	Check lab results of folic acid levels. Report to doctor any patient use of over the counter (OTC) nonprescription folic acid supplements
and vitamin D	Dilantin and phenobarbital can cause vitamin D deficiency that affects calcium absorption needed for bone growth	Monitor lab serum calcium levels. Teach need for diet high in calcium and vitamin D
Cephalosporins and vitamin K	Cefotan, Cefobid, Moxam can cause vitamin K deficiency by destroying intestinal flora that produce the vitamin	Monitor prothrombin time. Observe for signs and symptoms of increased bleeding tendencies
Digoxin preparations and magnesium	Digoxin increases magnesium excretion. Deficiency in magnesium can cause drug toxicity	Monitor lab magnesium levels. Teach adolescents to avoid alcohol
Diuretics and vitamin B_1	Loop diuretics can increase excretion of vitamin B_1 causing a deficiency	Report signs of muscle weakness, tenderness, fatigue, depression, and edema
Isoniazid preparations and vitamin B_6	Anti-TB medications can inhibit absorption of vitamin B_6	Monitor closely for signs of peripheral neuropathy. Teach adolescents to avoid alcohol
Accutane and vitamin A	Iso Retinoin combines with vitamin A to cause vitamin A toxicity	Teach adolescents on this acne medication to avoid vitamins containing vitamin A. Monitor for headaches, hair loss and fissured skin
Lithium products and sodium	Lithium toxicity can occur if sodium is low. Lithium malabsorption can occur with high sodium intake	Teach adolescents on lithium to maintain normal sodium intake in their diets and avoid foods such as chips
Methotrexate products and folic acid	Antineoplastic drugs can decrease folic acid absorption	Monitor and report signs of anemia
Pentamidine and folic acid	Some drugs used for HIV-positive patients can cause folic acid deficiency	Monitor and report signs of anemia
Pyrimethamine and folic acid	Patients treated for toxoplasmosis with this drug can develop folic acid deficiency	Monitor and report signs of anemia
Septra-Bactrim and folic acid	These drugs restrict the enzyme necessary for folic acid utilization	Monitor for signs of anemia and compliance with OTC supplements

Adapted from Cerrato, P. (1993, June). OTC interactions, vitamins and minerals. *RN, 56*(9). Copyright © 1993 Medical Economics, Montvale, NJ. Reprinted by permission.

vitamin, and vitamin C, found in citrus fruits, are also valuable. Dietary practices influence the development of cavities (Table 15–11), and parents are encouraged to limit the *frequency* of sugar intake.

In the past, total carbohydrate consumption was thought to be the most important dietary consideration for dental health. Today more attention is given to the frequency with which sweets are eaten and how long they stick to the teeth. Sticky retentive foods have more caries (cavity) potential than do sugared drinks that are quickly cleared from the mouth. Oral care after eating sticky foods is recommended. Foods that can be recommended as snacks include cheese, peanuts, milk, sugarless gum, and raw vegetables. Items to be avoided include sugared gum, dried fruits, sugared soft drinks, cakes, and candy.

Of most importance in preventing caries is the administration of fluoride by mouth after 6 months of age. Ideally, fluorides may be present naturally in the water supply or may be added to it. The fluoride content of city water or prepared formula may decrease the need for fluoride supplements. When necessary, systemic fluorides can be offered until the last permanent tooth erupts at about the age of 13 years. Many fluoride preparations are available, often incorporated with vitamins. These tablets are obtained by prescription and should not be interchanged among children of various ages, as too much fluoride may cause the teeth to become "mottled" *(Fluorosis)*. Fluoride may also be applied directly to the teeth by the dentist.

Another aspect of tooth care is the prevention of *bottle-mouth caries (nursing caries syndrome)*. This

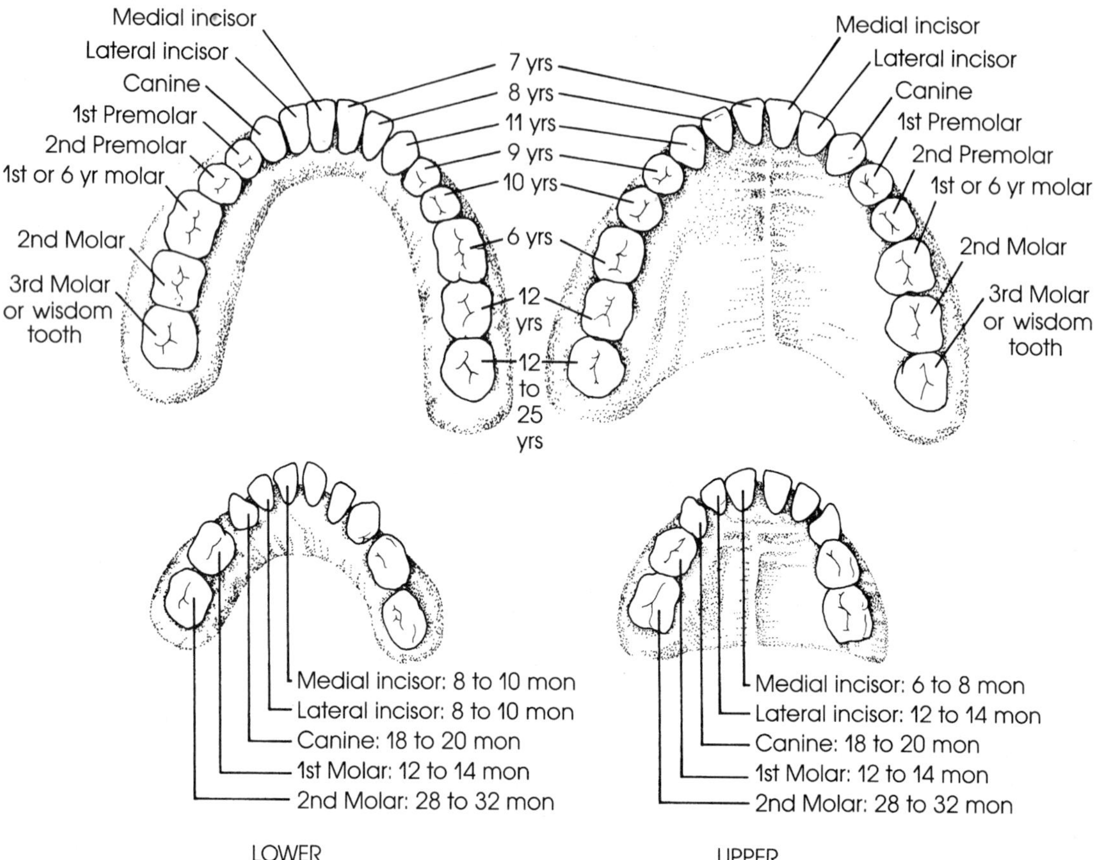

Figure 15–10. • Permanent and deciduous teeth and age of eruption.

Table 15–11
DEVELOPMENTAL DENTAL HYGIENE

Age	Dental Hygiene Practice
1st year of life	A clean wash cloth can be used by parents to wipe the teeth; no toothpaste necessary (baby may not like foaming action or taste and the fluoride in the toothpaste should not be swallowed). Child is not put to bed with bottle of milk or juices. If baby must have a bottle, water is used
2–3 yr	Parents introduce soft brush and toothpaste. Only a pea-sized amount of toothpaste is used to minimize fluoride ingestion
3–6 yr	Deciduous teeth erupt, and toward end of this period, baby teeth start to exfoliate (fall out). Parents assist children and remind them to brush and floss until at least 8 years of age. Small, soft toothbrush is used. Bedtime routine of brushing is established, as salivary flow rates slow during sleep, reducing natural protective mechanisms. Parents are advised to brush for the child at least once a day and to clean teeth that are in contact with each other with dental floss. Number of sweets eaten per day is monitored
6–12 yr	First permanent molars appear. The pits and fissures of molars make them primary site for caries. Sealants (plastic coating) professionally applied to molars provide a mechanical barrier against bacteria. Parents continue with fluorides, flossing, reducing *frequency* of exposure to carbohydrates. Adolescent gingivitis (*gingi,* "gum," and *itis,* "inflammation of") characterized by redness, swelling, and bleeding is common in children and adolescents and may be aggravated by hormonal changes at puberty. Motivating the adolescent to assume responsibility for dental care may be complicated by rebellion against authority and some incapacity to appreciate long-term consequences. Topical fluorides and fluoride toothpastes are available. Orthodontic treatments place adolescent at high risk for gingivitis and caries around appliances or braces. Mouth protectors should be used to prevent dental injuries from contact sports

Data from Griffen, A., & Goepferd, S. (1991). Preventive oral health care for the infant, child and adolescent. *Pediatric Clinics of North America, 38.*

occurs when an infant is put to bed with a bottle of milk or sweetened juice. Sugar pools within the oral cavity, causing severe decay. It is seen most often in children between 18 months and 3 years of age. Eliminating the bedtime bottle or substituting water is recommended.

The maintenance of good oral health is an integral portion of comprehensive care for a sick or disabled pediatric patient. Education, prevention, and referral in the home, school, or hospital setting must be part of the child's plan of care. Untreated dental caries or malposition of erupting teeth can cause periodontal disease in later years if not treated promptly. Delayed or early eruption of teeth can be indicative of some endocrine disorders or other pathology and should be recorded and reported. Parents and caretakers should avoid "tasting" baby food fed to infants and young children as the transmission of acid producing bacteria from their mouths can be passed on to the food or feeding utensils and contribute to tooth decay in the infant. Regular toothbrushing can start with tooth eruption. Children should brush before bedtime (Fig. 15–11) because the protective bacteriocidal effects of saliva decrease during sleep and bacterial growth can cause tooth decay.

Parents and children should be educated concerning the care of the toothbrush in order to provide maximum effectiveness of the tooth brushing activity:

- Replace toothbrush every 3 months
- Replace toothbrush after a viral illness
- Avoid rinsing bristles in hot water
- Do not use a closed container for toothbrush storage
- Avoid sharing toothbrushes among children

Dental flossing should be done with an up-and-down motion. A back-and-forth "sawing" motion can cause injury to gingival tissues. Children need assistance and supervision with flossing until at least 8 years of age. The proper size toothbrush will aid in developing good toothbrushing technique.

Trauma to the teeth occurs often in school-age children. Appropriate protective devices can prevent injury during sports activities. If a primary tooth is knocked out (avulsed) due to trauma, the child should be referred to a dentist for a "spacer" that will maintain tooth alignment until the permanent tooth erupts. If a permanent tooth is avulsed due to trauma, the tooth should be immersed in milk and brought with the child to the dentist for immediate care. Open wounds to oral tissues may require tetanus prophylaxis or antibiotics. All tooth fractures should be referred to a dentist for evaluation and treatment.

Dental problems that occur often with adolescents include puberty gingivitis; gingivitis associated with oral contraceptive use; drug related gingivitis, and hyperplastic gingivitis associated with orthodontic therapy. Temporomandibular joint problems (TMJ) and malocclusion due to missing teeth require dental referral. Orthodontic appliances such as fixed braces can trap plaque and food and increase tooth decay. Meticulous oral hygiene, brushing, flossing and fluoride applications are part of comprehensive orthodontic care.

A team approach to dental care for the child receiving chemotherapy or radiation therapy includes the dentist, doctor, nurse, parent, and patient. Brushing and flossing when the platelet count is over 20,000/mm^3 or using moist gauze when platelet count is under 20,000/mm^3 is advised to prevent infection and bleeding. The use of chlorhexidine may be prescribed to reduce oral lesions.

Disabled children can master independent toothbrushing by modifying the toothbrush. Using padded tongue depressors to visualize the oral cavity and an aspirating catheter attached to the toothbrush and connected to a suction machine can assist in providing dental care for a severely disabled child.

PLAY

Play is the business of children. Observing the child at play can assist in assessing growth and development and understanding the child's relationship with family members. Any plan of care for a hospitalized child of any age should include a play activity that will either encourage growth and development or encourage expression of thoughts and feelings. Playrooms in the hospital pediatric unit can be used for children who are not communicable. Medications and treatments should not be carried out in the playroom setting. Play can also be therapeutic, assisting in the recovery process. An example of *therapeutic play* is the game of having the child "blow out" the light of a flashlight as if it were a candle, to promote deep breathing. Table 15–12 reviews age-appropriate play behaviors.

Nursing Tip

When a tooth is "knocked out" or avulsed traumatically, the tooth should be gently cleansed of obvious dirt under running water or saline and placed in milk until dental care is obtained.

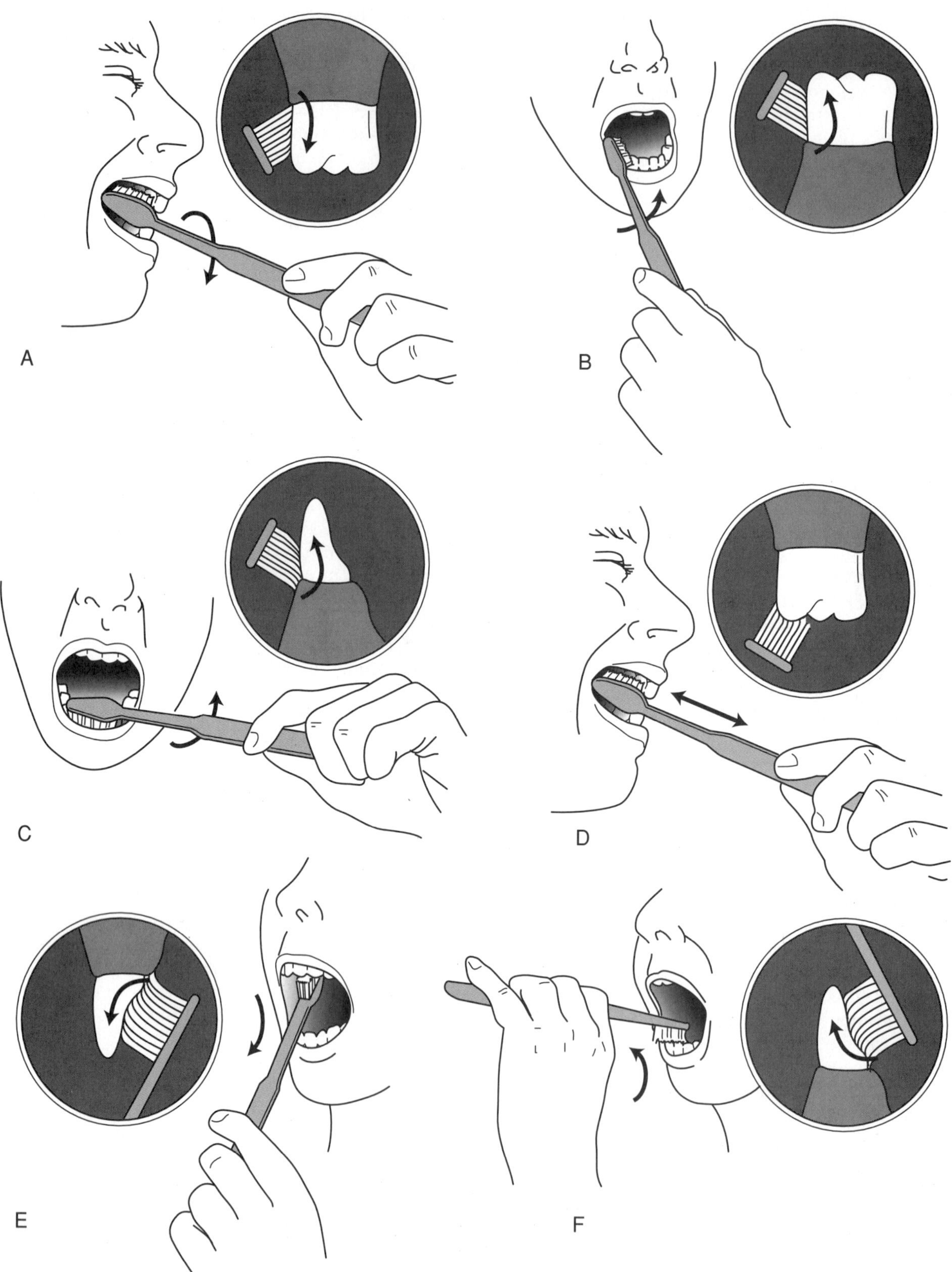

Figure 15–11. • Mechanical and chemical plaque control. The Bass technique showing the placement of the bristles and toothbrush at 45° angle to the long axis of the teeth and the back and forth vibratory brushing actions. **A,** Place brush where teeth and gums meet. **B,** Keep brush where teeth and gums meet. **C,** Use short, careful strokes. **D,** Use same method on inside surfaces. **E,** Brush up and down. **F,** Keep strokes short.

Table 15–12
DEVELOPMENT OF PLAY

Age Group	Type of Play	Suggested Play Activity
Infants	Explore, imitate	Provide visual stimuli for newborns; touch stimuli for infants and toys involving manipulation for 1-year-olds
1–2 years	Parallel play	Children play next to each other but not with each other. Provide each child with toys that reflect activities of daily living
3–5 yr	Cooperative play	Children play with each other, each taking a specific role. "You be the mommy and I'll be the daddy"
	Creative play	A simple box can become a train to a 3-year-old
5–8 yr	Symbolic group play; secret clubs	Secret codes. "Knock Knock" jokes; rhymes are popular at this age
8–10 yr	Competitive play	Children at this age can accept competition with structured rules and high interactive physical activity
13–19 yr	Fantasy play; cliques	Leadership activities such as babysitting or tutoring is popular Daydreaming occurs Board games are popular Interactive social activities in "cliques" occur at and after school

Art is an appropriate play activity at almost any age and provides an avenue of experimentation as well as creative expression and feeling of accomplishment in the child. Computer programs are popular at all age groups, providing problem solving games, manipulative skills, as well as opportunities for new learning. Both these activities need to be balanced with active play experiences. Nursing interventions should focus on encouraging optimal play activities and experiences that are age appropriate. Parents need guidance concerning the value of play that may not always be a neat and clean activity. Helping parents to select appropriate toys that are safe as well as appropriate to the illness is essential. For example, a stuffed animal may not be the toy of choice for an asthmatic child. In the health care setting, a blood pressure cuff can give the child a "hug." The child can play with equipment he or she will see in his or her environment to provide stress relief.

KEY POINTS

- Growth and development are orderly and sequential, although there are spurts and plateaus.
- Cephalocaudal development proceeds from head to toe.
- Children are susceptible to nutritional deficiencies because they are in the process of growth and development.
- Abraham Maslow depicted human development on the basis of a hierarchy of needs.
- Freud's theories view personality development as phases of psychosexual development.
- Piaget describes phases of cognitive development.
- Erick Erikson described eight stages of psychosocial development from birth to adulthood.
- Developmental theories can serve as guides to nursing intervention; however, each child grows and develops at an individual pace.
- A family is one or more persons that interact together.
- Parent–child interactions affect positive growth and development.
- Deciduous teeth are baby teeth. The proper care of the teeth depends on caretaker supervision and the child's physical level of development and mastery.
- Optimal nutrition is essential to physical and neurological growth and development.
- Motor development follows a predictable sequence.
- Nutritional practices of early childhood will persist through adulthood.
- The nurse is responsible to counsel and teach positive nutritional practices that are acceptable to the family's culture, religion, and lifestyle.
- The availability of age-appropriate toys enhances physical, emotional, and mental development in infants, children, and adolescents.

- Computer games can foster problem solving, cognitive development, and motor coordination but should be balanced with active play activities.
- Many hospitals have playrooms that must be kept safe from painful or invasive experiences.
- A nurse is an advocate, educator, and collaborator in a family-centered care environment.

MULTIPLE-CHOICE REVIEW QUESTIONS

Choose the most appropriate answer.

1. How many erupted teeth would you expect an 8-month-old infant to have?
   a. 2
   b. 4
   c. 6
   d. 8
2. During the 1st week of life, the newborn's weight
   a. increases about 5% to 10%.
   b. decreases about 5% to 10%.
   c. stabilizes.
   d. fluctuates widely.
3. Adding sugar or salt to babyfood
   a. increases taste and acceptance.
   b. is a firm cultural practice.
   c. may predispose to excessive weight gain.
   d. should be determined by parent preference.
4. To meet the needs as described by Erikson of a school-aged child diagnosed with diabetes, the nurse should
   a. explain carefully to the mother the need to rigidly adhere to dietary modifications.
   b. allow the child to eat whatever he wants and administer insulin to maintain optimum glucose levels.
   c. allow the child to perform his own accuchecks and administer his own insulin.
   d. perform accuchecks four times a day and at bedtime.
5. It is most appropriate to first introduce competitive games at
   a. 3 to 5 years of age.
   b. 7 to 8 years of age.
   c. 9 to 10 years of age.
   d. 12 to 15 years of age.

BIBLIOGRAPHY AND READER REFERENCE

Bartholmey, S. (1994). Infant rice cereal: A simple ORT solution. In *Pediatric Basics.* Fremont, MI: Gerber Products Co.

Behrman, R., Kleigman, R., & Arvin, A. (1996). *Nelson's textbook of pediatrics* (15th ed.). Philadelphia: Saunders.

Bomar, P. (Ed.). (1996). *Nurses and family health promotion: Concepts, assessment, and interventions.* (2nd ed). Philadelphia: Saunders.

Bowden, V., Dickey, S., & Greenberg, C. (1998). *Children and their families: The continuum of care.* Philadelphia: Saunders.

Cookfair, J. (1996). *Nursing care in the community.* St. Louis, MO: Mosby.

Levine, M. D., Carey, W. B., & Crocker, A. C. (1992). *Developmental-behavioral pediatrics* (2nd ed.). Philadelphia: Saunders.

Mahan, L. K., & Escott-Stump, S. (1996). *Krause's food, nutrition and diet therapy* (9th ed.). Philadelphia: Saunders.

Public Health Service, U.S. Department of Health and Human Services, and NHLBI. (1993). National Cholesterol Education Program (NCEP): *Report of the expert panel on detection, evaluation, and treatment of high blood cholesterol in adults* (NIH Publication No. 88-2925). Washington, DC: U.S. Government Printing Office.

Smilkstein, G. (1984, Fall). The physician and family functions. *Family Systems Medicine,* 263–279.

Swanson, J., & Nies, M. (1997). *Community health nursing: Promoting the health of aggregates* (2nd ed.). Philadelphia: Saunders.

U.S. Department of Health and Human Services (1992). *Child health USA '91.* Washington, DC: U.S. Government Printing Office.

Wong, D. (1995). *Whaley & Wong's nursing care of infants and children* (5th ed.). St. Louis, MO: Mosby.

chapter 16

The Infant

Outline

Objectives

On completion and mastery of Chapter 16, the student will be able to

- Define each vocabulary term listed.
- Describe the physical and psychosocial development of infants from 1 to 12 months, listing age-specific events and guidance when appropriate.
- Discuss the major aspects of cognitive development in the first year of life.
- Discuss the nutritional needs of growing infants.
- Describe how to select and prepare solid foods for the infant.
- List four common concerns of parents about the feeding of infants.
- Discuss the development of feeding skills in the infant.
- Identify the approximate age for each of the following: posterior fontanel has closed; central incisors appear; birth weight has tripled; child can sit steadily alone; child shows fear of strangers.
- Describe normal vital signs for a 1-year-old infant.
- Discuss safety issues in the care of infants.
- Discuss the approach and care of an infant with colic.
- Identify age-appropriate toys and their developmental or therapeutic value.
- Discuss principles of safety during infancy.
- Discuss the development of positive sleep patterns.

Vocabulary

colic
extrusion reflex
grasp reflex
milestones
norms
object permanence
oral stage
parachute reflex
pincer grasp
posterior fontanel
prehension
satiety
separation anxiety
Washington Guide
weaning

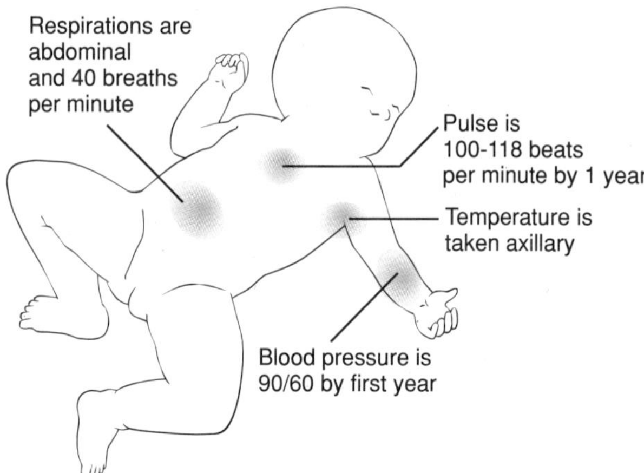

Figure 16–1. • Average vital signs of the infant.

Physical, emotional, and cognitive growth and the development of motor abilities occur rapidly during the first year of life. *Milestones* of growth and development describe general patterns of achievements at various stages of infancy. These milestones, or patterns, are referred to as *norms.* Norms can vary greatly for the individual child, but the nurse must understand the normal range for milestone achievement to assess the progress of growth and development of the infant and initiate early referral for follow-up care.

During the neonatal phase of development, the chief tasks mastered were the establishment of effective feeding patterns and a predictable sleep–wake cycle. Infants who have unmet hunger needs can become irritable, may not perceive feeding as pleasurable, and may fail to develop trust in the caregiver. Parental bonding and social interaction begin in the neonatal phase but heighten when the infant begins to respond with a social smile, making the caregiver feel "loved."

By the time the infant is 4 to 6 months old, the positive parental interaction with the infant should be obvious during clinic visits. If the parent does not appear to enjoy the developmental changes in the infant at this age or does not appear relaxed during interactions with the infant, further follow-up of possible family dysfunction or social or mental stresses should be initiated.

By 9 months of age, control of feeding may become an issue of conflict between parent and infant. The parent needs to "let go" to introduce the infant to finger foods and initiate drinking from a cup. As the infant reaches toward autonomy, offering limited choices can reduce conflict. If the nurse notices an overly neat and orderly approach during feeding, parental guidance may be necessary. *Separation anxiety* (see p. 520 Chapter 21), can be expected by the 9th-month clinic visit, and the nurse should expect to spend some time playing with and getting to know the infant to establish the rapport necessary for a successful physical assessment. Repetition is the key to successful parent teaching and counseling by the nurse.

Children, unlike adults, are in the process of growing while they are hospitalized. To provide total patient care, the nurse must be able to recognize a patient's needs at various stages of growth and development. The pulse rate, respiration, and blood pressure that are normal for an infant are not normal for the adult patient (Fig. 16–1). The nurse must try to meet individual needs effectively and to administer the specialized nursing care required for the particular patient. *The most common cause for concern about a child is a sudden slowing, not typical for age, of any aspect of development.*

GENERAL CHARACTERISTICS

Oral Stage. Sucking brings the infant comfort and relief from tension. This *oral stage* of personality development is important for the infant's physical and psychological development. The nurse, knowing the importance of sucking to the baby, holds the baby during feedings and allows sufficient time to suck. Infants who are warm and comfortable associate food with love. The baby who is fed intravenous fluids is given added attention and a pacifier to ensure the necessary satisfaction of sucking (Fig. 16–2). When the teeth appear, the infant learns to bite and enjoys objects that can be chewed. Gradually, the baby begins to put fingers into the mouth. When babies can use their hands more skillfully, they will not suck their fingers as often and will be able to derive pleasure from other sources.

Motor Development. The *grasp reflex* is seen when one touches the palms of the infant's hands and flexion occurs. This reflex disappears at about 3 months. *Prehension,* the ability to grasp objects between the fingers and the opposing thumb, occurs slightly later (5–6 months) and follows an orderly sequence of development (Fig. 16–3).

By 7 to 9 months, the *parachute reflex* appears. This is a protective arm extension that occurs when an infant is suddenly thrust downward when prone. By 1 year, the *pincer grasp* coordination of index finger and thumb is well established.

Emotional Development. Love and security are vital needs of infants. They require the continuous affection of their parents. If trust is to develop, consistency must be established. Parents are assured that they need not be afraid of spoiling infants by attending promptly to their needs. Infants who are consistently picked up in response to crying show less crying episodes when they are toddlers and less aggressive behavior at 2 years of age. Loving adults affirm that the world is a good place in which to live. Each day the infant becomes impressed by parental actions and learns to imitate and trust caretakers. A sense of trust is vital to the development of a healthy personality. Many consider it to be the foundation of emotional growth. The child who does not develop a sense of trust learns to mistrust people, which could have a permanently negative effect on personality development.

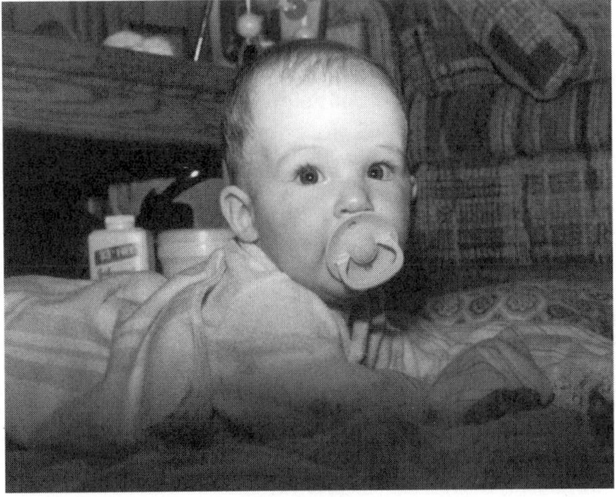

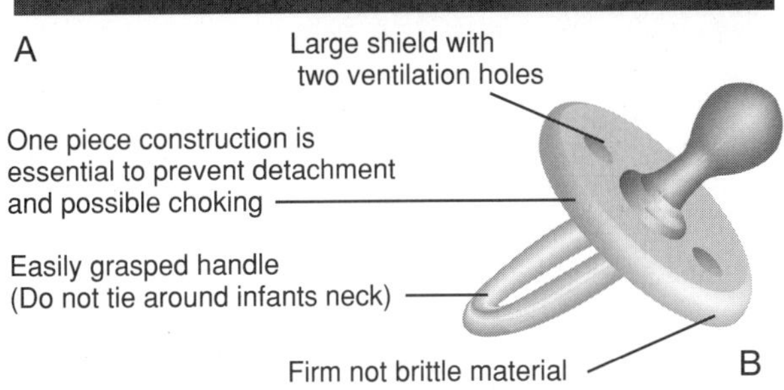

Figure 16–2. • **A** and **B.** Pacifier. Pacifiers provide nonnutritive sucking to meet the needs of the oral phase of infancy. A safe pacifier is illustrated **(B)**.

Parents are taught to talk, sing, and touch their babies while providing care. They should not expect too much or too little from them. Babies will easily accomplish various activities if they are not forced before they reach maturity. When an infant shows readiness to learn a task, parents should provide encouragement.

Need for Constant Care and Guidance. The full-time caretaker needs and deserves the understanding of and kind support from relatives at home and from the nurse in the hospital. Pediatrics involves family-centered care. A short break from pressures provides renewed energy with which to enjoy the baby. A trip to the store or a stroll with the baby in the carriage affords stimulation and a change of environment for the baby and the caretaker. The infant who is constantly left in a crib or playpen and is not introduced to a variety of learning experiences may become shy and withdrawn. *Sensory stimulation is essential for the development of the baby's thought processes and perceptual abilities.*

If a mother is unable to room-in with her hospitalized infant, personnel should try to imitate her care by promptly fulfilling the infant's physical and emotional needs. In the nursery, the nurse first feeds the baby who appears hungry, rather than delaying feeding to adhere to a specific routine. Wet diapers are changed as soon as possible. The crying child is soothed. The exactness of time or method of bathing or feeding the infant is less important than the care with which it is done. The baby easily recognizes warmth and affection or the lack of them.

DEVELOPMENT AND CARE

Table 16–1 is a guide to infant care from the 1st month to the 1st year. Some of the aspects of care (e.g., safety measures) are important throughout the entire year. The nurse explains to parents that physical patterns cannot be separated from social patterns and that abrupt changes do not take place with each new month. Human development cannot be separated into specific areas any more than the body's structure can be separated from its function. *No two infants are just alike at a certain age. Table 16–1 is just a guide!* However, individual variations range about central norms that serve as guidelines in the evaluation of an infant's or child's progress. The addition of the various solid foods to the diet and the time of immunizations vary slightly, depending

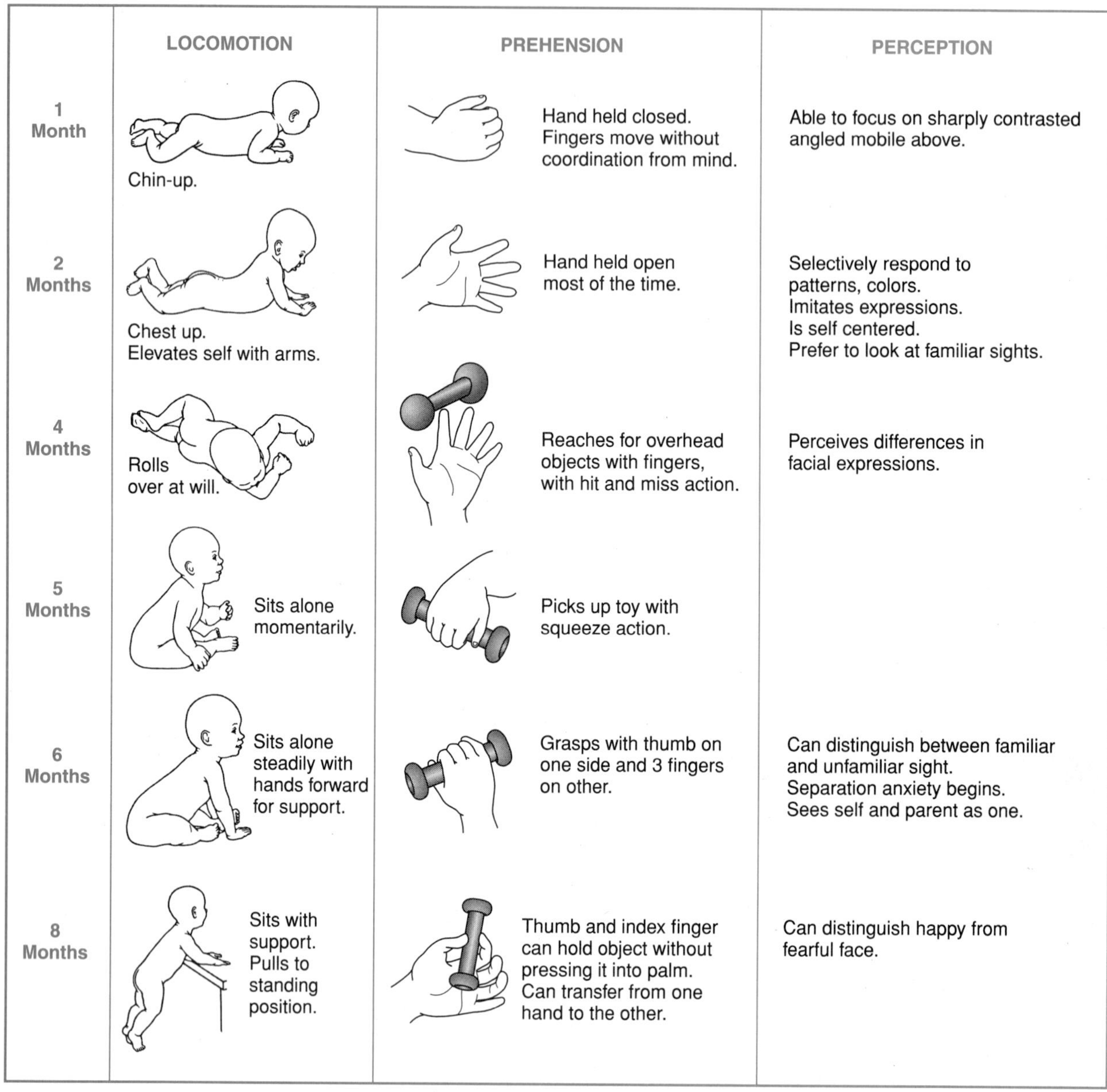

Figure 16–3. • The development of locomotion, prehension, and perception.

Illustration continued on following page

on the baby's health and the physician's protocol. Table 15–5, p. 396 outlines the parental tasks involved in guiding the infant through the stages of growth and development.

HEALTH MAINTENANCE

The prevention of disease during infancy is of the utmost importance and includes all measures that improve the physical health and psychosocial adjustment of the child. The concept of periodic health appraisal is not new. In the late 1800s, "milk stations" were established in various localities throughout the United States to provide safe water and milk for babies in an effort to reduce the number of deaths from infant diarrhea.

Community-Based Care

Parenting skills can be impaired by several socioeconomic factors, as well as physical and mental problems. A prime responsibility of the nurse in the

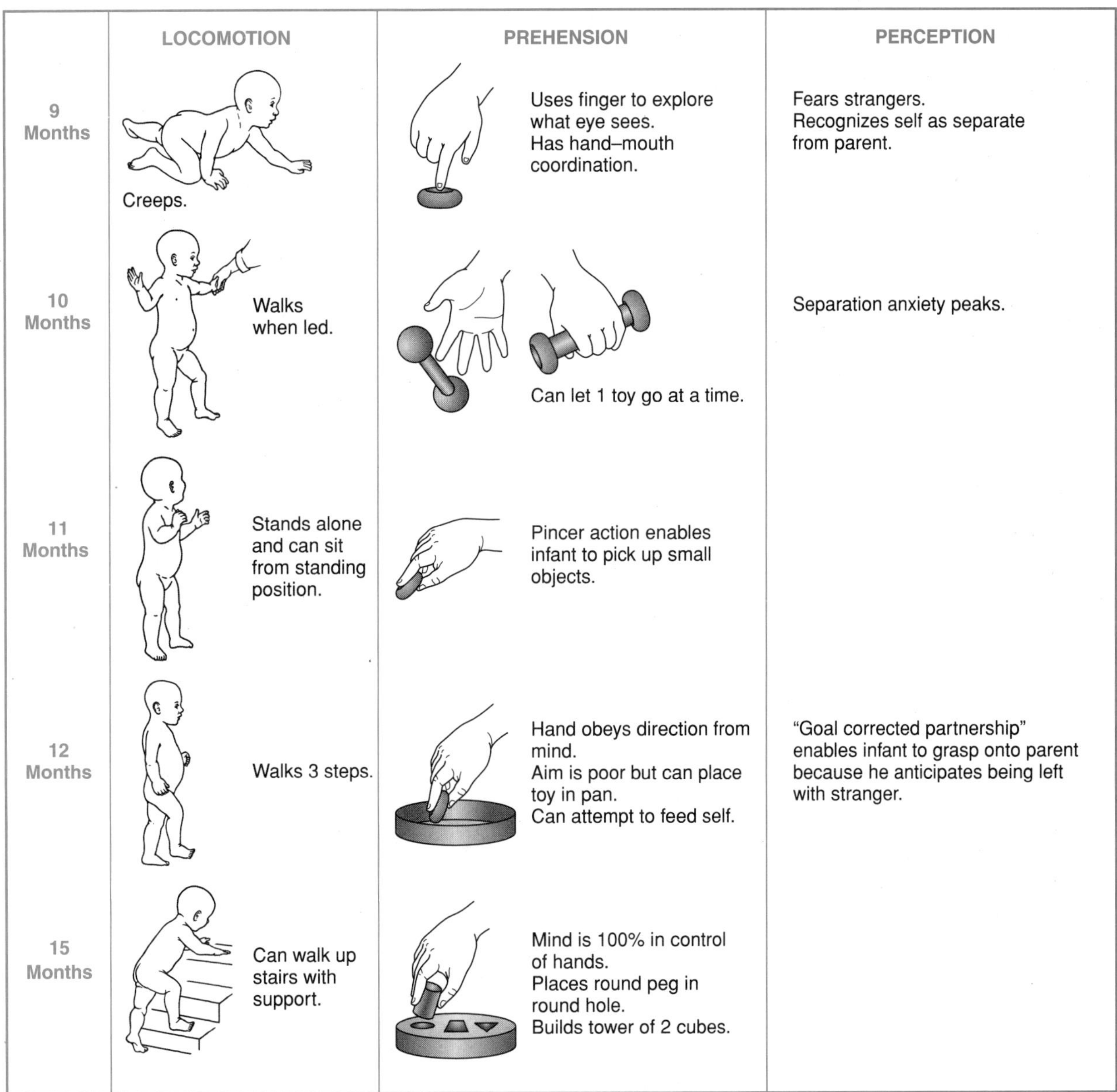

Figure 16–3. • *Continued*

community-based clinic is to guide the parent and assist in the development of skills necessary to ensure the proper growth and development of their child. The nurse can provide encouragement and explanations of strategies that will enable parents to be successful in coping with various infant behaviors.

The nurse is the important link in the initiation of referral to the multidisciplinary health care team, follow up of progress, and maintenance of communication between the family and the health care team members. A home-based infant stimulation program can use a teacher, nurse, occupational or speech therapist or physical therapist depending on the specific need of the infant, to directly stimulate the infant and teach the parents how to provide the care.

A day care nursery school can be utilized and the public school system offers special classes and tutoring for school-aged children in need. Counseling, behavior management techniques and cognitive therapy can be provided by a psychologist. Neurodevelopmental therapy (NDT) can be provided by a professional or occupational or physical therapist. Speech therapy and auditory testing are also available within the community. The social

(Text continued on p. 420)

Table 16–1
PHYSICAL DEVELOPMENT, SOCIAL BEHAVIOR, AND CARE AND GUIDANCE OF INFANTS

1 Month

Physical Development

Weighs approximately 8 lb. Has regained weight lost after birth. Gains about 1 inch in length per month for the first 6 months. Lifts head slightly when placed on stomach. Pushes with toes. Turns head to side when prone. Head wobbles. Head lags when infant pulled from lying to sitting position. Clenches fists. Stares at surroundings

Vaginal discharge in girls and breast enlargement in boys and girls from maternal hormones received in utero are not unusual and disappear without treatment

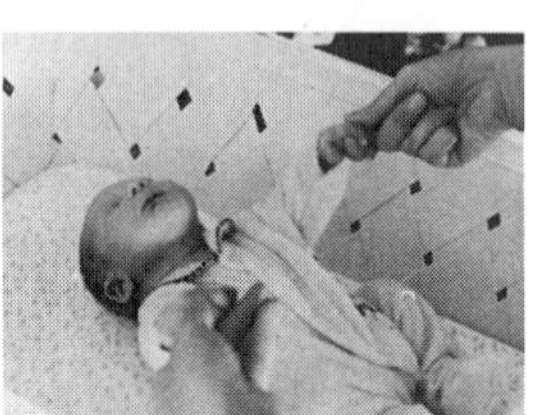

Note head lag of 1 month old.

Protect baby from sun and insects with sunscreen or protective clothing

Social Behavior

Makes small throaty noises. Cries when hungry or uncomfortable. Sleeps 20 out of 24 hr. Awakes for 2 AM feeding

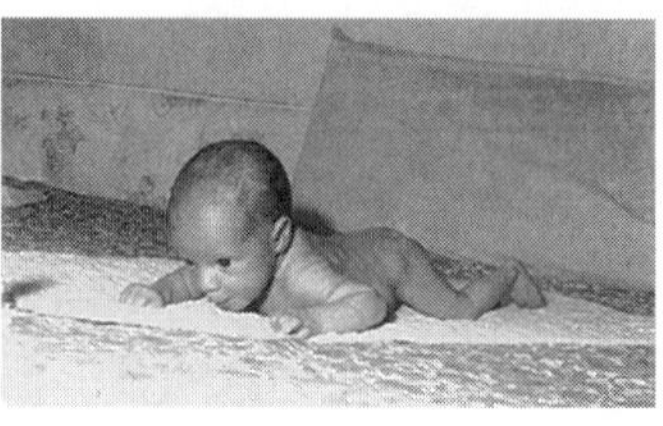

1 month of age.

Care and Guidance

Sleep. Back; if side-lying position, support back with blanket roll. Use a firm, tight-fitting mattress in a crib with bars properly spaced so that the baby's head cannot be caught between them. Raise crib rails. Do not use a pillow

Diet. Breast milk every 2 to 3 hr or iron-fortified formula every 4 hr as baby indicates need. Vitamin D (400 IU/day) in dark-skinned infants, breast-fed babies, or infants who are not regularly exposed to sunlight. Burp baby well

Exercise. Allow freedom from the restraints of clothing before bath. Provide fresh air and sunshine whenever possible. Support head and shoulders when holding infant. Attend promptly to physical needs. Provide colorful hanging toys for sensory stimulation out of infant's reach

2 Months

Physical Development

Posterior fontanel closes. Tears appear. Can hold head erect in midposition. Follows moving light with eyes. Holds a rattle briefly. Legs are active

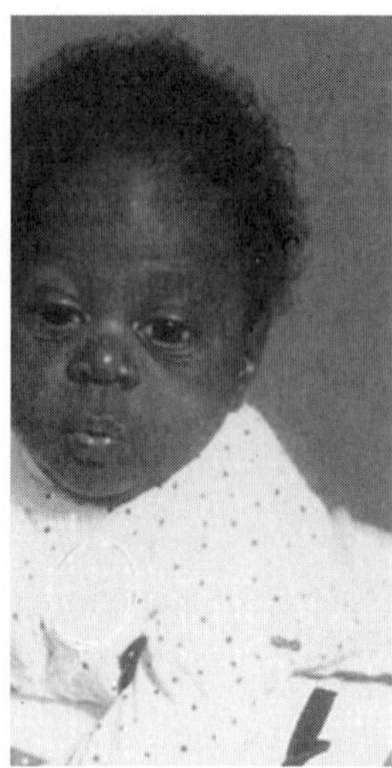

The 2-month old can hold head erect in midline for brief periods of time.

Social Behavior

Smiles in response to mother's voice. Knows crying brings attention. Awakes for 2 AM feeding

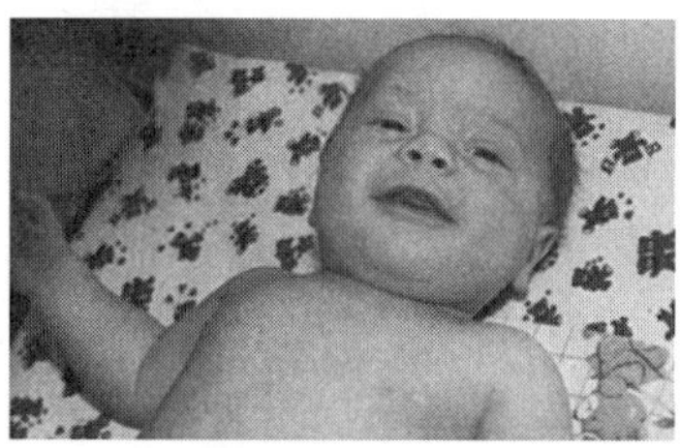

The smile of the 2-month old delights parents.

Care and Guidance

Sleep. Develops own pattern; may sleep from feeding to feeding

Diet. Breast milk or formula

Exercise. Provide a safe, flat place to kick and be active. Do not leave baby alone, particularly on any raised surface. Physical examination by the family doctor, well-baby clinic, or pediatrician

Immunization. First DTP, an inoculation against diphtheria, whooping cough, and tetanus. Oral polio vaccine (OPV), *Haemophilus influenzae* type b (HbCV), and second HBV vaccine. Still completely depends on adults for physical care. Needs a flexible routine throughout infancy and childhood

Pacifier. If used, select for safety. Choose one-piece construction and loop handle to prevent aspiration (see Fig. 16–2).

Hiccups. Are normal and subside without treatment. Small amounts of water may help

Colic (paroxysmal abdominal pain, irritable crying). Usually disappears after 3 mo. Place baby prone over arms (Fig. 16–4). Use pacifier. Massage back. Relieve caretaker periodically

Table 16–1

PHYSICAL DEVELOPMENT, SOCIAL BEHAVIOR, AND CARE AND GUIDANCE OF INFANTS *(Continued)*

3 Months

Physical Development

Weighs 12–13 lb. Stares at hands. Reaches for objects but misses them. Carries hand to mouth. Can follow an object from right to left and up and down when it is placed in front of face. Supports head steadily. Holds rattle

Social Behavior

Cries less. Can wait a few minutes for attention. Enjoys having people talk to him. Takes impromptu naps

Care and Guidance

Sleep. Yawns, stretches, naps in mother's arms

Diet. Mother's milk or formula

Exercise. May have short play period. Enjoys playing with hands

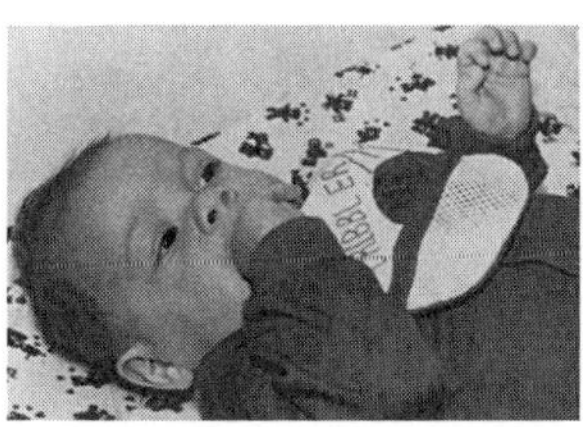

The 3-month old carries his hand to his mouth.

4 Months

Physical Development

Weighs about 13–14 lb. Drooling indicates appearance of saliva and beginning of teething. Lifts head and shoulders when on abdomen and looks around. Turns from back to side. Sits with support. Begins to reach for objects he or she sees. Coordination between eye and body movements. Moves head, arms, and shoulders when excited. Extends legs and partly sustains weight when held upright. Rooting, Moro, extrusion, and tonic neck reflexes are no longer present

Social Behavior

Coos, chuckles, and gurgles. Laughs aloud. Responds to others. Likes an audience. Sleeps through the night

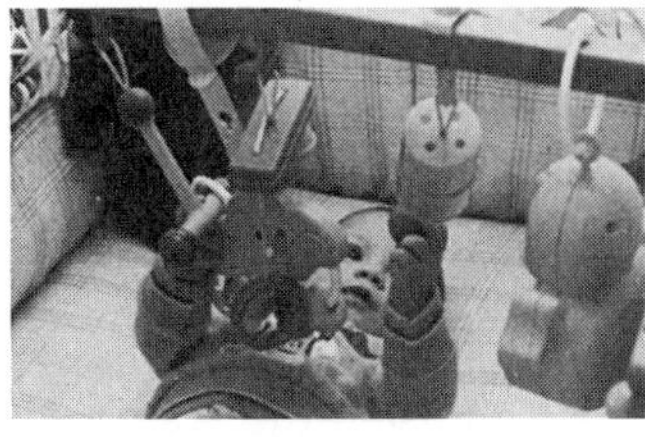

Visual stimulation is important to the growing infant. The 4-month old reaches for objects.

Care and Guidance

Sleep. Stirs about in crib. Sleeps through ordinary household noises

Diet. Mother's milk or formula

Exercise. Plays with hand rattles and dangling toys. Start acquainting with a playpen, where baby can roll with safety

Immunization. Second DTP, OPV, and HbCV

Elimination. One or two bowel movements per day. May skip a day

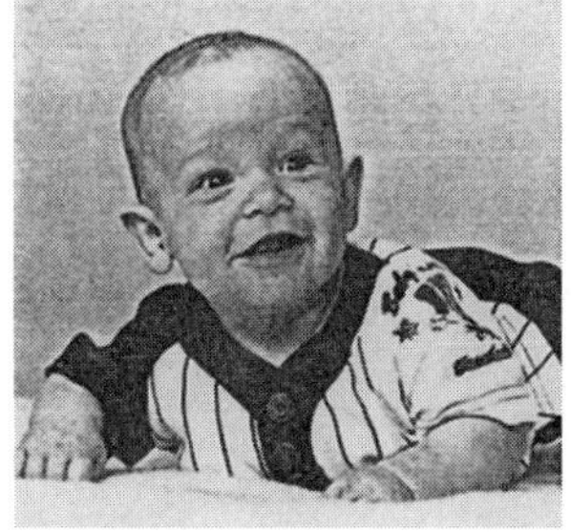

While on his abdomen the 4-month old can lift his head and shoulders and look around.

5 Months

Physical Development

Sits with support. Holds head well. Grasps objects offered. Puts everything into mouth. Plays with toes

Social Behavior

Talks to himself. Seems to know whether persons are familiar or unfamiliar. May sleep through 10 PM feeding. Tries to hold bottle at feeding time

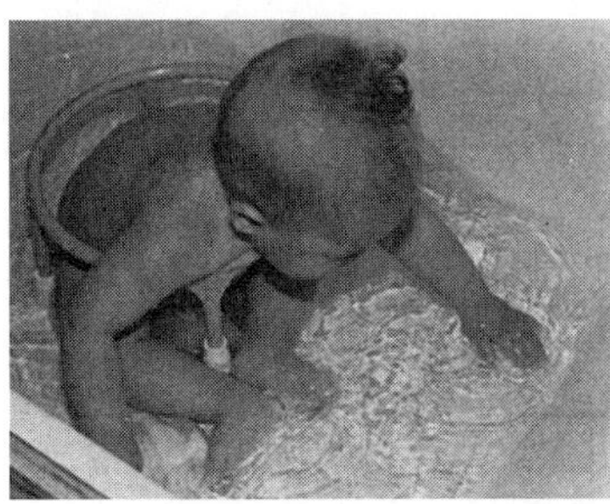

At 5 months, infant enjoys water play. Do not leave unattended in tub.

Care and Guidance

Sleep. Takes two or three naps daily in crib

Diet. Mother's milk or formula

Exercise. Provide space to pivot around. Makes jumping motions when held upright in lap

Safety. Check toys for loose buttons and rough edges before placing them in playpen

Table continued on following page

Table 16–1
PHYSICAL DEVELOPMENT, SOCIAL BEHAVIOR, AND CARE AND GUIDANCE OF INFANTS *(Continued)*

6 Months

Physical Development
Doubles birth weight. Gains about 3–5 oz/wk during next 6 mo. Grows about a half inch per month. Sits alone momentarily. Springs up and down when sitting. Turns completely over. Hitches (moves backward when sitting). Bangs table with rattle. Pulls to a sitting position. Chewing more mature. Approximates lips to rim of cup

Social Behavior
Cries loudly when interrupted from play. Increased interest in world. Babbles and squeals. Sucks food from spoon. Awakes happy

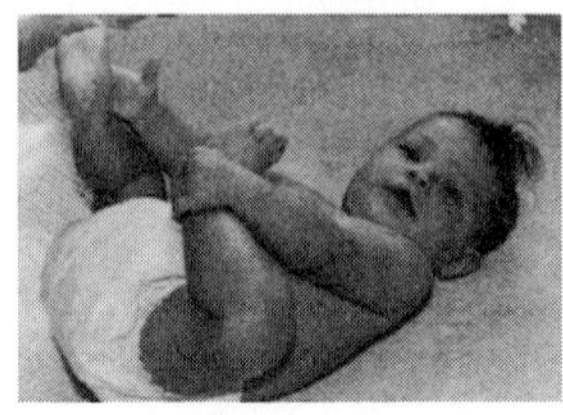

Infant plays with his feet.

Care and Guidance
Sleep. Needs own room. Should be moved from parents' room if not previously done. Otherwise, as baby becomes older, may become unwilling to sleep away from them
Diet. Introduce first solid foods, usually rice cereal fortified with iron. See Figure 16–5 for progression
Exercise. Grasps feet and pulls toward mouth
Immunization. DTP, HbCV, and HBV
Safety. Remove toxic plants. Provide a chewable object, such as a teething ring, for enjoyment

7 Months

Physical Development
Two lower teeth appear. These are the first of the deciduous teeth, the central incisors. Begins to crawl. Moves forward, using chest, head, and arms; legs drag. Can grasp objects more easily. Transfers objects from one hand to the other. Appears interested in standing. Holds an adult's hands and bounces actively while standing. Struggles when being dressed

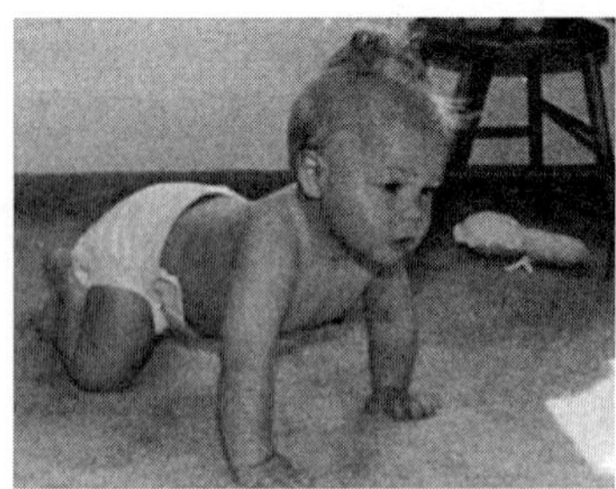

Infant begins to get around.

Social Behavior
Shifts moods easily—crying one minute, laughing the next. Shows fear of strangers. Anticipates spoon feeding. Sleeps 11–13 hr at night

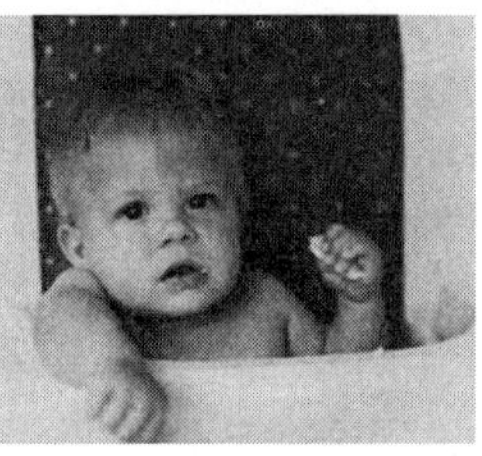

At 7 months infant enjoys finger foods.

Care and Guidance
Sleep. Fretfulness due to teething may appear. This is generally evidenced by lack of appetite and wakefulness during the night. In most cases, merely soothing and offering a cup of water are sufficient
Diet. Add fruit. Add finger foods, such as toast or zwieback
Exercise. Primitive locomotion

Table continued on following page

worker can assist with social and environmental problems.

Skilled health services today encompass periodic health appraisal; immunizations; assessment of parent–child interaction; counseling in the developmental processes; identification of families at risk (e.g., for child abuse); health education and anticipatory guidance; referrals to various agencies; follow-up services; appropriate record-keeping; and evaluation and audit by peers. They are provided in a variety of health care facilities. Ideally the infant is seen in the clinic at least five times during the 1st year at specific intervals (2 months, 4 months, 6 months, 9 months, and 1 year). Private group practice, hospital-based clinics, and neighborhood health centers are examples of health care settings. These visits are as important for parents as they are for the baby. They provide caretaker support and reassurance as well as information and anticipatory guidance for the many developmental changes of the infant's 1st year. A common concern, diaper rash, is outlined in Nursing Care Plan 16–1.

Table 16–1

PHYSICAL DEVELOPMENT, SOCIAL BEHAVIOR, AND CARE AND GUIDANCE OF INFANTS *(Continued)*

8 Months

Physical Development

Sits steadily alone. Uses index finger and thumb as pincers. Pokes at object. Enjoys dropping article into a cup and emptying it

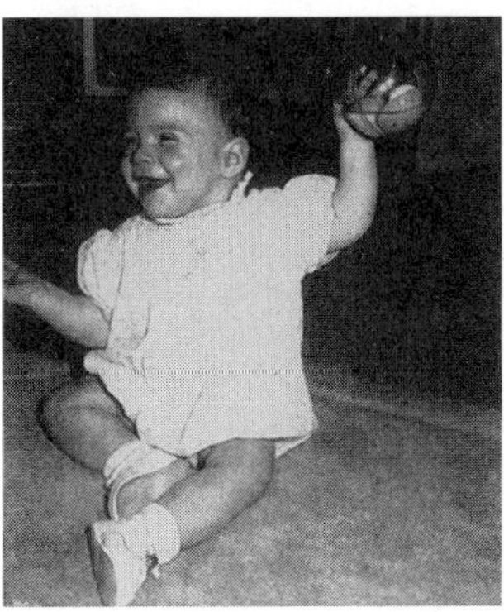

Infant can sit steadily.

Social Behavior

Plays pat-a-cake. Enjoys family life. Amuses self longer. Reserved with strangers. Indicates need for sleep by fussing and sucking thumb. Impatient especially when food is being prepared

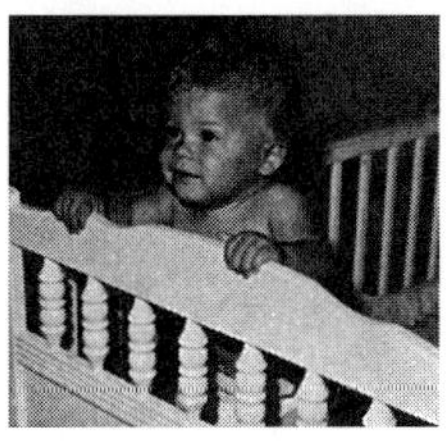

Infant shows increased interest in standing.

Care and Guidance

Sleep. Takes two naps a day

Diet. Add vegetables. Continue to add new foods slowly, observing for reactions

Exercise. Enjoys jump chair. Rides in stroller. Stuffed toys or those that squeak or rattle are appropriate

Safety. Remain with baby at all times during bath in tub. Protect from chewing paint from window sills or old furniture. Paint containing lead can be poisonous. Safety-lock doors to ovens, dishwashers, washing machines, dryers, and refrigerators

9 Months

Physical Development

Shows preference for use of one hand. Can raise self to a sitting position. Holds bottle. Creeps. (Carries trunk of body above floor but parallel to it. More advanced than crawling)

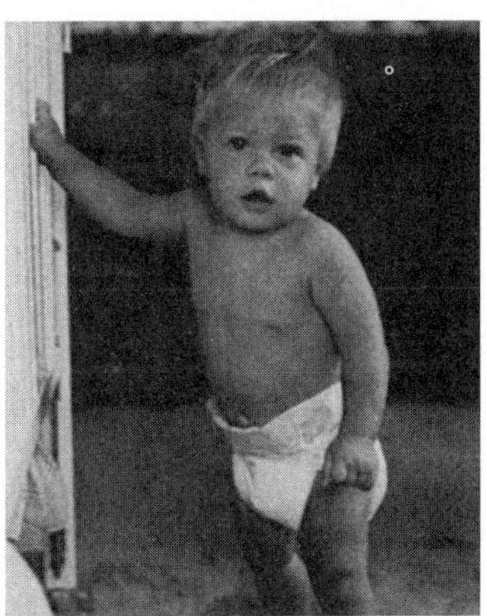

Infant cruises around holding on to furniture.

Social Behavior

Tries to imitate sounds, e.g., says "ba-ba" for bye-bye. Cries if scolded. Drops food from highchair at mealtime. May fall asleep after 6 PM feeding

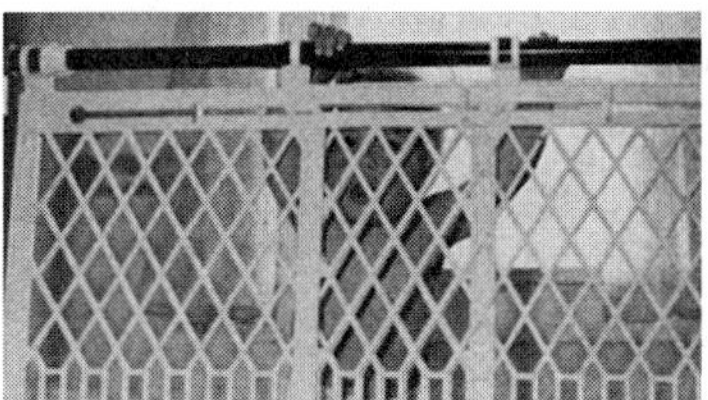

Stairway gates prevent falls.

Care and Guidance

Sleep. Has generally begun to sleep later in the morning

Diet. Add meat, beans. Introduce chopped and mashed foods. Place newspaper beneath feeding table. Use unbreakable dishes. Allow baby to pick up pieces of food by hand and put them into mouth

Safety. Keep a supply of syrup of ipecac on hand. Know phone number of nearest poison control center. Avoid tablecloths with overhangs baby could reach

Exercise. Is busy most of the day exploring surroundings. Provide sufficient room and materials for safe play. Help baby to learn. Distract curious child from danger. In this way punishment is limited—avoid excessive spankings and "nos"

Table continued on following page

During routine clinic visits, a careful health history is obtained. Growth grids during infancy include measures of weight, length, and head circumference. The reading and recording of growth charts are described on page 383. There are numerous developmental screening tests. The *Denver Developmental Screening Test,* which is widely used, is discussed in Chapter 15 (Fig. 15–5). The *Brazelton*

Table 16–1
PHYSICAL DEVELOPMENT, SOCIAL BEHAVIOR, AND CARE AND GUIDANCE OF INFANTS *(Continued)*

10 Months

Physical Development

Pulls to a standing position in the playpen. Throws toys to floor for parent to pick up. Cries when they are not returned. Walks around furniture while holding on to it

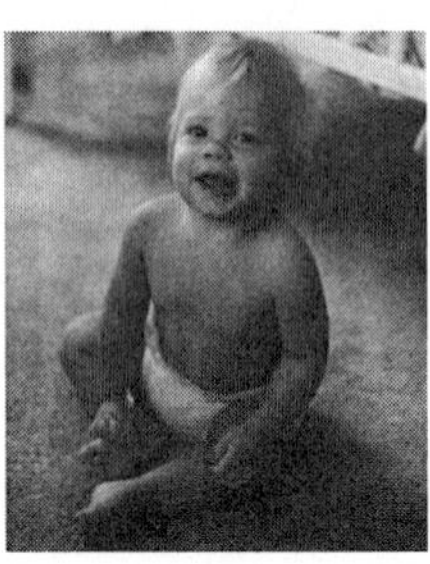

Note the lower tooth.

Social Behavior

Knows name. Plays simple games such as peek-a-boo. Feeds himself a cookie. May cry out in sleep without waking

Care and Guidance

Sleep. Avoid strenuous play before bedtime. A night light is convenient for parent and makes baby's surroundings more familiar. Pajamas with feet are warm, as baby becomes uncovered easily

Diet. Takes juice and water from cup. Solid foods in general are taken well

Exercise. Tours around room holding adult's hands. Daytime clothing should be loose so as not to interfere with movement

11 Months

Physical Development

Stands upright holding on to adult's hands

Social Behavior

Understands simple directions. Impatient when held. Enjoys playing with empty dish and spoon following meals

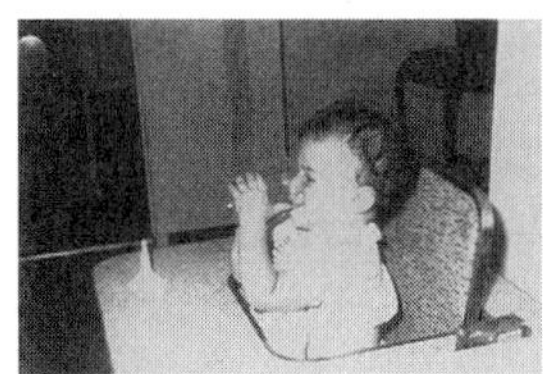

Drinking from cup is easy but spills occur.

Care and Guidance

Sleep. Greets parents in morning with excited jargon

Diet. Still spills from cup. Enjoys blowing bubbles

Exercise. Plays with toys in tub. Enjoys gross motor activity. Kicks, pulls self up

Safety. Cover electrical outlets with tape. Put household cleaners and medicines out of reach if not previously done. Needs to be sat down in playpen at times, since tends to stand until becoming exhausted

12 Months

Physical Development

Pulse 100–140 beats/min. Respirations 20–40/min. Triples birth weight. Height is about 29 inches. Stands alone for short periods. May walk. Puts arm through sleeve as an aid to being dressed. Six teeth (four above and two below). Drinks from a cup, eats with a spoon with supervision. Pincer grasp is well established. Handedness (the preference for the use of one hand), although not fully established, may be evidenced

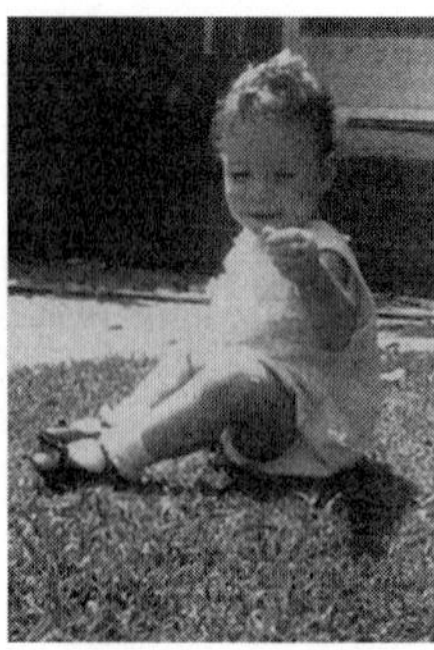

Pincer grasp enables infant to pick up small leaf.

Social Behavior

Friendly. Repeats acts that elicit a response. Recognizes "no-no." Verbalization slows because of concentration on getting about. Enjoys rhythmic music. Shows emotions such as fear, anger, and jealousy. Reacts to these emotions from adults. Plays with food, removes it from mouth

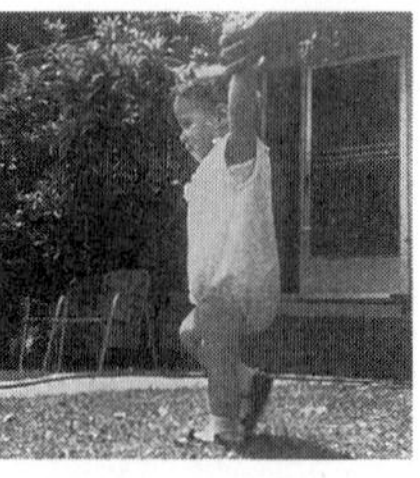

At 12 months can stand alone and walk with assistance.

Care and Guidance

Sleep. May take one long nap daily

Diet. Gradually add egg white and fish (baked, steamed, or boiled). Add orange juice. Add well-cooked table foods. Interest in eating dwindles

Exercise. Enjoys putting objects in a basket and then removing them. Places objects on head. Distraction is an effective way to deal with determination to do what baby wants regardless of outcome

> **Nursing Tip**
>
> The American Academy of Pediatrics recommends a supine or side-lying position for infants to avoid sudden infant death syndrome (SIDS). Care should be taken to use a sturdy mattress and avoid soft pillows that inhibit breathing.

Neonatal Behavioral Assessment Scale is of particular value during the newborn period; it helps to describe the emerging personality of the baby and includes evaluation of infant reflexes, general activity, alertness, orientation to spoken voice, and response to visual stimuli. Although not a screening test per se, the *Washington Guide to Promoting Development in the Young Child* is also useful in evaluating the child's functional ability in such areas as feeding, sleep, toilet training, play, and motor activity. Expected tasks for each area are listed along with ideas for parental guidance. Although scoring is omitted, it provides a tool for systematic observation of the development of the infant and child from birth through 5 years of age.

The physical examination is adapted to the needs of the infant. Routine assessments of hearing and vision are an integral part of the examination. In the newborn period, loud noises should precipitate the *startle,* or *Moro, reflex.* Localization of sound during infancy can be roughly ascertained by standing behind the child seated on the mother's lap and ringing a bell or repeating voice sounds. The baby's response is compared with the average for that age level. Vision is mainly assessed by light perception. The examiner shines a penlight into the eyes and notes blinking, following to midline, and other responses. Laboratory tests may include a hemoglobin or hematocrit to detect anemia and a urinalysis. Screening tests for a variety of asymptomatic diseases are assuming greater importance; examples of these are the phenylketonuria (PKU) test, tuberculin test, and sickle cell test.

Colic. *Colic* is characterized by periods of unexplained irritability and crying in a healthy, well-fed infant. Although the exact cause is unknown, it is thought to be a combination of infant, parental, and environmental factors. Colic can interfere with parent–infant interactions if the infant is not soothed by holding or carrying and parental fatigue and guilt grow. Providing parents of colicky babies periods of rest and "breaks" can prevent a cycle that may lead to child abuse. Figure 16–4 illustrates the "colic carry." Holding the infant close to the body while supporting the abdomen and providing a gentle rocking motion often soothes the colicky infant.

Coping with the Irritable Infant

One of the goals of early parent–infant interaction is to promote a calm, alert infant that can

NURSING CARE PLAN 16–1

Selected Nursing Diagnosis for the Infant with Diaper Rash

Nursing Diagnosis: High risk for impaired skin integrity and perineal area irritation possibly related to improper cleansing and infrequent diaper change

Goal	Nursing Interventions	Rationale
Skin will remain dry; there will be no signs of redness, irritation, or oozing	1. Suggest frequent diaper changes	1. Diaper dermatitis is caused by prolonged and repeated exposure to urine, feces, soaps, detergents, ointments, and friction; changing a wet or soiled diaper promptly eliminates this problem; exposing skin to light and air facilitates drying and healing
	2. Demonstrate how to cleanse the diaper area thoroughly and how to dry between skin folds; have parent return demonstration. Review "wiping from front to back"	2. After soiling, perineal area is cleansed with plain water and, if needed, a mild soap; disposable wet "wipes" can aggravate a diaper rash if infant is sensitive to an ingredient in product; moisture between skin folds prevents healing
	3. Review changes in diet	3. Addition of new foods or a change from breast milk to formula may be related to rash
	4. Evaluate finances of family	4. Socioeconomic factors have a bearing on parent compliance

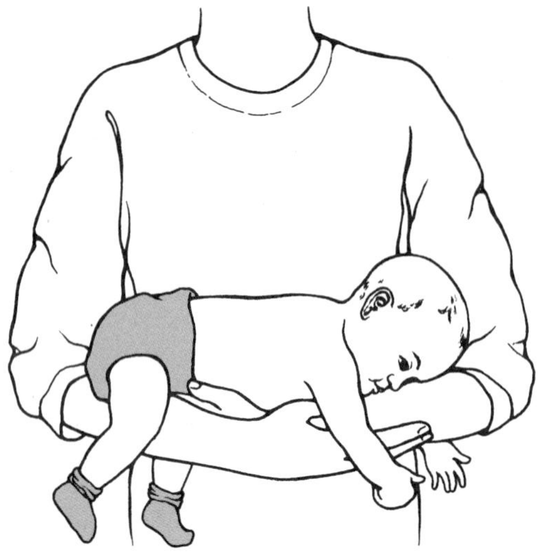

Figure 16–4. • The colic carry.

respond to parents and the environment. Success in this area promotes a feeling of competence in the parent. Some infants cannot tolerate environmental stimulation and handling and start to cry during diaper changes, feeding, and rocking. Lights, sound, and movement cause some infants to become irritable. Some techniques to cope with these problems include:

- Shield infant's eyes from bright light.
- Sit quietly with infant. Do not talk or sing.
- Eliminate noise from radio and TV.
- Talk in soft voice.
- Change position of infant slowly.
- If the infant turns away, squirms, grimaces, or puts the hands in front of the face, stop interaction and reduce environmental stimuli.
- Swaddle infant snugly in a light blanket with extremities flexed and hands near face.

NURSING CARE PLAN 16–2

Selected Nursing Diagnosis for the Infant with Colic

Nursing Diagnosis: Altered family process related to fussiness of infant

Goals	Nursing Interventions	Rationale
Parents will demonstrate increased coping behaviors by 1 wk Parents will verbalize feelings of increased confidence in caring for the baby	1. Educate parents about common manifestations of colic.	1. No one cause has been established for colic; infant appears otherwise healthy but demonstrates cramplike pain, drawing legs to abdomen and demonstrating irritable cry; it is time limited to about 3 months
	2. Determine whether other causes have been ruled out by physician	2. Intestinal obstruction and infection may mimic symptoms of colic; bowel movements are not abnormal with colic
	3. Review caretaker's history and usual day with infant	3. This helps to determine if colic is related to type of feedings, diet of breastfeeding mother, passive smoking, milk allergy, activities of family members while baby is being fed, etc.
	4. Identify soothing measures used by parents and their effectiveness	4. Environment may be overstimulating infant; parents may not know how to soothe baby
	5. Suggest abdominal massage, wind-up swing, car rides	5. These measures may help to relieve symptoms; burping before and after feedings and placing in an upright position after feedings may also decrease distress
	6. Demonstrate "colic carry" (Fig. 16–4)	6. This may comfort infant by applying a little extra pressure on abdomen
	7. Suggest periods of free time for parents	7. Constant crying by infants produces a great deal of frustration in family members; caution against shaking infant, which can be harmful to the head and neck
	8. Emphasize that colic is not a reflection on parenting skills	8. First-time parents may feel anxious and incompetent; nurse provides reassurance and support and builds on their strengths

- Provide nonnutritive sucking.
- Rock infant slowly and gently. Avoid sudden movements.
- Cradle infant firmly in lap during feeding and remain still during sucking efforts.

Repetitious banging of toys on a table by an infant may be perceived by the parent as an irritating type of behavior. Counseling may be required to help parent to understand that this is a developmental phase of motor activity and should be encouraged!

Coping with a Lethargic Infant. Stimulation, interaction, and nourishment are essential for optimum infant growth and development. Some infants respond to an excessively stimulating environment by "shutting down" and sleeping. Some coping strategies for dealing with this infant include:

- Avoid bright lights.
- Move and handle infant slowly and gently.
- Talk in a calm voice.
- Sit infant upright at intervals.
- *Slowly* dress and undress infant.

Developing Positive Sleep Patterns

Most newborns sleep at 4-hour intervals and increase their sleep intervals to 8 hours by 4 to 6 months of age. Synchronizing the circadian rhythm of the infant to the family routine is a learned behavior. Parents need to be alert to the infant's individual rhythm and promote activities that will foster a stable synchronized pattern (Table 16–2).

Until 6 months of age, infants will rely on parents to soothe them back to sleep when they awake during the night. If the parent resorts to midnight pacing or car rides, the infant will learn to rely on the parent to get them back to sleep after 6 months of age also. Following the guidelines listed in Table 16–2 will assist the infant to develop "self-soothing" behaviors so the infant can roll over, grasp his pacifier, and return to sleep on his own. Helping the infant to achieve this ability will also make parents feel more confident in their parenting skills and less fatigued and frustrated.

Immunizations

Health personnel must repeatedly stress to parents the importance of immunizations. A delay can lead to undue risks of serious illness, sometimes with fatal complications.

The nurse can stress to working parents that an unprotected child may become sick, making it necessary for them to lose valuable working hours. Immunization also prevents numerous doctor and hospital expenses and is required before school entry. A delay or interruption in a series does not interfere with final immunity. It is not necessary to restart any series, regardless of the length of delay. Accurate records prevent confusion. A detailed discussion of immunizations and common childhood communicable diseases is in Chapter 31.

Nutrition Counseling

The nutritional needs of infants reflect rates of growth, energy expended in activity, basal metabolic needs, and the interaction of the nutrients consumed (Mahan & Escott-Stump, 1996). The baby is born with a rooting reflex, which assists in finding the nipple. The sucking reflex is present at birth. There is a forward and backward movement of the tongue. As the infant grows, neuromaturation of

Table 16–2
ENCOURAGING GOOD SLEEP PATTERNS

Discourage	Encourage
Middle-of-the-night feedings Unrealistically early bedtime Active play prior to bedtime	Maintaining consistent routines for feeding, play, and bedtime Recognizing signs of sleepiness Providing quiet activities before bedtime and then expecting infant to accept being placed into bed
Rocking infant to sleep or allowing infant to fall asleep nursing or bottlefeeding. (prolonged contact between milk and tooth enamel can cause *nursing caries*)	Putting infant to bed sleepy but awake
Skipping daytime naps	Avoiding overtiring infant
Placing infant in family bed to quiet infant Pacing the floor and carrying infant to encourage sleep	Checking and gently patting the crying infant during the night but do not feed, play with, or rock infant to sleep. Using a favorite blanket or pacifier in crib of infant to encourage "self-soothing"
Loud noises in environment	Using "white noise" (monotonous recording of motor or static) to block out noises in the room

the cheeks and tongue enables advancement to a more mature sucking pattern that utilizes negative pressure to obtain milk. At about the 3rd to 4th month, the *extrusion reflex* (protrusion), which pushes food out of the mouth to prevent intake of inappropriate food, disappears.

The digestive system continues to mature. By 6 months, it can handle more complex nutrients and is less susceptible to food allergens. The stomach capacity expands from 10 to 20 ml at birth to 200 ml by 12 months. This expansion enables the infant to consume more food at less frequent intervals. As the pincer grasp becomes more developed, the baby can pick up food with tiny fingers and place it in the mouth. By 2 years, the child masters spoon feeding.

Parental Concerns. Parents have many concerns about feeding their infant during the 1st year of life. This is a period when readiness to receive nutritional education is usually high; therefore, the nurse looks for opportunities to provide accurate information. Assessment of parental knowledge; infant development, behavior, and readiness; parent-child interaction; and cultural and ethnic practices is important. Nutritional care plans based on developmental levels assist parents in recognizing changes in feeding patterns. The components of a nutritional assessment are discussed in Chapter 15.

A suggested parental guide to determining the adequacy of the diet includes:

- The infant has gained 4 to 7 oz/wk for the first 6 months.
- The infant has at least six wet diapers per day.
- The infant sleeps peacefully for several hours following feedings.

Monitoring of weight, height, head circumference, and skin fold thickness determines if the diet is adequate; therefore, the value of periodic well-baby examinations is stressed. Bottle-fed infants are usually fed at 3 to 4-hour intervals. Breastfed infants may require feedings at 2- to 3-hour intervals because breast milk is more easily digested. A flexible, but regular, schedule that provides a rest period between feedings is best for parent and infant. The nurse reassures parents that most children eat enough to grow normally, although intake is seldom constant and varies in quantity and quality. Forced feedings are not appropriate.

Breastfeeding and Bottle Feeding. Infants, in proportion to their weight, require more calories, protein, minerals, and vitamins than do adults. Their fluid requirements are also high. Human milk is the best food for infants under 6 months of age. It contains the ideal balance of nutrients in a readily digestible form. Breastfeeding soon after birth helps to promote bonding and stimulates milk production. It protects the infant from certain bacteria, and allergic reactions are minimal.

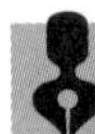

Nursing Tip

Whole milk and "imitation milk" should not be given to infants until after 1 year of age.

Nutritious infant formulas are also available. Many pediatricians recommend iron-fortified formulas because maternal iron stores decrease by 6 months of age. A baby who cannot tolerate milk-based formulas may be placed on a soy-based formula. These formulas are nutritionally sound. Whole cow's milk is not recommended for infants under 1 year of age, as the tough, hard curd is difficult to digest. This type of milk may also contribute to iron-deficiency anemia by increasing gastrointestinal blood loss. Formula preparation is discussed in Chap. 9, p. 250. Table 16–3 reviews the advantages of the various types of milk available. Box 16–1 reviews how to heat formula in a microwave oven.

It is suggested that infants remain on human milk or iron-fortified formula for the 1st year of life. Parents are sometimes unsure of when their baby has had enough formula. It is important to explain *satiety* behavior at the various ages, as depicted in Table 16–4. Coaxing babies to finish the last drop in a bottle is unnecessary. Infants who are breastfed longer than 6 months gain less weight by 1 year of age than bottle-fed infants.

Taste cells develop during the 8th week of gestation and the fetus begins to respond to flavors when swallowing amniotic fluid. At birth, the infant demonstrates a preference for certain tastes, preferring sweet and rejecting sour. Breast milk may supply flavor experiences based on the mother's diet. Infants should be given an opportunity to develop their own personal tastes by being offered a variety of foods when solid foods are introduced. Figure 16–5 illustrates how feeding skills develop in infants and toddlers.

Addition of Solid Foods. Parents often wonder when to begin adding solid foods. The addition of

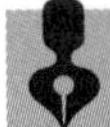

Nursing Tip

Honey should not be included in the diet of infants under 2 years of age to prevent the development of botulism.

Table 16–3
COMMON MILK PREPARATIONS FOR THE FIRST YEAR

	Advantages	Disadvantages
Human breast milk	No preparation needed, nonallergenic, provides antibodies	Lifestyle or illness of mother may influence availability
Prepared, ready-to-feed formula	No preparation needed, no refrigeration needed before opening the bottle	Expensive
Formula concentrate	Easy to prepare, can prepare one bottle at a time or a maximum of one day's feeding at a time	Must be refrigerated after preparation Must use accurate proportions. Safe water supply must be used to dilute the concentrate. (Water from a natural well may have a high mineral concentrate)
Formula powder	Least expensive formula, lasts up to 1 mo once opened	Needs accurate measurement. Needs safe water supply. Needs to be shaken thoroughly to dissolve powder

solid food at about 6 months is recommended as this is when the tongue extrusion reflex disappears and the gastrointestinal tract is mature enough to digest the foods. There are a number of commercially prepared brands of baby foods. Parents should be instructed to read the labels on the jars to obtain nutrition information. Home-prepared foods may also be utilized (Box 16–2).

BOX 16–1

HEATING REFRIGERATED FORMULA IN A MICROWAVE OVEN

Most formula can be fed at room temperature. If a formula has been refrigerated, it can be warmed by running warm water over the bottle. Microwave warming is not recommended because it can produce "hot spots" within the formula. However, because microwaving is a popular current practice, the nurse should explain the proper technique. Microwaving frozen breast milk may destroy some immune properties and is not advisable.

1. Heat only one portion at a time.
2. Keep the bottle in upright position and uncovered.
3. Heat a 4-oz. bottle for a *maximum* of 30 seconds.
4. Heat an 8-oz. bottle for a *maximum* of 45 seconds.
5. Replace nipple and invert bottle several times.
6. Test formula temperature before feeding by placing a few drops on your wrist.

Adapted from Bush, G., & Anentheswaran, R. (1992). Microwave heating of infant formula: A dilemma resolved. *Pediatrics, 90*(3), 414.

Between 4 and 6 months, sucking becomes more mature, and munching (up-and-down chopping motions) commences. Rice cereal is often recommended as the first solid food because it is less allergenic than others.

Only small amounts are offered at first (1 teaspoonful). A small amount of food is placed on the back of the tongue. Cereal may be diluted with formula or water. The consistency is thickened and amounts of solid foods are gradually increased as the infant becomes more familiar with them. A small bowl and a spoon with a long, straight handle is suggested. Single-ingredient foods are introduced (green beans rather than mixed vegetables), as it is easier to determine food allergies this way. Only one new food is offered in a 4-day to 1-week period to determine tolerance.

If the baby refuses a certain food, it is temporarily omitted. Mealtime is kept pleasant. The baby is allowed to try new foods, even the ones that parents dislike. New foods should not be introduced when the baby is ill because adverse responses may not be effectively assessed. The amount of food consumed varies with the child. Fruit juices are generally offered at about 5 to 6 months of age, when the infant begins to drink from a cup. An exception is the addition of orange juice, which is withheld until the baby is 1 year old, especially when family members have known allergies. Other highly allergenic foods that may be delayed include fish, nuts, strawberries, chocolate, and egg whites.

A spouted plastic cup is helpful at first. The juice is initially diluted. Then the quantity is gradually increased to 3 to 4 oz a day. Baby food can be prepared in a food grinder, electric blender, or food mill or by mashing the food to the desired texture. The infant's height and weight should increase at approximately the same rate.

Recommended Fat Intake during Infancy. Fat contains more calories than carbohydrates and pro-

Table 16–4
GROWTH AND DEVELOPMENT OF MEALTIME BEHAVIOR

Age	Hunger Behavior	Communication	Feeding Behavior	Satiety	Parental Guidance
Birth–3 mo	Cries. Hands fisted. Body tense	Roots in search of nipple	Strong suck reflex. Needs to be burped	Falls asleep when full. Hands relaxed. Body relaxed. Withdraws head from nipple	Burp frequently. Avoid over/underfeeding. Recognize signs of satiety
3–5 mo	Grasps and draws bottle to mouth. Tongue protrudes in anticipation of nipple. Fusses. Mouths hands	Reaches with open mouth to receive nipple	Strong suck. Holds nipple firmly. Preference for tastes. Pats bottle	Tosses head back. Ejects nipple. Distracted easily by surroundings. Plays with nipple	Provide predictable routine. Allow infant to gain experience with varied textures of fingers/toys
6–9 mo	Reacts to food preparation. Reaches for bottle	Vocalizes hunger. Pulls spoon to mouth. Holds bottle	Picks up small food with raking then pincer action. Draws food from spoon with lips. Chewing begins	Changes posture. Closes mouth. Plays with utensils. Shakes head "no"	Offer 1 new food at a time at spaced intervals to assess responses. Include familiar favorites
10–12 mo	Vocalizes. Grasps utensils. Fussy	Attempts to feed self. Purses lips to cup's edge	Skilled pincer action to pick up pieces of food and place in mouth. Drinks from cup. Chews food	Shakes head "no." Sputters food. Throws food to floor	Allow infant to assist with feeding. Introduce foods with varied textures. Avoid foods that can be aspirated

Note: Parents who are alert to infant's communication of hunger and satiety help the infant develop self-regulation and communication skills.

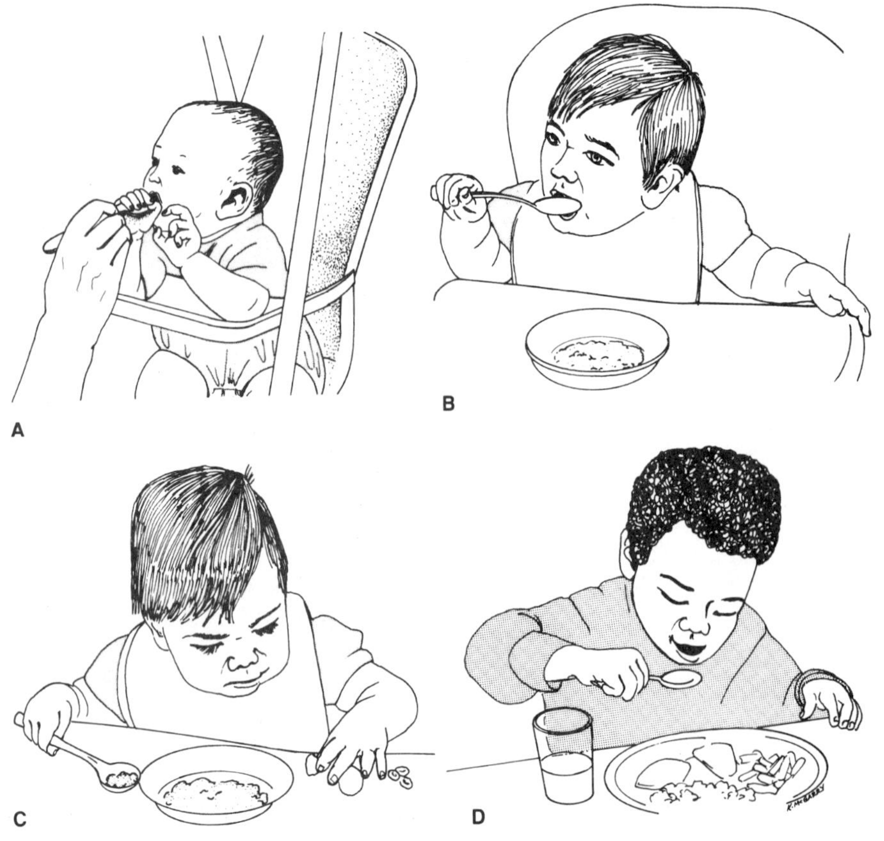

Figure 16–5. • Development of feeding skills in infants and toddlers. **A,** At 7 months, this child begins to reach for the spoon. **B,** At 9 months, this little girl begins to use her spoon independently, although she is not yet able to keep food on it. **C,** The 9-month-old shows a refined pincer grasp to pick up food. **D,** The 2-year-old is much more skillful at self-feeding and has the ability both to rotate the wrist and to elevate the elbow to keep food on the spoon. (Modified from Mahan, L. K., & Escott-Stump, S. [1996]. *Krause's food, nutrition and diet therapy* [9th ed., p. 190]. Philadelphia: Saunders.)

BOX 16–2

DIRECTIONS FOR HOME PREPARATION OF INFANT FOODS

1. Select fresh, high-quality fruits, vegetables, or meats.
2. Be sure all utensils, including cutting boards, grinder, and knives, are thoroughly clean.
3. Wash hands before preparing the food.
4. Clean, wash, and trim the food in as little water as possible.
5. Cook the foods until tender in as little water as possible. Avoid overcooking, which may destroy heat-sensitive nutrients.
6. Do not add salt. Add sugar sparingly. Do not add honey to food for infants less than 1 year of age. (Botulism spores have been reported in honey, and young infants do not have the immune capacity to resist this infection.)
7. Add enough water so that the food can be easily puréed.
8. Strain or purée the food with an electric blender, food mill, baby food grinder, or kitchen strainer.
9. Pour purée into ice cube tray and freeze.
10. When food is frozen hard, remove the cubes and store in freezer bags.
11. Unfreeze and heat (in water bath or microwave oven) in serving container the amount of food that will be consumed at a single feeding.

From Mahan, L. K., & Escott-Stump, S. (1996). *Krause's food, nutrition and diet therapy* (9th ed.). Philadelphia: Saunders.

teins. Since infants have a limited stomach capacity and a high caloric need, fats in easily digestible forms are needed to meet their caloric needs for growth and development and for brain development. Infants have a high basal metabolic rate (BMR) and require almost three times more calories per kilogram of weight than adults do to maintain their rapid growth and development in the first year of life. In the young infant, breast milk and infant formulas provide the necessary fats that the infant is able to digest. *Feeding infants under 2 years of age a low-fat diet will compromise growth and development.*

Nursing Tip

Cereal and baby food should *not* be mixed in a bottle with formula.

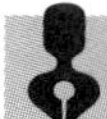

Nursing Tip

New solid foods should be introduced *before* the milk feedings to encourage the infant to try the new experience.

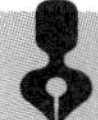

Nursing Tip

As solid food intake increases, the amount of formula or milk should decrease to avoid overfeeding.

The fat and cholesterol contents of foods designed for infant consumption are therefore not usually labeled as adult foods are. By 6 months of age, amylase and lipase are present in the digestive tract to aid in digesting fat content present in solid foods. A well-balanced diet will provide appropriate fat and cholesterol intake. Evaluating the height and weight of infants on a growth chart during clinic visits is an essential assessment of growth and development. Whole cow's milk can be introduced after 1 year of age, and low-fat milk can be introduced after 2 years of age.

Buying, Storing, and Serving Foods. Baby foods stored in jars are vacuum-packed. Parents are taught to check safety seals before purchase. (Directions are generally indicated on the jar, e.g., to reject product if safety button is up.) The expiration date of the product should be checked. Dates are usually found on the caps of jars and on the sides of cereal and bakery items. Unopened jars of baby food and juices are stored in a dry, cool place. Jars are rotated, and those on hand the longest are used first.

When a jar is opened, a definite "pop" is heard as the vacuum seal is broken. Food is transferred to a serving dish. One should not feed out of the jar or return leftovers to the jar because saliva may turn certain foods to liquid by digesting them in the jar. Unused portions may be stored in the refrigerator in the original jar. Special precautions are taken

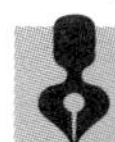

Nursing Tip

Human milk and properly prepared formula supply adequate fluid for the infant under normal conditions. During illness or hot, humid weather, the infant may require additional water.

when food is heated in the microwave, as sometimes food heats unevenly.

Weaning. *Weaning* is defined as substituting a cup for a bottle or breastfeeding. Since sucking is a major source of pleasure in the first year of life, weaning is a major step in growth and development. Signs of readiness to wean can be seen in the infant who eagerly looks forward to new tastes and textures found on the spoon. The infant may not want to be held close during feedings and may start to "bite" the nipple as teeth erupt. The approaching stage of autonomy provides the child with motivation to manipulate the cup. Imitation of older siblings or parents also contributes to readiness. Weaning should be very gradual and start with daytime feedings. Weaning is usually completed by 2 years of age but may continue longer in some cultures.

Infant Safety

Car Safety. Infant seats should be used for all infants traveling in automobiles. A rear-facing infant seat should be used for infants under 1 year of age and be located in the center of the rear seat of the automobile. Cars with passenger-side safety air bags pose a danger to infants in infant seats who are placed in the front seat. The infant seat should be firmly anchored to the vehicle by the car seat belt (see Fig. 17–10, p. 448).

Preventing Falls. Never leave an infant on a flat surface, such as a changing table, unattended. Newborn infants have crawling reflexes that can cause them to fall off a changing table. Infants under 4 months of age have rounded backs and can accidentally roll off a flat surface. Infants over 4 months of age can voluntarily roll over. Crib rails should be raised and securely locked. Infants should be secured in high chairs or swings. An infant seat should not be placed on a table or high surface. The crawling infant should be protected from stairways and heavy or unsturdy furniture should not be available for an infant to use to pull themselves to a standing position.

A safe environment for a crawling infant includes storage of poisonous items out of the sight and reach of the infant. Cabinet locks are available. Plants, batteries, pool areas, plugs, loose hanging wires, and pets can be hazardous to an infant. Close supervision at all times is essential to the safety of any environment.

Toy Safety. Selection of toys should be appropriate for the age and diagnosis, but safety is the most important feature involved in toy selection. Infants put everything into their mouths, so choking is a major problem if a toy has small or removable parts. When the pincer skill is developed, infants will be able to pick up small objects such as pins and put them in their mouths. Toys appropriate for older siblings can be dangerous to infants. For example, if an infant drinks the glue from a model airplane set an older sibling is playing with, the results can be deadly. Constant supervision is essential. Toys should nurture growth and development (Table 16–5). A child's response to a toy can indicate readiness to learn new skills. An infant who is able to reach for and pick up a toy evidences readiness for communication.

Summary of Major Developmental Changes in First Year

- Weight doubles by 6 months, triples by 1 year of age.

Table 16–5
TOYS FOR THE FIRST YEAR

Age	Visual Stimulation	Auditory Stimulation	Sensorimotor Stimulation
0–2 mo	Black-and-white contrasting mobiles placed at midline of infant's vision	Talk Music Ticking clock	Cuddle, rock
3–5 mo	Unbreakable mirrors. Infant seat positioned to view the room	Talk to infant, provide rattles	Cradle gym, infant swing
6–9 mo	Play Peek-a-boo (teaches object permanence). Encourage imitation of facial expression	Use appropriate names for objects. Speak clearly	Introduce various textures for infant to touch. Use teething toys
10–12 mo	Large picture books. Take for shopping trips. Soft blocks. Nested boxes	Read, sing nursery rhymes. Imitate sounds of animals	Push-pull toys. Activity boxes

Note: Toys for each age group should be varied to stimulate sight, touch, sound and movement. Safety for age and diagnosis is of utmost importance in selection of a play activity or toy.

- Height increases by 1 inch per month for first 6 months to 29 inches (74 cm) by 1 year of age (increase is mainly in the trunk of the body).
- Head circumference increases 0.6 inches (1.5 cm) each month for the first 6 months and is 18 inches, or 46 cm, by 12 months of age.
- Head circumference and chest circumference are equal by the first year of life.
- Closure of the posterior fontanel occurs by 2 months.
- Closure of the anterior fontanel occurs by 18 months.
- Primitive reflexes are replaced by voluntary movements.
- Maternal iron stores decrease by 6 months of age.
- Digestive processes increase functioning at 3 months of age. Amylase and lipase are deficient until 6 months of age, decreasing ability to digest fats found in solid foods.
- Tooth eruption begins at 6 months of age when "biting" activities start.
- Binocular vision is established by 4 months of age.
- Depth perception begins to develop at 9 months of age.
- Between 5 and 6 months of age infants can voluntarily roll over.
- By 1 year of age infants can take some independent steps.
- *Separation* (of self from others), *object permanence* (objects exist even if they are out of visual field), and *symbols* (saying bye-bye means someone is leaving) are major aspects of cognitive development in the first year of life.

KEY POINTS

- A development of a sense of trust begins in infancy and is vital to a healthy personality.
- Breast milk or formula is the most desirable food for the first 6 months of the baby's life, followed by gradual introduction of a variety of solid foods.
- Sensory stimulation is essential for the development of the infant's thought processes and perceptual abilities.
- Health maintenance visits are essential during the 1st year to detect variations from normal growth patterns, to provide immunizations, and to educate and support parents.
- The nurse must stress to parents the value of immunizations for infants and children.
- Human milk and properly prepared formula supply an adequate fluid intake for the infant under normal conditions. During illness or very hot, humid weather, the infant may require additional water.
- Feeding an infant a low-fat diet before 2 years of age will compromise growth and development.
- The most common cause of concern is an atypical for age slowing of any aspect of development.

MULTIPLE-CHOICE REVIEW QUESTIONS

Choose the most appropriate answer.

1. The startle reflex is also known as the
   a. Moro reflex.
   b. rooting reflex.
   c. pincer reflex.
   d. grasp reflex.
2. A car seat for an infant under 1 year of age
   a. is not needed if the infant is held securely in the lap of an adult.
   b. should be placed close to the driver in the front passenger seat.
   c. should face the rear and be placed in the center of the back seat.
   d. should face forward and be placed on the driver's side of the back seat.
3. To detect allergies when feeding new foods,
   a. introduce single-ingredient foods.
   b. mix the food with one the infant likes.
   c. mix the food with formula.
   d. offer two new foods at a time.
4. The nurse is discussing home safety with the mother of a 4-month-old infant. Which of the following is a priority topic:
   a. Placing locks on cabinet doors that contain cleaning supplies
   b. Covering electrical outlets
   c. Raising and securing crib siderails
   d. Encouraging reading and talking to infant
5. A mother expresses concern that her 1-year-old infant is overweight. She states that her family has a tendency to be overweight and wishes to discontinue formula feedings and start the infant on low-fat milk. The nurse assesses the present weight of the infant is 24 pounds. Birth weight was 8 pounds, 2 ounces. The best response of the nurse would be
   a. to place the infant on low-fat milk as the infant is slightly overweight at this time.
   b. to place the infant on regular whole milk as the infant's weight is appropriate for his age.
   c. to indicate that the infant is underweight for his age and needs to have supplemental formula added to the diet.
   d. to note that infancy is a period of rapid growth and weight loss will occur as the infant becomes more active.

BIBLIOGRAPHY AND READER REFERENCE

Alexander, M., & Kuo, K. (1997). Musculoskeletal assessment of newborns. *Orthopedic Nursing, 16*(1), 124.

Behrman, R., Kleigman, R., & Arvin, A. (1996). *Nelson's textbook of pediatrics.* (15th ed.). Philadelphia: Saunders.

Bowden, V., Dickey, S., & Greenberg, C. (1998). *Children and their families: A continuum of care.* Philadelphia: Saunders.

Brazelton, T. B. (1993). *Touchpoints: Your child's emotional and behavioral development.* Reading, MA: Addison-Wesley.

Bush, G., & Anentheswaran (1992). Microwave heating of infant formula: A dilemma resolved. *Pediatrics, 90*(3), 414.

Crawley, T. (1996). Childhood injury significance and prevention strategies. *Journal of Pediatric Nursing,* 2(4), 225.

Dewey, K., et al. (1993). Breastfed infants are leaner than formula-fed infants at 1 year of age: The Darling study. *American Journal of Clinical Nutrition, 57*(2), 140–145.

Eichner, R. (1994). Circadian Rhythms. *Sports Medicine, 22*(10), 82.

Erhardt, R. P. (1993). Finger feeding: A comprehensive developmental perspective. *Pediatric Basics, 66,* 2–6.

Fleisher, D. (1998). Coping with colic. *Contemporary Pediatrics, 15*(6), 144.

Health alert: Air bag/child seat warning label. (1994). *AAP News, 19*(4), 22.

Kleinman, R. (1994). Build to a variety of foods. *Pediatric Basics, 69,* 4.

Lauer, R. (1994). Babies need fat. *Pediatric Basics, 69,* 14.

Levine, M. D., Carey, W. B., & Crocker, A. C. (1992). *Developmental-behavioral pediatrics* (2nd ed.). Philadelphia: Saunders.

Mahan, L. K., & Escott-Stump, S. (1996). *Krause's food, nutrition & diet therapy* (9th ed.). Philadelphia: Saunders.

Neifert, M. (1996). Early assessment of breastfeeding infant. *Contemporary Pediatrics, 13*(10), 142.

Peckenpaugh, N. J., & Poleman, C. M. (1996). *Nutrition essentials and diet therapy* (7th ed.). Philadelphia: Saunders.

Pokorni, J., & Stanga, J. (1996). Cognitive strategies for young infants born to women with history of substance abuse and other risk factors. *Journal of Pediatric Nursing, 22*(6), 540.

Schmitt, B. (10/93). Characteristics of newborn babies. *Contemporary Pediatrics, 10*(10), 107.

Schmitt, B. (1993). The first weeks at home with your baby. *Contemporary Pediatrics, 10*(11), 77.

Sullivan, S., & Birch, L. (1994). Infant dietary experience and acceptance of solid foods. *Pediatrics, 93*(2), 271–277.

Wong, D. (1995). *Whaley and Wong's nursing care of infants and children* (5th ed.). St. Louis, MO: Mosby.

Wolfson, A., Lacks, P., & Fullerman, A. (1992). Effects of parent training on infant sleeping patterns, parent stress, and perceived parental competence. *Journal of Consulting and Clinical Psychology, 60*(1), 41–48.

chapter 17

The Toddler

Outline

GENERAL CHARACTERISTICS
- Physical Development
- Sensorimotor and Cognitive Development
- Speech Development

GUIDANCE AND DISCIPLINE

DAILY CARE

TOILET INDEPENDENCE

NUTRITION COUNSELING

DAY CARE

INJURY PREVENTION

TOYS AND PLAY

Objectives

On completion and mastery of Chapter 17, the student will be able to

- Define each vocabulary term listed.
- Describe the physical, psychosocial, and cognitive development of children from 1 to 3 years of age, listing age-specific events and guidance when appropriate.
- Describe the task to be mastered by the toddler according to Erikson's stages of growth and development.
- List two developmental tasks of the toddler period.
- Discuss speech development in the toddler.
- Discuss how adults can assist small children in combating their fears.
- Identify the principles of toilet training (bowel and bladder) that will assist in guiding parents' efforts to provide toilet independence.
- List two methods of preventing the following: automobile accidents, burns, falls, suffocation and choking, poisoning, drowning, electric shock, and animal bites.
- Describe the characteristic play and appropriate toys for a toddler.
- Discuss principles of guidance and discipline for a toddler.
- Describe the nutritional needs and self-feeding abilities of a toddler.

Vocabulary

autonomy
behavior
cariogenic
cooperative play
defecate
Denver II
egocentric
mastery
negativism
object permanence
parallel play
ritualism
separation anxiety
temper tantrum
timeout
toddler

GENERAL CHARACTERISTICS

Children between the ages of 1 and 3 years are referred to as *toddlers.* They are able to get about by using their own powers and are no longer completely dependent persons. By this time, they have generally tripled their birth weight and gained control of their head, hands, and feet. The remarkably rapid growth and development that took place during infancy begins to slow down. The toddler period presents different challenges for the parents and the child.

The toddler is in Erikson's stage of Autonomy versus Shame and Doubt, which is based on a continuum of trust established during infancy (see p. 396). The challenging tasks to be mastered by the toddler include increasing independence, toilet training, self-feeding, self-dressing, speech development, and a curiosity to explore their widening environment. One major parental responsibility is to maintain safety while allowing the toddler the opportunity for social and physical independence. Another major parental responsibility is to maintain a positive self image and body image in the child whose behavior is inconsistent and often frustrating. Toddlers alternate between dependence and independence. They test their power by saying "no" frequently. This is called *negativism.* Offering limited choices and the use of distraction can be helpful tools in handling toddlers (too many choices can confuse the toddler). Developing self control and socially acceptable outlets for aggression and anger are important factors in the formation of personality and behavior. *Ritualism* is another characteristic of toddler behavior. By making rituals of simple tasks, toddlers increase their sense of security, and so their rituals should be respected. Table 17–1 summarizes the toddler's physical development, social behavior, and care at various ages.

Table 17–1
PHYSICAL DEVELOPMENT, SOCIAL BEHAVIOR, AND CARE AND GUIDANCE OF TODDLERS

	Social	Fine Motor	Gross Motor	Language	Cognition
12–16 months	Imitates adults' activities, seeks alternate methods of achieving solitary play	Drinks from cup, holds spoon, builds tower of 2 blocks, prefers finger feeding	Begins to walk	Uses words. Activity oriented. Follows simple commands	Classifies objects with function. Object permanence begins to develop
16–18 months	Curious, parallel play	Places objects in appropriately shaped openings	Walks alone, can walk backwards	Use symbolic language ("bye-bye")	Can imitate from memory
	Ritualistic behavior	Improved self-feeding		Is able to point to familiar objects	Begins to realize cause/effect

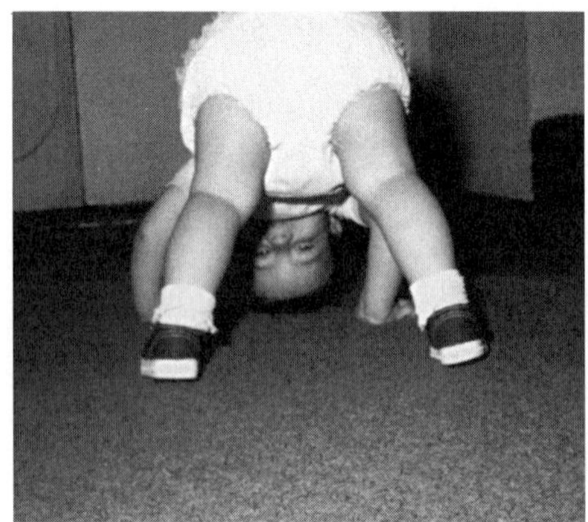

The toddler examines the environment from all angles.

Table 17–1

PHYSICAL DEVELOPMENT, SOCIAL BEHAVIOR, AND CARE AND GUIDANCE OF TODDLERS *(Continued)*

	Social	Fine Motor	Gross Motor	Language	Cognition
24 months	Increased independence Egocentric—everything is "mine" Increased autonomy, can say "no"	Builds tower of 6–7 blocks Turns pages of book Can undress self	Runs, throws ball Climbs steps Imitates oral hygiene. Jumps with both feet	Uses plural words Uses words to tell story Names familiar objects	Continuous investigation and exploring Develops likes and dislikes
36 months	Establishes toilet independence. Identifies sexual roles. Begins to share. May have imaginary playmate	Holds cup by handle and spoon with 2 fingers. Copies a circle	Balances. (Hops) Jumps on 1 foot. Use tricycle Climbs stairs using alternate feet	Can hold conversation Frequently asks why and how. Says full name	Can understand one idea or concept at a time. Knows 2 colors. Imitates parental roles

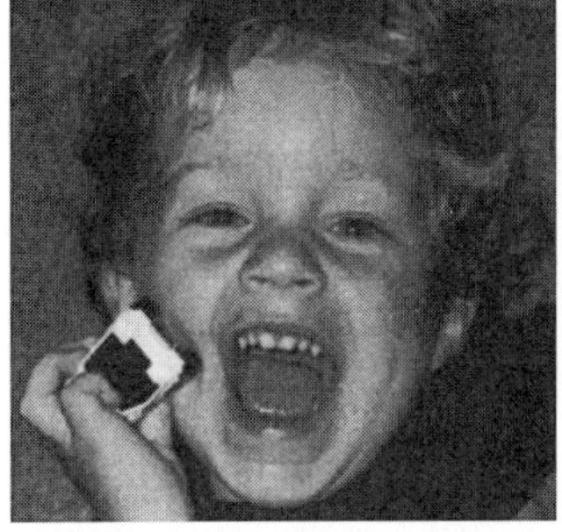

The 2½-year-old has all of his or her deciduous teeth.

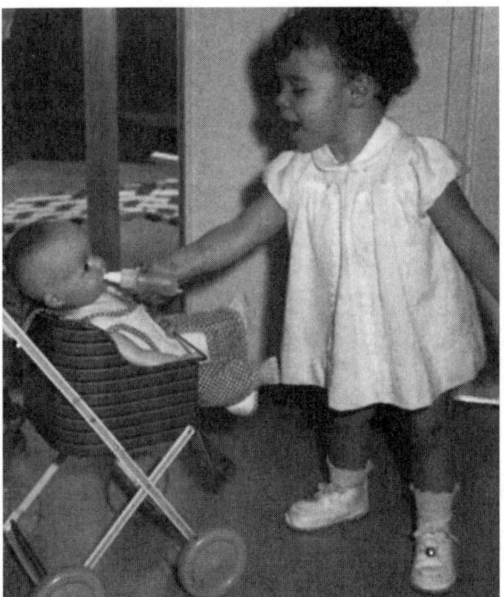

Imitating parental behaviors can help the toddler to prepare for the arrival of a new sibling.

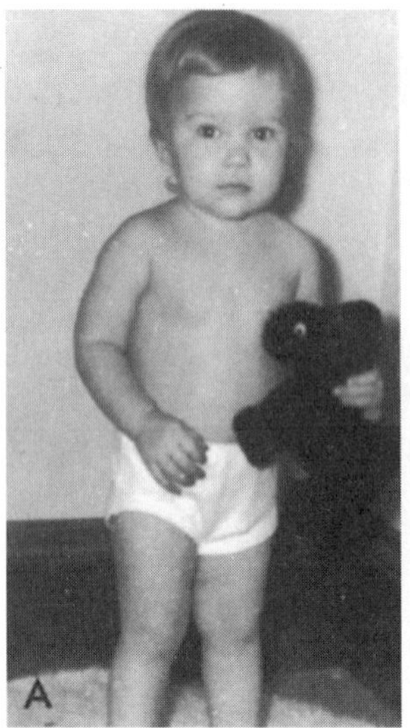

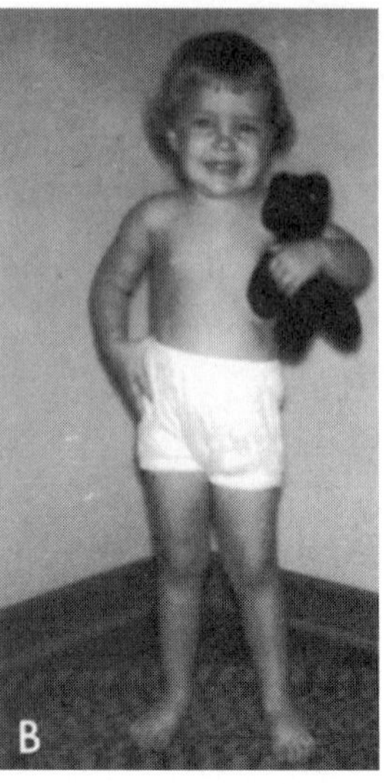

Figure 17–1. • Compare the growth and development of the child of 20 months **(A)**, and the child of 2½ years **(B)**.

Physical Development

The toddler's body changes proportions (Fig. 17–1). The legs and arms lengthen through ossification and growth in the epiphyseal areas of the long bones. The trunk and head grow more slowly. The average weight of a 2-year-old is 27 pounds. The toddler gains 4 to 6 pounds (1.8–2.7 kg) per year. The birth weight has quadrupled by 2½ years of age. The toddler grows 3 inches (7.5 cm) per year in height. The average height of a 2-year-old is 34 inches (86.6 cm). The height of a 2-year-old is thought to be one half of the potential adult height of that child. The height and weight are plotted carefully on a growth chart during each clinic visit to reflect the steady pace of growth and development.

The rate of brain growth decelerates. The increase in head circumference during infancy is 10 cm (4 inches), whereas during the 2nd year of life it is only 2.5 cm (1 inch). Chest circumference continues to increase. After the second year, the child appears leaner because the chest circumference begins to exceed the abdominal circumference. The protuberant abdomen flattens when the muscle fibers increase in size and strength.

Myelination of the spinal cord is practically complete by 2 years, allowing for control of anal and urethral sphincters. Bowel and bladder control is usually complete by 2½ to 3 years of age.

Respirations are still mainly abdominal but shift to thoracic as the child approaches school age. The toddler is more capable of maintaining a stable body temperature than is the infant. The shivering process, in which the capillaries constrict or dilate in response to body temperature, has matured.

The skin becomes tough as the epidermis and dermis bond more tightly, protecting the child from fluid loss, infection, and irritation. The defense mechanisms of the skin and blood, particularly phagocytosis, are working more effectively than they were during infancy. The lymphatic tissues of the adenoids and tonsils enlarge during this period. The eustachian tube continues to be shorter and straighter than in the adult. Tonsillitis, otitis media, and upper respiratory infections are common problems. Eruption of deciduous teeth continues until completion at about 2½ years (see Chapter 15).

The blood pressure of a toddler may average 90/56, and the respiratory rate slows to 25 per minute and continues to be abdominal breathing. The pulse of a toddler slows to a range of 70 to 110 beats per minute. Digestive processes and the volume capacity of the stomach increase to accommodate a three-meal-a-day schedule.

Sensorimotor and Cognitive Development

The senses and motor abilities of the toddler do not function independently of one another. Two-year-old toddlers reach, grasp, inspect, smell, taste, and study objects with their eyes. Their attention becomes centered on characteristics of their surroundings that capture their interest. Binocular vision is well established by the age of 15 months. By 2 years, visual acuity is about 20/40.

As memory strengthens, toddlers can compare present events with stored knowledge. They assimilate information through trial and error plus repetition. They try alternative methods of accomplishing a goal. Thought processes advance, preparing the way for more complex mental operations. The sensorimotor and preconceptual phase of development described by Piaget develop rapidly between the ages of 1 and 3 years and affect the behavior of the toddler.

Separation anxiety (consisting of protest, despair, and detachment), which was developed in infancy, continues throughout toddlerhood. Toddlers are able to tolerate longer periods of separation from parents to explore their environment. They become aware of cause and effect. Often they correlate a type of object with its function. For example, if their toys are stored in a paper bag, they will gleefully open any paper bag they see, expecting to find toys.

If the bag contains garbage or drugs, they can be injured and may be punished. This can be confusing to the toddler and frustrating to the parents.

The concept of spatial relationships develops, and toddlers are able to fit square pegs in the square hole and round pegs in a round hole. Toys should be selected to promote this ability. *Object permanence* continues to develop, and the toddler becomes aware that there may be fun items behind closed doors and in closed drawers. The toddler's curiosity and ability to explore make it important to educate parents to keep dangerous objects out of their reach. The toddler begins to internalize standards of behavior as evidenced by saying "no-no" when tempted to touch a forbidden object.

The toddler copies the words and the roles of the models seen in the home. The toddler may "help mommy clean" or "help daddy shave." By 2 years of age there is a recognition of sexual differences.

Toddlers may confuse essential with nonessential body parts. Expelling feces and flushing it down the toilet can be upsetting to some toddlers as they may feel they expelled a part of themselves that has disappeared. The toddler's body image and self-esteem may be impaired if they are scolded in a way that makes them feel *they* are bad rather than their *behavior.* The nurse must help the parents to develop skills that will enable toddlers to feel they are loved even though the specific behavior is unacceptable.

Speech Development

Language development parallels cognitive growth. The increase in the level of comprehension is particularly striking and exceeds verbalization. By 3 years of age, the child has a rather extensive vocabulary of about 900 words. Speech is more than 90% intelligible (Table 17–2).

At about the end of the 1st year, the baby begins to make noises that sound like "bye-bye," "ma-ma" and "da-da." When toddlers see the happy response to these sounds, they repeat them. This is true throughout the toddler period. To want to learn to talk small children must have an appreciative audience.

At first, children refer to animals by the sounds the animals make. For example, before saying "dog," the toddler repeats "bow-bow." Soon the child can say short phrases such as "Daddy gone car." Toddlers also respond to tone of voice and facial expression. If an adult sounds threatening, the toddler may answer "no" and then again in a louder voice.

Sometimes adults scold the child merely for being too young to understand what is requested. Imagine yourself being punished in a foreign country because you could not speak or comprehend the language well enough to defend yourself. Adults who show empathy to the small child can help to minimize their frustrations.

Table 17–2
LANGUAGE MILESTONES

Expressive Language	Age (mo)	Receptive Language	Age (mo)
Social smile	2	Alerts	1
Coos	3	Recognizes mom	2
Laughs	4	Orients to voice	4
Razzes	5	Orients to bell	5
"Ah-goo"	5	Looks directly at bell	9
Babbles	6	Understands "no"	9
Dada/Mama		Plays gesture games	9
nonspecific	8		
specific	10		
1st word	11	Follows one-step command	
		with gesture	12
		without gesture	16
2nd word	12	Knows one body part	18
Jargon	15	Points to one picture	18
4–6 words	16	Follows two-step command	24
2-word phrases	21	Points to seven pictures	24
2-word sentences	24	Follows prepositional commands	36
Pronouns	36		
Plurals	36		

Note: This table of language milestones is a guide to assessing normal language development. Although most mentally retarded children are language delayed, not all language-delayed children are mentally retarded. Some normal children also are late talkers.

Adapted by Montgomery, T. (1994). When not talking is the chief complaint. *Contemporary Pediatrics, 11*(9), 49.

Table 17–3

WHEN A CHILD WITH A COMMUNICATION DISORDER NEEDS HELP

Age	Behavior
0–11 months	Before 6 months, the child does not startle, blink, or change immediate activity in response to sudden loud sounds
	Before 6 months, the child does not attend to the human voice and is not soothed by his or her mother's voice
	By 6 months, the child does not babble strings of consonant + vowel syllables or imitate gurgling or cooing sounds
	By 10 months, the child does not respond to his or her name
	At 10 months, the child's sound making is limited to shrieks, grunts, or sustained vowel production
12–23 months	At 12 months, the child's babbling or speech is limited to vowel sounds
	By 15 months, the child does not respond to "no," "bye-bye," or "bottle"
	By 15 months, the child will not imitate sounds or words
	By 18 months, the child is not consistently using at least six words with appropriate meaning
	By 21 months, the child does not respond correctly to "Give me . . .," "Sit down," or "come here" when spoken without gestural cues
	By 23 months, two-word phrases have not emerged that are spoken as single units ("Whatzit," "Thank you," "Allgone")
24–36 months	By 24 months, at least 50% of the child's speech is not understood by familiar listeners
	By 24 months, the child does not point to body parts without gestural cues
	By 24 months, the child is not combining words into phrases ("Go bye-bye," "Go car," "Want cookie")
	By 30 months, the child does not demonstrate understanding of on, in, under, front, back
	By 30 months, the child is not using short sentences ("Daddy went bye-bye")
	By 30 months, the child has not begun to ask questions, using where, what, why
	By 36 months, the child's speech is not understood by unfamiliar listeners
At any age, the child is consistently dysfluent (not clear) with repetitions, hesitations, blocks, or struggles to say words. Struggle may be accompanied by grimaces, eye blinks, or hand gestures.	

From Behrman, R., & Kleigman, R. (1994) *Nelson's essentials of pediatrics* (2nd ed.). Philadelphia: Saunders.

When parents are concerned about the child's delayed speech (Table 17–3), they can discuss it with their doctor during one of the child's routine physical examinations so that it can be evaluated in the light of total physical growth and development. Many late talkers are perfectly normal children who prefer listening over active participation.

GUIDANCE AND DISCIPLINE

Discipline for the toddler involves guidance. The goal is to teach, not to punish. Teaching the toddler self-control with positive self-esteem is desirable rather than encouraging a completely submissive, "obedient" child. The toddler who scribbles on the wall needs to be given the opportunity to scribble on paper, a more socially acceptable outlet.

Temper tantrums often occur during the toddler years, and parent responses reinforce to the child the desirability or risks involved in such behavior. Expectations need to be commensurate with the child's physical and cognitive abilities. Toddlers get into many situations over their heads. When adults make firm decisions, the problem is resolved, at least for the time being. The child feels secure.

Limit setting should include praise for desired behavior as well as disapproval for undesired behavior. A *timeout* period in a safe place helps the child to develop self-regulation. Timing should not begin until the child has settled down. The child is praised once calm. Timing for timeout is usually based on 1 minute per year of age.

Children, like adults, seek approval. It is effective and helps to increase their self-confidence (Fig. 17–2). The positive approach should be taken as often as possible. One assumes that the toddler is going to be good rather than bad. "Thank you, Johnny, for giving me the matches" will make them arrive in your hand more quickly than "Give me those matches right now," said in a threatening tone. The use of fear or physical aggression should not be part of discipline as it does not foster self-control and can lead to physical or mental abuse.

Fear is a valuable emotion to the child if it does not become too intense. Unfortunately, many children fear many situations that are not in themselves dangerous, and this sometimes deprives them of activities that otherwise would be enjoyable. When a toddler begins to ride a tricycle, if the parent warns, "be careful—don't fall," the toddler may develop a fear of the risk taking that may be involved in experiencing new activities.

The physical and mental health of the child at the time of a fear-provoking experience affects the extent of the reaction. Also, if the child is alone, fear may be greater than if someone such as a parent or nurse is present. Once a fear has been learned, it is more difficult to eliminate. Favorite possessions and repetitive rituals are *self-consoling behaviors* for the toddler, particularly at bedtime and during separation from parents.

Stress increases fear of separation. Adults should attempt to control their own fears in the presence of young children. Respect and understanding should always be accorded to children who are afraid. Making fun of the fear or shaming the child in front of others is detrimental to their self-esteem.

Many toddlers who independently explore the clinic examining room while waiting to be examined may cling to the parent when the stranger, who is the health care examiner, enters the room and approaches the child. The toddler who does not seek the parent during stressful situations or turns to a stranger for comfort reflects a need for closer evaluation of the parent–child relationship.

The "terrible two's" with negativistic behavior predominating, is the start of the disciplinary pattern of the family that will carry throughout the childhood years and affect the personality of the child. Corporal punishment, involving spanking is accepted in many traditional cultures as the mainstay of discipline. However, regular spanking reflects a desperate effort by the parent to gain control over a toddler exercising his or her beginning autonomy and developing negativism. Potential injury, child abuse, and reciprocal aggressive behavior in the child can be avoided with careful parental guidance concerning alternative techniques of discipline. Timeout, limit setting, clear communication, and frequent rewards/approval for positive behavior are effective noncorporal techniques of discipline.

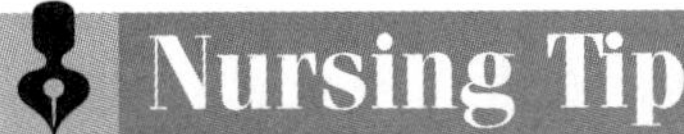

Caregivers need to provide safe areas for the toddler to explore. They need to watch carefully before saying "no."

Communicating love and respect to the child with a clear message that it is the *behavior* not the *child* that is disapproved by the adult, are the keys to effective discipline. Behavior problems that can occur during early childhood are detailed in Table 17–4.

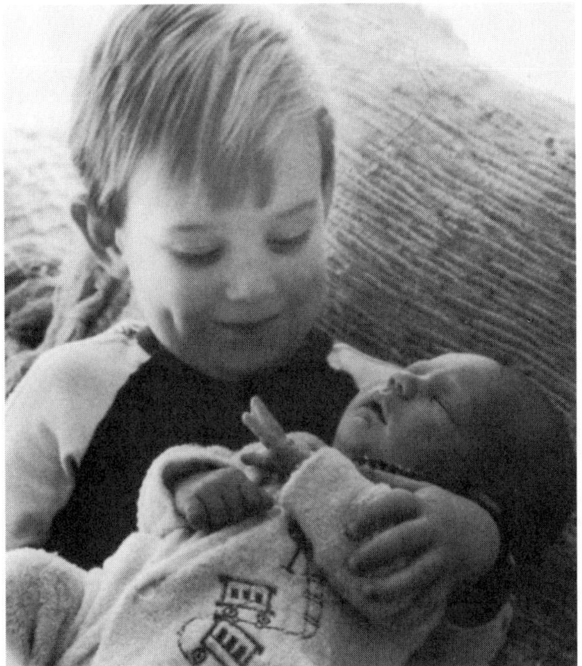

Figure 17–2. • Note the pride on this toddler's face as he holds his new sister.

DAILY CARE

Nutrition, dentition, and oral care are discussed in Chapter 15. When talking to the toddler, the adult should be at eye level with the child. This way, the adult seems less overwhelming. This is of particular importance when the child is in a fear-provoking environment, such as the hospital. A flexible schedule organized about the needs of the entire household is best for the toddler. The toddler needs a consistent routine, but it can differ for special occasions.

The clothing of toddlers should be simple and easy for them to put on and take off. Pants with elastic waists are convenient for them to pull down when they use the toilet. All clothing must be fairly loose to provide freedom of movement for jumping and other strenuous activities. Sunburn protection with clothing or sunscreen is necessary to prevent skin damage (Fig. 17–3).

The toddler wears shoes mainly for protection. They should fit the shape of the foot and be ½ inch longer and ¼ inch wider than the foot. The heels must fit securely. Children should wear their usual shoes at their periodic checkups because these show how the shoes have been worn, which indicates to the doctor how the children are using their

Table 17–4

BEHAVIOR PROBLEMS DURING EARLY CHILDHOOD, NORMAL EXPECTATIONS, AND PARENTAL GUIDANCE

Behavior	Normal Expectations	Child Factors Contributing to Problem	Parental Guidance
Sleep disorders	Occasional nightmares beginning at about 36 months Ritual bedtime routine; attempt to delay sleep peaks between 2 and 3 years	Excessive napping during the day Insufficient adult interaction during the day, leading to use of bedtime as opportunity to gain adult attention	Provide 1 nap a day until end of 2nd year when naps can be eliminated Use of bedtime rituals, such as a quiet activity or bedtime stories, are helpful
	Head banging and rocking between 1 and 4 years provide release of tension	Unusual fears related to darkness, being left alone	Use of favorite toy or blanket in the bed can ease insecurities involved in separation Provide environment conducive to sleep Avoid scary TV shows
		Discomfort of wet diapers Illness	Restrict fluids before bedtime
Temper tantrums	Tantrums peak at 2 years of age, decreasing in frequency and intensity until they rarely occur by about 4 years of age. Usually occur in response to frustrated desires of a child, such as wanting a toy that cannot be purchased	Used as a manipulative device to gain control of parental behavior Insufficient positive interaction with adults, leading to use of tantrums to gain attention	Use simple explanations of behavior expectations. Use time out responses (1 minute per year of age) Maintain consistency of expectations from both parents Reward good behavior
Toilet training and bed wetting	Has full physiologic capacity for day control by 3 years, night control by 4 years	Fears and anxiety in response to negative toilet training	Use positive rewards for successful toileting. Ignore accidents
	Daytime and nighttime "accidents" occur throughout early childhood, decreasing in frequency by 4 years	Used as an attention-getting device if positive means of gaining attention are lacking	Recognize signals of need to use toilet Restrict fluids before bedtime
	Regression occurs with environmental or social changes, such as arrival of sibling, moving, divorce	May use constipation as a control mechanism Excessive fluid intake before bedtime	Use clothing that toddler can easily remove for self-toileting
Aggressive or quarrelsome behavior, sibling rivalry	Ability to play cooperatively begins to emerge at 3–5 years. Before this age, is seldom able to share toys; often wants toys that another child has	Insufficient positive adult attention leads to deliberate use of aggression to gain adult attention	Prepare toddler for the separation and change involved in the arrival of a new sibling Provide for any changes involved 1–2 months before arrival of sibling (e.g., change to a new bed or room)
	Predominant use of physical hitting, shoving to express displeasure; verbal abilities begin to emerge	Aggression may arise from actual or perceived adult preference for sibling or playmate	Provide toddler with doll to imitate parental behaviors Provide for special individual time with toddler each day
Inability to separate; excessive shyness	Can separate easily by 3 years if surroundings are consistent, predictable, positive	Inadequate establishment of self-concept, leading to lack of confidence even in familiar surroundings	Prepare toddler for anticipated separation
	Continues to protest separation if environment changes or if confronted by total strangers	Uses protest of separation as a manipulative control device	Refer to time using concrete terms ("I will return after lunch" rather than "I will return at 1 PM")
	Shy in new and strange surroundings, relaxed and spontaneous in familiar surroundings	Fear of being abandoned	Avoid radiating parental anxiety at the planned separation Spend time with toddler and in new environment or with new caretaker before leaving

From Chinn, P., Leitch, C. (1979). *Child health maintenance* (2nd ed.). St. Louis, MO: Mosby-Year Book.

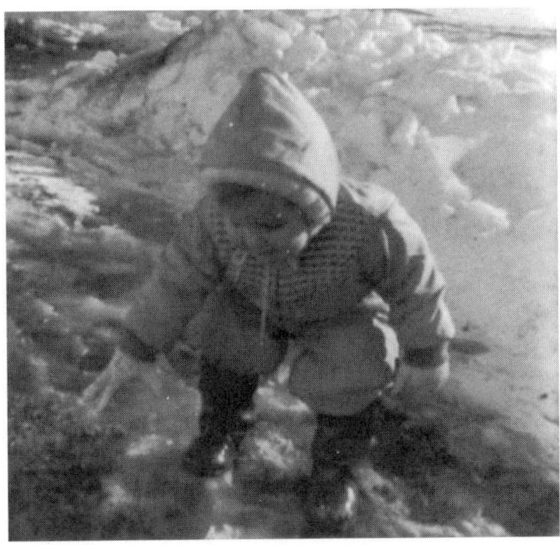

Figure 17–3. • The toddler needs security, but she also needs opportunities to explore her world. She must be dressed suitably for the weather. Touching cold snow or experiencing the movement of water at a beach are new experiences for a toddler.

bodies. Whenever safe and possible, the toddler may go barefoot, since this strengthens the foot muscles. Socks must be large enough that they do not flex the toes. The toddler should be taught to pull socks free from the toes before putting on shoes.

Good posture is the result of proper nutrition, plenty of fresh air and exercise, and sufficient rest. The toddler's mattress must be firm. The chair and play table are adapted to size. In some cases, this can be easily accomplished by placing a rolled-up blanket or pad in the seat of the chair. A sturdy small stool placed in the bathroom will bring the child to the proper height for brushing their teeth. As in all areas of learning, the child's posture is greatly influenced by that of other members of the family. The toddler who is happy and is allowed gradually increasing independence develops a sense of security, which is reflected in the posture (Fig. 17–4). Slouching is sometimes seen in children who are insecure and lack self-confidence.

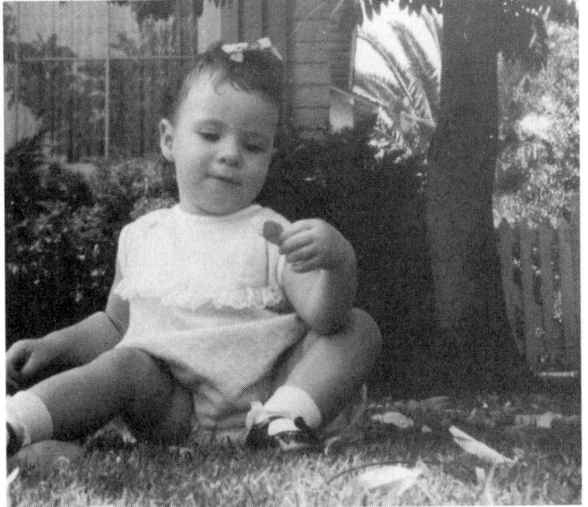

Figure 17–4. • The toddler uses all senses to explore the outside world.

TOILET INDEPENDENCE

There are many approaches to toilet training. Much depends on the temperament of both the individual child and the person guiding the child. Readiness is important. Voluntary control of anal and urethral sphincters occurs at about 18 to 24 months. The child's waking up dry in the morning or from naptime is an indication of maturity. Children must be able to communicate in some fashion that they are wet or need to urinate or defecate. They must be willing to sit on the potty for at least 5 to 10 minutes.

Toddlers seek approval and like to imitate the actions of parents. They wander into the bathroom and are curious about what is taking place there. If a parent feels that the child will respond to training at this time, the child might first be put in training pants or pull-up diapers. These can be removed quickly and easily, and the child becomes more aware of being wet.

The use of a child's potty chair or a device that attaches to an adult seat is a matter of personal preference. A potty chair may make the toddler feel more secure, for it is small (Fig. 17–5). It should support the back and arms of the child. The feet should touch the floor. If a potty seat is not available, the child can be placed on the standard-size toilet, facing the toilet tank. This method may increase feelings of security. The toddler can use a regular toilet with a bench to support the child's feet.

Bowel training is generally attempted first; however, some toddlers become bladder trained during the day because they enjoy listening to the "tinkle" in the potty. If toddlers have bowel movements at the same time each day, they may progress fairly rapidly. They should not be left on the potty chair for more than a few minutes at a time.

Demands and threats do more damage than good. Life is smoother for all if the parent remains

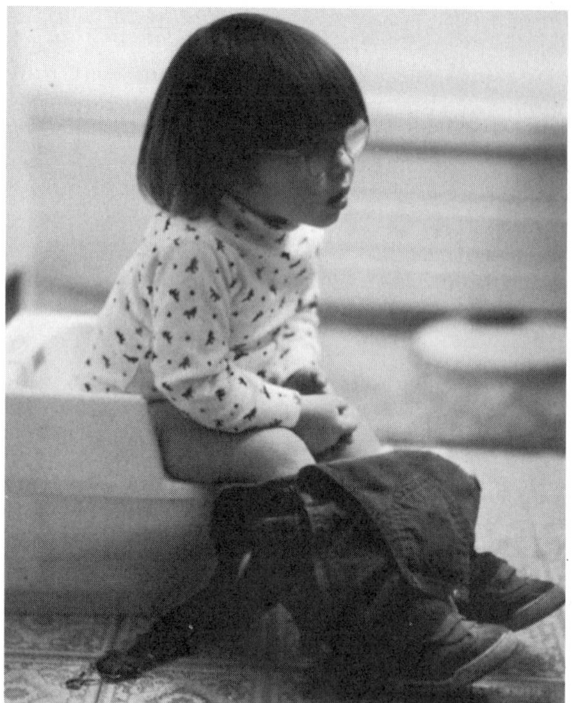

Figure 17–5. • Toilet training should be a nonstressful experience for the toddler. Nurses can help parents to identify readiness for toilet independence. The nurse assesses the parents' expectations, family and cultural pressures, and developmental readiness of the child before instruction begins.

patient and keeps this new adventure pleasant. Training should not be undertaken when the family or child is under stress, such as during illness or a move to a new location.

Bladder training is begun when the toddler stays dry for about 2 hours at a time. One morning a parent may discover that the toddler has gone the entire night without wetting. It is then logical to put the child on the potty chair and to praise success. Bladder training varies widely, particularly during the night. Restricting fluids before bedtime may help. Placing the half-asleep child on the potty chair accomplishes little.

Most children continue to have occasional accidents until the age of 4 years. If the toddler has a mishap, parents should accept it matter-of-factly and merely change the clothes. When adults show continuous affection to their children and accept both bad and good days, children benefit.

Nursing Tip

Nurses can help parents to identify readiness for toilet independence.

The word that toddlers use to signal defecation or urination should be one that is recognized by others besides the immediate family. Sometimes, a parent may forget to inform the baby-sitter or nursery school teacher of the word that the child uses. This causes the toddler unnecessary frustration because those about them cannot understand what they are trying to say.

Toddlers who are toilet trained at home should continue to use the potty in the hospital setting. They may be acutely embarrassed by wetting the crib. Nurses regularly consult the child's nursing care plan to maintain continuity of care as well as promote growth and development of the toddler. Although regression of bowel and bladder training is common during hospitalization, personnel often contribute to it by not taking time to investigate the child's needs.

NUTRITION COUNSELING

Caloric requirements per unit of body weight decline in the toddler from 120 cal/kg during infancy to 100 cal/kg. Children need an adequate protein intake to cover maintenance needs and to provide for optimum growth. Milk should be limited to 24 oz a day. Too few solid foods can lead to dietary deficiencies of iron. Children between the ages of 1 and 3 years are high-risk candidates for anemia.

The toddler who is well nourished shows steady proportional gains on height and weight charts and has good bone and tooth development. The diet history should be adequate with excessive calories and large amounts of vitamins avoided.

The toddler is noted for having a fluctuating appetite with strong food preferences. The nurse reminds parents that any nutritious food can be eaten at any meal; for example, soup for breakfast and cereal for supper. Serving size is important (Table 17–5). Too-large servings are discouraged because they may overwhelm the child and can lead to overeating problems. One tablespoon of solid food per year of age serves as a measurement guide. A quiet time before meals provides an opportunity for the child to "wind down." The toddler's refusal to eat may be due to fatigue or not being particularly hungry. The toddler may eat one food with vigor one week and refuse it the next. A flexible schedule designed to meet the needs of the toddler and the rest of the family must be worked out by the individual family. Forcing toddlers to eat only creates further difficulties. They are

Table 17–5

APPROXIMATE SERVING SIZES PER MEAL

	1 Year of Age	2–3 Years of Age
Bread	½ slice	1 slice
Cereal	½ oz	¾ oz
Rice/pasta	¼ cup	⅓ cup
Vegetables	2 tbsp	3 tbsp
Fruit	⅓ cup	½ cup
Milk	¼ cup	⅓ cup
Meat, beans	2 tbsp	3 tbsp

Note: Approximate serving sizes per meal for a toddler. For food pyramid see p. 398.

quick to sense parents' frustration and may use mealtime to obtain attention by behaving poorly and refusing to eat. Discipline and arguments during mealtime only upset everyone's digestion.

Toddlers are fond of ritual. This is frequently seen at mealtime. They want a particular dish, glass, and bib. It is best to go along with the wishes, as long as they do not become too pronounced. It gives them a sense of security and in the long run, saves time and energy for the adult.

Toddlers have a brief attention span. They may try to stand in the highchair or wander away from the table. If they have eaten a fair amount of the meal, they may be excused; otherwise distraction of some type is necessary. Toddlers who regularly feed themselves may enjoy being helped by mommy or daddy. Some restaurants that cater to families provide crayons and special placemat to keep the small child occupied until adults finish their dinners. In the hospital, the toddler who is fed in a highchair wears a jacket restraint, and the nurse remains with the child.

The toddler's food is chopped into fine pieces. A variety of foods are offered, and one should try to plan contrast of colors and textures. A 2-year-old likes finger foods. Foods are served at moderate temperatures. Candy, cake, and soda between meals are to be avoided. See page 403 for nutritional guide.

Children like colorful dishes, which must be made of an unbreakable substance. Washable plastic bibs, placemats, and protection for the floor around the highchair are advisable. Silverware should be small enough that it can be handled easily. Seating equipment should be adjusted so that the child is comfortable and maintains good posture. Figure 17–6 illustrates the self-feeding skills of the toddler of 18 months.

Nursing Tip

Determining Size of Portions

Toddlers and young children should be offered 1 tablespoon of solid food per year of age or ¼ of adult portion of a food item.

DAY CARE

Family life has changed dramatically since the 1970s. Today many more children are cared for in community settings outside of the home. Since 1992 the fastest growing group of persons in the labor force were women with infants. Not only were more mothers working, but they were also returning to the work force sooner after the child was born. It was clear that alternative methods of child care were necessary. These arrangements must meet families' personal preferences, cultural perspectives, and financial and special needs. Parents must take an active role in ensuring high-quality care (Fig. 17–7). Nurses need to be resource persons and family advocates because finding adequate day care can be stressful.

The decision to place a toddler in the care of others while parents work can be difficult and produce feelings of guilt in the parent. The concept of such care is not new. Many cultures, such as the Israeli's, have traditionally placed toddlers in day care while working on a "kibbutz." The hours of care extend from early morning to the dinner time hour. Successful alternate child care arrangements depend on specific guidelines in selecting the facility (see p. 463), frequent visits to the facility, and close communication and conferences with the staff in the facility. Day care for the toddler differs somewhat from the preschool child because of the toddler's shorter attention span, the tendency to *parallel play* rather than group play, and the need for closer supervision to maintain safety.

There are a variety of types of child care. Many children today can be cared for by relatives (Fig. 17–8), friends, neighbors, or those who have advertised such services. However, there is little research on these types of home arrangements, and few standards of quality control. Most licensed day care centers are private businesses run for profit. They are subject to state regulations about physical layout, number of children per caretaker, education of personnel, and so on. Parents have to plan ahead for times when the child is sick and unable to attend. A few innovative programs for in-home care of sick children have been developed. Employer-supported child care is a rapidly growing area. These programs are very diverse. Some companies provide family day care (care of the child in the

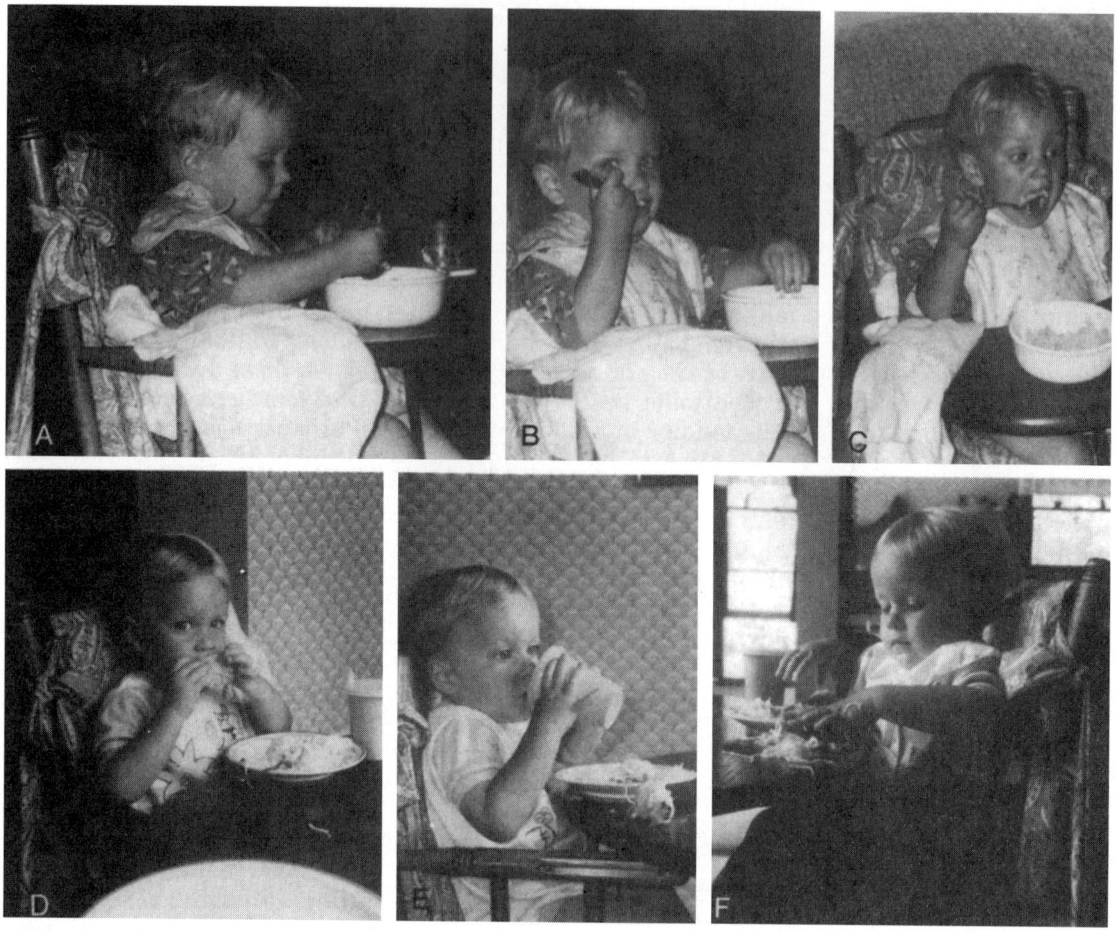

Figure 17–6. • At 18 months the toddler can hold a spoon **(A)**, can bring food to the mouth **(B)**, does not yet have the ability to rotate the wrist and elevate the elbow to keep food on the spoon **(C)**, manages finger foods **(D)**, drinks well from a cup **(E)**, and enjoys playing with food **(F)**.

provider's home) as well. Other employers assist parents through reimbursement, referral programs, or support of existing child care programs in the community.

For low-income and some middle-income families, the cost of child care is difficult, if not impossible, to maintain. Some form of continued or expanded government assistance or private funding is necessary. Inspection and monitoring of child care facilities to ensure compliance with health (physical and mental) and safety standards are paramount. Ideally, all day care programs would include comprehensive health services and health education programs. Criteria for selecting a day care center are similar to those discussed for nursery schools (see p. 463).

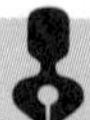

Nursing Tip

A major task for parents is to "let go" and allow toddler to interact with influences outside the family, in day care centers, or preschools.

INJURY PREVENTION

Accidents kill and cripple more children than any disease known and are *the leading cause of death* in childhood. Unfortunately, we do not have a preventive for this, but we do have a defensive weapon. This weapon is knowledge. If parents understand their child's activities at certain ages, they can prevent many serious injuries by taking necessary precautions (Table 17–6).

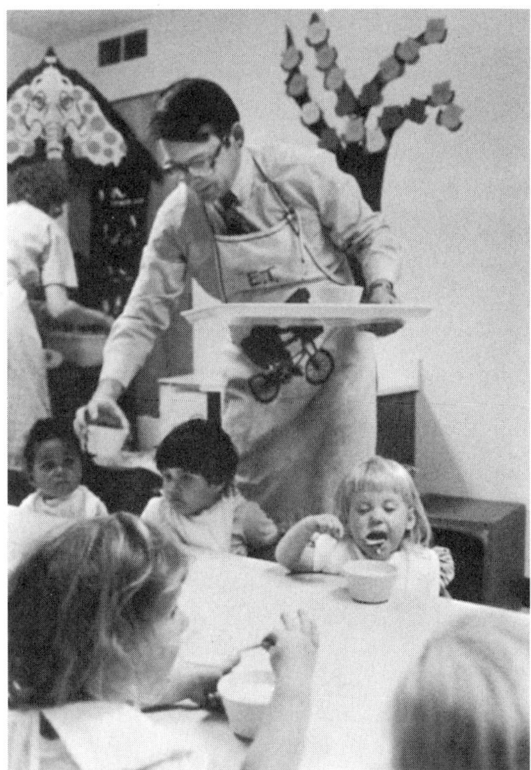

Figure 17–7. • Parents must take an active role in ensuring high-quality day care. An indication of a good program is the child's degree of happiness while attending the day care center. (Courtesy of Blank Memorial Hospital for Children, Des Moines, IA.)

Nurses have an important responsibility to review injury prevention with parents during each clinic visit. The normal behavior characteristics of a toddler, including curiosity, mobility, and negativity make the toddler prone to injuries, which often occur in and around the home (Fig. 17–9).

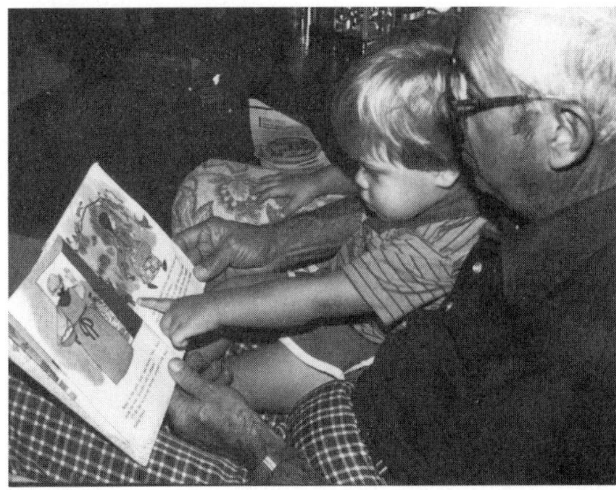

Figure 17–8. • Active and involved grandparents benefit all three generations.

Car safety is important. The use of seatbelts are effective if worn properly. A shoulder strap that extends across the neck or a lap belt that fits high on the abdomen or waist area can be harmful rather then helpful. A child seat placed in the front car seat close to the passenger air bag can be dangerous. Table 17–6 correlates hazards that are frequently associated with the toddler age group.

Nurses demonstrate safety measures to their patients and their families. This is most effectively done by good example. Measures pertinent to the pediatric unit are discussed on page 538. Nurses in the community can often contribute indirectly to the welfare of others by the example set and by being aware of emergency medical facilities available in the community.

Consumer Education

The federal government and concerned private agencies have attempted to regulate some of the variables that cause injuries. A few examples are ensuring the use of nonflammable material for children's sleepwear, child-proofing caps on medicine bottles and certain household products, and establishing maximum temperatures for home hot-water heaters. Smoke detectors in homes and public places are commonplace. In 1974 the United States Consumer Product Safety Commission established regulations for crib slats, locks, and latches and crib mattress size and thickness. Safety warnings on the crib's carton advise buyers to use a snug mattress only. This type of information should be reinforced by the nurse.

Laws have been passed in virtually all states that require infants and small children to be restrained while riding in automobiles (Fig. 17–10). These restraints must follow standards established by the Federal Motor Vehicle Safety Department. Rental cars also loan child seat restraints. The use of car seats begins with the first ride home from the hospital.

New homes are required to have smoke detectors. Consumers who live in older homes and apartment complexes are also encouraged to install them. Various other safety codes are mandatory for public buildings, with additional measures required for buildings specifically for the handicapped. The problems of surveillance and upkeep nevertheless are considerable. Many children live in substandard housing with little supervision. The education of parents is of monumental importance in decreasing death and disability (Figs. 17–11 and 17–12).

Table 17–6
HOW TO PREVENT HAZARDS CAUSED BY THE BEHAVIORAL CHARACTERISTICS OF TODDLERS

Behavioral Characteristics	Hazard and Prevention Strategies
Automobile	
Impulsive, unable to delay gratification, increased mobility, egocentric	Teach child street safty rules Teach child the meaning of red, yellow, and green traffic lights Caution children not to run from behind parked cars or snowbanks Use car seat restraints appropriately Hold toddler's hand when crossing the street Supervise tricycle riding Do not allow children to play in the car alone Driver must look carefully in front and behind vehicles before accelerating Teach children what areas are safe in and around the house Supervise child under 3 years at all times
Burns	
Fascination for fire Toddler can reach articles by climbing, pokes fingers in holes and openings; can open doors and drawers; is unaware of cause and effect	Teach the child the meaning of "hot" (one mother taught this by allowing the child to touch beach sand warmed by the sun) Put matches, cigarettes, candles, and incense out of reach and sight Turn handles of cooking utensils toward the back of the stove Beware of hot coffee; avoid tablecloths with overhang Keep appliances such as coffee pots, electric frying pans, and food processors and their cords out of reach Test food and fluids heated in microwave ovens to ensure that center is not too hot Beware of hot charcoal grills Use snug fireplace screens Mark children's rooms to alert fire fighters in emergency Keep a pressure-type fire extinguisher available, and teach all family members who are old enough how to use it Practice what to do in case of fire in your home Install smoke detectors Cover electrical outlets with protective caps Check bath water temperature before placing child in water Do not allow child to handle water faucets Protect child from sun with sunscreen and clothing
Falls	
Toddlers like to explore different parts of the house. They can open doors and lean out open windows. Their depth perception is immature. *Their capabilities change quickly.* Although they may seem quite grown up at times, they still require constant supervision at home and on the playground	Teach children how to go up and come down stairs when they show a readiness for this task Fasten crib sides securely and leave them up when child is in the crib Use side rails on a large bed when child graduates from crib Lock basement doors or use gates at top and bottom of stairs Mop spilled water from floor immediately Use window guards Use car seat restraints appropriately Keep scissors and other pointed objects away from the toddler's reach Use childproof door knobs and drawer closures Secure child in shopping cart at store Supervise climbing child in playground Clothing and shoelaces should be appropriate to prevent tripping
Suffocation and choking	
Explores with senses, likes to bite on and taste things. Eats on the run	Do not allow small children to play with deflated balloons, as these can be sucked into windpipe Inspect toys for small or loose parts Remove small objects such as coins, buttons, pins from reach Avoid popcorn, nuts, small hard candies, chewing gum or large chunks of meat, such as hot dogs Debone fish, chicken Learn Heimlich maneuver Inspect width of crib and playpen slats Keep plastic bags away from small children; do not use as mattress cover If child is vomiting, turn him or her on side Avoid nightclothes with drawstring necks Discard old refrigerators and appliances or remove doors

Table continued on following page

Table 17–6

HOW TO PREVENT HAZARDS CAUSED BY THE BEHAVIORAL CHARACTERISTICS OF TODDLERS *(Continued)*

Behavioral Characteristics	Hazard and Prevention Strategies
Poisoning	
Ingenuity increases, can open most containers. Increased mobility provides child access to cupboards, medicine cabinets, bedside stands, interior of closets. Looks at and touches everything. Learns by trial and error. Puts objects in mouth.	Store household detergents and cleaning supplies out of reach and in a locked cabinet Do not put chemicals or other potentially harmful substances into food or beverage containers Keep medicines in a locked cabinet; put them away immediately after using them Use child-resistant caps and packaging Flush old medicine down toilet Follow physician's directions when administering medication Do not refer to pills as "candy" Educate parents as to when and how to use ipecac syrup Explain poison symbols to child and to parents not fluent in English Keep telephone number of poison control center available When painting, use paint marked "for indoor use" or one that conforms to standards for use on surfaces that may be chewed by children Wash fruits and vegetables before eating Obtain and record name of any new plant purchased Alert family of location and appearance of poisonous plants on or around property or frequently encountered when camping Use childproof locks on cabinets Use dishes that do not have high lead content
Drowning	
Lacks depth perception. Does not realize danger. Loves water play	Watch child continuously while at beach or near a pool Empty wading pools when child has finished playing Cover wells securely. Wear recommended life jackets in boats Begin teaching water safety and swimming skills early Lock fences surrounding swimming pools Supervise tub baths; be aware that a young child can drown in a very small amount of water
Electric shock	
Pokes and probes with fingers	Cover electrical outlets. Cap unused sockets with safety plugs. Water conducts electricity; teach child not to touch electrical appliances when wet; keep appliances out of reach Keep electrical appliances away from tub and sink area
Animal bites	
Immature judgment	Teach child to avoid stray animals Do not allow toddler to abuse household pets Supervise closely
Safety	
Easily distracted Trusting of others Falls frequently	Teach toddler stranger safety Do not personalize clothes Do not allow toddler to eat or suck lollipops while running or playing Keep sharp edged objects out of reach Keep sharp-edged furniture out of play area

Keep first aid chart and emergency numbers handy. Know location of and how to get to nearest emergency facility

TOYS AND PLAY

In 1970 the Child Protection and Toy Safety Act was passed in an effort to halt the distribution of unsafe toys. In addition, parents must be taught to inspect toys purchased and to buy toys suitable for the age, skills, and abilities of the individual child. Some labels now give safety information and intended age. Parents are also taught to inspect toys routinely for damage.

Notification of recall for a specific toy is generally announced on radio and television as well as published in newspapers and consumer journals. Toy boxes and toy chests are also a potential hazard. The most serious injuries caused by a box or chest are the result of the lid's falling on a child or a child's being trapped inside. A parent can report a product hazard by writing the United States Consumer Product Safety Commission, Washington DC 20207.

Play is the work of a toddler. Through play, toddlers learn how to manipulate and understand

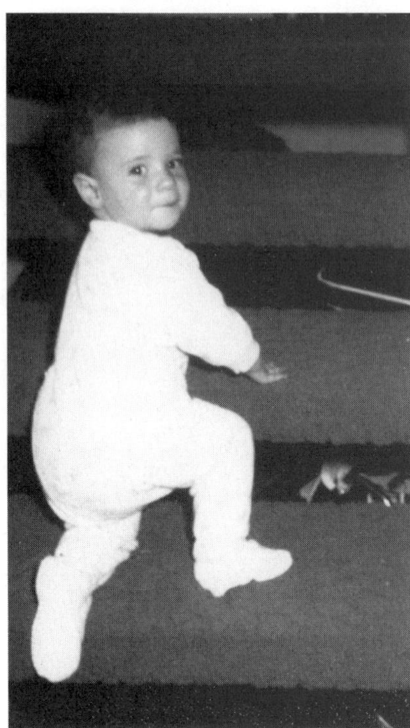

Figure 17–9. • The toddler is able to climb stairs and requires close supervision to maintain safety.

their environment, socialize, and learn about their world. High-priced toys are not necessary. Pots and pans from the kitchen, supervised water play, dancing to music, crayons or finger paint and paper are preferred by toddlers. Often a picture book reviewed while on the lap of a family member can be enjoyed over and over again. Tricycles can be adapted to the size and ability of the toddler. Objects that can be pushed or pulled are preferred to wind-up toys for this age group. The sense of touch can be stimulated by providing materials such as fur, sandpaper, felt and nylon. Colors can be taught while having the toddler aid in sorting the laundry. Memory can be stimulated by pointing to familiar pictures in a book, newspaper or magazine. Counting can be taught while climbing stairs. Supervision and maintenance of safety are the keys to a positive play experience for the toddler.

As toddlers become aware of their expanding environment, their social development takes form. *Egocentric thinking* in which children relate everything to themselves predominates. They engage in *parallel play,* playing next to, but not with, their peer. They gradually develop *cooperative play* that involve imagination and sharing skills.

Nurses must closely assess children with special needs for safety precautions. Children with handicaps such as visual, motor, or intellectual impair-

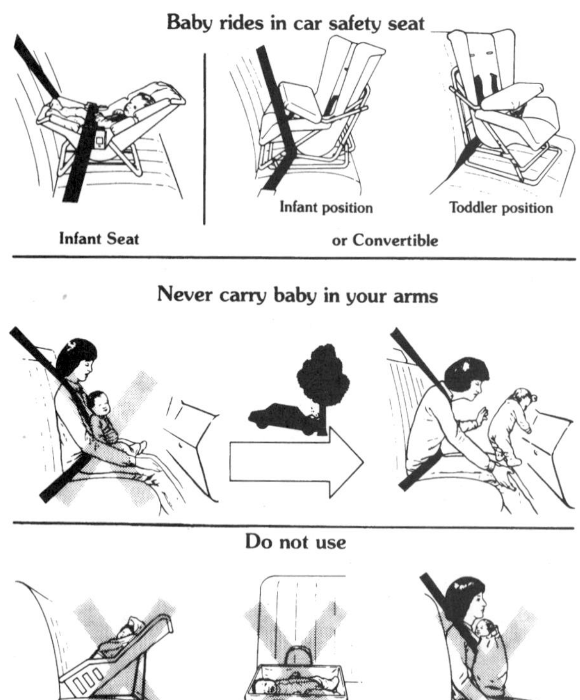

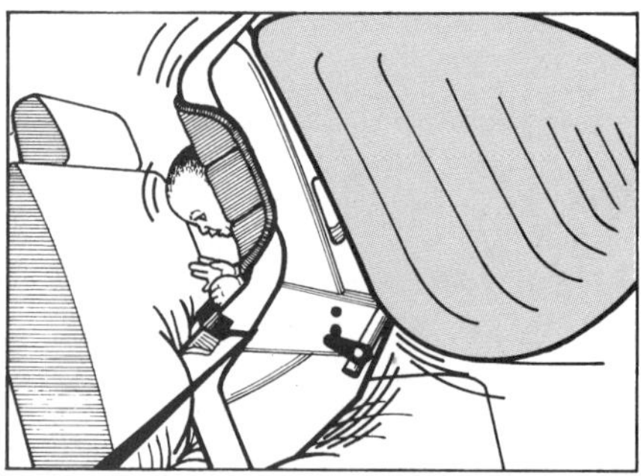

Figure 17–10. • **A,** Infants and children should ride in a car safety seat for all car trips. The seat is ideally placed on the center rear seat of the car and secured with the car's seatbelt. The infant should face the rear until 1 year of age and at least 20 lbs. The back should be flat against the car seat, and the head and body of a small infant should be supported with rolled cloth diapers or blankets. The seat's harness should be fastened snugly. Household carriers and travel beds that are not crash-tested are *unsafe* to use as car safety devices. The infant should never be carried in one's arms. (Adapted courtesy of Evenflow Juvenile Furniture Company, Los Angeles, CA.) **B,** A front passenger-side air bag can strike the back of the safety seat, and the impact could seriously injure a baby's neck and head. To prevent this injury, always place the baby in the back seat. (From American Academy of Pediatrics. [1993, Spring]. *Safe Ride News.*)

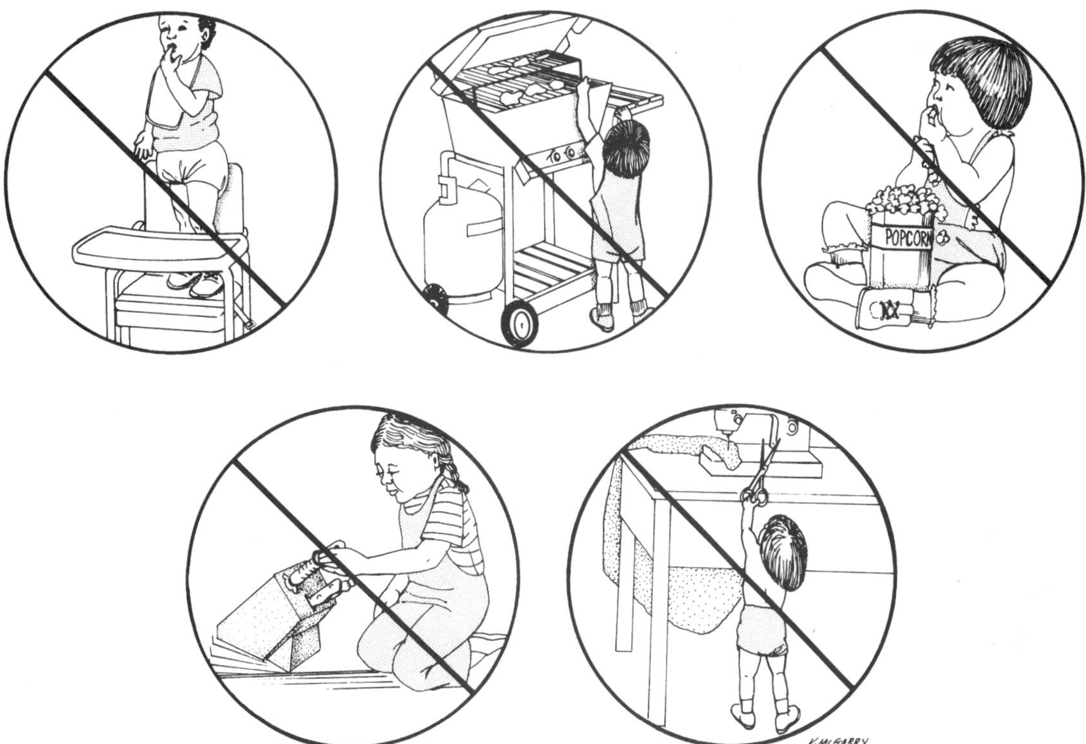

Figure 17–11. • Safety measures are taken to protect toddlers from these hazards.

ments; convulsive disorders; or diabetes, require extended instruction according to the child's particular needs. Immobile children need to be protected from sunburn and wind or rainy weather. Adults must also guard these children from mosquitoes and other vectors. Control of the agent of injury involves some of the methods mentioned in the discussion of consumer education, such as child-proof caps on medication containers and regulations for children's furniture (Fig. 17–13).

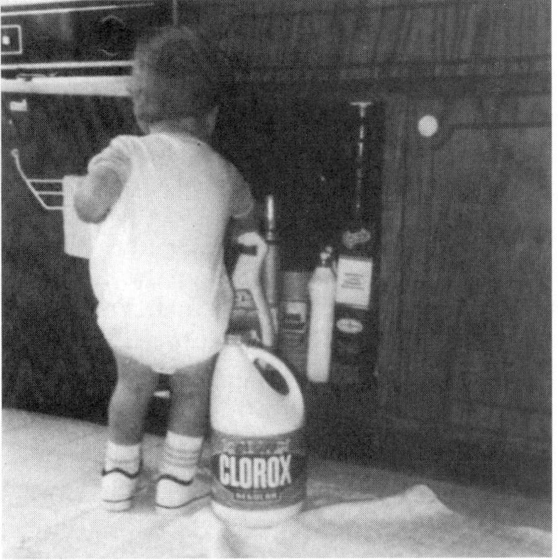

Figure 17–12. • Poisoning prevention is particularly important for toddlers between the ages of 1 and 4 years.

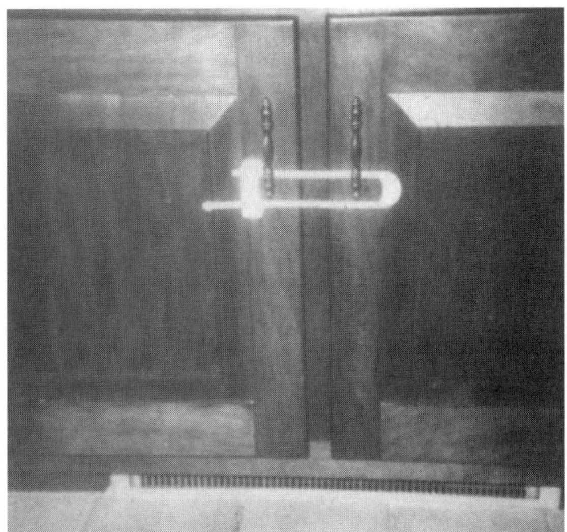

Figure 17–13. • Inexpensive safety devices, such as these plastic door handle devices, limit access to materials that are dangerous to the inquisitive toddler.

KEY POINTS

- The birth weight has quadrupled by 2½ years of age.
- Physical changes of the toddler include the acquisition of fine and gross motor skills, including increased mobility and increased eye–hand coordination.
- The digestive volume and processes of the toddler increase to accommodate a three-meal-a-day schedule.
- Complete bowel and bladder control is usually achieved by 2½ to 3 years of age.
- Erickson refers to the toddler stage as one in which the child's task is to acquire a sense of autonomy (self-control) while overcoming shame and doubt.
- The most evident cognitive achievements of the toddler are language and comprehension.
- Some important self-regulatory functions mastered by the toddler include toilet independence, self-feeding, tolerating delayed gratification, separation from parents, and perfecting newfound physical skills and speech.
- Separation anxiety includes the stages of protest, despair, and detachment.
- Parental guidance is needed to deal with the negativism, temper tantrums, and sibling rivalry that is characteristic of this age group.
- Discipline for the toddler should be designed to teach rather then punish.
- Some methods of dealing with the inconsistencies of the toddler include distraction, ignoring minor infractions, reward and praise, and timeout in a safe place.
- Accidents and poisoning are the leading causes of death in the toddler age group.
- Infants and children should ride in a car safety seat for all car trips.

MULTIPLE-CHOICE REVIEW QUESTIONS

Choose the most appropriate answer.

1. The term used to denote the toddler's concentration on self is
   a. ritualism.
   b. negativism.
   c. egocentric thinking.
   d. egomania.
2. The nurse assesses the vital signs of a 2-year-old. A normal respiratory rate (per minute) would be:
   a. 18–20.
   b. 25–30.
   c. 35–40.
   d. 45–50.
3. Which statement by the parent would indicate a need for further guidance.
   a. I use a car seat for my toddler whenever we are in the car and he is right beside me as I drive so I can keep an eye on him.
   b. I use a car seat for my toddler whenever we are in the car and secure it onto the rear seat of the car.
   c. I use a car seat for my toddler that is designed to hold children up to 40 pounds.
   d. I use a car seat for my toddler that is designed to fasten with the car seatbelt.
4. A mother tells the nurse that her 2-year-old toddler often has temper tantrums when at the family dinner table and asks how to handle the behavior. The best response of the nurse would be:
   a. Temper tantrums are normal for a 2-year-old and she will grow out of it.
   b. The toddler should be removed from the family dinner table until he is old enough to behave.
   c. Strict discipline and corporal punishment are appropriate to help the child to gain self-control.
   d. Parents should agree on a method of discipline, such as timeout, and use it when the child misbehaves.
5. One of the developmental tasks of the toddler that is most hazardous to safety is
   a. brief attention span.
   b. need for ritual.
   c. fluctuating appetite.
   d. need to explore.

BIBLIOGRAPHY AND READER REFERENCE

Ashwill, J., & Droske, S. (1997). *Nursing care of children: Principles and practices.* Philadelphia: Saunders.

Ball, J., & Bindler, R. (1995). *Pediatric nursing.* Norwalk, CT: Appleton & Lange.

Behrman, R., & Kleigman, R. (1994). *Nelson's essentials of pediatrics* (2nd ed.). Philadelphia: Saunders.

Blum, N. J., et al. (1995). Disciplining young children: The role of verbal instructions and reasoning. *Pediatrics, 96*(1), 336.

Bowden, V., Dickey, S., & Greenberg, C. (1998). *Children and their families: The continuum of care.* Philadelphia: Saunders.

Levine, M. D., Carey, W. B., & Crocker, A. C. (1992). *Developmental-behavioral pediatrics* (2nd ed.). Philadelphia: Saunders.

Mahan, L. K., & Escott-Stump, S. (1996). *Krause's food, nutrition and diet therapy* (9th ed.). Philadelphia: Saunders.

McFadden, E. A. (1994). Equipment safety for infants and children. *Journal of Pediatric Nursing, 9*(5), 335.

Montgomery, T. (1994). When not talking is the chief complaint. *Contemporary Pediatrics, 11*(9), 49.

Socolar, R. R., & Stein, R. E. (1995). Spanking infants and toddlers: Maternal belief and practice. *Pediatrics, 95*(1), 105.

Ulione, M. S. (1997, June). Health promotion and injury prevention in a child developmental center. *Journal of Pediatric Nursing, 12*(13), 148.

Wong, D. (1995). *Whaley & Wong's nursing care of infants and children* (5th ed.). St. Louis, MO: Mosby.

chapter 18

The Preschool Child

Outline

Objectives

On completion and mastery of Chapter 18, the student will be able to

- Define each vocabulary term listed.
- List the major developmental tasks of the preschool-age child.
- Describe the physical, psychosocial and spiritual development of children from 3 to 5 years of age, listing age-specific events and guidance when appropriate.
- Describe the development of the preschool child in relation to Piaget, Erikson and Kohlberg theories of development.
- Discuss the characteristics of a good nursery school.
- Discuss the value of play in the life of a preschool child.
- Designate two toys suitable for the preschool child, and provide the rationale for each choice.
- Describe the speech development of the preschool child.
- Discuss the value of the following: time-out periods, consistency, role modeling, rewards.
- Describe the developmental characteristics that predispose the preschool child to certain accidents, and suggest methods of prevention for each type of accident.
- Discuss the development of positive bedtime habits.
- Discuss the approach to problems such as enuresis, thumb-sucking, and sexual curiosity in the preschool child.
- Discuss one method of introducing the concept of death to a preschool child.

Vocabulary

animism
associative play
art therapy
centering
echolalia
egocentrism
enuresis
identification
play therapy
preconceptual stage
preoperational phase
ritualism
separation anxiety
symbolic functioning
therapeutic play
timeout

GENERAL CHARACTERISTICS

The child from 3 to 5 is often referred to as the *preschool child.* This period is marked by slowing of the physical growth process and mastery and refinement of the motor, social, and cognitive abilities that will enable the child to be successful in his or her school years.

The major tasks of the preschool child include preparation to enter school, development of a cooperative type play, control of body functions, acceptance of separation, and increase in communication skills, memory, and attention span. Dentition and nutrition are discussed in Chapter 15.

Physical Development. The infant who tripled his or her birth weight at 1 year has only doubled the 1-year weight by age 5. For instance, the baby who weighs 20 pounds on the first birthday will probably weigh about 40 pounds by the fifth. The child between ages 3 and 6 grows taller and loses the chubbiness seen during the toddler period. Between 3 and 5 years of age, there will be an increase of 3 inches in height, mostly in the legs, that contributes to the development of an erect, slender appearance. Visual acuity is 20/40 at 3 years and 20/30 at 4 years of age. All 20 primary teeth have erupted. Hand preference will be developed by 3 years of age, and efforts to change a left-handed child to a right-handed child can cause a high level of frustration. Appetite fluctuates widely. The normal pulse rate is 90 to 110 beats/min. The rate of respirations during relaxation is about 20/min. The systolic blood pressure is about 85 to 90 mm Hg; the diastolic is about 60 mm Hg.

Preschool children have good control of their muscles and participate in vigorous play; they become more adept at using old skills as each year passes. They can swing and jump higher. Their gait resembles that of an adult. They are quicker and have more self-confidence than they did as toddlers.

Cognitive Development. The thinking of the preschool child is unique. Piaget calls this period the *preoperational phase.* It comprises the ages of 2 to 7 years and is divided into two stages, the *preconceptual stage,* age 2 to 4 years, and the *intuitive thought stage,* age 4 to 7 years. Of importance in the preconceptual stage is the increasing development of language and symbolic functioning. Symbolic functioning is seen in the play of children who pretend that an empty box is a fort; they create a mental image to stand for something that is not there.

Another characteristic of this period is *egocentrism,* a type of thinking in which children have difficulty seeing any point of view other than their own. Because children's knowledge and understanding are restricted to their own limited experiences, misconceptions arise. One misconception is *animism.* This is a tendency to attribute life to inanimate objects. Another is *artificialism,* the idea that the world and everything in it are created by people.

The intuitive stage is one of prelogical thinking. Experience and logic are based on outside appearance (the child does not understand that a wide glass and a tall glass can both contain four ounces of juice). A distinctive characteristic of intuitive thinking is *centering,* the tendency to concentrate on a single outstanding characteristic of an object while excluding its other features.

With time and experience, more mature conceptual awareness is established. The process is highly complex, and the implications for practical application are numerous. Interested students are encouraged to explore these concepts through further study. Table 18–1 summarizes some major theories of personality development for the preschooler.

Effects of Cultural Practices. Cultural practices can influence the development of a sense of initiative in families that practice authoritarian-type parenting styles that put a great value on obedience and conformity. Parents and older siblings are models for language development and the mastery of sounds proceeds in the same order around the world. Some parents speak both English and a native language in the home. Studies have shown that young children adapt quickly to a bilingual environment. Cultural preferences related to dietary practices are discussed in Chapter 15.

Language Development. The development of language as a communication skill is essential for success in school. Delays or problems in language expression can be caused by physiological, psychological, or environmental stressors. Early detection and referral before 5 years of age can prevent school problems.

Table 18–1
PRESCHOOL GROWTH AND DEVELOPMENT

	Intelligence	Emotional	Language	Play	Parental Guidance
3 years	Piaget's preoperational phase Understands time in relation to concrete activities Knows own sex Attention span is approximately 15 minutes, easily distractible	Freud's phallic stage Oedipus complex may develop in boys Erikson's stage of initiative versus guilt Wishes to please parents Ritualism provides security Egocentric (unable to see viewpoint of others)	Vocabulary of approximately 300–800 words Uses plurals Forms 3-word sentences Can repeat 3 numbers Understanding occurs before expressive ability	Kohlberg: beginning moral development Identifies with same-sex parent Develops understanding of good/bad Explains different emotions in pretend play Starts to engage in group play Highly imaginative	Child usually wants to please parents Guidance techniques are based on this principle Overprotection during this stage of initiative can thwart the development of a coping mechanism in the child Self-esteem will be enhanced by having child "help" the parent
4 years	Can count to 5 Knows simple songs Sexual curiosity is high Attention span is approximately 20 minutes Adds logic to thinking Understands feelings are connected to actions	May use tantrums to relieve frustrations and if successful, may become a coping mechanism Has mood swings Is highly imaginative Asks many questions Likes to "show off" accomplishments Experiments with masturbation	Has vocabulary of 1500 words Uses 4 to 5 word sentences Experiments with language and words May use offensive words without understanding the meaning	Engages in rough and tumble play Learns how much he can control Demonstrates sibling rivalry	Minimize passive activity, such as doing puzzles *for* the child Repetition of words without comprehension should be referred for follow-up care (*echolalia*) Teach self-control through limit setting Guide parent in discipline techniques Provide nutritious snacks Answer questions truthfully
5 years	Beginning concept of past, present, and future although time is evidenced in activity rather than hour Knows days of the week Attention span reaches 30 minutes Can count to 10 Knows name and address Behaviors that result in rewards are considered right, behaviors that result in punishment are considered wrong	Less egocentric and beginning awareness of outside world Enjoys activities with parents of same sex	Has vocabulary of 2000 words Can name 4 colors Uses 6- to 8-word sentences with pronouns, etc.	Wants to play "by the rules," but cannot accept losing Can copy sample shapes and print first name Preference for hand use is established	Child can participate in own care Teach front to back wiping after bowel movements Provide information concerning vision and hearing assessment facilities in community Review immunization status Prepare parent for separation and entrance of child to school

Table 18–2 lists the language, cognitive and perceptual abilities required for success in school. Problems detected and treated during the preschool years can prevent many school problems in later years. Table 18–3 describes the clinical symptoms of typical language disorders. Evaluating language development must be done together with an assessment of problem-solving skills.

Table 18–2

SELECTED PERCEPTUAL, COGNITIVE, AND LANGUAGE PROCESSES REQUIRED FOR ELEMENTARY SCHOOL SUCCESS

Process	Description	Associated Problems
Perceptual		
Visual analysis	Ability to break a complex figure into components and understand their spatial relationships	Persistent letter confusion (e.g., between *b, d,* and *g*); difficulty with basic reading and writing and limited "sight" vocabulary
Proprioception and motor control	Ability to obtain information about body position by feel and unconsciously program complex movements	Poor handwriting, requiring inordinate effort, often with overly tight pencil grasp; special difficulty with timed tasks
Phonologic processing	Ability to perceive differences between similar sounding words and to break down words into constituent sounds	Delayed receptive language skills; attention and behavior problems secondary to not understanding directions; delayed acquisition of letter–sound correlations (phonetics)
Cognitive		
Long-term memory, both storage and recall	Ability to acquire skills that are "automatic" (i.e., accessible without conscious thought)	Delayed mastery of the alphabet (reading and writing letters); slow handwriting, inability to progress beyond basic mathematics
Selective attention	Ability to attend to important stimuli and ignore distractions	Difficulty following multistep instructions, completing assignments, and behaving well; peer interaction problems
Sequencing	Ability to remember things in order, facility with time concepts	Difficulty organizing assignments, planning, spelling, and telling time
Language		
Receptive language	Ability to comprehend complex constructions, function words (e.g., if, when, only, except), nuances of speech, and extended blocks of language (e.g., paragraphs)	Difficulty following directions, wandering attention during lessons and stories, problems with reading comprehension; problems with peer relationships
Expressive language	Ability to recall required words effortlessly (word finding), to control meanings, varying position and word endings to construct meaningful paragraphs and stories	Difficulty expressing feelings and using words for self-defense, with resulting frustration and physical acting out: struggling during "circle time" and in language-based subjects (e.g., English)

From Behrman, R., Kleigman, R., & Arvin, A. (1996). *Nelson's textbook of pediatrics* (15th ed., p. 57.). Philadelphia: Saunders.

Table 18–3

NOT TALKING: A CLINICAL CLASSIFICATION

When Parents Say	Classify the Symptoms as
"I'm the only one who understands what she says."	Articulation disorder
"She'll do what I say, but when she wants something, she just points."	Expressive language delay
"He can't play 'show me your nose,' and the only word he says is Mama."	Global language delay
"He never made those funny baby sounds or said Mama and Dada, and now he just repeats everything I say."	Language disorder
"He used to say things like Joey go 'bye bye,' but now he doesn't talk at all."	Language loss

From: Montgomery, T. (1994). When children do not talk. *Contemporary Pediatrics, 11*(9), 49.

Spiritual Development. Preschoolers learn about religious beliefs and practices from what they observe in the home. The preschooler cannot yet understand abstract concepts. Their concept of God is concrete, sometimes treated as an imaginary friend. Preschool children can memorize bible stories and related rituals, but their understanding of the concepts are limited. Observing religious traditions practiced in the home during a period of hospitalization (such as before meal or bedtime prayers) can help the preschool child to deal with stressors.

Sexual Curiosity. When guiding parents concerning sexual education of young children, the nurse should use the principles of teaching and learning common to other clients:

- First assess the knowledge base of the child, then assess what specific information the child is asking for.
- Be honest and accurate in providing information at the child's level. Although the child may not understand completely at first, the child's re-

peated questions and explanations will form the basis of later learning and understanding.
- Use correct terminology so that misinformation or misinterpretation can be avoided.
- Provide sex education at the time the child asks the question. The asking of the question often indicates readiness to learn.
- Parents need to understand that sexual curiosity starts as an inquiry into anatomical differences. Perhaps differences in urinating later becomes the focus. A general understanding of babies coming from mommy's tummy precedes the more mature concept of sexual organs and functioning.

Preschool children are as matter-of-fact about sexual investigation as they are about any other learning experience and are easily distracted to other activities. Sexual curiosity displayed in the form of masturbation or "playing doctor" should be approached in a positive manner. The appropriate touch or dress can be taught without generating a "bad" or "dirty" concept of the activity. Teaching socially acceptable behavior must be in the form of guidance rather than discipline.

Masturbation. Masturbation is common in both sexes during the preschool years. The child experiences pleasurable sensations, which lead to repetition of the behavior. It is beneficial to rule out other causes of this activity, such as rashes or penile or vaginal irritation. Masturbation in the preschool child is considered harmless if the child is outgoing, sociable, and not preoccupied with the activity.

Education of the parents consists of assuring them that this behavior is a form of sexual curiosity and is normal and not harmful to the child, who is merely curious about sexuality. The cultural and moral background of the family must be considered in assessing the degree of discomfort about this experience. A history of the time and place of masturbation and the parental response is helpful. Punitive reactions are discouraged, as these can potentially harm the child. Parents are advised to ignore the behavior and distract the child with some other activity. The child needs to know that masturbation is not acceptable in public; however, this must be explained in a nonthreatening manner. Children who masturbate excessively and who have experienced a great deal of disruption in their lives benefit from ongoing counseling.

Bedtime Habits. The development and reinforcement of optimum bedtime habits is important in the preschool years. Parents should be guided to engage the child in quiet activities before bedtime, to maintain specific rituals that signal bedtime readiness such as storytelling, and to verbally state "after this story, it will be bedtime." The use of a nightlight, a favorite bedtime toy, or a glass of water at the bedside is an option. Attention-getting behavior that results in taking the child into the parent's bed should be discouraged, as it rewards the attention-getting behavior and defeats the objectives of the bedtime ritual. The nurse should be aware that specific cultures encourage "family beds," where children regularly sleep with siblings and parents. Understanding cultural practices is essential before preparing a teaching plan.

PHYSICAL, MENTAL, EMOTIONAL, AND SOCIAL DEVELOPMENT

The Three-Year-Old

Three-year-olds are a delight to their parents. They are helpful and can assist in simple household chores. They obtain articles when directed and return them to the proper place. Three-year-olds come very close to the ideal picture that parents have in mind of their child. They are living proof that their parents' guidance during the trying 2-year-old period has been rewarded. Temper tantrums are less frequent, and in general the 3-year-old is less erratic. Of course, they are still individuals, but they seem to be able to direct their primitive instincts better than previously. They can help to dress and undress themselves, use the toilet, and wash their hands. They eat independently, and their table manners have improved.

Three-year-olds talk in longer sentences and can express thoughts and ask questions. They are more company to their parents and other adults because they can talk about their experiences. They are imaginative, talk to their toys, and imitate what they see about them. Soon they begin to make friends outside the immediate family. The type of play typical of this period is both *parallel* and *associative.* Children play in loosely associated groups. Their play is often similar (Fig. 18–1). Because they can now converse with playmates, they find satisfaction in joining their activities. Three-year-olds play cooperatively for short periods. They can ask others to "come out and play." If 3-year-olds are placed in a strange situation with children they do not know, they commonly revert to "parallel play" because it is more comfortable.

Preschoolers begin to find enjoyment away from mom and dad (Fig. 18–2), although they want them nearby when needed. They begin to lose some of their interest in their mother, who up to this time has been more or less their total world. The father's prestige begins to increase. Romantic attachment to

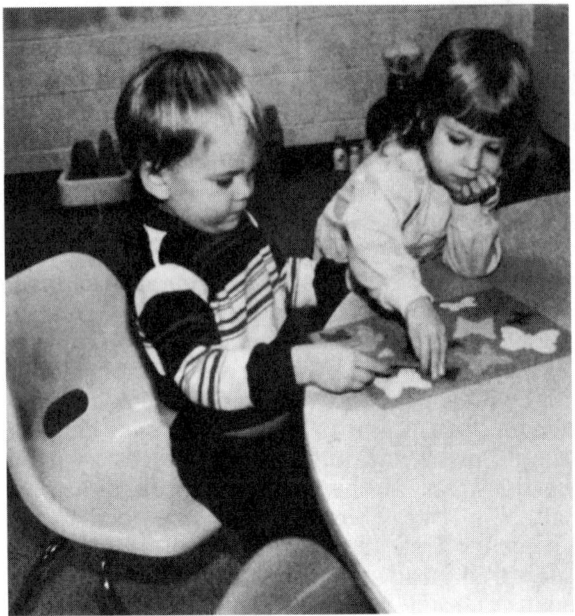

Figure 18–1. • Preschoolers enjoy both parallel and associative play.

the parent of the opposite sex is seen during this period. A daughter wants "to marry Daddy" when she grows up. Children also begin to identify themselves with the parent of the same sex.

Preschool children have more fears than the infant or the older child because of increased intelligence, which enables them to recognize potential dangers; development of memory; and graded independence, which brings them into contact with many new situations. Toddlers are not afraid of walking in the street, because they do not understand its danger. Preschool children realize that trucks can injure, and they worry about crossing the street. This fear is well founded, but many others are not.

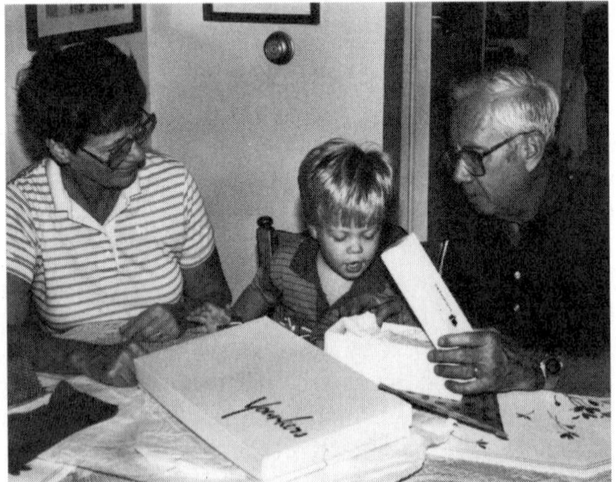

Figure 18–2. • Happy birthday, Grandpa! The preschool child's world begins to extend outward, and he or she finds enjoyment away from mom and dad.

The fear of bodily harm, particularly the loss of body parts, is peculiar to this stage. The little boy who discovers that baby sister is made differently may worry that she has been injured. He wonders if this will happen to him. Masturbation is common during this stage as children attempt to reassure themselves that they are all right. Other common fears include fear of animals, fear of the dark, and fear of strangers. Night wandering is typical of this age group.

Preschool children become angry when others attempt to take their possessions. They grab, slap, and hang on to them for dear life. They become very distraught if toys do not work the way they should. They resent being disturbed from play. They are sensitive, and their feelings are easily hurt. Much of the unpleasant social behavior seen during this time is normal and necessary to the child's total pattern of development.

The Four-Year-Old

Four-year-olds are more aggressive and like to show off newly refined motor skills. They are eager to let others know they are superior, and they are prone to pick on playmates. Four-year-olds are boisterous, tattle on others, and may begin to swear if they are around children or adults who use profanity. They recount personal family activities with amazing recall, but forget where their tricycle has been left. At this age, children become interested in how old they are and want to know the exact age of each playmate. It bolsters their ego to know that they are older than someone else in the group. They also become interested in the relationship of one person to another. Timmy is a brother, but also Daddy's son.

Four-year-olds can use scissors with success. They can lace their shoes. Vocabulary has increased to about 1500 words. They run simple errands and can play with others for longer periods. Many feats are done for a purpose. For instance, they no longer run just for the sake of running. Instead, they run to get someplace or see something. They are imaginative and like to pretend they are doctors or firefighters. They begin to prefer playing with friends of the same sex.

The preschool child enjoys simple toys and common objects (Fig. 18–3). Raw materials are more appealing than toys that are ready-made and complete in themselves. An old cardboard box that can be moved about and climbed into is more fun than

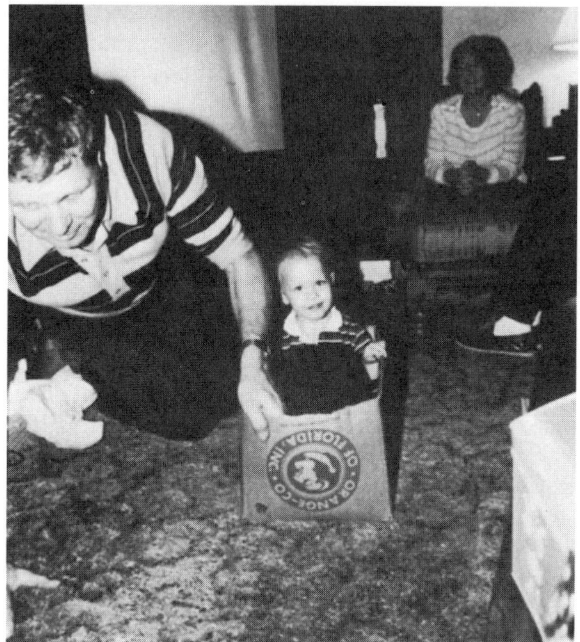

Figure 18–3. • Expensive toys are not necessary for growth and development. Here a simple box stimulates the imagination of the child.

a doll house with tiny furniture. A box of sand or colored pebbles can be made into roads and mountains. Parents should avoid showering their children with ready-made toys. Instead, they can select materials that are absorbing and that stimulate the child's imagination.

Stories that interest young children depict their daily experiences. If the story has a simple plot, it must be related to what they understand to hold their interest. They also enjoy music; they like records they can march around to, music videos, and simple instruments they can shake or bang. (Make up a song about their daily life, and watch their reaction.)

The Concept of Death. Between 3 and 4, children begin to wonder about death and dying. They may be the hero who shoots the intruder dead, or they may witness a situation in which an animal is killed. Their questions are direct. "What is 'dead'? Will I die?" The view of the family is important to the interpretation of this complex phenomenon.

Perhaps children can become acquainted with death through objects not of particular significance to them. For instance, the flower dies at the end of the summer. It does not bloom anymore. It no longer needs sunshine or water, for it is not alive. Usually young children realize that others die, but they do not relate death to themselves. If they continue to pursue the question of whether or not they will die, parents should be casual and reassure them that people do not generally die until they have lived a long and happy life. Of course, as they grow older they will discover that sometimes children do die. The underlying idea, nevertheless, is to encourage questions as they appear and gradually help them accept the truth without undue fear. There are many excellent books for children about death. Two that are appropriate for the preschool child are *Geranium Mornings* by S. Powell, and *My Grandpa Died Today* by J. Fassler.

The Five-Year-Old

Five is a comfortable age. Children are more responsible, enjoy doing what is expected of them, have more patience, and like to finish what they have started. Five-year-olds are serious about what they can and cannot do. They talk constantly and are inquisitive about their environment. They want to do things correctly and seek answers to their questions from those who they consider to "know" the answers. Five-year-old children can play games governed by rules. They are less fearful because they feel their environment is controlled by authorities. Their worries are less profound than at an earlier age.

The physical growth of 5-year-olds is not outstanding. Their height may increase by 2 to 3 inches, and they may gain 3 to 6 pounds. They may begin to lose their deciduous teeth at this time. They can run and play games simultaneously, jump three or four steps at once, and tell a penny from a nickel or a dime. They can name the days of the week and understand what a week-long vacation is. They usually can print their first name.

Five-year-olds can ride a tricycle around the playground with speed and dexterity. They can use a hammer to pound nails. Adults should encourage them to develop motor skills and not continually remind them to "be careful." The practice children experience will enable them to compete with others during the school-age period and will increase confidence in their own abilities. As at any age, children should not be scorned for failure to meet adult standards. Overdirection by solicitous adults is damaging. Children must learn to do tasks themselves for the experience to be satisfying.

The number and type of TV programs that parents allow the preschool child to watch are topics for discussion. Although children enjoyed TV at 3 or 4 years of age, it was usually for short periods. They could not understand much of what was going on. The 5-year-old has better comprehension and may want to spend a great deal of time watching TV. The plan of management differs with each family. Whatever is decided needs to be discussed with the child. For example, TV should not be allowed to interfere with good health habits, sleep, meals, and physical activity. Most parents find that children do not insist on watching TV if there is something better to do.

GUIDANCE

Discipline and Setting Limits

Much has been written on the subject of discipline, which has changed considerably over time. Today, authorities place much importance on the development of a continuous, warm relationship between children and their parents. They believe this helps to prevent many problems. The following is a brief discussion that may help the nurse in guiding parents.

Children need limits for their behavior. Setting limits makes them feel secure, protects them from danger, and relieves them from making decisions that they may be too young to formulate. Children who are taught acceptable behavior have more friends and develop good self-esteem. They live more enjoyably within the neighborhood and society. The manner in which discipline or setting limits are carried out varies from culture to culture. It also varies among different socioeconomic groups. Individual differences occur among families and between parents and vary according to the characteristics of each child.

The purpose of discipline is to teach and to gradually shift control from parents to the child, that is, self-discipline or self-control. Positive reinforcement for appropriate behavior has been cited as more effective than punishment for poor behavior. Expectations must be appropriate to the age and understanding of the child. The nurse encourages parents to try to be consistent because mixed messages are confusing for the learner.

Timing and Timeout. Most researchers agree that to be effective, discipline must be given at the time the incident occurs. It should also be adapted to the seriousness of the infraction. The child's self-worth must always be considered and preserved. Warning the preschool child who appears to be getting into trouble may be helpful. Too many warnings without follow-up, however, lead to ineffectiveness. Spankings, for the most part, are not productive. The child associates the fury of the parents with the pain rather than with the wrong deed, because anger is the predominant factor in the situation. Thus, the real value of the spanking is lost. Beatings administered by parents as a release for their own pent-up emotions are totally inappropriate and can lead to child abuse charges. In addition, the parent serves as a role model of aggression. Whether a parent is affectionate, warm, or cold (uncaring) also plays a role in the effectiveness of child rearing.

Time out periods, *usually lasting 1 minute per year of age,* with the child sitting in a straight chair facing a corner is considered an effective discipline technique. There should be no interaction or eye contact during the time out period and a timer with a buzzer should be used. Often a child will attempt interaction during this period by asking "how much more time is left." The child should learn that any interaction starts the timer at zero. Using the child's room or a soft comfortable chair for timeout is not effective, as the child will either fall asleep or engage in another activity and the objective of timeout is defeated. Timeout should be preceded by a short (no longer than 10 word) explanation of the reason and followed by a short (no more than 10 word) restatement of why it was necessary. Longer explanations are not effective for young children. If the child knows the rules and the behavior that will precipitate a timeout and receives no more than one warning that there will be a timeout if the undesirable behavior continues, then the child will learn self-control. Consistency is the key to helping the child to learn acceptable behavior. Parents need to be taught to resist using power and authority for their own sake. As the child matures and understands more clearly, privileges can be withheld. The reasons for such actions are carefully explained.

Reward. Rewarding the child for good behavior is a positive and effective method of discipline. This can be done with hugs, smiles, tone of voice, and praise. Praise can always be tied with the act: "Thank you, Suzy, for picking up your toys." "I appreciate your standing quietly like that." The encouragement of positive behavior eliminates many of the undesirable effects of punishment.

Rewards should not be confused with bribes. The parent may offer a child a reward if he behaves in a specific situation *before* an incident occurs. For example, the parent may say "you may pick out one small toy after we are finished shopping if you behave during this trip." If this agreement is not made *prior* to an incident, and the child misbehaves and *then* is offered one small toy to behave, this is a bribe that serves to reinforce the bad behavior and is not a desirable technique of behavior management.

Consistency and Modeling. Being consistent is difficult for parents. Realistically, it is only an ideal to strive for—no parent is consistent all the time. Consistency must exist *between* parents as well as within each parent. It is suggested that parents establish a general style for what, when, how, and to what degree punishment is appropriate for misconduct. Parents who are lax or erratic in discipline and who alternate it with punishment have children who experience increased behavioral difficulties.

The influence of modeling or good example has been widely explored. Studies show that adult models significantly influence children's education. Children identify and imitate adult behavior, verbal and nonverbal. Parents who are aggressive and repeatedly lose control demonstrate the power of action over words. Those who communicate, show respect and encouragement, and set appropriate limits are more positive role models. Finally, parents need assistance in reviewing parental discipline during their own childhood to recognize destructive patterns that they may be repeating.

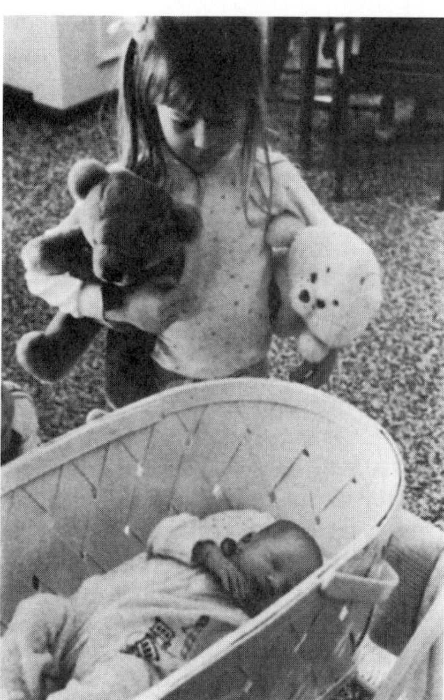

Figure 18–4. • The arrival of an additional family member creates a lot of new feelings for the preschooler.

Jealousy

Jealousy is a normal response to actual, supposed, or threatened loss of affection. Children or adults may feel insecure in their relationship with the person they love. The closer children are to their parents, the greater is their fear of losing them. Children envy the new baby. They love the sibling but resent its presence. They cannot understand the turmoil within themselves (Fig. 18–4). Jealousy of a new baby is strongest in children under 5 years of age and is shown in various ways. Children may be aggressive and may bite or pinch, or they may be rather discreet and may hug and kiss the baby with a determined look on their face. Another common situation is children's attempt to identify with the baby. They revert to wetting the bed or want to be powdered after they urinate. Some 4-year-olds even try the bottle, but it is usually a big disappointment to them.

Preschool children may be jealous of the attention that their mother gives to their father. They may also envy the children they play with if they have bigger and better toys. There is less jealousy in an only child, who is the center of attention and has a minimum number of rivals. Siblings of varied ages are apt to feel that the younger ones are "pets" or that the older ones have more special privileges.

Parents can help to reduce jealousy by the early management of individual occurrences. Preparing young children for the arrival of the new baby minimizes the blow. They should not be made to think that they are being crowded. If the new baby is going to occupy their crib, it is best to settle the older child happily in a large bed before the baby is born. Children should feel that they are helping with care of the infant. Parents can inflate their ego from time to time by reminding them of the many activities they can do that the new baby cannot.

If it is convenient, the new baby is given a bath or a feeding while the older child is asleep. In this way, the older sibling avoids one occasion in which the mother shows the newborn affection for a relatively long time. Some persons think that giving the child a pet to care for helps. Many hospitals offer sibling courses that assist parents in helping the child to overcome jealousy.

If the child tends to hit the baby or another child, both children must be separated, but the one who has caused or is about to cause the injury needs as much attention as the victim, if not more. Similar aggressiveness is seen when the child is made to share toys. It is even more difficult to learn to share Mother, so the child must be given time to adjust to new situations. Children are assured that they are loved but told that they cannot injure others.

Thumb-Sucking

Thumb-sucking is an instinctual behavioral pattern that is considered normal. It is seen by sonogram about the 29th week of embryonic life. Although the cause is not fully understood, it satisfies and comforts the infant. Nonnutritive sucking in the form of thumb-sucking or use of a pacifier have several documented benefits in the first year of life when the infant is in the oral phase of development. Increased weight gain, decreased crying, the development of self-consoling ability and increased behavioral organization have been documented in infants who have been allowed to suck unrestrained. If a pacifier is used, safe construction is essential (see Fig. 16–2, p. 415). The pacifier causes less dental problems than the rigid finger and is more easily relinquished. Parents need guidance in the safe use of pacifiers. Cleanliness is essential as often the pacifier falls onto a dirty surface.

Finger- or thumb-sucking will not have a detrimental effect on the teeth as long as the habit is discontinued before the second teeth erupt. Most children give up the habit by the time they reach school age, although they may regress during periods of stress or fatigue. Management includes education and support of the parents to relieve their anxiety and prevent secondary emotional problems in their children. The child who is trying to stop thumb-sucking is given praise and encouragement.

Enuresis

Description. Enuresis is the involuntary urination after the age at which bladder control should have been established. The term *enuresis* is derived from the Greek word *enourein,* "to void urine." Bedwetting has existed for generations and affects many cultures. There are two types: primary and secondary. Primary enuresis refers to bedwetting in the child who has never been dry. Secondary enuresis refers to a recurrence in a child who has been dry for a period of 1 year or more. *Diurnal,* or daytime, wetting is less common than *nocturnal,* or nighttime, episodes. It is more common in boys than in girls; and there may be a genetic influence. In many children, a specific cause is never determined. By the age of 5 years, about 92% of children achieve daytime dryness. By 12 to 14 years of age, approximately 98% of children remain dry during the night. Sometimes enuresis is the result of inappropriate toilet training. Parents who demand early toilet training can cause a child to rebel and defy them by continuing to wet the bed. Parents who are not alert to the needs of the child may not recognize readiness to toilet train and therefore thwart the child's efforts to master this developmental task. Stressful events can precipitate bedwetting.

In some cases, organic causes of nocturnal enuresis include urinary tract infections, diabetes mellitus, diabetes insipidus, seizure disorders, obstructive uropathy, abnormalities of the urinary tract, and sleep disorders. Maturational delay of the nervous system and small bladder capacity have also been suggested as causes.

Treatment and Nursing Care. A detailed physical and psychological history is obtained. Such factors as the pattern of wetting, number of times per night or week, number of daytime voidings, type of stream, dysuria, amount of fluid taken between dinner and bedtime, family history, stress, and reactions of parents and child are documented. The nurse also determines any medications that the child may be taking and the extent to which social life is inhibited by the problem, such as the inability to spend the night away from home. Developmental landmarks, including toilet training, are reviewed. If there appears to be an organic cause, appropriate blood and urine studies are undertaken. In most cases, physical findings are negative.

Education of the family is extremely crucial to preventing secondary emotional problems. Parents are reassured that many children experience enuresis and that it is self-limited in nature. Power struggles, shame, and guilt are fruitless and destructive. Reassurance and support by the nurse are of great help.

It is essential that the child be the center of the management program. The positive approach of rewarding dry nights and charting the progress is very helpful. *Liquids after dinner should be limited and the child should routinely void before going to bed.*

When the child does not respond to routine management, other techniques include counseling, hypnosis, behavior modification, and pharmacotherapy. Moisture-activated conditioning devices are also commercially available (an alarm rings when the child wets). These have had limited success. Bladder-training exercises, in which the child is asked to withhold the urine for as long as possible, may stretch the bladder and increase its size. The child's bedroom should be as close to the bathroom as possible, and a night-light employed.

The nurse prepares the parents for relapses, which are common. The response to various therapies is highly individual. Overzealous treatment is to be avoided. A nonpunitive, matter-of-fact attitude is most prudent. Imipramine hydrochloride (Tofranil) has been found to decrease enuresis. It is administered before bedtime. Imipramine has a variety of side effects, including mood and sleep disturbances and gastrointestinal upsets. Overdose can lead to cardiac arrhythmias, which may be life-threatening. Dosage and administration should be closely supervised. It is not recommended for children under age 6. Desmopressin (DDAVP) nasal spray, has been used with some success but is expensive.

NURSERY SCHOOL

The change from home to nursery school is a big step toward independence. At this age, children are adjusting to the outside world as well as to the family. Some children have the complicating factor of a new baby in the house.

Many parents work outside the home and find it necessary to provide alternate care settings for their children. Some parents who have only one child seek preschool experiences for their child to enhance their growth and development by providing experience with playmates. Nurses can provide guidance to parents in selecting an appropriate preschool to meet their child's needs. A *family day care center* provides child care for small groups of children for 6 or more hours of a 24-hour day. Work-based group care may be provided by some employers as a convenience to their employees. *Preschool programs* provide structured activities that foster group cooperation and the development of coping skills. The child can gain self-confidence and a positive self-esteem in a good preschool program. Qualified preschool teachers are objective in their interaction with the child and often can detect problems that can be followed up before the child enters kindergarten. Parents may need guidance in selecting a preschool for their child.

The following is a list of suggestions to guide the nurse in helping parents to select a facility appropriate for their child:

- A state licensing agency should be contacted for a list of local day care centers or preschools.
- The accreditation criteria for preschools can be obtained by writing the National Association for the Education of Young Children, 1834 Connecticut Avenue, NW, Washington DC 20009.
- Teachers prepared in early childhood education should staff the preschool.
- The student-to-staff ratio should be reviewed.
- The philosophies of the facility, including discipline procedures, environmental safety, sanitary provisions, fee schedules, and facilities for snacks, meals, and rest time should be reviewed.
- Schedules and facilities for active/passive and indoor/outdoor play should be reviewed.
- The school should routinely require a personal history of the child before admission to the program.
- The parent should visit the preschool and personally observe the environment. Talking with parents of other children attending the school is helpful. Children are accepted into nursery schools between the ages of 2 and 5 years. Most sessions last about 3 hours.

DAILY CARE

The child between 3 and 6 years of age does not require the extensive physical care given to a baby but still needs a bath each day and a shampoo at least once a week. It is best to keep hairstyles simple. Dental hygiene and nutrition are discussed in Chapter 15.

Clothing. Clothes should be loose enough to prevent restriction of movement and allow for active play without stepping on hems. Clothes should be washable. Simple clothes make it easy for preschoolers to dress themselves. A hook nailed to the door within reach is helpful. These children should dress and undress themselves as much as they can. Mother or Father can assist but should not take over.

Shoes should be sturdy and supportive. Protective gear such as helmets for bicycling should be a natural part of dressing for play activities. Dressing appropriately for the weather encountered is essential. Flame retardant sleepwear is available in most stores. Waterproof tablecloths may be advisable during mealtimes.

Accident Prevention. Accidents are still a major threat during the years from 3 to 5. At this age, children may suffer injuries from a bad fall. Preschool children hurry up and down stairs. They climb trees and stand up on swings. They play hard with their toys, particularly those that they can mount. Stairways must be kept free of clutter. Shoes should have rubber soles, and new ones are bought when the tread becomes smooth. When buying toys, parents must be sure they are sturdy and age appropriate. Preschool children should not be asked to do anything that is potentially dangerous, such as carrying a glass container or sharp knife to the kitchen sink.

Automobiles continue to be a threat. Children are taught where they can safely ride their tricycle and where they can play ball, and they should not be allowed to use sleds on streets that are not blocked off for this purpose. They must not play in or around the car or be left alone in the car. The use of *car seats* or *seatbelt restraints* continues to be important.

Burns that occur at this age are frequently due to the child's experimentation with matches. Children are also intrigued by fancy cigarette lighters. Hot

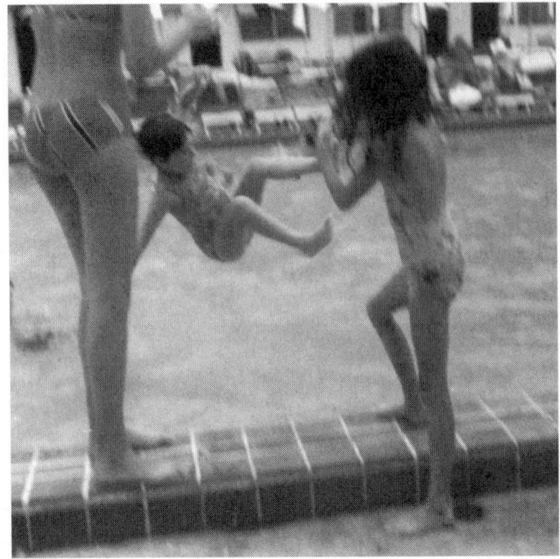

Figure 18–5. • Unsupervised water play can quickly lead to unexpected injuries.

coffee burns are also common. These items are common hazards for this age group; they should be kept well out of reach and their dangers should be explained to the child.

Poisoning is still a danger. Children try to imitate adults and are apt to sample pills, especially if they smell good. Their increased freedom brings them into contact with many interesting containers in the garage or basement.

Preschool children are also taught the dangers of talking to or accepting rides from strangers. If they are stopped by a driver, they should run to the house of people they know. Parents should make it clear to children in nursery school that they will never send a stranger to call for them. Children must know the dangers of playing in lonely places and of accepting gifts from strangers. Children should always know where to go if Mother or Father or baby-sitter cannot be found. Preschool children still require a good deal of indirect supervision to protect them from dangers that arise from their immature judgment or social environment (Fig. 18–5).

PLAY IN HEALTH AND ILLNESS

Value of Play

Play is important to both healthy and sick children's physical, mental, emotional, and social development (Fig. 18–6). Children climbing on a jungle gym develop coordination of their muscles and exercise all parts of their bodies. They use energy and develop self-confidence. Their imagination may take them to the jungle, where they swing from limb to limb. They face imagined fears and solve problems that would be much more trying, if not impossible, in reality. They communicate with other children and take a further step in developing moral values, that is, taking one's turn and considering others. Other types of play help children to learn colors, shapes, sizes, and textures and can teach creativity. This natural and readily available outlet must be tapped by nursing and health care personnel. Children may be unfamiliar with every facet of the hospital, but they know how to play, and playing is a good way for the nurse to establish rapport with them.

The Nurse's Role

Some hospitals have well-established playroom programs supervised by play therapists. *Play therapy* is an important part of every pediatric nursing care plan. It is not necessary to be an expert in manual dexterity, art, or music; rather one must understand the needs of the child. Play is not just the responsibility of those assigned to it, nor is it confined to certain times or shifts.

Many factors are involved in providing suitable play for children of various ages in the hospital.

The patient's state of health determines the amount of activity in which he or she can participate. The nurse can provide many activities that relieve stress and provide enjoyment for the patient on bed rest. Overstimulation, nevertheless, would

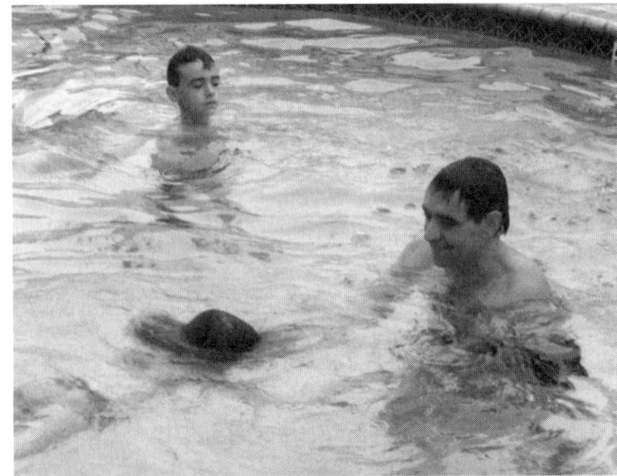

Figure 18–6. • Teaching the preschooler swimming skills and rules is important to prevent injuries.

be hazardous for some severely ill children. Nurses are always on guard for signs of fatigue in patients and use their judgment accordingly.

The diagnosis of the hospitalized child should also be considered when choosing an appropriate toy. For example, a friction toy is inappropriate for a child in an oxygen-rich environment. Sparks from the toy can cause an explosion. A stuffed animal may not be an appropriate toy for an asthmatic child who may be allergic to the contents of the stuffing. A washable laundry bag tied to the bed of a hospitalized child can be used to store the child's own toys neatly and safely. Following discharge of the child from the hospital, toys may be taken home with the child, discarded, or resterilized for reuse.

Safety must be considered in selecting an appropriate toy. Toys should be safe, durable, and suited to the child's developmental level. Toys should not be sharp or have parts that are easily removed and swallowed. Too many toys at one time are confusing to the child. Complicated toys are frustrating and disappointing. Well-selected toys, such as crayons, blocks, and dolls, are useful throughout the years. Each child needs sufficient time to complete an activity. In general, quiet play should precede meals and bedtime for both well and sick children. Investigations have shown that the toys enjoyed by boys and those enjoyed by girls are more similar than dissimilar.

During routine procedures, the nurse can entertain the child with nursery rhymes, stories, nonsense games, songs, finger play, or puppets (Fig. 18–7). Often the other children on the unit can be included for "I'm thinking of something blue, red, and green," and so forth. Simple crafts are fun. The nurse may find various instructions from children's magazines or the local public library. Scrapbooks are entertaining. Children may even enjoy making a storybook about their hospital experience. The nurse involved in enrichment programs for children can make a definite contribution. Surprise boxes in which a gift is opened every day provide anticipation for the patient. Collections of scraps containing bright ribbons, bits of string, pipe cleaners, paper bags, newspapers, or bits of cotton can be started. Because the turnover of patients is rapid, many projects can simply be repeated with different children.

Music is provided by radio, recorders, VCRs, and piano. Older children enjoy sending messages to friends via a tape deck. Special children's recordings and videotapes are available. The services of a music therapist are available in some institutions. Drawing materials, finger paints, and modeling clay foster expression and creativity. They require merely a flat surface, such as the overbed table, and a particular medium. The bedridden child can participate in messy projects, too. The bed is simply protected with newspapers or plastic. Children in cribs need adequate back support for such projects. This is done by elevating the mattress or using pillows. Simple computer games may be available in the hospital setting.

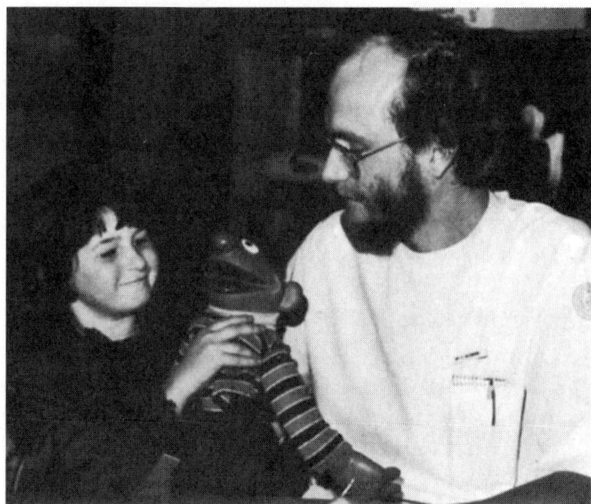

Figure 18–7. • Puppets are universal means of communicating with children. (Courtesy of the New Hampshire Vocational-Technical College, Claremont, NH.)

Playmates may be limited in the hospital setting if the child has a condition that is communicable. However, surgical and orthopedic patients can play together in a playroom with appropriate supervision. The nurse should guide the parents to play *for* a child who is fatigued or weakened by illness. The child can maintain the role of observer.

Types of Play

Preschool children need playmates to promote social development. The play characteristic of each age group is shown in Table 15–12, p. 411. The preschool-age child gradually moves from parallel and associative play to cooperative play with playmates.

The play of preschool children should be noncompetitive. The healthy preschool child requires active play activities that are supervised for safety. Large construction sets, number or alphabet games, crayons, play tools, housekeeping toys, musical toys, pop-up books, large puzzles, and clay are examples of suitable toys for the preschool-age child. Active play can involve simple climbing,

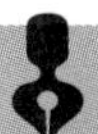

Nursing Tip

Imaginary playmates are common and normal during the preschool period and serve many purposes, such as relief from loneliness, mastery of feats, and scapegoat.

sliding, and running activities. Imaginary friends are common to the preschool-age child. They serve many purposes in helping the child to adjust to an expanding world and increased independence. Parents can acknowledge the presence of the imaginary friend as part of pretend play, but the responsibilities of reality do not include the pretend friend. Parents should not intervene in play groups. Allowing the child to master frustration and develop social skills is essential to growth and development.

Play and the Mentally Retarded or Handicapped Child. The child who is mentally handicapped needs more stimulation through play than the child who is not. The nurse must consider the mental age of the child rather than the chronologic age when guiding parents about the selection of toys. The environment should be as colorful and bright as possible. The child may be introduced to objects of various sizes and textures. Play with other children must be supervised because the poorer-judgment of mentally handicapped children may get them into difficulty. They may be aggressive and may not realize their own strength. Adequate space in which to run is necessary. These children should be brought into group play gradually. Materials are presented one at a time.

Mentally handicapped children may have to be taught how to play, since they may not have had the preschool play experience of the unaffected child. Repetition of play experiences is necessary. Equipment and play materials need to be altered to accommodate the child's size and yet be suitable for the mental age. The nurse or teacher needs to improvise games and songs to meet the special needs of this group. For a more complete discussion of the growth and development and care of the mentally handicapped or retarded child, see Chapter 23.

Therapeutic Play. Play and toys can be of *therapeutic* value in retraining muscles, improving eye–hand coordination, and helping children to crawl and walk (push–pull toys). A musical instrument, such as the clarinet, promotes flexion and extension of the fingers. Blowing is an excellent prerequisite for speech therapy. Therapists supervise such activities. They leave specific instructions if they wish their work to be reinforced on the unit. Blowing out the light of a flashlight as if it were a candle is therapeutic play for a postoperative preschool child.

Play Therapy. The nurse may also hear the term *play therapy* used. This technique is used for the child under stress. A well-equipped playroom is provided. Children are free to play with whatever articles they choose. A counselor may be in the room observing and talking with the child, or the child may be observed through a one-way glass window. By using these as well as other methods, the therapist obtains a better understanding of the patient's struggles, fears, resentments, and feelings toward self and others. When children act out their feelings through "dramatic play," the feelings are externalized, which relieves tension. The interpretation of child behavior is complex and requires a great deal of time, study, and sensitivity to be fully understood.

Art Therapy. *Art therapy* is useful in communicating with children and adults. It is becoming more widely utilized. The art therapist is especially trained to assist children to express their feelings and communicate through drawings, clay, and other media. Some hospitals with inpatient mental health units have art therapy departments.

NURSING IMPLICATIONS OF PRESCHOOL GROWTH AND DEVELOPMENT

The nurse should anticipate parental concern with nutritional problems in the preschool child. Daily appetites may fluctuate widely but the weekly pattern will probably show stability to meet the child's growth needs. During clinic visits the parents should be guided to provide age-appropriate foods at mealtimes in appropriate portions. The child's developing self-regulatory mechanism will determine how much he or she will eat, based on feelings of hunger or satiety. Efforts to control the preschool child's intake may result in power struggles or over- or undereating patterns.

Safety is a high priority in this active age range. "Child-proofing" the home and the need for adequate supervision and safety equipment during sports activities should be emphasized. Preschoolers who will be given immunizations via a "shot" will be calmed by giving pretend "shots" to their doll and having a parent present to comfort them. Explanations such as "the shot will hurt just a little but will prevent them from getting sick" is beyond the Piaget preoperational level of understanding of the preschool child. The ability to understand detailed explanations is not yet present in preschool-age children, even if verbal ability is high. The preschool-age child may have unfounded fears that will respond best to reassurance and "protection" by parents, rather than reasoning why the fear is unfounded. The nurse should provide parental guidance concerning the changing behavior patterns of the preschool-age child. The characteristic alternating dependence and independence can be frustrating for parents. Parents who do not volunteer any positive comments about their child during conversations may require further investigation and interview. Problems with day care and discipline must be discussed. The use of corporal punishment (spanking) as a major disciplinary technique can lead to child abuse. The use of timeout and alternative methods of discipline (p. 460) should be stressed.

Hospitalization can be frightening to a preschool child who is egocentric and prone to magical thinking. Because the preschool child cannot fully understand cause and effect, he may perceive hospitalization as punishment for his behavior. The preschool child may feel abandoned by the parents and continues to be subject to *separation anxiety.* Separation anxiety is manifested by the stages of protest, despair, detachment, and regression to earlier behaviors. Bedwetting is common in the hospitalized preschool child, and parents should be encouraged to be patient and positive. Assigning a consistent caregiver and providing age-appropriate diversional activities are essential for a hospitalized preschool child.

The nurse who is with children daily can describe their behavior. It is important to describe good and poor behavior, conversations that seem pertinent, and the child's relationships with other children in the hospital. What is the approach to play? Do they join in freely or linger outside the group? Do they prefer active or quiet activities? Do they seem to tolerate frustrations? Can they talk with their playmates and convey their ideas? What kind of attention span do they have? These observations and charting are meaningful and promote better understanding and appropriate interventions by nurses and other personnel.

KEY POINTS

- The child from 3 to 5 is often referred to as the "preschool child." During this period, the child grows taller and loses the chubbiness of the toddler period.
- The major tasks of the preschool child include preparation to enter school, the development of a cooperative type play, control of body functions, acceptance of separation, increase in communication skills, memory and attention span.
- Gross and fine motor skills become more developed, as evidenced by participation in running, skipping, and drawing pictures.
- Piaget refers to the preschool period as one in which symbolic thought processes and language emerge.
- Erikson's preschool stage involves the development of initiative. Kohlberg's theory concerning preschoolers refers to the moral development and the beginning awareness of needs of others.
- Language ability develops rapidly, and the child is able to construct rather complicated sentences by the end of this period.
- The many questions of the preschool child need to be listened to carefully and answered thoughtfully and truthfully.
- Play is the business of children. It contributes to physical and mental well-being by encouraging communication, socialization, and outlets for energy.
- Cooperative and highly imaginative play is characteristic of the preschool child.
- Social issues of the preschool period include learning to share and to control impulses.
- Common concerns of parents during this period include how to set limits, to handle jealousy, and to respond to thumb-sucking and masturbation.
- Corporal punishment of the preschool child can nurture rebellion and aggression. Appropriate discipline techniques can assist the child to develop self-control.
- Careful evaluation of day care and nursery school programs is important to ensure high-quality care.

- Accidents are still a major hazard for preschool children because of their immature judgment and increased locomotive skills.
- During the preschool years the parents need guidance to understand the developmental roadmap of physical, emotional, and cognitive growth to help the child to meet life's challenges and goals and to enrich family interaction.
- Primary enuresis refers to bedwetting in a child who has never been dry. Secondary enuresis refers to bedwetting in a child who has been dry for a period of 1 year or more.

MULTIPLE-CHOICE REVIEW QUESTIONS

Choose the most appropriate answer.

1. When selecting play activities for a healthy 4-year-old, the parent should be guided to understand that the 4-year-old:
   a. enjoys solitary play, sitting next to a friend.
   b. enjoys cooperative play with friends.
   c. enjoys competitive play with teams.
   d. enjoys observing rather than participating.
2. Masturbation is
   a. uncommon during preschool years.
   b. common in both sexes during the preschool years.
   c. a sign of extreme anxiety in the preschool child.
   d. a sign of incompetent parenting.
3. The nurse is guiding a parent concerning techniques of dealing with a child with enuresis. The most appropriate suggestion by the nurse would be:
   a. Wake the child in the middle of the night and take him to the bathroom to void.
   b. Limit liquids after dinner and have the child void before going to bed.
   c. Use a consistent technique of discipline whenever the bed is wet.
   d. Keep the child in diapers until bedwetting is no longer a problem.
4. The appropriate amount of time to use in timeout period for a 3-year-old child is:
   a. 1 minute.
   b. 3 minutes.
   c. 5 minutes.
   d. 10 minutes.
5. A 4-year-old child is in Erikson's stage of:
   a. autonomy
   b. industry
   c. initiative
   d. identity

BIBLIOGRAPHY AND READER REFERENCE

AAP Committee on Children with Disabilities. (1994). Screening infants and young children for developmental disabilities. 5:863.

Ashwill, J., & Droske, S. (1997). *Nursing care of children: Principles and practice.* Philadelphia: Saunders.

Behrman, R. E., Kleigman, R., & Arvin, A. (1996). *Nelson's textbook of pediatrics* (15th ed.). Philadelphia: Saunders.

Blum, N. J., et al. (1995). Disciplining young children: The role of verbal instruction and reasoning. *Pediatrics, 96*(2), 336.

Bowden, V., Dickey, S., & Greenberg, C. (1998). *Children and their families: A continuum of care.* Philadelphia: Saunders.

Brazelton, T. (1993). *Touchpoints: Your child's emotional and behavioral development.* Reading, MA: Addison-Wesley.

Byrd, R. (1998). School readiness: More than a summers work. *Contemporary Pediatrics, 15*(5), 39.

Crawley, T. (1996). Childhood injury: Significance and prevention strategies. *Journal of Pediatric Nursing, 11*(4), 225.

Eichner, R. (1994). Circadian rhythms. *Sports Medicine, 22*(10), 82.

Hauck, M. R. (1991). Cognitive abilities of the preschool child: Implications for nurses working with children. *Journal of Pediatric Nursing, 6*(4), 230.

Leung, A., & Robson, W. (1993). Childhood masturbation. *Clinical Pediatrics, 32*(4), 238.

Levine, M. D., Carey, W. B., & Crocker, A. C. (1992). *Developmental-behavioral pediatrics* (2nd ed.). Philadelphia: Saunders.

Montgomery, T. (1994). When children do not talk. *Contemporary Pediatrics, 11*(9), 49.

Nelms, B. (1993). Discipline: What do you recommend. *Pediatric Health Care, 7*(1), 1–2.

Rappaport, L. (1992). Enuresis. In M. D. Levine, W. B. Carey, & A. C. Crocker, *Developmental-behavioral pediatrics* (2nd ed.). Philadelphia: Saunders.

Thomas, R. M. (1996). *Comparing theories of child development.* Pacific Groves, CA: Brooks-Cole.

Ulione, M. (1997). Health promotion and injury prevention in a child developmental center. *Journal of Pediatric Nursing, 12*(13), 148.

Wong, D. (1997). *Whaley & Wong's Essentials of pediatric nursing* (5th ed.). St. Louis, MO: Mosby.

chapter 19

The School-Age Child

Outline

GENERAL CHARACTERISTICS
- Physical Growth
- Gender Identity
- Sex Education

INFLUENCES FROM THE WIDER WORLD
- School-Related Tasks
- Play
- Latchkey Children

PHYSICAL, MENTAL, EMOTIONAL, AND SOCIAL DEVELOPMENT
- The Six-Year-Old
- The Seven-Year-Old
- The Eight-Year-Old
- The Nine-Year-Old
- Preadolescence
  - Eleven- and Twelve-Year-Olds

GUIDANCE AND HEALTH SUPERVISION
- Pet Ownership

Objectives

On completion and mastery of Chapter 19, the student will be able to

- Define each vocabulary term listed.
- Describe the physical and psychosocial development of children from ages 6 to 12, listing age-specific events and type of guidance where appropriate.
- Discuss how to assist parents in preparing a child for school.
- List two ways in which school life influences the growing child.
- Contrast two major theoretical viewpoints of personality development during the school years.
- Discuss accident prevention in this age group.
- Discuss the value of pet ownership for the healthy school-age child and the family education necessary for the allergic or immunocompromised child.
- Discuss the role of the school nurse in providing guidance and health supervision for the school-age child.

Vocabulary

age of industry
androgynous
concrete operations
latchkey child
preadolescent
sexual latency
SIECUS
tooth avulsion

GENERAL CHARACTERISTICS

School-age children from 6 to 12 differ from preschool children in that they are more engrossed in fact than in fantasy and are capable of more sophisticated reasoning. School-age children develop their first close peer relationships outside of the family group, and their first affiliation with adults outside of their family who will influence their lives in a significant way (Table 19–2).

As a result of the increased contact with the world outside of the family and increased cognitive abilities, school-age children begin to understand how others evaluate them. School-age children are often judged by their performance—good grades or athletic feats. The sense of industry and the development of a positive self-esteem are directly influenced by the child's ability to become an accepted member of a peer group and meet the challenges in the environment. The school-age child must be able to pay attention in class (with at least a 45-minute attention span), understand language and progress from the *skill* of writing or reading to *understanding* what is written or read (Fig. 19–1). To be successful in school, the child needs to work toward a delayed reward and risk being unsuccessful in his or her efforts. However, parents must be guided to understand that multiple unsuccessful experiences for their child can lead to the development of a fear of trying in the future. New experiences for the school-age child include the first night sleeping away from home at a friend's house or camp, successes that are formally celebrated, chores that are dependably performed, conflict resolution with peers and the selection of adult role models.

BOX 19–1

FEATURES OF MAJOR THEORIES OF DEVELOPMENT DURING LATER CHILDHOOD

Sigmund Freud

- Child is in period of sexual latency.
- Child's repression of sexuality makes it possible to form same-sex friendships; child assumes role of leader or follower.
- Child is heavily influenced by parents and teachers, who can bolster self-image or more deeply repress sexuality.

Erik Erikson

- Child's development is heavily influenced by others.
- Child's leadership abilities and popularity depend on successfully controlling environment.
- By learning to be productive, self-directing, and accepted at school and in society, child gains positive self-concept.

Jean Piaget

- Child can concentrate on more than one aspect of a situation at a time.
- Child becomes capable of abstract reasoning, but thought is still limited to own experience.
- Child understands cause and effect.

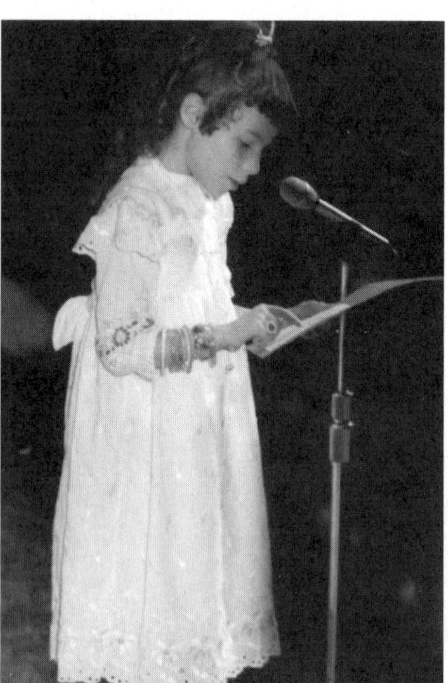

Figure 19–1. • The school-age child first learns the skill of reading and then refines the understanding of what is read.

School-age children have an ardent thirst for knowledge and accomplishment. They tend to admire their teachers and adult companions. They use the skill and knowledge they obtain to attempt to master the activities they enjoy, including music, sports, and art. Thus, this phase is referred to by Erikson as the *age of industry.* Unsuccessful adaptations at this time can lead to a sense of inferiority. Participation in group activities heightens. Romantic love for the parent of the opposite sex diminishes, and children identify with the parent of the same sex. Freud refers to this period as a time of *sexual latency* (Box 19–1). The type of acceptance school-age children receive at home and at school will affect the attitudes they develop about themselves and their role in life. Piaget refers to the thought processes of this period as *concrete operations.*

Concrete operations involves logical thinking and an understanding of cause and effect. The egocentric view of the preschool child is replaced by the ability to understand the point of view of another person. They can understand the origin or consequence of an event they are experiencing. By 10 years of age, the child understands that people do not always control events in life, such as death, spirituality, or the origin of the world (Box 19–1; see also Table 15–3).

Between 6 and 12 years of age, children prefer friends of their own sex and usually prefer the company of their friends to that of their brothers and sisters. Outward displays of affection by adults are embarrassing to them. Although they are now too big to cuddle on their parents' laps, they still require much love, support, and guidance.

Physical Growth

Growth is slow until the spurt directly before puberty. Weight gains are more rapid than are increases in height. The average gain in weight per year is about 5.5 to 7 pounds (2.5–3.2 kg). The average increase in height is approximately 2 inches (5.5 cm). Growth in head circumference is slower than before because myelinization within the brain is complete by 7 years of age. Between the ages of 5 and 12 years, the head circumference increases from 20 to 21 inches. At the end of this time, the brain has reached approximately adult size. (Dentition and nutrition is discussed in Chapter 15.)

Muscular coordination is improved, and the lymphatic tissues become highly developed. The skeletal bones continue to ossify and the body has a lower center of gravity. The body is supple, and sometimes skeletal growth is more rapid than is growth of muscles and ligaments. The child may appear "gangling." There is a noticeable change in facial structures as the jaw lengthens. The sinuses are frequently sites of infection. The 6-year molars (the first permanent teeth) erupt. The loss of baby teeth begins at about 6 years of age and about 4 permanent teeth erupt per year. The gastrointestinal tract is more mature, and the stomach is upset less often. Stomach capacity increases and caloric needs are less than in preschool years. The heart grows slowly and is now smaller in proportion to body size than at any other time of life.

The shape of the eye changes with growth. The exact age at which 20/20 vision occurs, once believed to be about the age of 7, is now believed to be sometime during the preschool years. The capabilities of the child's sense organs, including hearing, have an important bearing on learning abilities.

The vital signs of the child of school age are near those of the adult. Temperature is 98.6°F (37°C); pulse is 85 to 100 beats/min, and respiration is 18 to 20/min. The systolic blood pressure ranges from 90 to 108 mm Hg, and the diastolic from 60 to 68 mm Hg. Boys are slightly taller and somewhat heavier than girls until changes indicating puberty appear. The differences among children are greater at the end of middle childhood than at the beginning.

The changes in body proportions help the child to prepare for activities commonly enjoyed in school. However, size is not correlated with emotional maturity and a problem is created when a child faces higher expectations because he is taller and heavier than his or her peers. Sedentary activities and habits in the school-age child are associated with a high risk of developing obesity and cardiovascular problems in later life.

Gender Identity

The sex organs remain immature during the school-age years, but interest in gender differences progress to puberty. Sex role development is greatly influenced by parents through differential treatment and identification. These two interdependent processes are at work in the family and in society. In infancy, boys and girls are often wrapped in pink or blue blankets. Later, their dress, the kinds of toys and games chosen for them, television, and the attitudes of family members may serve to fortify gender identity, although unisex dress and play are currently popular.

The influence of the school environment is considerable. The teacher can directly foster stereotyping in the assignment of schoolroom tasks, the choice of textbooks, and disapproval of behavior that deviates from the child's sex role. Aggressive behavior is sometimes overlooked in boys but is discouraged in girls.

Some adults develop a sex role concept that incorporates both masculine and feminine qualities, sometimes termed *androgynous.* Because healthy interpersonal relationships depend on both assertiveness and sensitivity, the incorporation of traditionally masculine and feminine positive attributes may lead to fuller human functioning.

Sex Education

Sex education is a lifelong process. Parents convey their attitudes and feelings about all aspects of life, including sexuality, to the growing child. Sex education is accomplished less by talking or formal instruction than by the whole climate of the home, particularly the respect shown to each family member.

Children's questions about sex should be answered simply and at their level of understanding. Correct names should be used to describe the genitals. The hospitalized child who complains, "My penis hurts," is understood by all. Private masturbation is normal and is practiced by both males and females at various times throughout their lives. It does not cause acne, blindness, insanity, or impotence. The young boy needs to be prepared for erections and nocturnal emissions (wet dreams), which are to be expected and are not necessarily due to masturbation. The young girl is prepared for menarche and is provided with the necessary supplies. This is particularly important to the early maturer because an elementary school may not provide dispensing machines in the restrooms. (See discussion of menstrual cycle in Chapter 2.)

Both sexes are concerned during the school years with the disproportion of their bodies, and they may be self-conscious when undressing. They may compare themselves with their friends. They need reassurance about their awakening sexuality, which affects their thoughts and behavior.

Factual knowledge concerning sex and drugs is an essential component of sex education both in the home and at school. School nurses can assist in preparing sex education programs, but participation of parents is valuable. Sex education can be taught in the context of the normal process and function of the human body. Facts must be provided. Value clarification can be added and influenced by parents in the home. If children realize that parents are uncomfortable with discussing the subject, they may turn to peers, who often supply erroneous and distorted information. The Sex Information and Education Council of the United States, (SIECUS, 130 W. 42nd Street, Suite 350, New York, NY 10036) maintains that every sex education program should present the topic from six aspects: biologic, social, health, personal adjustment and attitudes, interpersonal associations, and establishment of values.

Regardless of the practice setting, nurses can help parents and children with sex education through careful listening and anticipatory guidance. They can teach decision-making skills and responsibility. Nurses should review normal developmental behavior and explain age-specific information. They provide families with useful written information that stresses sexuality as a healthful rather than as an illness-related concept. The nurse should always consider cultural differences when counseling (Table 19–1).

Table 19–1
USING THE NURSING PROCESS IN SEX EDUCATION OF THE SCHOOL-AGE CHILD

Intervention	Observation
Data collection, history taking	Readiness to learn is indicated by asking questions concerning sex, menstruation, "wet-dreams," and pregnancy
Assessment	Observe parent–child interactions and determine level of communication
	Observe peer interaction to determine child's self-image, self-confidence, and ability to communicate
	Observe parent's knowledge and ability to discuss issues pertaining to sex education
	Assess child's understanding of sexual development and body changes
Plan/implement	Discuss growth and development with parent and child
	Reinforce teaching techniques and opportunities with parents
Evaluate	With each clinic or home visit, evaluate results of parent–child interaction concerning sex education

AIDS Education. Education concerning sexually transmitted diseases and AIDS prevention should be presented in simple terms. The school nurse is a vital link in the education of the child and the parents. There are audiovisual materials designed for the school-age child. Factual information about AIDS and concrete information on how to say "no" to sexual intercourse and drugs is an essential component in AIDS education of the preadolescent. The nurse can help to implement educational programs in the school, clinic, church, and other community organizations. The facts concerning the harmful effects of drugs and unprotected sex should be communicated to the child without using scare tactics.

Nursing Tip

When discussing sexuality with school-age children, it is necessary to review slang or street terms. Most children hear the terms but may be confused about their meaning.

INFLUENCES FROM THE WIDER WORLD

School-Related Tasks

Schools have a profound influence on the socialization of children. Children bring to school what they have learned and experienced in the home. Although some children come from healthy, intact families who are financially secure, many do not. The child may be disabled, retarded, or abused or may suffer from a chronic illness. Parents may be alcoholics, substance abusers, unemployed, or may suffer from numerous other physical or stress-related conditions. Nurses must remember these factors because they surface continually with this population. In addition, children may be unable to verbalize their needs; therefore, caretakers must become particularly astute in their observations. Table 19–2 reviews expected growth and development.

A holistic attitude of child care must focus not only on intellectual achievement and test scores but also on such qualities as artistic expression, creativity, joy, cooperation, responsibility, industry, love, and other attributes. The sensitive nurse can assist parents by affirming the individuality of children and by encouraging parents to share with their children the pride they are experiencing as the children learn and progress through the elementary grades. Box 19–2 is a summary of parental guidance that the nurse may find useful in preparing children for the beginning of school.

The nurse assesses patterns of communication between parents and child and assists with specific behavioral problems. The transition to junior high school or "middle schools" generally means multiple classrooms, a series of teachers, and a change of buildings. The child is developing adult characteristics and has new feelings about the body and about parents, teachers, and peers. Anticipatory guidance includes a review of normal physiology and how it changes with puberty. Information concerning sexuality is reviewed, and the child is encouraged to ask questions at the time they arise.

A warm, ongoing relationship between parents and child helps to provide a safe atmosphere of caring. Adults should develop a heightened awareness for such things as school attendance problems, tardiness, and signs of loneliness or depression. They should continue to encourage children to discuss their school problems, feelings, and worries. Parents and children must set realistic goals. A good question for adults to contemplate periodically is, "When was the last time this child had a success?" Homework should be the child's responsibility, with a minimum of assistance from parents. For some children, visits to the nurse's office may be their only continuous contact with a health care worker. The nurse may be instrumental in establishing positive health patterns that may be carried into adulthood.

The school nurse can guide the parents in determining health care requirements for the school-age child. Schools provide some health screening, but the financial resources of the family may prevent adequate follow-up care, clothing, or transportation. School lunch programs are available in most schools for the child identified in need.

Safety is an important issue for the school-age child. The rules of the road should be taught before the child walks to school. Car safety and the use of seatbelts must be a regular ritual. Caution in play is essential, although a child must not be made to feel afraid to try new activities or skills.

Table 19–2

GROWTH AND DEVELOPMENT OF THE SCHOOL-AGE CHILD IN SCHOOL-RELATED TASKS

Child's Task	Parent's Task	Nursing Intervention
Adapt to differences in expectations of teachers	Communicate with teacher to maintain consistency in expectations and discipline	School nurse should be contacted to facilitate parent–teacher–child interaction
Compete with 30 or more peers for adult attention	Praise child's accomplishments Avoid comparisons to other children	Evaluate parent–teacher interactions and provide guidance and positive support
Learn to accept criticism from peers and teachers without losing self-esteem	Supervise peer activities. Provide constructive activities	Provide teacher–parent guidance
Assimilate peer values with family values	Maintain open communication. Encourage peer activity. Introduce and accept other cultures in community	Provide anticipatory guidance in dealing with behavior problems Observe and deal with signs of prejudice
Find satisfaction in achievements at school	Allow children to achieve. Do not complete tasks for them	
Participate in group activities	Encourage child to join a group or club and actively participate as a member	Refer to community agencies such as churches, organizations, and club activities as needed
Learn self control. Handle prejudice from others in a positive way	Encourage participation in activities away from home and with peers. Have faith in child's problem-solving abilities. Discuss coping with prejudices of others	Encourage parents to "let go" and provide guidance while encouraging independence

BOX 19–2

PARENTAL GUIDANCE FOR CHILDREN STARTING SCHOOL

Encourage parents to

- Review normal growth and development of 5- to 6-year-olds.
- Anticipate regression such as thumb-sucking, clinging behavior, occasional soiling.
- Encourage children to express what they think school will be like.
- Arrange for children to meet others who will be entering school with them.
- Tour school with child.
- Introduce child to school crossing guard, bus driver.
- Teach child family name and telephone number.
- Teach safety precautions about crossing street, strangers, "blue star" homes (community-established "safe homes" for children in an emergency. Such houses are designated by a blue star or other symbol).
- Allow sufficient time in the morning to prepare for school.
- Provide a cheerful send-off.
- Instruct child as to where to go in case of emergency at home, such as neighbor or relative.
- Walk to school until the child understands the route, or designate a bus stop.
- Listen to child at end of day; become interested in school life.
- Get to know the child's teacher; take an interest in the school.
- Inform the teacher of sudden or unusual stress in the child's life.

Data from Rogers, F., & Head, B. (1983). *Mister Rogers talks with parents.* New York: Berkley Books; and other sources.

Play

Play activities in the school-age child involves increased physical and intellectual skills and some fantasy. The sense of belonging to a group is very important, and conformity to "be just like my friends" is of vital importance to the child. The culture of the school-age child involves membership in a group of some kind. If parents do not provide a club, scout, or church group, the child may find a group of his or her own, which may be a gang.

Teams are important to growth and development and competition is a new challenge (Fig. 19–2).

Nursing Tip

Caution parents about the safe storage of firearms. Since 1979, more than 50,000 children in the United States have died from gunshot wounds. Most of these deaths occurred in the home, not on the streets.

Rituals such as collecting items and playing board games are enjoyable quiet activities for the school-age child. TV is often considered to be a "babysitter" when overused, but many educational and exciting programs are offered during prime time hours. Computer and video games challenge intellect and skill and are healthy outlets as long as they do not completely replace active physical play. Play enables the child to feel powerful and in control, and mastering new skills helps them to feel a sense of accomplishment that is necessary to successfully achieve Erikson's phase of "industry."

Latchkey Children

Latchkey children in the United States are children who are left unsupervised after school because parents are away from home or at work and extended family are not available to care for them.

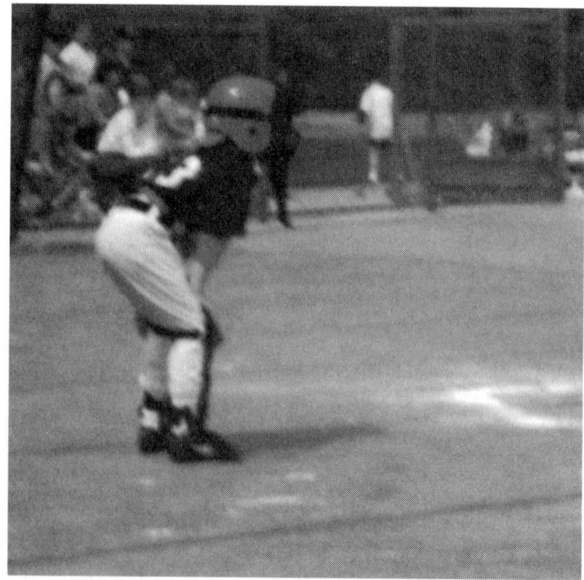

Figure 19–2. • Membership on a team, participation in sports, and the experience of competition are important in the growth and development of the school-age child.

These children are subject to a higher rate of accidents and are at risk of feeling isolated and alone. Some latchkey children, however, enjoy the independence and become skilled in problem solving and self-care. A back-up adult should be available to the child in case of emergencies. Many latchkey children do not participate in after-school social and sports activities and may be slower to identify themselves as belonging to a group. The school nurse can be a key source for providing information about the needs of the school-age child and quality after-school care programs that may be available in the community.

Box 19–3 shows parental and child guidance for latchkey children. Nurses should be aware of local resources, such as "Prepared for Today," a program sponsored by the National Boy Scouts of America, and Young Men's Christian Association (YMCA) and Young Women's Christian Association (YWCA) after-school activities. They can also assist in developing innovative programs such as cooperative baby-sitting, in which parents exchange child care services. The nurse must spend time with parents, lend support, and help them to explore their options.

BOX 19–3

GUIDANCE FOR LATCHKEY FAMILIES

Teach child about safety

- Do not enter the house if the door is ajar or anything looks unusual.
- Do not display keys; keep door locked.
- Teach how to answer the telephone (parents are busy, not "out").
- Teach first-aid techniques.
- Review fire safety rules and route of escape; walk through procedure with child.
- Teach cooking rules.
- Review safe bathing methods (no electrical appliances around water); necessary when older children are watching younger children.
- Address weather-related safety (e.g., tornadoes, thunderstorms)
- Caution about the dangers of garage door openers.

Teach parents to

- List emergency numbers and post near telephone.
- Designate a neighbor who is usually home for help in emergencies.
- Teach child own name, telephone number, address, and parents' name.
- Leave work number with child.
- Lock up firearms or remove from house.
- Prepare a first-aid kit and designate location.
- Address street safety with child when returning from school; include precautions with strangers.
- Consider obtaining a pet for child.
- Be home on time or call child.
- Leave tape-recorded message to decrease loneliness of child, recommend specific activities rather than TV.
- Help child to feel successful and appreciated.
- Assess home and neighborhood for hazards specific to their locale.

Data from McClellan, M. (1984). On their own: Latchkey children. *Pediatric Nursing,* 10, 2000.

PHYSICAL, MENTAL, EMOTIONAL, AND SOCIAL DEVELOPMENT

The Six-Year-Old

Children of 6 years burst with energy and are on the go constantly. They soon become overtired, and it is necessary to limit their activities. They like to start tasks, but do not always finish them, for their attention span is fairly brief. They tend to be bossy, sometimes rude, and experiment with language, but they are very sensitive to criticism. Their conscience is active, and they find it difficult to make decisions.

One of the most obvious physical changes at this age is the loss of the temporary teeth (Fig. 19–3). The important 6-year molars also erupt. Children can jump-rope, throw and catch a ball, tie shoelaces, and perform numerous other feats that require muscle coordination. Their language differs from that of the preschool child. They use it for a purpose rather than for the pure joy of talking. Their vocabulary consists of about 2500 words. They require 11 to 13 hours of sleep a night.

Boys and girls play together at this age, although they begin to prefer to associate with children of the same sex. Most children enjoy collecting objects such as shells, leaves, or stones. Play at this time usually reflects events that occur in the immediate environment.

Six-year-old children need time and support to help them to adjust to school. If they have nursery school or kindergarten experience, the transition may be more comfortable. Most children go to

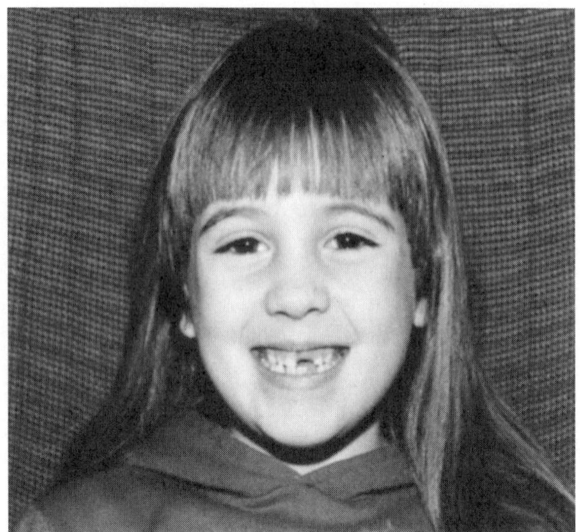

Figure 19–3. • One of the most obvious physical changes of the 6-year-old is the loss of primary teeth.

school expecting the same reception that they are accustomed to at home. If parents are critical or overprotective, children will assume that the teacher will be, too. When the teacher's response differs markedly from their expectations, they feel insecure and may even be hostile toward the teacher. Parents need to observe children for signs of fatigue and stress. Not all children are ready for school merely because they reach the proper age. Even those who are ready need time and support from parents and teachers before they can settle down to the job at hand. Being in school exposes the child to infection more frequently than being at home. Preschool immunizations and a physical examination are indicated. (See Immunizations in Chapter 31.)

The Seven-Year-Old

The 7-year-old is a quieter child, and some educators have noted that second graders are the easiest children to teach. They set high standards for themselves and for their families. They have a good sense of humor, tend to be somewhat of a "tease" (wiggle loose teeth to annoy adults), and are a little more modest than at an earlier age. They enjoy being active, but also appreciate periods of rest. The second grader may have a "crush" on a friend of the opposite sex.

These children know the months and seasons of the year and begin to tell time. They have a beginning concept of arithmetic, can count by twos and fives, and know that money is valuable. Their hands are steadier. Interest in God or heaven may be heightened.

Active play is still important to both sexes. The boys are more apt to tease the girls than to participate in games such as jump-rope or tag. Both sexes enjoy bike riding and table games. Realistic toys, such as dolls that can be bathed and fed and trains that back up and whistle, appeal to the 7-year-old. Comic books are also popular. Becoming increasingly independent, the children imagine themselves accomplishing feats more adventurous than those of their parents. They cannot understand how Mom and Dad ever chose to lead such "dull lives."

The Eight-Year-Old

The 8-year-old wants to do everything and can play alone for longer than the 7-year-old. The work of an 8-year-old is usually creative. They enjoy group activities, such as Brownies and Cub Scouts, and prefer companions of the same sex. They become interested in group fads. Eight-year-olds like to be considered important, particularly by adults. They may behave better for company than for the family. Hero worship is evident.

The arms and hands of the 8-year-old seem to grow faster than the rest of the body. The large and small muscles are better developed, and movements are smoother and more graceful. The child can write rather than print and understands the number of days that must pass before special events such as Christmas, birthdays, and discharge from the hospital.

The 8-year-old enjoys competitive sports but is generally a poor loser (Fig. 19–4). Long, involved

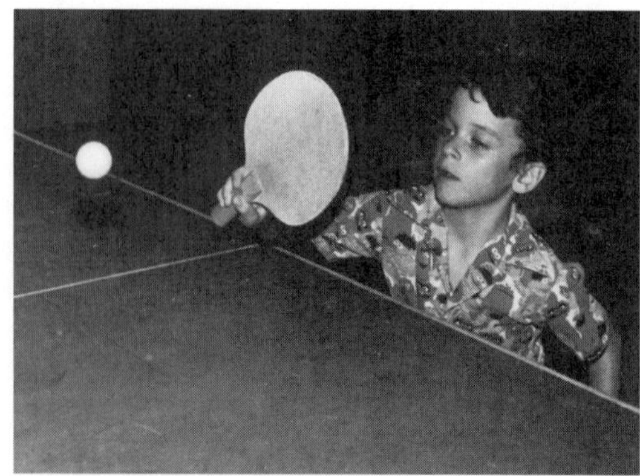

Figure 19–4. • School-age children enjoy active competition.

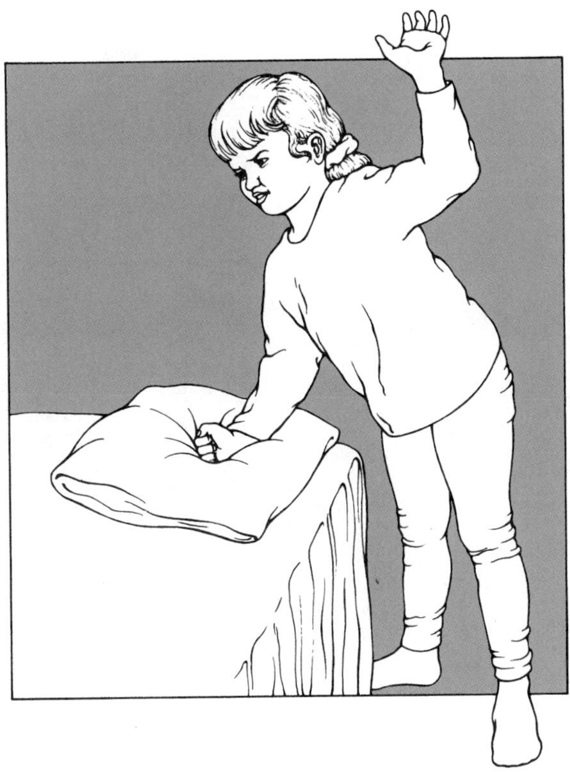

Figure 19–5. • Punching a pillow is a good way for the child to release anger without hurting others.

arguments frequently occur. A healthy way to teach a child to express anger is to have the child pound on a pillow (Fig. 19–5). Wrestling is frequent, and dramatic play is popular. Most children like to be the hero or heroine of their favorite program. Neighborhood secret clubs are organized, and all members must strictly adhere to the rules.

The Nine-Year-Old

The 9-year-old is dependable, shows more interest in family activities, assumes more responsibility for personal belongings and for younger brothers and sisters, and are more likely to complete tasks (Fig. 19–6). They resist adult authority if it does not coincide with the opinions or ideals of the group. However, they are more able to accept criticism for their actions. Individual differences are pronounced.

Worries and mild compulsions are common. Nervous habits, sometimes referred to as tics, may appear and may vary widely. Eye blinking, facial grimacing, and shoulder shrugging are but a few

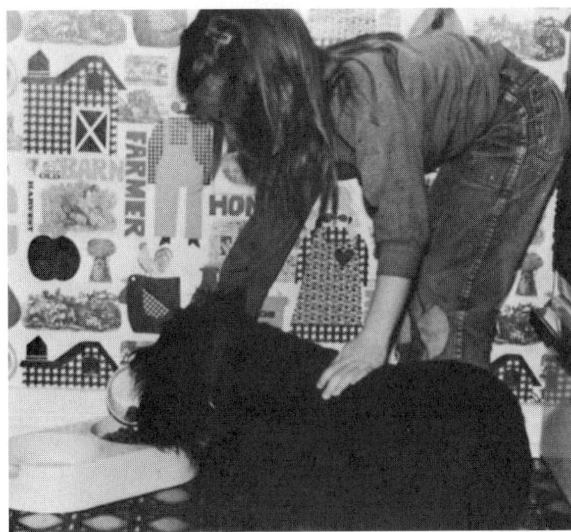

Figure 19–6. • The 9-year-old is capable of caring for the family pet.

examples. The child cannot help such actions and should not be scolded for them because they are mainly due to tension; they usually disappear when home and social life become more relaxed.

Hand and eye coordination is well developed, and manual activities are managed with skill. The child works and plays hard and becomes overtired. About 10 hours of sleep a night are needed. The permanent teeth are still erupting.

Competitive sports are still popular, as are reading, listening to the radio, watching TV, and playing computer games. Sports programs that take into consideration the limitations of children at various ages should be encouraged. Teaching proper techniques and the use of adequate safety devices is essential (Fig. 19–7). As the child approaches puberty, boys develop more muscle mass than girls and therefore competitive contact sports should have separate teams for boys and girls (Fig. 19–8).

Girls play for long periods of time with dolls. An interest in music is shown, and the child may desire to take lessons (Fig. 19–9). Children know the date, can repeat months of the year in order, can multiply

Nursing Tip

Mutual respect involves accepting the child's feelings. When helping children to identify feelings, start with the terms *mad, glad, sad,* or *scared.*

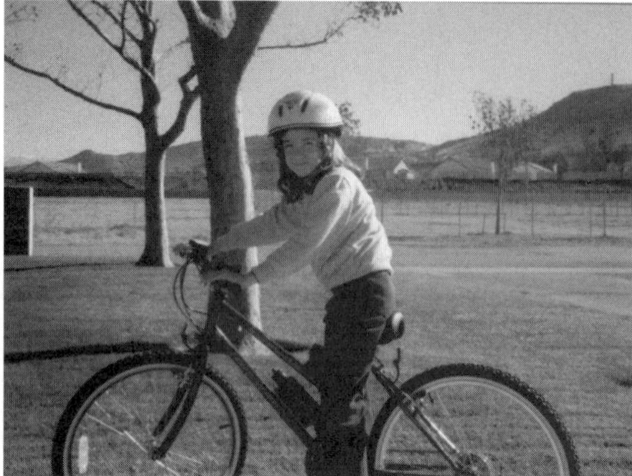

Figure 19–7. • Protective clothing is necessary for potentially hazardous play. Provide protective equipment appropriate for any sport the child plays (e.g., helmets for bicycling, skateboarding, ice hockey).

and do simple division and are ready for more complex math. They take care of their bodily needs, and by now their table manners are considerably improved.

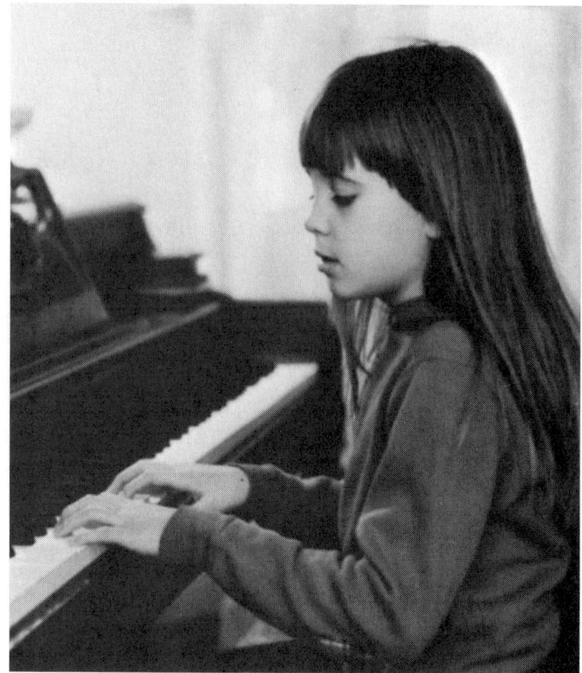

Figure 19–9. • Outlets such as music help the child to express feelings in a positive way.

Preadolescence

The Ten-Year-Old

Age 10 marks the beginning of the preadolescent years. Girls are more physically mature than boys. The child begins to show self-direction, is courteous to adults, and thinks clearly about social problems and prejudices. The 10-year-old wants to be independent and resents being told what to do but is receptive to suggestions. The ideas of the group are more important than individual ideas. Interest in sex and sex investigations continue.

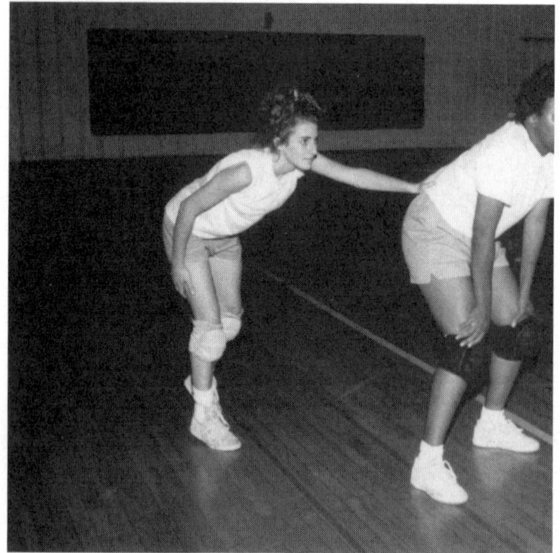

Figure 19–8. • Being a member of a team and an active player is important to school-age children. Preadolescents should have separate teams for girls and boys.

In general, girls are more poised than boys. Both sexes are fairly reliable about household duties (Fig. 19–10). Slang terms are used. The 10-year-old can write for a relatively long period of time and maintains good writing speed. The child uses fractions and knows abstract numbers. Boys and girls begin to identify themselves with skills that pertain to their sex role. They are intolerant of the opposite sex. The play enjoyed by the 10-year-old is similar to that enjoyed by the 9-year-old. In addition, the child takes more interest in personal appearance.

Eleven- and Twelve-Year-Olds

Adjectives that describe 11- and 12-year-olds include intense, observant, all-knowing, energetic, meddlesome, and argumentative. This period before the onset of puberty is one of complete disorganization. It begins earlier in some children; the onset and rate of physical maturity vary greatly. Before the end of this period, the hormones of the body begin to influence physical growth. Posture is poor. There are 24 to 26 permanent teeth.

The child has an overabundance of energy and is on the go every minute. Girls become "tomboyish" in their actions. Table manners are a thing of the past, and the refrigerator is constantly emptied. Children at this age are less concerned with their appearance. They seem to be often preoccupied, and this, along with physical activities and numerous anxieties, accounts for some of the decline seen in school grades. Ability to concentrate decreases, and parents complain that the child "never hears anything." When asked to do a new task, these children moan and groan.

Group participation is still important. They enjoy being a team player. Preadolescent children are not ready to stand alone, but they cannot bear the thought of depending on parents. They must overcome the problems they confront without parental help. Their attitude implies, "Can't you see that I'm not a child anymore?"

During preadolescence, children are interested in their bodies and watch for signs of growing up. Girls look forward to menstruation and wearing their first bra. Boys and girls tend to ignore the opposite sex, but really they are very much aware of them. There is a tendency to tease one another. Their descriptions of each other are far from complimentary: "stupid," "crazy," and "nerd." Both sexes enjoy earning money by obtaining odd jobs. The preadolescent often seeks an adult friend of the same sex to idolize.

Guiding preadolescents is not easy. They need freedom within limits and recognition that they are no longer babies. They should know why parents make a decision. They should not be expected to follow household rules blindly. Their conscience enables them to understand and accept reasonable discipline. They ignore constant verbal nagging. They should be provided constructive opportunities to release pent-up emotions and energy. One can more easily accept their irritating behavior by realizing that much of it is indeed "just a phase."

The American Academy of Pediatrics Committee on Sports Medicine and School Health recommends teaching motor skills and fitness exercises in the school setting to promote positive attitudes toward exercise in later life. The focus should be on mastering the skill of the sport and enjoying the exercise rather than winning a game. Selecting students for teams based on athletic prowess is inappropriate for the preadolescent child. Ceremonies should recognize all participants rather than star players. In the gym class, discipline for misbehavior should not be in the form of assigned extra pushups or extra laps of running on the track. Such discipline measures foster a negative attitude toward healthy exercise.

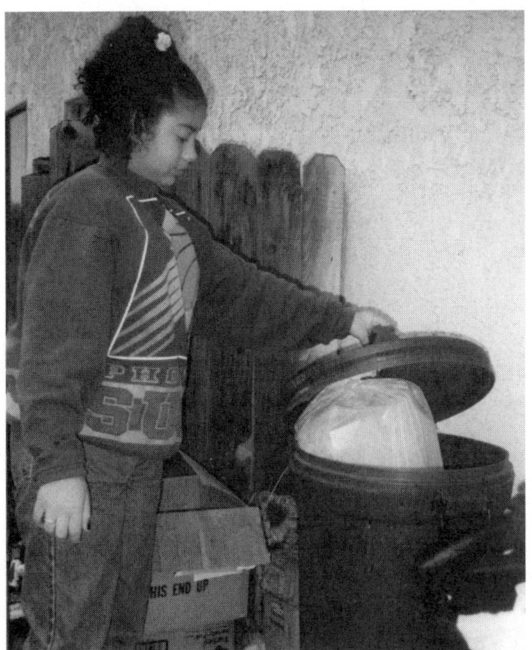

Figure 19–10. • The school-age child contributes to the smooth running of the household by performing household chores. (Reminders are frequently necessary!)

GUIDANCE AND HEALTH SUPERVISION

Health Examinations. The yearly preschool physical examination is given in the spring preceding school admission. This allows time to correct any problems that are found. Booster immunizations are given as needed; the child's teeth are examined and dental work is completed. (See Immunizations in Chapter 31.) Good dental hygiene and regular professional dental care are essential as the permanent set of teeth erupts. Dental health and nutrition are discussed in Chapter 15.

School health programs aimed at maintaining and promoting health are provided in most school systems. Nurses and other professional persons who take part in such programs can play an important role in counseling parents. They also help to meet the needs of disabled children enrolled in their schools. A carefully taken health history provides the nurse with much-needed information (Fig. 19–11). Table 19–3 reviews development of the school-age child.

I. GENERAL INFORMATION
Name ______________________ Date ______________
Age and birth date ______________ Language ______________
Grade ______________ Informant ______________
Sex ______________ Parents' home and business,
Religion ______________ phones ______________

II. FAMILY PROFILE (health history of family members)
Mother ______________
Father ______________
Siblings ______________
Paternal grandparents ______________
Maternal grandparents ______________
Life change events: death, divorce, new baby, moves of family, illness, separation, etc.
____
____

III. CHILD PROFILE
Newborn status: Did baby leave hospital with you? ______________
Birth defects ______________
Developmental history: Age for crawling ______________ sitting ______________
walking ______________ speech ______________ toilet training ______________
Immunizations ______________
Habits, general behavior in school ______________ Home ______________
Sleeping patterns ______________ Fears ______________
Exercise ______________ Friends ______________
Interests ______________ Special skills ______________
____
Previous illness or accidents ______________
Is child taking any medications? ______________
Hearing aid ______________ Glasses ______________
Dental care ______________ Allergies ______________
Typical foods consumed:
breakfast ______________
lunch ______________
supper ______________
snacks ______________
Eating problems ______________ Elimination ______________
Menses ______________ Sexual maturation ______________
Sex education ______________ Personal hygiene ______________
Review of systems ______________
____

IV. NURSE'S OBSERVATIONS AND COMMENTS
General physical description ______________
____
Results of screening procedures: vision ______________ audiometer ______________
Scoliosis ______________ Other ______________
Individual health education and guidance ______________
____
Problem-solving plan ______________
____

Interviewer ______________

Figure 19–11. • Health assessment summary of the school-age child.

Table 19–3
SUMMARY OF SCHOOL-AGE CHILD GROWTH AND DEVELOPMENT AND HEALTH MAINTENANCE

Age (years)	Physical Competency	Intellectual Competency	Emotional-Social Competency	Nutrition	Play	Safety
General: 6–12	Gains an average of 2.5–3.2 kg/yr (5.5–7 lb/yr). Overall height gains of 5.5 cm (2 in)/yr; growth occurs in spurts and is mainly in trunk and extremities Loses deciduous teeth; most permanent teeth erupt Progressively more coordinated in both gross and fine motor skills Caloric needs increase during growth spurts	Masters concrete operations Moves from egocentrism; learns he or she is not always right Learns grammar and expression of emotions and thoughts Vocabulary increases to 3000 words or more Handles complex sentences	Central crisis; industry versus inferiority; wants to do and make things Progressive sex education needed Wants to be like friends; competition important Fears body mutilation, alterations in body image; earlier phobias may recur; nightmares; fears death. Nervous habits common	Fluctuations in appetite due to uneven growth pattern and tendency to get involved in activities Tendency to neglect breakfast in rush of getting to school. Although school lunch is provided in most schools, child does not always eat it	Plays in groups, mostly of same sex; gang activities predominate Books for all ages Bicycles important. Sports equipment Cards, board and table games Most of play is active games requiring little or no equipment	Enforce continued use of seat belts during car travel Bicycle safety must be taught and enforced Teach safety related to hobbies, handicrafts, mechanical equipment
6–7	Gross motor skill exceeds fine motor coordination Balance and rhythm are good—runs, skips, jumps, climbs, gallops Throws and catches ball Dresses self with little or no help	Vocabulary of 2500 words. Learning to read and print Begins concrete concepts of numbers, general classification of items Knows concepts of right and left; morning, afternoon, and evening; coinage; intuitive thought process Verbally aggressive, bossy, opinionated, argumentative Likes simple games with basic rules	Boisterous, outgoing, and a know-it-all Whiny; parents should sidestep power struggles, offer choices Becomes quiet and reflective during 7th yr; very sensitive Can use telephone Likes to make things; starts many, finishes few Give some responsibility for household duties	Preschool food dislikes persist. Tendency for deficiencies in iron, vitamin A, and riboflavin, 100 ml/kg of water/day, 3 gm/kg protein daily	Still enjoys dolls, cars, and trucks. Plays well alone but enjoys small groups of both sexes; begins to prefer same-sex peer during 7th yr Ready to learn how to ride a bicycle Prefers imaginary, dramatic play with real costumes Begins collecting for quantity, not quality Enjoys active games such as hide-and-seek, tag, jump rope, roller skating, kickball	Teach and reinforce traffic safety Still needs adult supervision of play Teach to avoid strangers, nerver take anything from strangers Teach illness prevention and reinforce continued practice of other health habits Restrict bicycle use to home ground; no traffic areas; teach bicycle safety. Wear helmet Teach and set examples about harmful use of drugs, alcohol, smoking

Table continued on following page

Table 19–3
SUMMARY OF SCHOOL-AGE CHILD GROWTH AND DEVELOPMENT AND HEALTH MAINTENANCE *(Continued)*

Age (years)	Physical Competency	Intellectual Competency	Emotional-Social Competency	Nutrition	Play	Safety
8–10	Myopia may appear Secondary sex characteristics begin in girls Hand–eye coordination and fine motor skills are well established. Movements are graceful, coordinated Cares for own physical needs completely Constantly on the move; plays and works hard; enforce balance in rest and activity	Learning correct grammar and to express feelings in words. Likes books he or she can read alone; will read funny papers, scan newspaper. Enjoys making detailed drawings Mastering classification, seriation, spatial, temporal, and numeric concepts Uses language as a tool; likes riddles, jokes, chants, word games. Rules guiding force in life now Very interested in how things work, what and how weather, seasons, and the like are made	Strong preference for same-sex peers; antagonizes opposite-sex peers Self-assured and pragmatic at home; questions parental values and ideas Has a strong sense of humor Enjoys clubs, group projects, outings, large groups, camp Modesty about own body increases over time; sex-conscious Works diligently to perfect skills he or she does best Happy, cooperative, relaxed, and casual in relationships Increasingly courteous and well mannered with adults Gang stage at a peak; secret codes and rituals prevail Responds better to suggestion than to dictatorial approach	Needs about 2100 calories/day; nutritious snacks. Tends to be too busy to bother to eat Tendency for deficiencies in calcium, iron, and thiamine Problem of obesity may begin now Good table manners Able to help with food preparation	Ready for lessons in dancing, gymnastics, music Restrict TV time to 1–2 hr/day Likes hiking, sports Enjoys cooking, woodworking, crafts Enjoys cards and table games Likes radio and records Begins qualitative collecting now	Stress safety with firearms. Keep them out of reach and allow use only with adult supervision Know who the child's friends are; parents should still have some control over friend selection Teach water safety; swimming should be supervised by an adult

Table continued on following page

The eating habits of a child of this age should be basically sound, as long as a variety of nutritious foods are offered. Food preferences occur. A nutritious breakfast is important. The federal government has established the school breakfast program in many areas. The National School Lunch Program has been ongoing. Summer lunch programs are also available. These lunches must provide certain nutritional standards (the goal is to provide one-third of the recommended daily allowance of foods).

Children who are inattentive at school should be screened for vision or hearing deficits, language or learning disabilities before being diagnosed as attention deficit disorders (ADD). Increasing structure and decreasing distractions is the first step in helping any child with a school problem. Emphasis

Table 19–3
SUMMARY OF SCHOOL-AGE CHILD GROWTH AND DEVELOPMENT AND HEALTH MAINTENANCE *(Continued)*

Age (years)	Physical Competency	Intellectual Competency	Emotional-Social Competency	Nutrition	Play	Safety
11–12	Vital signs approximate adult norms Growth spurt for girs; inequalities between sexes is increasingly noticeable; boys greater physical strength Eruption of permanent teeth complete except for third molars Secondary sex characteristics begin in boys Menstruation may begin	Able to think about social problems and prejudices; sees others' points of view Enjoys reading mysteries, love stories Begins playing with abstract ideas Interested in whys of health measures and understands human reproduction Very moralistic; religious commitment often made during this time	Intense team loyalty; boys begin teasing girls and girls flirt with boys for attention Best-friend period Wants unreasonable independence, rebellious about routines; wide mood swings; needs some time daily for privacy Very critical of own work. Hero worship prevails Facts-of-life chats with friends prevail Masturbation increases Appears under constant tension	Male needs 2500 cal/day; female needs 2250 (70 cal/kg/day); both need 75 ml/kg of water/day; 2 gm/kg protein daily	Enjoys projects and working with hands Likes to do errands and jobs to earn money Very involved in sports, dancing, talking on phone Enjoys all aspects of acting and drama	Continue monitoring friends Stress bicycle and roller blade safety on streets and in traffic and use of helmet and other protective gear

From Betz, C., Hunsberger, M., & Wright, S. (1994). *Family centered nursing care of children* (2nd ed.). Philadelphia: Saunders.

should be placed on producing successful experiences and increasing complexity slowly. Realistic demands need to be balanced by unconditional support during successes and failures of the developing child. The school nurse should be aware of parenting styles that demonstrate difficulty in "letting go" and parenting styles that demonstrate excessive pressure, if the development of behavior problems are to be averted.

Active play with family members is important to the school-age child (Fig. 19–12). Divorce, separation, domestic violence, and neighborhood gangs can negatively affect the progress of development in the school-age child. The school nurse can initiate appropriate referrals to community agencies.

Health supervision should include assessment of physical activity and school performance. A child who avoids activities that may reveal his physical appearance, such as changing into gym clothes or cooperating in health exams, may have a negative perception of his or her own physical appearance. Parents need guidance to understand the difference between participation in sports activities that help to develop skill, teamwork, and fitness, and high-stress activities that increase the risk of skeletal injury and focus on winning as a central theme. Often a 6-year-old with an advanced athletic ability who is guided into early competition and experiences outstanding commendations, loses self-esteem when he is 12 years old and the ability of peers develops to, or exceeds, his or her level and he or she no longer experiences the spotlight. The school-age child can understand simple explanations of his or her illness but sometimes can revert to believing illness is "punishment" for behavior or thoughts.

School children need time and a place to study. They require a desk in their own room or at least a private area of the house where they can concentrate. Their furniture should be of the proper size; lighting should be adequate. They must learn to take responsibility for their assignments and school

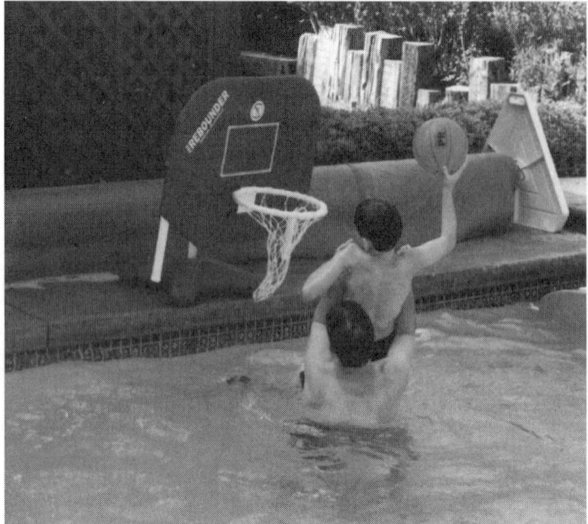

Figure 19–12. • Active play with family members is important to the school-age child.

supplies. Parents can encourage school children by showing interest in what they are learning, by joining parent–teac her organizations, and by visiting periodically with the teacher. Parents should be encouraged to vote on civic matters that will benefit the school system in their community.

At this age, an allowance or at least a means of earning money provides children with opportunities to learn its value. It takes time and encouragement for them to learn to spend money wisely. Such experiences aid in making the school-age child a more responsible person.

Pet Ownership

Pet ownership is a common practice in families with children. After 7 years of age, children can be responsible for caring for the needs of a family pet. Pets that have close contact with children have the potential of transmitting disease (Table 19–4). Studies have documented the positive influence of pet ownership in improving the medical and psychological outcome after illness or surgery. Handicapped children especially benefit from interacting with pets (increased self-esteem and positive attitudes). Pets allow the ill person who feels separated from other people to feel companionship and acceptance. Shy children often find pet ownership eases the path to socialization with others who initiate contact because of the pet.

The age of the child, the presence of allergies, or an immunocompromised family member are major factors that influence the desirability of pet ownership. Toddlers and young children may not understand limitations in handling pets that can respond by biting or scratching (Fig. 19–13). Certain breeds of dogs have a greater tendency to bite, such as Chows, German Shepherds, St. Bernards, Pit Bulls, Bull Terriers, Akitas, Rottweilers, Dobermans, Chihuahuas, and Daschunds should be avoided as pets for young children.

Table 19–4

DISEASES THAT CAN BE TRANSMITTED BY PETS TO HUMANS

Vector	Disease
Dog bites	Cellulitis, septicemia
Geckos	*Salmonella*
Dogs, cats, birds, farm animals	*C. Campylobacter* (gastroenteritis, Guillain-Barré syndrome)
Cats, dogs, ferrets, racoons, skunk, bats, foxes, and wolves	Rabies
Reptiles, rodents, cats, dogs	Cryptosporidiosis (gastroenteritis)
Dogs, cats	Parasites, pneumonia, hypereosinophilia, toxocariasis
Dogs, cats	Fungal skin infections
Dogs, cats, reptiles, turtles	Leptospirosis
Blood contact during birth of animals	Brucellosis, Q fever
Kittens	Cat scratch disease (lymphodenopathy and preauricular adenitis)
Cats	Toxoplasmosis*
Birds, farm animals, cats	Q fever
Birds	Psittacosis, cryptococcosis, histoplasmosis
Fish	Fish tank granuloma (related to *M. tuberculosis* organism that causes ulcerated skin lesions after cleaning the fish tank)

*Toxoplasmosis can cause congenital malformations in the fetus. Pregnant females are urged to avoid contact with litter boxes.

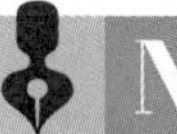

Nursing Tip

Emergency Treatment of an Avulsed Tooth

When a permanent tooth is accidentally knocked out of the socket, the tooth should be picked up by the crown to avoid damaging the root area. Place the tooth in milk until the child and tooth arrive at a dentist's office.

Immunocompromised children are at risk of contracting illness that is spread by some animals. Box 19–4 explains methods advised to minimize risks to immunocompromised children. Birds, rodents, turtles, and reptiles are not recommended as pets because they cannot be screened for potential pathogens, have few vaccines, and are most likely to transmit disease. Risk factors in pet ownership of cats and dogs can be further reduced if children are cautioned not to kiss pets, not allow them to sleep in bed with the child, avoid exposure to animal feces, and encourage handwashing after handling a pet. Families and pets can benefit by taking obedience courses available at low cost in most communities.

Having an allergy to animal dander does not always rule out having a pet. Parent education concerning pet selection and hygiene can assist the family in making a decision that is best for all family members. Toddlers who spend most of their time indoors and babies born in winter months are more likely to have a cumulative exposure to allergens that increases a sensitivity response. Cats are most often the allergen offender as allergens are secreted by sebaceous glands onto the cat hair and skin and in the saliva. Cats shed their hair and dander and electrostatic properties enable the allergens to adhere to carpets and walls, making allergy-proofing of the house a difficult challenge. The Poodle breed of dog does not have a shed cycle and so may be the least offensive pet for the allergic child.

Shar Pei, Terriers, Labradors, and Pit Bulls may release more allergens because they are very susceptible to atopic conditions that cause scratching. Young neutered female dogs produce less allergens than older unneutered males. If an allergenic pet is already part of the family, risks can be minimized by frequent bathing and keeping the pet outdoors or at least out of the child's bedroom. A 3% tannic

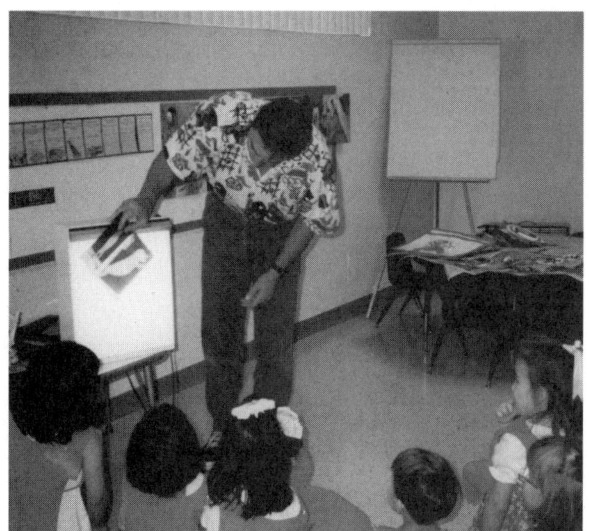

Figure 19–13. • A veterinarian talks to a school class about his career and the care of pets.

BOX 19–4

TEN WAYS TO PROTECT IMMUNOCOMPROMISED CHILDREN FROM PET-TRANSMITTED DISEASE

1. Choose a healthy animal (preferably a dog or cat) older than 1 year of age to reduce the likelihood of colonization with human pathogens.
2. Neuter the pet at an early age to minimize roaming activity and interaction with animals in the wild.
3. Feed pets only cooked meat and foods unlikely to be contaminated with animal feces to minimize gastrointestinal colonization with potential pathogens.
4. Keep the animal indoors as much as possible to limit interaction with other animals and reduce exposure to disease.
5. Treat the animal for fleas monthly during flea season to prevent transmission of disease by these ectoparasites.
6. Do not keep birds, reptiles, turtles, or rodents as pets because they are more likely to carry unusual human pathogens, cannot be immunized, and are difficult to screen for transmissible diseases.
7. Make sure a pet dog or cat receives booster immunizations for rabies, distemper, canine hepatitis, leptospirosis, parovirus, and feline leukemia virus.
8. Have a veterinarian test the pet's stools annually for *Salmonella, Campylobacter, Giardia,* and *Cryptosporidium* and screen the animal for dermatophytes, which are transmissible to humans.
9. Have cats tested annually for feline leukemia since positive animals are more likely to acquire human infectious agents such as cryptosporidiosis.
10. Avoid exposure to farm animals and petting zoos unless the animals have been carefully screened for human pathogens.

Adapted from Steele, R. (1997). Sizing up the risks of pet transmitted diseases. *Contemporary Pediatrics, 14*(9), 65.

acid spray to carpets and furniture can reduce the allergen potential of cat dander. Desensitization of the child by an allergist is also an option. Except for bite injuries, where secondary infection is common, the benefits of pet ownership often outweigh the risks. Education concerning the approach to and handling of pets is beneficial to children whether or not they own pets, as they are likely to come in contact with pets in their neighborhood or at their friend's house. Infection can occur via contact with saliva, feces, fecal droppings, urine and/or inhalation or skin contact with organisms.

KEY POINTS

- School age, from 6 to 12 years, is a time of increased independence when the child begins to incorporate, perfect, and process skills and information gained in earlier years.
- Erikson calls this stage the *stage of industry* or accomplishment.
- Freud describes this period as the sexual *latency stage,* when the child's energy is directed toward cognitive and physical skills.
- Major changes occur in the child's cognitive-perceptual patterns. Piaget refers to this stage as the *concrete operational stage.*
- Growth is slow until the spurt directly before puberty.
- School has an important influence on the socialization of children.
- The child acquires a positive self-concept from the ability to be productive, self-directed, and accepted.
- Peers range from same-sex friends in the early years to opposite-sex friends around puberty. Group acceptance is important.
- Both sexes need accurate information and reassurance in advance about changes of puberty and reproduction.
- The availability of junk food hampers efforts to provide proper nutrition. Meals may be sporadic because of activities of the child and the parents' working schedules.
- Accident prevention is still extremely important. These children are prone to injuries from motor vehicles, bicycles, skateboards, swimming, and their tendency to be overactive and distracted.
- Language development during the school-age years develops and expands the ability to communicate. The school-age child experiments with words without fully understanding the meaning.
- Moral development includes an understanding of rules, fairness, values, and knowledge of right and wrong.
- After-school daycare in relation to developmental needs is a concern of working parents.
- Pet ownership can nurture a sense of responsibility and encourage socialization in a shy child. Selection of an appropriate pet for the child and family is essential.
- The school nurse plays an important role in providing anticipatory guidance, health assessment, and community referral.

MULTIPLE-CHOICE REVIEW QUESTIONS

Choose the most appropriate answer.

1. The pulse of the school age child is approximately
   a. 100–120 beats/min.
   b. 95–120 beats/min.
   c. 85–100 beats/min.
   d. 60–80 beats/min.
2. By age 12, the brain
   a. decreases in circumference.
   b. reaches approximately adult size.
   c. reaches approximately child size.
   d. divides into the cerebrum and cerebellum.
3. While playing in school, a 9-year-old child suffers a mouth injury that causes his tooth to be knocked out of his mouth. The teacher or school nurse should
   a. place the tooth in a cup of clean water and send the child home.
   b. place the tooth in a cup of milk and call parent to take the child to the dentist.
   c. wrap the tooth in a clean cloth and call parent to take the child to the dentist.
   d. rinse the child's mouth and place the tooth in an envelope for the child to show his parent.
4. The parent of an 8-year-old child seeks advice from the nurse because her child is overweight. The nurse would advise the parent to
   a. provide a reward for the child when he avoids between-meal snacks for a full week.
   b. limit privileges when the child eats sweets or junk food.
   c. include the child in meal planning and preparation.
   d. limit party-going activities where sweets will be served.
5. Sandra, age 9, is practicing the piano. She continues to have difficulty in playing the theme song from a popular movie. She starts to pound on the piano keys in frustration. You would enter the room and say
   a. "Just what do you think you're doing? That piano costs money!"
   b. "That's not difficult. Pull yourself together or you'll never amount to anything."
   c. "That piece sounds hard. I can see how you could be discouraged."
   d. "Here, let me show you how to play that."

BIBLIOGRAPHY AND READER REFERENCE

American Academy of Pediatrics. (1994). Diseases transmitted by animals. In G. Peters (Ed.), *Report of Committee on Infectious Diseases* (p. 614). Elk Grove, IL: Author.

American Academy of Pediatrics Committee on Injury and Poison Prevention. (1995). Bicycle helmets. *Pediatrics, 4,* 609–610.

Ashwill, J., & Droske, S. (1997). *Nursing care of children: Principles and practice.* Philadelphia: Saunders.

Barba, B. E. (1995). The positive influence of animals: Animal assisted therapy in acute care. *Clinical Nurse Specialist, 9,* 199.

Barrett, D., & Sleasman, J. (1997). Pediatric AIDS: So now what do we do. *Contemporary Pediatrics, 14*(16), 111.

Bass, J. W., Vincent, J. M., & Person, D. A. (1997). The expanding spectrum of Bartonella infections: II cat-scratch disease. *Pediatric Infectious Disease Journal, 16,* 163.

Beck, A. M., & Meyers, N. M. (1996). Health enhancement and companion animal ownership. *American Review of Public Health, 17,* 247.

Behrman, R. E., Kleigman, R., & Arvin, A. (1996). *Nelson's textbook of pediatrics* (15th ed.). Philadelphia: Saunders.

Betz, C., Hunsberger, M., & Wright, S. (1994). *Family-centered nursing care of children* (2nd ed.). Philadelphia: Saunders.

Bowden, V., Dickey, S., & Greenberg, C. (1998). *Children and their families: The continuum of care.* Philadelphia: Saunders.

Bush, R., Fodal, R., & Van Metre, T. (1995). Taming your patient's animal allergies. *Patient Care, 29*(7), 71.

Byrd, R. (1998). School readiness: More than a summers work. *Contemporary Pediatrics, 15*(5), 39.

Center for Disease Control and Prevention USPHS/IDSA. (1995). Guidelines for prevention of opportunistic infections in persons with HIV: A summary. *MMWR, 44,* RR-8.

Connelly, K. (1997). Advising families about pets. *Contemporary Pediatrics, 14*(2), 71.

Finan, S. L. (1997). Promoting healthy sexuality: Guidelines for the school-age child and adolescent. *Nurse Practitioner, 22*(11), 62–72.

Gaedeke, M. K. (1992). Emergency treatment for tooth avulsion. *Nursing 92,* 33.

Gershman, K. A., Socks, J., & Wright, J. (1994). Which dogs bite? A case controlled study of risk factors. *Pediatrics,* 93-913.

Hart, B., & Hart, L. (1985). Selecting pet dogs on the basis of cluster analysis of breed behavior profiles and gender. *Journal of American Veterinary Medicine Association, 180*(11), 1181.

Department of Health and Human Services. (1991). *Healthy People 2000: National Health Promotion and Disease Prevention Objectives.* DHHS Publication No. (PHS) 91-50213. Washington, DC: Government Printing Office.

Huston, C. (1997). Dental luxation and avulsion. *American Journal of Nursing, 97*(9), 48.

MacBriar, B., et al. (1995). Development of a health concerns inventory for school-age children. *Journal of School Nurses, 11*(3), 25.

Mahan, L. K., & Escott-Stump, S. (1996). *Krause's food, nutrition and diet therapy.* Philadelphia: Saunders.

Matzen, J. (1995). Assessment of HIV/acquired immunodeficiency syndrome audiovisual materials designed for grades 7–12. *Journal of Pediatric Nursing, 10*(2), 114.

National Association of State Public Health Veterinarians, Inc. (1997). Compendium of Animal Rabies Control. *MMWR, 46*(RR4), 1.

Plaut, M., Zimmerman, E., & Goldstein, R. A. (1996). Health hazards to humans associated with domestic pets. *American Review of Public Health, 17,* 221.

Seigel, J. M. (1995). Pet ownership and the importance of pets among adolescents. *Anthrozoos, 8*(4), 217.

Shor, E. (1998). Guiding the family of a school aged child. *Contemporary Pediatrics, 15*(3), 75.

Steele, R. (1997). Sizing up risks of pet transmitted diseases. *Contemporary Pediatrics, 14*(9), 43–68.

Wong, D. (1995). *Whaley & Wong's nursing care of infants and children* (5th ed.). St. Louis, MO: Mosby.

chapter 20

The Adolescent

Outline

GENERAL CHARACTERISTICS

GROWTH AND DEVELOPMENT
- Physical Development
- Psychosocial Development
- Cognitive Development
- Peer Relationships
- Career Plans
- Responsibility
- Daydreams
- Sexual Behavior
- Sex Education

PARENTING

HEALTH EDUCATION AND GUIDANCE
- Nutrition
- Vegetarian Diets
- Sports and Nutrition
- Nutrition and School Exams
- Personal Care
- Safety
- Health Assessment

COMMON PROBLEMS OF ADOLESCENCE
- Substance Abuse
- Depression

THE NURSING APPROACH TO ADOLESCENTS

Objectives

On completion and mastery of Chapter 20, the student will be able to

- Define each vocabulary term listed.
- Identify two major developmental tasks of adolescence.
- Discuss three major theoretic viewpoints on the personality development of adolescents.
- List five life events that contribute to stress during adolescence.
- Describe menstruation to a 13-year-old girl.
- Describe Tanner's stages of breast development.
- Identify two ways in which a person's cultural background might contribute to behavior.
- List three guidelines of importance for the adolescent participating in sports.
- Summarize the nutritional requirements of the adolescent.
- Discuss the importance of peer groups, "cliques," and best friends in the developmental process of an adolescent.
- Discuss two main challenges during the teen years that the adolescent must adjust to.
- List a source for planning sex education programs for adolescents.

Vocabulary

abstract thinking	growth spurt
adolescence	homosexual
androgen	intimacy
asynchrony	lesbian
cliques	menarche
epiphyseal closure	puberty
estrogen	self-concept
formal operations	SIECUS
gay	SMR
gender	Tanner's stages

GENERAL CHARACTERISTICS

Adolescence is defined as the period of life beginning with the appearance of secondary sex characteristics and ending with cessation of growth and emotional maturity. The term comes from the word *adolescere,* meaning "to grow up." Adolescence is often divided into early, middle, and late periods because the teenager of 13 varies a great deal from the 18-year-old. Middle adolescence appears to be the time of greatest turmoil for most families. Perhaps one of the most characteristic features of adolescence is its uncertainty. It is a period of life that in our culture lasts a comparatively long time and involves a great number of adjustments. The major tasks of adolescence include establishing an identity, separating from family, initiating intimacy and career choices for economic independence. Some of the major theories of development are summarized in Box 20–1.

Life is never dull when there are adolescents in the family. The surge toward independence becomes more and more pronounced, making it practically impossible for adolescents to get along with their parents, who represent authority. When adolescents submit to parental wishes, they may feel humiliated and childish. If they revolt, conflicts arise within the family. Parents and teenagers have to weather the storm together and try to come up with solutions that are relatively satisfactory to all.

Numerous other factors account for the restlessness of adolescents. Their bodies are rapidly changing, and they experience intense sexual drives. They want to be accepted by society, but they are not sure how to go about it. Adolescents question life and search to find what psychologists call their sense of identity, they ask: "Who am I?" "What do I want?" This is followed by the intimacy stage, in which teenagers must learn to avoid emotional isolation. They must face the fear of rejection in shared activities such as sports, in close friendships, and in sexual experiences. The older adolescent thinks about the future and is generally idealistic. Jean Piaget and other investigators indicate that during this time teenagers reach the final stages of *abstract reasoning,* logic, and other symbolic forms of thought, which increases sophistication in moral reasoning.

These facts sound complicated in themselves, but they are intensified by a world that is constantly changing. *Gender roles* are less well defined in many households and parents may not be traditional role models for their children. Many adolescents are living in single-parent homes or with working relatives, where little, if any, supervision is available.

Conformity is one of the strongest needs of the adolescent in society. Today, with electronic technology bringing common experiences to people all over the world via radio, TV, and computers, the strength of conformity often overrides cultural or

BOX 20–1

FEATURES OF MAJOR THEORIES OF DEVELOPMENT DURING ADOLESCENCE

Sigmund Freud

- Adolescent is in genital stage, the final stage of psychosexual development
- Self-love (narcissism) disappears; love for others (altruism) develops
- Peers and parents are less influential than before, but still provide love and support

Erik Erikson

- Adolescent's main concerns are self-definition and self-esteem
- Adolescent experiences identity crisis brought on by physical (including sexual) changes and conflict about future choices and expectations of others
- Adolescent must adapt to these changes and develop a new self-concept and appropriate vocational choices
- Adolescent learns to understand self in relation to others' perceptions and expectations

Jean Piaget

- Adolescent is in stage of formal operations, so has ability to reason logically and abstractly
- Adolescent is oriented toward problem solving

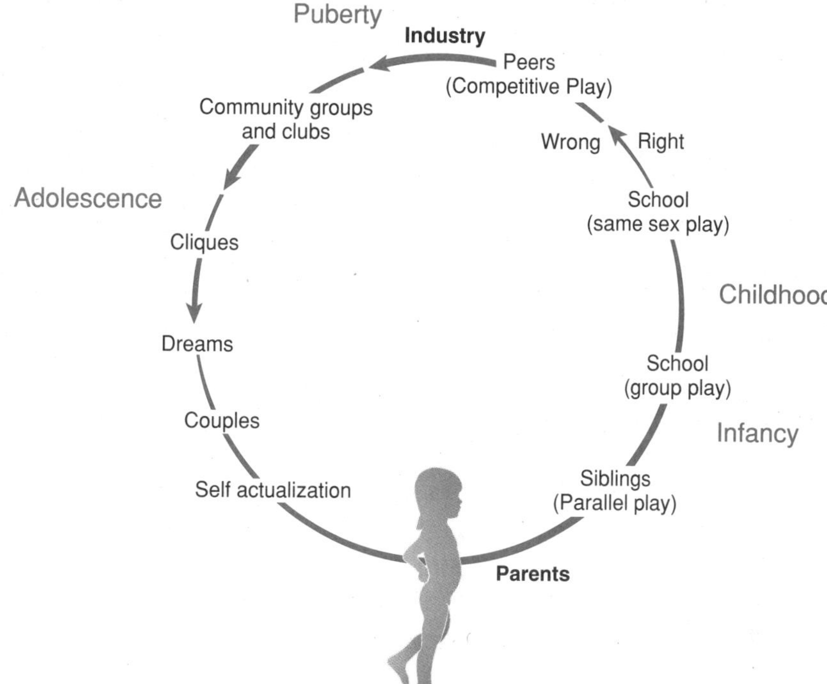

Figure 20–1. • Roadmap of social interaction. In infancy and early childhood, the child's focus is on parents. As the child grows, peers replace parents in importance. When adolescents mature, they return to the family with new respect, independence, and cooperation.

traditional practices. Assimilation is beginning to occur via technology.

The needs of the family often compete with the needs of the teen when parents try to push the teen into an activity or career that meets the parent's own personal need or dreams. Parents must be guided to enjoy the interests and activities of the teen without imposing their personal desires. The main challenges of the teen years include adjusting to rapid physical and physiological changes, maintaining privacy, coping with social stresses (Figs. 20–1 and 20–2) and pressures, maintaining open communication, and developing positive health care practices and lifestyle choices.

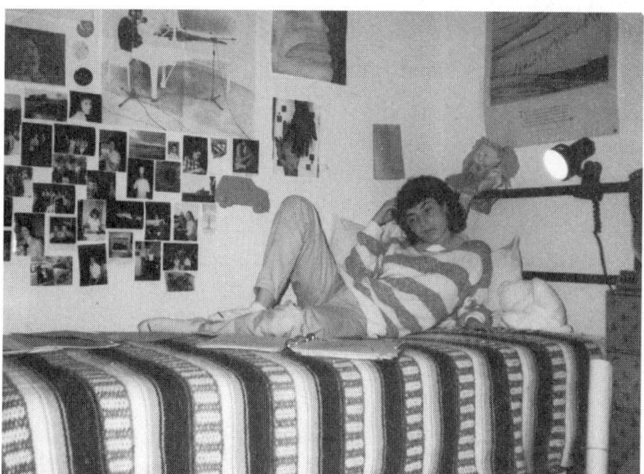

Figure 20–2. • Adolescents need privacy.

GROWTH AND DEVELOPMENT

Physical Development

Preadolescence is a short period immediately preceding adolescence. In girls it comprises the ages of 10 to 13 years and is marked by rapid changes in the structure and function of various parts of the body. It is distinguished by puberty, the stage at which the reproductive organs become functional and secondary sex characteristics develop. Both sexes produce male hormones, *androgens,* and female hormones, *estrogens,* in comparatively equal amounts during childhood. At puberty, the hypothalamus of the brain signals the pituitary gland to stimulate other endocrine glands—the adrenals and the ovaries or testes—to secrete their hormones directly into the bloodstream in differing proportions (more androgens in the boy and more estrogens in the girl).

The age of puberty varies and is somewhat earlier for girls than for boys. The final 20% of mature height that occurs during adolescence is called the *growth spurt* and usually occurs by 18 years of age. The major cause of weight gain is the increase in skeletal mass. Understanding the implications of

Nursing Tip

A rapid period of growth in which a body reaches adult height and weight before 18 years of age is known as a *growth spurt*.

growth and development for nursing assessments is shown in Figure 20–3.

General appearance tends to be awkward, that is, long-legged and gangling; this growth characteristic is termed *asynchrony* because different body parts mature at different rates. The sweat glands are very active, and greasy skin and acne are common. Both sexes mature earlier and grow taller and heavier than in past generations (Fig. 20–4). Because of the gross motor development that occurs during adolescence, teenagers can gain satisfaction from sports. Table 20–1 outlines the growth and development of adolescents.

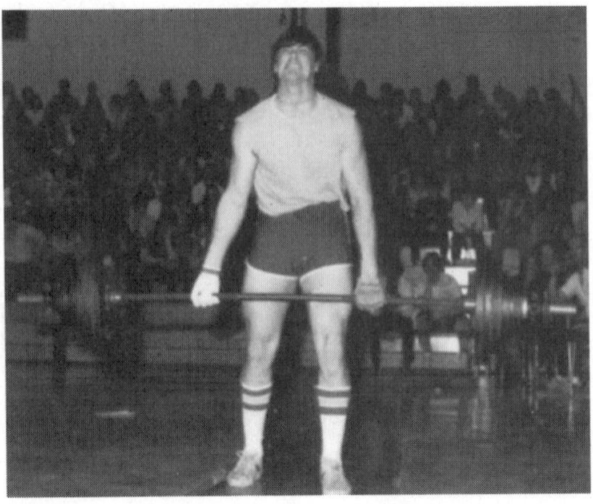

Figure 20–4. • Young people today mature earlier than in past generations, and they are also taller and heavier. Many develop high levels of physical competence.

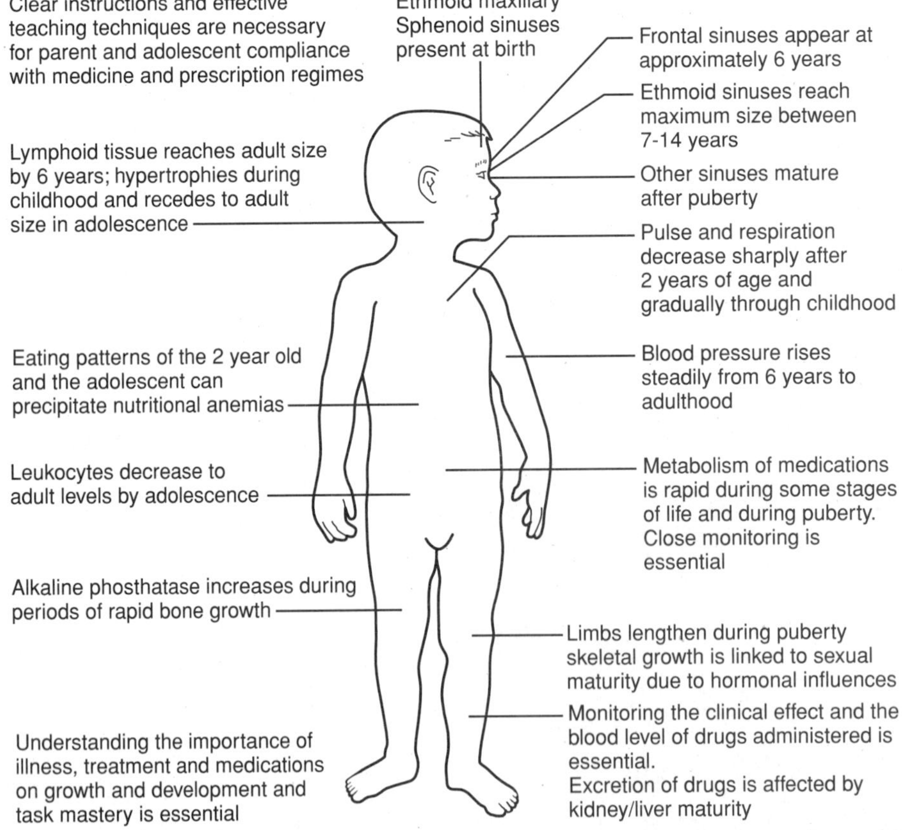

Figure 20–3. • There are many developmental changes that take place between infancy and adolescence. The nurse must understand the implications of growth and development for nursing assessments.

Boys. During fetal life the placental chorionic gonadotropin stimulates leydig cells to secrete testosterone. Thus week 8 to 12 of fetal life is important in the sexual development of the male (XY) child. The Luteinizing hormone (LH) maintains testosterone levels. One to two years before puberty, serum levels of LH increase during sleep. The secretion of gonadotropins stimulate gonad enlargement and the secretion of sex hormones. The interaction between the hypothalamus, pituitary, and gonads supports the development of puberty. In boys, puberty begins with hormonal changes between 10 and 13 years of age. Enlargement of the testicles and of internal structures and pigmentation of the scrotum are followed by enlargement of the penis. Erections and nocturnal emissions take place. The production of sperm begins between 13 and 14 years of age. The shoulders widen, and the pectoral muscles enlarge. The voice deepens. Hair begins to grow on the chest, axillae, pubic areas, and face (Fig. 20–5 and Box 20–2).

An athletic scrotal support (jock strap) is necessary for boys participating in sporting events, for dancers, and the like. It supports and protects the genitals and also prevents embarrassment from exposure. A support is purchased by size. Good personal hygiene is necessary because heat and friction may lead to jock itch, a fungal infestation of the groin. Sharing athletic supporters is discouraged.

The American Cancer Society recommends that boys examine their testes during or after a hot bath or shower. Each testicle is examined using the index and middle fingers of both hands on the underside of the testicle and the thumbs on the top of the testicle. The testicles are gently rolled between the thumb and the fingers. Testicular and scrotal self-examinations are performed once a month. If a lump is discovered, it should be reported immediately to a health care provider.

Girls. Pubertal changes occur 6 months to 2 years before boys. Puberty is easily recognized in girls by the onset of menstruation (Fig. 20–6). The first menstrual period is called the *menarche.* It commonly occurs about age 12 or 13, but this varies. It may occur as early as 10 or as late as 15 years of age. Secondary sex characteristics become more apparent before the menarche. Fat is deposited in the hips, thighs, and breasts, causing them to enlarge. See Box 20–2.

Table 20–1
GROWTH AND DEVELOPMENT OF THE ADOLESCENT

	Early (10–13 yr)	Middle (14–16 yr)	Late (17–21 yr)
Physical growth	Secondary sex characteristics appear	Spurt in height growth occurs	Growth slows
Body image	Self-conscious Adjusts to pubertal changes	Experiments with different "images" and "looks"	Accepts body image Personality emerges
Self-concept	Low self-esteem Denial of reality	Impulsive Impatient Identity confusion	Positive self-image Empathetic Independent thinker
Behavior	Behaves for rewards	Behaves to conform	Responsible behavior
Sexual development	Sexual interest	Sexual experimentation	Sexual identity emerges Develops caring relationships
Peers	"Cliques" of unisex friends Has "best friend" Hero worship Has adult "crushes"	Dating begins Has need to please significant peer Develops heterosexual peer group	Individual relationships valued Partner selection
Family	Ambivalent to family Strives for independence	Struggles for autonomy and acceptance Rebels/withdraws Demands privacy	Achieves independence Reestablishes family relationships
Cognitive development	Concrete thinking Here and now is important	Early abstract Daydreams, fantasizes Starts inductive and deductive reasoning	Abstract thinking Idealistic
Goals	Socializing is priority Goals are unrealistic	Identifies skills/interests Becomes a superachiever or dropout	Identifies career goals Work or college
Health concerns	Concerned about normalcy	Concerned about experimenting drugs or sex	Idealistic Decision making for lifestyle choice
Nursing interventions	Convey limits Encourage verbalization	Help them solve problems from choices Use peer group sessions Provide privacy	Discuss goals Allow participation in decisions Provide confidentiality

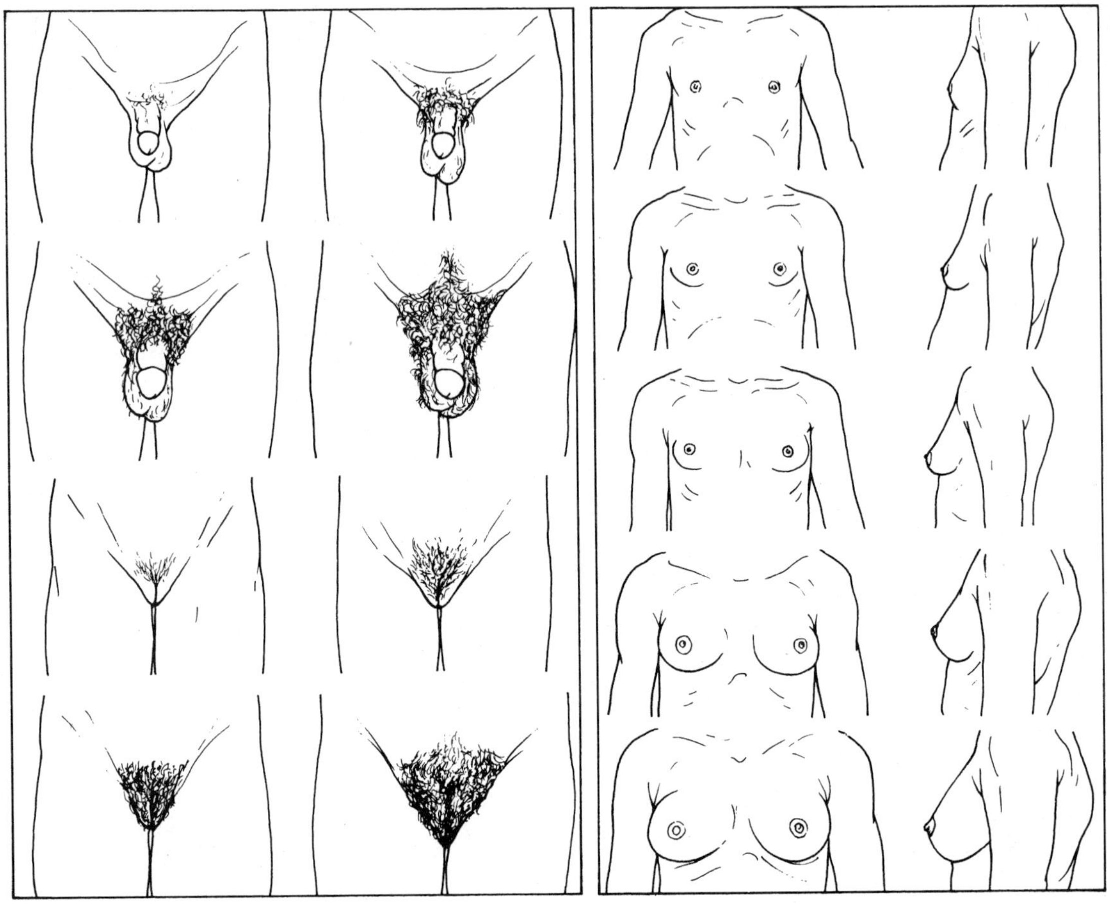

Figure 20–5. • **A,** Sex maturity ratings (SMR) of pubic hair changes in adolescent boys and girls. **B,** Sex maturity ratings of breast changes in adolescent girls. (Redrawn from photographs of J. M. Tanner, M.D., Institute of Child Health, Department of Growth and Development, University of London, England.) Bone growth is closely correlated with SMR because epiphyseal closure is controlled by hormones.

At this time, the teenager may need to be fitted for a bra. The lingerie department of a store has fitting rooms. Measurements need to be ascertained and various styles tried on for comfort. Straps should fit so that they do not continually fall from the shoulders. Cups need to be large enough to support fullness near the underarms. The garment needs to fit across the back so that it is not uncomfortably tight. Teenagers generally like attractive undergarments that have some type of lace trim. Sports bras are available for girls who participate in active sports. Puberty is a good time to begin to teach breast self-examination (see Box 11–1, p. 277). Informational materials are available through the American Cancer Society.

The external genitals grow. Hair develops in the pubic area (see Fig. 20–5 and Box 20–2) and the underarms. It is important to note that ballet dancers, runners, gymnasts, and adolescents engaged in other athletic activities that involve a lean body and high level of physical activity can alter the mechanisms affecting puberty and cause a delay in the onset of menarche. Energy balance, activity, and nutrition are important factors to evaluate when menstruation is delayed. When the ends of the long bones knit securely to their shafts *(epiphyseal closure)*, further growth can no longer take place. For a detailed discussion of physiology of reproductive organs, see Chapter 2.

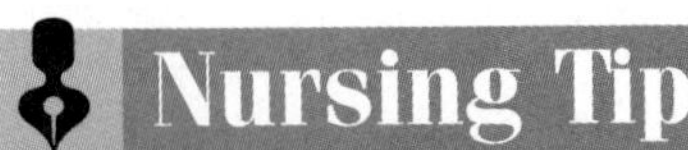

Young women are taught breast examination, and young men should be instructed in examination of the testes.

Psychosocial Development

Sense of Identity. Physical growth and sexual interest correlate with sexual maturity. Cognitive growth and social changes correlate with chronological age and placement in school. Stresses can increase when physical growth and cognitive growth occur at different rates in the same adolescent. Although the early maturing male often finds positive social adjustment and acceptance, early maturing females are often embarrassed and develop low self-esteem. The teenager's desire for freedom and independence is extremely important and necessary for developing individuality. To accomplish this, young persons must reject their childhood self and often the people most closely associated with it. Erikson identifies the major task of this group as *identity versus role confusion.* Emancipation is a critical element in the establishment of identity.

Adolescents want to be people in their own right, and they "try on" different roles. *Self-concept* (one's view of oneself) fluctuates during this time and is molded by the demands of parents, peers, teachers, and others. Interaction with others helps teenagers to determine who they are and in what direction they want to proceed. This process is more difficult for low-income minorities and is complicated by many factors, such as illness, broken homes, and the extent of formal education. Young persons who are unable to master confusion and establish an identity may become rigid in their actions, bewildered, or depressed, or they may cling to the conformity of peer groups long after the need should have passed. Some show an inordinate need for something "new and exciting." They may experience low self-esteem and alienation, and they may confront many other difficulties on entering the adult world.

BOX 20–2

TANNER'S STAGES OF SEXUAL MATURITY

Sex maturity ratings (SMR) range from 1 to 5. A score of 1 represents the prepubertal child; 5 corresponds to adult status.

Boys: Genital Development

Stage 1. Preadolescent; testes, scrotum, and penis are of about the same size and proportion as in early childhood

Stage 2. Enlargement of scrotum and testes; skin of scrotum reddens and changes in texture; little or no enlargement of penis at this stage

Stage 3. Enlargement of penis, which occurs at first mainly in length; further growth of testes and scrotum

Stage 4. Increased size of penis with growth in breadth and development of glands; testes and scrotum larger, scrotal skin darkened

Stage 5. Genitalia adult in size and shape

Girls: Breast Development

Stage 1. Preadolescent: elevation of papilla only

Stage 2. Breast bud stage: elevation of breast and papilla as small mound; enlargement of areolar diameter

Stage 3. Further enlargement and elevation of breast and areola, with no separation of their contours

Stage 4. Projection of areola and papilla to form a secondary mound above the level of the breast

Stage 5. Mature stage: projection of papilla only due to recession of the areola to the general contour of the breast

Both Sexes: Pubic Hair

Stage 1. Preadolescent; vellus over the pubes is not further developed than that over the abdominal wall, that is, no pubic hair

Stage 2. Sparse growth of long, slightly pigmented, downy hair, straight or curled, chiefly at the base of the penis or along the labia

Stage 3. Considerably darker, coarser, and more curled; hair spreads sparsely over the junction of the pubes

Stage 4. Hair now adult in type, but area covered is considerably smaller than in the adult; no spread to the medial surface of thighs

Stage 5. Adult in quantity and type with distribution of the horizontal (or classically "feminine") pattern; spread to medial surface of thighs, but not up linea alba or elsewhere above the base of the inverse triangle (spread up linea alba occurs and is rated stage 6)

Data from the standard illustrations in Tanner, J. M. (1962). *Growth of adolescence* (2nd ed.). Oxford: Blackwell Scientific.

1. The *pituitary gland* is a small gland at the base of the brain. It sends out chemical messengers through the blood to various parts of the body. These messengers, or hormones, are responsible for many steps of growth and change as we develop. When a girl reaches the age of puberty, the pituitary gland sends out a new hormone that affects the functions of a group of organs concerned with menstruation.

3. The *ovaries* are two small female organs that manufacture human egg cells. When a girl reaches the age of puberty, these little cells receive a signal from the pituitary gland and begin to grow. Each month a cell escapes from an ovary and starts to travel along a passageway—one of the fallopian tubes. This movement of the egg cell is called ovulation. If one of these cells becomes fertilized by a male cell, it can develop into a baby.

4. The *fallopian tubes,* into which the egg cells pass, lead toward the uterus.

5. The *uterus* is also called the womb. This is where the egg cell develops if it has been fertilized. Each month a soft, thick lining (the endometrium) of tissue and blood vessels forms inside the uterus.

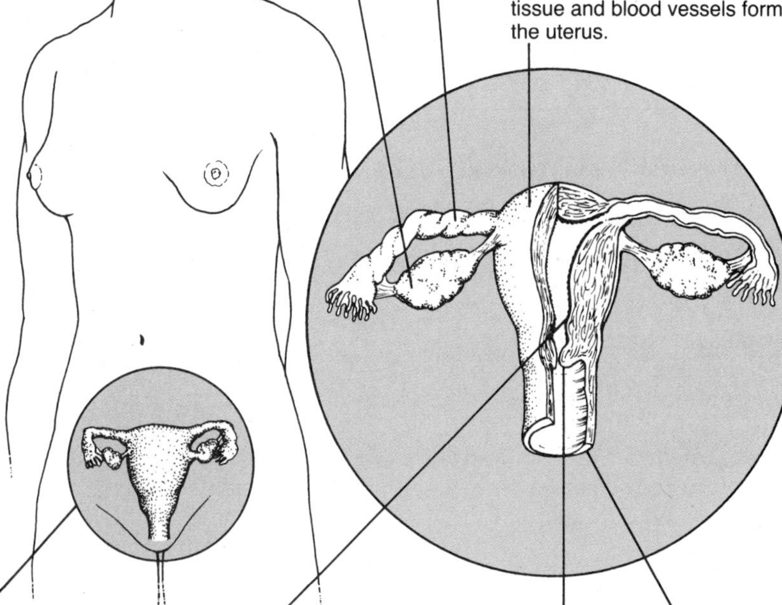

2. The *pelvic area* is located in the lower part of the body in the region of the hips. It is here that the organs associated with menstruation are located.

7. The *cervix* is the lower part of the uterus, which connects it with the vagina.

6. The *endometrium,* or uterus lining, serves as a warm nest to shelter and nourish the unborn child until it has grown enough to be ready to come into the world as a baby. But unless an egg cell has been fertilized and a baby started on its way toward birth, there is no need for the cell or for the blood and tissues of the endometrium. And so they are passed from the body.

8. The *vagina,* a passageway leading to the outside of the lower part of the body, carries away these materials in a flow of blood. This is called menstrual flow. When it occurs, it lasts for several days each month and is known as menstruation.

Figure 20–6. • Menstruation.

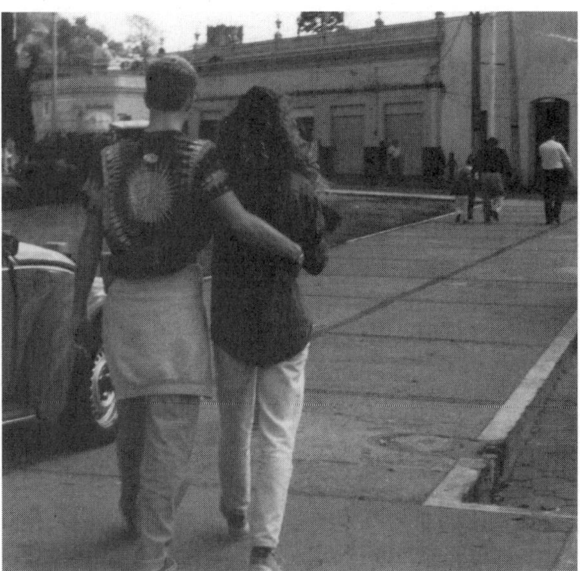

Figure 20–7. • As adolescents move toward young adulthood, they become ready to take the risks of close affiliations and friendship and to establish relationships with members of the opposite sex.

Sense of Intimacy. Developing intimacy is closely entwined with resolving one's sense of identity. As adolescents move toward young adulthood, they become ready to take the risks of close affiliations and friendships and to establish relationships with the opposite sex (Fig. 20–7). Avoidance of this may lead to a deep sense of isolation. Adolescence is a period of trying and testing. Disagreements with parents often revolve around dating, the family car, money, chores, school grades, choice of friends, smoking, sex, and use of social drugs. The young person questions parental values and morals and is particularly sensitive to hypocrisy.

Adults who associate with teenagers should try to create an atmosphere of interest and understanding. Adolescents must know that adults care. They need practice in making decisions, which need to be respected even if they make mistakes. Parents should set limits and expect them to be challenged but adhered to. Parents and nurses who see other people's intrinsic worth, feel good about themselves, and do not see the teenager's behavior as a reflection on their parenting or nursing, provide a more secure environment for growth. Loving detachment is not easy, but it is an effective tool in dealing with adolescents.

Nursing Tip

In adolescence, dependency creates hostility. Parents who foster dependence invite unavoidable resentment. Wise parents make themselves increasingly dispensable. Their language is sprinkled with such statements as "The choice is yours." "You decide about that." "If you want to." "It's your decision."

Cultural and Spiritual Considerations. Americans are multicolored, multicultural, and multilingual. The value of independence as a goal of maturational and emotional development may not be adopted by all. Many immigrants and Americans of Asian-American background come from societies that are patriarchal, highly structured and have distinct social roles. The good of the family takes precedence over personal goals. The protection of family image and neighborhood reputation is essential. The traditional Chinese do not recognize the period of adolescence. There is no word for it in their language. As part of a search for their identity, adolescents focus on the values and ideals of the family and decide to embrace them or separate from them. Adolescents often perceive that their feelings and thoughts are unique and therefore do not express their feelings freely. Adolescents can understand abstract concepts and symbols, and exposure to religion and religious practices other than those experienced within their own traditional family can help them to stabilize their group identity. The nurse's awareness of these and other cultural influences on the adolescent's behavior will help to provide holistic care (Fig. 20–8).

Realistic Body Image. In early adolescence, the young person must adjust to the dramatic changes of puberty. The focusing on bodily development during early and middle adolescence is one factor contributing to egocentrism, or self-centeredness. Young persons create what has been termed an "imaginary audience." They believe everyone is looking at them. This preoccupation with self is normal and accounts for the constant hair-combing and makeup-repairing frequently observed in a group of teenagers (Fig. 20–9). Young adolescents may try to hide their changing body or to advertise it. They may take pride in their abilities or feel frustrated when their actual abilities do not match their perceived abilities.

Nursing Tip

Every culture is unique. Adolescent behavior problems and expectations differ in different areas of the world and must be respected.

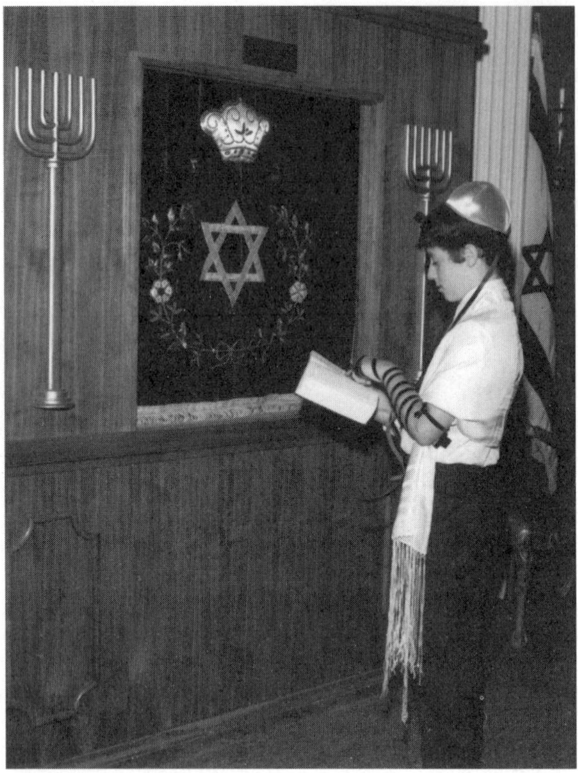

Figure 20–8. • Adolescents can understand abstract concepts and symbols and religious traditions can help to stabilize identity. The Bar Mitzvah is a spiritual rite of passage into adulthood.

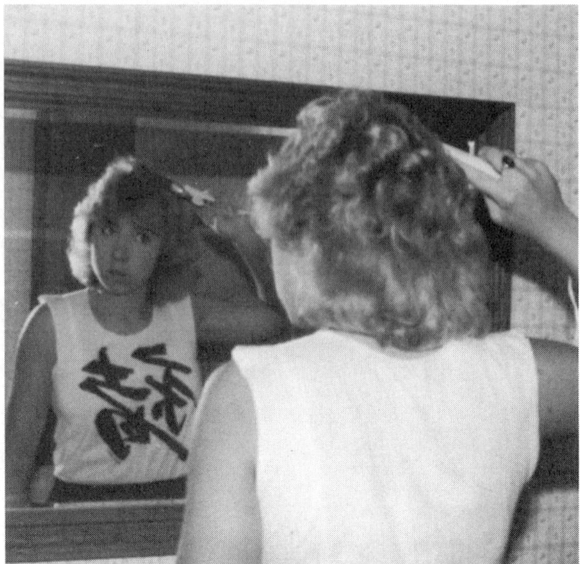

Figure 20–9. • The teenager's self-esteem is influenced by how far her body image deviates from the mythic (body ideal).

In early adolescence every effort is made to be just like their peers. A pimple on the skin or a disability is disastrous to the young adolescent. By late adolescence, most have completed their growth and are less self-conscious and enjoy their individual skills, abilities, and interests. Chronic illness or eating disorders (see Chapter 32) may complicate or exacerbate unresolved problems of body image.

Cognitive Development

Piaget's theory of cognitive development states that development is systematic, sequential, and orderly. Young adolescents are still in the *concrete phase* of thinking. They take words literally. A young teenage girl, if asked by the nurse, "Have you ever slept with anyone?" may not connect the question with a vaginal infection or sex. By middle adolescence, the ability to think abstractly has increased. Piaget calls this the stage of *formal operations.*

Older adolescents can see a situation from many viewpoints and can imagine or organize unseen or unexperienced possibilities. *Abstract thinking* emerges. The adolescent is able to sympathize and empathize. They can understand their own values and actions and also understand and accept differing values and actions of people from other cultures.

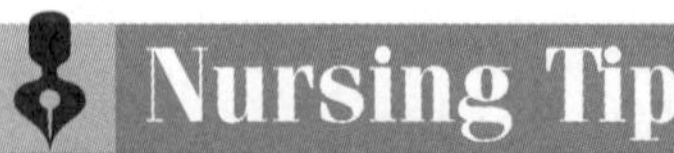

Maintaining open communication is an important key to avoiding a stormy adolescent phase.

Peer Relationships

Peer groups held adolescents to feel that they "belong" and make it possible to experiment with social behaviors (Fig. 20–10). School assumes an important role in the psychological development of the adolescent by providing the focus for initiating social interaction. Small, exclusive groups called *cliques* form. These unisex groups are made up of adolescents with similar interests, values, and tastes. Belonging to the group is of utmost importance to the young adolescent.

Within the "clique" the adolescent often develops a close personal relationship with one peer of the same sex. This *best friend* interaction supports social development by enabling adolescents to experiment with behaviors together and listen and care about each other (Fig. 20–11). Stable "best friend" experiences often precede successful heterosexual relationships in later life.

The peer group serves as a mirror for "normality" and helps to determine where one "fits in." It is vitally important in helping adolescents to define themselves. Acceptance by one's friends helps to decrease the loneliness and sense of loss many teenagers experience on the road to adulthood.

The social norms and pressures exerted by the group may cause problems. The selection of friends and allegiance to them may bring about confrontations within the family. Parents need help in understanding that the teenager's exaggerated conformity is necessary to moving away from dependence and obtaining approval from persons outside the nuclear family. Failure to develop social competence may produce feelings of inadequacy and low self-esteem.

Nurses can assist the family by supporting them and by educating them in the dynamics of this age group. They can direct them to such groups as peer helpers (for the adolescent) and community educational programs sponsored by various agencies. Organizations such as Parents without Partners might be another avenue.

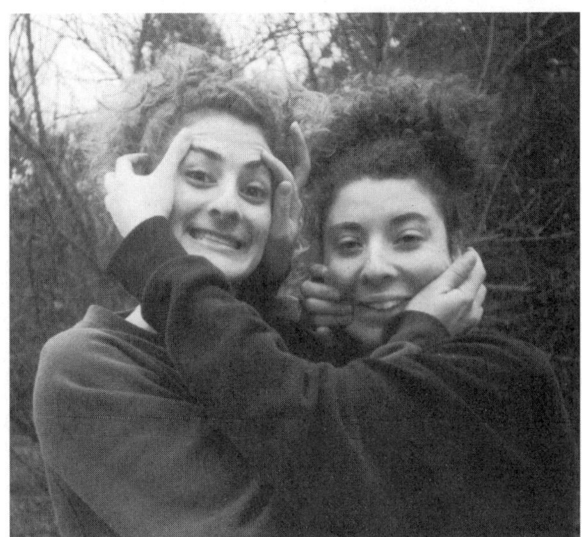

Figure 20–11. • Adolescents practice facial expressions and try out new hair arrangements. "Best friend" interaction supports social development by enabling adolescent to experiment with behavior and care about each other.

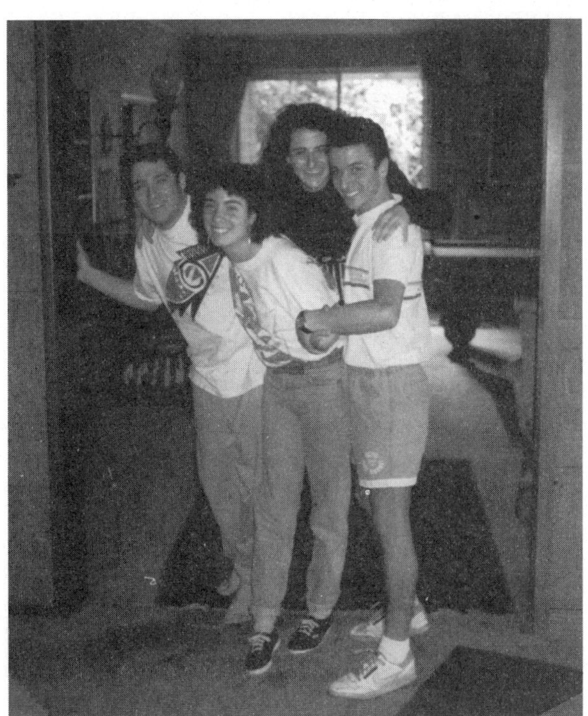

Figure 20–10. • Immersion into a peer group helps adolescents to free themselves from childhood dependence.

Career Plans

Some adolescents graduate from high school with a definite idea of what they would like to do. Many, however, are unsure of what they want. To choose a career that is best suited for them, teenagers must first know themselves. What particularly interests them? What are they good at? What are their shortcomings?

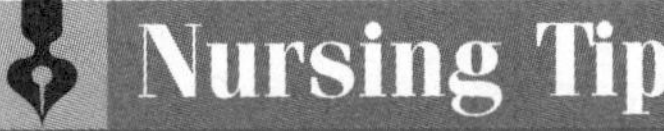

Nursing Tip

Psychosocial milestones that must be accomplished during adolescence include the 5 "I"s:

- Image of self
- Identity
- Independence
- Interpersonal relationships
- Intellectual maturity

Adapted from Cohall, A. (1997). What's normal and what's not. *Patient Care, 31*(11), 84.

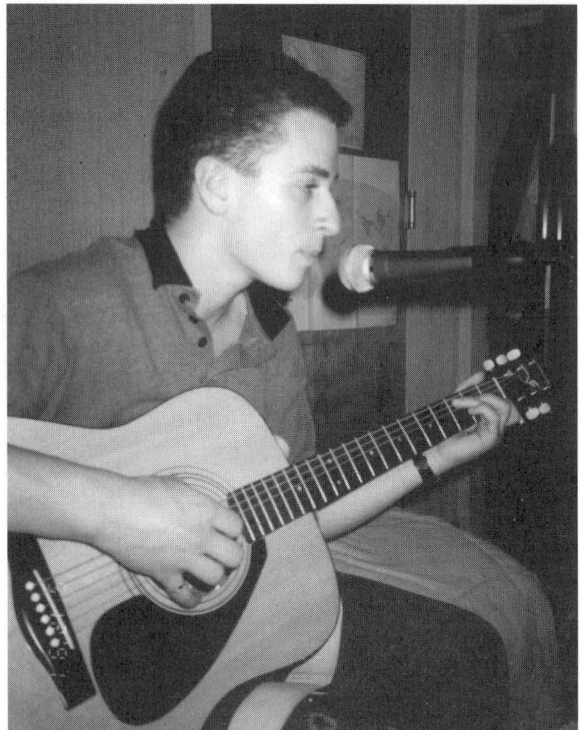

Figure 20–12. • Parents should encourage adolescents to take advantage of their talents. Singing, playing a musical instrument, or developing mechanical skills is part of adolescent life.

By this time, adolescents have already taken some definite steps toward a goal. Choice of high school curriculum and grades determine eligibility for college or preparation for a specific vocation. Parents should observe the interests of their children and encourage them to take advantage of their talents (Fig. 20–12). Whenever possible, a teenager should investigate various fields by talking to people who are involved in them.

Valuable information can also be obtained by career exploration, which is available at most colleges, and by pamphlets from professional organizations, the government, and other sources. The school guidance counselor administers aptitude tests as an additional guide and can work with the teenager to expose them to as wide a selection of careers as possible (Fig. 20–13). The teenager must make the final decision. To be happy in their work, the teenager must choose it of their own free will, and not because their parents expect them to follow in their footsteps.

The job market today is extremely competitive and almost nonexistent for some people without skills or education. Productive employment needs to fit young people's life framework and offer an opportunity for personal growth. Some positive aspects of employment include helping to build self-esteem, promoting responsibility, testing new skills, constructively channeling energies, providing money for increased independence, engaging the young person in interactions with adults, and allowing them to assume an active rather than a passive role. In contrast, when adolescents are forced to take a job because of economic or personal pressures, they may have to drop out of school. With few skills and no experience, they may remain locked in low-level employment. This is often perpetuated from one generation to another.

Responsibility

Adolescents look forward to challenges. Parents must encourage their children to take on new responsibilities. The adolescent is often humiliated by being placed in a dependent role, such as when a parent or sibling drives them to school. Driving a car or a bicycle or walking provide a sense of independence and responsibility. Even routine jobs can be made more inspiring if youths are taught to see them in relation to a longer-term objective.

Young adolescents must also be taught the value of money. An allowance helps them to learn financial management. If money is simply handed out as requested, it is more difficult to develop responsibility for finances. Allowances should be increased from time to time to comply with the age and needs of the teenager.

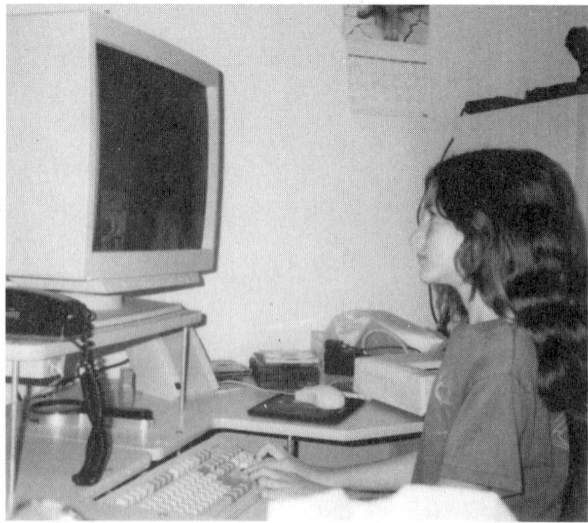

Figure 20–13. • The computer is an integral part of the adolescent's learning process. There are on-line opportunities for homework assistance and career opportunities.

Middle and older adolescents who have jobs can be taught to use a checkbook and a savings account. Many find satisfaction in purchasing their own clothes. A teenager who buys an old car soon discovers that it takes money to insure, run, and repair it. Such experiences provide valuable lessons in finance. Among younger teenagers, a common means of earning money is baby-sitting. Many boys and girls begin to assist with baby-sitting at about 12 or 13 years of age. Baby-sitting courses are valuable because young people need to be prepared for this important responsibility.

Daydreams

Adolescents spend a lot of time daydreaming in the solitude of their rooms or during a biology lecture. Most of this behavior is normal and natural for this age group. Daydreaming is usually considered harmless if the young person continues the usual active pursuits. It also serves several purposes. Adolescence is a lonely, in-between age; daydreaming helps to fill the void. Imaginatively acting out what will be said or done in various situations prepares teenagers to deal with others, so that they are better able to cope with real situations. Daydreams are also a valuable safety valve for the expression of strong feelings.

Sexual Behavior

Adolescents need to meet and become acquainted with members of the opposite sex. This may begin by admiration from afar, which is accompanied by daydreams as the young person attempts to attract the other's attention.

Group dates for structured school or church functions are followed by double dating and then single-couple dating. Popular dancing provides an opportunity for symbolic expression of sexual urges without physical contact. Slow dancing provides a mode of close physical contact in public that is socially acceptable. Long telephone conversations link the teen with peers when they are at home or feeling alone (Fig. 20–14). "Crushes" or feelings of attachment to a person of the opposite sex who is popular or possesses qualities important to the adolescent is a common occurrence. Competition and rivalry may be keen, but often long-term commitment and deep romantic attachments are not present.

Sexual experimentation often occurs as a response to peer pressure; as a means for momentary pleasure; as a learning experience to satisfy curiosity; or as a means of gaining a feeling of being loved and cared about. Sexual behavior can affect the growth and development of the adolescent. Unplanned pregnancies or sexually transmitted diseases are two major complications of adolescent sexual interaction.

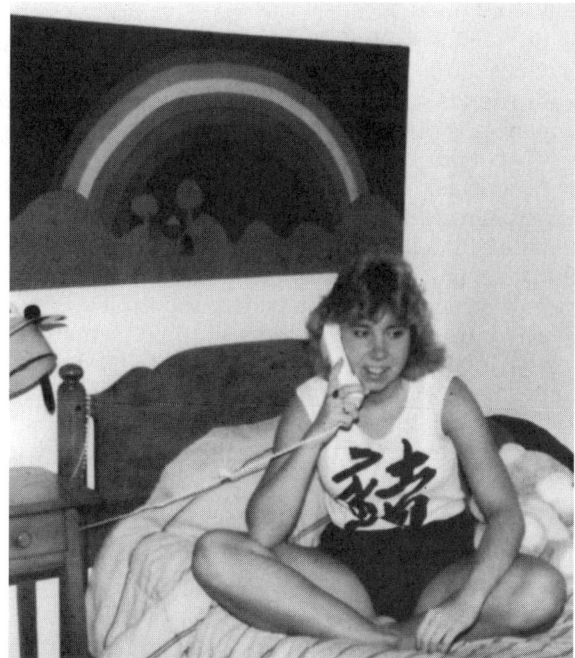

Figure 20–14. • The teenager often finds that those who understand her best are age mates. Communicating by telephone provides needed peer support.

The adolescent's cultural background influences patterns of dating. Conflict often arises when the teenager wants to be independent and quickly adopts American norms of dating while parents insist on strict traditional values. This is particularly noticeable with daughters.

Dating is one of the early social aspects of growing up. Attending the high school prom is a ritual of adolescence. As such, it may become a battleground for the struggle for independence. Parental opposition is often based on their unspoken fears of rejection. They may also fear sexual experimentation, pregnancy, or AIDS. Parents may respond by imposing strict restrictions, such as curfews, chaperones, and limitations on use of the car. When these problems are not discussed openly, the adolescent may react by rebelling sexually or by other means to test injunctions of control, rather than for the prohibited act itself.

Sexual curiosity and masturbation are common among adolescents. There is also a need for the intimacy of close personal friendships. Seeking one person of the opposite sex to share confidences and feelings may lead to sexual intimacies. This may produce guilt feelings and can lead to isolation from friends and family. The breaking up of such romances is often a source of great emotional pain.

Most of our knowledge about the sexual behavior of Americans comes from the pioneering efforts of Alfred Kinsey. Although his studies had flaws, they provided much in-depth information. A wide variety of sexual behavior is freely discussed and depicted in movies, in magazines, and on TV. Music directed toward young people often centers on sexual themes. Premarital sexual activity has become much more widespread, and teenagers are initiating their sexual activity at increasingly younger ages. One out of ten pregnancies occurs between the ages of 15 and 19 annually, and approximately 68% of teenagers have had sexual relationships before age 15.

Sex Education

Sex education for the adolescent is a challenge. Nurses must put aside their own attitudes and biases, understand society, cultural, and moral values, and incorporate a broad understanding of physical and psychological growth and development to prepare an effective school or clinic program. TV, movies, magazines, and computer "chat rooms" or "web sites" provide a source of sex education for the adolescent that may or may not be accurate and helpful to the young adult.

The increasing incidence of AIDS (acquired immunodeficiency syndrome) and of other sexually transmitted diseases (STDs) was a factor resulting in the formalized incorporation of sex education in schools. In the past, sex education in the public schools tended to concentrate on the physiology of sex, on the reproductive systems, and on sexually transmitted diseases. Information about personal values concerning sexuality, facts about contraception, safe sex, and peer pressure were sorely lacking. However, this is changing because of the AIDS crisis. Formal structured comprehensive sex education programs are available from SIECUS (Sexuality Information and Education Council of the United States, 130 W. 42nd Street, Suite 350, New York, NY 10036) and other community agencies. These types of programs are geared to kindergarten through grade 12 and present information about all aspects of health, such as nutrition, dental care, how to avoid drugs, and STDs. These courses should be presented as age-appropriate. The physiology of the reproductive systems can be taught at about grade 5. By grade 8 such topics as coping skills for dating and sexuality, pregnancy, and birth can be reviewed. Abstinence and contraception are discussed.

Decision-making is emphasized. Flowcharts should show the possible consequences of certain actions. The high school units can include how to handle teenage pregnancy, prenatal and postnatal care, and effective parenting techniques. A unit on intimate relationships can be presented as a series of discussions and activities designed to help students to think about the nature of love. It can cover ideas such as compromise, problem solving, and communication skills. It should emphasize the many reasons why teenagers should say "no" to casual sex.

Factual and sensitive information provided by concerned parents is, of course, the ideal. However, too often peers provide erroneous material or parents postpone education until a crisis arrives. Children need to be told what bodily changes to expect and why these changes occur. *Two years too soon is better than 1 day too late!* Parents who have answered their children's questions truthfully throughout childhood offer a secure and natural foundation to build on. Studies have shown that teens who obtain early sex education information from caring parents or well-informed adults do *not* have a higher rate of sexual activity.

Concerns about Being "Different." Adolescents have certain concerns that are specific to puberty. The girl who begins to experience physical changes at about the age of 10 may feel self-conscious, for she towers over her friends or has to wear a bra. She may be teased because she is different. The other extreme is the late-comer who feels abnormal and unattractive because her friends look more feminine.

Such problems are not limited to girls. Of particular concern is the boy on a slow schedule of development. Still a "shrimp" at 15, he is unable to compete for placement on school teams because of his size. He sees his male friends being admired for their height and strength, and this is a threat to him. Such fears are natural and usually are alleviated by reassurance that although boys begin to grow later than girls their growth spurt lasts longer. During assessment the nurse has an opportunity to support the adolescent concerned about normal growth and development.

Traditional sex stereotypes define being "male" by activity and achievement and being "female" by sensitivity and interpersonal competence. Society's current trends toward equality of the sexes may affect these roles. Nevertheless, few adolescents escape the social pressures that dictate acceptable sexual attitudes and behavior for each gender.

Table 20–2
USING THE NURSING PROCESS IN PLANNING SEX EDUCATION FOR THE ADOLESCENT

Data collection	Discuss level of knowledge concerning puberty and body changes Discuss peer acceptance Discuss sexual practices and outlets such as masturbation Discuss use of drugs/alcohol, cigarettes
Assessment	Assess body image and understanding concerning body changes Assess for signs of abuse Assess for risk factors involving sexual behavior and substance abuse Assess sexual practices, including contraception Assess for sexual variation or deviation
Planning	Provide a private area and nonjudgmental environment for teaching Discuss safe sex practices and personal views and values of teen Teach techniques and value of self-breast/testicular exam Discuss contraceptive choices if appropriate Teach need for regular follow-up health care
Evaluation	Follow-up during return home or clinic visits concerning problems identified or teaching completed

Homosexuality. When a person has an attraction for a person of their own gender, that person is referred to as *homosexual.* A *lesbian* is a female who prefers other females as sexual partners. A male is called *gay* when he prefers another male as his sexual partner. Homosexuality in adolescence is not uncommon. *This experimentation is not a positive predictor of adult sexual preference;* rather, it may merely indicate a desire to explore alternative lifestyles. However, most homosexuals do report having had homosexual experiences during adolescence. Many theories about the origins of homosexuality have been presented. These include a genetic basis, hormonal influences, and psychological and sociologic factors. None have been proved. Gay and lesbian youths, in addition to handling the usual adolescent tasks, face problems of "coming out," rejection, and other issues.

Nurses must be sensitive to these issues when obtaining histories and working with young people. They must also be aware of their personal biases to determine their potential effectiveness with this population. Support groups for parents and friends of gay and lesbians are available. Those who question their sexual orientation are referred to counselors and health agencies that can respond to their needs. An example of the use of the nursing process in planning sex education for the adolescent is seen in Table 20–2.

PARENTING

Parenting an adolescent requires major adaptations on the part of the parents. At times it is difficult for parents to cope with adolescents. The shift in parenting philosophies, from the rigid rules of discipline, to permissiveness, or a current middle-of-the-road position, often leads to confusion. Some parents are unsure of their own opinions and may hesitate to exert authority. Others refuse to "let go" or change any of their beliefs to accommodate today's youth. Issues of privacy and trust abound, and conflict occurs as the adolescent desires more adult liberties. Adolescents may need time alone to separate themselves from family and search for their identity.

Teenagers need to talk about their fears, such as school exams or how they will look with a certain haircut. They need assistance in sorting out confused feelings. A confidential accepting atmosphere will promote quality communications (Fig. 20–15). Physical symptoms, such as stomach aches, insomnia, and headaches, surface in relation to anxiety. Bizarre behavior may be a call for long-overdue help.

Some approaches to such problems are presented in Table 20–3. As adolescents try to separate themselves from their family they may reject some family traditions such as family outings or dress codes. When parents respond to this behavior negatively, the separation widens and tension grows. Often

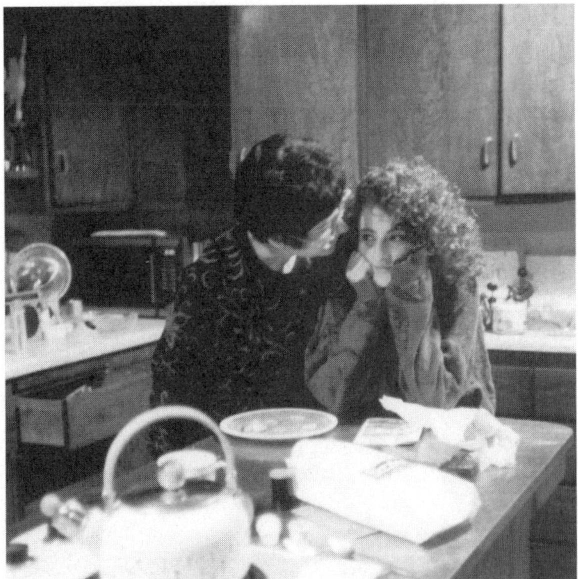

Figure 20–15. • Listening is an important tool for establishing rapport. A confidential accepting atmosphere will promote quality communications.

Table 20–3
EFFECTIVE APPROACHES TO PROBLEMS

Approach	Purpose	Example
Reflective listening	Showing you understand teenager's feelings. Used when teenager "owns" problem	"You're very worried about the semester exam?" "Sounds like you're feeling discouraged because the job's so difficult."
"I" message	Communicating your feelings about how teenager's behavior affects you. Used when you own problem	"When I'm ill and the dishes are left for me to do, I feel disrespected because it seems no one cares about me." "When you borrow tools and don't return them, I feel discouraged because I don't have the tools I need when there's a job to do."
Exploring alternatives	Helping teenagers decide how to solve problems they own	"What are some ways you could solve this problem?" "Which idea appeals to you most?" "Are you willing to do this until . . . ?"
	Negotiating agreements with teenager when you own problem	"What can we do to settle this conflict between us?" "Are we in agreement on that idea?" "What would be a fair consequence if the agreement is broken?"
Natural and logical consequences	Permitting teenagers, within limits, to decide how they will behave and allowing them to experience consequences	*Natural:* Teenager who forgets coat on cold days gets cold; teenager who skips lunch goes hungry
	Natural consequences apply when teenager owns problem. Logical consequences apply when either parent or teenager owns problem	*Logical:* Teenager who spends allowance quickly does not receive any more money until next allowance day; teenager who neglects to study for a test gets low grade

Source: Systematic Training for Effective Parenting of Teens, Parenting Teenagers, © 1990 by Don Dinkmeyer and Gary D. McKay.

adolescents search for adults outside of the family as role models and confidants. Coaches or scout leaders can fulfill this role and serve as positive outlets for gaining a sense of "belonging" when there are conflicts at home.

The teenager who is the subject of heavy concentrations of parental attention can become overanxious. As adolescents mature, they become more secure and are able to develop a new and more satisfactory relationship with their parents. In the meantime, one must keep the lines of communication open, promote respect and trust, and provide confidentiality and a sense of privacy. In spite of the problems parents face with their teenagers throughout adolescence, the family continues to play a major role in socialization (Fig. 20–16).

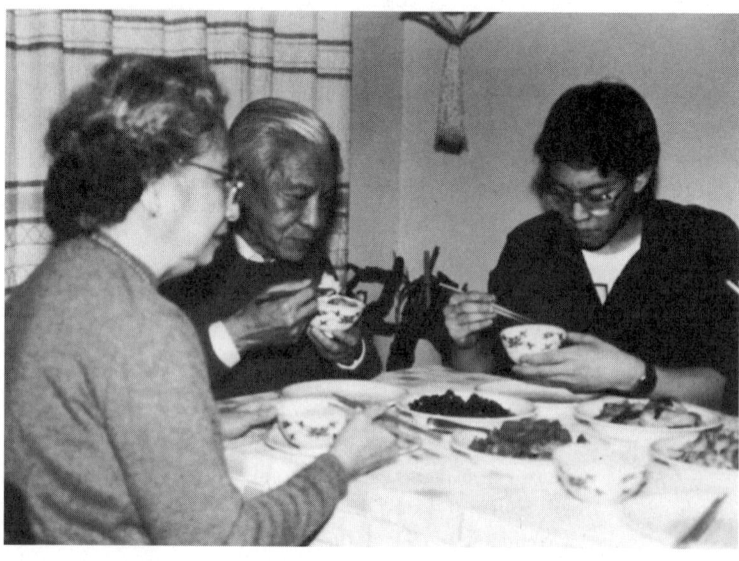

Figure 20–16. • The family continues to be an important agent of socialization for the adolescent. (From Foster, R., Hunsberger, M., & Anderson, J. J. [1989]. *Family-centered nursing care of children* (p. 620). Philadelphia: Saunders.)

Nursing Tip

Privacy and confidentiality are essential when communicating with adolescents.

HEALTH EDUCATION AND GUIDANCE

Nutrition

Teenagers grow rapidly; therefore, they need foods that provide for their increase in height, body cell mass, and maturation. Adolescents appear to be "always hungry" because their stomach capacity is too small to meet the increased caloric and protein requirements of their rapid growth spurt. Frequent meals are needed. Dietary deficiencies are more likely to occur at this age because of this acceleration and because eating patterns become more irregular. Nutritional requirements are more strongly correlated with sex maturity ratings (SMR; see Box 20–2) than with age. Girls at SMR 2 and boys at SMR 3, for example, are close to their peak growth velocities. They require adequate intake of nutrients and calories, regardless of chronologic age.

The most noticeable changes in the adolescent's eating habits are skipped meals, more between-meal snacks, and eating out more often. Breakfast and lunch are often omitted. Part-time jobs, school activities, and socialization may result in the teenager's eating little or nothing during the day and then "catching up" in the evening. Fast-food restaurants are inexpensive and provide food quickly for the busy adolescent. These foods tend to be high in calories, fat, protein, sugar, and sodium and low in fiber. Most food chains have added salads and other more healthy foods, which is applauded. Carbonated drinks often replace milk, resulting in low intakes of calcium, riboflavin, and vitamins A and D. The few fruits and vegetables eaten provide insufficient fiber.

Foods should be selected from the basic food pyramid (see Fig. 15–7, p. 398). In estimating calories, variables such as physical activity and gender must also be considered. The minerals most likely to be inadequately supplied in the adolescent's diet are calcium and iron. Zinc is known to be essential for growth and sexual maturation and is therefore of great importance in adolescence. Good sources of zinc include meat, liver, eggs, and seafood, particularly oysters. Sources for vegetarians include nuts, beans, wheat germ, and cheese.

Calcium has a key role in bone formation. In both girls and boys, the daily recommended dietary allowance (RDA) for calcium increases from 800 mg at age 10 to 1200 mg during the growth spurt. The primary source of calcium is dairy products.

The need for iron increases in both sexes at this time. This increased need is primarily due to increases in muscle mass and blood volume in boys and, to a lesser degree, in girls. A menstruating female loses 15 to 30 mg of iron per cycle. Iron absorption varies in individuals. Good sources of iron include liver, poultry, fish, dried beans, vegetables, egg yolk, and enriched breads. Adolescents need guidance in proper food selection in and out of the home to prevent obesity and the detrimental effects of high cholesterol levels. Calorically dense food that provides little nutrient value should be avoided. The RDAs for adolescents are listed in Table 20–4.

Vegetarian Diets

A number of young people are becoming vegetarians. Lacto-ovo vegetarians include eggs and dairy products in their diets and generally have adequate nutrient intakes. This is one of the most common types of vegetarian diet.

However, total vegetarians (vegans), who eat no animal protein, eggs, or dairy products are at particular risk of developing deficiencies in protein, vitamin B_{12}, calcium, iron, iodine, and possibly zinc. A total vegetarian diet is adequate only if it is carefully planned.

Sports and Nutrition

The best training diet is one that contains foods from each of the basic food groups in sufficient quantities to meet energy demands and nutrient requirements. What to eat and when to eat it in relation to muscle exercise is vital to successful athletic performance. Athletes exhaust reserves of muscle glycogen. Carbohydrates (CHO) that can be rapidly converted to blood glucose and transported to muscles will provide the rapid recovery of muscle glycogen necessary for maintaining prolonged intense muscle activity. Eating a glucose source that is absorbed slowly will prevent the development of chronic low muscle energy stores. To hasten muscle energy recovery, the young athlete should consume at least 50 g of a rapidly used carbohydrate within 4 hours after exercise. Food high in fat and protein will prolong carbohydrate metabolism. Carbohydrates that provide both energy and other nutrients are best for athletes. Therefore fruits and fruit juices are a better choice than sugar-rich soft drinks and candy. The fat content in candy will slow carbohydrate absorption. Some foods that provide a rapid supply of carbohydrates to muscles include corn flakes, bagels, raisins, maple syrup, potatoes, and rice. Some foods that supply a slow release of carbohydrates to muscles include apples, pears, green peas, chick peas, skim milk, and plain yogurt. Fluids lost by sweat must be replaced by drinking small amounts of fluid during a workout. Thirst is one guide for intake.

Caffeine and alcohol deplete body water and are to be avoided. Anabolic steroids, used by some athletes to gain weight and increase strength, are detrimental to bone growth. Iron is particularly necessary for female athletes, who may be borderline or deficient in their intake of this mineral.

Nutrition and School Exams

The role of diet in the treatment of illness has become traditional practice. The role of nutrition in health is becoming prominent in health education today. Nutritional practices are the focus of weight control programs, and special nutritional supplements are available for athletes, pregnant women, and the elderly. Studies have shown that foods can affect behavior, moods, and alertness.

For the adolescent who is scheduled to take an important school examination, the nurse can offer nutritional guidance as part of the exam preparation. Carbohydrates such as pancakes and syrup, breakfast pastries, or a muffin and jelly increase serotonin in the brain that results in a soothing, sleepy response. Bacon and eggs are high in fat and cholesterol and are therefore slow to digest, diverting blood from the brain during the digestion process, resulting in decreased alertness. More than 4 cups of a caffeine-containing beverage such as coffee can cause overstimulation and nervousness. However, protein-rich meals increase amino acids and tyrosine, which will break down into norepinephrine in the brain and result in increased alertness. Fish, soy, peanuts, and rice increase choline and acetylcholine in the brain, which results in increased memory. Therefore, a "proper" meal before a big school test may help the adolescent's achievement as well as their health.

Fad Diets, Anorectic Drugs. Fad diets, although popular with the teenager, provide little long-term success. Unsupervised weight loss can be dangerous. Anorectic drugs (sympathomimetic agents, diuretics, hormones) have limited effect on weight loss and can be harmful. The potential for stimulant-type drug abuse among teenagers is high, which makes avoidance of such self-medication even more important. Most fad diets tend to be monotonous. Liquid-protein diets can lead to a serious electrolyte imbalance. Diets that promote special food combinations tend to be

Table 20–4
RECOMMENDED DIETARY ALLOWANCES FOR THE ADOLESCENT, 11–18

	11–14 Years		15–18 Years	
Nutrient	**Males**	**Females**	**Males**	**Females**
Kilocalories	2500	2200	3000	2200
Protein (g)	45	46	59	46
Vitamin A (μg RE)	1000	800	1000	800
Vitamin D (μg)	10	10	10	10
Vitamin E (mg TE)	10	8	10	8
Vitamin C (mg)	50	50	60	60
Folate (μg)	150	150	200	180
Niacin (mg)	17	15	20	15
Riboflavin (mg)	1.5	1.3	1.8	1.3
Thiamine (mg)	1.3	1.1	1.5	1.1
Vitamin B_6 (mg)	1.7	1.4	2	1.5
Vitamin B_{12} (μg)	2	2	2	2
Calcium (mg)	1200	1200	1200	1200
Phosphorus (mg)	1200	1200	1200	1200
Iodine (μg)	150	150	150	150
Iron (mg)	12	15	12	15
Magnesium (mg)	270	280	400	300
Zinc (mg)	15	12	15	12
Selenium (μg)	40	45	50	50

Source: National Academy of Sciences-National Research Council. (1989). *Recommended dietary allowances* (10th ed.). Washington, DC: Author.
Abbreviations: RE, retinol equivalent; TE, tocopherol equivalent.

unbalanced and expensive and difficult to maintain over time. *Prolonged fasting can be life-threatening.*

A balanced weight reduction plan based on the food pyramid (see Fig. 15–7, p. 398) is best for losing weight gradually and maintaining the weight loss. It teaches the young person how to select nutritious foods and helps to establish patterns that can be lifelong. Behavior modification techniques, such as keeping food diaries and learning to eat more slowly, and nonfood rewards, such as clothing and flowers, have also proved successful when combined with sensible eating. Weight reduction programs should also include an increase in regular physical activity. Group participation provides an opportunity for peer contact, acceptance, and support.

Personal Care

Sleep. Sleep requirements vary from individual to individual. Adolescents may obtain the 8 hours generally suggested, but often at irregular hours. Many employed young people have to work very late hours, particularly in the summer months. This necessitates sleeping later in the morning. Another trend is for the young people who have worked long hours during the day to try to make up for lost sleep after work. They seem either to sleep all the time or to burn the candle at both ends! Complaints of fatigue are heard more often at home than elsewhere. If teenagers stay up late at night, they will be tired in the morning. This is called "learning by natural consequences."

Exercise. Exercise has many benefits. One does not have to participate actively in sports per se to derive the benefits from a brisk walk, bike ride, or swim. Many teenagers who are not athletes can benefit from a less sedentary lifestyle. These patterns, when carried over into adulthood, contribute to good health.

Hygiene. The adolescent needs personal hygiene information because body changes require more frequent bathing and the use of deodorants. The nurse can help the young person to sort out the various claims of reliability for hair removal, menstrual hygiene, and cosmetics products and procedures. The practice of body-piercing, a popular teenage fad, should be performed by an experienced person using sterile instruments. The skin around the point of insertion of the body ring should be regularly inspected for signs of infection. Swapping of body rings is discouraged. Teenagers are warned not to use another's razor, particularly in light of the risk for AIDS.

Dental Health. The prevalence of tooth decay has substantially decreased. This is believed to result from the widespread use of fluorides, including community fluoridation, and dental products containing fluorides. Teenagers are nonetheless at risk for dental caries because of inadequate dental maintenance and frequent snacking on sucrose-containing candies and beverages. When dental hygiene is neglected, the period of greatest tooth decay in the permanent teeth is from ages 12 to 18 years. Lack of oral hygiene (inadequate brushing, flossing, and rinsing, particularly after meals) fosters the accumulation of plaque and food debris. Missing, aching, or decayed teeth contribute to poor nutrition. Young people with unattractive teeth may suffer from low self-esteem. Corrective orthodontic appliances are often worn during adolescence and meticulous oral hygiene is essential to prevent discoloration of tooth enamel and other complications (see Chapter 15).

Healthy, white teeth are synonymous with popularity and sex appeal, according to media hype. Regular dental visits during adolescence must be maintained as a priority in health care teaching of adolescents and their families. See Chapter 15 for detailed discussion of dental health.

Sunbathing. Adolescents respond to movie and magazine pictures of the ideal "healthy suntanned body" as an attractive aspect of a body image. The young adult looks forward to sunbathing on the beach or at the pool during summer vacations and often prepare their bodies by trying to obtain a tanned appearance by artificial means. The nurse plays a vital role in educating the adolescent concerning the danger of the sun's rays and the need for skin protection with a sun protective factor (SPF) of at least 15. Protection of the eyes from the sun is also essential. Excessive sunlight and the use of artificial tanning machines can cause serious long-term reactions.

Safety

The chief hazard to the adolescent is the automobile (Fig. 20–17). Road and off-road vehicle accidents kill and cripple teenagers at alarming rates. Some schools now offer driver training courses as an integral part of the educational program. Students learn how to drive and the accompanying responsibilities; however, this does not ensure compliance. Preventing motor vehicle accidents is of utmost importance to every community. Adolescents who ride motorcycles, motor scooters, or motorbikes should know the rules of the road and wear special safety equipment, such as helmets.

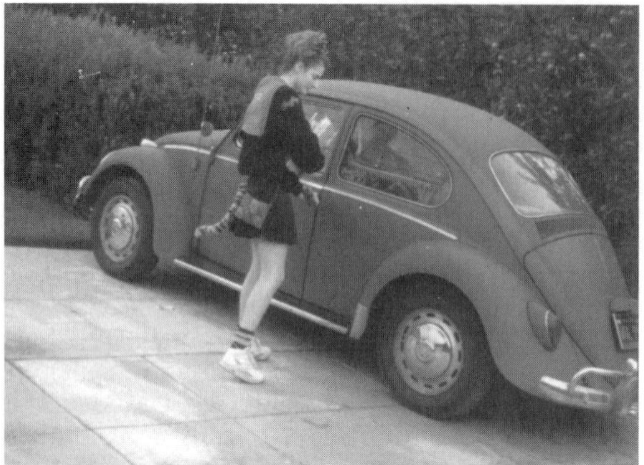

Figure 20–17. • Teenagers look forward to getting their driver's license. The search for independence also brings responsibilities.

Young people should learn how to swim and swimming safety. Accidents result from diving into unsafe areas, from using alcohol or drugs while swimming, and from unsafe use of jet skis. If adolescents are interested in hunting or similar sports that require a gun, they must be instructed in the proper safeguards.

Sports Injuries. Sports involving body contact can be hazardous to the adolescent. Sports teams separated by age only are a special problem since adolescents of one specific age group can vary in size, weight, and muscle strength. Protective gear should be worn by team players in any contact sport. The feeling of strength and the need to show off can motivate the adolescent to participate in risky behavior. The school nurse can play a key role in safety education by working closely with school coaches and parents.

Health Assessment

The prevention of illness in this age group, as in all others, is of primary importance. Annual physical examinations are recommended for adolescents. This is often a requirement for the young person wishing to enter a certain sport. Pre-sports physical examinations can vary greatly in their thoroughness. Immunizations need to be reviewed and updated, including Varivax (a vaccine for the prevention of chicken pox), hepatitis B, and tuberculin testing (see Chapter 31 for immunization protocols). A rubella titer should be obtained from all girls. Those found to lack protective levels should be immunized, regardless of any history of infection or immunizations. The young woman is instructed to avoid pregnancy for at least 2 months after immunization. Cholesterol, urine analysis, and other screening programs are conducted in the school and community. Deficits of vision and hearing, scoliosis, or high blood pressure may be detected.

> **Nursing Tip**
>
> Obtaining a driver's license, graduating high school, and reaching the legal drinking age are American rites of passage through adolescence. Other cultures offer specific ceremonies to mark phases of development.

COMMON PROBLEMS OF ADOLESCENCE

Substance Abuse

The growing drug trade and the increase in vandalism and crime expose adolescents to unprecedented assaults in their schools and in their neighborhoods. Gang-related deaths from guns and knife wounds have escalated greatly. To parents and all who provide services to children, this growing menace is a source of great frustration and concern.

When adolescents experiment with different types of behavior in a search for their identity, they may experiment with drugs. The best weapon against addiction to drugs is education. Drugs are often made available in the schools and in the streets of the neighborhood where adolescents congregate. The need to conform, the need to be accepted, peer pressure, and the emotional depression often occurring in the turmoil of adolescent adjustments are strong influences for drug use. Education concerning the dangers of drug use is essential in the home and in the school.

Adolescents are prone to mood swings as they try to adjust to the many physical and psychological changes that are occurring in their lives. The present may feel overwhelming and the future blurs. The PACE interview (Schwartz, 1987) can assist in distinguishing the drug-free adolescent from one who may be experimenting with drugs and requires follow-up referral:

P—Parents, peers, and pot. Question the adolescent concerning his parents, relationships with peers, and his attitude and exposure to marijuana.

A—Alcohol, automobiles. Question the adolescent concerning alcohol use (e.g., beers at parties) and his driving record.

C—Cigarettes. Discuss smoking history.

E—Education. Discuss attitude and performance in school.

If two or more of the PACE letters are problem areas, the adolescent may be at high risk for drug abuse and require professional referral. Follow-up care may involve a contract with the adolescent to be drug free, education, teaching coping skills, and parental referral to a support group such as Tough Love Groups or the National Federation of Parents for Drug Free Youth (Silver Springs, MD).

Depression

Sometimes an adolescent who appears to be adjusted and performing well in school may become depressed. Drug use can precede the development of depression. Working parents and busy teachers can easily overlook slowly changing behaviors. A change in school performance, in appearance, or in behavior can be a warning sign of depression, which if left untreated can lead to suicide. A threat of suicide is a call for help that must be taken care of without delay. The school nurse can help the adolescent by recognizing the depression, encouraging open communication, posting the numbers of available hotlines, identifying appropriate coping mechanisms, and providing professional referrals.

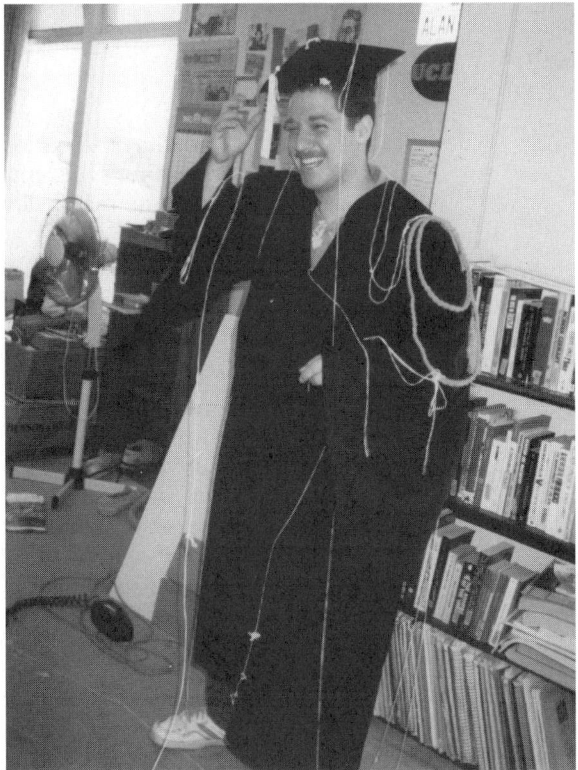

Figure 20–18. • Graduation from high school is the self-actualization of the adolescent. Peers and family share the joy with the new graduate.

THE NURSING APPROACH TO ADOLESCENTS

The nurse must open lines of communication with adolescents and enable them to feel at ease before initiating care or teaching. A sense of humor is helpful. Providing privacy and ensuring confidentiality and respect are basic to adolescent communication. The nurse must be careful not to behave like a teen because the adolescent may perceive that behavior as "phoney." Adolescent hostility may be evidence of fear of the unknown and rebellion may be an effort at grasping independence. The nurse should guide the parents concerning the need to listen, understand, and share with teens. Helping parents to distinguish between normal problems of adolescence and problems that require referral and follow-up is essential. For example, demands for privacy are normal, but overall withdrawal requires referral and follow-up care.

Health care teaching should include nutrition, dental care, personal care, body piercing, accident prevention, substance abuse, self-control, risk-taking behavior, money, and time management. Open-ended questions concerning common problems of adolescence may encourage discussion of a topic adolescents may not initiate by themselves.

Graduation from high school is self-actualization for the adolescent (Fig. 20–18). Getting a job that will provide for self-support or going to college, which may involve leaving home, is the first step of entrance into independent adulthood (Fig. 20–19).

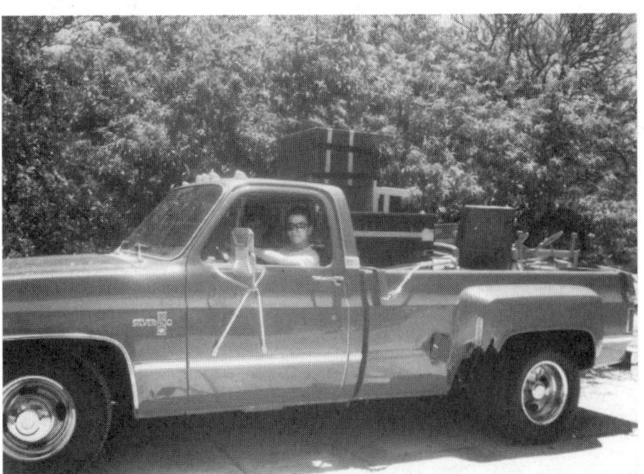

Figure 20–19. • Moving away from home and going away to college mark entrance into adulthood.

KEY POINTS

- Adolescence is defined as the period of life beginning with the appearance of secondary sex characteristics and ending with emotional maturity and the cessation of growth.
- According to Erikson, the major developmental task of adolescence is to establish a sense of identity.
- Other major tasks of adolescence include separating from family, initiating intimacy, and making career choices.
- Freud considered adolescence as the last stage of psychosexual development. He termed this the *genital stage.*
- Jean Piaget suggests that the cognitive development during adolescence reflects abstract reasoning and logic. He calls this stage the period of *formal operations.*
- The physical development seen during this period is distinguished by puberty, the stage at which the reproductive organs become functional and secondary sex characteristics develop.
- Adolescents vary in their rate of physical and social maturation and their ability to resolve conflicts concerning self-esteem and autonomy.
- A nonjudgmental, confidential, adult role model can help to avoid a crisis for the adolescent.
- SIECUS is an example of a national organization that assists in the development and implementation of sex education programs.
- Some main challenges of the teen years include adjusting to rapid physical changes, maintaining privacy, coping with stresses and pressures, maintaining open communication and developing positive lifestyle choices.
- Peer groups help the adolescent to separate from the family and experiment with social behaviors.
- A "clique" affords the adolescent the opportunity to "belong" and to develop close personal relationships with others who have similar interests and values.
- The first menstrual period is called the *menarche.*
- The teenager struggles with the development of a realistic body image.
- The epidemic of AIDS creates new demands for accurate, safe, and timely sex education.
- Adolescence is a time of conflict with parental authority and values. The influence of peers and heterosexual relationships increase.
- Motor vehicle accidents, homicide, and drownings are leading causes of mortality in this age group.

MULTIPLE-CHOICE REVIEW QUESTIONS

Choose the most appropriate answer.

1. One of the tasks of adolescence as defined by Erikson is
   a. finding an identity.
   b. sexual latency.
   c. heterosexuality.
   d. concrete operations.
2. When teaching an adolescent concerning safety, which of the following concepts of adolescent behavior should be considered?
   a. The typical adolescent understands teaching, respects, and usually follows the advice of adults.
   b. Growth and development are complete in the adolescent and muscle coordination and skills lessen risks for injury.
   c. Safety concerns at this age mostly focus around sports injuries.
   d. Adolescents are risk takers and tend to experiment with potentially dangerous outcomes.
3. Puberty can most accurately be defined as the period of life characterized by the
   a. occurrence of sexual maturity and appearance of secondary sex characteristics.
   b. substitution of adult interests and value systems for child interests.
   c. most rapid rate of physical and mental growth and development.
   d. awakening of sexual feelings and the initiation of sexual experience.
4. Pat, age 16, towers over her companions. This bothers her, and she confides in you and says, "I just hate school—everyone is always staring at me." Your best response would be
   a. "Don't pay any attention to it."
   b. "You just don't know how lucky you are to be tall."
   c. "This will resolve itself in time. Don't worry."
   d. "Tell me more about how this embarrasses you."
5. Which of the following action is most important when planning the management of obesity in adolescents?
   a. Planning a low-calorie diet
   b. Incorporating favorite or fad foods into the diet
   c. Encouraging a positive attitude toward obesity
   d. Offering rewards for self-control

BIBLIOGRAPHY AND READER REFERENCE

Alan Guttmacher Institute. (1994). *Sex and America's Teenagers.* New York: Guttmacher Institute.

Armstrong, M. (1994). Adolescents and tatoos: Marks of identity or deviation? *Dermatology Nursing, 6*(2), 119–124.

Behrman, R. E., Kleigman, R., & Arvin, A. (1996). *Nelson's textbook of pediatrics* (15th ed.). Philadelphia: Saunders.

Bonny, A., & Biro, F. (1998). Recognizing and treating STD's in adolescent girls. *Contemporary Pediatrics, 15*(3), 119.

Cohall, A. (1997). What's Normal What's Not. *Patient Care, 31*(11), 82.

Finan, S. (1997). Promoting healthy sexuality. Guidelines for the school-age child and adolescent. *Nurse Practitioner, 22*(11), 62–72.

Friedman, R., & Downey, J. (1994). Homosexuality. *New England Journal of Medicine, 331*(14), 923–930.

Futterman, D., Hein, K., & Kunins, H. (1993). Teens and AIDS. *Contemporary Pediatrics, 10*(9), 55.

Gidwane, G. (1997). Menstruation and the athlete. *Contemporary Pediatrics, 14*(1), 27.

Hatcher, J., et al. *Contraceptive technology* (16th ed.). New York: Livingston.

Healthy People 2000: National health promotion and disease prevention objectives. (1991). U.S. Department of Health and Human Services. PHS 91-50213. Washington, DC: Government Printing Office.

Kay, L. E. (1995). Adolescent sexual intercourse: Strategies for promoting abstinence in teens. *Postgraduate Medicine, 97*(6), 121–134.

Levine, M. D., Carey, W. B., & Crocker, A. C. (1992). *Developmental behavioral pediatrics* (2nd ed.). Philadelphia: Saunders.

Mahan, L. K., & Escott-Stump, S. (1996). *Krause's food nutrition and diet therapy* (9th ed.). Philadelphia: Saunders.

Orr, D. (1998). Helping the adolescent toward adulthood. *Contemporary Pediatrics, 15*(5), 55.

Porter, C. P., Oakley, D., Rones, D., et al. (1996). Pathways of influence on 5th and 8th graders' reports about having had sexual intercourse. *Research Nurse and Health, 19:* 193–204.

Schor, E. (1998). Guiding the family of the school aged child. *Contemporary Pediatrics, 15*(3), 75.

Schwartz, R. (1987). Are you ready to deal with the pot smoking patient. *Contemporary Pediatrics, 11*(4), 85.

Shelow, S., Baron, M., Beard, L., et al. (1995). Sexuality, contraception and the media. *Pediatrics, 95,* 298–300.

Stevens-Simon, C. (1997). Reproductive health care for your adolescent female patients. *Contemporary Pediatrics, 14*(2), 35.

Swartz, M. (1994). Promoting helmet use in recreational sports. *Journal of Pediatric Health Care, 8*(3), 138–139.

Tanner, S. (1993). Weighing the risks: Strength training for children and adolescents. *Sports Medicine, 21*(6), 104.

Turecki, S., & Wernick, S. (1994). *The emotional problems of normal children and how parents can understand and help.* New York: Bantam.

Wong, D. (1996). *Whaley & Wong's essentials of nursing care of infants and children* (5th ed.). St. Louis, MO: Mosby.

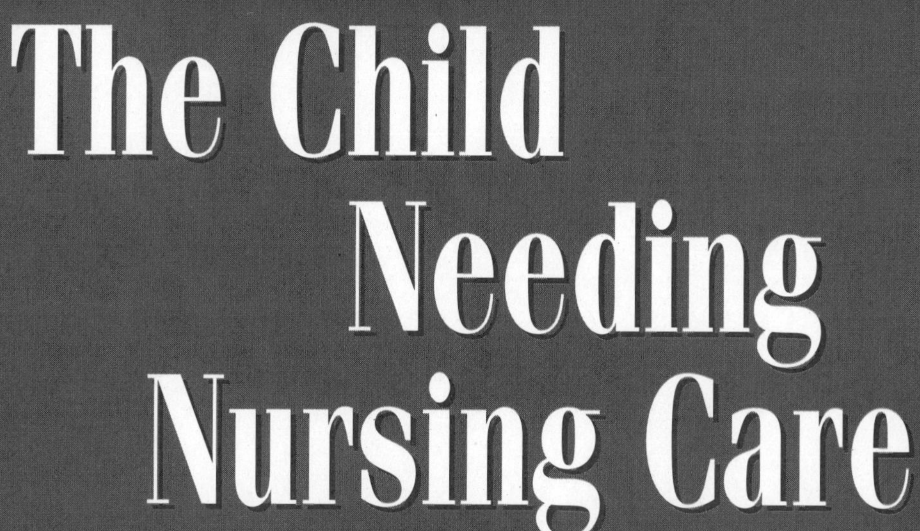

The Child Needing Nursing Care

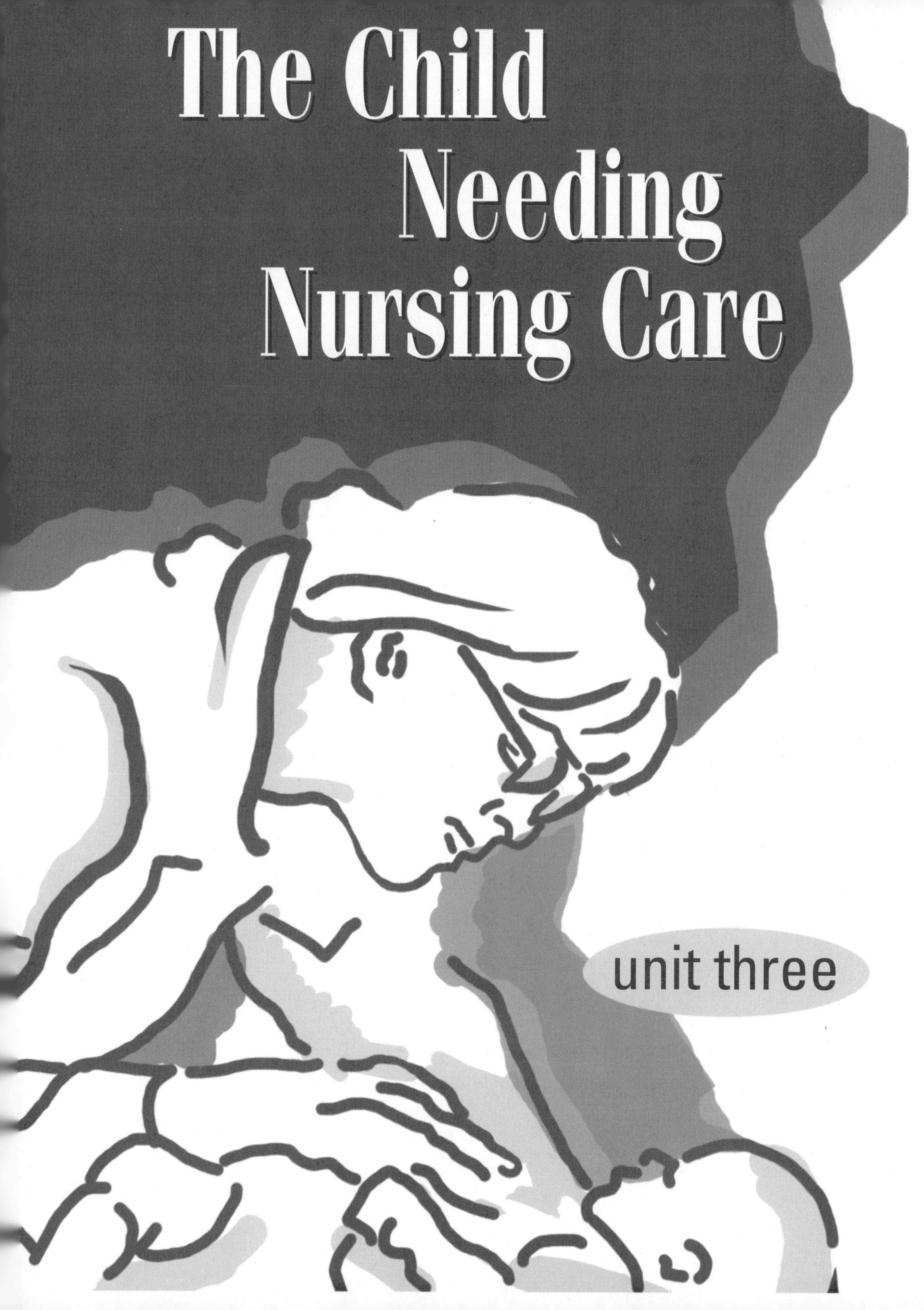

unit three

chapter 21

The Child's Experience of Hospitalization

Outline

Objectives

On completion and mastery of Chapter 21, the student will be able to

- Define each vocabulary term listed.
- Describe three phases of separation anxiety.
- Identify two problems confronting the siblings of the hospitalized child.
- List two ways in which the nurse can lessen the stress of hospitalization for the child's parents.
- List four ways of providing sensorimotor activities for the infant.
- Describe two ways to prepare the child emotionally for surgery.
- Describe two milestones in the psychosocial development of the preschool child that contribute either positively or negatively to the adjustment to hospitalization.
- Contrast the problems of the preschool child and school-age child facing hospitalization.
- List three strengths of the teenager that the nurse might utilize when formulating nursing care plans.
- Interpret a clinical pathway for a hospitalized child.
- Organize a nursing care plan for a hospitalized child.
- Identify various health care delivery settings.

Vocabulary

care map
clinical pathway
emancipated minor
narcissistic
nursing care plan
peer
personal space
rapport
regression
respite care
separation anxiety
transitional object

HEALTH CARE DELIVERY SETTINGS

Outpatient Clinic

Many hospitals today have well-organized outpatient facilities and satellite clinics for preventive medicine and care of the child who is ill. The advent of Medicaid and of other such programs has made these services available to low-income families. Within clinics, there may be specialty areas (particularly at children's facilities), such as well-child clinics, asthma clinics, cardiac clinics and orthopedic clinics. In some institutions, information is distributed and brief classes are held for waiting parents.

Types of Outpatient Clinics

Satellite clinics are convenient and offer families flexible coverage. Some are located in shopping malls. Parents may browse with children and be contacted by a beeper when it is their turn to see the physician. This eliminates confining children in a small area and is less frustrating to caretakers. In many cities, a group of pediatricians practice in an office removed from the hospital, which aids in the distribution of health services and provides evening and weekend health coverage.

In many offices, the pediatricians or their nurses are available at certain hours of each day to answer telephone inquiries. The pediatric nurse practitioner may visit patients in the home, give routine physical examinations at the clinic, and otherwise work with the physician, so that a higher quality of individual care may be attained. The nurse practitioner is frequently the primary contact person for children in the health care system.

Another area of outpatient care is the pediatric research center, such as the one at St. Jude's Hospital in Memphis, Tennessee. This type of institution offers highly specialized care for patients with particular disorders, often at little or no expense to the patient. In the outpatient clinic, as in all other settings, documentation and record review are important parts of nursing assessment.

Outpatient Surgery Clinic. Elective outpatient surgery for patients with uncomplicated conditions, such as a herniorrhaphy or tonsillectomy, offer the advantage of lower cost, reduced incidence of nosocomial infection, and recuperation at home in familiar surroundings. These outpatient clinics eliminate the need to separate the child from the family, and the treatment and the emotional impact of the illness are reduced. Careful preparation must be given, and assurance must be obtained that the child's home environment is adequate to meet recovery needs.

Promoting a Positive Experience

The attitude of nurses, receptionists, and other personnel in the clinic, office, or hospital unit, is of the utmost importance. It can make the difference between an atmosphere that is warm and kindly and one in which the patient is made to feel dehumanized. As more and more medical care is instituted in outpatient clinics, there will be an even greater reduction in the number of children who require hospitalization. For many, the only exposure to medical personnel will be through brief clinic appointments. We should all, therefore, make the encounters positive ones for patients and families.

Home

Because hospitalization is now brief for most children, the choice is not either hospital or home care but a combination of the two. They are becoming interdependent. Dramatic technical improvements and research in specific disease entities are also helping to advance the movement to home care (e.g., cryoprecipitate for hemophiliacs, Broviac catheters for chemotherapy, heparin locks, glucometers). Home care, however, is broader than in years past. It is not merely a matter of supplying appliances and nursing care, but it includes assessment of the total needs of children and their families. Families need to be linked to a wide variety of network services. This ideally involves a multidisciplinary approach headed by the physician or medical center.

The hospice concept for children has received accolades from parents who have benefited from its service. Local and national support groups for specific problems afford opportunities for families to share and support one another and to learn from others' successes and failures. Special groups and camps for children with chronic illnesses are also well established. Group therapy for children under stress is equally important in preventing mental health problems (e.g., groups for children whose parents are divorced, Alateen for children of alcoholics). These and other programs not only have the potential for improving life for the child and family but also may help to reduce the high cost of medical care. Currently, reform is resulting in dramatic changes in the delivery of health care to children and families. These changes will impact the role and responsibilities of the nurse working both in wellness centers providing preventative care and in hospitals or homes treating illness.

Children's Hospital Unit

The children's unit differs in many respects from adult divisions. The pediatric unit or hospital is designed to meet the needs of children and their parents. A cheerful, casual atmosphere helps to bridge the gap between home and hospital and is in keeping with the child's emotional, developmental, and physical needs. Patients often wear their own clothing while they are hospitalized, and nurses wear colorful smocks or pastel uniforms. Colored bedspreads and wagons or strollers for transportation are also more homelike.

The physical structure of the division includes furniture of the proper height for the child, soundproof ceilings, and color schemes with eye appeal. There is a special treatment room for the doctor to examine the patient. In this way, the other children do not become disturbed by the proceedings. Some hospitals have a schoolroom. When this is not available, it is necessary for the teacher to visit each child individually. Today's modern general hospitals have separate waiting rooms for children. This is more relaxing for parents, since they do not have to worry about whether their child is disturbing adult patients, and it is less frightening to the child.

Most pediatric departments include a playroom (Fig. 21–1). It is generally large and light in color. Bulletin boards and blackboards are within reach of the patients. Mobiles may be suspended from the ceiling. Some playrooms are equipped with an aquarium of fish and blossoming plants because children love living things. A variety of toys suitable for different age groups are available. This room may be under the supervision of a child life specialist, a play therapist, or nursery school teacher. Parents usually enjoy taking their children to the playroom and observing the various activities.

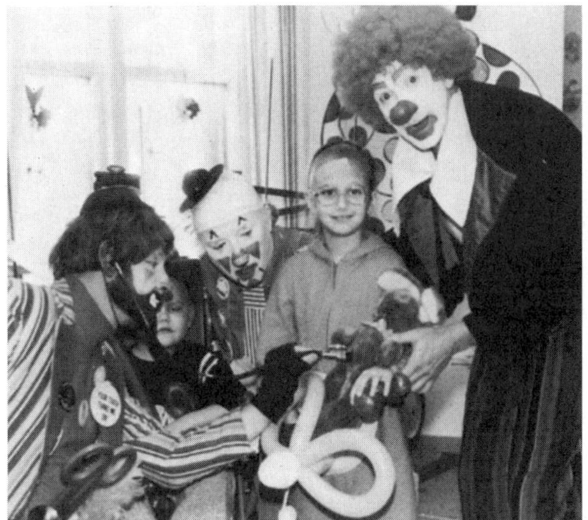

Figure 21–1. • Special visitors to the playroom. (Courtesy of Blank Memorial Hospital for Children, Des Moines, IA.)

When the child is not able to be taken to the playroom because of the diagnosis or physical condition, bedside play activities appropriate to the developmental level and diagnosis of the child should be provided (Fig. 21–2). The daily routine of the pediatric unit emphasizes parent rooming-in, the provision of consistent caregivers, and flexible schedules designed to meet the needs of growing children.

THE CHILD'S REACTION TO HOSPITALIZATION

The child's reaction to hospitalization depends on many factors such as age, amount of preparation given, security of home life, previous hospitaliza-

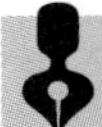 **Nursing Tip**

Play is an important part of a nursing care plan for children.

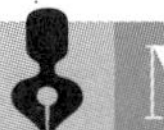 **Nursing Tip**

Familiar rituals and routines must be incorporated into the plan of care for a hospitalized child.

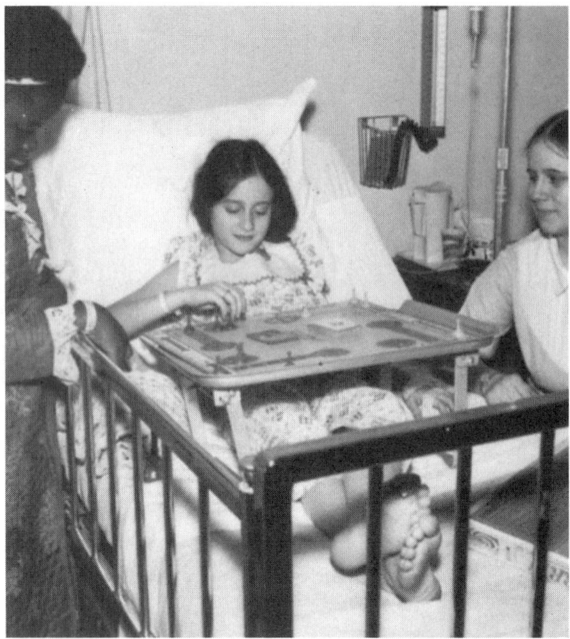

Figure 21–2. • Establishing good communication between patient and nurse takes time and effort. (Courtesy of Rivier College/St. Joseph Hospital School of Practical Nursing, Nashua, NH.)

tions, support of family and medical personnel, and child's emotional health. Many children cannot grasp what is going to happen to them even though they have been well prepared. At a time when children need their parents most, they may be separated from them, placed in the hands of strangers, and even fed different foods. Add to this a totally new environment and tummyache, and you have one frightened and unhappy child.

Each child reacts differently to hospitalization. One is demanding and exhibits temper tantrums, whereas another becomes withdrawn. The "good" child on the unit may be going through greater torment than the one who cries and shows feelings outwardly. The best prepared nurse cannot replace the child's parents. However, hospitalization can be a period of growth rather than just an unpleasant interlude. Children may see the nurse as someone who cares for them physically, as their parents would, and as a source of security and comfort.

The major causes of stress for children of all ages are separation, pain, and fear of body intrusion. They are influenced by the patient's developmental age, the maturity of the parents, cultural and economic factors, religious background, past experiences, family size, state of health on admission, and other factors.

Separation Anxiety

Separation anxiety occurs in infants 6 months and older and is most pronounced in the toddler age. There are three stages of separation anxiety. These include *protest, despair,* and *denial* or *detachment.* Unless infants are extremely ill, their sense of abandonment is expressed by a loud *protest.* Toddlers may watch and listen for their parents. Their cry is continuous until they fall asleep in exhaustion. Toddlers may call out "mommy" repeatedly, and the approach of a stranger only causes increased screaming. The crying gradually stops and the second stage of *despair* sets in. Children appear sad and depressed. They move about less and withdraw from strangers who approach. They do not play actively with toys. In the third stage of *denial* or *detachment,* children appear to deny their need for the parent and become detached or uninterested in their visits. They become more interested in their surroundings, their toys, and their playmates. On the surface, it appears the child has adjusted to the separation.

However, it is important for the nurse to understand that the child is using a coping mechanism to detach and reduce the emotional pain. If the detachment stage is prolonged, an irreversible disruption of parent–infant bonding may occur. Health care workers who do not understand the stages of separation anxiety may label the crying protesting child as "bad" and the withdrawn depressed child in despair as "adjusting," and the child who is in the detachment phase as a "well-adjusted" child. This misinterpretation can prevent health care workers from providing desperately needed assistance and guidance to child and family.

The nurse must understand that the child who is

Nursing Tip

The achievement of developmental tasks should be part of the plan of care for the hospitalized child.

Nursing Tip

The stages of separation anxiety includes protest, despair, and detachment or denial.

Nursing Tip

Any time toddlers are left by their mother or primary caretaker, they experience some degree of separation anxiety, for example, when they are left with day care personnel, baby-sitters, or relatives.

in despair reverts back to the protest stage when the parent arrives for a visit. This is good! The child who has reached the detached phase appears unmoved and uninterested in the parent's arrival. Nursing interventions are needed in this case to preserve and heal parent–infant relationships. The nurse should help the parents to understand they should not deceive the child into believing they will stay and "sneak out" while the child is distracted. This can tear the bond of trust.

Pain

The negative physical and psychological consequences of pain are well documented. Patients in pain secrete higher levels of cortisol, have compromised immune systems, more infections, and delayed wound healing. Nurses must maintain a high level of suspicion for pain when caring for children. Infants cannot show the nurse where it hurts, and frequently a child's report of pain is not given the credibility of an adult's report. Also, children may not realize they are supposed to report pain to the nurse. If children feel they will receive an injection to be more comfortable, they may refrain from complaining. Family members also experience emotional pain.

Nonpharmacological techniques, such as drawing, distraction, imagery, relaxation, and cognitive strategies as well as analgesia provide necessary relief from symptoms. The child may draw "how the pain feels" and where it is located. Distractions such as story telling, quiet conversation, and puppet play are effective. Imagery techniques, such as having children imagine themselves in a safe place, relieves anxiety. Slowing down breathing and listening to relaxation tapes is effective in reducing pain in adolescents. Cognitive (thinking) techniques such as "thought stopping" are also helpful in older patients. In this technique, the patient is instructed to repeat the word "stop" in response to negative thoughts and worries. A backrub or hand massage is also relaxing, depending on the child's age and diagnosis. Pain assessment and pharmacological responses of infants and children are discussed in Chapter 22.

Fear

Intrusive procedures, such as intravenous (IV) lines and blood tests, are fear provoking. They disrupt the child's trust level and threaten self-esteem and self-control. They may require restriction of activity. *Care must be taken to respect the modesty, integrity, and privacy of each child.* Hospital personnel can provide an environment that supports the child's need for mastery and control. These interventions are discussed according to age in this chapter and throughout the text. Selected nursing diagnoses for the hospitalized child and family are presented in Nursing Care Plan 21-1.

Regression

Regression of growth and development during hospitalization can be expected. *Regression* is the loss of an achieved level of functioning to a past level of behavior that was successful during earlier stages of development. Examples of regression include demanding a bottle in a child who usually drinks from a cup, or refusal to use a "potty" chair in a child who has achieved bowel and bladder control, or demanding to be "carried" by a child who had been walking independently. Regression can be minimized by an accurate nursing assessment of the child's abilities and the planning of care to support and maintain growth and development. However, regression should not be punished. Nurses can guide parents to praise appropriate behavior and ignore regressions. When the child is free of the stress that caused the regression, praise will motivate the achievement of appropriate behavior.

Cultural Needs

Showing culturally sensitive attitudes toward families with hospitalized children decreases anxiety. Flexibility and careful listening are necessary to understand them. Studies of children in many different societies show that American middle-class culture is different from childhood environments derived from other traditions. Nurses must also be aware of their own cultural biases and how they might affect the assessment. In some cases, a translator may be required.

NURSING CARE PLAN 21-1

Selected Nursing Diagnosis for Hospitalized Child and Family

Nursing Diagnosis: Anxiety, related to hospitalization of child as evidenced by restlessness, facial tension, insomnia, crying, clinging behavior, regression to previous stage of growth and development, or maladaptive behaviors

Goals	Nursing Intervention	Rationale
Child/family will experience decreased anxiety as demonstrated by ability to relax, present a calm demeanor, and ability to effectively participate in child's care	1. Assess child/family's knowledge as to reason for hospitalization	1. Provides information to the nurse as to what areas need clarification and reinforcement of correct information
	2. Explain routines usually followed on unit and orient the child and parent to the unit, including play room	2. Helps to decrease level of anxiety for the child and parents
	3. Suggest that parents or family members bring in a photograph, favorite toy, or favorite music tape/CD for child	3. These items help to provide a link to home and help to promote a sense of security in the child
	4. Recognize and teach the parent about age-appropriate separation anxiety	4. The age of the child is a major factor to consider in adjusting to separation from familiar people and surroundings
	5. Instruct parents to explain to the child when they will return in an age-appropriate manner (e.g., "After *Sesame Street*" is over" or "When Reading Rainbow starts" or "before dinner")	5. Establishes a sense of trust that the child has not been abandoned. Also, toddlers and young children do not fully understand the concept of time. By using a favorite show or a meal time as a marker, helps to lessen the degree of anxiety the child may feel
	6. Provide for consistency in personnel assigned to child, as much as possible	6. Consistency is necessary to develop a sense of trust; although maladaptive behaviors may be normal in unfamiliar circumstances, if consistency and support are not given, coping abilities decrease
	7. Support parents by showing a willingness to be available to them to listen, and/or to answer questions	7. Nurse's availability to show interest in parents and answer questions shows concern, prevents the potential for misunderstanding of prescribed treatments, and helps to lessen the anxiety of family members
	8. Maintain child's contact with family; involve family in child's care when appropriate	8. Increases sense of security in child and provides a sense of purpose for the family

The nurse must create a bridge between the health care system of the United States and the diverse people that system serves. Effective utilization of health care service and compliance with treatment plans is enhanced when the nurse's approach is compatible with cultural needs and beliefs. Teaching will be effective only if the parents or child understand the language used. Interpreters should be used as needed. Nonverbal cues and body language are important in intercultural communication. Nurses should take the time to learn what their gestures and movements mean to the family from another culture.

In some developing countries, the energies of parents are focused on survival rather than promoting growth and development or intellectual skills. These practices become ingrained in the child-rearing practices handed down from generation to generation. For example, within these cultures, parents may believe that an ill infant must be near the caretaker's body at all times. Therefore, in the Western hospital, the nurse may find it a challenge to coax parents to allow the infant to remain in the crib, separated from them, and enveloped by an oxygen tent.

Crying may be interpreted by some cultures as a signal of an organic upset or illness. Since diarrhea is a frequent cause of infant death in developing countries, frequent feeding in response to crying is a survival response. When families from these developing countries using these survival practices move to the United States, where survival threats decrease, it takes generations to change the child care practices and focus on promoting growth and development and fostering intellectual abilities.

One cultural group may prize autonomy and initiative in their children, whereas another tolerates only complete obedience. Protective amulets or charms placed on wrists or clothing of infants must be respected. In the gypsy culture, the color red and the number 3 are positive symbols. Therefore a red-colored medicine to be given three times a day will receive more compliance than a white-colored medication prescribed two times a day. Respecting cultural and religious beliefs will enhance compliance.

The nurse must be careful to separate survival practices from cultural beliefs. It may be advantageous to change care practices based on survival when the threat to survival is no longer present; however, if the practice is based on cultural belief, then the practice must be respected and no attempt should be made to change. *The nurse must assess the family through the eyes of its culture to avoid labeling a family who is "different" as dysfunctional.*

Fostering Intercultural Communication

Personal Space. *Personal space* is defined as an imaginary circle that surrounds us. The size of that space is determined by culture. We can observe the space by watching two friends of the same culture talk to each other. Some people stand close to each other. Nurses who invade that "personal space" can be thought of as "pushy" or suspect and the parent who retreats can be thought of by the nurse as "cold."

Smiling. A smiling nurse may not be received by varying cultures as a "friendly" nurse. In Russia, a smile indicates happiness and is inappropriate in a serious or sad situation. Nurses may interpret a nonsmiling Russian as "unfriendly" if they are unaware of this cultural difference. The Vietnamese, however, smile in all circumstances. Their smile is a show of respect. When they are reprimanded, they smile to show they did not mind being reprimanded.

Eye Contact. In the United States, eye-to-eye contact with the person you are communicating with is considered a show of respect and attention. In the Asian culture however, eye-to-eye-contact is seen as disrespect. Native Americans consider staring at a speaker rude behavior. Eye contact is acceptable for short periods only. The cultural term the *evil eye* originates from cultures who interpret eye-to-eye contact as disrespectful.

Touch. In the United States, touch is often considered a gesture of friendliness. However, touch can give misleading messages. A pat on the head may infer superiority of the person touching the head. In the Vietnamese culture, touching the head is thought to rob those being touched of their souls.

Focus. Some cultures are receptive to communication or teaching if the focus is on the problem. Some cultures deal with the problem by focusing on its future impact on the family or life of the child. Teaching strategies need to be designed to approach the topic from the perspective appropriate to that culture.

When teaching infant and child care, the nurse must always assess the values of the cultural practice of the family before imposing a "standardized" process. Avoiding cultural conflict is essential to the successful outcome of parent and child teaching. Culture evolves and is not static. However, most families from varying cultures strive to maintain their cultural identities while adapting to Western practices. The nurse should support maintaining the individual cultural identity of that family. Culturally sensitive health care is also discussed in Chapter 15.

THE PARENTS' REACTIONS TO THE CHILD'S HOSPITALIZATION

When children are hospitalized, the whole family is affected. The parents of the hospitalized youngster need others to show interest in their physical and emotional needs as well. If they are frightened and tense, the child soon senses it.

Parents may feel that they are to blame for the child's illness; they may feel that they should have recognized the symptoms earlier or that they could have prevented an accident by closer supervision. Immunizations and other types of preventive care may also have been neglected. These feelings can cause a sense of guilt, helplessness, and anxiety.

Parents seldom are the cause for direct hospital admission of a child. Even in cases of child abuse or neglect, nothing is gained by blaming the parents. The nurse must remain objective and empathetic. The nurse listens carefully to parental concerns and acknowledges the legitimacy of their feelings, for example, "It is understandable that you feel this way; everything happened so fast." Parents also frequently express feelings of helplessness at the loss of the parental role as protector. The nurse encourages and supports parents and other family members, stresses their importance to the child's recovery, and encourages their participation in the care of the child. The admission of a child to the hospital is anxiety producing. The uncertainty of the situation can become overwhelming, causing feelings of panic. However, these feelings are usually temporary. The nurse should remain relaxed, reassure the parents, and reinforce positive parenting. Information about the child's condition and treatment plan is given. Needs are assessed and interventions planned to meet specific needs.

Poor communication results in unnecessary fears. The nurse should explain in simple terms some of the equipment being used and facilities available on the unit. The nurse listens attentively and tries to clear up misconceptions. Rooming-in may alleviate some anxieties of parents. However, the nurse must continue to promptly and cheerfully tend to the needs of the child, to indicate to the parents that their child is in good hands. Parental involvement in a child's care offers the nurse the opportunity to assess the relationship and to provide guidance and teaching as needed.

Parents may have to take time from work, especially if treatment involves travel to special centers. Ronald McDonald homes offer lodging and other familiar amenities at no cost for parents of patients with life-threatening illness. The availability of these facilities is explored with the family. The social service worker may be of help in such instances. The care and welfare of other children at home while one parent is at work and the other is rooming-in with the ill child should be discussed. Parents should be advised that pain control techniques are available and will be used to minimize painful experiences for the ill child.

Parents may ventilate their feelings and stresses through anger, crying, or body language. Behavior is not only a response to the current situation but often involves attitudes resulting from early childhood experiences. The nurse must not pass judgment on individuals whose behavior may seem demanding or unreasonable. *An understanding and acceptance of people and their problems are essential for the successful pediatric nurse.*

Nursing Tip

When a child is admitted to the hospital, every family member is affected.

Siblings are also affected when a brother or sister is hospitalized. They may feel left out, guilty, or resentful of the attention focused on the ill child. Suitable interventions by the nurse include directing some attention to the siblings, supporting their efforts to comfort the family member, and engaging them in play or drawing pictures, such as "How it feels to have an ill brother or sister." They may also make cards and pictures for the patient.

THE NURSE'S ROLE IN HOSPITAL ADMISSION

As members of the nursing team, nurses are often called on to admit new patients. Besides performing the procedure skillfully, they must be prepared to meet the emotional needs of those involved. The impression the nurse gives, whether good or bad, definitely affects the patient's adjustment. Empathy in responding to the fears of the child and family members makes the admission procedure stimulating and educational—a positive experience for all.

A child should be prepared for hospitalization when possible. Ideally, the child and parents should tour the pediatric unit before admission. This enables the parents to meet the people who will care for their child. Children and their families may be overwhelmed by the size of the institution and the fear of becoming lost.

Between ages 1 and 3, children are worried about being separated from their parents. After age 3, children may become more fearful about what is going to happen to them. Parents should try to be as matter-of-fact about this new experience as possible. Unless they have been hospitalized before, children can only try to imagine what will happen to them. It is not necessary to go into much detail, since the child's imagination is great and giving information that is beyond comprehension may create unnecessary fears. It is logical to dwell on the more pleasant aspects, but not to the extent of saying that hospitalization involves no discomforts. For example, one might mention that meals will be served on a tray, that baths will be taken from a basin at the bedside, and that the child will be with other children. The fact that there is a buzzer for calling the nurse may add to the child's sense of security. The parents may plan with the child what favorite toy or book to bring.

Perhaps more important than explaining certain occurrences is listening to how the child feels and encouraging questions. Parents should prepare them a few days, but not weeks, in advance. Parents should never lure children to the hospital by pretending that it is some other place. In emergency situations, there is little time for preparation. The entire medical team must try to give added emotional support to the child in such cases. The initial greeting should show warmth and friendliness—smile and introduce yourself.

Some hospitals allow the patient to be taken to the playroom for a short time before going to the room. When the parent tells the nurse the child's name, associating it with a familiar person who has the same name will help the nurse to remember it. It creates a much warmer feeling to speak of "John" or "Susy" than "your little boy" or "your daughter."

When the child and parents are taken to the child's room, the nurse introduces them to the other children. The parent is seated comfortably. Explain the admission procedure carefully. Avoid discussing in front of children information that they will not understand. The parent is encouraged to do as much for the child as possible, for example, remove clothes. The nurse tries not to appear rushed. A matter-of-fact attitude must be maintained regardless of the patient's condition. A soft voice and quiet approach are less frightening to the child. A nurse's looking anxious causes unnecessary worry for everyone concerned. A troubled look may have nothing to do with the patient. Taking one step at a time is advised. Calmness is catching. The nurse remains available to answer questions that might arise. When there is a good relationship between parent and nurse, the child benefits from higher-quality care.

When children are hospitalized, the nurse should be aware of the developmental history as well as the medical history. A developmental history includes:

- Family relationships and support systems
- Cultural needs that may affect care and hospital routine
- Nicknames, rituals, routines
- Developmental level and abilities
- Communication skills
- Personality, adaptability, coping skills
- Past experiences, divorce, new siblings, extended family
- Previous separation experiences—vacations or hospitalizations
- Impact of current health problem on growth and development
- Preparation given the child
- Previous contact with health care personnel

Whenever invasive or painful procedures are performed, adequate restraints should be applied to allow the procedure to be completed as quickly as possible. Comforting, rewards, and praise should follow every painful or frightening procedure.

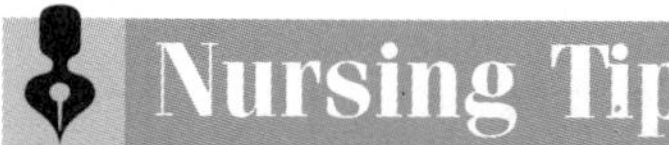

When explaining procedures to children, it is helpful to identify the child's role in the event: for example, "You will be asked to step on the scale."

DEVELOPING A PEDIATRIC NURSING CARE PLAN

Developing the pediatric *nursing care plan* is similar to developing an adult care plan. The care plan is the result of the nursing process. It states specifically what is to be done for each child and keeps the focus on the child, not on the condition or therapy. An established list of accepted nursing diagnoses is available and in use (see Appendix C). These serve as a standard for organizing data collection. They also serve as a vehicle by which one nurse can communicate with another. A nursing diagnosis for a pediatric patient may require some modification. Assessing the child includes a knowledge of growth and developmental processes. It also includes evaluating the primary caretaker, who has a direct role in the safety and maintenance of the child's health. Nursing care plans are guides that need continual evaluation and reevaluation to determine whether the goals for the individual child are being met. Some hospitals use a Kardex system (Fig. 21–3). Figure 21–4 shows a nurse entering assessment data, for later retrieval, into the unit computer.

CLINICAL PATHWAYS

Clinical pathways are used in acute care settings as well as alternate care settings. The clinical pathway is an interdisciplinary plan of care that displays progress of the entire treatment plan for the patient. The main difference between a clinical pathway and a nursing care plan is that the nursing care plan focuses on the nurse's role in the care of the patient, and the clinical pathway focuses on the broader view of the entire multidisciplinary health care team and general outcome goals of care. Un-

12-1

DIET 1800 calorie
Constant Carbohydrate

Self Select X Evenflo ___ Warm ___
Cup ___ Playtex ___ Cold ___

Intake ✓
doctor's order 12-1
Output ✓
doctor's order 12-1

IV's Heparin lock for blood draws

Date started 12-1
IV site Ⓛ hand
Needles #20 jelco
Tubing Change —

Activity
Bedrest ___
Bathroom Priv. ___
May be held ___
Up ad lib X 12-1
Playroom ___
Other Pt to be up and dressed
Interim Summary 12-5

Bath
Complete ___
Partial ___
Tub/Shower 12-1
Shampoo ___
Special Instructions:

Safety Precautions
Crib Net ___
Restraints ___
Seiz. Prec. ___
ID band on 12-1
Name Tag on Crib ___
Siderail release ___

Vital Signs 12-1
TPR Routine
BP Routine
Neuro Check —
Growth Chart —
OFC —
Weight daily

Special Equipment
Glucometer

Allergies
none Known

Resp. Therapy

Routine Lab Orders

Therapy Schedule
Exercise 1000 and 1400

STANDING	MEDICATIONS	DATE	TREATMENTS
12-1	Sliding Scale Insulin Sub-q Give the following! 5units Regular insulin acetone large 3units Regular insulin acetone moderate 1unit Regular insulin acetone small	12-1	Blood glucose tests to be done at 0700, 1100, 1600, 2100, 0200 using dextrostix or chemstrips unless patient has own meter. Patient or parent to do testing except at 0200
		12-1	Call resident if blood sugar is less than 50 or greater than 240
		12-1	Acetest all urines until negative or blood sugar below 240
PRN			
12-1	Tylenol 325mg q 3°-4° prn headache.	12-1	Oral treatment of insulin reaction 15grams carbohydrate (6oz. of orange juice) Repeat if signs or symptoms persist after rechecking.

Room	Name	Diagnosis	Assoc. Nurse	Primary Nurse	Doctor
364-1	Cory Johnson	Newly diagnosed diabetes mellitus	Peg T	Craig J	Roberts

Figure 21–3. • The Kardex serves as a reference to patient problems that require nursing intervention.

Illustration continued on following page

derstanding the nursing process and the nursing care plan is essential to understand the nurse's role in the clinical pathway.

Clinical pathways are also called *critical pathways, care maps, multidisciplinary action plans (MAPs),* and *anticipated recovery paths (ARPs).* They are used for patients with a predictable course of illness to identify appropriate timing of interventions that will facilitate early recovery.

An RN case manager develops the clinical pathway, coordinates, evaluates the progress, and documents any deviations or variances that may be caused by unexpected complications. The pathway can be used as a patient education tool to help the

PEDIATRIC NURSING CARE PLAN

Date	Patient Problems/Teaching Needs	Expected Outcomes	Nursing Orders	Initials
12-2	Knowledge deficit related	Patient and patient's	① Show patient and family new	
	to newly diagnosed diabetes	family will discuss	equipment A. Syringes	
	mellitus	disease and its	B. Insulin	
		treatment.	C. Glucometer	
			D. Dextrosticks	CR
			② Allow patient time to	
			begin excepting disease	CR
			③ Discuss resources outside hospital	
			A. ADA	
			B JDF	CR
			④ Be supportive to patient	
			and family during learning	
			process	CR

Age 13	Birth Date 2-12-72	Hospital # 7391-85	Religion Methodist	Service PEDS	Admission Date 12-1-85	Time 1200

NURS 372 4/80 632034462

Figure 21–3. • *Continued*

patient to anticipate interventions by the multidisciplinary health care team. The student nurse or float nurse can identify where they fit into the total plan of care for this one patient.

Communication among departments is enhanced by the clinical pathway, which sets timelines for the achievement of specific goals. Some hospitals are beginning to use clinical pathways in the clinic and have the pathway continue with the patient through hospitalization and extend to home care follow-up. This ideal of the outcome-based plan of care is not yet nationally utilized. Pictorial pathways (Fig. 21–5) have been used and are especially valuable in patient education and anticipatory guidance. Clinical pathways for children with specific conditions are presented in various chapters of this book.

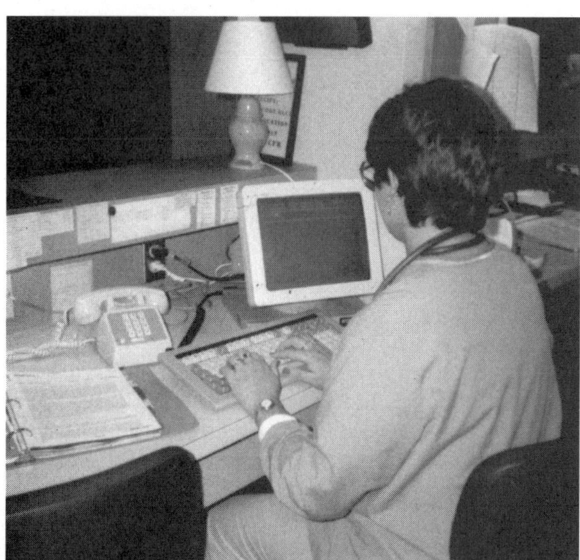

Figure 21–4. • The nurse enters assessment data and retrieves information about the patient's progress on the unit computer. (Courtesy of Columbia/HCA Portsmouth Regional Hospital, Portsmouth, NH.)

THE HOSPITALIZED INFANT

Hospitalization is frustrating for infants. During infancy rapid physical and emotional development takes place. Infants are used to getting what they want when they want it, and they show their displeasure quickly when illness restricts the satisfaction of their desires. Babies who were breastfed at home may be unable to continue this regimen. They miss the continuous affection of their parents. Their daily schedule is upset. The infant who drinks well from a cup at home may refuse it entirely at the hospital.

Nursing personnel must try to meet the needs of these little patients by protecting them from excess frustration. It is not wise to expect them to develop new habits when they need energy to cope with their illness and the strange environment. One of the nurse's major goals during this period is to assist with the parent–infant attachment process and to promote sensorimotor activities. This can be fostered by providing means for the infant and

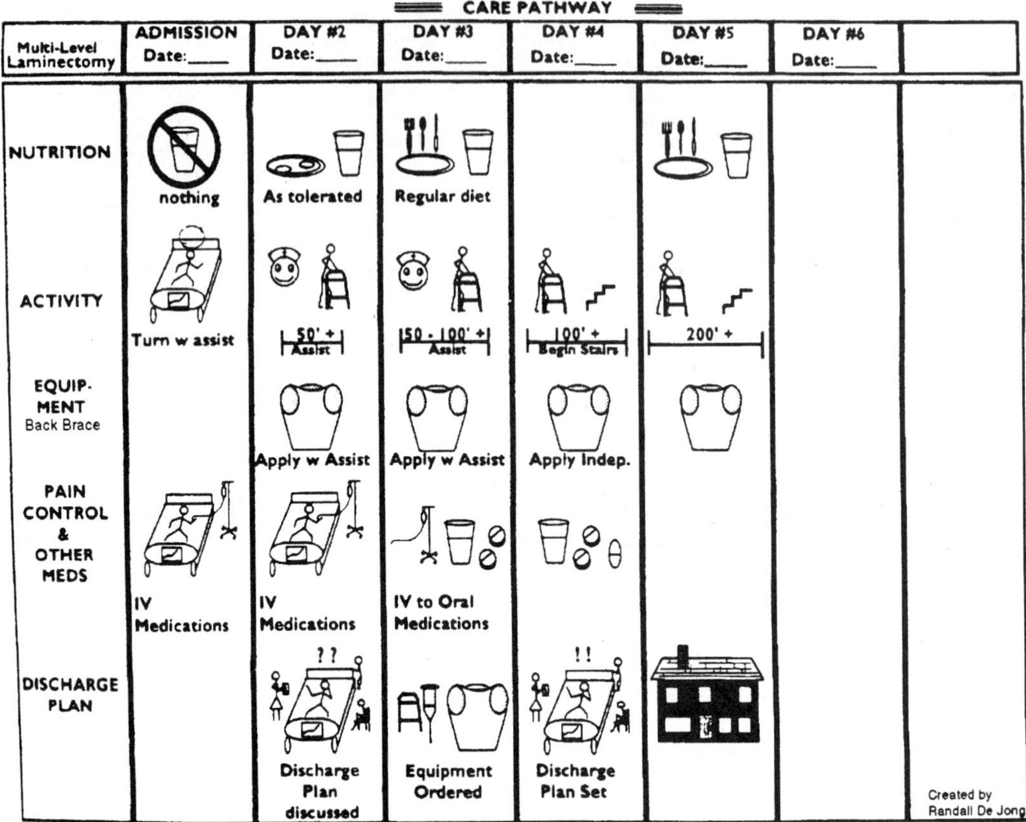

Figure 21–5. • Pictorial clinical pathway. (Courtesy Providence General Medical Center, Everett, Washington. Created by Randall De Jong.)

significant other to interact and by attempting to ease the tension of the parents. The nurse can serve as a role model by performing activities with the baby, such as cuddling, rocking, talking, and singing. A swing, a bath with squeeze toys, a pacifier, and a hanging mobile are also appropriate as the infant's condition permits.

Because the infant cannot understand explanations, the nurse administers uncomfortable procedures as gently as possible and returns the infant to the parents for consolation (Fig. 21–6). Liberal visiting hours are essential. When parents are not available, soothing support and gentle touch are provided; otherwise, the infant may learn to associate only pain with nursing care. Consistency in caretakers is also important at this stage of development.

THE HOSPITALIZED TODDLER

The toddler's world revolves around the parents, particularly mother (or significant caretaker). Hospitalization is a painful experience for toddlers. They cannot understand why they are separated from mother, and they become very distressed. Toddlers who have a continuous, secure relationship with mother react more violently to separation because they have more to lose. Nursing goals in the care of the hospitalized toddler are presented in Box 21–1.

The stages of separation anxiety are at its peak (see page 520). The nurse who comprehends the various separation stages sees parental visits as essential, even though the process of separation and reunion is painful. A cohesive staff is essential to help to tolerate the constant angry protest of these children. Education of the parents helps to promote their continued visits and to decrease feelings of inadequacy. Ritualistic patterns of care that involve structure are appropriate for children in this age group.

Repetitive games that deal with disappearance and return are helpful. Peekaboo and hide-and-seek serve such a purpose. The use of a *transitional object,* such as a blanket or a favorite toy, promotes security. Pictures of the family and tape recordings of favorite stories are other measures that help the child to remain connected with the family. When the nurse or mother leaves, she explains when she will return in terms of the toddler's experience, for example, after naptime or lunch, and then she returns promptly at that time. A loving hug, good-bye, and prompt exit are then necessary. Parents should not wait until a child falls asleep to depart. This avoids confrontations but disturbs the child's sense of trust. The nurse assures the parents that she will remain with the child to comfort her. The continued reappearance of the parents as promised is of value in reducing the child's anxiety and reestablishing his or her sense of trust.

Rooming-in is highly desirable. When rooming-in is impossible, consistent caregivers should be assigned to care for the child and the mother. The nurse indicates by her approach that she considers the mother's contributions extremely important to the child's well-being. She interprets the stages of separation anxiety to the mother. The nurse must also realize that the mother is under stress and should not be asked to assume responsibilities beyond her capabilities. The nurse observes parents for signs of fatigue and suggests appropriate interventions.

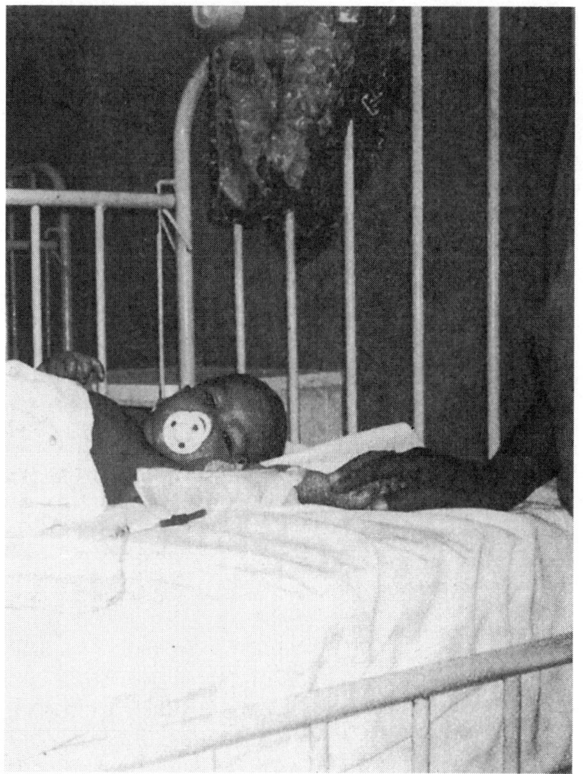

Figure 21–6. • Having a mother nearby and a pacifier comfort this hospitalized child.

BOX 21–1

NURSING GOALS IN THE CARE OF HOSPITALIZED TODDLERS

- Reassure parents, particularly the child's primary caregiver.
- Maintain the toddler's sense of trust.
- Incorporate home habits of the child into nursing care plans, for example, transitional objects.
- Allow child to work through or master threatening experiences through soothing techniques and play.
- Provide individualized, flexible nursing care plans in accordance with child's development and diagnosis.

Occasionally parents do not choose to care for their child; for example, "We feel that since we are paying for this, we should just be able to entertain him." In such instances, the parents' wishes are respected. Referral to the clinical nurse specialist might also be appropriate to facilitate communication and to understand better the underlying dynamics of the situation.

The home habits of the toddler are recorded and utilized. A potty chair is provided if the child is trained. Some regression in behavior is to be expected. If the toddler still prefers bottles to cups, one should not attempt to change this in the hospital. Familiar toys and books are important. A steady, calm voice communicates safety (Figs. 21–7 and 21–8). Toddlers are in the stage of autonomy. Loss of a small amount of the self-control they have achieved usually results in resistance and negativism.

Children are forewarned about any unpleasant or new experience that they may have to undergo while in the hospital. This is done in keeping with their level of understanding. Being truthful about things that may hurt prevents the child from feeling betrayed. Preparation and explanation are done immediately before a procedure so that the child does not worry needlessly for an extended time. Crying and protesting when told about certain procedures are healthy expressions of feelings and relieve tension. Distractions such as blowing bubbles, looking through a kaleidoscope, and pop-up toys may help to reduce anxiety and pain.

Supervised playroom activity contributes to intellectual, social, and motor development. Treatments in the playroom are avoided. Toddlers are

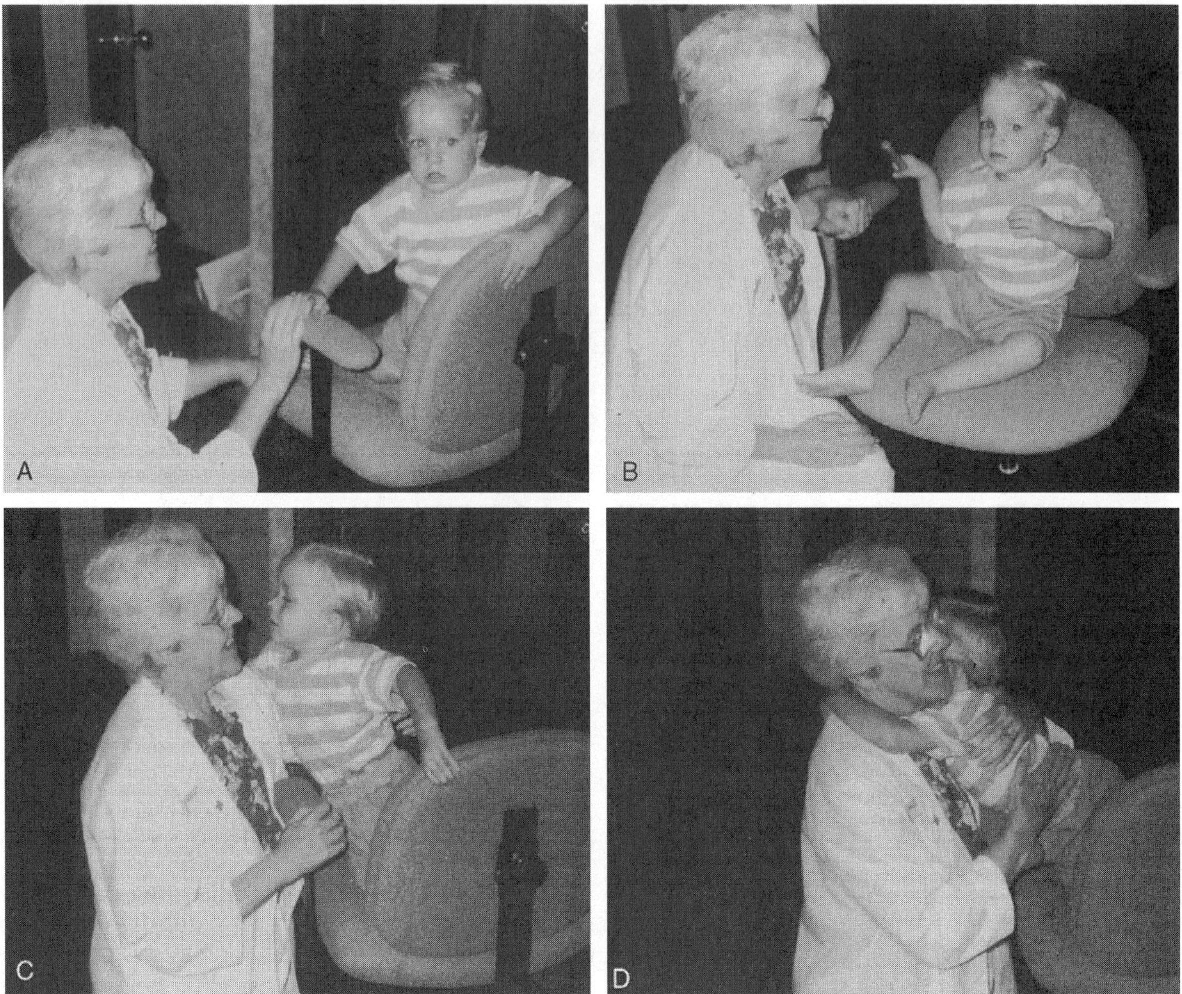

Figure 21–7. • The clinical nurse specialist approaches the small child calmly, slowly, and at eye level. **A,** child's apprehension; **B,** contemplation; **C,** gaining of control; and **D,** beginning of trust.

encouraged to play with safe equipment used in their care, such as bandages, tongue blades, and stethoscopes. Whenever possible, they are allowed out of their cribs, as confinement is frustrating for little ones who have just begun to enjoy walking. Playtime establishes rapport and is an important part of the nursing care of children.

There are indications that restraining the child's mobility by surgical and medical procedures involving splints, IV therapy, burn dressings, and so on may contribute to the development of emotional or personality problems or to speech and learning difficulties (Behrman & Kleigman, 1996). Therefore, when restraint is required, it must be accompanied by increased emotional support such as rooming-in, additional attention from nurses, and suitable diversion.

It is common for children to experience changes in behavior on their return home. They may be demanding and may cling to mother every minute. "He just won't let me out of his sight" is a common description. The mother should give the toddler extra attention and reassurance until trust is regained.

THE HOSPITALIZED PRESCHOOLER

The experience of hospitalization may be easier for preschool children who have had outside contact, such as nursery school and kindergarten, than for those who have never been separated from their parents. Because children of this age operate with concrete thinking, they can understand more and they can be better prepared for hospitalization. Explanations must be made in realistic terms as preschool children cannot understand abstract explanations. They are made to realize that hospitalization is not a punishment for something they have done wrong. Children may feel guilty, particularly if an accident happens because of some mischief on their part, as in the case of burns or falls.

Preschool children are distressed when their mothers prepare to leave them, but unlike the toddler, they can understand time relationships through activities—at breakfast, after lunch, and the like. The nurse and parents must not tell the child that they will return unless they intend to do so.

At this age, the child is afraid of bodily harm, particularly invasive procedures. The surgical patient needs to be shown the part of the body that requires surgery. The nurse can sketch a body outline and draw a circle around the operative site, giving simple information about the system that will be affected. It is stressed that only this area of the body will be involved. Children in this age group engage in magical thinking and fantasy. Fantasizing the unknown can be frightening to a young child. The preschooler needs clear, understandable, truthful explanations. Compliment children who ask questions; listen to them and correct any misinterpretations that they may have. Help the child to increase self-esteem through praise. The child relieves tension through role playing. Tongue depressors, adhesive bandages, and other materials related to everyday hospital life are relished by the sick child.

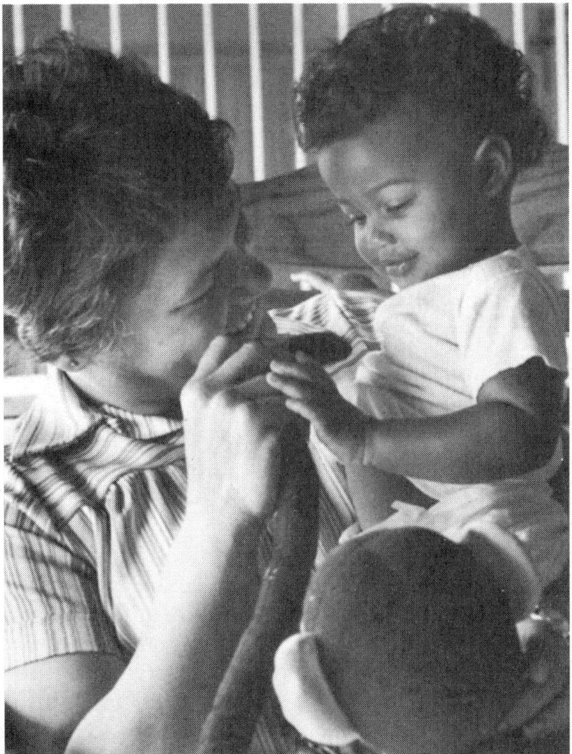

Figure 21–8. • Establishing rapport with the hospitalized toddler. (Courtesy of Blank Memorial Hospital for Children, Des Moines, IA.)

Parents are faced with a disrupted home life throughout the child's hospitalization. The mother cannot cope with everyday tasks when she is lonely for and worried about her child. The frequent trips to the hospital interfere with her daily routine and other children in the family may resent them. Contact with the physician is needed. Parents have a legal and ethical right to be informed of the benefits and risks of therapy and to be included in the decision-making process. When the child is finally discharged, he or she may be demanding and irritable. Parents need the kind support of hospital personnel to enable them to make informed decisions and meet these added strains.

THE HOSPITALIZED SCHOOL-AGE CHILD

Children of school age can endure separation from their parents if it is not prolonged. Children who have been cherished from birth can tolerate brief interruptions in their lives more easily than can those who have been denied a secure environment. The school-aged child is in a stage of industry and independence. Forced dependency in the hospital (such as immobilization) can result in a feeling of loss of control and loss of security. School-age children need to feel "grown up." They can participate in their care and be offered simple choices to foster their feeling of independence. They can choose their menus within appropriate restrictions, "help the nurse" in various activities, and can keep busy with age-appropriate toys.

Knowledge of growth and development in the school-age child assists in anticipatory guidance. Nurses can also enlist parents to determine what, if any, successful approaches they use in guiding the child. Behavioral problems may be addressed by a team conference. Nurses who work with children should keep abreast of current trends and guidance approaches. Positive direction and consistency are tools of particular importance to the pediatric nurse.

The education of the school-age child must continue throughout any illness. This gives the child a sense of continuity with the outside world, provides periods of socialization, reinforces weak academic areas, and reassures the child that he can

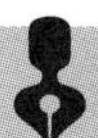

Nursing Tip

Observation of nonverbal clues, such as facial grimaces, squirming about, and finger tapping, is important in determining pain relief and support for the child.

return to his peers after discharge. The parents may act as liaisons between school and hospital. The teacher needs to be informed of the child's physical and emotional health to be effective. The nurse provides children with opportunities to study undisturbed so that they will be prepared for classes. Diagnostic tests and treatments should be scheduled around established school routines whenever possible. Many school districts have individual tutors for homebound or hospitalized school-aged children.

It is common for school-age children to be "brave," showing little, if any, fear in situations that actually upset them a good deal. Observation of body language may provide some clues to emotional states. The nurse's presence during unfamiliar procedures is comforting. Following treatments the nurse should encourage children to draw and talk about their drawings or to act out their feelings through puppet play.

THE HOSPITALIZED ADOLESCENT

Adolescents, in particular, experience feelings of loss of control during hospitalization. Daily routines are disrupted, and dependence–independence issues come to the foreground. When feelings of independence, self-assertion, and identity are threatened, the adolescent may respond by withdrawal, noncompliance, or anger. Care plans need to be designed to incorporate choice, privacy, and understanding.

Early Adolescence

Nursing care plans need to be oriented to the adolescent's age. Illness during early adolescence, approximately 10 to 13 years of age, is seen mainly as a threat to body image. There is a *narcissistic* concern about height, weight, and sexual development. Patients are aware of heightened body sensations and often have numerous physical complaints. Intense relationships with members of one's own sex are prevalent; they precede heterosexual involvement. Patients in this age group are anxious about how the illness will affect their physical appearance, functioning, and mobility; however, they are not usually overwhelmed by forced dependence. Self-portrait drawings are effective at this time. Maintaining privacy and same-sex room assignments are essential.

Middle Adolescence

During middle adolescence, approximately 14 to 16 years of age, teenagers are anxious about their ability to appeal to the opposite sex and to meet sex role expectations. Physical growth is practically complete. The peer group assumes greater importance in determining acceptability and behavior. During middle adolescence, the struggle for emancipation from the family, although erratic, is at its peak. It is disturbing not only to the teenager but also to parents, who must relinquish much of their control to hospital personnel. Incorporating choice, privacy, appropriate hair and cosmetic appearance, and opportunity for peer visitors is important during hospitalization.

Late Adolescence

Late adolescents, approximately 17 to 21 years of age, are mainly concerned with the task of education, career, marriage, children, community, and style of life. The dating partner becomes the person of primary importance. Hospitalization may pose the threat of postponement of career and future plans. Contact with school personnel, counselors, and teachers is important to prevent long-term impact on the education and development of the teenager.

Adjustment to Illness. The adolescent has many intellectual strengths, including the ability to think abstractly and to solve problems. Adolescents can understand the implications of their disease both in the present and in the future, and they are capable of participating in decisions related to treatment and care. The nurse who recognizes these skills and encourages their practice helps patients to gain confidence in their intellectual abilities, thus increasing their sense of independence and self-esteem.

Roommate Selection. Roommate selection, although frequently overlooked, is extremely important for this age group. Teenagers usually do better with one or more roommates than in single rooms. Because few community hospitals have adolescent wings, it is helpful if the patients participate in the decision as to whether they are admitted to the pediatric or the adult unit. A few adjoining rooms at the ends of these units will suffice. One should avoid placing the teenager next to a senile, dying, or severely debilitated patient in the adult unit or an infant in the pediatric unit.

ADMISSION TO THE PEDIATRIC UNIT

On the child's arrival at the unit, the nurse introduces the child to the staff; reviews routines, including any specific rules; and provides the child and parent with an information booklet. The nurse repeats the information periodically and has the child verbalize his or her understanding of it. The nurse acquaints the child and parents with the mechanics of the unit, for example, how to raise and lower the bed and use the call system, television, VCR, and intercom. Children and their parents are helped to locate the bathroom, kitchen, and recreational facilities. The telephone and dialing system is explained. They generally prefer their own clothes; however, some adolescent units keep scrub pants and tops in the unit, and the teenager may prefer them to conventional hospital garb. Children with conditions that require long-term immobilization (such as traction) should not be placed in a room with a child who has a viral illness to prevent nosocomial infections.

The nurse keeps children and their parents informed as to what to expect. This includes personnel they will see and upcoming tests. Time is allowed for questions and for the expression of feelings. The physician should discuss with the child and family just what is wrong and what can be expected of therapy in age-appropriate terms. When the prognosis is not predictable, the nurse shares uncertainty honestly while emphasizing that everyone is working together for the best possible outcome.

Surgery

Surgical patients need preoperative information. This includes such matters as what, if any, area of the body is to be shaved, why this needs to be done, and the likelihood of enemas, dietary restrictions, and medications. When possible, a visit to the recovery room is made to orient patients to postoperative surroundings. They are prepared in advance for waking up surrounded by life-support systems, bandages, casts, traction, or other apparatus following specific surgery. Also, one must explain to the patient and family the hospital's feedback system that will keep them informed of progress immediately following the operation. The inclusion of family and the sharing of feelings and ideas are extended throughout the confinement.

Behavioral Considerations

Skillful management of childhood behavior is best achieved through careful selection of nursing staff members. The nurses working with young people must be *flexible.* Often their patients compete for attention and can be manipulative.

The nurse's role should be that of the person to whom the child can relate in time of need. Working with children of various ages is a unique experience that carries its own rewards. The nurse who understands this and who is knowledgeable about the developmental and psychosocial considerations of childhood contributes greatly to the child's adjustment and recovery.

Confidentiality and Legality

Respecting the confidentiality of children is important to establishing trust. In general, information should not be divulged or shared without consent. Many problems can be avoided if the confidentiality of the relationship is clearly defined during initial meetings. Patient records must be carefully monitored to avoid loss or observation by unauthorized personnel. The nurse must avoid giving private information about any client to telephone callers or visitors. Appointment books in an office are kept closed rather than open on the clerk's desk.

An *emancipated minor* generally refers to an adolescent younger than 18 years of age who is no longer under the parent's authority. Married minors or minors in the military are automatically considered emancipated and may give consent for medical treatment for themselves and their children.

In some parts of the United States, the young adolescent may receive medical assistance without parental awareness for certain conditions, such as sexually transmitted diseases, contraception, pregnancy, abortion, and drug abuse. These laws are designed to afford the young person immediate medical help without fear of reprisal. However, some laws are being challenged in the courts. In a medical emergency, a minor can be treated without the consent of parents if the situation is life-threatening. Most states require that an individual be 18 or over to give blood.

Because laws vary from state to state, nurses must keep abreast of policies and legislation within their practice. Such information is available from the local medical or state nursing licensing boards. Most states do not specifically address the subject of responsibility for payment of medical care. In general, if the teenager is the sole consenter to a procedure, he or she has implied responsibility for payment.

DISCHARGE PLANNING

Preparation for the patient's discharge ideally begins on admission, for the goal of hospitalization is to return a healthier and happier child to the parents. An approach directed only toward good physical care of the patient's disease is not sufficient. The nurse must also consider the emotional growth of the child and the education of the patient and family. This will provide a positive learning experience for all involved.

If a patient requires specific home treatment, such as hyperalimentation, colostomy care, crutches, special diet, or insulin therapy, instructions are given to the parents gradually throughout their child's hospitalization. The instructions are written so that they may be referred to as needed. If the older child is to administer any self-treatment, careful explanations and supervision will be required until both patient and parents are confident that they can carry out the procedure safely at home. This may require the home health services.

Parents also must be prepared for behavioral problems that may arise following hospitalization. Severe stress may be obvious during the patients' stay. The services of a children's counselor are helpful if nightmares and regression continue. Guidance suggestions include:

- Anticipating behaviors such as clinging, regression in bowel and bladder control, aggression, manipulation, and nightmares
- Allowing the child to become a participating family member as soon as possible
- Taking the focus off the illness. Praising accomplishments unrelated to it
- Being kind, firm, and consistent with misbehavior
- Building trust by being truthful
- Providing suitable play materials such as clay, paints, and doctor and nurse kits
- Allowing time for free play
- Listening to and clarifying misconceptions about the illness
- Avoiding long periods of separation until a sense of security is regained
- Allowing the child to visit hospital staff during routine clinic visits if desired

Whenever possible, parents are given at least 1 day's notice of their child's discharge from the hospital so that they can make necessary arrangements. This is particularly important if both parents work or if transportation is a problem. The physician writes the discharge order. The approximate hour of dismissal is relayed to the parents. The child is weighed and dressed, and all personal belongings are collected. Parents are given a written return appointment card when indicated. They are informed of any new habits the patient may have acquired during hospitalization. Necessary medications or materials that the parents have paid for are rendered.

Parents sign a release form and visit the hospital business office according to hospital procedure. The nurse accompanies the child and parents to the hospital exit to say goodbye. According to condition, the child is placed in a hospital wagon, wheelchair, or stretcher for transport. The nurse assists the patient into the car seat or assists in fastening seatbelts. Charting includes when and with whom the patient departed, patient's behavior (smiling, alert, crying, and so on), method of transportation from the division, patient's weight, and any instructions or medications given to the patient or parents.

HOME CARE

Many teenagers with acute and chronic conditions are being cared for in the home. Home health care and other community agencies work together to provide holistic care. *Respite care* provides trained workers who come into the home for brief periods to relieve parents of the responsibility of caring for the child. This enables the parents to shop, do business transactions, or simply take a much-needed vacation. The school systems also share in the responsibility of care, which is crucial if a family is to be successful in home care. The health care worker assisting in the home should:

- Observe how the parents interact with the child.
- Observe facial expressions and body language.
- Post signs above the bed denoting special considerations, such as "Never position on left side" and "Do not feed with plastic spoon."
- Listen to the parents and observe how they attend to the physical needs of the youngster.
- Do not be afraid to ask questions or discuss apprehensions the parents may have about their ability to care for the child.
- Be attuned to the needs of other children in the home.
- Be creative in exploring avenues for socialization, as these children are seldom invited to birthday or slumber parties.
- Explore community facilities or support groups that might benefit the family.

KEY POINTS

- The care of sick children can take place in a variety of settings.
- Play is an important part of a nursing care plan for children.
- Nursing care plans for hospitalized children should include measures to minimize negative impact on growth and development.
- Three major causes of stress for children of all ages are separation, pain, and fear of bodily harm.
- Separation anxiety is most pronounced in the toddler.
- The three stages of separation anxiety are protest, despair, and detachment.
- When a school-age child requires hospitalization, a school, home, or hospital teacher should be requested by the nurse to prevent loss of grade status.
- Nurses caring for children must maintain a high level of suspicion for pain because children are often unable to verbalize discomfort.
- Techniques such as drawing, distraction, imagery, relaxation, and cognitive strategies as well as analgesia provide relief from pain.
- A culturally sensitive attitude toward families with hospitalized children decreases anxiety.
- Avoid treatments in the playroom.
- The surgical patient needs to be shown the part of the body that will be operated on. Children are assured that this is the only area of the body that will be involved.
- Respecting the confidentiality of the teenager is important to establishing trust.
- The pediatric nursing care plan is the result of the nursing process applied to the child.
- Clinical Pathways are a multidisciplinary plan of care with outcome goals that involve timelines.
- The developmental level of the child influences specific needs during the hospitalization experience.
- The age, sex, developmental level, and diagnosis of the child are factors that influence placement on a unit.
- Discharge planning begins on the day of admission.

MULTIPLE-CHOICE REVIEW QUESTIONS

Choose the most appropriate answer.

1. The stages of separation anxiety in the toddler are
   a. protest, despair, denial.
   b. denial, dependence, submission.
   c. protest, sadness, despair.
   d. despair, anxiety, regression.
2. An object such as a blanket or favorite toy is referred to as
   a. a transitory item.
   b. a transitional object.
   c. a transitional task.
   d. a cuddly.
3. The best way to minimize separation anxiety in a hospitalized infant is to
   a. explain routines carefully.
   b. encourage parent to room-in.
   c. provide age-appropriate roommates.
   d. provide an age-appropriate toy.
4. Which of the following statements by the parent of a hospitalized 4-year-old child indicates an understanding of the child's needs?
   a. "I am going to buy him a box of new toys to keep him busy while in the hospital."
   b. "I am going to bring some of his favorite toys from home for him to play with while in the hospital."
   c. "I'm glad there is a television in the room for him to watch all day."
   d. "I will stay every day until he falls asleep and then I will go home."
5. A 4-year-old hospitalized child wets his bed. The parents tell the nurse that the child was completely toilet trained. The nurse should understand that
   a. the parents are denying a problem exists.
   b. the child may be developmentally delayed.
   c. the child may be experiencing regression.
   d. the child is probably "punishing" the parents.

BIBLIOGRAPHY AND READER REFERENCE

Behrman, R. E., & Kleigman, R. (1998). *Nelson's essentials of pediatrics* (3rd ed.). Philadelphia: Saunders.

Beyea, S. (1996). *Critical pathways for collaborative nursing care.* Philadelphia: Saunders.

Coyne, I. (1995). Partnership in care: Parents' view of participation in their hospitalized child's care. *Journal of Clinical Nursing, 4*(2), 71–79.

French, G. M., Painter, E., & Courty, D. (1994). Blowing away shot pain: A technique for pain management during immunization. *Pediatrics, 93*(3), 384–388.

Ignatavicius, D., & Hausman, K. (1995). *Clinical pathways for collaborative practice.* Philadelphia: Saunders.

Kachoyeanos, M., & Friedhoff, M. (1993). Cognitive and behavioral strategies to reduce children's pain. *MCN: American Journal of Maternal Child Nursing, 18,* 14–19.

Maikler, V. (1998). Pharmacologic pain management in children. A review of intervention research. *Journal of Pediatrics Nursing, 1*(1), 3.

McCarthy, A., Cool, V., & Hanrahan, K. (1998). Cognitive behavioral interventions in children during painful procedures: Research challenges and program development. *Journal of Pediatric Nursing, 13*(1), 55.

Terndrup, T. (1996). Pediatric pain control. *Annals in Emergency Medicine, 27*(4), 466–470.

Tester, M., Holzemer, W., & Savedra, M. (2/98). Pain behaviors: Postsurgical responses of children and adolescents. *Journal of Pediatrics Nursing, 13*(1), 41.

Wong, D. (1997). *Whaley & Wong's essentials of pediatric nursing.* (5th ed.). St. Louis, MO: Mosby.

Wilkenson, J. (1996). *Nursing process: A critical thinking approach.* Reading, MA: Addison-Wesley.

chapter 22

Health Care Adaptations for the Child and Family

Outline

Objectives

On completion and mastery of Chapter 22, the student will be able to

- Define each vocabulary term listed.
- List five safety measures applicable to the care of the hospitalized child.
- Describe the principles for using restraints for children.
- Devise a nursing care plan for a child with a fever.
- Position an infant for a lumbar puncture.
- Contrast the administration of medicines to children and adults.
- Discuss two nursing responsibilities necessary when a child is receiving parenteral fluids and the rationale for each.
- Summarize the care of a child receiving oxygen.
- List the adaptations necessary when preparing a pediatric patient for surgery.
- Illustrate techniques of transporting infants and children.
- Plan the basic daily assessment of hospitalized infants and children.

(Continued)

Objectives (Continued)

- Identify the normal vital signs of infants and children at various ages.
- Discuss the technique of obtaining urine and stool specimens from infants.
- Demonstrate techniques of administering oral, eye, and ear medications to infants and children.
- Compare the preferred sites for intramuscular injection for infants and adults.
- Discuss pain management in infants and children.
- Calculate dosage of a medicine that is in liquid form.

Vocabulary

auscultation	mummy restraint
Broviac catheter	nomogram
BSA	O.D.
clean catch	O.S.
conscious sedation	O.U.
deltoid	parenteral
dimensional analysis	patient-controlled analgesia
dorsogluteal	phototoxicity
drops	subcutaneous
elixir	TPN
gastrostomy button	tracheostomy
heparin lock	tympanic thermometer
intramuscular	vastus lateralis
low-flow oxygen	venous access devices
lumbar puncture	ventrogluteal
mist tent	

ADMISSION TO THE PEDIATRIC UNIT

Informed Consent

When the child is admitted to the pediatric unit, a written *informed consent* is obtained for treatments that are given. An informed consent implies that the parent or legal guardian is capable of understanding information given to them, including the purpose and risks of the procedure, and voluntarily agrees to that procedure. The consent must be signed by the parent, the doctor who provides the information, and a witness. The nurse acts as a patient advocate in ensuring proper consent has been signed before a procedure and that the child is also given age-appropriate information concerning what to expect.

Identification

Every child admitted to the pediatric unit must have an identification bracelet applied. The identification (ID) of the patient should be checked before medications are administered or treatments carried out. Often a bracelet that was applied on admission will be taken off by the child or may fall off. Identification should be verified and a new bracelet reapplied (Fig. 22–1). The bracelet should be snug enough to prevent voluntary removal by the child.

Essential Safety Measures in the Hospital Setting

The nurse must be especially conscious of safety measures on the children's division. *Accidents are a major cause of death among infants and children.* By demonstrating concern about safety regulations, the nurse not only reduces unnecessary accidents

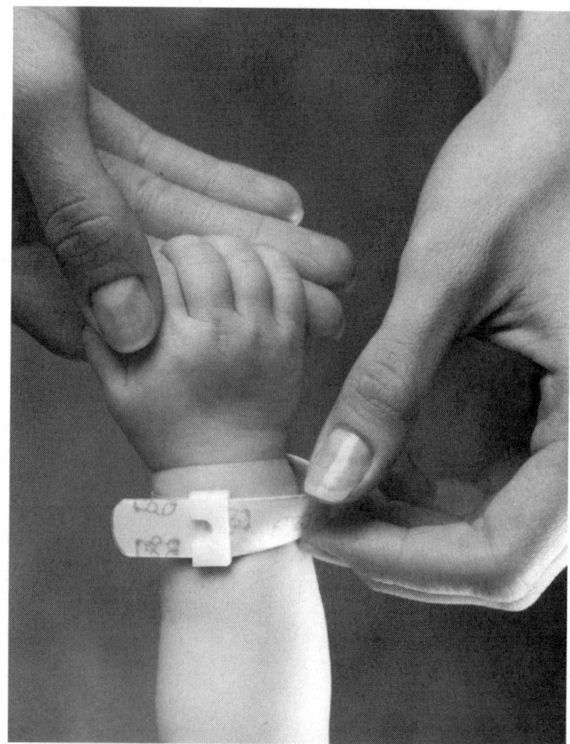

Figure 22–1. • ID bracelet. All hospitalized children must have an identification bracelet that is checked prior to administering medications or providing care. (Courtesy of Precision Dynamics Corporation, San Fernando, CA.)

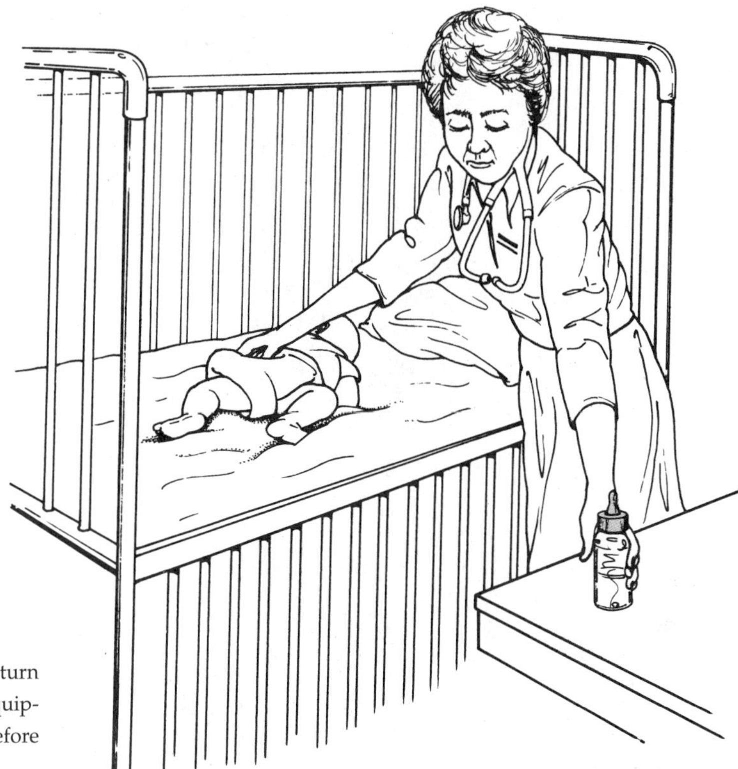

Figure 22–2. • Maintain hand contact if you must turn your back on the infant or toddler. If you need equipment that is out of reach, raise the side of the crib before leaving the infant or child.

but also sets a good example for parents. Although the physical layout of each institution cannot be altered by personnel, many simple safety measures can be carried out by the entire hospital team. The following is a list of measures applicable to the children's unit.

DOs

- Keep crib sides up at all times when the patient is unattended in bed (Fig. 22–2).
- Wash your hands before and after caring for each patient.
- Identify child by bracelet, not room number.
- Check wheelchairs and stretchers for flaws before placing patients in them.
- Use a bubble-top or plastic-topped crib for infants and children capable of climbing over the crib rails (Fig. 22–3).
- Place cribs so that children cannot reach sockets and appliances.
- Inspect toys for sharp edges and removable parts.
- Apply restraints correctly to prevent constriction of a part.
- Keep medications and solutions out of reach of the child.
- Lock the medication cabinet when not in use.
- Identify the patient properly before giving medications.
- Keep powder, lotions, tissues, baby wipes, disposable diapers, safety pins, and so on out of infant's reach.
- Remain with the small child while taking the temperature.
- Prevent cross-infection. Diapers, toys, and materials that belong in one patient's unit should not be borrowed for another patient's use.
- Restrain children in highchairs.
- Take proper precautions when oxygen is in use.
- Handle infants and small children carefully. Use elevators rather than stairs. Walk at the child's pace.
- Locate fire exits and extinguishers on your unit and learn how to use them properly. Become familiar with your hospital's fire manual.

DON'Ts

- Don't prop nursing bottles or force-feed small children. There is danger of choking.
- Don't allow ambulatory patients to use wheelchairs or stretchers as toys.
- Don't remove dressings or bandages unless specifically instructed.
- Don't leave an active child in a baby swing, feeding table, or highchair unattended.
- Don't leave a small child unattended when out of the crib.

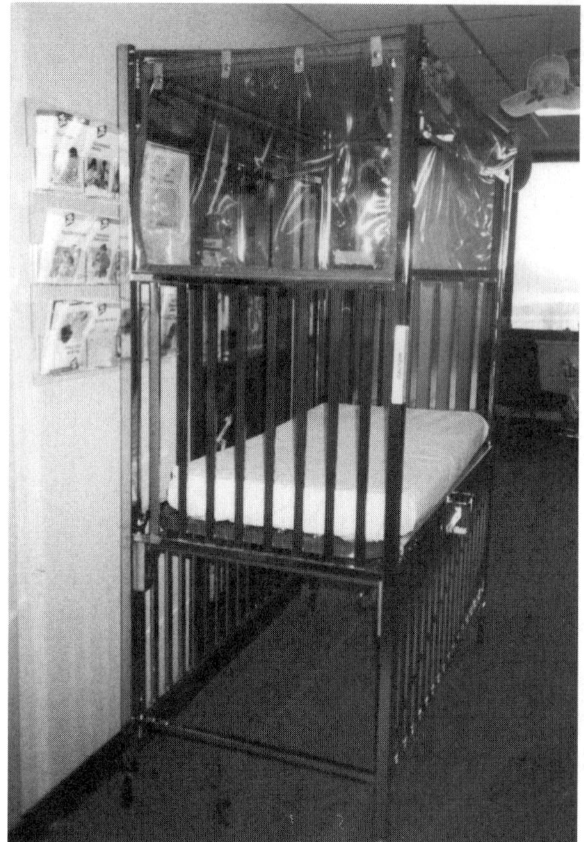

Figure 22–3. • One type of crib used in the hospital to protect toddlers and small children from falls. (Courtesy of Columbia/HA Portsmouth Regional Hospital, Portsmouth, NH.)

- Remain with the child who uses the bathtub.
- Don't leave medications at the bedside.

Many other safety measures must be carried out as each nurse becomes more familiar with the hazards of individual units. Nurses must use their eyes to see with, not just to look at, and then must take the necessary precautions.

Transporting, Positioning, and Restraining the Infant

The means by which the child is transported within the unit and to other parts of the hospital depends on age, level of consciousness, and how far one has to travel. Older children are transported in the same way as adults. Younger children are often transported in their cribs, in a wagon or wheelchair, or on a stretcher. The side rails on a stretcher are raised during transport. The nurse ensures that the patient's identification band is secured before leaving the division. A notation is made as to where the child is being taken and for what purpose.

Figure 22–4 depicts three safe methods for holding a baby. Head and back support are necessary for young infants. The movements of small children are often random and uncoordinated; therefore, they must be held securely. The football hold is useful when one hand needs to be free, such as for bathing the baby's head. Box 22–1 lists the principles for using restraints for children.

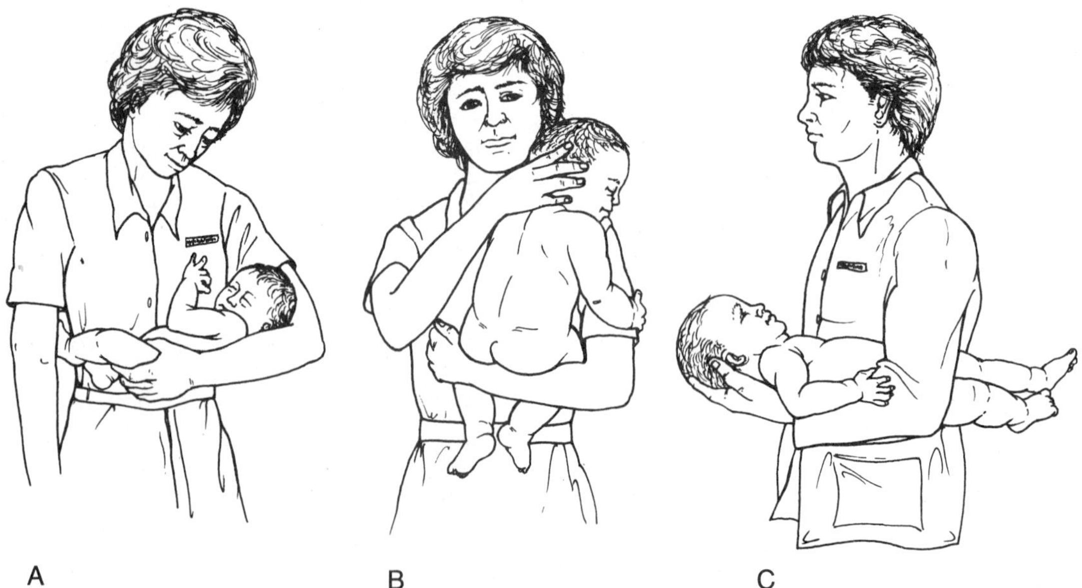

Figure 22–4. • **A,** The cradle position. **B,** The upright position. **C,** The football position.

BOX 22–1

PRINCIPLES OF USING RESTRAINTS FOR CHILDREN

Restraints may be used for infants and children to facilitate examinations or treatments and to maintain safety. The reason for the restraint must be explained to the parents and the child. Restraints are used *only when necessary, are not a substitute for close observation and should involve the fewest joints possible* in order to enable free movement that is necessary for growth and development. Excessive restraints can result in the infant or child fighting the restraint, thereby wasting energy and increasing oxygen consumption needs. Parents should be taught the importance of fastening safety straps on infants who are in highchairs, shopping carts and infant seats.

The Mummy Restraint

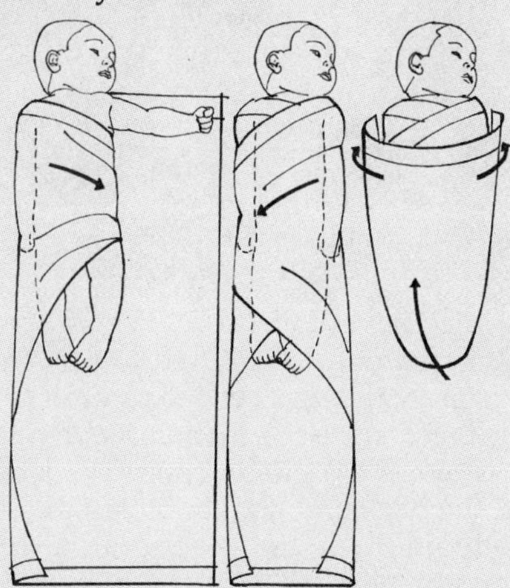

(From Leifer, G. [1982]. *Principles and techniques in pediatric nursing*, 4th ed. Philadelphia: Saunders, p. 78.)

- Place a small light blanket flat on the bed with the top at infant's shoulders.
- Fold the blanket over the body and under the arm at the opposite side, tucking in the excess under the infant.
- Place the other arm at the side, and fold the blanket over the body tucking the excess under the infant. The weight of the infant holds the restraint in place.
- Separate the bottom of the blanket, fold upward toward the shoulder, tucking the sides under the infant's body.

The arms should be in anatomical position. This restraint provides a feeling of snug security for the infant. It may be used for jugular venipunctures, nasogastric tube insertion and other procedures.

The Elbow Restraint

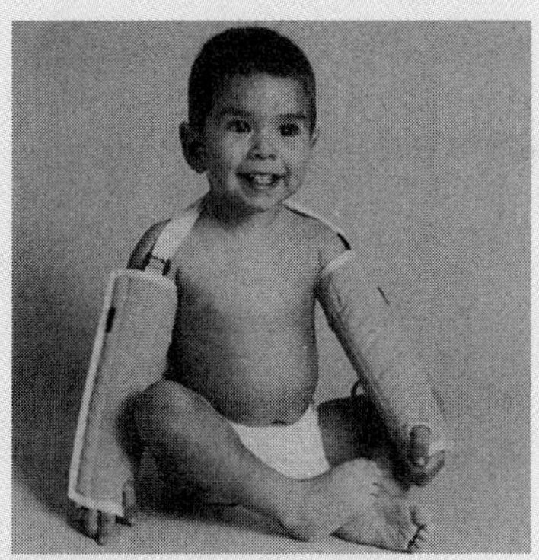

(Courtesy of Medi-Kid Co., Hemet, CA.)

The elbow restraint prevents flexion of the elbow but otherwise allows free movement. It is used during treatments such as scalp vein infusions, during post-op cleft lip surgery or to prevent scratching in children with skin lesions. It is well tolerated by infants and children. The restraint should be removed frequently for range of motion exercise of the joint and assessment for brachial nerve injury. A neurovascular check of the fingers should document color, warmth, movement, sensation, and pulse at frequent intervals.

Box continued on following page

ASSESSING THE CHILD

Children are different from adults both anatomically and physiologically. A nursing assessment is done to determine the level of wellness, the response to medication or treatment, or the need for referral.

The Basic Assessment

The *basic assessment* involves casual observation without touching. The child's general appearance will indicate if he is seriously ill or within normal limits. Generally, if the child is not alert and responsive to the environment, serious illness may be

BOX 22-1

PRINCIPLES OF USING RESTRAINTS FOR CHILDREN *(Continued)*

Clove Hitch Restraint

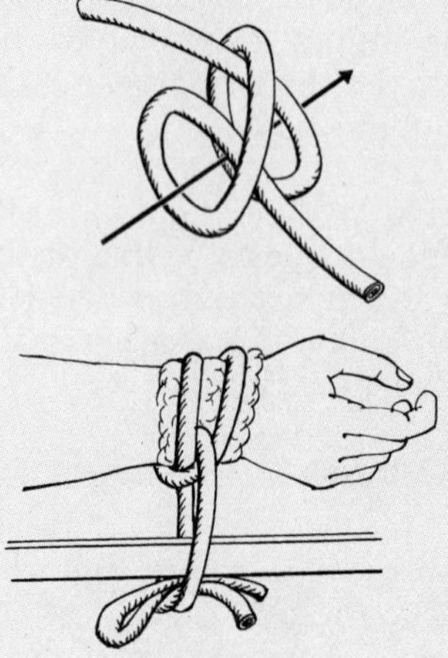

(From Leifer, G. [1982]. *Principles and techniques in pediatric nursing*, 4th ed. Philadelphia: Saunders, p. 81.)

The clove hitch restraint is used to restrain one or more limbs, usually for the prevention of self injury. The clove hitch knot will not tighten and impair circulation as the child pulls against the restraint, if it is applied properly. Padding the skin is essential. Frequent release, range of motion exercise and assessment of the skin should be documented. The arrow shows the loops that are placed together before the wrist is inserted. The ends should be tied to the mattress spring and not the crib sides to avoid excessive pressure if the cribside is lowered.

Jacket Restraint

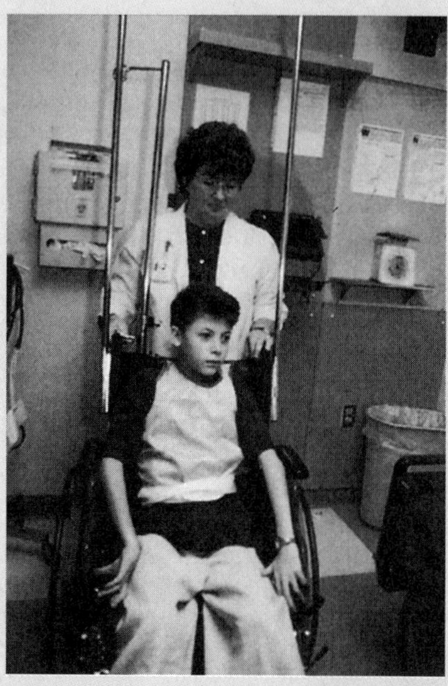

(From Bowden, V. R., Dickey, S. B., Greenberg, C. S. [1998]. *Children and their families: The continuum of care.* Philadelphia: Saunders, p. 489.)

The jacket restraint can be used to prevent the child from crawling over the siderail of the bed or highchair or to maintain body alignment when in bryants traction. The jacket ties in the back and should be secured to the bedframes and not the bedrail to prevent excess tightening if the bedrail is lowered. Infants and children can wriggle out of the jacket restraint and therefore must be watched closely to avoid injury. Frequent changes of position are necessary to prevent complications of prolonged immobility.

suspected. If the child is lethargic, prompt intervention by a physician or health care provider is essential. Applying knowledge of basic growth and development will enable the nurse to determine whether the activities and behavior of the child are age-appropriate. A child who has not mastered age-appropriate milestones should be referred for follow-up care. The presence of bruises on the body of the child that may be in different stages of healing, the lack of body cleanliness or appropriate dress, and the interaction or lack of interaction between parent and child are also areas that may require prompt referral for follow-up care. Is the child tipping his head? Rubbing the ears? Is the child maintaining a rigid body position to breathe? To avoid movement of an extremity? Is the child coughing, wheezing, vomiting? Is the skin pale, flushed, or cyanotic? Are there signs of respiratory distress, such as flaring of the nares, substernal or intercostal retractions, rapid respiratory rate? If stridor or grunting sounds are heard during respiration, prompt referral should be made.

The History Assessment

The *history assessment* affords the nurse the opportunity to teach parents about the child's needs and prevention of injury and illness. The immunization record should be reviewed and plans for future immunizations discussed. Encouraging safe environment that includes the use of car seats and protective gear for sports activities should be part of every teaching plan.

The Physical Assessment

The *physical assessment* includes a head-to-toe assessment that should be completed, at minimum, once each shift, or once each clinic visit, even if the clinic visit is for a specific problem. Assessment of vital signs is a priority. Often the first sign of shock or body stress in infants or children is tachycardia (a rapid heartbeat). However, a fall in blood pressure may be a *late* sign of shock in children because of a compensatory mechanism that is activated early. Therefore, hypotension in an infant or child is considered an acute emergency. Extreme irritability or pupils that are unequal in response to light should be reported immediately. The anterior fontanel, which is usually open until 18 months of age, should be palpated. A *sunken* fontanel may indicate dehydration, whereas a *bulging* fontanel indicates increased intracranial pressure (ICP). A fontanel that feels *flat* to the contour of the head is normal. Increased intracranial pressure in the older child and adult is manifested by a rise in systolic blood pressure and a widening pulse pressure, irregular respirations, and bradycardia. In the infant, however, the open fontanels allow for brain swelling to occur without these classic signs and a decreased level of consciousness may be the only manifestation of ICP.

Bradycardia (a slow heartbeat) is always treated as a medical emergency in infants and young children. Unlike adults, infants and children cannot increase the stroke volume of their heart for a more effective cardiac output when the heart slows and must rely on increased rate alone to increase output. Therefore, fatigue and heart failure may result. Mottling of the skin of the extremities may be normal in infants because of their immature temperature control mechanisms. Maintaining warmth during assessment is essential for infants. Because of their large body surface area and high metabolic rate they are prone to fluid loss and hypothermia as well as cold stress.

An accurate weight should be recorded (Chapter 12, Fig. 12–11) because the dosage of medications for infants and children are prescribed based by milligram per kilogram weight. The temperature of infants may be taken via axilla, or in the ear (Fig. 22–6). Fever is defined as a temperature over 100.4° F (38° C) in infants under 3 months or above 100° F (37° C) in children over 3 months.

Because dehydration is a problem in infants and young children, assessment of skin turgor (Chapter 12, Fig. 12–13) is part of any total assessment. The lungs should be clear to auscultation and the chest should move symmetrically. Bowel sounds should be active in all four quadrants and the abdomen should not be distended or tender to palpation. The skin should be observed for rashes or lesions.

Pulse and Respirations

The nurse counting a pulse feels the wave of blood as it is forced through the artery. The pulse rate varies considerably in different children of the same age and size. The pulse rate and respiratory rate of the newborn are high (Tables 22–1 and 22–2). Both pulse and respiratory rates gradually slow down with age until adult values are reached.

The pulse of the older child is taken just like that of an adult. Apical pulses are advised for children under age 5 years. The apical pulse is heard through a stethoscope at the apex of the heart. The

Table 22–1
AVERAGE PULSE RATES AT REST

Age	Lower Limits of Normal (Per Minute)		Average (Per Minute)		Upper Limits of Normal (Per Minute)	
Newborn	70		125		190	
1–11 mo	80		120		160	
2 yr	80		110		130	
4 yr	80		100		120	
6 yr	75		100		115	
8 yr	70		90		110	
10 yr	70		90		110	
	Girls	**Boys**	**Girls**	**Boys**	**Girls**	**Boys**
12 yr	70	65	90	85	110	105
14 yr	65	60	85	80	105	100
16 yr	60	55	80	75	100	95
18 yr	55	50	75	70	95	90

From Behrman, R. E., & Kliegman, R., Arvin S., (1996). *Nelson's textbook of pediatrics* (15th ed.). Philadelphia: Saunders.

Table 22–2
NORMAL RESPIRATORY RANGES FOR CHILDREN

Age	Rate per Minute
Birth to 1 mo	30–40
1 mo to 1 yr	26–40
1–2 yr	20–30
2–6 yr	20–30
6–10 yr	18–24
Adolescent	16–24

nurse counts the rate for 1 full minute. Another common site is the radial pulse (at the thumb side of the wrist just above the radial artery). The temporal pulse may be assessed if the child is asleep. Actually, the pulse may be assessed in any area where a large artery lies close to the skin, especially if the artery runs across a bone and has little soft tissue around it. The following are the most common sites: radial, temporal (just in front of the ear), mandibular (on the lower jawbone), femoral (in the groin), and carotid (on each side of the front of the neck). The carotid pulse may not be appropriate in infants with chubby necks.

The child's respirations are counted in the same way as the adult's. For 1 minute the nurse notes the number of times the chest or abdomen rises and falls. The rate and character of respirations are important in determining the patient's general condition.

Blood Pressure

Blood pressure is defined as the pressure of the blood on the walls of the arteries. It is an index of elasticity of arterial walls, peripheral vascular resistance, efficiency of the heart as a pump, and blood volume. Common sites for measuring blood pressure in children are the brachial artery, popliteal artery, and posterior tibial artery (Fig. 22–5). There are several old and new methods for measuring blood pressure in newborns and children.

Auscultation. This is done as for an adult, but with a pediatric stethoscope and cuff. The cuff should be long enough to encircle the extremity. The width of the cuff should cover two-thirds of the upper arm. The following sizes are suggested: birth to 1 year, 1½ inches; 2–8 years, 3 inches; 8–12 years, 4 inches. Pressure is normally higher in the lower extremities. The American Heart Association designates the muffled tone as the most accurate index of diastolic pressure but recommends recording both that and the final distinct sound as the complete record; thus 120/80/78. Nurses should clarify this with the physician or the institution employed to ensure uniformity. To determine *pulse pressure,* the diastolic reading is subtracted from the systolic. This usually varies from 20 to 50 mm Hg. Widening pulse pressure may be a sign of increased intracranial pressure.

Palpation. Palpation is one of the oldest methods. The cuff is applied and inflated above the expected pressure. The fingers are placed over the brachial or radial artery. The systolic pressure is recorded at the point when the pulse reappears. Diastolic pressure is unobtainable. This method is useful in newborns.

Electronic or Ultrasonographic (Doppler) Measurement. This is a noninvasive type of blood pressure monitoring that ultrasonically detects motion of the arterial wall. A transducer with an attached cuff is secured over an artery, usually the brachial,

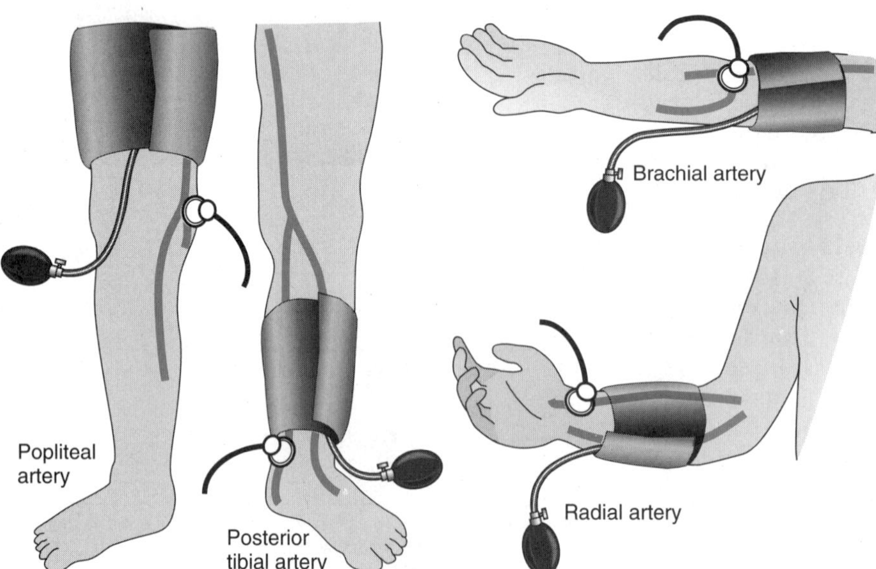

Figure 22–5. • Common sites for measuring blood pressure in children: brachial artery; popliteal artery; posterior tibial artery. Blood pressure may be taken with a manometer and stethoscope or by oscillometry (dinamap) using a cuff with a sensor connected to a machine that provides a digital readout of the blood pressure. A stethoscope is not necessary when this method is used.

femoral, or popliteal. The cuff is inflated above systolic pressure and then gradually reduced. The transducer transmits vascular sounds, and the measurement appears on a digital readout. Both systolic and diastolic pressure are recorded. Electronic blood pressure machines do not require auscultation with a stethoscope. A cuff is applied, the machine is turned on, and a digital reading is obtained usually in less than 1 minute.

Some hospitals require blood pressure measurements for all children and others only for the older child. The nurse explains what is about to happen, for example, "This will hug your arm and feel tight for a few seconds." The child is allowed to examine the sphygmomanometer and cuff.

Blood pressure is lower in children than in adults. If a patient needs to have blood pressure measurements taken throughout hospitalization, the nurse observes the previous readings before charting the current one. Many factors account for variations in blood pressure. Included are time of day, sex, age, exercise, pain, and emotion. A blood pressure taken when a child is frightened or crying is not accurate. If a significant change is observed, recheck the blood pressure. Abnormal readings are charted and reported to the nurse in charge. Tables 22–3 and 22–4 show normal blood pressure readings for boys and girls (ages 1–18).

Temperature

Body temperature measurement can be oral, rectal, axillary, or tympanic. There are several types of thermometers. The electronic thermometer, the plastic strip thermometer, and the tympanic membrane sensor are commonly used in the pediatric unit. The electronic thermometer works quickly and is ideal because the plastic sheath is unbreakable. The plastic strip changes color according to sensed temperature changes. Tympanic thermometers (Fig. 22–6) have a blunt tip that is covered with a disposable cover and can be inserted into the ear. It records temperature from the tympanic membrane (eardrum) by an infrared emission. This site is of importance because both the hypothalamus (temperature-regulating center) and the eardrum are perfused by the same circulation.

Oral Temperature. The procedure is the same as for adults.

Rectal Temperature. The patient is placed in a comfortable position, either on the side with the knees slightly flexed or on the stomach. Infants may be in the supine position with their legs firmly held around the ankles. This is not recommended for toddlers because they are stronger and the feet are in a good kicking position. Insert the lubricated thermometer a maximum of 1 inch. Electronic thermometers register within 15 seconds or less. The rectal temperature is taken last because it may make the child cry, which influences pulse rate, respiratory rate, and blood pressure. Because this is an intrusive procedure with risk of injury as well as cross-contamination, *most institutions use only axillary or tympanic temperatures for children unless contraindicated.* Table 22–5 shows normal temperature ranges.

Table 22–3
NORMAL BLOOD PRESSURE READINGS FOR BOYS

	Systolic Blood Pressure Percentile					Diastolic Blood Pressure Percentile				
Age in Years	**5th**	**10th**	**50th**	**90th**	**95th**	**5th**	**10th**	**50th**	**90th**	**95th**
1	71	76	90	105	109	39	43	56	69	73
2	72	76	91	106	110	39	43	56	68	72
3	73	77	92	107	111	39	42	55	68	72
4	74	79	93	108	112	39	43	56	69	72
5	76	80	95	109	113	40	43	56	69	73
6	77	81	96	111	115	41	44	57	70	74
7	78	83	97	112	116	42	45	58	71	75
8	80	84	99	114	118	43	47	60	73	76
9	82	86	101	115	120	44	48	61	74	78
10	84	88	102	117	121	45	49	62	75	79
11	86	90	105	119	123	47	50	63	76	80
12	88	92	107	121	126	48	51	64	77	81
13	90	94	109	124	128	45	49	63	77	81
14	93	97	112	126	131	46	50	64	78	82
15	95	99	114	129	133	47	51	65	79	83
16	98	102	117	131	136	49	53	67	81	85
17	100	104	119	134	138	51	55	69	83	87
18	102	106	121	136	140	52	56	70	84	88

From the Second Task Force on Blood Pressure Control in Children, National Heart, Lung and Blood Institute, Bethesda, MD. Tabular data prepared by Dr. B. Rosner, 1987.

Table 22–4
NORMAL BLOOD PRESSURE READINGS FOR GIRLS

Age in Years	Systolic Blood Pressure Percentile					Diastolic Blood Pressure Percentile				
	5th	10th	50th	90th	95th	5th	10th	50th	90th	95th
1	72	76	91	105	110	38	41	54	67	71
2	71	76	90	105	109	40	43	56	69	73
3	72	76	91	106	110	40	43	56	69	73
4	73	78	92	107	111	40	43	56	69	73
5	75	79	94	109	113	40	43	56	69	73
6	77	81	96	111	115	40	44	57	70	74
7	78	83	97	112	116	41	45	58	71	75
8	80	84	99	114	118	43	46	59	72	76
9	81	86	100	115	119	44	48	61	74	77
10	83	87	102	117	121	46	49	62	75	79
11	86	90	105	119	123	47	51	64	77	81
12	88	92	107	122	126	49	53	66	78	82
13	90	94	109	124	128	46	50	64	78	82
14	92	96	110	125	129	49	53	67	81	85
15	93	97	111	126	130	49	53	67	82	86
16	93	97	112	127	131	49	53	67	81	85
17	93	98	112	127	131	48	52	66	80	84
18	94	98	112	127	131	48	52	66	80	84

From the Second Task Force on Blood Pressure Control in Children, National Heart, Lung and Blood Institute, Bethesda, MD. Tabular data prepared by Dr. B. Rosner, 1987.

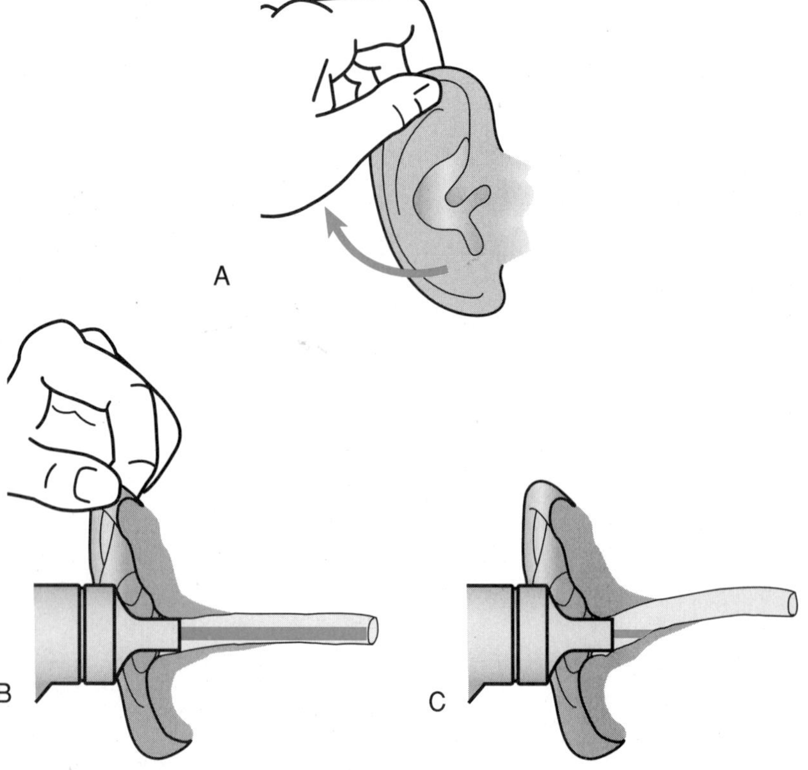

Figure 22–6. • **A,** Pulling the pinna of the ear up and back before inserting the ear thermometer in children over 3 years of age. **B,** Straightens the auditory canal so that the infrared ray reaches the tympanic membrane. **C,** If the auditory canal is not straightened, the infrared ray will reach the walls of the ear canal providing an inaccurate *body* temperature.

Table 22–5
NORMAL TEMPERATURE RANGES FOR CHILDREN

Method	Range
Oral	36.4–37.4°C (97.6–99.3°F)
Rectal	37.0–37.8°C (98.6–100.0°F)
Axillary	35.8–36.6°C (96.6–98.0°F)
Ear	36.9–37.5°C (98.4–99.5°F)

Axillary Temperature. Axillary temperatures are usually taken on newborns and/or according to unit policy. The thermometer is held in the axilla with the baby's arm pressed against the side. Traditionally, an axillary temperature is considered 1° F lower than an oral temperature. The nurse always records the route used.

Assessing Body Temperature. The tympanic thermometer measures core body temperature by detecting the infrared energy emitted from the tympanic membrane. (Core body temperature is the estimated temperature of the internal body organs.) The tympanic temperature is generally 0.2 to 1.2° C lower than the rectal temperature. The tympanic technique is accurate for all ages. However, some brands of tympanic thermometers have ear probes that do not fit well into the auditory canal of infants under 3 months of age. These thermometers should be used for infants over 3 months of age. Gently pulling the pinna (earlobe) down and back in infants *under 3* years of age and slightly up and back in children, straightens the auditory canal and provides a more accurate temperature reading. The probe of the thermometer should be aimed at the opposite eyebrow. The accuracy of the tympanic temperature is not affected by illness such as otitis media. A table of Celsius and Fahrenheit temperature equivalents appears in Appendix E.

Weight

Weight must be accurately recorded on admission (Chap. 12, Fig. 12–11). The weight of a patient provides a means of determining progress and is necessary to determine the dosage of certain medications. The way in which the nurse weighs the child depends on the age.

The infant is weighed completely naked in a warm room. A fresh diaper chux or scale paper is placed on the scale. This prevents cross-contamination, that is, the spread of germs from one infant to another. The scale is balanced to compensate for the weight of the diaper. The infant is placed gently on the scale. The nurse's left hand is held slightly above the infant to prevent falling. Once the exact weight appears on the digital readout, the infant is removed from the scale, wrapped in a blanket, and soothed. The weight is immediately recorded. The scale paper is disposed of in the proper receptacle.

The older child is weighed in the same manner as an adult. A paper towel is placed on the scale for the patient to stand on. The patient is generally weighed in a hospital gown. The shoes are removed. If the child is unable to stand on the scales, it may be necessary for the nurse to hold the child and read the combined weights. The nurse is then weighed and subtracts that number from the combined weight to obtain the patient's weight. Occasionally, a child is weighed while wearing a cast. The nurse records this as, for example, "weight 34 pounds with cast on right arm." It is often desirable to record the weight in pounds as well as kilograms. Some parents find pounds a more familiar term. Kilograms is used to calculate safe dosages of medications.

Height

The child's height is measured along with weight. The infant's height must be measured while the infant is lying on a flat surface alongside a metal tape measure or yardstick. The knees should be pressed flat on the table. The measurement is taken from the top of the head to the heels and recorded (see Chapter 15, Fig. 15–2).

Head Circumference

Head circumference increases rapidly during infancy as a result of brain growth. It is generally measured on infants and toddlers and on all children with neurologic defects. The tape measure is placed around the head slightly above the eyebrows and ears and around the occipital prominence of the skull (see Chapter 12, Fig. 12–4). The measurement is recorded.

COLLECTING SPECIMENS

Urine Specimens

A urine specimen is obtained from the newly admitted patient. Certain general principles of collecting specimens are observed:

- Explain the procedure to the patient (as age appropriate).
- Use a clean container or urine collection device.
- Check frequently for results.

- Label all specimens clearly and attach the proper laboratory slip.
- Record in nurses' notes and on intake and output sheet.

Figures 22–7 and 22–8 show how to apply newborn and pediatric urine collectors and how to recover a specimen.

In small infants, a cotton ball may be placed at the opening of the collector. When the infant voids into the cotton ball, the small volume of urine can be retrieved by aspirating the cotton ball with a syringe. Urine collected directly from ultra absorbent disposable diapers may yield inaccurate protein pH and specific gravity measurements because of the chemicals in the diaper.

Obtaining a Clean-Catch Specimen. Special sterile containers are available for *clean-catch* specimens; the manufacturer's directions should be followed. All require cleansing of the perineum with an antiseptic. Rinsing and drying of the perineum are important in order to prevent contamination of urine from the antiseptic. Wiping is done from front to back. After the urine stream has started, the

NURSING CARE PLAN 22–1

Selected Nursing Diagnoses for the Child with a Fever

Nursing Diagnosis: Fluid volume deficit: potential for dehydration due to increased metabolic rate

Goals	Nursing Interventions	Rationale
Child does not become dehydrated as evidenced by good skin turgor, moist mucus membranes, no weight loss	1. Increase fluid intake; offer juice, water, popsicles, yogurt, as age appropriate	1. Body's metabolic rate increases with fever; children have a higher proportion of body water; therefore, more water can be lost rapidly; body systems such as the kidneys are immature at some ages
Child's temperature will be between 36.5 and 37.4° C (97.4 and 99.4° F)	1. Administer tepid sponge bath for fever of 40.0° C (104.0° F)	1. Tepid baths help to reduce fever and may make patient more comfortable
	2. Assess vital signs prior to sponge bath	2. Provides baseline data
	3. Retake vital signs 30 min after procedure	3. Retaking of vital signs will determine if fever is decreasing
	4. Expose skin to air following procedure, prevent shivering	4. Promotes evaporation and cooling of skin
	5. Administer antipyretic medications according to physician's instructions	5. Frequently child with a fever also has a headache and painful joints; antipyretic medications will relieve these discomforts as well as reduce fever
Child does not injure self as evidenced by absence of bruises	1. Keep side rails raised	1. Side rails provide safety from falls
	2. Observe child frequently	2. Frequent observation will detect subtle changes and possibly reduce complications
	3. Remain with child if tub bath is given	3. Threat of drowning is always present with small children and water
Parent understands and verbalizes nature and treatment of fever Parent verbalizes understanding of how to read a thermometer	1. Explain nature of fever (not always bad); too-vigorous control may mask signs of illness	1. Potential benefits of fever have been cited; it is thought to enhance the body's defense mechanisms and to increase antibody activity
Parent verbalizes understanding of potential for convulsion	2. Emphasize removal of clothes when child has fever	2. Removal of clothing cools child
Parent knows how to give appropriate care during a convulsion	3. Call physician if child looks sick or acts in a way different from normal	3. Degree of fever does not always reflect the severity of disease
	4. Demonstrate how to read a thermometer	4. This gives parents a sense of control; accuracy of fever will be ensured on discharge
	5. Discuss with parent potential for convulsion	5. Only a small number of children convulse with fever; however, discussion is advisable
	6. Review management of a convulsion	6. Knowledge allays anxiety
	7. Discourage use of alcohol sponge baths, which may reduce temperature too fast, leading to convulsions	7. Alcohol sponge bath may still be suggested by older relatives
	8. Discourage use of cold water	8. Cold water may cause shivering and raise body temperature

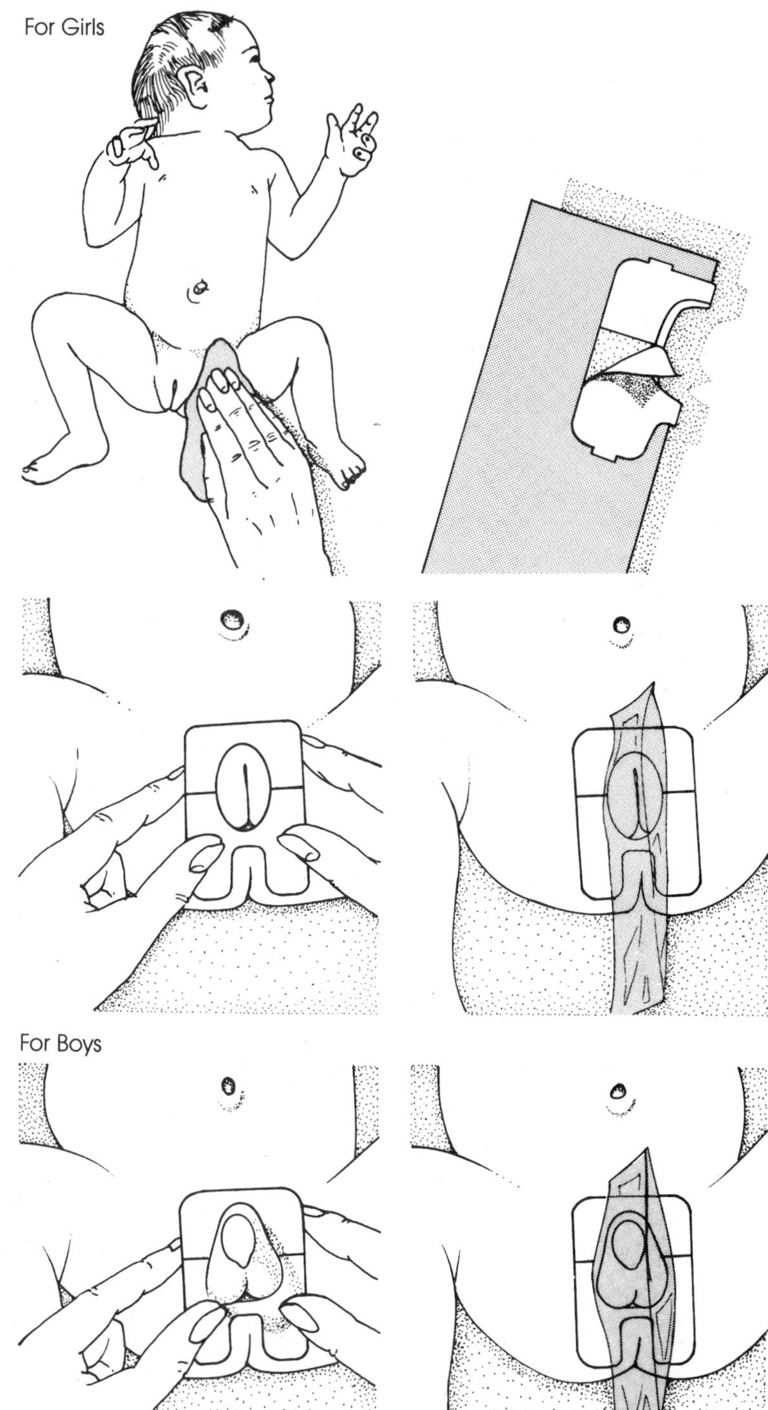

Figure 22–7. • Applying newborn and pediatric urine collectors. Two key points are as follows: (a) The skin must be clean and perfectly dry. Avoid oils, baby powders, and lotion soaps, which may leave a residue on the skin and interfere with the ability of the adhesive to stick. (b) Application must begin on the tiny area of skin between the anus and the genitals. The narrow "bridge" on the adhesive patch keeps feces from contaminating the specimen and helps to position the collector correctly. (Permission to reproduce this copyrighted material has been granted by the owner, Hollister, Inc., Libertyville, IL.)

midstream specimen is caught in the sterile container. The nurse's participation is either direct or supervisory, depending on the child's age or the availability of a parent. Adolescents, who may be embarrassed by carrying a urine specimen through the halls, may be given a bag or other suitable camouflage. The specimen should be sent to the laboratory promptly.

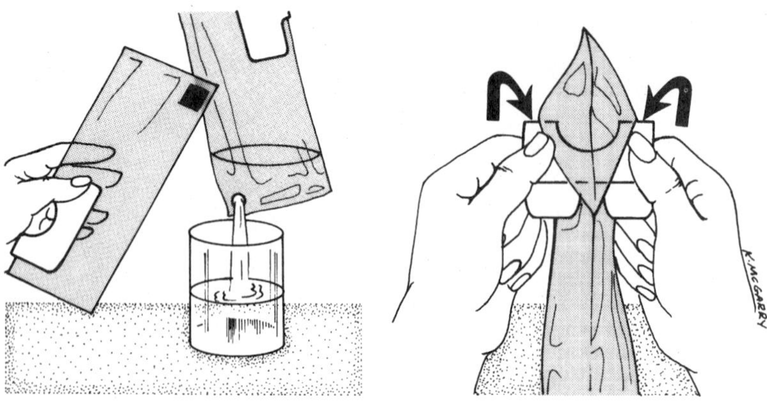

Figure 22–8. • Recovering the specimen. You can drain the urine bag collector into a clean beaker or specimen bottle by removing the tab in the lower corner, or you can seal the specimen inside the collector itself by folding the sticky adhesive sides together. Then place the collector with specimen into a paper or plastic cup. (Permission to reproduce this copyrighted material has been granted by the owner, Hollister, Inc., Libertyville, IL.)

Obtaining a 24-Hour Specimen. At times a 24-hour urine specimen may be requested to determine the rate of urine production and measure the excretion of specific chemicals from the body. The nurses on each shift must closely supervise this test to maintain its accuracy, as lost specimens necessitate restarting the test. Problems can arise if the collection device does not adhere to the skin properly; therefore, the nurse must be alert for this occurrence. Diversions suitable to the child's age are employed. A sign is attached to the infant's crib to alert personnel of a 24-hour urine collection. The average daily amount of urine excreted, by age, is given in Table 22–6.

Testing for Albumin. The nurse working in a doctor's office or clinic may also be requested to test urine for albumin, that is, protein. Normally, little or no albumin is found in the urine of a healthy child. Reagent strips especially intended for this purpose are available. The nurse dips the end of the strip into urine and compares the strip with a special color chart. Specific instructions accompany test materials.

Stool Specimens

Stool specimens are obtained from older children as from adults. This is embarrassing for most children, who are "turned off" by the suggestion. The ambulatory child can use a bedpan placed beneath a toilet seat. It is difficult for a child to tell the nurse that the sample has been collected. The nurse can acknowledge these feelings by giving the child permission to express them without being critical, for example, "I know this must be embarrassing for you. It is for grown-ups too, but we need this because . . ." and so on. An infant's stool specimen can be obtained from the infant directly from the diaper by scraping the specimen from the diaper with a tongue depressor and placing it in the specimen container. Most specimen containers contain a level of liquid. The label indicates a "fill line." The amount of infant stool needed for a specimen is the amount which, when placed into the container, results in the fluid level rising to the "fill line."

Some specimens must be sent to the laboratory while they are warm. The specimen container is labeled properly, placed in a plastic bag, and the laboratory slip is attached. The nurse charts the time, color, amount, and consistency of the stool; the purpose for which it was collected, that is, blood, ova, parasites, or bacteria; and any related information.

Table 22–6
AVERAGE DAILY EXCRETION OF URINE

Age	Fluid Ounces	Milliliters
1st and 2nd days	1–2	30–60
3rd to 10th days	3–10	100–300
10th day to 2 mo	9–15	250–450
2 mo to 1 yr	14–17	400–500
1–3 yr	17–20	500–600
3–5 yr	20–24	600–700
5–8 yr	22–34	650–1000
8–14 yr	27–47	800–1400

Blood Specimens

Positioning the Child. Positioning the child for blood drawings is extremely important. The nurse is often asked to assist in these procedures. Figures 22–9 and 22–10 depict how to position the patient for jugular and femoral venipuncture. Both the jugular and the femoral veins are large; therefore, the patient is frequently checked to ensure that there is no bleeding. These sites are used mainly when other areas have been exhausted. The baby is soothed accordingly, as crying and thrashing may precipitate oozing. The nurse charts the site utilized, name of blood test, and any untoward developments.

Lumbar Puncture

The nurse sometimes assists the physician with a *lumbar puncture,* which is also referred to as a *spinal tap.* It is done to obtain spinal fluid for examination or to reduce pressure within the brain in such conditions as hydrocephalus or meningitis. Disposable lumbar puncture sets are used.

Normal spinal fluid is clear like water. The pressure ranges from 60 to 180 mm Hg. It is somewhat lower in infants. The procedure for children is essentially the same as for adults. The main difference lies in the patient's ability to cooperate with positioning. The nurse explains that the child must lie quietly and will be helped to do this. Sensations during a lumbar puncture include a cool feeling when the skin is cleansed and a feeling of pressure when the needle is inserted. The way in which the child is held can directly affect the success of the procedure.

The patient lies on the side with the back parallel to the side of the treatment table. The knees are flexed, and the head is brought down close to the flexed knees. The nurse can keep the child in this position by placing the child's head in the crook of one arm and the knees in the crook of the other arm. The nurse's hands are then clasped together at the front of the child. The nurse leans forward, gently placing the chest against the patient (Fig. 22–11).

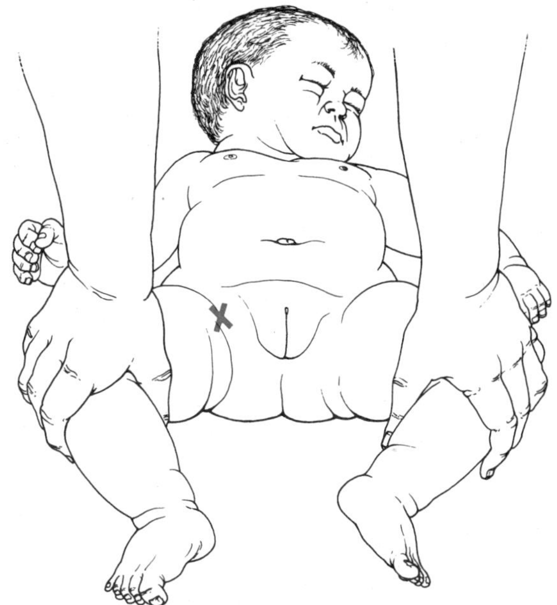

Figure 22–10. • An infant positioned for femoral venipuncture. This position exposes the groin area.

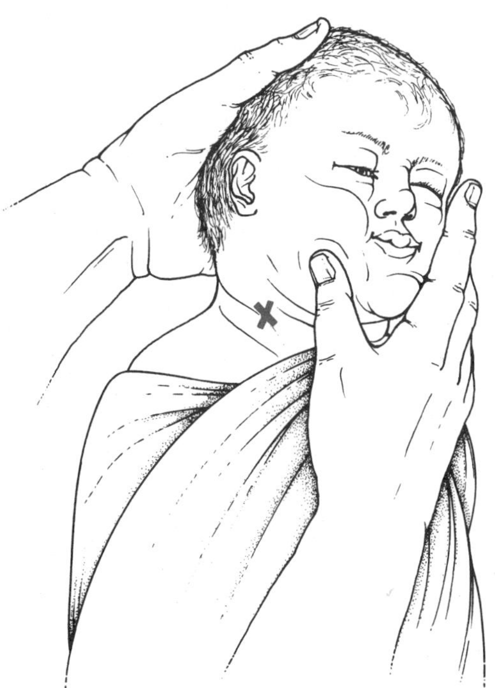

Figure 22–9. • An infant prepared for jugular venipuncture. The head and shoulders are extended over a table or pillow.

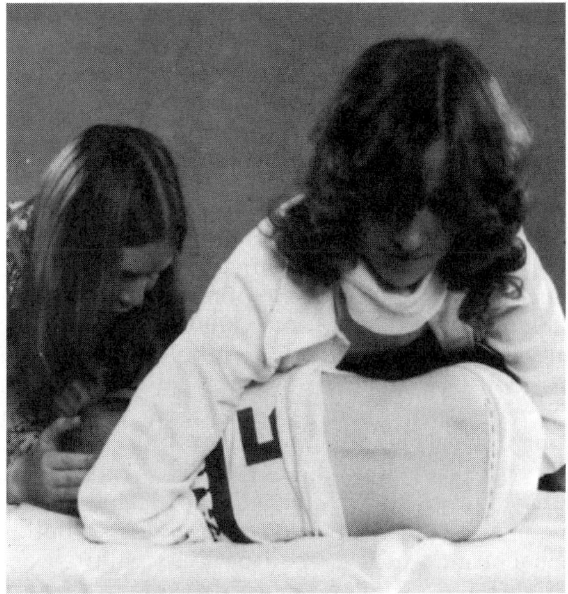

Figure 22–11. • A child positioned for a lumbar puncture. Although the nurse may appear to be placing her weight on the child, the weight is actually placed on the nurse's elbows. If the parents are present during this procedure, they can give the child emotional support. (From Betz, C., Hunsberger, M., & Wright, S. [1994]. *Family-centered nursing care of children* [2nd ed.]. Philadelphia: Saunders.)

Once the child is positioned, the doctor prepares the lower back using sterile technique. A vial of 1% procaine hydrochloride (Novocain) may be necessary unless this is provided in the sterile setup. The top of the vial is cleansed with an alcohol sponge. Once the area has been locally anesthetized, the doctor inserts a special hollow needle into the patient's lower back and collects the spinal fluid in two or three test tubes. When the procedure is completed, a sterile Band-Aid is placed over the injection site and the child is comforted. Specimens are labeled and taken to the laboratory with the appropriate requisition form.

The adolescent may avoid postlumbar puncture headache by lying flat for some time. The nurse charts the date and time of the lumbar puncture and the name of the attending physician. Also charted are the amount of fluid obtained; its character, for example, cloudy or bloody; whether or not specimens were sent to the laboratory; and the patient's reaction to the procedure.

ADMINISTERING MEDICATIONS TO INFANTS AND CHILDREN

Medication administration is a primary responsibility of the nurse. It is important for the nurse to understand that the responses of infants differ from those of children and that the responses of infants and children differ from those of adults. These concepts must also be communicated to the parents who often administer over-the-counter medications to their growing child. The most common over-the-counter medication administered by parents to infants and children is acetaminophen (Tylenol®). A physician or health care provider may advise the parents to "give a teaspoon of acetaminophen to their young child." However, the parents who purchase the medication may choose Tylenol *drops* instead of Tylenol *elixir.* The one teaspoon dose of Tylenol *elixir* is the dose ordered. However, 1 teaspoon of Tylenol *drops* is a massive overdose and can harm the young child. These kind of accidents can be prevented by parent education. Understanding the differences in drug absorption, distribution, metabolism, and excretion between children and adults is essential to provide safe pediatric nursing.

Physiological Responses to Medications in Infants and Children

Age is the most important variable in predicting response to any drug therapy. The functions of various organs in the body mature as the child grows and develops.

Absorption of Medications in Infants and Children

Gastric Influences. In the neonate there is an absence of free hydrochloric acid in the stomach. The acid content of the stomach reaches adult levels by 2 years of age. The administration of medications that require an acid medium in the stomach to be absorbed, such as phenobarbital or Dilantin (phenytoin), therefore may not be completely absorbed before 2 years of age. The administration of such medications near the time of formula feedings will further decrease acid content of the stomach. After 2 years of age, the ingestion of orange juice increases gastric acidity, causing more effective absorption of medication that requires an acid medium to absorb.

Intestinal Influences. Children under 5 years of age have a more rapid intestinal transit time than adults. Medication may have moved out of the small intestines before it is completely absorbed. Therefore, delayed or timed-release oral medication may not be fully absorbed by children younger than 5 years. The presence of pancreatic enzymes may be low under 1 year of age. Some medications depend on pancreatic enzymes to help to absorb the drug.

Topical Medications (ointments). Pediatric patients have a thin stratum corneum that allows topical medications to be absorbed. The larger skin surface area also increases the amount of absorption of topical medication as compared to adults. The use of a plastic diaper can also cause increased absorption of a topically applied medication in the diaper area of the skin. Hydrocortisone and Hexachloraphene may produce adverse systemic responses when applied to the buttocks and covered with a plastic diaper.

Parenteral Medications (IM). Poor peripheral perfusion in the young infant will slow intramuscular drug absorption. IM drugs administered to infants and children under 4 years of age should be water soluble to prevent precipitation. In neonates, medication may pass through the blood–brain barrier more easily than in older children and adults. Therefore medications that depress respiration may have a more powerful effect on neonates than in adults.

Metabolism

Most medications are metabolized in the liver. Since the liver and enzymes are not functioning at a mature level until 2 to 4 years of age, drugs generally metabolize slower in the infant and young child than in the adult. Medications given at frequent intervals to infants and children may result in toxic levels and responses.

Excretion

Many medications such as penicillin and digoxin depend on the kidney for excretion. The immature kidney function prevents effective excretion of drugs from the body in infants under 1 year of age.

The combination of slow stomach emptying that delays medication from being absorbed, rapid intestinal transit time that may prevent the full amount of medication from being absorbed, unpredictable liver function that may impair metabolism of the drug, and inability to effectively excrete medications via the kidney result in altered responses to medication and a high risk for toxicity.

NURSING RESPONSIBILITIES IN ADMINISTERING MEDICATIONS TO INFANTS AND CHILDREN

It becomes a legal and ethical responsibility of the nurse to understand that growing children differ in their ability to respond to medications. Nurses *must observe for toxic symptoms* whenever medications are administered and *document positive and negative responses.* Close attention must be paid to pediatric dose calculations. *Every* medication administered should have the *safety* of the dose prescribed *calculated* before administration. The official sources for safe dosage levels for various age groups is provided by the manufacturer's pocket insert or the PDR *(Physician's Desk Reference)*, which is published yearly. One method of determining safe dosage for infants and children is described in Box 22–2 (p. 556). Parent teaching is essential to ensure compliance when the child is sent home. Instructions should include:

- The importance of administering the medicine.
- The importance of completing the prescribed course.
- Techniques of measuring amount of medication to give in each dose. The use of the teaspoon in the home is not advisable when administering medication to infants and children. Inexpensive accurate measuring devices are available in pharmacies.
- Techniques of administering medications to their infant or child:
    - Using a dropper or syringe or measured cup
    - Not mixing medication with formula, food, or water
    - Shaking medication before administering
    - Refrigerating unused portions of medication
- Techniques of encouraging child compliance:
    - Allowing toddler and young child autonomy of assisting with taking his own medication—by squirting the contents into his or her own mouth or drinking it from the cup
    - Providing praise for cooperation and perhaps a chart of stars or stickers for compliance
    - Providing good tasting liquid or ice-pop *following* administration of a medication that has a "bad taste"
- The importance of writing a schedule and documenting the administration to avoid "forgetting" or "double-dosing."

Selected tips in giving medication to children at various ages is described in Table 22–7.

Selected Drug–Drug Interactions

The nurse should be alert to possible interactions between drugs prescribed and between prescription drugs and drugs that parents may purchase without a prescription. Table 22–8 is a partial list of some common drug–drug interactions.

Selected Drug–Food Interactions

The nurse should be aware that food and nutrients can influence the absorption, metabolism, and excretion of certain drugs. Foods that influence gastrointestinal motility or the pH of gastric secretions can affect absorption, lessening the drug's therapeutic value. Table 22–9 lists some drug–food interactions.

Selected Drug–Environment Interactions

Some medications can cause skin reactions when the child is exposed to the sun *(phototoxicity)*. Parents should be advised to keep their child protected from the sun while he or she is taking these medications. Drugs that decompose when exposed to the air or light are dispensed in darkened bottles. These drugs should not be purchased in the large economy size as deterioration might occur to tablets before all are used up. Table 22–10 lists some examples of drug–environment interactions.

Calculating Pediatric Drug Dosages

Most pediatric medications are prescribed in milligrams per kilogram of body weight per 24 hours. A hospital drug formulary is usually available on the unit to enable the nurse to determine the safety of a particular dose. If there is any question, one should consult the charge nurse, the physician who wrote the order, or the hospital pharmacist. The nurse should be undisturbed when preparing medications.

The physician calculates a particular dosage of a medication for each child. One method, calculation by *body surface area (BSA)*, is considered to be the most accurate. In this method, a *nomogram* is used (Fig. 22–12).

The child's height is located on the left scale, and the weight on the right scale. A line is drawn between the two points. The point at which the line transects the surface area (SA) gives the body surface area (BSA) of the individual child. If the patient's size is roughly average, the surface area can

Table 22–7
SELECTED AGE-APPROPRIATE TECHNIQUES OF GIVING MEDICATIONS TO CHILDREN

Age	Consideration
Infant	Apply bib Support and elevate head and shoulders Plastic disposable syringe is accurate and safe for oral medications Depress chin with thumb to open mouth Slowly insert medication along the side of the infant's mouth; this helps to prevent gagging Allow time for swallowing The recommended site for intramuscular (IM) injections is the vastus lateralis muscle Avoid use of buttocks, as gluteal muscles are undeveloped in infants; danger of injury to sciatic nerve As a rule of thumb, give no more than 1 ml of solution in a single site; if in doubt, confer with another nurse or physician Soothe infant
Toddler	May require help of another person May require some type of restraint if no assistance is available Let child explore an empty medicine cup Explain reasons for medication Crush tablets if it is not chewable If child is cooperative, may hold medicine cup Allow child to drink at own pace When giving IM medications, carry out injection quickly and gently Be prepared to find that resistive behavior is at its peak, particularly kicking, crying, and thrashing about Be prepared to be surprised, as some toddlers are very cooperative
Preschool	Chewable tablets and liquids are preferred Regression in pill taking may be seen Watch for loose teeth that may be swallowed Avoid prolonged reasoning Involve parents if appropriate Provide puppet play to help child express frustrations concerning injections Praise child following procedure
School Age	Can take pills and capsules; instruct child to place pill near back of tongue and immediately swallow water Emphasize swallowing of fluid to distract the child from swallowing the pill Some children continue to have a difficult time swallowing pills, and other forms of the medication should be explored (many come in suspensions); never ridicule child Child can be unpredictable from day to day in their cooperation; allow more time for giving pediatric medication Always ascertain that child is fully awake (particularly after nap time and during night shift) Always inform child of what you are about to do Remain with fearful child after procedure until child regains composure When this is not possible or appears prolonged, enlist help of auxiliary personnel
Adolescent	Prepare patient with explanations suitable to level of understanding Always ensure privacy Teach adolescent what side effects to report Identify adolescents on contraceptives to avoid drug interactions (may have been too embarrassed to provide information during history or may be attempting to keep secret from significant others) Remain with patient until medication is consumed (particularly if patient has a behavior disorder) Anticipate mood swings in compliance Consider possibility of adolescent addiction (drugs, alcohol) even though this may not be a presenting problem; many medications would be altered by such conditions

Table 22–8
SELECTED DRUG–DRUG INTERACTIONS

Drug	Interacts with	Interaction
Antacids	Steroids	Decreased absorption
	Digoxin	Decreased absorption
	NSAIDs	Decreased absorption
	Tetracycline	Decreased absorption
	Theophylline	Increased toxicity
Barbiturates	Oral contraceptives	Decreased protection
	Steroids	Decreased steroid effectiveness
	Influenza vaccine	Barbiturate toxicity
	Theophylline	Decreased theophylline effect
Bleomycin	Oxygen	Increased lung toxicity
Erythromycin	Phenytoin	Decreased phenytoin effect
	Theophylline	Increased theophylline toxicity
Isoniazid	Antacid	Decreased absorption
	Phenytoin	Increased phenytoin toxicity
	Valproate	Hepatic and CNS toxicity
Phenytoin	Alcohol	Acute toxicity
	Antacid	Decreased phenytoin effect
	Antidepressants (tricyclic)	Increased phenytoin toxicity
	Contraceptives	Decreased protection
	Steroids	Decreased steroid effect
	Digoxin	Decreased digoxin effect
	Folic acid	Decreased phenytoin effect
	Isoniazid	Increased phenytoin toxicity
	Theophyllin	Decreased effect of both medications
	Valproate	Increased phenytoin toxicity

also be estimated from the weight alone by using the enclosed area of Figure 22–12. The results are inserted into a formula. The average adult BSA is approximately 1.7 m^2:

$$\frac{\text{BSA (child)}}{\text{BSA (adult)}} \times \text{Average Adult Dose} = \text{Child's Dose.}$$

Calculating the Safe Drug Dose

Mg/kg. For adults, most medications have an "average dose." There is no average dose in pediatrics because the weight of the child can vary between 2 pounds to 150 pounds, and at different ages the ability to metabolize and excrete drugs may be limited. Therefore it is necessary for the nurse to calculate if the dose ordered is safe. When calculating safe dosage for an infant or child, the mg/kg protocol can be used by the nurse. For example, the doctor orders 25 mg of a medication to be administered. The nurse checks the PDR or other drug book and finds that the safe dose for that medication is 2 to 4 mg/kg. This child weighs 7 kg. Using the highest safe dose, the nurse inserts the actual weight of the child (kg) to the formula so that the formula now reads: the safe dose of *this* medication for *this* child is 4 mg × 7 kg, or 28 mg. Since

Table 22–9
SELECTED DRUG–FOOD INTERACTIONS

Drug	Interacts with	Interaction
Aminoglycosides gentomycin Penicillin Tetracycline	Any food	Decreased absorption rate
Theophylline	High protein Low CHO diet	Decreased time of drug activity in body
MAO inhibitors (Nardil, Parnate, Marplan)	Tyramine containing foods such as yogurt, processed meats, beer	Possible hypertensive crises
Iron supplements	Starch, egg yolks	Decreased iron absorption
Antihypertensives	Licorice or natural licorice extract	Can counteract effect of antihypertensive drugs
Vitamin C	Foods high in Vitamin B_{12}	Decreased absorption of vitamin B_{12} if both vitamins are taken together

Table 22–10

DRUG–ENVIRONMENT INTERACTIONS

Drugs	Interacts with	Interaction
Tofranil, phenothiazines, griseofulvin, tetracyclines, Diuril	Sun	Skin rash when child is exposed to the sun
Vitamin C	Air	Decomposes when exposed to air

the doctor's order does not exceed 28 mg, the dose that the doctor ordered is safe to give. If the doctor's order had exceeded the computed safe dose, the nurse would call his or her supervisor or the doctor.

Dimensional Analysis. *Dimensional analysis* is one method of calculating dosages, using basic arithmetic and algebra (Box 22–2).

Example. A doctor orders 0.025 g of a drug. Each

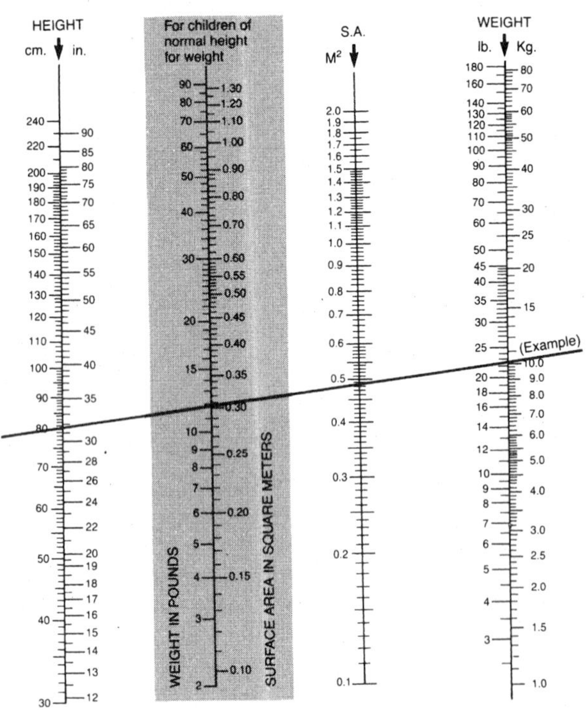

Figure 22–12. • Nomogram for estimating surface area. The body surface area of the child is indicated where a straight line that connects the height and weight levels intersects the surface area column. If the patient is of average size, the surface area can be deduced on the basis of weight alone (see shaded box). (Nomogram modified from data of E. Boyd by C. D. West.) (From Behrman, R., & Kleigman, R. [1998]. *Nelson's essentials of pediatrics* [3rd eds., p. 805]. Philadelphia: Saunders.)

BOX 22–2

FORMULA FOR DIMENSIONAL ANALYSIS

$$\frac{\text{Unit}}{\text{Dosage on hand}} \times \frac{\text{Dosage wanted}}{\text{Unit to give}}$$

tablet is 12.5 mg. How many tablets will you give? You know that 1000 mg = 1 g. Therefore,

$$\frac{1000 \text{ mg}}{1 \text{ g}} \times \frac{0.025 \text{ gm}}{? \text{ mg}} = 1000 \times 0.025 = 25 \text{ mg}$$

You would give 25 mg. Remember that each tablet is 12.5 mg:

What you have		**What you want to give**
$\frac{1 \text{ (tab)}}{12.5 \text{ mg}}$	$\times$	$\frac{25 \text{ mg}}{? \text{ tab}} = 2$ tablets

You would give two tablets.

Another Example of Dimensional Analysis. A doctor orders 5 mg of a drug. The label reads 10 mg/2 cc. How many cc are you going to give?

$$\frac{\text{Unit}}{\text{Dosage}} \frac{2 \text{ cc}}{10 \text{ mg}} \frac{5 \text{ mg}}{? \text{ cc}} = \frac{10}{10} = 1 \text{ cc}$$

Give 1 cc.

Determining Whether a Dose is Safe for an Infant. A doctor orders 200 mg Q 6 h. The PDR states that a 40-mg/kg dose is a safe dose for infants. This infant weighs 12 pounds.

$\frac{200 \text{ mg}}{\text{Dose}}$	$\times$	$\frac{2.2 \text{ lbs}}{1 \text{ kg}}$	$\times$	$\frac{1 \text{ infant}}{12 \text{ lbs}}$	=	36.6-mg/kg dose
(Dose ordered)		(convert pounds to kg)		(Weight of child)		(What child is receiving)

Since the 36.6-mg does not exceed the stated safe dose of 40 mg/kg/dose, the dose ordered is safe for this child.

Besides knowing the correct amount and route of a drug, the nurse must also be aware of the toxic side effects that might occur. The absorption, distribution, metabolism, and excretion of drugs differ substantially in children, who also react more quickly and violently to medication. Drug reactions are therefore not as predictable as they are in adult patients. The drug's impact on normal growth and development must be considered. Drug circulars must be read carefully to determine the suitability of a particular drug for children. *Drugs should be given only by the route indicated.*

Double-checking with another nurse may be required in some hospitals when administering drugs such as digoxin (Lanoxin), insulin, or heparin. *The child should be correctly identified by using the hospital identification band. The nurse must always know what medications the patient is receiving, whether or not the nurse personally administers them.* See Table 22–7 for further age-appropriate techniques of administering pediatric medications.

Administering Oral Medications

The administration of medication by mouth is preferred in children, but is not always possible because of vomiting, malabsorption, or refusal. Children younger than 5 years find it difficult to swallow tablets or capsules. Most pediatric medications are available in liquid, suspension, or chewable tablets. Only scored tablets should be divided. Suspensions must be fully shaken before use.

Medication may have to be disguised in a pleasant-tasting medium, when the medication is bitter or otherwise unpalatable. Cherry syrup or jelly may be used. The use of important sources of nutrients, foods, or liquids, such as orange juice, for this purpose is discouraged because the child may develop a distaste for them. The medication is never referred to as "candy." Medication is administered slowly, especially if the child is crying. *The patient's head and shoulders are elevated to prevent aspiration.* Toddlers may attempt to push the medicine cup away. In anticipation of this response, the nurse holds the child, with hands restrained, in the nurse's lap in a semisitting position (Fig. 22–13). "Chasers" of water, fruit juice, frozen ice pops, or carbonated beverage are appreciated. In choosing a chaser, the patient's age and diet are considered.

If a nasogastric tube is in place, the nurse tests for proper placement of the tube before pouring medication into the funnel. A small amount of water is administered afterward to cleanse the tube. The procedure is recorded on the intake and output (I & O) sheet.

For infants, an oral syringe is an excellent device for measuring small quantities (Figs. 22–14 and 22–15). It is easily transported, and medication can be given directly from the syringe. The syringe is placed midway back at the side of the mouth. A bib is placed on an infant before performing the procedure. Medication should not be placed in a bottle of juice or water; if some of the contents are refused, there is no way to determine how much of the drug was consumed. A medibottle, device that consists of a syringe attached to a nipple can be used for infants who will suck the medication from the nipple as the plunger of the syringe is slowly depressed (Fig. 22–15).

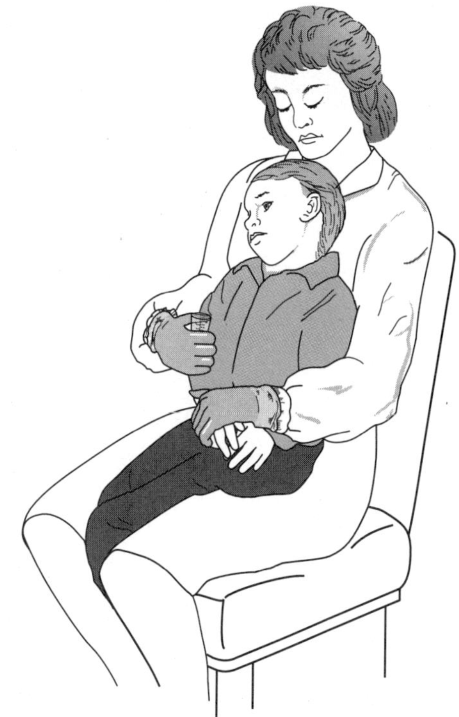

Figure 22–13. • The cup method of administering medication. The nurse may hold the child on her lap and restrain the child's hands as shown, to prevent spilling of the medication. Note that the child's legs are restrained between the knees of the nurse.

A plastic medicine dropper is useful, and the drug manufacturer may provide one with the medication. It is used only for the medication specified—it is not intended for measuring other liquids. A drug ordered in teaspoons should be measured in milliliters to ensure accuracy (5 ml = 1 teaspoon). The nurse administering medications on the pediatric unit must keep the medicine tray or cart in sight at all times. This prevents other patients from upsetting or ingesting the contents.

Administering Parenteral Medications

Nose, Ear, and Eye Drops

Except for a few differences, the principles for administering nose, ear, and eye drops to children are essentially the same as for adults. Infants and

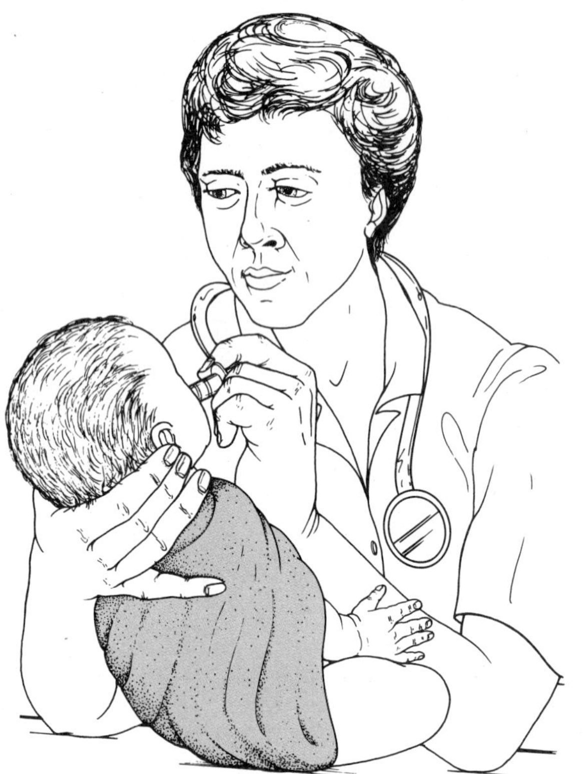

Figure 22–14. • Medications can be administered to the infant with an oral syringe. The head of the infant must be elevated when oral medications are given.

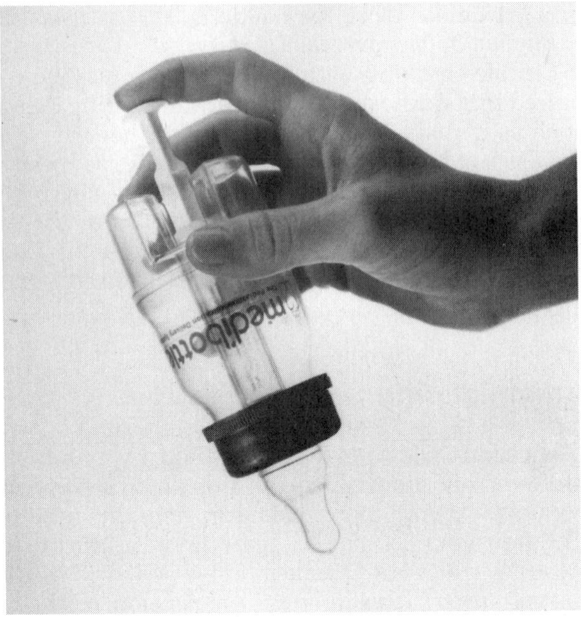

Figure 22–15. • The Medibottle may be attached to the syringe so that the infant can suck on the nipple to consume the medication. The nurse controls the flow with gentle pressure on the syringe barrel. (Photo courtesy of the Medicine Bottle Co., 175 W. Jackson Boulevard, Chicago, IL 60604.)

small children need to be restrained in a *mummy restraint* (Box 22–1 on p. 541).

Nose Drops. The procedure for administering nose drops to a small child is listed in Procedure (at right).

Ear Drops. The doctor may prescribe a drug to be instilled into the ear to relieve pain. If the drops were refrigerated, they are allowed to warm to room temperature. In the child *under 3 years,* the infected ear is drawn down and back to straighten the canal, and the correct number of drops are instilled. In *the older child,* the *ear lobe is pulled upward and backward* to obtain the same result. Gentle massage of the area in front of the ear may facilitate entry of the drops. The patient remains supine for a few minutes to permit the fluid to be absorbed. The nurse charts the following: time, name of drug, number of drops administered, area (right or left ear), untoward reactions, and whether or not the patient obtained relief.

Eye Drops/Creams. Ophthalmic medication is administered to a child in the same manner as for

Procedure Technique for Administering Nose Drops to the Small Child

Equipment

Sheet for restraint
Nose drops
Tissues, clean gloves

Method

1. Immobilize the infant with mummy restraint.
2. Wipe excess mucus from nose with a tissue.
3. Place infant on back with head over the side of the mattress or neck extended over a pillow.
4. Encircle infant's cheeks and chin with left arm and hand to steady.
5. Instill drops with right hand.
6. Keep infant in this position for ½ to 1 min to allow the drops to reach the proper area.
7. Remove restraints. Make infant comfortable.
8. Chart the following: time, name of nose drops, strength, number of drops instilled, how the patient tolerated the procedure, and untoward reactions.

the adult. The child is informed of the need for the medication. The patient is identified, and orders and the label on the bottle are checked for correct medication and concentration. The nurse ascertains which eye requires treatment, that is, right eye (O.D.), left eye (O.S.), or both eyes (O.U.). The hands are washed before and after the procedure. With the thumb and index finger, gentle pressure is applied in opposite directions to open the eye. The older child is instructed to "look up." Supporting the hand on the patient's forehead, the medication is instilled into the center of the lower lid (conjunctival sac) (Fig. 22–16). The child is instructed to close the eye but not to squeeze it, as this could expel some of the solution.

Ointment is applied in the same conjunctival sac as eye drops. When only one nurse is available and the patient is an infant, the mummy restraint is applied. Occasionally, children refuse to open their eyes. The nurse must use ingenuity to coax a reluctant patient. It may help to involve parents.

Rectal Medications

Some drugs, such as sedatives and antiemetics, come in the form of suppositories. Children's suppositories are long and thin in comparison with the cone-shaped types administered to adults. The nurse, wearing a rubber glove or finger cot, inserts the lubricated suppository well beyond the anal sphincter about half as far as the forefinger will reach. The nurse applies pressure to the anus by gently holding the buttocks together until the child's desire to expel the suppository subsides.

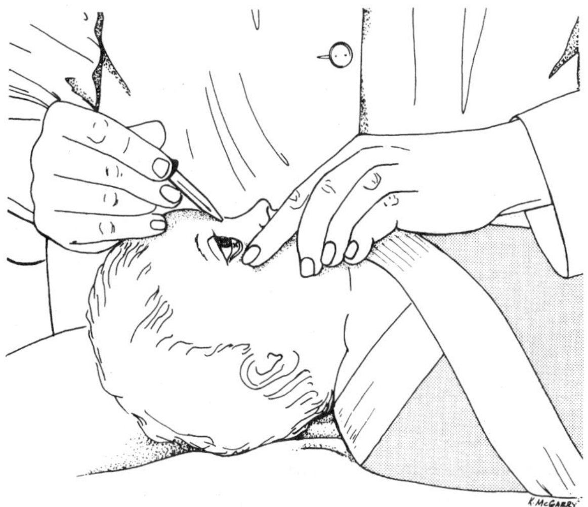

Figure 22–16. • Technique of instilling eye drops. The eye drops should fall in the center of the lower conjunctival sac, never directly on the eyeball. Gloves are worn as there may be infection or drainage from the eyes.

Nurses administer medications via the nasal spray, transdermal patches, and implanted ports as well as the traditional oral, intramuscular, or subcutaneous route.

Intramuscular and Subcutaneous Injections

Most medications given to infants and children are given by the oral or intravenous route. However, some medications must be given by the *subcutaneous route (SC),* such as insulin for diabetic children. Some medications must be given via the *intramuscular route (IM),* such as immunizations or vitamin K to newborn infants. The site and technique of injection can affect the absorption rate and the effect of the drug on the child.

The Subcutaneous Route. In SC injections, absorption occurs by slow diffusion into the capillaries. If a medication such as epinephrine is given IM instead of SC, a life-threatening cardiac arrhythmia could occur. If the SC site is exercised immediately before or after an SC injection, the absorption rate will be increased. (If insulin is the drug injected, hypoglycemia could occur because of the rapid absorption.) Sites should be rotated. Irritating solutions should not be injected SC.

The Intramuscular Route. An IM injection places medication into the skeletal muscle below the subcutaneous tissue. The medication spreads among the muscles elastic fibers and absorbs rapidly. Aspirating the plunger after injection and observing for a flashback of blood will confirm muscle placement of the needle. Accidental injection into a vein can cause a toxic response. Accidental injection into the subcutaneous tissue can cause tissue necrosis.

Intramuscular Sites. Intramuscular injections are given into the *vastus lateralis* muscle of the thigh in all infants (see Fig. 22–17). The site is free of major nerves and blood vessels, but small nerve endings can cause the injection to be painful. The *ventrogluteal* site places the medication into the gluteus medius and minimus muscles that are free of major nerve and blood vessels. This site can be used in children after they have been walking for 1 year. The *dorsogluteal* site is a high risk for sciatic nerve injury or piercing of a major blood vessel. This site is small and poorly developed in infants and is not used for IM injections. The *deltoid* site in the upper arm has a small muscle mass that limits the amount of medication that can be injected at one time. There are major blood vessels and the radial nerve can be injured. The deltoid muscle is not a preferred site

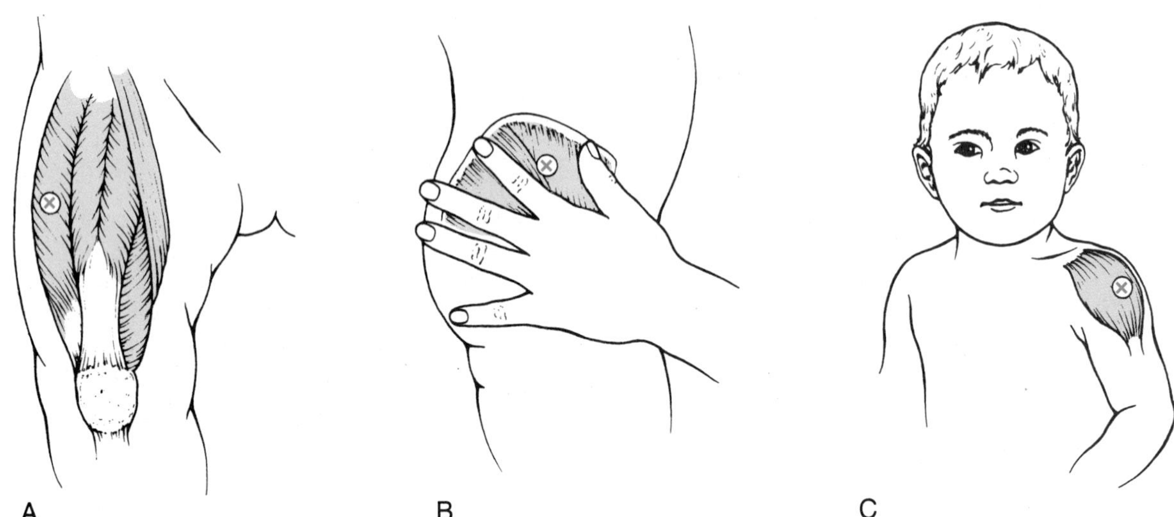

Figure 22–17. • Appropriate sites for intramuscular injection in children. **A,** The thigh. **B,** Ventrogluteal. **C,** Deltoid. The vastus lateralis (A) is preferred in children under 3 years.

EMLA® CREAM (lidocaine 2.5% and prilocaine 2.5%)

INSTRUCTIONS FOR APPLICATION OF EMLA CREME

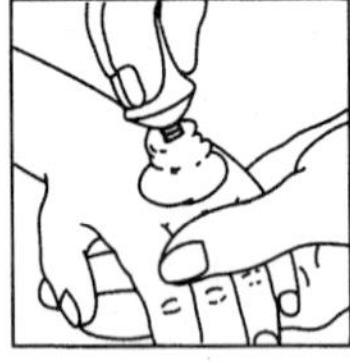
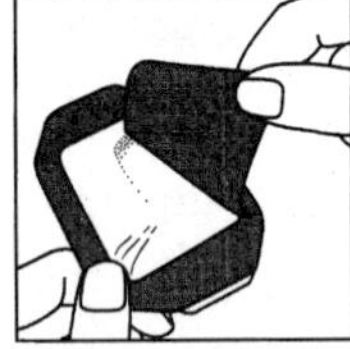
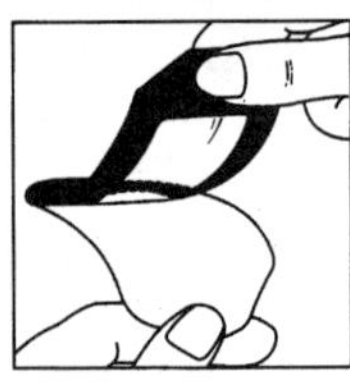
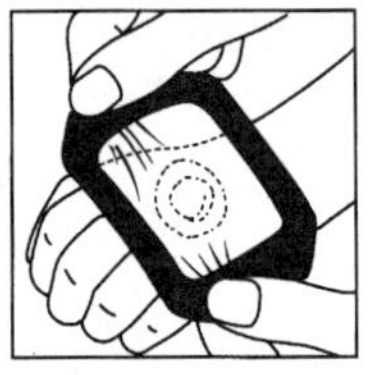
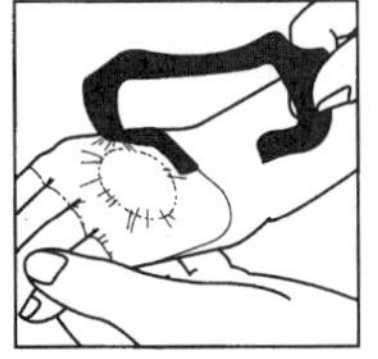
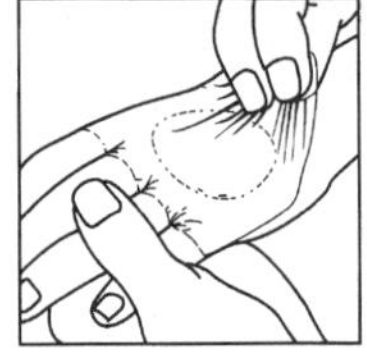

1. In adults, apply 2.5 g of cream (1/2 the 5 g tube) per 20 to 25 cm^2 (approx. 2 in. by 2 in.) of skin in a thick layer at the site of the procedure. For pediatric patients, apply as prescribed by your physician.

2. Take an occlusive dressing (provided with the 5 g tubes only) and remove the center cut-out piece.

3. Peel the paper liner from the paper framed dressing.

4. Cover the EMLA® Cream so that you get a thick layer underneath. Do not spread out the cream. Smooth down the dressing edges carefully and ensure it is secure to avoid leakage. (This is especially important when the patient is a child.)

5. Remove the paper frame. The time of application can easily be marked directly on the occlusive dressing. EMLA® must be applied at least 1 hour before the start of a routine procedure and for 2 hours before the start of a painful procedure.

6. Remove the occlusive dressing, wipe off the EMLA® Cream, clean the entire area with an antiseptic solution and prepare the patient for the procedure. The duration of effective skin anesthesia will be at least 1 hour after removal of the occlusive dressing.

PRECAUTIONS

1. Do not apply near eyes or on open wounds.
2. Do not use in children under one month of age.
3. Keep out of reach of children.

Manufactured by:
Astra Pharmaceutical Production, AB
Södertälje, Sweden

ASTRA®
Astra USA, Inc.
Westborough, MA 01581

021700R01

Figure 22–18. • Emla Creme: a topical anesthetic can be used prior to an invasive procedure to reduce the pain involved in piercing the skin. (Courtesy of Astra Pharmaceutical Products, Inc., Westborough, MA.)

for children under 6 years in most cases. However, absorption of medication is more rapid in the deltoid than in the buttock or the thigh.

Reducing the Pain of Injections. Nurses can take the time to reduce the discomfort associated with injections. *Positioning* the patient properly can minimize muscle tenseness and ease the procedure. The child can be face down or on the side with the upper leg placed in front of the lower one to relax the muscles. For a vastus lateralis injection, the child's toes should be turned so that the hip rotates internally. The child can flex the elbow and support the arm for a deltoid injection. A *topical anesthetic* such as Emla® (see Fig. 22–18) can be used when the time of injection can be planned in advance. Storing alcohol sponges in the refrigerator or rubbing the site with an *ice cube* prior to injection will numb the site. The current design of many syringes for the purpose of minimizing accidental needle punctures to the caregiver that can spread infections and increase risk of HIV has made it impossible to change the needle on the syringe after drawing up the medication and before administering it. The needle should be inserted *rapidly* while the child is *distracted.* The medication is *injected slowly* to minimize the increasing pressure within the muscle. Rapid removal of the needle and mild massage or exercise of the extremity will increase absorption and comfort.

The size of the syringe and of the needle varies with the size of the child, volume of medication prescribed, amount and general condition of the muscle tissue, frequency of injections, and viscosity (thickness) of the drug. A small needle gauge, such as 25 to 27, and a length of 0.5 to 1 inch is commonly used. As a general rule, 1 ml is the maximum volume to be given in one site to infants and small children. Small or premature babies may tolerate even less. For volumes less than 1 ml, a tuberculin syringe or low-dose syringe is preferred. Some syringes are designed to automatically retract the needle into the syringe following injections or have a plastic sleeve (Fig. 22–19) pull over the needle after use. This eliminates the practice of "recapping" the needles and reduces the risk of accidental needle sticks.

The nurse should anticipate some protest from children about injections. Whenever possible, a second person should assist by distracting and restraining the child. The child's first injection is particularly important because it establishes the pattern for future reactions (Fig. 22–20). The school-age child may assist in selecting the site, if possible. This helps to increase feelings of mastery and control. Injections are more of a threat to toddlers and preschool children, who are too young to understand their necessity. Do not shame the uncooperative child. Fortunately, because most medications can now be given orally, by rectum, or intravenously, the necessity for administering intramuscular injections to children is decreasing.

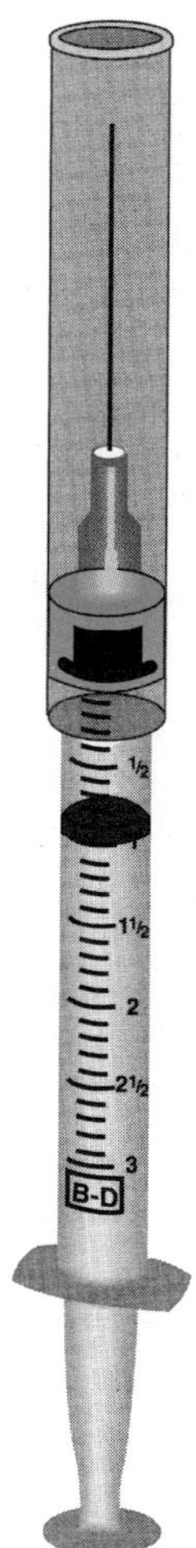

Figure 22–19. • This syringe has a plastic sleeve that covers the needle after medication is administered. This helps to protect the nurse from an accidental needle stick. (Redrawn from Becton Dickinson and Company, Franklin Lakes, NJ.)

Intravenous Medications

The Intravenous Route. An IV injection places the drug directly into the bloodstream in a faster, more predictable timeframe.

Medications given by the intravenous (IV) route are being administered routinely in pediatric pa-

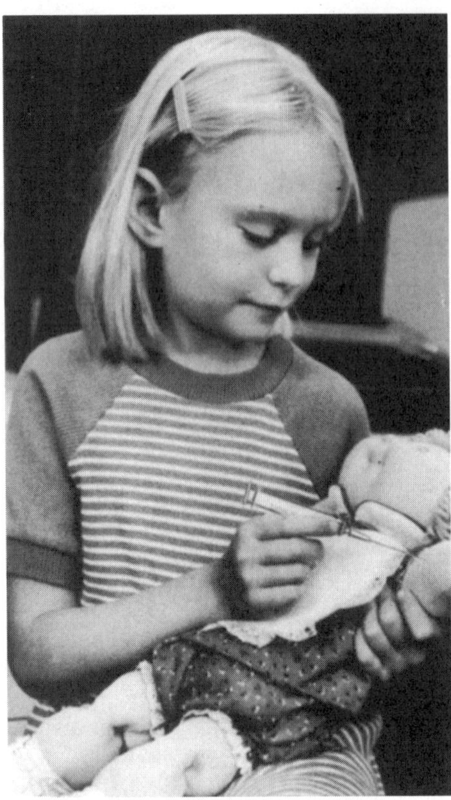

Figure 22–20. • By giving injections to dolls or puppets, children can be prepared for this procedure and may be less frightened by it. (Copyright 1985, *American Journal of Nursing Company*. Reprinted with permission from Meer, P. [1985]. Using play therapy in outpatient settings. *MCN: American Journal of Maternal Child Nursing, 10,* 379.)

tients. In some cases it prevents repeated intramuscular injections, which are unpleasant. Other drugs are effective only if given by this method. The medication is also absorbed more rapidly, which is of value. Each hospital has its own policies about who may start IV lines or add medications to an established line. The nurse assesses the IV line carefully for infiltration, inflammation, and patency.

Intravenous medications can cause phlebitis and the nurse must assess the child's IV site hourly for reddened areas or signs of inflammation. Infiltration is a risk for children who are active, and the site should be assessed hourly as children cannot communicate the burning or pain that may accompany infiltration. Leakage at the IV site, a tense tissue turgor, and cool blanched skin around the IV site may indicate infiltration and the nurse manager should be notified. Since the medication reaches the heart and brain within seconds, adverse reactions can occur quickly. The nurse must be aware of the side effects associated with the drug administered. A rapid rate of flow of the IV solution can cause fluid overload (manifested by increased pulse or blood pressure, distended neck veins, and puffy eyes) or a slow rate of infusion can result in clot formation that obstructs the patency of the IV. The nurse should monitor the rate of the IV flow, refill the burettes hourly (Fig. 22–21), observe the condition of the IV site, and assess the responses of the child.

Sites for IV infusion in children are illustrated in Figure 22–22. A pediatric armboard is used (Fig. 22–23) to restrain the extremity used for IV access and the insertion site is secured and covered to prevent tampering by the child or parents. The child with an IV in the extremity or the scalp will benefit from being held and rocked and need not

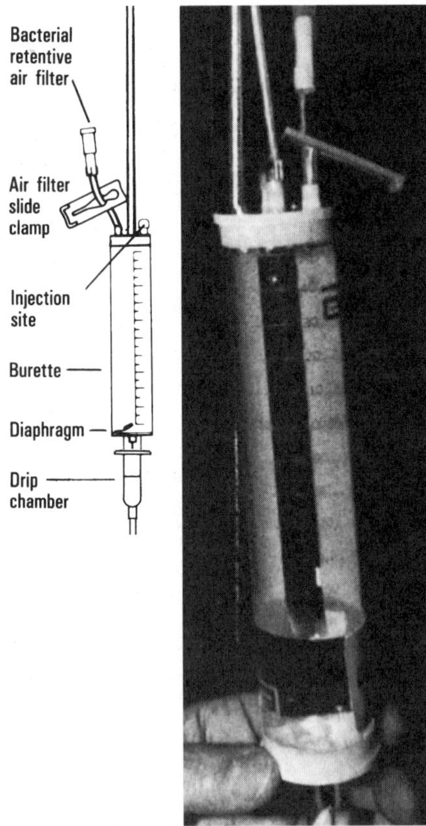

Figure 22–21. • The graduated control (burette) chamber delivers "micro" drops, making it easier to calculate the rate and amount of fluids absorbed. (Photograph from Betz, C., Hunsberger, M., & Wright, S. [1994]. *Family-centered nursing care of children* [2nd ed.]. Philadelphia: Saunders; drawing modified with permission of Abbott Laboratories.)

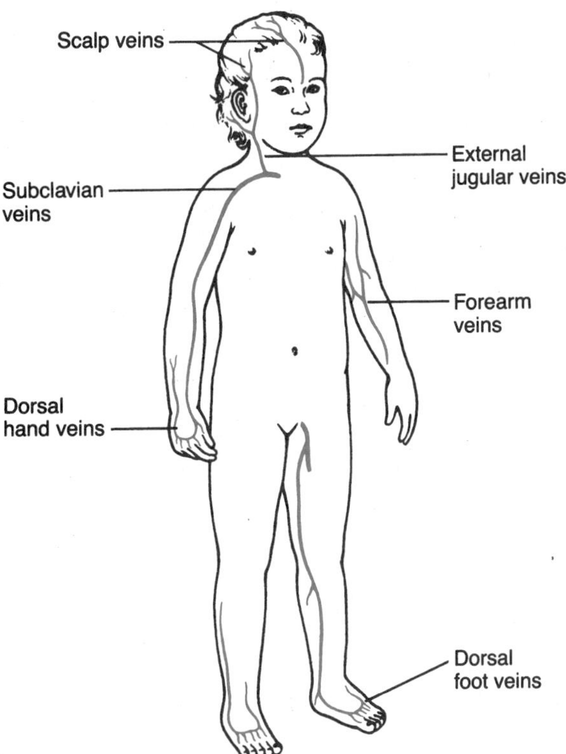

Figure 22–22. • Sites for intravenous infusion in children.

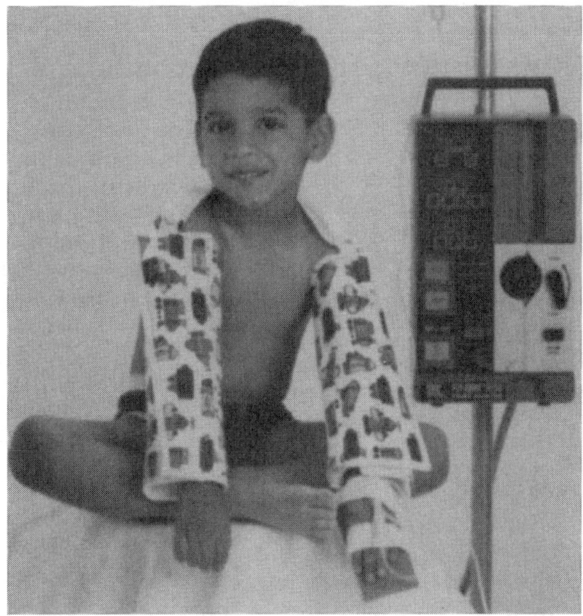

Figure 22–23. • The armboard immobilizes the arm during IV therapy and permits movement. (Courtesy of the Medi-Kids Co., Hemet, CA.)

have his or her whole body immobilized. Infusion pumps are used in pediatrics to control the administration of small volumes of fluid and to prevent changes in rate due to changes in position or activity of the infant or child. A pacifier should be provided for infants who are placed on NPO (nothing by mouth) to fulfill their developmental need for sucking.

Long-Term Venous Access Devices (VAD)

Peripheral Devices (VAD)

Heparin Lock. A *heparin lock* is a device that keeps a vein open for long-term intermittent medicine administration. It allows children to be more ambulatory because they are free of IV tubing. When a patient has a heparin lock in place, repeated "sticks" can be avoided. The apparatus consists of an IV needle attached to a 3¼-inch plastic tube that is plugged by a resealable rubber insert. This rubber top allows the insertion of a needle so that blood can be drawn or medications administered. The original needle remains in place and is periodically flushed with heparin or saline to prevent clotting.

Central Venous Access Devices. A peripherally inserted central catheter (PICC) is inserted for moderate-length therapy. The median, cephalic, or basilic vein is used in the antecubital area and threaded into the superior vena cava. Specially trained RNs may insert the PICC line. Dressings are changed frequently, the insertion site assessed, and care is taken to prevent dislodgement during this procedure.

Long-Term Central Venous Access Devices

Hickman, Groshong, and Broviac Catheters. Hickman, Groshong, and Broviac catheters are tiny, flexible rubber tubes that can be inserted into a vein in the chest to establish a long-term IV site. Medications, chemotherapy, IV fluids, and blood products can be given through the catheter. They can also be utilized for hyperalimentation (see p. 564). The pediatric *Broviac catheter* is used for children. The line is inserted while the patient is under local or general anesthesia. It remains in the patient from 1 month to 1 year, or even longer. The child or parents are taught how to care for the catheter during hospitalization so that they may continue the procedure at home under supervision of home care nurses. Some catheters are flushed daily or weekly with heparin or saline. Activities of daily living are not curtailed; however, the physician should be contacted about any unusual change in activity. The exit site should be kept dry. The patient or family must participate in the home care and the presence of the catheter may impact the child's self-image. A light shirt with a pocket, worn inside out, provides a place for any excess tubing and covers the area, protecting it from the fingers of a curious child. If a catheter leak occurs, the tubing should be taped, a clamp applied and medical intervention obtained.

Implanted Ports. Infusion ports that can be implanted under the skin are also available (port-A-Cath, MediPort, Infuse-A-Port, Groshong venous port). These small plastic devices are generally implanted under the chest skin beneath the clavicle. A small catheter is threaded from the port into a large central vein. The procedure is done under local or general anesthesia. Blood samples can be obtained, and medicines injected by a puncture through the skin into the port. Special needles are provided by the manufacturer. The use of a local or topical anesthetic makes the skin puncture painless. The advantage is that nothing protrudes from the body that can be dislodged, and it is less apparent. This is especially important for the self-conscious young person. Activities such as swimming may not be curtailed because the skin is intact. Vigorous contact sports are curtailed and the child should be cautioned not to play with the bulge. Removal requires minor surgery.

Nursing Care of a Child Receiving Parenteral Fluids. *Parenteral* (*para*, "beside or apart from," and *enteron*, "intestine") fluids are those given by some route other than the digestive tract. They are necessary when sickness is accompanied by vomiting or loss of consciousness or when the gastrointestinal system requires rest. The extremity in which the IV is inserted is restrained on an armboard, and the insertion site is secured and covered. If the infant is NPO (nothing by mouth) a pacifier should be offered. Diversional therapy will prevent the child from focusing on the IV tubing and using it as a toy. The infant should be picked up, rocked, and played with. IV pumps such as the IVAC pump prevent change in IV infusion rate when positions or activity change. The IV pump allows the administration of microdrops of intravenous solution so that a slow rate of infusion can be maintained. Adult IV sets administer 15 drops per 1 ml. Pediatric IV sets administer 60 drops per ml. A burette (Figure 22–21) is attached between the IV tubing and the pump and enables the nurse to fill the burette with the amount of solution to be administered in 1 hour. The infusion pump alarms to alert the staff that the burette must be refilled, allowing the nurse to monitor the IV site hourly. The nurse observes the child hourly for

- The rate of flow of the solution
- Swelling at the needle site
- Low volume in the bag or Soluset or the need to refill the burette
- Pain or redness at the site of insertion
- Moisture at or around the site

An accurate intake and output record is kept for all children receiving IV fluids. Nursing guidelines for intravenous therapy at various stages of development are described in Table 22–11.

Total Parenteral Nutrition (TPN). *Total parenteral nutrition (TPN)* is also known as *hyperalimentation* and provides the total nutritional needs for infants and children who cannot use the GI tract for nourishment for a prolonged period (Fig. 22–24). It allows highly concentrated solutions of proteins, glucose, and other nutrients to infuse directly into a large vessel such as the superior vena cava. These concentrated solutions are not currently given through peripheral veins. The nursing responsibilities are similar to those for other IV infusions. The solution is prepared by the pharmacist and is sterile. Monitoring vital signs, intake and output, and lab reports are essential nursing responsibilities.

Hypoglycemia, hyperglycemia, and electrolyte imbalances can occur. Prior to discontinuing TPN therapy, the rate is *gradually* decreased and the child monitored for adverse responses. Parents may need extensive teaching and return demonstrations if they are expected to care for their child receiving TPN treatment at home. Community agencies should be contacted to aid and support the family.

ADAPTATION OF SELECTED PROCEDURES TO CHILDREN

Nutrition, Digestion, and Elimination

When an infant cannot take food or fluids by mouth, but the gastrointestinal tract can function, a gavage feeding may be ordered. A *gavage* feeding places nutrients into the stomach so that natural digestion can occur. This can be accomplished by placing a nasogastric tube into the stomach via the nose and securing it in place with tape or using the oral route, reinserting a new tube with each feeding. When long-term feeding is required, a gastrostomy may be performed and a tube inserted directly into the stomach (see Fig. 22–25).

Gastrostomy

A *gastrostomy* (*gastro*, "stomach," and *stoma*, "opening") is made to introduce food directly into the stomach through the abdominal wall by means of a surgically placed tube or button. It is used in infants or children who cannot have food by mouth because of anomalies or strictures of the esophagus or who are severely debilitated or in coma. Cleansing of the skin around the tube will prevent irrita-

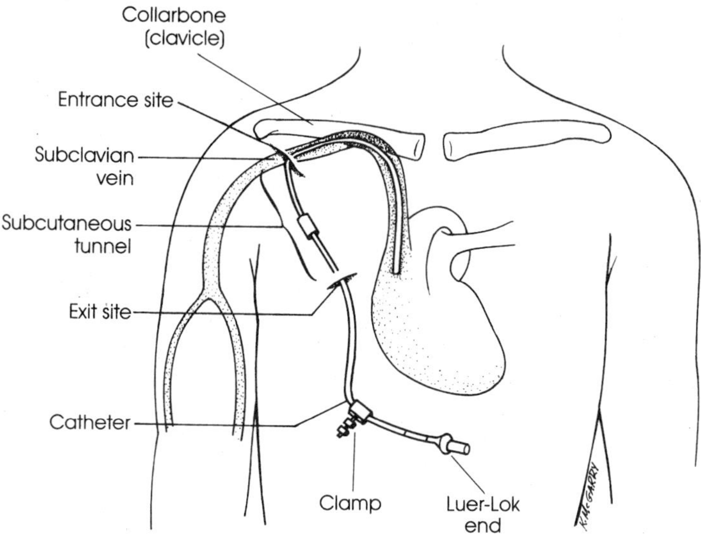

Figure 22–24. • Catheter placement for total parenteral nutrition.

Nursing Tip

One way of determining fluid loss in infants is to weigh the dry diaper, mark the weight on the outside of the diaper, and then weigh the wet diaper. Subtract the weight of the dry diaper from the weight of the wet diaper and record results on the intake and output record. Include both urine and liquid stools (1 g = 1 ml of output).

tion from formula or gastric secretions. The nurse observes and reports vomiting or abdominal distention. Brown or green drainage may indicate that the tube has slipped through the pylorus into the duodenum. This could cause an obstruction and is reported immediately (Procedure, p. 566. Gastrostomy Tube Feeding).

Enema

Administering an enema to a child is essentially the same as for adults; however, the type, amount, and the distance for inserting the tube require modifications. In addition, a child's bowel is more easily perforated under pressure (Betz, Hunsberger, & Wright, 1994). An isotonic solution (saline) is used in children. Tap water enemas are contraindicated. Plain water is hypotonic to the blood and could cause rapid fluid shift and overload if absorbed through the intestinal wall. The type of solution intended is always ascertained. Commercial enemas specific for the child are commonly used. The amount of fluids varies somewhat in procedure recommendations. The smaller the child, the less solution is used.

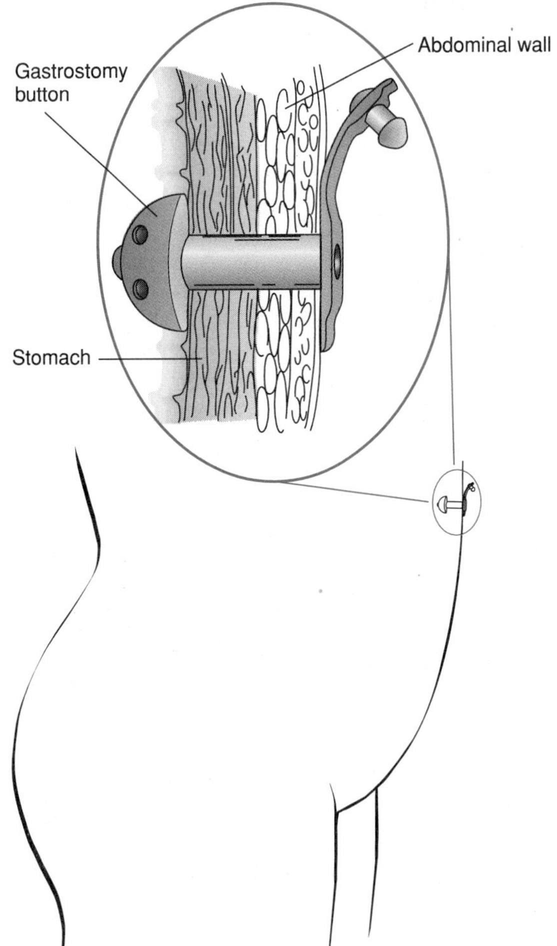

Figure 22–25. • The gastrostomy button allows feedings to be administered directly into the stomach through the abdominal wall.

Procedure Gastrostomy Tube Feeding

Equipment

Tray, gloves
Warmed formula
Funnel or syringe barrel
Syringe for aspiration
15 to 30 ml of water to flush tube as ordered
Note: Equipment should be sterile for preterm and newborn infants.

Method

1. Position child comfortably either flat or with head slightly elevated if not contraindicated. Provide pacifier to relax baby.
2. Check residual stomach contents by attaching syringe to gastrostomy tube and aspirating. If amount of residual is large (10–25 ml for newborns, over 50 ml for older children), replace residual and decrease present formula by equal amount or delay feeding for a short time. (This may vary according to the pediatrician's protocol.) Overloading the stomach can cause reflux and increases the danger of aspiration. If residual continues or increases, report this to the physician. If no residual is obtained, inject 2 to 5 cc of air into the tubing while listening via the stethoscope placed on the abdomen for a "whoosh" sound indicating that air has entered the stomach.
3. Attach the syringe barrel (if not already present for continuous elevation) to the gastrostomy tube. If the tube has more than one lumen, be sure to use the port *labeled for food or formula.* Fill with formula. Remove clamp. This prevents air from entering the stomach and causing distention.
4. Elevate the receptacle. Allow the formula to flow slowly by gravity—*force should not be used.*
5. Continue to add formula to the syringe before it empties completely (to prevent excess air from entering the tubing).
6. Clamp the tube as the final formula or water is passing through the lower part of the syringe. (*Note:* In infants, some physicians may prefer that the gastrostomy tube remain open at all times to produce a safety valve in the event that the baby vomits. In such cases, the tube is elevated above the patient's body.)
7. Whenever possible, hold the patient quietly after feeding. Reposition in the Fowler's position or on right side to promote gastric emptying.
8. Record the type (gastrostomy feeding), the amount given, the amount and characteristics of residual, and how the child tolerated the procedure. Record input and output on the chart.

The exact amount for infants should be prescribed by physician order. Guidelines range from a low of 50 ml for infants to a high of 500 to 750 ml for the adolescent. The nurse consults the procedure manual for the institution's guidelines. The tube is inserted from 1 to 4 inches, according to the size and age of the child. Infants and small children may be unable to retain the solution; therefore, it may be necessary to hold the buttocks together for a short time.

Oil-Retention Enema. When giving an *oil-retention enema,* use the prescribed amount, generally 60 to 100 ml of oil at 37.8° C (100° F). Apply gentle pressure over the anal area to prevent the oil from being expelled. A cleansing enema (saline) generally follows in 30 to 45 minutes later.

These are invasive procedures; therefore, careful age-appropriate explanations are necessary. Other invasive procedures related to the gastrointestinal tract include barium enema, intestinal biopsy, endoscopy, and colonoscopy. These are performed by the gastroenterologist. Currently, rectal suppositories are used more frequently than enemas.

Respiration

Tracheostomy Care

A *tracheostomy* is a surgical procedure in which an opening is made in the trachea to enable the patient to breathe. This artificial airway may be necessary in emergency situations, may be an elective procedure, or may be combined with mechanical ventilation. Some of the childhood conditions that may require tracheostomy are acute epiglottitis, head injury, and burns. Nursing care is indispensable to the survival of the patient, as blockage of the tube by mucus or other secretions can lead to suffocation. In many hospitals, the patient is placed in the ICU immediately following surgery because this is a critical period requiring frequent suctioning and close observation. The patient is placed on heart and respiratory monitors. When the child's condition stabilizes, the patient is transferred to another unit.

The child is placed in an area of high visibility. This is important because small children communicate their needs by crying and the tracheostomy prohibits vocalization. Whenever possible, one person is assigned to the child and to work with the parents. The nurse reinforces preoperative teaching and explains what happened: for example, "You were having a lot of trouble breathing. This operation is called a tracheostomy and helps you to breathe more easily. A small opening has been made in your neck. A hollow tube was inserted to keep the area open. It is frightening not to be able to speak. When you are better, the hole will close by itself and your voice will return." An explanation of suction might be, "We have to keep the area in your neck open. This tube goes into the throat and clears it." Use of suction can be shown in a glass of water. The child is prepared for the unfamiliar sound. "You might feel like gagging, but afterward you will feel better. I know this is difficult for you and I'm sorry."

The nursing care of the child with a tracheostomy is a significant responsibility. The anatomic differences between children and adults and the small child's inability to communicate through writing increase the need for close observation. In addition toddlers often have short, stubby necks that become easily irritated. It may be helpful to place a reminder on the intercom at the clerk's desk or in other suitable areas, indicating that this patient cannot cry or speak. The nurse's touch and quiet voice and the presence of significant others help to make the child feel secure. Routines are incorporated by repeating familiar stories. A favorite article, such as a blanket or toy, is kept nearby. A supply of teaching aids and of dramatic play material is made available. Puppets are particularly valuable.

Room temperature should be comfortably warm. Moisture and humidity may be added by a *mist tent* (Fig. 22–26), a special tracheostomy collar, or direct attachment to a mechanical ventilator. This is necessary because the nose and mouth no longer warm and moisten the inspired air. Adequate fluids are provided.

Tracheostomy Tube. Maintaining patency of the tracheostomy tube is of utmost importance. Plastic or silastic tubes are generally used because they are flexible and reduce crust formation. They are lightweight and disposable, and most do not have inner cannulas. Cuffed tubes are not usually necessary in infants and small children, as their air passages are smaller and the tracheostomy tube provides a sufficient seal. The surgeon chooses a tracheostomy tube that is appropriate for the patient's neck size and condition. Administering oxygen by manual resuscitator (bagging) prior to or following the procedure helps to prevent hypoxia.

Suctioning. Selection of a suction catheter is important. The nurse chooses one that does not block the tube during suctioning. The diameter should be about one-half the size of the tracheostomy tube. Hands are washed before proceeding. The nurse uses sterile gloves for the procedure, and all equipment used in the care of a tracheostomy should be sterile. Suction is applied as the catheter is *withdrawn.* The tube is rotated to allow removal of secretions on all sides. With Y-tube technique, suction is achieved by closing the port with the thumb. A drop of saline may be inserted before suctioning to aid in loosening secretions. Because variations in this procedure exist and modifications are frequently required, one must understand what is intended for the particular patient. The nurse asks for clarification and specific procedures of the institution where employed.

Suctioning is done periodically and when necessary. Indications for suctioning include noisy breathing, bubbling of mucus, and moist cough or respirations. During suctioning, patients can rapidly become hypoxic. Suctioning is limited to approximately 15 seconds. To judge timing, some nurses hold their own breath. Two or three breaths for reoxygenation are allowed between suctioning. The depth of suctioning is important. In general, suctioning is limited to the length of the tracheostomy tube or slightly beyond to stimulate coughing. The catheter is cleared with sterile water between insertions. Unnecessary suctioning is avoided. The suction catheter is discarded after use. Disposing of water after suctioning prevents the growth of *Pseudomonas* organisms.

Tracheal Stoma. The tracheal stoma is treated as a surgical wound. The area is kept free of secretions and exudate to minimize the risk of infection. Cotton-tipped applicators dipped in half-strength hydrogen peroxide can be utilized to remove crusted mucus. Tapes around the child's neck should be loose enough to allow one finger to be easily inserted. The knot is placed to the side of the neck. The condition of the skin beneath the tape is assessed. The tape is changed as necessary. Two people are used for this procedure, one to hold the outer cannula and the other to change the tape. When feeding the infant, the nurse covers the tracheostomy with a bib or moist piece of gauze to prevent aspiration of food particles.

Observing for Complications. The nurse observes the patient for such symptoms as restlessness, rising pulse rate, fatigue, apathy, dyspnea, sternal retractions, pallor, cyanosis, and inflammation or drainage around the incision. Possible complications include tracheoesophageal fistula, stenosis, tracheal ischemia, infection, atelectasis, cannula occlusion, and accidental extubation. Baseline assessment of the patient is done on each shift and prior to suctioning. The patient's mental status, respirations, pulse rate and rhythm, and chest

Table 22–11

NURSING GUIDELINES FOR PEDIATRIC IVS AT VARIOUS STAGES OF CHILD'S DEVELOPMENT

Developmental Characteristics*	IV Placement (Ideal Sites)†	Preparation of Child	Family Involvement
Infant (1st Year)			
Dependent on others for all needs. Needs to feel physically safe through close relationship with one caretaking person (usually the mother). Trust develops through needs being met consistently. Mistrust and anxiety develop when needs are met inconsistently. Stranger anxiety begins at approximately 6–8 mo	Scalp vein (best site); foot, hand, forearm	Best not to feed infant immediately before IV insertion (vomiting and aspiration possible)	Prepare family about need for IV therapy, insertion procedure, appearance of infant with IV, and fluid needs. Encourage family to continue providing baby with tactile and verbal stimulation, and tender, loving care. Demonstrate safe ways to hold an infant with an IV. Encourage questions and clarify misconceptions
Toddler (Ages 1–3)			
Discovers and explores self and surrounding world. Enjoys new mobility skills. Develops egocentric thinking and need for parallel play. Tolerates short separations from mother. Transitional objects (security blanket, special toy) provide some comfort. Oppositional syndrome ("no" stage). Separation anxiety an important problem in hospitalized toddlers separated from mother, ages 8–24 mo	Hand, arm, foot. Important: From this age group on, the less dominant extremity should be used for the IV whenever possible. Determine handedness prior to IV insertion	Prepare child immediately before procedure (child has limited attention span and is likely to become more anxious if prepared sooner). Give very simple explanation in concrete terms. Show equipment to be used. Do not offer choice. See preparation for preschool age (below) and assess ability of each child to understand	Prepare family as to need for IV therapy, insertion procedure, and appearance of child with IV. Whether parents remain with the child during the procedure varies. If they stay with the child their role is to comfort rather than to assist with restraining. Demonstrate to parents how to safely handle child with IV
Preschool (Ages 4–6)			
Magical thinking, based on what the child would like to believe. Cannot always distinguish fantasy from reality. Fears intrusive procedures. Castration fears common. Develops conscience (guilt), while asserting independence and mastering new skills. Learning to share	Hand, forearm (less dominant)	Prepare child just prior to procedure. Using small bottle, tubing, and doll or stuffed animal, explain in literal terms the need for IV and insertion procedure. Allow child to see and touch equipment. Explain how child can help with procedure by cleaning site, opening packages, taping, and so on. Allow some degree of control in the situation. Say you will help child to hold still and that it is O.K. to cry	As with toddlers, parents may or may not stay with the child during the procedure. If they stay, they should provide comfort and support, but they should not be asked to restrain the child for IV insertion. Reinforce child's need for honest, simple explanations. Reassure parents that child can still play and be active, even with IV

sounds are of particular importance. Accurate recording of observations is essential to evaluation. The time and frequency of suctioning, the character of secretions, the relief afforded the patient, the behavior, the appearance of the wound, and other pertinent data are recorded.

A sterile hemostat is kept at the bedside for emergency use. Accidental *extubation,* or expulsion of the tube, although uncommon, can occur from severe coughing if the tapes are too loose. Patency of the airway is maintained by spreading the edges of the wound with the sterile clamp until a duplicate tube is inserted. An extra tracheostomy tube and the equipment needed for its replacement are always kept in a visible, easily reached area at the bedside for use in such emergencies. As the child's condition improves, he or she is weaned from the tube. The opening gradually closes by granulation.

Table 22–11

NURSING GUIDELINES FOR PEDIATRIC IVS AT VARIOUS STAGES OF CHILD'S DEVELOPMENT *(Continued)*

Related Nursing Actions	Protection of IV Site†	Mobility Considerations‡	Safety Needs
Restrain during insertion. Comfort and cuddle during and after insertion. Observe carefully during insertion for problems of vomiting, aspiration, and so on. Firmly restrain extremity with IV (see next column). Use of pacifier diminishes stress, especially for infants given nothing by mouth (NPO)	IV may be secured with tape and is wrapped. Extremity may be restrained by using a small arm board, a sandbag, or wrist and ankle restraints	Keep restraints as loose as possible to allow for motion. Release any restrained extremities hourly for range of motion (ROM). Mitten hands with cotton and stockinette to prohibit infant's grasping IV. Restraining all extremities is *rarely* necessary. Remember infant's need for sensory stimulation	Maintain strict intake and output (I & O). Secure IV tubing out of range of kicking legs and flailing arms. Check restraints frequently for effectiveness and presence of adequate circulation
Restraining the toddler for an IV usually requires more than one person. Reassure child through verbal and tactile stimulation during procedure. Provide toys such as pegs to hammer, for therapeutic expression of anger, after procedure and throughout hospitalization	See that for infant (above). A securely anchored IV is essential for the normally active toddler. Even the best site protection will not remain effective unless it is coupled with close nursing supervision and distracting activities for the child	Toddlers cope with the world and learn about it through action. Therefore, minimum restraints should be used, and tying the child in bed is to be avoided. Parental presence during waking hours permits the child to be constantly supervised and makes restraints unnecessary in many cases. However, be careful to avoid setting up a situation in which the child associates parent's departure with punishment by restraint	Child is unaware of danger at this age; will not know that movement of IV causes pain. Constant supervision needed when out of bed. Remind frequently not to touch IV, but do not expect compliance. Distracting activities accomplish much more than does a scolding for handling the IV. Tape connections on tubing if child continues to handle tubing. Keep tubing clamps out of reach
Tell child IV is not being given as punishment. *Never* bribe or threaten with IVs (e.g., "Drink, or you'll get another IV.") Praise for cooperation or any efforts in that direction. Maintain patient privacy. Do not start an IV in view of other patients, visitors, or staff. Child needs support to cope with intrusiveness of this procedure. Show understanding	See that for infant (above). As with toddlers, securely anchored IVs are essential, but inadequate unless coupled with close supervision and age-appropriate activities	Preschoolers need maximum mobility to master surroundings. Provide a range of out-of-bed activities whenever possible	Child will be curious about IV. Is capable of understanding instructions to not touch it but needs frequent reminders. IV clamps should be out of reach or taped over. Constant supervision needed when out of bed. Child is liable to take off down the hall, heedless of pole, bottle, and so on. Short attention span limits duration of cooperation with instructions

Table continued on following page

Children whose tubes must remain in place for a longer time require periodic tube changes.

Additional Nursing Measures. Additional nursing measures include frequent change of position, use of elbow restraints, oral feedings unless contraindicated, and careful bathing to prevent water from entering the tube. Range-of-motion exercises are a must for long-term patients, and in acute cases arm restraints are removed one at a time to allow for passive exercises. The diet is ordered by the physician. Although patients may initially have nothing by mouth, as the condition improves they progress to a soft or normal diet. The Fowler position is preferred during feedings. The older child

Table 22–11

NURSING GUIDELINES FOR PEDIATRIC IVS AT VARIOUS STAGES OF CHILD'S DEVELOPMENT *(Continued)*

Developmental Characteristics*	IV Placement (Ideal Sites)†	Preparation of Child	Family Involvement
School Age (Ages 7–11)			
Struggles between mastery of new skills and failure. Enjoys school, learning skills, games with rules. Needs to succeed. Fears body mutilation. May feel need to be brave. Can understand hospital rules. World now expanding beyond family. Peer group becomes important. Competitiveness	Hand, forearm (less dominant)	Prepare child ahead of time but on same day of insertion. Carefully explain and demonstrate equipment and reasons for IV therapy, letting patient watch you or help set up equipment. Ask child for questions about need for IV and procedure. Give child choices and let child help in procedure whenever possible. Tell child crying is O.K. because needles hurt, and you will help in holding still	Whenever possible, family and child should be prepared together so that family can reinforce what the child has been told. Stress to family the child's need for some independence in activities of daily living, even with an IV. Parental presence or participation in IV insertion may be appropriate, but child's preference should be considered primary
Adolescent (Ages 12–18)			
Vacillates between needs for independence and dependence. Adult cognitive abilities, deductive reasoning. Coping mechanisms: rationalization, intellectualization. Peer acceptance very important. Egocentric, rebellious at times, especially against parents and authority figures. Very concerned with body image, body changes, sexuality, and role. Searching for "who I am"	Hand, forearm (less dominant)	Prepare patient several hours to a day before procedure, if possible. Needs time between preparation and insertion to absorb explanations and ask questions. For most adolescents, approach discussions on an adult level. Explain need for IV therapy and expected duration, and show equipment. May need much support for acceptance of therapy	Explain therapy needs and duration as with patient. Decision regarding parental presence during procedure should be patient's, not parents'. Stress to family participation in decisions affecting child's care

can cooperate by holding the head flexed with chin down. This decreases swallowing difficulties, as the esophagus opens and the airway narrows.

Discharge. Certain patients are discharged with a tracheostomy (Fig. 22–27). This is anticipated, and instruction and demonstration for the parents begin early. Parents who are comfortable with the procedure during hospitalization will feel more secure when the child returns home. Information about parent groups and visiting nurse and other referrals are made prior to discharge.

Oxygen Therapy

Table 22–12 reviews selected considerations for the child receiving oxygen. See Chapter 13 for care of a child in an incubator.

Safety Considerations. All equipment used for oxygen therapy must be inspected periodically. Combustible materials and potential sources of fire are kept away from oxygen equipment. These materials are essentially the same as for adults; for the child, however, friction toys are also to be avoided because the sparks they can create could cause ignition. Nylon or wool blankets are not to be used. One should know where the nearest fire extinguisher is located. Parents are alerted to the precautions and presence of "no smoking" signs.

Infection control is extremely important. It is imperative that cross-infection via unclean equipment be prevented. Humidifiers and nebulizers, which are warm and moist, serve as an excellent medium for the growth of disease-producing organisms. Although most masks, tents, and cannulas that come into direct contact with the child are disposable, other pieces of mechanical equipment cannot be discarded. *They require periodic cleansing if therapy is extended and terminal cleansing according to product direction.* The respiratory therapy department should be contacted as necessary.

Prolonged exposure to high oxygen concentrations can be toxic to some body tissues, such as the retina in preterm infants and the lungs in the general population, but particularly in children with pulmonary diseases such as asthma or cystic fibrosis. It is therefore necessary to measure oxygen

Table 22–11
NURSING GUIDELINES FOR PEDIATRIC IVS AT VARIOUS STAGES OF CHILD'S DEVELOPMENT *(Continued)*

Related Nursing Actions	Protection of IV Site†	Mobility Considerations‡	Safety Needs
Approach child expecting cooperation (this age group likes to please adults), but expect that child will need help holding still. Allow the child to clean the site with alcohol swab and to cut tape prior to insertion. Praise cooperative efforts. Give child step-by-step explanation of procedure as it progresses. Child may like to take some responsibility in keeping I & O	Will need less protection than younger children owing to interest in making IV work correctly. May naturally protect extremity with IV. Some children appreciate a warning sign—"Hands Off," on a piece of tape over the IV as a reminder. Utilize the child's natural curiosity and interest in learning. Tell child the rules of safe IV handling	Show patient and family how to safely manipulate IV for out-of-bed activities (walking in hall with pole, keeping tubing out of wheelchair wheels, and so on)	Remind patient periodically about necessary caution with IV. Show patient the clamps, and caution against handling them. Teach patient signs of IV problems. Enlist child's help in the interest of good compliance, but do not entirely depend on it. Tape tubing connections. Child may forget about IV. Emphasize need for caution in some activities, especially if play includes other children
Be aware of IV adding to patient's dependency status and need for some control. Encourage child to keep own I & O, help in counting drip rate, and so on	See that for school age (above). If patient is very active, will need well-protected, well-anchored IV, as movements may be more forceful and strength greater than those of younger patients	See that for school age (above). Encourage mobility as much as possible as a means of independence for the adolescent	Be aware of possibility of adolescent rebellion showing itself in lack of cooperation with therapy. These patients may rebel if feeling threatened, and may be very manipulative in testing behaviors. Consistent limits, clearly communicated to patient, parents, and staff, are needed. Instruct patient as to signs of infiltration, phlebitis, and so on

Modified from Guhlow, L.J., & Kolb, J. (1979). Pediatric IVs: Special measures you should take. *RN*, 42, 40. Published in RN, the full-service nursing journal. Copyright © 1979 Medical Economics Company Inc, Oradell, NJ. Reprinted by permission.

*Each stage builds on the earlier ones, and during hospitalization many children regress to behaviors appropriate to earlier levels of development.

†No child should be restricted to bed simply because of having an IV!

IV refers to intravenous line, throughout table.

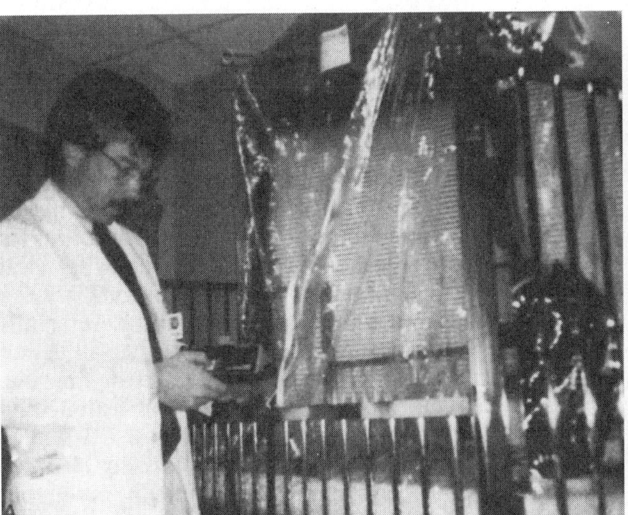

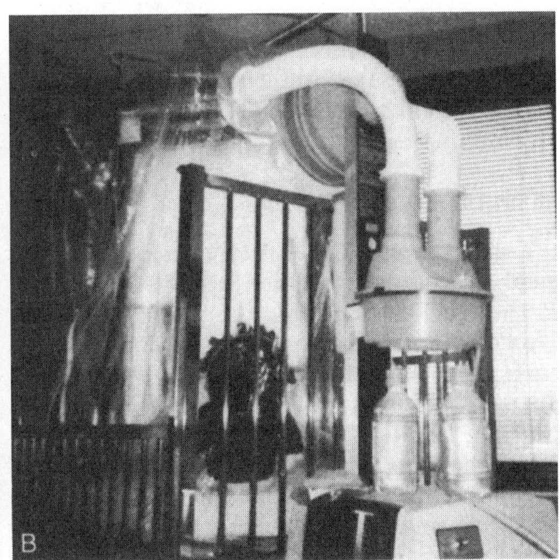

Figure 22–26. • **A,** The respiratory therapist measures the oxygen concentration in the tent by an oxygen analyzer. **B,** The working unit of the mist tent. (Courtesy of Columbia/HCA Portsmouth Regional Hospital, Portsmouth, NH.)

concentrations at regular intervals with an *oxygen analyzer* (see Fig. 22–26). This is usually done by the respiratory therapist; however, the nurse needs to ensure that the procedure is carried out on assigned patients. Readings are obtained close to the child's head. The amount of oxygen administered depends on the child's arterial oxygen concentration. Blood gas determinations (Po_2 and Pco_2) ensure safe and accurate therapy. Noninvasive pulse oximeters that measure blood oxygen tension via the skin are available (see Chapter 13, Figure 13–6).

Oxygen is a dry gas and requires the addition of moisture to prevent irritation of the respiratory tree. High-humidity concentrations may be achieved by the use of jet humidifiers on several oxygen units. *Compressed air rather than oxygen* may also be used for this purpose. *Oxygen therapy is terminated gradually.* This allows the patient to adjust to *ambient* (environmental) oxygen. The nurse slowly reduces liter flow, opens air vents in Isolettes, or opens zippers in croup tents. The child's response is constantly monitored. An increase in restlessness and in pulse and respirations indicates that the child is not tolerating withdrawal from the oxygen-enriched environment.

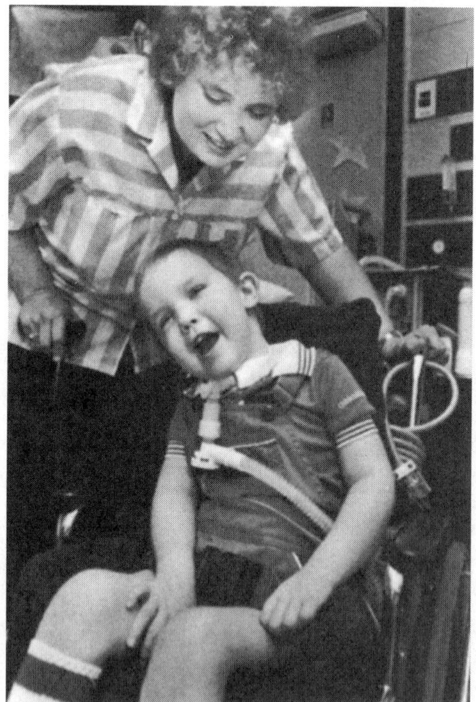

Figure 22–27. • Tracheostomy. The acuity level of discharged patients is more intense today and necessitates education and support of family members in all aspects of care. This child is being discharged with a tracheostomy in place. (Courtesy of Blank Memorial Hospital for Children, Des Moines, IA.)

Methods of Administration. Oxygen is administered to children as age-appropriate via Isolette, nasal cannula, mask, hood, or tent. Regardless of the method used, the child is observed frequently to determine the effectiveness of the oxygen therapy. *The desired goals include decreased restlessness and improved breathing, vital signs, and color.* The highest concentrations of oxygen can be delivered by way of a plastic hood (see Chapter 13, Figure 13–5). Warmed, humidified oxygen is delivered directly over the child's head. It may be used in a warming unit.

Mist Tent. A mist tent (Fig. 22–26) provides an atmosphere of fine particles of water suspended in a cool air or oxygen environment. The zippered openings in the clear plastic canopy facilitates easy access and observation of the child. A nebulizer can be attached to provide medicated inhalation therapy. The child should be dressed warmly when inside the tent to prevent hypothermia. The oxygen concentration should be checked periodically and a pulse oximeter assessment of oxygen saturation should be monitored.

Often a physician's order will read "keep O_2 saturation at 93%." This means that if the O_2 saturation on the pulse oximeter reads above 93% the oxygen liter flow can be lowered and the child carefully monitored. If the O_2 saturation level reads below 93% the liter flow can be gradually increased and the child closely monitored until the reading reaches 93% (see Chapter 13 for pulse oximeter). A parent at the bedside stroking the infant through the zippered opening in the canopy can have a calming effect. Keeping a child dry in a high-humidity tent can be a challenge. Frequent linen and clothing changes are essential.

Low-Flow Oxygen. *Low-flow oxygen* (Fig. 22–28) is a method of oxygen delivery used for children with chronic lung disease (such as cystic fibrosis) who are oxygen dependent for prolonged periods. These children react poorly to high oxygen concentrations. About 1 or 2 liters per minute of oxygen are administered via nasal cannula or a "blow-by" catheter that is placed on the upper lip just below the nostrils. Since this type of oxygen delivery is used for prolonged periods, parent teaching concerning home management is a nursing responsibility.

Management of Airway Obstruction

An emergency treatment known as the *Heimlich maneuver* is recommended to dislodge food or foreign bodies from the airway. This technique works on the principle that forcing the diaphragm up

Table 22–12
SELECTED CONSIDERATIONS FOR THE CHILD RECEIVING OXYGEN

Age	Comment
General Considerations: Signs of respiratory distress include an increase in pulse and respiration, restlessness, flaring nares, intercostal and substernal retractions, and cyanosis. In addition, children with dyspnea frequently vomit, which increases the danger of aspiration. Maintain a clear airway by suctioning if needed. Organize nursing care so that interruptions are kept at a minimum. Observe children carefully, as your vision may be obstructed by mist, and young children are unable to verbalize their needs	
Newborn	Oxygen may be provided via hood, which may be used in warming unit Oxygen may be provided via Isolette; keep sleeves closed to decrease oxygen loss Oxygen needs to be warmed to prevent neonatal stress from cold Analyze concentration carefully to avoid retrolental fibroplasia or pulmonary disease Parents are primary focus of preparations; help to develop good parenting skills and self-confidence in their ability to care for the child who is ill
Infant	Nose may need to be suctioned by bulb syringe to remove mucus Child may benefit from use of infant seat; secure seat to bed frame, watch for slumping in seat *Make sure crib sides are up; a canopy often gives the illusion of safety* Avoid the use of baby oil, A and D ointment, petroleum jelly (Vaseline) or other oil- or alcohol-based substances Anticipate stranger anxiety at around 6–8 mo; baby clings to parents, turns away from nurse An extremely irritable baby may benefit from comforting in parent's lap followed by sleeping in tent; clarify at report time Frequently, children can be removed from oxygen for bathing and eating; determine before proceeding
Toddler	Anticipate that a toddler will be distressed by a tent Anticipate regression When child is restless and fussy, she may pull tent and covers apart Toddler cannot tell nurse if tent is "too hot" or "too cold" Change clothing and bed linen when damp Child may be comforted by transitional object such as blanket Parents may have suggestions as to how to keep child happy in tent
Preschool	Tent plastic distorts view Because thought processes are immature in preschool children, reality and fantasy are inseparable Prepare child for all procedures to decrease fear Anticipate that child will feel lonely and isolated Child will enjoy stories, puppets, dramatic play If extremely restless and anxious, child may benefit from holding parent's hand through small opening in zippers Helpful if child can be out of tent for meals
School Age	School children usually are less frightened by tent; fears center around body mutilation and loss of control Preparation information continues to focus on what the child will see, hear, feel, and be expected to do Child may benefit from writing a story about the experience; nurse reviews story with child and clarifies misconceptions; posting story on unit affirms child's self-esteem and mastery (always ask permission to post) Allow child to make realistic choices before, during, and after procedures Draw "what it feels like to be in a tent" and discuss
Adolescent	Adolescent needs more time to process information, needs to know the results of blood studies and other tests Nurse remains available to the patient to answer questions as they arise Trust is extremely important as adolescent attempts to move beyond the nuclear family Anticipate problems of being restricted by apparatus May feel weird when visited by peers; wavers between feeling self-confident and feeling ineffective Reiterate no smoking and other safety precautions with patient and peers Include patient in therapy, may be able to manage own oxygen needs Review safe use of oxygen in the home if required for comfort and survival

causes residual air in the lung to be forcefully expelled resulting in "popping" the obstruction out of the airway.

Older Child Standing or Sitting. Stand behind the standing or sitting victim and wrap your arms around the victim's waist, with one hand made into a fist (Fig. 22–29). The thumb side rests against the victim's abdomen, slightly above the navel and well below the tip of the sternum (xyphoid process). Grasp the fist with the other hand and press into the victim's abdomen with a quick upward thrust. Six to ten thrusts may be necessary to dislodge the object. Each thrust should be a separate and distinct movement.

Older Child Lying Down (Conscious or Unconscious). Position the child on his back. Kneel at the child's feet if the child is on the floor or stand at the child's feet if the child is on a table. Place the heel of one hand on the child's abdomen in the midline, slightly above the navel and well below the rib cage. Grasp the fist with the other hand and press into the victim's abdomen with a quick upward thrust. Repeat six to ten thrusts as needed. Direct thrusts upward into the midline and not to either side of the abdomen. The smaller the child, the gentler the procedure should be.

Infant. Determine airway obstruction. If the object is visualized, remove it, trying not to push the object deeper into the throat. If this approach is unsuccessful, position the child prone with the head lower than the trunk. (Support head and neck with one hand and straddle the infant face down over your forearm supported on your thigh, as shown in Figure 22–29). Resting the infant on the thigh, perform five forceful back blows between the shoulder blades with the heel of one hand. After delivering the back blows, place the free hand on the infant's back, so that the victim is sandwiched between the two hands, and turn the infant on his or her back, with the head still lower than the trunk. Deliver five thrusts in the mid-sternal region in the same manner as for external chest compressions, but at a slower rate (3–5 seconds). Repeat until the foreign body is expelled. Do not perform abdominal thrusts as this may cause injury to the infant's abdominal organs. When the airway is cleared, conventional cardiopulmonary resuscitation (CPR) can be initiated. Since all nurses are required to have basic CPR certification, the technique is not reviewed at this time.

The Throat-E-Vac. Some hospitals and ambulance services use equipment specifically designed for removal of food from the airway. One such device in the Throat-E-Vac (Fig. 22–30). The patient is positioned with the head slightly hyperextended. The correct size mouthpiece from the Throat-E-Vac kit is placed on the end of the tube on the pump and inserted into the child's mouth over the tongue. The nurse uses her hand to seal the mouthpiece. The nose is closed with a nose clip. The nurse pumps with quick strokes and watches the gauge for any rise in vacuum. When the blockage is dislodged, the vacuum gauge will suddenly drop to zero. A finger sweep clears the airway. Resuscitation measures can then be initiated. The unit is designed for use in complete airway obstruction. If pumping fails to produce a rise in the level of the vacuum gauge, then the airway is not completely obstructed and other resuscitative measures may be initiated until a physician is available.

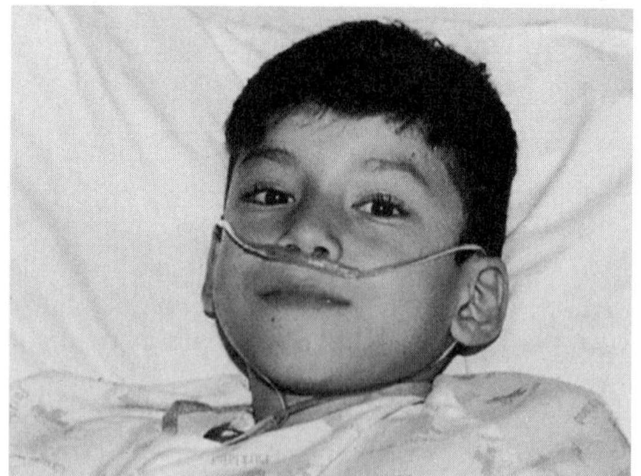

Figure 22–28. • Child receiving blow-by oxygen therapy via nasal route. (Photograph from Ashwill, J. & Droske, S. [1997]. *Nursing care of children. Principles and Practice.* Philadelphia: Saunders.)

Preoperative and Postoperative Care

Children are particularly fearful of surgery and require both physical and psychological preparation at the child's level of understanding. Listening to the child is especially valuable to clarify misunderstandings. The child is asked to point to the operative site on a body outline. "Show me what they are going to fix." Explain anesthesia and allow the child to play with a mask (Fig. 22–31). Children and adults need reassurance. Nursing interventions following surgery are aimed at assisting the child to master a threatening situation and minimizing physical and psychological complications. Table 22–13 and 22–14 summarize preparation for surgery and postoperative care.

When adults are prepared for surgery they are usually kept NPO (nothing by mouth) from the midnight prior to the scheduled surgery date. The surgery may be done in the morning or the afternoon. Infants should not be maintained on NPO status for longer than 4 to 6 hours because of the high risk for dehydration. It is a nursing responsibility to check that the test procedure or surgery is scheduled as early as possible in the morning to avoid a prolonged wait. Pacifiers should be provided to infants who are on NPO status to meet their developmental need for sucking.

Pain Management

Freedom from pain is a basic need and a right of the infant and child. However, the infant and child cannot always express pain and therefore assertive observation and assessment by the nurse are essential. Distraction, relaxation, music, explanations, hand holding, and stroking are methods of relieving pain that do not involve medications. A child who is old enough to understand and cooperate can assist in determining strategies that can minimize

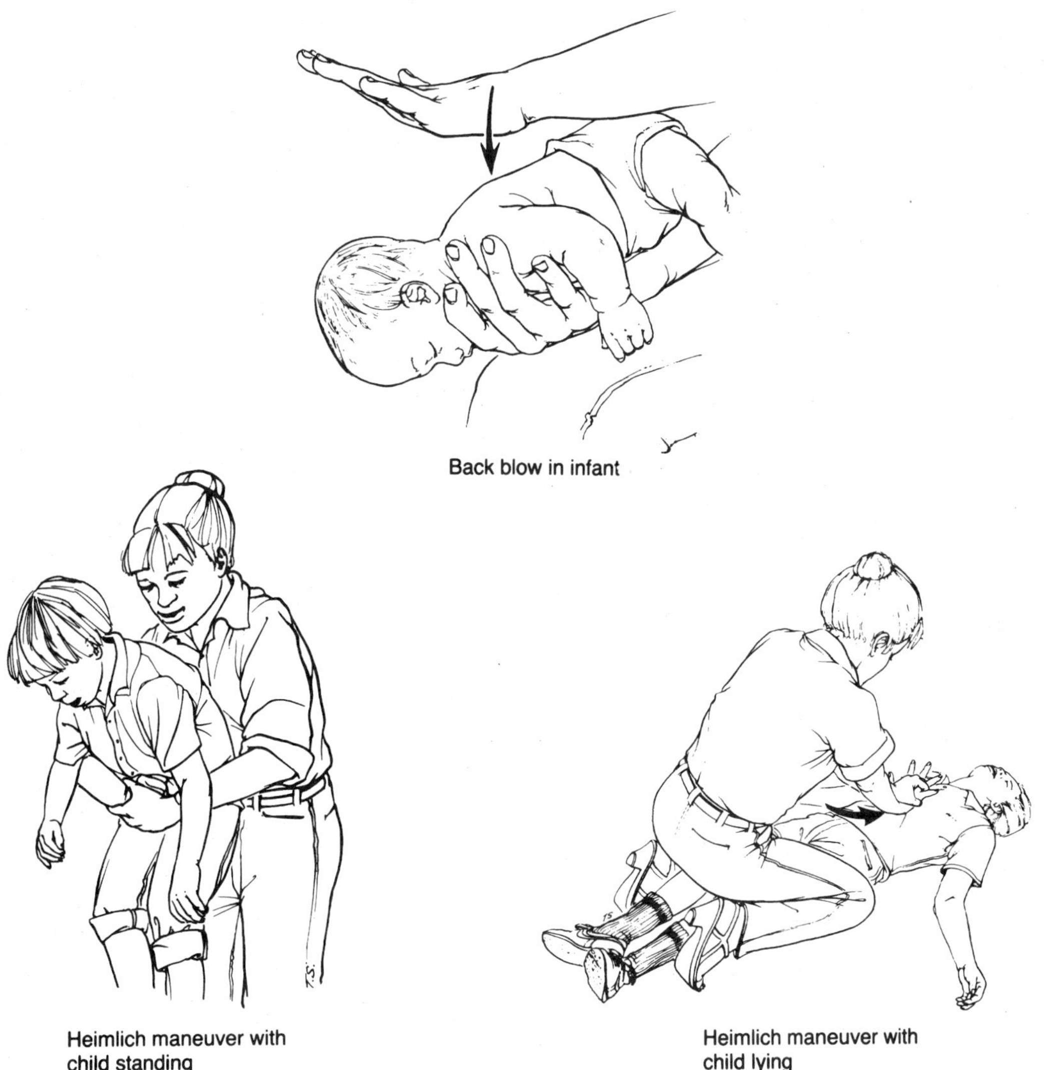

Figure 22–29. • Procedures for clearing an airway obstruction. (From Guidelines for cardiopulmonary resuscitation and emergency cardiac care [1992]. *JAMA, 268,* 2171–2302. Copyright 1992, American Medical Association.)

or relieve pain. Opioids are drugs used to relieve pain and should be given as needed. Topical medications can prevent pain during invasive procedures and should be used (see Fig. 22–18).

Figure 22–32 lists 4 pain assessment tools. When a child is in pain, the family shares that pain on an emotional level. Prevention of pain, assessment of pain, and relief of pain in infants and children are primary nursing responsibilities.

Patient-controlled analgesia (PCA) allows the patient to press a button attached to an IV analgesic infusion to administer a bolus of medication. Parents and children as young as 7 years of age can be taught to use PCA. A built-in lockout interval prevents accidental overdosing. Any child receiving opioid analgesic drugs should be observed closely for side effects, such as respiratory depression.

When a low-dose analgesic is administered around the clock on a regular schedule, rather than PRN more effective pain relief at lower doses may be achieved. However, "breakthrough pain" can occur and additional doses of an analgesic may need to be given. This type of pain management is called preventative pain control.

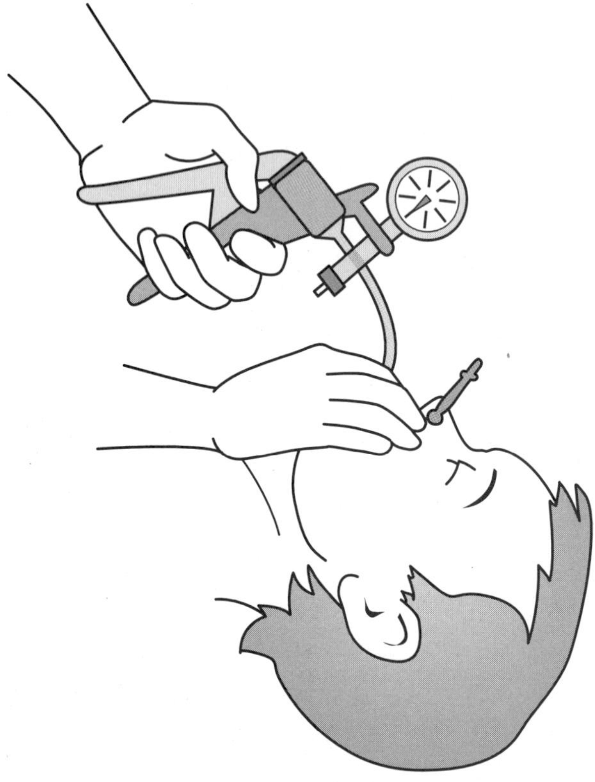

Figure 22–30. • The Throat-E-Vac. (From Leifer, *Principles and techniques in pediatric nursing.* Philadelphia: Saunders.) (Courtesy of Prism Enterprises, San Antonio, TX.)

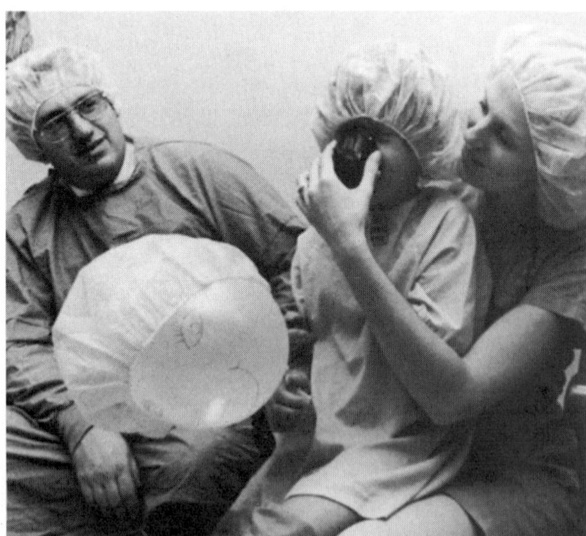

Figure 22–31. • Preparing the child for the sights and sounds of surgery. (Courtesy of Blank Memorial Hospital, Des Moines, IA.)

Table 22–13
SUMMARY OF PREPARATION OF THE CHILD FOR SURGERY

Procedure	Adult	Child	Modification
Consent	Yes	Yes	Parent or legal guardian
Blood work	Yes	Yes	Age-appropriate restraint
Urinalysis	Yes	Yes	Age-appropriate collection (U-bag) Assist school child Age-appropriate instructions
Evaluate for respiratory infection, nutritional status	Yes	Yes	Utilize more objective observations in infants and toddlers because of child's limited verbal skills
Allergies	Yes	Yes	Indicate clearly on chart
Nothing by mouth (NPO)	Yes	Yes	Increase fluids prior to NPO Length of time may vary with age and type of surgery (6–12 hr) If surgery is late, place appropriate notice on child: "Do not feed me" Remove goodies from bedside stand No gum Supervise hungry ambulatory patients carefully
Vital signs	Yes	Yes	Approach child carefully, explain, demonstrate Allow more time
Void before surgery	Yes	Preferred	Not always possible in infants and toddlers
Bath	Yes	Yes	Hospital gown, may wear underwear or pajama bottoms depending on age, type of surgery
Identification	Yes	Yes	Identification bracelet
Teeth	Yes	Yes	Check for loose teeth, orthodontic appliance
Skin preparation	Yes	Possible	May be done in operating room
Nails	Yes	Yes	Trim, remove nail polish
Glasses or contact lenses	Yes	Yes	Have children and adolescents remove glasses or contact lenses
Enemas	Possible	Possible	Not routine
Transportation	Yes	Yes	Crib or stretcher Parents may accompany to operating room door
Emotional preparation	Yes	Yes	Preoperative tour Group and individual puppet play Body drawings of parts involved Play selected by child as mode of expression Support parents during surgery
Sedation	Yes	Yes	Usually 20 min prior to surgery
Record all pertinent data	Yes	Yes	Essentially the same with pediatric modifications as indicated by the above

Conscious Sedation

Conscious sedation is the administration of intravenous drugs to a patient to impair consciousness but retain protective reflexes, the ability to maintain a patent airway and the ability to respond to physical and verbal stimuli. Conscious sedation is used to perform therapeutic or diagnostic procedures outside the traditional operating room setting. A skilled registered nurse is required to continuously monitor the patient in an area where emergency equipment and drugs are accessible for resuscitation.

Discharge criteria include stable vital signs, age-appropriate motor and verbal abilities, adequate hydration, and a presedation level of responsiveness and orientation. Parents are instructed concerning diet, home care, and follow-up visits.

Table 22–14
SUMMARY OF POSTOPERATIVE CARE OF THE CHILD

Procedure	Adult	Child	Modification
Return from recovery room	Yes	Yes	Notify parents Smaller patients generally in crib Age-appropriate safety precautions
Note general condition, alertness	Yes	Yes	Infant and toddler cannot verbalize fear or pain
Vital signs	Yes	Yes	Every 15–30 min until stable Blood pressure is sometimes omitted for infant
Evaluate for shock	Yes	Yes	Essentially same
Assess operative site for bleeding, dressing intactness	Yes	Yes	Essentially same Elevate casted extremities Circle drainage
Restraints	Possible	Probable	May be necessary to protect IV Remove periodically for range of motion
Connect dependent drainage (urinary catheter, Levin tubes, oxygen)	Yes	Yes	Prepare child for sight and noises of equipment; draw pictures to clarify purpose
Position patient	Yes	Yes	Prop on side unless contraindicated, no pillow
Intravenous (IV)	Yes	Yes	Should have pediatric adapting device and infusion pump Monitor rate meticulously, as infants and small children respond quickly to fluid shifts Measure and record intake and output
Assess elimination	Yes	Yes	Bowel and bladder
Relief of pain	Yes	Yes	Hold, comfort small children unless contraindicated Be sensitive to behavioral changes such as increase in irritability, crying, regression, nail biting, passivity, withdrawal Administer pain relievers Involve parents in care Provide transitional object such as blanket, favorite toy, pacifier Be aware of transcultural considerations that provide familiarity and comfort
Nothing by mouth (NPO)	Yes	Yes	Until fully awake Babies are started on clear fluids by bottle unless contraindicated Avoid brown or red liquids, which may be confused with old or fresh blood Monitor bowel sounds
Consider diet	Yes	Yes	Advance from clear to full liquids to soft to regular diet
Observe for complications	Yes	Yes	Turn, cough, deep-breathe, dangle feet, ambulate early; less of a problem in children Splint operative site with hands when child coughs

1. Visual analog scale
   Child points to where the pain falls on the scale.

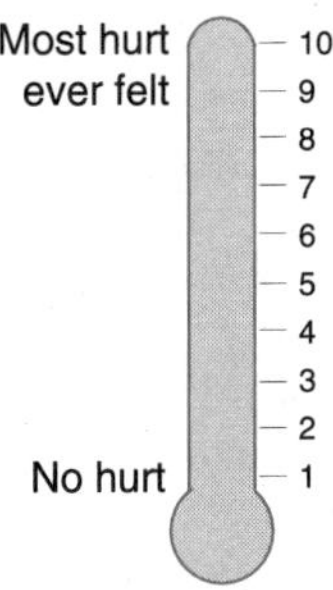

2. Descriptive word scale
   Child chooses the word that describes the pain.

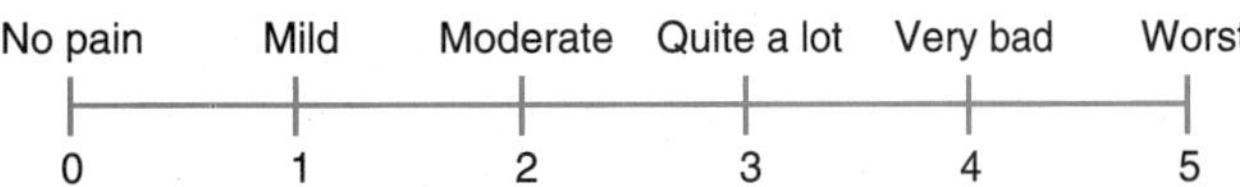

3. Faces (Oucher) scale
   Child tells which face represents the pain at that moment.

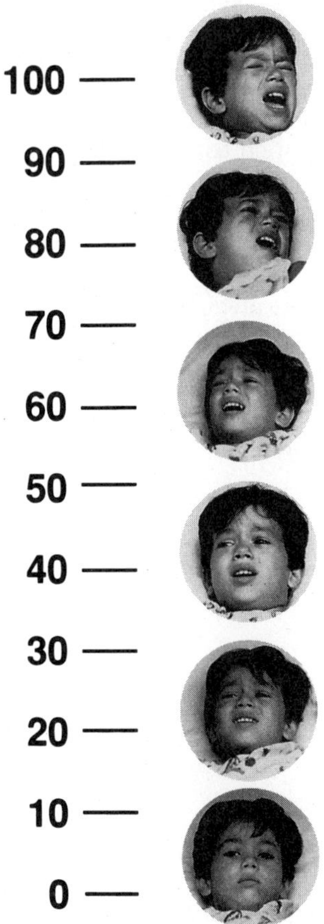

4. Poker chip
   a. Use 4 red poker chips (color variations have also been cited)
   b. Place horizontally in front of child
   c. Say "These are pieces of hurt—one piece is a little, and four pieces are a lot."
   d. Ask "How many pieces of hurt do you have right now?"
   e. Record number on flow sheet (no pain equals zero)

Figure 22–32. • Four pain assessment tools for children. (Oucher scale reproduced courtesy of Antonia M. Villarruel, Ph.D., R.N., and Mary J. Penyes, Ph.D., R.N., © 1990.)

KEY POINTS

- The nurse must be especially conscious of safety measures on the children's division, particularly of keeping crib sides up when the child is unattended, careful application of restraints, safe transport, and proper identification of the child.
- Include the parents in both planning and implementing care. Children are prepared for and encouraged to express their feelings about treatments.
- Weights must be accurate because medication is often estimated by the child's weight.
- The correct-size blood pressure cuff must be used for children to obtain an accurate reading. It should cover two-thirds of the upper arm.
- Special urine collection devices are used for newborns and infants.
- Positioning of the child for jugular and femoral puncture is important. Because these are large veins, the infant is frequently checked for bleeding following these procedures.
- Medications for children have to be adapted to size, age, and body surface. The absorption, distribution, metabolism, and excretion of drugs differ substantially in children. Their reactions to drugs are less predictable.
- The recommended intramuscular injection site for children under 3 years of age is the vastus lateralis.
- Careful observation of the child receiving intravenous fluids is necessary because overload of fluids in an infant can lead to cardiac failure. IV pumps such as the IVAC pump are used to monitor infusions. Intake and output sheets must be accurate.
- When administering ear drops to children under 3 years of age, the pinna of the ear is pulled down and back to straighten the ear canal. In the older child, the pinna of the ear is pulled up and back.
- The nurse must monitor the rate of the IV flow, refill the burettes, observe the condition of the IV site, and assess the response of the child.
- A pacifier should be offered to infants who are placed on nothing by mouth.
- Weighing a wet diaper and subtracting the dry weight of a similar diaper is one method of recording the output of infants.

MULTIPLE-CHOICE REVIEW QUESTIONS

Choose the most appropriate answer.

1. Which of the following approaches is best when administering an oral medication to a young child:
   a. "Would you please take your medicine now, David."
   b. "Look how good Johnny took his medication. Can you do that too, David?"
   c. "You must take your medicine now if you want to get better."
   d. "It's time for your medication David, would you like water or juice after it?"
2. The preferred site for an intramuscular injection in infants is
   a. dorsogluteal.
   b. ventrogluteal.
   c. vastus lateralis.
   d. deltoid.
3. The doctor orders 10 mg of Demerol for an infant following surgery. The label reads: 50 mg/1 ml. You would administer
   a. 10 minims.
   b. 8 minims.
   c. 6 minims.
   d. 3 minims.
4. When preparing an enema for a young child, the nurse would select which of the following solutions
   a. tap water.
   b. saline.
   c. oil retention.
   d. Fleet's solution.
5. The best method to reduce the pain of a scheduled injection for a pediatric patient is to
   a. administer oral analgesics prior to the scheduled time of injection.
   b. use distraction techniques such as music.
   c. apply topical medication, such as EMLA, prior to scheduled time of injection.
   d. reassure the child that it won't hurt for very long.

BIBLIOGRAPHY AND READER REFERENCE

Behrman, R., & Kleigman, R. (1998). *Nelson's essentials of pediatrics* (3rd ed.). Philadelphia: Saunders.

Betz, C., Hunsberger, M., & Wright, S. (1994). *Family centered nursing care of children* (2nd ed.). Philadelphia: Saunders.

Bowden, V., Dickey, S., & Greenberg, C. (1998). Children and their families: a continuum of care. Philadelphia: Saunders.

Braun, S., Preston, B., & Smith, R. (1998). Getting a better read on thermometry. *RN, 61*(3), 57.

Carrol, P. (1998). Closing in on safer suctioning. *RN, 61*(5), 22.

Kirkpatrick, J., Alexander, J., & Cain, R. (1997). Recovering urine from diapers: Are test results accurate? *MCN: American Journal of Maternal Care Nursing, 22*(1), 96.

Maikler, V. (1998). Pharmacologic pain management in children. *J Ped Nursing, 13*(1), 3.

Metheny, N., Wehrle, M., & Wiersemal, C. (1998). Testing feeding tube placement: auscultation vs. ph method. *AJN, 98*(5), 37.

Niederhauser, V. (1997). Prescribing for children: Issues in pediatric pharmacology. *Nurse Practitioner, 22*(3), 16.

Olson, J., Ablon, L., & Giangrasso, A. (1995). *Medical dosage calculations.* Reading, MA: Addison-Wesley.

Peters, K. (1998). Bathing premature infants: Physiological and behavioral consequences. *Critical Care, 7*(2), 90.

Rodman, J. (1994). Pharmicokinetic variability in the adolescent: Implication of body size and organ function for dosage regime design. *Journal of Adolescent Health, 15*(8), 654–662.

Thomas, D. (1996). Assessing children: It's different! *RN, 59*(4), 38.

Varella, L., Jones, E., & Meguid, M. (1997). Drug–nutrient reactions in enteral feeding: A primary care focus. *The Nurse Practitioner, 22*(6), 98.

Wells, N., King, J., Hedström, C., & Youngkins, J. (1995). Does tympanic temperature measure up. *MCN, 20*(2), 95.

Williams, R. (1996). How to give medicine to children. *FDA Consumer Magazine.* Publication #FDA 96–3223.

Wong, D. (1997). *Whaley & Wong's essentials of pediatric nursing.* St. Louis, Mo: Mosby.

Zenk, K. (1994). Challenges in providing pharmaceutical care to pediatric patients. *American Journal of Hospital Pharmacy, 51,* 668–694.

chapter 23

The Child with a Sensory or Neurologic Condition

Outline

Objectives

On completion and mastery of Chapter 23, the student will be able to

- Define each vocabulary term listed.
- Discuss the prevention and treatment of ear infections.
- Outline the nursing approach to serving the hearing-impaired child.
- Discuss the cause and treatment of amblyopia.
- Compare the treatment of paralytic and nonparalytic strabismus.
- Review the prevention of eyestrain in children.
- Discuss the functions of the 12 cranial nerves and nursing interventions for dysfunction.
- Describe the symptoms of meningitis in a child.
- Discuss the various types of epilepsy and the nursing responsibilities during a seizure.
- Describe four types of cerebral palsy and the nursing goals involved in care.
- Outline the prevention, treatment, and nursing care for the child with Reye's syndrome.
- Formulate a nursing care plan for the child with a decreased level of consciousness.
- Prepare a plan for success in the care of a mentally retarded child.
- Describe three types of posturing that may indicate brain damage.
- Describe signs of increased intracranial pressure in a child.
- Describe the components of a "neurologic check."
- State a method of determining level of consciousness in an infant.
- Identify the priority goals in the care of a child who experienced near drowning.

Vocabulary

amblyopia	mental retardation
athetosis	myringotomy
aura	neurologic check
clonic	nystagmus
concussion	otoscope
cryosurgery	papilledema
dyslexia	paroxysm
encephalopathy	partial seizures
enucleation	petit mal
generalized seizures	postictal
grand mal	posturing
humoral	retinoblastoma
hyperopia	sepsis
hyphema	shaken baby syndrome
idiopathic	sign language
intracranial pressure (ICP)	status epilepticus
	strabismus
ketogenic diet	tonic

THE EARS

The ear, which can be considered a part of the nervous system, contains the receptors of the eighth cranial nerve (acoustic). The ear performs two main functions: hearing and balance. Figure 23–1 summarizes ear, eye, and neurologic differences between children and adults. The three divisions of the ear are depicted in Figure 23–2. In the newborn, the tympanic membrane is almost horizontal and is more vascular than in the adult. It has a dull and opaque appearance and an inconsistent light reflex. The eustachian tube is shorter and straighter in the infant than in the adult. Three functions of the eustachian tube are *ventilation* of the middle ear, *protection* from nasopharyngeal secretions and sound pressure, and *drainage.* Middle-ear infections are common during childhood.

When nurses examine the ear, they observe both its exterior and its interior. Ear alignment is observed. The top of the ear should cross an imaginary line drawn from the outer canthus of the eye to the occiput. Low-set ears may be associated with kidney disorders and mental retardation. The outer ear and the area around it are inspected for cleanliness and drainage. The inner ear is inspected with an *otoscope.* One method of restraint used when assisting with the examination of the inner ear is to lay the child on a table with the arms held alongside the head, which is turned to the side. Another method of positioning a child for an ear exam:

Nursing Tip

Before instilling eardrops in *infants,* gently pull the pinna of the ear *down and back.* In *children,* gently pull the pinna of the ear *up and back* to straighten the external auditory canal.

- Child is placed in adult's lap.
- Hold head firmly against adult's chest.
- One arm of child is placed behind adult.
- One arm is restrained by adult across child's abdomen.
- Child's legs are held between adult's thighs.

Ear Hygiene. Teach parents to cleanse the ear with a wash cloth. Never probe the ear with sharp objects or swabs. If wax (cerumen) is hard it can be softened with a commercial product such as Debrox® (carbamide peroxide 6.5%). If wax is persistent, consult with the physician. If a child inserts an object into the ear, professional removal is advised to avoid wedging the object farther into the ear.

Otitis Externa

An acute infection of the external ear canal is called *otitis externa* and is often referred to as *swimmer's ear* because prolonged exposure to moisture is often the precipitating factor. Pain and tenderness on manipulating the pinna or tragus of the ear (see Fig. 23–2) are specific signs. The ear canal may be erythematous, but the tympanic membrane is normal. A foreign body, cellulitis due to diabetes, or herpes zoster should be ruled out. Irrigation and topical antibiotics are the treatment of choice. The doctor may insert a loose cotton gauze wick into the outer third of the ear canal. The wick is kept moist with frequent drops of a medicated solution.

Otitis Media

Description. Otitis media (*ot,* "ear," *itis,* "inflammation of," and *media,* "middle") is an inflammation of the middle ear. The middle ear is a tiny cavity in the temporal bone. Its entrance is guarded by the sensitive tympanic membrane, or eardrum, which transmits sound waves through the "oval

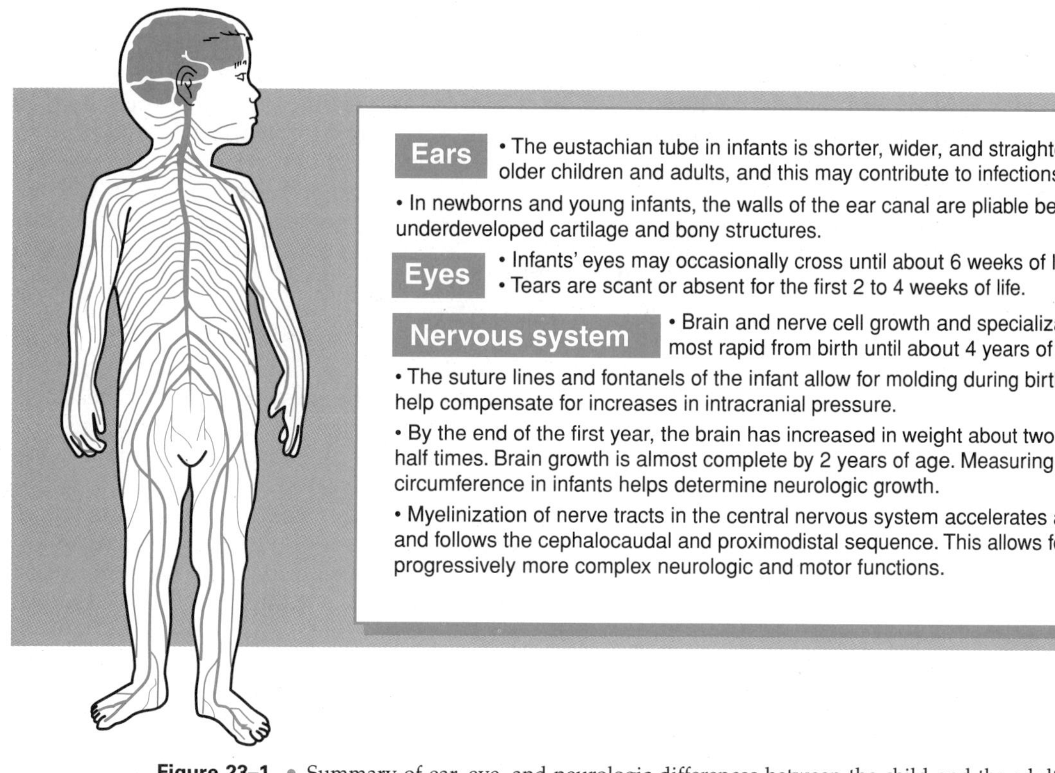

Figure 23–1. • Summary of ear, eye, and neurologic differences between the child and the adult.

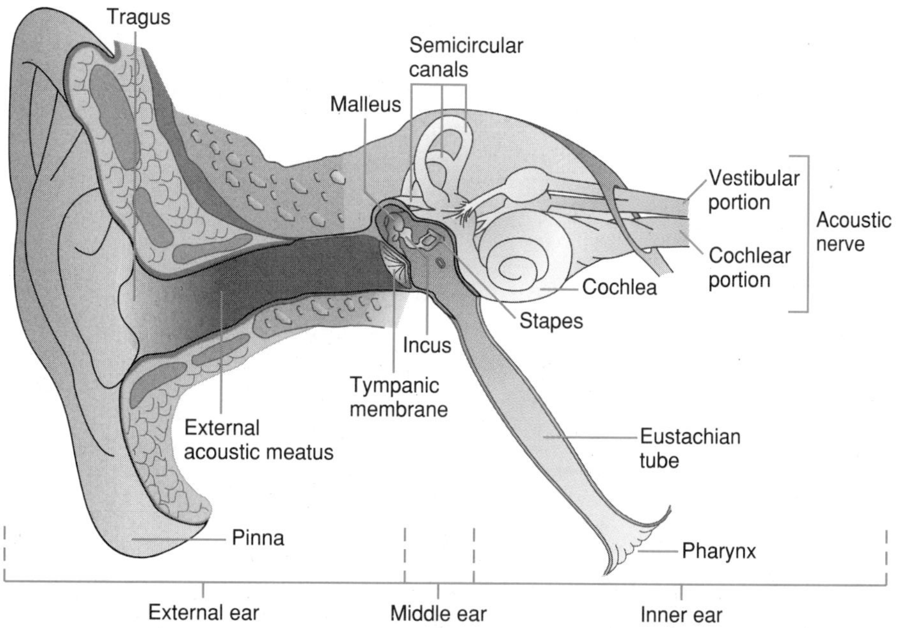

Figure 23–2. • There are three divisions of the ear, the outer ear, the middle ear, and the inner ear. In the newborn, the mastoid process and bony part of the external canal are not fully developed, leaving the *tympanic membrane* vulnerable to injury. Newborns can hear as soon as amniotic fluid is drained by the first sneeze. In infants the *eustachian tube* is shorter, wider, and straighter than in adults. Pooling of fluids such as milk in the throat of an infant who falls asleep with a bottle of milk can contribute to ear infections.

window" to the inner ear, which contains the organs of hearing and balance. The middle ear opens into air spaces, or sinuses, in the mastoid process of the temporal bone. It is also connected to the throat by a channel called the eustachian tube. These structures—the mastoid sinuses, the middle ear, and the eustachian tube—are lined by mucous membranes. As a result, an infection of the throat can easily spread to the middle ear and mastoid. The eustachian tube also protects the middle ear from nasopharyngeal secretions, provides drainage of middle-ear secretions into the nasopharynx, and equalizes air pressure between the middle ear and the outside atmosphere. These protective functions are diminished when the tubes are blocked. Unequalized air within the ear creates a negative pressure that allows organisms to be swept up into the tube.

Otitis media may be secondary to an upper respiratory tract infection or may be a complication of a communicable disease. Otitis media occurs most often in children between 6 and 24 months of age and in early childhood. It is more prevalent in young males. It is caused by a variety of organisms, of which *Strepococcus pneumoniae* and *Haemophilus influenzae* are the most common.

Infants are more prone to middle-ear infections than older children and adults because their eustachian tubes are shorter, wider, and straighter (Fig. 23–3). When babies lie flat for long periods, microorganisms have easy access from the eustachian tube to the middle-ear. Feeding methods may have a bearing on middle-ear infection when pooling of fluids, such as milk in the throat of an infant who falls asleep with a bottle of milk, provides a source for growth of organisms. The infant's *humoral* (*humor,* "body fluid") defense mechanisms are immature. Children in passive smoking environments have more respiratory infections because of the effect of secondary smoke on the protective cilia that line the nose. Day care attendance can contribute to the risk of upper respiratory infections and otitis media because of increased exposure to ill children.

Manifestations. The symptoms of otitis media are pain in the ear, which is often very severe, irritability, and diminished hearing. Fever, which may ran as high as 104° F (40° C), headache, vomiting, diarrhea, and febrile convulsions may also occur. Earaches in infants may be manifested by general irritability, frequent rubbing or pulling at the ear, and rolling of the head from side to side. The older child can point to the place that is tender. Some children are asymptomatic. An otitis media detector is an instrument that can help to diagnose otitis media in children.

If an abscess forms, a rupture of the eardrum may result, and drainage from the ear may be evident. When this happens, the pressure is relieved and the child is more comfortable. Some amount of hearing loss may result from the rupture. Otitis media is considered chronic if the condition persists for more than 3 months. Recurrent attacks can lead to serious complications. Chronic otitis media can lead to *cholesteatoma* (*chole,* "bile," *steato,* "fat," and *oma,* "tumor"), a cystlike sac filled with keratin debris. This may occlude the middle ear and erode adjacent ossicle bones, causing hearing loss. This con-

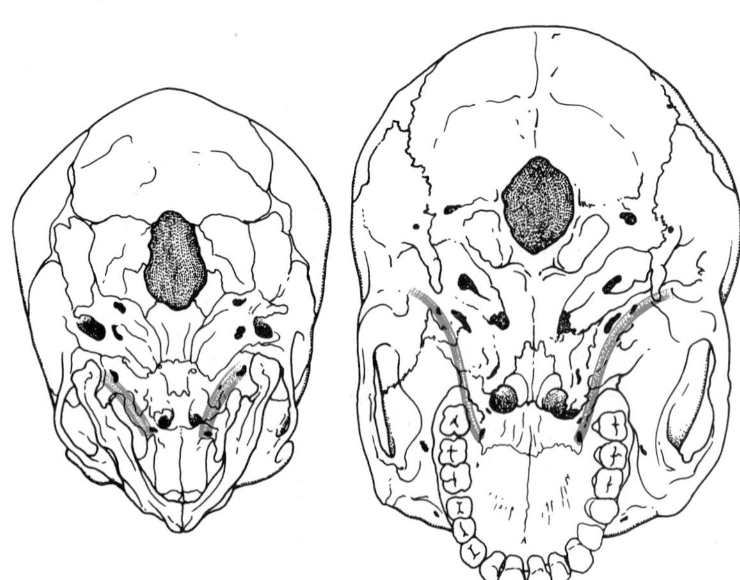

Figure 23–3. • Position and direction of the eustachian tube in the infant and adult. The infant's eustachian tube is shorter, wider, and straighter.

Nursing Tip

Signs and Symptoms of ear infection *can include:*

- Rubbing or pulling at the ear
- Rolling head from side to side
- Hearing loss
- Loud speech
- Inattentive behavior
- Articulation problems
- Speech development problems

dition is best treated by an otolaryngologist. Other complications of an ear infection include mastoiditis, deafness, and meningitis. Prevention lies in prompt recognition and treatment of upper respiratory infections.

Treatment. When an infection is evident, treatment is directed toward finding the causative organism and relieving the symptoms. A throat culture may be taken to determine the specific organism. Broad-spectrum antibiotics may be given orally and should be continued until the prescribed amount of medication is taken. Analgesics are given to relieve pain.

Surgical Treatment. Surgical intervention may be necessary when medical treatment is unsuccessful. The physician may incise the tympanic membrane to relieve pressure and to prevent a tear by spontaneous rupture. This is called a *myringotomy* (*myringa,* "eardrum," and *otomy,* "incision of"). A *tympanic (TM)* button or tympanostomy ventilating tube (PE pressure equalizer) may be inserted. This may fall out spontaneously within 6 to 12 months. In some children, tubes may need to be reinserted to continue ventilation. Care is taken to avoid getting water in the ears while bathing or showering. All children should be followed to make sure that the condition is resolved and to evaluate any hearing loss that may have occurred.

Comfort Measures. A warm compress may be applied locally. If the eardrum has ruptured, the child is placed on the affected side. Cold may also be beneficial. An ice pack may be prescribed to reduce edema and pressure. The skin around the ears must be kept clean and protected from any drainage to prevent tissue breakdown. Parents are instructed not to use cotton swabs in the ears.

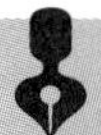

Nursing Tip

Instruct caretakers that the child's condition may improve dramatically after a few days on antibiotics. To prevent recurrence, they must continue to administer the medication until the prescribed amount is completed.

Hearing Impairment

Description. About 1 in 1000 newborns is born with some type of hearing impairment. This number may increase to 2 in 1000 for hearing loss occurring during childhood. Hearing-impaired children present special challenges to the health care team. Hearing loss can affect speech, language, social and emotional development, as well as behavior and academic achievement. The nurse should have a basic understanding of how to approach and work with a hearing-impaired child.

The inner ear is fully formed during the early months of prenatal life. If an expectant mother contracts German measles or another viral infection during this period the child may be born with a hearing loss, which is termed *congenital deafness.* Deafness can also be *acquired.* Infectious diseases, such as measles, mumps, chickenpox, or meningitis, can result in various degrees of hearing loss. The common cold, some medications, exposure to loud noise levels, certain allergies, and ear infections may also be responsible. Hearing problems can also be temporary if they are due to wax accumulation. Some rattles and squeaky toys can emit sounds as loud as 110 decibels. (Above 80 decibels can cause damage.) These type of toys should not be held close to the infant's ear.

Early diagnosis and treatment of hearing-impaired children are important to prevent adverse physical and mental complications from developing. Members of the health care team concerned with the child who is hearing impaired include the physician, otologist (ear specialist), audiologist, speech therapist, specially trained teacher, social

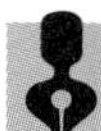

Nursing Tip

When addressing a hearing-impaired child, the nurse should

- Be at eye level with the child
- Be face to face with the child
- Establish eye contact
- Talk in short sentences
- Avoid using exaggerated lip or face movement

worker, psychologist, school nurse, and members of the child's family.

The various degrees of hearing loss range from complete *bilateral* (which affects both ears) to a loss so mild that the problem is never discovered. Hearing loss can be from defects in transmission of sound to the middle ear, from damage to the auditory nerve or ear structures, or from a mixed hearing loss that involves both a defect in nerve pathways and interference with sound transmission. If hearing loss is complete, the child misses all the pleasures of sound and has difficulty in communication, since children learn to talk by imitating what they hear. Behavior problems arise because these children do not understand directions. They may become aggressive with other children in their attempt to communicate. If they are ridiculed by playmates, personality development will be affected Unless these children are helped, they may become socially isolated.

Partial bilateral deafness may be responsible for behavior problems and poor progress in school. It may be caused by chronic ear infections, such as otitis media, or by blockage of the eustachian tube. Children who have hearing losses in one ear are less affected if hearing in the other ear is normal.

Diagnosis and Treatment. Early diagnosis and prompt treatment are primary requisites, regardless of the child's age. Complete bilateral deafness is usually discovered during infancy. Partial deafness may be unrecognized until the child begins school. Many hearing problems are detected by the school nurse administering standard hearing tests. School-aged children should have hearing tests every 3 years.

Response deficits of the infant to sounds, music, or the *startle reflex,* in infants under 4 months of age are the first signs that may alert the parents or nurse to the possibility of hearing impairment. A *crib-o-gram* is an automated system that senses the motor response of an infant to sound. The test results may not be accurate in infants who are ill or agitated. *Tympanometry* measures ear pressure but is difficult to perform adequately on an active infant or small child. A tuning fork is used to evaluate for air conduction (Rinne test) or bone conduction (Weber test). This type of test requires the child to be cooperative and able to communicate what they heard or felt. The *evoked otoacoustic emissions (OAE)* test is a preferred method for neonatal testing. The *brainstem auditory evoked response (BAER)* test records brain wave responses generated by the auditory system.

Many hearing defects are amenable to medical or surgical treatment. Hearing aids can amplify sound waves. Surgically placed *cochlear implants* are now used for some children with nerve damage. Children who suffer a severe loss of hearing need more extensive help from personnel at an auditory training center. These children need to begin treatment as soon as the hearing loss is discovered.

Role of the Nurse. Various methods are used to bring the child into the world of sound. Lip reading, sign language, writing, visual aids, and amplified sound are but a few examples. The parents are instructed in means of communication that coincide with those used by the teachers.

The nurse must be aware of the symptoms of deafness in the child. Newborns are observed for their response to auditory stimuli. The Brazelton Neonatal Behavioral Assessment Scale evaluates the infant's orientation response to the sound of a voice. The persistence of the Moro reflex beyond 4 months may also be an indication of deafness. The infant who makes no verbal attempts by 18 months of age should undergo a complete physical examination. Indifference to sound, behavior problems, or poor school performance may also be signs of deafness. The nurse inquires into the facilities that are available in the community for such a child.

The hearing-impaired child in the hospital needs the same opportunities to communicate as the child who does not have this handicap. The nurse smiles when approaching the child. Body language communicates a lot, especially if there is a severe communication problem. The nurse faces the child when speaking and is positioned at eye level with the child. The nurse must ensure that the child saw her or him before touching to avoid startling the child. *Sign language* is the use of hand signals that correspond to words and assist in communication with a deaf child. Previously developed speech patterns may regress during hospitalization. Visual aids, writing, or drawing can be used to enhance communication.

If a hearing aid is indicated, the child is equipped with one and taught how to use it. Regular check-ups ensures that the aid is working properly. A hearing aid is expensive and invaluable to the child. It is put in a safe place when not in use. When the child goes to surgery, it is given to the parents or placed in the hospital safe. The pockets of hospital gowns are checked before the gowns are placed in the laundry.

The National Hearing Aid Center provides information about hearing aids. Hearing aids are designed to fit in the ear, behind the ear, on eyeglass frames, or on the body with wires to the ear. The nurse should check ear hygiene and be sure hairs are not caught on the end of the hearing aid to

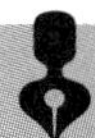

Nursing Tip

Signs of Ear Problems

- Pulling at the ear
- Discharge from the ear
- Hearing loss
- Swelling around ear
- Vertigo, falling, stumbling
- Nystagmus of eyes
- Ringing in the ears
- Facial paralysis

ensure a proper fit and to minimize noise and whistling problems. Teaching safe battery handling and storage and promoting self-care are important nursing responsibilities.

Home care of the hearing-impaired child should include speech therapy. Flashing lights should be installed in the home to alert the child to doorbells and other sound-based devices. Telecommunication devices for the deaf (TDD) are available to enable telephone communication. Closed captioning devices for TV are available to the child who can read.

The school nurse can help the family to nurture socialization skills. Some hearing-impaired children attend special schools for the deaf, and some are mainstreamed into the general school population. Each hearing-impaired child and each family unit should be followed by the multidisciplinary health care team.

Barotrauma

Today, many children travel with their family via airplanes and may react to a change in altitude and barometric pressure. During airplane descent, children should be encouraged to yawn or chew on gum to promote swallowing. Infants should be bottle-fed juice or water to promote swallowing, which produces autoinflation and relief of symptoms. Systemic decongestants can be taken before air travel and timed so that peak effectiveness occurs during airplane descent.

Nursing Tip

- Emphasize to parents the need to supervise the care and storage of hearing aid batteries to prevent accidental ingestion.
- When inserting the ear piece of a hearing aid, be sure that the ear canal is free of hair.

Teenagers may participate in recreational underwater diving that can cause barometric pressure stress to the ear, resulting in severe earaches and other serious problems. Underwater diving should be slow during the descent phase to minimize negative pressure buildup. Sensory hearing loss and vertigo with nausea and vomiting may be early signs of decompression sickness when it occurs during the ascent phase of diving. The diver should be referred for medical care. Upper respiratory infections or tympanic membrane perforation are contraindications to diving as vertigo, nausea, vomiting, and disorientation can occur with dangerous results.

THE EYES

The eye is the organ of vision. The anatomy of the eyeball is depicted in Figure 23–4. The eyes begin to develop as an outgrowth of the forebrain in the 4-week-old embryo. The newborn's sight is not mature, but the newborn can see. Visual acuity is estimated to be in the range of 20/400. This improves rapidly and may reach 20/30 to 20/20 by the age of 2 or 3 years (Behrman, Kleigman, & Arvin, 1996). The shape of the newborn's eye is less spherical than the adult's eye. The eyes may appear crossed in the early weeks of life, but alignment and coordination are usually achieved by 3 to 6 months of age. Tears are not present until 1 to 3 months of age. *Depth perception does not begin to develop until about 9 months.* In the United States, about 64 per 100,000 children have serious vision deficits and approximately 100 per 100,000 children have mild visual problems.

On physical examination, the nurse observes the eyes to see if they are symmetric and an equal distance from the nose. Epicanthal folds (*epi,* "upon," and *canthus,* "angle") are folds of skin that extend on either side of the bridge of the nose that covers the inner eye canthus. Some folds are broad covering a large portion of the inner eye, causing the eye to appear crossed. Large epicanthal folds occur as part of some chromosomal anomalies. Pupils are observed for size, shape, and movement. Their reaction to light is observed by shining a penlight into the eye and quickly removing it. The healthy pupil constricts (gets smaller) as the light approaches and dilates (gets larger) as it disappears (Fig. 23–15, p. 612). Older children are given explanations concerning the examination. They are al-

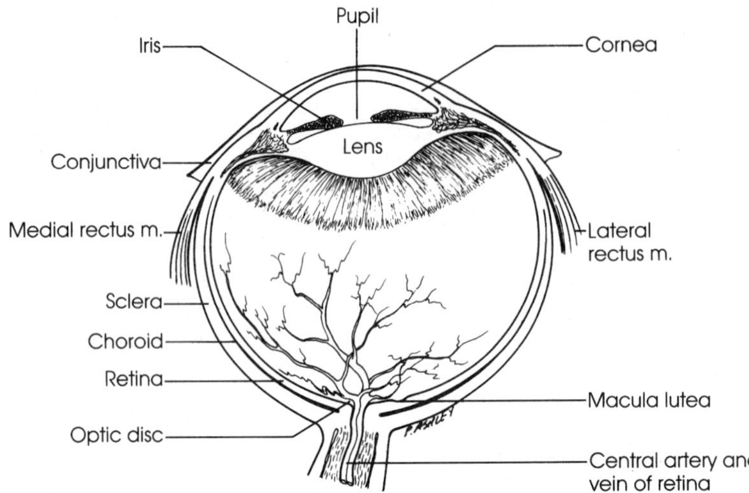

Figure 23–4. • Structure of the eyeball. (From Marlow, D. R., & Redding, B. A. [1988]. *Textbook of pediatric nursing* [6th ed., p. 102]. Philadelphia: Saunders.)

lowed to hold the ophthalmoscope and to turn it off and on.

Visual Acuity Tests

The ability of an infant to fixate and focus on an object can be demonstrated by 6 weeks of age. The object should not emit a sound, to be sure the infant is turning toward a sight stimulus rather than a sound stimulus. Visual acuity can be tested by 2½ to 3 years of age.

There are a variety of visual acuity charts (Fig. 23–5). The Snellen alphabet chart, and the Snellen E version for preschoolers who have not learned the alphabet, are commonly used to assess the ability to see near and far objects. Picture cards are also useful for children who do not know letters.

The Titmus machine is frequently used for school children and adolescents. Directions for testing are standardized and must be carefully adhered to for proper results. Computerized tests, such as the random-dot stereogram, also show promise in the visual screening of children. Visual acuity is important in the learning process. Retinopathy of the premature (ROP) is discussed on page 336.

Dyslexia

Dyslexia (*dys* "difficult," and *lexis* "diction") is a reading disability that involves a defect in the cortex of the brain that processes graphic symbols.

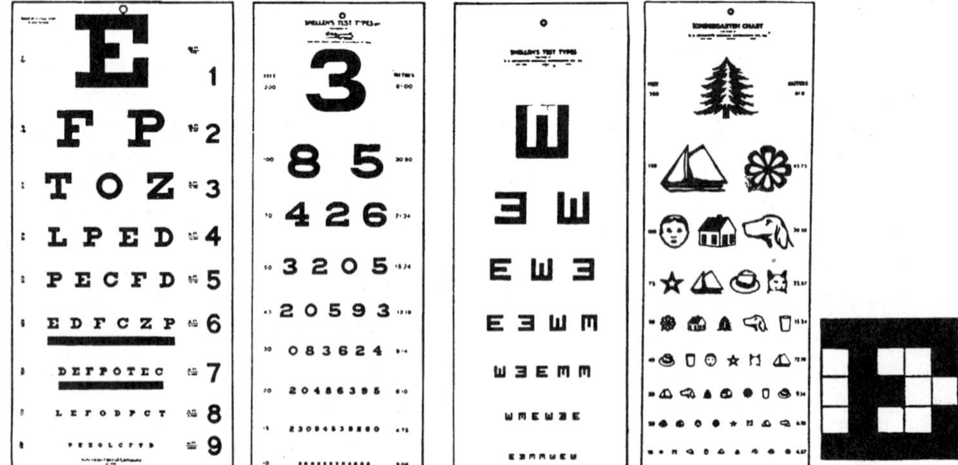

Figure 23–5. • Various types of visual acuity charts. (From Behrman, R. E., & Kliegman, R. M. [1992]. *Nelson's textbook of pediatrics* [14th ed.]. Philadelphia: Saunders.)

Although eye evaluation is recommended when a child has mirror vision or word reversal, the problem does not involve any local eye defect. Correcting vision problems will aid in optimal visual function. A treatment for dyslexia involves remedial instruction.

Amblyopia

Description. *Amblyopia* (lazy eye) is a reduction in or loss of vision that usually occurs in children who strongly favor one eye. If both retinas do not receive a clearly defined image, bilateral amblyopia may result. However, it is more common for one eye to be affected. When abnormal binocular interaction occurs (such as crossed eyes or strabismus), the prognosis depends on how long the eye has been affected and on the age of the child when treatment begins. The earlier the treatment, the better the results. One commonly accepted diagnostic sign is that vision in the normal eye is at least two Snellen lines (E charts) better than that in the affected eye. There are various types of amblyopia. *Strabismus* is the most common; however, dissimilar refractory errors can also result in this condition. Since amblyopia occurs as a result of sensory deprivation of the affected eye, children are at risk for developing the problem until visual stability occurs, usually by 9 years of age.

Treatment and Nursing Care. Early detection and prompt treatment are essential. The goal of treatment is to obtain normal and equal vision in each eye. Treatment consists of eyeglasses for significant refractive errors (hyperopia, myopia) and patching (occlusion) of the *good eye.* The good eye is patched to force the use of the affected eye. Daytime patching may be instituted. In some cases, part-time occlusion is sufficient. Occlusion therapy is often difficult to maintain. The nurse can be of help by explaining the importance of the procedure and by offering support. The child is often subjected to teasing by peers. Providing a safe place to express feelings is important to promoting a healthy self-image. In selected cases, an opaque contact lens or a contact lens of sufficiently high power to blur the vision in the better eye is used (Behrman et al., 1996).

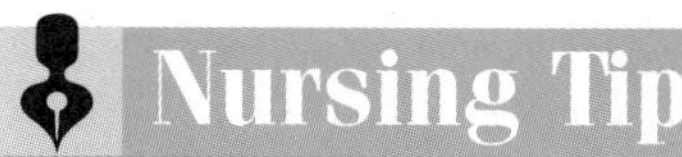

At birth the quiet, alert infant will respond to visual stimuli by cessation of movement. Visual responsiveness to the mother during feeding is noted. The infant's ability to focus and follow objects in the first months of life should be documented. Coordination of eye movements should be achieved by 3 to 6 months of age.

Strabismus

Description. *Strabismus* (cross-eye), also known as *squint,* is a condition in which the child is not able to direct both eyes toward the same object. There is a lack of coordination between the eye muscles that direct movement of the eye. When the eyes cannot coordinate sight together, the brain will disable one eye to provide a clear image. The disabled eye can develop permanent visual impairment due to sensory deprivation (amblyopia). Normal binocular vision is the goal that must be accomplished by early intervention *before the eye matures.*

There are several kinds of strabismus. *Nonparalytic strabismus* (concomitant) involves a constant deviation in the gaze related to the faulty insertion of the eye muscle. One eye always looks crossed. The extraocular muscles are normal. *Paralytic strabismus* (nonconcomitant) involves a paralysis or weakness in the extraocular muscle. Double vision is experienced. Deviation of the gaze occurs with movement, when the eye attempts to focus. To avoid double vision *(diplopia)* the child will tilt his head or squint when focusing on an object. Strabismus may be present at birth or may be acquired after a disease or injury. This type of strabismus can occur following head trauma or a neurologic disease. It is important to note that epicanthal folds can give a false impression of strabismus.

Treatment. In nonparalytic strabismus the refractory error is usually corrected with eyeglasses. When paralytic strabismus is seen during early infancy, the doctor may recommend that the unaffected eye be covered by a patch until the baby is old enough to wear glasses. The affected eye may improve through use and often becomes normal. Eye exercises and glasses are effective ways of treating the condition medically. If they do not help, surgery should be considered. It is generally performed when the child is 3 or 4 years old. Early correction is necessary to prevent amblyopia. If strabismus is left untreated, blindness may result in the affected eye because the brain tends to obliterate the confusing double image.

Nursing Care. The child undergoing surgery for strabismus may be hospitalized for only a brief period. The surgery involves structures outside the eyeball; therefore, the child is allowed to be up and about postoperatively. Eye dressings are kept at a

Nursing Tip

Symptoms of strabismus include:

- Eye "squinting" or frowning to focus
- Missed objects reached for
- Covers one eye to see
- Tilts head to see
- Dizziness, headache

minimum, and elbow restraints may be sufficient to keep the child from touching the dressings.

Prevention of Eyestrain. Children who are beginning to read need books with large type in which the letters are spaced far apart. The lighting must be adequate and without glare. Chairs and desks must be of the proper height.

Symptoms that may indicate eyestrain include inflammation, aching or burning of the eyes, squinting, a short attention span, frequent headaches, difficulties with schoolwork, or inability to see the blackboard. It is important for the nurse to *assess* the child for eyestrain, to *teach* proper eye care, *prevent* complications of eyestrain or strabismus, *refer* as needed for follow-up care and assist in *rehabilitation.*

Conjunctivitis

Conjunctivitis (*conjungere,* "to join together," and *itis,* "inflammation") is an inflammation of the conjunctiva or the mucous membrane that lines the eyelids. It is caused by a wide range of bacterial and viral agents, allergens, irritants, toxins, and systemic diseases (Fig. 23–6). Conjunctivitis that occurs with viral exanthems such as measles are usually self-limiting. It is common in childhood and may be infectious or noninfectious. The acute infectious form is commonly referred to as *pinkeye.* Conjunctivitis can also result from an obstruction of the lacrimal duct. The common forms of conjunctivitis generally respond to warm compresses and topical antibiotic eye drops or eye ointments. Ointments blur vision and are not generally used during daytime hours in the ambulatory child.

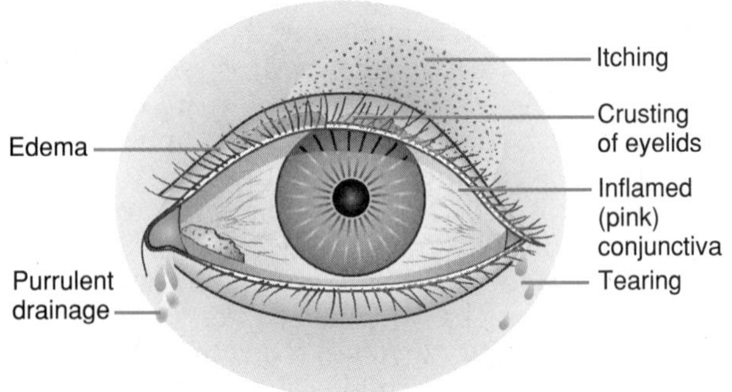

Figure 23–6. • Signs of conjunctivitis.

The nurse instructs parents to administer the drops for the prescribed time to prevent recurrence. Parents and older children are taught to wipe secretions from the *inner canthus downward and away from the opposite eye.* Because conjunctivitis spreads easily, affected children should use separate towels and be instructed to wash their hands frequently. *Ophthalmia neonatorum,* an acute conjunctivitis in the newborn, is discussed on page 241. Allergic conjunctivitis is often associated with allergic rhinitis (*rhin,* "nose," and *itis,* "inflammation") in children with hay fever. Symptoms include itching, tearing of one or both eyes, and edema of the eyelids and periorbital tissues. The child may appear distracted and irritable. The technique for instilling eyedrops is discussed in Chapter 22.

Hyphema

Hyphema, the presence of blood in the anterior chamber of the eye, is one of the most common ocular injuries. It can occur from either a blunt or a perforating injury. Blows from flying objects, such as a baseball or snowball, or forceful coughing or sneezing can cause this condition. These accidents are common among active school children. Hyphema appears as a bright-red or dark-red spot in front of the lower portion of the iris.

Treatment includes bed rest and topical medication. The head of the bed is elevated 30 to 45 degrees to decrease intraoccular pressure and decrease intracranial pressure if there is an associated head injury. The condition generally resolves itself without residual problems.

Retinoblastoma

Description. *Retinoblastoma* is a malignant tumor of the retina of the eye. There are hereditary and spontaneous forms. The average ages at diagnosis are 12 months for bilateral tumors and 21 months for unilateral tumors (Behrman et al., 1996). Gene-mapping techniques have shown chromosome 13 to be affected in hereditary forms. Chromosome 13 is also known to cause other congenital defects.

Manifestations. A yellowish-white reflex is seen in the pupil because of a tumor behind the lens.

This is called the *cat's eye reflex* or *leukokoria* (*leuk,* "white," and *kore,* "pupil"). This may be accompanied by loss of vision, strabismus, hyphema, and in advanced tumors, pain. In unilateral tumors, metastasis to the unaffected eye is common. When retinoblastoma is suspected in children, an examination under anesthesia is performed so that the pediatric opthamologist may carefully examine the fundus of the eye.

Treatment and Nursing Care. The standard treatment for unilateral disease is *enucleation* (removal) of the eye. Irradiation may be used if the tumors are very small, but it is less common. Other treatments include *cryosurgery* (freezing the tumor to kill cells) and *photocoagulation* by laser to destroy the blood vessels supplying the tumor. On return from surgery for enucleation, the child has a large pressure dressing on the eye. Elbow restraints may be necessary to prevent removal of the dressing. The bandage is observed for bleeding and vital signs are assessed. In a few days, the surgeon removes the dressing and an eye patch is applied. Other structures of the eye, such as the lids, lashes, and tear glands, are not affected. An eye prosthesis is fitted when the socket has healed. Instructions for care of the prosthesis are provided at the time of final fitting. Providing education and emotional support of the child and family and referral to the multidisciplinary health care team is essential.

THE NERVOUS SYSTEM

The nervous system is the body's communication center; it receives and transmits messages to all parts of the body. It also records experiences (memorization) and integrates certain stimuli (learning). The anatomy of the nervous system is depicted in Figure 23–7. Neural tube development occurs during the 3rd to 4th week of fetal life. This eventually becomes the central nervous system (CNS). The fusing process of the neural tube is critical. Its failure to fuse may lead to such congenital conditions as spina bifida or anencephaly (Chapter 14). Most neurologic disabilities in childhood result from congenital malformation (birth defects), brain injury, or infection. The twelve cranial nerves and their functions are shown in Figure 23–8.

Central nervous system (CNS) dysfunction may be detected by *a neurologic check* (see pp. 611–612 and Table 23–6), skull x-ray films, ultrasound brain waves, computed tomography (CT), magnetic resonance imaging (MRI), electromyography, and other methods. The reflexes of the newborn are good indicators of neurologic health. In the ill child, a decreased level of consciousness may be an indication of a neurologic problem. Box 23–1 describes causes of altered level of consciousness. In the finger–nose test used to determine coordination, the child is asked to extend the arm and then to touch his or her nose with the index finger. This is done with the eyes opened and closed. The inability to balance on one foot in a school-age child would be assessed. Cranial nerve assessment, selected dysfunction, and nursing interventions are described in Table 23–1.

BOX 23–1

CAUSES OF ALTERED LEVEL OF CONSCIOUSNESS (LOC)

- A fall to 60 mm Hg or below of PaO_2
- A rise above 45 mm of $PaCO_2$
- Low blood pressure causing cerebral hypoxia
- Fever (1-degree rise in fever increases oxygen need by 10%)
- Drugs (sedatives, antiepileptics)
- Seizures (postictal state)
- Increased intracranial pressure (ICP)

Reye's Syndrome

Description. Reye's syndrome is an acute noninflammatory *encephalopathy* (pathology of the brain) and *hepatopathy* (pathology of the liver) that follows a viral infection in children. There may be a relationship between the use of aspirin (acetasalycilic acid) during a viral flu or illness such as chickenpox (varicella) and the development of Reye's syndrome. For this reason, aspirin is generally contraindicated for the pediatric population. Some studies show that a genetic metabolic defect triggers Reye's syndrome when the stress of a viral illness produces vomiting and hypoglycemia.

Pathophysiology and Manifestations. Liver cell pathology causes an accumulation of ammonia in the blood. Toxic levels of ammonia causes cerebral manifestations, such as cerebral edema and in-

Nursing Tip

Discourage the use of aspirin and other medications that contain *salicylates* in children with flulike symptoms. Advise parents to read labels of medication carefully to determine ingredients.

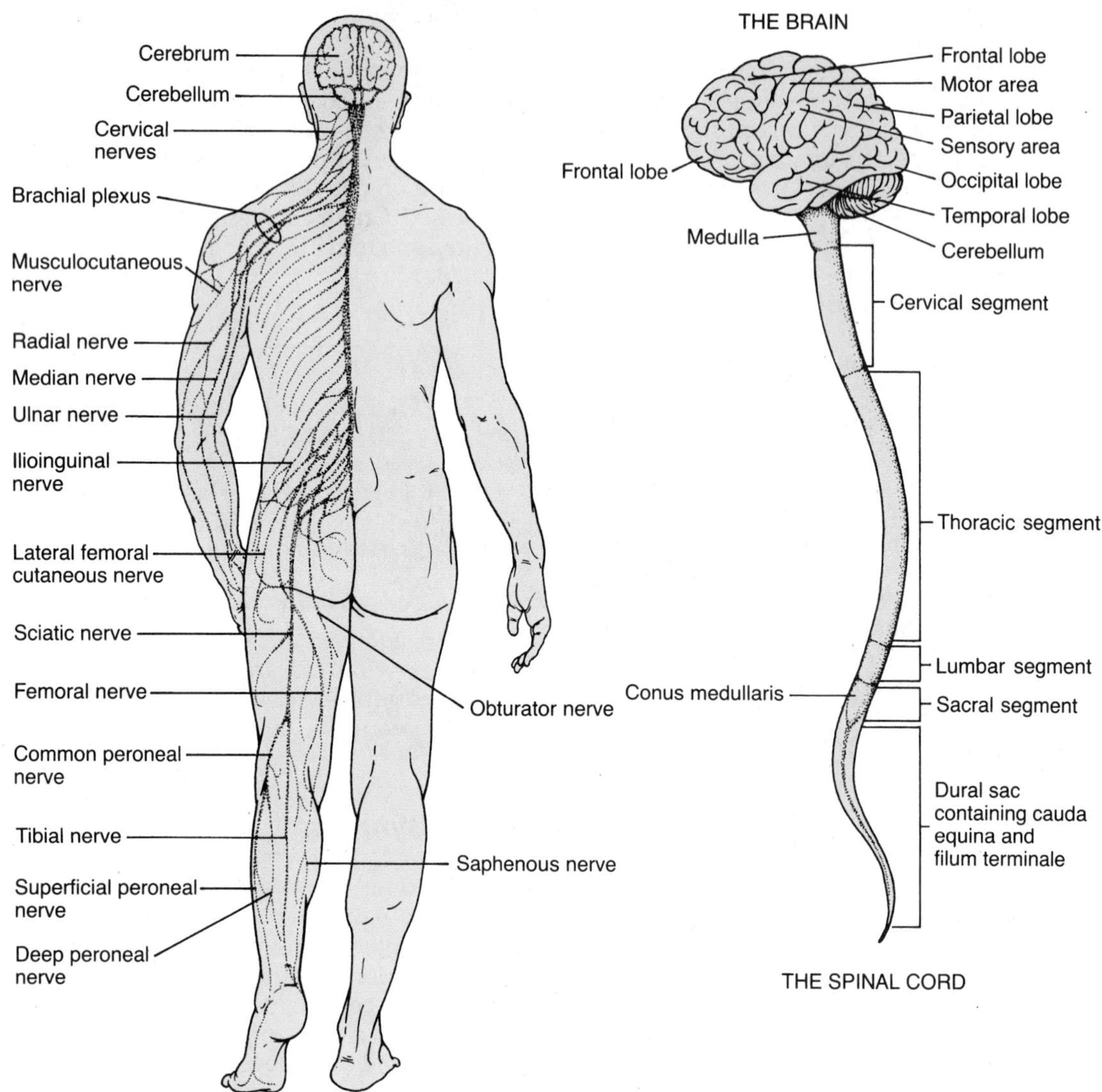

Figure 23–7. • The nervous system consists of the brain, spinal cord, sense organs, and nerves. The nervous system is the principal regulatory system.

creased intracranial pressure (ICP), which results in neurologic signs such as altered behavior, altered level of consciousness, seizures, and coma.

In children the sudden onset of effortless vomiting, and altered behavior (such as lethargy or combativeness) or altered level of consciousness following a viral illness are characteristic of Reye's syndrome. The results of blood tests assessing liver function will be abnormal. In infants, diarrhea, hypoglycemia, tachypnea with apneic episodes, and seizures may occur approximately 1 week following a respiratory illness. See Box 23–2 for the characteristic signs and symptoms of Reye's syndrome.

Prevention. The education of the public concerning the dangers of using salicylate containing medications during viral illnesses, such as varicella, in children may have contributed to the decline in the occurrence of Reye's syndrome. The availability of varicella vaccine may also have an impact on the reduction of the incidence of Reye's syndrome. The national Reye's Syndrome Foundation in Bryon, Ohio, supports research and provides educational materials on this disorder.

Treatment. Early treatment can result in complete recovery. However, progression to the acute stage is often rapid and unpredictable. The goals of treatment include reducing ICP and maintaining a patent airway, cerebral oxygenation, and fluid and electrolyte balance (see Nursing Care Plan 23–1).

Frequent assessment of vital signs and a careful assessment of neurologic status are *essential.* Observation for signs of bleeding is important because liver dysfunction causes blood clotting abnormalities. Parental education and support are necessary. Encouraging parents to participate in their child's care helps to reduce the parent's and child's level of anxiety.

Sepsis

Sepsis *(bacteremia)* is bacteria in the bloodstream that cause severe systemic response (Box 23–3). Sepsis may follow an infection such as meningitis,

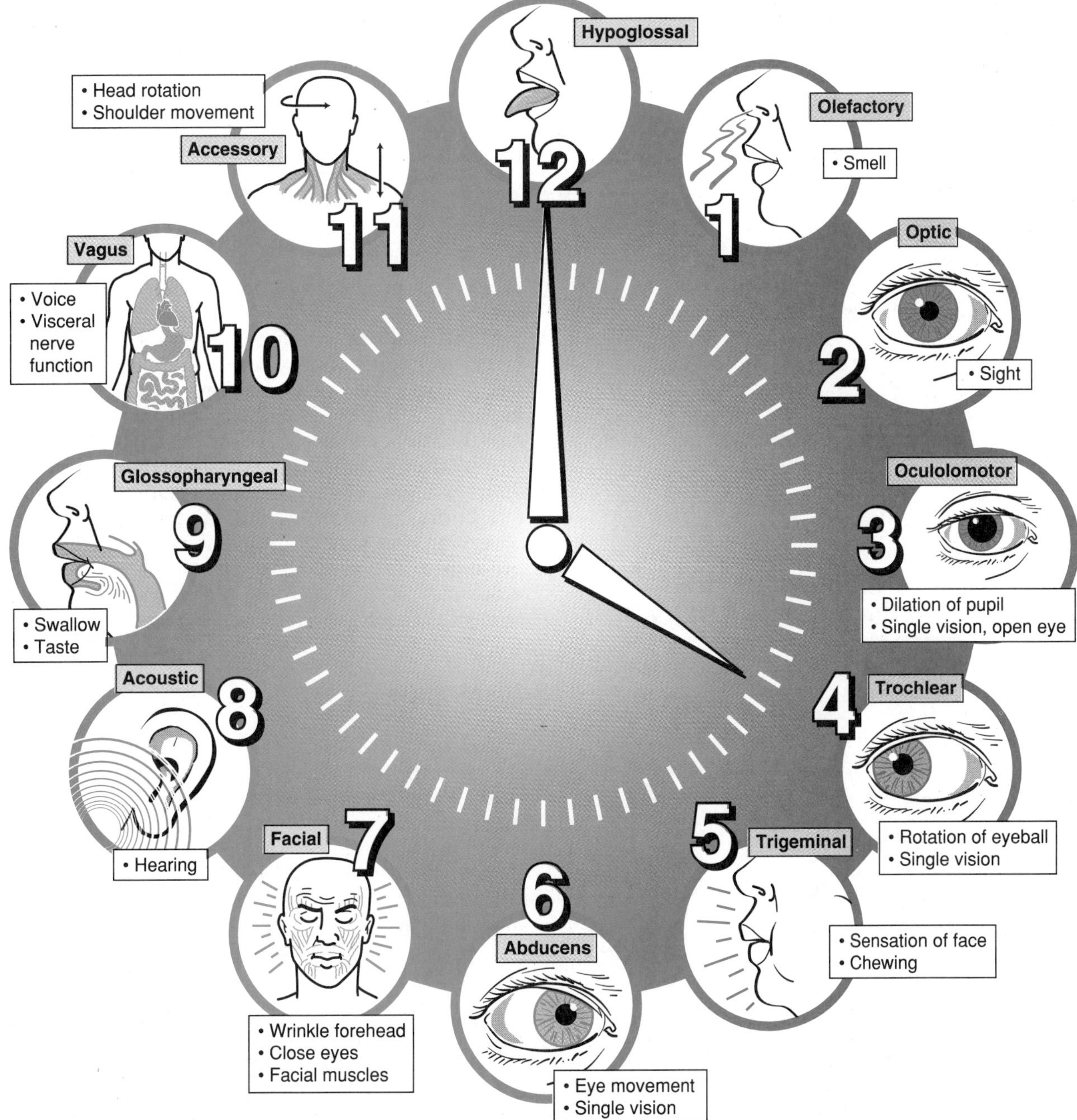

Figure 23–8. • The twelve cranial nerves and their functions.

Table 23-1
CRANIAL NERVE ASSESSMENT: SELECTED DYSFUNCTIONS AND NURSING INTERVENTIONS

Cranial Nerve	Dysfunction	Nursing Intervention
1. Olfactory	Inability to smell	Appetite may be suppressed—present food attractively
2. Optic	Inability to control pupil reflex	Protect eyes from glaring lights
3. Oculomotor	Double vision	Cover eyes
4. Trochlear	Inability to move eyes	When communicating, remain in child's view
5. Trigeminal	Difficulty in chewing	Provide soft foods
6. Abducens	Inability to control corneal reflex	Have eye ointment or eye patch on hand to protect cornea
7. Facial	Inability to close eye	Protect eyes with moist dressing
8. Acoustic	Inability to hear	Maintain body language for communication
9. Glossopharyngeal	Inability to taste or to control gag and cough reflexes	Provide visually attractive food Tracheotomy tray and suction at bedside
10. Vagus	Difficulty in talking or swallowing; visceral malfunction	Provide means of communication Assess for aspiration Assess body system functions and vital signs
11. Spinal accessory	Controls head, turn, and shrug shoulders	Provide position change and support
12. Hypoglossal	Controls tongue movement, thick speech	Have suction ready—observe ability to chew and swallow. Provide method of communication

or it may be from a primary infection. Children who are immunocompromised, have neutropenia, or the intensive care child receiving invasive therapy are at risk for developing sepsis. Sepsis causes a systemic inflammatory response syndrome (SIRS) as a reaction to the endotoxin of the bacteria that results in tissue damage. Complications of SIRS include shock and multiorgan system failure, leading to death.

Manifestations. Manifestations of sepsis include fever, tachypnea, tachycardia, hypotension, and neurologic signs such as lethargy. Lab tests may include positive blood cultures, reduced fibrinogen and thrombocyte levels and anemia. The presence of immature white blood cells and neutropenia are ominous signs. The nursing responsibilities include monitoring neurologic status and vital signs and observing for shock. Intravenous antibiotics are prescribed. *To prevent sepsis, immunization against* H. influenzae *type B is recommended for all children between the ages of 2 months and 4 years.*

BOX 23-2

CHARACTERISTIC MANIFESTATIONS OF REYE'S SYNDROME IN CHILDREN

A viral illness 1 week prior to presentation of symptoms such as:

- Persistent, effortless vomiting
- Diarrhea, hypoglycemia, lethargy, or combative behavior
- Tachypnea with apneic episodes in infants
- Absence of fever or jaundice
- Lab test results:
  - Elevated AST (SGOT) and ALT (SGPT)
  - Elevated serum ammonia
  - Elevated blood urea nitrogen (BUN) and creatinine (related to dehydration from vomiting)
  - Normal bilirubin levels
  - Hypoglycemia

A percutaneous liver biopsy is diagnostic, however, it may be difficult to do a biopsy if the child is gravely ill.

Meningitis

Description. Meningitis is an inflammation of the meninges (the covering of the brain and spinal cord). Various organisms can cause bacterial meningitis. Organisms may invade the meninges *indirectly* by way of the bloodstream (sepsis) from centers of infection such as the teeth, sinuses, tonsils, and lungs, or *directly* through the ear (otitis media) or from a fracture of the skull.

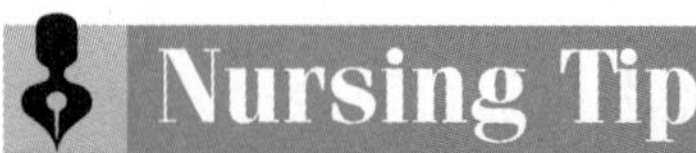

A rash with petechiae that develops in a child who is acutely ill and lethargic must be referred for immediate follow-up care.

Nursing Tip

When a spinal tap is planned, the infant can be sedated and Emla cream can be applied to the area to reduce discomfort during needle insertion.

Bacterial meningitis is often referred to as *purulent,* that is, pus-forming, because a thick exudate surrounds the meninges and adjacent structures. This can lead to certain sequelae, such as subdural effusion and, less frequently, hydrocephalus. The peak incidence for bacterial meningitis is between 6 and 12 months of age. Meningococcal meningitis is readily transmitted to others. Meningitis is less frequently seen in children older than 4 years. *Haemophilus influenzae* is the most common causative agent. Two *H. influenzae* type B vaccines are now available for infants. The approaches to nursing care for all types of meningitis are similar.

Manifestations. The symptoms of purulent meningitis result mainly from intracranial irritation. They may be preceded by an upper respiratory infection and several days of gastrointestinal symptoms such as poor feeding. Severe headache, drowsiness, delirium, irritability, restlessness, fever, vomiting, and stiffness of the neck (nuchal rigidity) are other significant symptoms. In infants, a characteristic high-pitched cry is noted. Convulsions are common. Coma may occur fairly early in the older child. In severe cases, involuntary arching of the back due to muscle contractions is seen (Fig. 23–9). This condition is called *opisthotonos* (*opistho,* "backward," and *tonos,* "tension"). The presence of *petechiae* (small hemorrhages beneath the skin) is suggestive of meningococcal infection.

Treatment. At the first indication of meningitis, the physician performs a spinal tap (lumbar puncture, see p. 551) to obtain a specimen of cerebrospinal fluid (CSF) for lab testing. In the early stages of the illness, the spinal fluid may be clear, but it rapidly becomes cloudy. The CSF pressure is increased, and further laboratory analysis indicates a high white cell count, an increase in protein, and a decrease in glucose.

The child is placed in isolation until 24 hours after antibiotic therapy. An intravenous (IV) line is established for the administration of antibiotics and to restore fluid and electrolyte balance. Antibiotics are selected on the basis of culture and sensitivity lab results. Antibiotics are usually administered for a minimum of 10 to 14 days. A sedative, such as phenobarbital, may make the child less restless. An anticonvulsant such as phenytoin (Dilantin) may also be required to decrease seizure activity.

Nursing Care. The isolation room is prepared in accordance with hospital protocol (see Appendix A). Nursing responsibility includes performing a neurologic assessment and maintaining an accurate recording of the child's vital signs and intake and output. The nurse should also organize care so that the child is disturbed as little as possible.

The child with meningitis may be overly sensitive to stimuli; therefore the room should be dimly lit and noise is kept to a minimum. The nurse carefully raises and lowers crib sides to avoid

BOX 23–3

SEPSIS

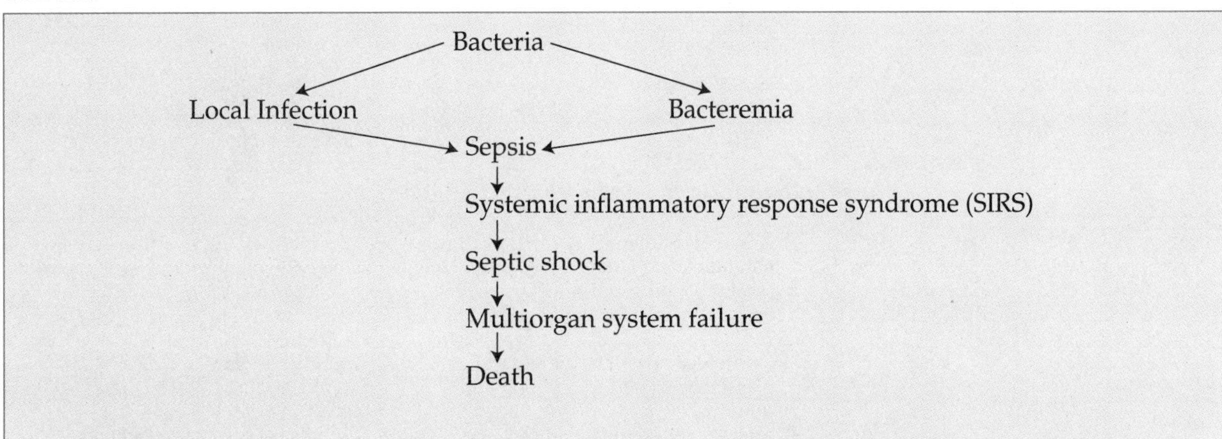

This chart shows the progression of primary bacteremia or local infection to sepsis and septic shock with complications. Early treatment of suspected sepsis can prevent these complications.

Adapted from Behrman, R., Kleigman, R., & Arvin, A. (1996). *Nelson's textbook of pediatrics* (15th ed., p. 705.) Philadelphia: Saunders.

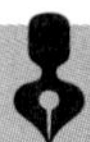

Nursing Tip

Encephalitis may occur as a complication of childhood diseases such as measles, mumps, or chicken pox. It is crucial that children receive the immunizations available for the diseases that are preventable.

jarring the bed. The nurse avoids startling the child by using a soft voice and gentle touch. These precautions are also explained to the parents.

Frequent monitoring of the child's vital signs is necessary. A slowed pulse rate, irregular respirations, and an increase in blood pressure are reported immediately, as they could indicate increased ICP. Fever may be controlled by antipyretics, sponge baths, or a hypothermia (cooling) mat-

NURSING CARE PLAN 23–1

Care of a Child with Altered Level of Consciousness

Nursing Diagnosis: High risk for ineffective airway/clearance/breathing pattern

Goals	Nursing Intervention	Rationale
Child will demonstrate effective airway clearance and breathing pattern, as evidenced by patent airway, age-appropriate respiratory rate (RR), lungs clear to auscultation, ability to breathe on his or her own without mechanical assistance	1. Assess airway for patency	1. Diminished oxygenation can lead to cerebral anoxia and/or death
	2. Assess for presence/absence of gag/swallow reflex, respiratory rate, rhythm, and effort, note any irregularities	2. Inability to protect the airway can lead to aspiration pneumonia. A marked increase or decrease in respiratory pattern can be a sign of impending respiratory failure
	3. Auscultate breath sounds, noting and reporting any adventitious breath sounds	3. Adventitious breath sounds are indicative of accumulated respiratory secretions, thereby increasing the risk for pneumonia or atelectasis
	4. Provide meticulous pulmonary toilet to prevent respiratory compromise	4. Good oral hygiene, suctioning of oral secretions, cleaning of buccal cavity, and turning child q2° will help to prevent respiratory problems.

Nursing Diagnosis: Potential for impaired skin integrity related to physical immobility

Goals	Nursing Intervention	Rationale
Child will maintain intact skin without signs or symptoms of tissue breakdown or decubitus	1. Assess all skin surfaces, noting areas of erythema, blanching, or edema. Pay particular attention to all bony prominences and areas in direct contact with the bed	1. Lying in one position for extended periods increases the risk of tissue breakdown and decubitus formation
	2. Reposition every 2 hours. Place child in prone position periodically (unless contraindicated by medical condition)	2. Repositioning helps to improve circulation and relieves pressure areas
	3. Bathe child daily and keep bedding free of wrinkles and crumbs	3. Bathing increases circulation due to the rubbing of the skin with the wash cloth. Having a bed free of wrinkles and crumbs prevents additional areas of potential skin breakdown and decubitus formation

Nursing Diagnosis: Ineffective parent/family coping

Goals	Nursing Intervention	Rationale
Parent/Family will demonstrate effective coping skills as evidenced by expressing a realistic understanding of child's illness and active participation in child's care.	1. Assess level of anxiety or concern of parent(s) and/or family members	1. Provides data to determine type of assistance or support that is needed
	2. Provide opportunities for instruction on how to care for the ill child	2. Enhances feelings of control/involvement in the health care of their child
	3. Reinforce and or clarify medical explanation of child's condition and prognosis	3. Ensures parent/family has a clear understanding of information received
	4. Identify community agencies and support services within the community available to the family	4. Provides family with sources of emotional and spiritual support in time of crises

tress. The nurse observes the child for additional or subtle signs of increased ICP, especially a change in alertness or muscle twitchings. The joints are also observed for swelling, pain, and immobility. Oxygen is given as ordered.

The child's intake and output are carefully observed and recorded. *Careful attention is given to maintaining the IV line.* Good oral hygiene is essential during this stage, when the child is receiving nothing by mouth. As the child's condition improves, the diet progresses from clear fluids to an age-appropriate diet. A special formula may be given when nasogastric feedings are necessary. During the convalescent period, oral fluids are encouraged, unless contraindicated. The nurse promptly reports a decrease in output of urine (oliguria), which could signal *urinary retention.* Bowel movements are recorded each day to detect constipation and avoid fecal impaction (an accumulation of feces in the rectum). The nurse continues to monitor neurologic status, recording and reporting findings, such as weakness of limbs, speech difficulties, mental confusion, and behavior problems. The child should be assessed for developmental deficiencies. When recovery is uneventful, the child may be discharged home and parents are taught principles of intermittent IV therapy that can be accomplished in the home setting with visits from a home health agency nurse.

Encephalitis

Description. *Encephalitis* (*encephalo,* "brain," and *itis,* "inflammation") is an inflammation of the brain. When the spinal cord is also infected the condition is known as encephalomyelitis (*myelo,* "spinal cord"). This disorder can be caused by "toga" viruses (RNA viruses) and herpes virus types 1 and 2; it can be the aftermath of disorders such as upper respiratory tract infections, German measles, or measles, or, rarely, an untoward reaction to vaccinations such as diphtheria, pertussis, and tetanus (DPT); or it may result from lead poisoning. Other etiologic agents include bacteria, spirochetes, and fungi.

Manifestations. The symptoms of encephalitis result from the CNS response to irritation. Characteristically, the history is that of a headache followed by drowsiness, which may proceed to coma. Because coma is sometimes prolonged, encephalitis is sometimes referred to as "sleeping sickness." Convulsions are seen, particularly in infants. Fever, cramps, abdominal pain, vomiting, stiff neck (nuchal rigidity), delirium, muscle twitching, and abnormal eye movements are other manifestations of the disease.

Treatment and Nursing Care. The treatment is supportive and is aimed at providing relief from specific symptoms. Sedatives and antipyretics may be prescribed. Seizure precautions are taken. Adequate nutrition and hydration are maintained. The nurse provides a quiet environment, good oral hygiene, skin care, and frequent changes of position. Oxygen is given as ordered, and the mouth and nose are kept free of mucus by gentle aspiration. Bowel movements are recorded daily, as the child may be constipated from lack of activity. Preventing the secondary effects of immobilization is paramount.

The nurse closely observes the child for neurologic changes. Fatality rates and residual effects are higher among infants than among older children. Speech, mental processes, and motor abilities may be slowed, and permanent brain damage and mental retardation can result. Growth and development

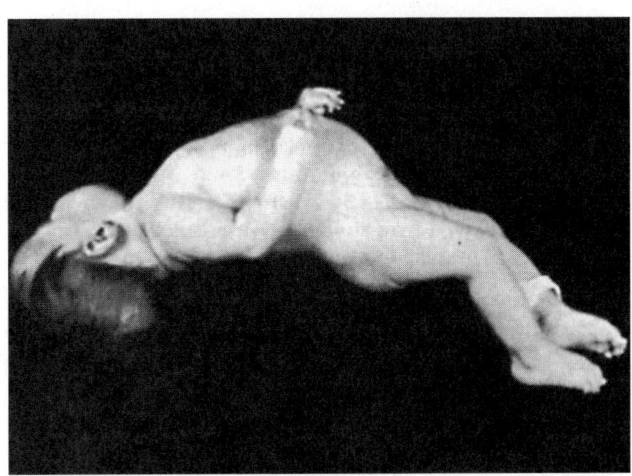

Figure 23–9. • The opisthotonos position. An involuntary arching of the back and extension of the neck are seen in children with meningeal irritation. (From Behrman, R., Kleigman, R., & Arvin, A. [1996]. *Nelson's textbook of pediatrics* [15th ed.]. Philadelphia: Saunders.)

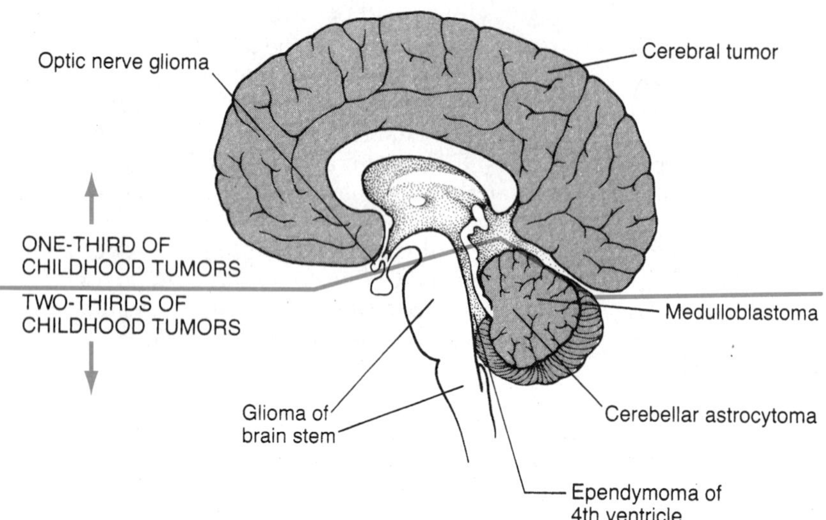

Figure 23–10. • Location of brain tumors in children.

and hearing evaluations should be monitored. Parents are encouraged to help with the care of the child as soon as the condition is stable. They are instructed about the nursing procedures for home care and any follow-up care required.

Brain Tumors

Description. Brain tumors are the second most common type of neoplasm in children (the first is leukemia). The majority of childhood tumors occur in the lower part of the brain (cerebellum or brain stem) (Fig. 23–10). The etiology of these tumors is unknown. They occur most commonly in school-age children.

Manifestations. The signs and symptoms are directly related to the location and size of the tumor. Most tumors create increased ICP with the hallmark symptoms of headache, vomiting, drowsiness, and seizures (Fig. 23–11). *Nystagmus* (constant jerky movements of the eyeball), strabismus, and decreased vision may be evidenced. *Papilledema* (edema of the optic nerve) may occur. Other symptoms include ataxia, head tilt, behavioral changes, and cerebral enlargement, particularly in infants. Deviations in vital signs are noticeable when the tumor presses on the brain stem.

Treatment and Nursing Care. Diagnosis is determined by clinical manifestations, laboratory tests, CT, MRI, and myelogram. Angiography is used to assist in the surgical approach by identifying the

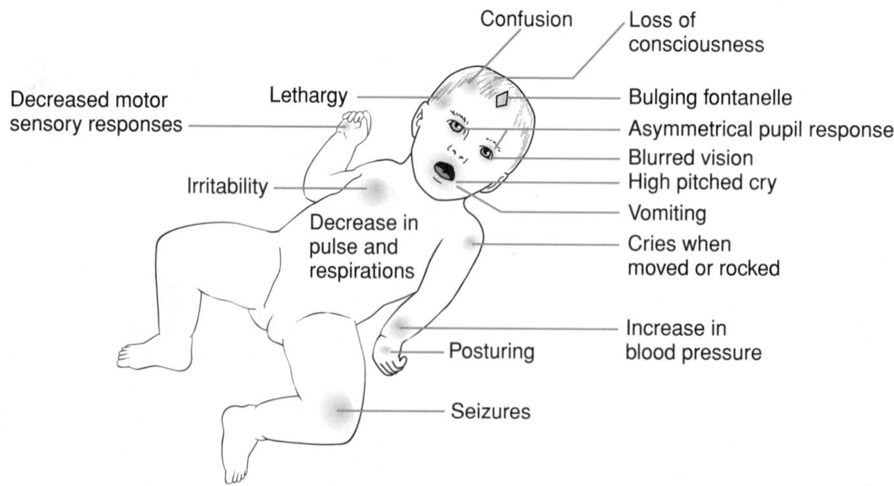

Figure 23–11. • Signs of increased intracranial pressure in infants and children.

Nursing Tip

The timing of information is important when preparing the child for various procedures.

tumor's blood supply. Preoperative emphasis is placed on carefully explaining various procedures and on familiarizing the child and family with the recovery room, ICU, and hospital personnel. The nurse explains that the child will have his or her head shaved. The size of the postoperative dressing is carefully explained. Applying a similar dressing to a doll may be helpful to the child.

Postoperative care is usually provided in the intensive care unit (ICU). Adjuncts to care may include using a hypothermia (cooling) blanket or a mechanical respirator. Parents must be prepared for the appearance of the child following surgery. Empathetic family support and appropriate referral are offered.

Radiation treatment may be prescribed. The radiologist outlines the areas to be treated on the child's head. *These marks are not washed off.* Small doses of radiation are given over a period of weeks. Chemotherapy regimens may follow radiation.

Seizure Disorders

Seizures are the most frequently observed neurologic dysfunction in children. The etiology varies (see Box 23–4). Seizures are sudden, intermittent episodes of altered consciousness lasting seconds to minutes and may include involuntary tonic and clonic movements. A *tonic movement* is a stiffening (contraction) of muscles. A *clonic movement* is an alternating contraction and relaxation of muscles.

Febrile Seizures

Febrile seizures is a transient condition affecting about 4% of children between the ages of 6 months to 5 years. There may be a genetic predisposition explaining why children in the same family present with this problem. The seizure occurs in response to a rapid rise in temperature often to a level of 101.8° F (38.8° C). Since the seizure lasts a short time and is no longer present when the child reaches a hospital, causes other than fever may need to be ruled out. Simple febrile convulsions are treated by teaching the parent to control the fever by appropriate use of antipyretics, such as acetaminophen, and cooling measures, such as removing heavy blankets and clothing. Parents should be reassured that the condition is self-limiting. The use of phenobarbital is not effective and may decrease cognitive function. Depakene (valproic acid) produces side effects and these drugs are not recommended for first-time treatment. Rectal or oral diazepam (Valium) for the duration of a febrile illness may be prescribed if febrile convulsions recur. Side effects such as lethargy, irritability or ataxia (lack of muscular coordination) should be reported. Febrile seizures rarely develop into epilepsy and have an excellent prognosis without residual problems.

Epilepsy

Description. The term *epilepsy* (chronic recurrent convulsions) comes from the Greek *epilepsia,* which means "seizure." In the past, words such as *fit, spell,* and *blackout* were used to describe this entity. These are nonspecific and tend to create confusion.

Epilepsy is a disorder manifested by a variety of symptom complexes. It is characterized by recurrent paroxysmal (sudden; periodic) attacks of unconsciousness *or* impaired consciousness that may be followed by alternate (tonic) contraction and (clonic) relaxation of the muscles *or* abnormal behavior. It is a disorder of the CNS in which the neurons or nerve cells discharge in an abnormal

BOX 23–4

CAUSES OF SEIZURES IN CHILDREN

Etiology of seizures can be
- Intracranial
  - Epilepsy
  - Congenital anomaly
  - Birth injury
  - Infection
  - Trauma
  - Degenerative diseases
  - Tumor
  - Vascular disorder
- Extracranial
  - Fever
  - Heart disease
  - Metabolic disorders
  - Hypocalcemia
  - Hypoglycemia
  - Dehydration and malnutrition
- Toxic
  - Anesthetics
  - Drugs
  - Poisons

Nursing Tip

No foreign object should be placed in the mouth during a seizure.

way. These discharges may be focal or diffuse. The site of general discharge can sometimes be ascertained by observing the child's symptoms during the attack. When the cause is unknown, the term *idiopathic* epilepsy is used.

The nurse observes and records the following: the child's activity immediately before the seizure; body movements; changes in color, respiration, or muscle tone; incontinence; and the parts of the body involved. When possible, the seizure is timed. The child's appearance, behavior, and level of consciousness following the seizure are also documented. Table 23–2 describes the first aid response and nursing responsibilities during a seizure.

Types of Epilepsy

Childhood epilepsy is classified into partial seizures and generalized seizures.

Generalized Seizures. *General seizures* involve loss of consciousness. The most common generalized seizure is *grand mal.* A grand mal epilepsy has three distinct phases. (1) An aura (subjective sensation), (2) a tonic/clonic seizure followed by (3) postictal lethargy, a short period of sleep. *Petit mal,* or absence seizures, often are recognized when an intelligent child is referred for medical evaluation because of unexplained failure to achieve in school. The reason for school failure is found to be absence seizures, that causes a temporary loss of awareness that results in a lack of continuity in the learning environment.

Partial Seizures. *Partial seizures* account for 40% of childhood convulsions. Consciousness may be intact or impaired. Partial seizures are often mistaken for alterations in behavior.

Treatment. Initially, treatment is aimed at determining the type, site, or cause of the disorder. Diagnostic measures include a complete history and physical and neurologic examinations. Skull radiography and CT are employed to establish the presence or absence of tumors, skull abnormalities, hematomas, and intracranial calcifications. MRI may be utilized. The EEG is also a valuable tool in diagnosing seizures. It is especially helpful in differentiating between an absence seizure and a complex partial seizure. Prolonged EEG monitoring (24 hours) is another diagnostic technique.

Laboratory studies such as complete blood count (CBC), determinations of serum calcium and blood urea nitrogen (BUN), and tests for lead poisoning or other metabolic disorders, are done. A spinal tap may be ordered when encephalitis or meningitis is suspected. If the seizure is related to any such underlying cause, appropriate therapy is initiated. When epilepsy is the diagnosis, anticonvulsant medications are prescribed (see Table 23–3).

The duration of therapy is based on the individual child. Initially, the doctor prescribes the lowest dose of anticonvulsant medication likely to control the seizures. Drowsiness, a common side effect of many anticonvulsants, may interfere with the child's activities. Careful recording of seizure activity and compliance to the drug regimen are of particular importance in determining a suitable program. Medication is given at the *same time each day,* generally with meals or at bedtime.

If it is necessary for the child to take medication during school hours, the parents sign a consent form so that the school nurse can monitor administration. Nurse and teacher response, particularly during and after a seizure, will have a significant effect on the attitude of classmates toward the child.

Abrupt withdrawal of anticonvulsant medications is the most common cause of *status epilepticus.* In the hospital, the nurse clarifies with the physician whether anticonvulsants are to be withheld if the child is NPO (nothing by mouth). As in any long-term drug therapy, periodic blood and urine tests are performed to detect therapeutic levels as well as subtle side effects. When children are old enough, they can assume responsibility for their own medications. *They should wear a medical identification bracelet.* During puberty and adolescence, dosages may have to be adjusted to meet growth needs. Premenstrual fluid retention in girls can sometimes trigger seizures. Surgery is being performed on children who are unresponsive to anticonvulsants and who have a well-defined focus of seizure activity in the brain.

The *ketogenic* diet is sometimes prescribed for children who do not respond well to anticonvulsant therapy. It is high in fats and low in carbohydrates and produces ketoacidosis in the body, which appears to reduce convulsive episodes. Reduction of fluid intake tends to increase the ketogenic effect. Use is limited because the diet is boring, requires strict adherence to intake, and compliance tends to be a problem.

Rebellion against medical routine is not uncommon during adolescence. Some states do not allow controlled epileptics to obtain a driver's license, which is disheartening to the child. Other states have stipulations as to the amount of seizure-free

Table 23–2
SEIZURE RECOGNITION AND FIRST AID RESPONSE

Seizure Type	What It Looks Like	Often Mistaken For	What to Do	What Not to Do
1. General Generalized tonic-clonic (also called *grand mal*)	Sudden cry (or aura), fall, rigidity, followed by muscle jerking; shallow, irregular breathing; possible loss of bladder or bowel control; usually lasts seconds to minutes, followed by some confusion, a period of sleep (postictal lethargy), and then return to full consciousness	Heart attack, stroke	Look for medical identification Protect from nearby hazards. Observe and record stages and manifestations Following seizure, maintain patent airway, turn on side, loosen clothing, reassure If multiple seizures, or if one seizure lasts longer than 5 min, call ambulance (911) If person is pregnant, injured, or diabetic, call for aid at once	Do not put any hard implement in the mouth Do not try to hold tongue; it cannot be swallowed Do not try to give liquids during or just after seizure Do not restrain
2. Absence (also called *petit mal*)	A blank stare, beginning and ending abruptly, lasting only a few seconds; most common in children; may be accompanied by rapid blinking, some chewing movements of the mouth; child is unaware of what is going on during the seizure, but quickly returns to full awareness once it has stopped; may result in learning difficulties if not recognized and treated	Daydreaming, lack of attention, deliberate ignoring of adult instructions	No first aid necessary, but if this is first observation of seizure(s), medical evaluation should be recommended	
A. Partial Simple partial (also called *Jacksonian*)	Jerking may begin in one area of body such as the arm, leg, or face; cannot be stopped, but child stays awake and aware; jerking may proceed from one area of the body to another and sometimes spreads to become a generalized seizure	Acting, out bizarre, behavior Hysteria Mental illness Psychosomatic illness Parapsychological or mystical experience	No first aid necessary unless seizure becomes generalized, then first aid as indicated; no immediate action needed other than reassurance and emotional support; medical evaluation should be recommended	
B. Simple partial (also called *sensory*)	Complains of a "funny" feeling in the stomach Motor activity with head turning and eye movement Lasts approximately 10 to 20 seconds	Tics, mental illness, psychosomatic illness	No action needed other than reassurance and emotional support	

Table continued on following page

time required before licensing. Excess intake of fluids, particularly alcoholic beverages, can trigger a seizure. Parents can obtain valuable information and support from the Epilepsy Foundation of America. Other major resources include the Department of Vocational Rehabilitation, the Department of Public Health, the Department of Social Services, and other community agencies. The greatest untapped resource for persons with epilepsy is often within themselves. In a comprehensive multidisciplinary treatment approach, team members help the child to mobilize their inner resources to deal with their lifelong treatment and to lead a fully productive normal life.

A fundamental principle of comprehensive epilepsy management is that the child become an active member of the health care team. The epileptic child can lead a normal life with a few safety

Table 23–2
SEIZURE RECOGNITION AND FIRST AID RESPONSE *(Continued)*

Seizure Type	What It Looks Like	Often Mistaken For	What to Do	What Not to Do
C. **Complex partial** (also called *psychomotor* or *temporal lobe*)	Usually starts with blank stare, followed by chewing, followed by random activity; person appears unaware of surroundings, may seem dazed and may mumble, is unresponsive; actions clumsy, not directed; may pick at clothing, pick up objects, try to take off clothes; may run, appear afraid; may struggle or flail at restraint; once pattern established, same set of actions usually occurs with each seizure; can last 1 to 2 minutes; no memory of actions or behavior	Disorderly conduct	Speak calmly and reassuringly to child and others Guide gently away from obvious hazards Stay with child until completely aware of environment Offer to help getting home	Do not grab hold unless sudden danger (such as a cliff edge or an approaching car) threatens Do not try to restrain Do not shout Do not expect verbal instructions to be obeyed
3. **Atonic seizures** (also called *drop attacks*)	More frequent occurrence in the morning with jerking motions on awakening; suddenly collapses; after 10 sec to 1 min, child recovers, regains consciousness, and can stand and walk again	Clumsiness, normal childhood stage; lack of good walking skills; drunkenness	No first aid needed (unless hurt during fall), but the child should be given a thorough medical evaluation	

guidelines. Restriction of physical activity is not necessary, but adult supervision during swimming or bathing is advisable. A family assessment is helpful in establishing rapport and setting realistic short-term and long-term goals. Too much attention to seizures by well-meaning adults can make control difficult. The child may learn to use the threat of a seizure to manipulate caretakers. Teaching should include first-aid treatment for seizures (Table 23–2), the importance of compliance with long-term medication regimes, and general reassurance that the child can lead a normal life. Medications used in the treatment of epilepsy are outlined in Table 23–3. The gum hypertrophy that occurs as a side effect of Dilantin will require meticulous oral hygiene and special care, especially if orthodontic treatment is necessary. Death or serious injury rarely occurs from a seizure, and it does not cause mental deterioration. The Individuals with Disabilities Education Act (IDEA) guarantees children with disabilities the right to publicly financed educational programs in the least restrictive environment. Most children under proper treatment can lead full and productive lives.

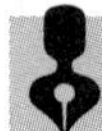

Nursing Tip

The nurse is responsible for maintaining seizure precautions for a child diagnosed with a seizure disorder:

- Side rails up
- Sharp or hard objects around bed padded
- Make sure child wears medical ID bracelet
- Supervision during potentially hazardous play, such as swimming
- Avoid triggering factors
- Teach importance of compliance with medication regime

Status Epilepticus

A prolonged seizure that can result in brain hypoxia and does not respond to treatment for 20 minutes or more, is called *status epilepticus.* A frequent cause is sudden stopping of epilepsy medication or generalized infection. Treatment includes managing airway, providing oxygen, observing and documenting details of the seizure, and providing IV therapy. Diazepam and phenytoin or a pentobarbital drug may be given IV. The child may need to be placed on a ventilator until seizures are controlled.

Other Conditions Causing Decreased Level of Consciousness

Several conditions are mistaken for epilepsy because they involve paroxysmal altered levels of

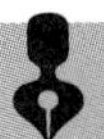

Nursing Tip

Common triggering factors for seizures

- Flashing of dark/light patterns
- Startling movements
- Hypoprotinemia
- Overhydration
- Photosensitivity

consciousness. *These conditions do not respond to antiepileptic drugs.*

Benign Paroxysmal Vertigo. This condition occurs in children under 3 years of age who develop ataxia and fall. Nausea, vomiting, and complaints of motion sickness and migraine headache follow. The condition responds to dimenhydrinate (Dramamine) medication.

Night Terrors. These occur in children between 5 and 7 years of age. The child may sleepwalk, thrash, scream, and is unaware of surroundings. A period of sleep follows. Brief treatment with diazepam (Valium) or imipramine (Tofranil) may be helpful, but family dysfunction should be investigated.

Breath-Holding Spells. Breath holding can result in cyanosis or extreme pallor. They are most frequent between 2 and 5 years of age. The child loses consciousness and parents are frightened. Counseling parents to avoid reinforcing the behavior by refusing to play or hold the child following the episode is helpful.

Cough Syncope. Cough syncopes are paroxysmal coughing spells, usually at night, that result in a diminished cardiac output, cerebral hypoxia, and loss of consciousness. The condition usually occurs in asthmatic children. Prevention involves avoidance of bronchoconstriction.

Prolonged QT Syndrome. A sudden loss of consciousness associated with vigorous exercise is caused by a heart problem and can result in loss of consciousness and death. It usually occurs during adolescence and arises from a defect in chromosome 11. Beta-blockers may be lifesaving. Knowledge of CPR and exercise restriction are essential.

Rage Attacks, or Episodic Dyscontrol Syndrome. Sudden recurrent attacks of violent physical behavior that appears out of control, followed by fatigue, remorse, and amnesia. The EEG is usually normal. This condition is often mistaken for partial seizure epilepsy.

Cerebral Palsy

Description. *Cerebral palsy* (CP) refers to a group of nonprogressive disorders that affect the motor centers of the brain. It is not fatal in itself, but at present there is no cure. It is one of the most common handicapping conditions seen in children, occurring in as many as 2 per 1000 live births. This

Table 23–3
PROPERTIES OF SELECTED ANTICONVULSANT DRUGS

Drug	Side Effects	Comments
Tegretol (carbamazepine)	Blurred vision, diplopia, drowsiness, vertigo	Few side effects, fewer sedative properties
Luminal (phenobarbital)	Drowsiness, irritability, hyperactivity	Safest overall medication; bitter, often combined with other drugs
Dilantin (phenytoin)	Ataxia, insomnia, motor twitching, gum overgrowth, hirsutism (hairiness), rash, nausea, vitamin D and folic acid deficiencies	Generally effective and safe; may cause cognitive impairment; regular massaging of gums decreases hyperplasia; used in combination with phenobarbital or primidone
Depakene (valproic acid)	Gastrointestinal disturbance, altered bleeding time, liver toxicity	Monitor blood counts; take with food or use enteric-coated preparations; potentiates action of phenobarbital and other drugs
Mysoline (primidone)	Ataxia, vertigo, anorexia, fatigue, hyperirritability, dermatitis	May be used alone or in combination; side effects minimized by starting with small amounts
Zarotin ethosuximide	Anorexia; gastrointestinal upset	
Valium (diazepam)	Headache, tremor, fatigue, depression	Used in combination or alone
Clonopin (clonazepam)	Behavior changes, ataxia, anorexia, nystagmus	Effective for most minor motor seizures
Felbamate (felbatol)	Blurred vision; rash, nausea	Can cause hepatic damage and blood dyscrasia
Gabapentin (neurotoxin)	Weight gain and somnolence	
Lamotrigine (lamictal)	Ataxia, rash, photosensitivity, angioedema and drowsiness	Given with valproic acid

Note: The physician determines the child's medication by the type of seizure and other factors. The goal is to achieve the best control with the minimum dosage and the least number of side effects. An important aspect of nursing intervention includes *reinforcing the need for drug supervision and compliance.*

disease is precipitated by many factors, some of which are birth injuries, neonatal anoxia, subdural hemorrhage, and infections such as meningitis and encephalitis. Studies indicate that more than one third of children with CP weighed less than 2500 grams at birth. Lead poisoning, head injuries, and febrile illness are sometimes responsible during the toddler period In some children, no single cause can be found, yet recent studies indicate that a congenital problem may exist.

Manifestations. The symptoms of cerebral palsy vary with each child and may range from mild to severe. Mental retardation sometimes accompanies this disorder; however, many children with CP have normal intelligence. The disease is suspected during infancy if there are feeding problems, convulsions not associated with high fever, and physical retardation. Developmental milestones are not achieved at the expected age level. Diagnostic tests may include spinal tap, EEG, pneumoencephalography, CT, and screening for metabolic disorders. Brain tumors must also be ruled out. Early recognition is important.

There are four types of cerebral palsy (Table 23–4). Two of the more common are those marked by spasticity and athetosis (Fig. 23–12). These conditions occur in about 75% of the cases. *Spasticity* is characterized by tension in certain muscle groups. The stretch reflex is present in the involved muscles. When the child tries to move the voluntary muscles, jerky motions result. Eating, walking, and other coordinated movements are difficult to accomplish. The lower extremities are usually involved. The legs cross and the toes point inward. The arms and trunk may also be affected. In *athetosis,* the child has involuntary, purposeless movements that interfere with normal motion. Speech, sight, and hearing defects and convulsions may be complications.

Treatment and Nursing Care. The goal of treatment of children with cerebral palsy is to assist them in making the most of their assets and to guide them in becoming well-adjusted adults, performing at their maximum ability. Both short-term and long-term goals must be realistic. Parents need help in accepting the child and should not be deceived into expecting miraculous cures from treatment. Early diagnosis can result in fewer physical and emotional problems.

Table 23–4
TYPES OF CEREBRAL PALSY

Type	Characteristics
Spastic	Involves damage to the cortex of the brain. Spasms occur upon movement. Related to cerebral asphyxia
Athetoid	Involves damage to the basal nuclei ganglion Continuous writhing involuntary movements. Often associated with hyperbilirubinemia
Ataxic	Uncoordinated movements and ataxia from a lesion in the cerebellum
Mixed	Usually a combination of spastic and athetoid

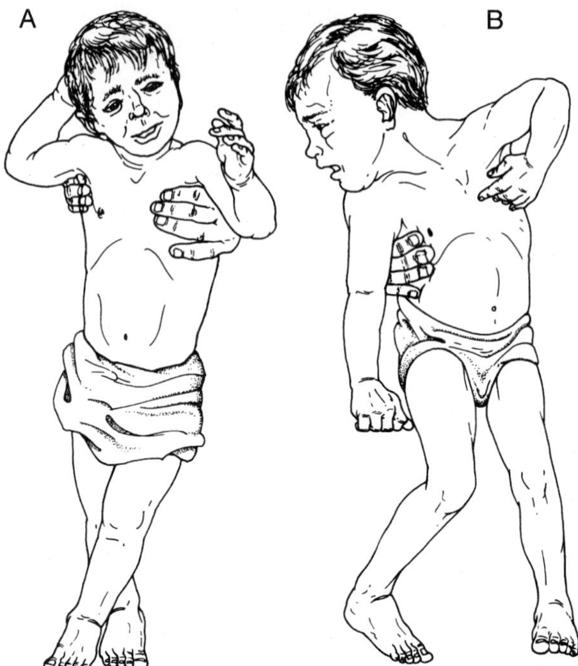

Figure 23–12. • Cerebral palsy. **A,** spasticity. **B,** athetosis.

Parents must be informed of community resources available to them. The family's religious affiliation should not be overlooked, as it can be a source of support and help during times of stress. The long course of this disability can place a financial burden on the family. Caretakers need respite care from time to time to enhance their coping skills.

The specific treatment is highly individualized depending on the severity of the disability. It is not uncommon for the parents of children with cerebral palsy to become the experts in caring for their child. Therefore, the parent should be an integral part of the health care team.

Good skin care is essential for the child with cerebral palsy. The nurse observes the skin for redness and other evidence of pressure sores. All precautions are taken to prevent the formation of *contractures* (degeneration or shortening of the muscles due to lack of use), which could result in permanent loss of function of the part involved, for example, leg, arm, or finger. The nurse encourages the children to do as much as they can for themselves. When they bathe, they are encouraged to put their muscles and joints through the normal range of motion. The nurse must use judgment in assessing the child's capabilities and assist only in those areas where the child is lacking.

Other measures necessary to prevent deformities include frequent change of position, the use of splints, and the carrying out of passive, range-of-motion, as well as stretching exercises. The nurse must also ensure that the child maintains good posture while in bed. This is done through the use of footboards and the proper positioning of pillows and other comfort devices.

Braces are frequently used to treat this disability. A brace is a mechanical aid that supports weakened muscles or limbs. All braces are routinely checked for correct alignment, loose or missing parts, and condition of straps and buckles. The child needs assistance to adjust to this unfamiliar device. Wheelchairs and crutches are designed to fit the child.

Orthopedic surgery may be indicated and may be followed by an extensive period of rehabilitation. The nurse must remember that the child is in a continuous state of psychological as well as physical growth during this period. Interest, or lack of it, may have a decided effect on the personality of the child in later years.

Feeding problems can lead to nutritional deficiencies. Vitamin, mineral, or protein supplements may be indicated for some children. Swallowing and sucking may be difficult. Vomiting is frequent because the gag reflex is overactive. The entire body may become tense. The nurse must be especially careful to feed the child slowly to prevent aspiration. It is difficult for these infants to adjust to solid foods, and it takes a great deal of patience on the part of parents and nurses to help them to adapt to this new experience (Box 23–5 and Fig. 23–13). As the children grow, they can be taught to manage special feeding equipment so that they are able to eat independently. They are also taught such activities as dressing and combing their hair. Dental care is discussed in Chapter 15.

The physically challenged child needs opportunities to play alone and with other children. Games suited to ability, such as finger painting, are fun and allow freedom of expression. Activities that require fine muscular movements of the hand cause frustration in the child whose arms and hands are affected by the disease. The nurse can learn a great deal from the parents about types of play the child enjoys. Children with cerebral palsy tire easily but find it difficult to relax. They use a great deal of energy to accomplish the simplest of tasks and they do not respond well to being hurried or overstimulated.

Educational opportunities geared to the child's abilities are essential. Public law 94–142 mandates that public schools provide education for handicapped children. The child's mental capacity is determined not just in the light of IQ itself but also by the demonstrated potential of the individual.

Preschools and summer camps for exceptional children are available. These programs vary in quality and extent of services. Parents are also referred to the United Cerebral Palsy Association, a national organization that provides education and

BOX 23–5

GENERAL MODIFICATIONS/PRECAUTIONS IN PEDIATRIC FEEDING TECHNIQUES FOR CHILDREN WITH CEREBRAL PALSY

1. Proper positioning and support of the head and back are essential prior to feeding solid foods.
2. Place small amounts of food on a spoon to avoid choking.
3. Avoid tilting the head back during feeding of solid foods as this will place the swallowing mechanisms out of alignment.
4. Do not touch the tip of the child's tongue with the spoon as this can activate the tongue extrusion reflex.
5. Use rubber-coated spoons for children with hyperactive bite reflex to protect teeth from injury.
6. Gently stroke the angle of the jaw below the ears to relax the bite of a child who has clamped down on a spoon.
7. Gently stroke, in a circular motion, the area under the chin to stimulate chewing when food is held in the mouth.
8. Gently press upward under the chin to stimulate swallowing when fluid is held in the mouth.
9. To help a handicapped child to drink from a cup, cut the top portion of the paper or plastic cup away to provide space for the nose. This will enable the cup to be tilted without the child's head being tilted back.
10. Avoid excessive pressure on the back of the head when positioning a handicapped child for feeding, to avoid reflex responses in body/torso position.

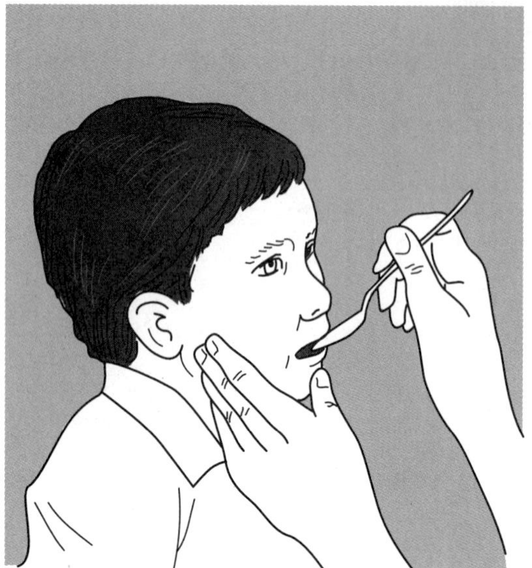
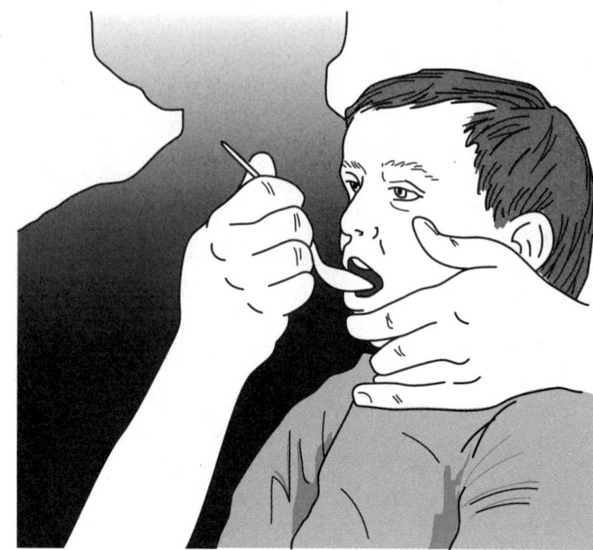

Figure 23–13. • Examples of two ways of feeding a handicapped child.

support services. The expanding role of nurses in the home and schools may further assist in mainstreaming these children into educational and social situations (Box 23–6).

Successful experiences help to improve a child's self-concept; repeated failures are demoralizing and may lower self-esteem. The health care team works to bring satisfaction to these children by making it possible for them to succeed. The amount of confidence and self-respect that a disabled child has depends a great deal on a supportive environment.

Mental Health Needs of the Physically Challenged Child. The requirements for good mental health in the physically challenged child do not differ from those of other children. They need to have their basic human drives satisfied and people who are genuinely interested in them. The disabled child needs to participate to the fullest extent in family, school, and community activities. Friendships with other handicapped and nonhandicapped peers are encouraged. Extended family and the community are important resources. Educational programs are integrating the handicapped more fully into the community. Barrier-free buildings and modifications that improve accessibility contribute positively to these efforts.

BOX 23–6

TREATMENT PROTOCOL FOR CEREBRAL PALSY

1. Establish communication.
2. Establish locomotion.
3. Utilize and optimize existing motor functions.
4. Provide intellectual stimulation.
5. Promote socialization.
6. Provide technology to encourage self-care and promote growth and development.
7. Provide multidisciplinary approach to care.

Mental Retardation

Mental retardation is defined as below-average mental functioning (IQ below 75) and a deficit in adaptive behavior (see Box 23–7) manifested during the developmental period (before 18 years of age).

Definition. Mental retardation has many descriptive labels. The specific terminology most often used in the medical field is *mental retardation,* or *cognitive impairment.* The education system most often uses *mentally handicapped, mentally deficient, mentally disabled, mentally impaired,* or *mentally challenged.* The educational system utilizes criteria for classroom placement and eligibility for available resources. U.S. Federal law provides for services from birth to 21 years of age. Public law requires providing the least restrictive environment for learning and mainstreaming with nonimpaired students whenever possible.

When a child is diagnosed as mentally retarded, correlating growth and development with mental functioning is important. For example, abstract

BOX 23–7

AMERICAN ASSOCIATION ON MENTAL RETARDATION (AAMR) DEFINITION OF MENTAL RETARDATION

- Two levels—mild or severe
- Intellectual functioning below IQ of 75
- Limitations in at least two of the following ten areas of adaptive behaviors:
    1. Communication
    2. Self-care
    3. Home living
    4. Social skills
    5. Community use
    6. Self-direction
    7. Health and safety
    8. Functional academics
    9. Leisure
    10. Work

thinking does not begin to appear before 12 years of age. *A child classified as mentally retarded is not necessarily retarded in all areas of mental functioning* (Box 23–8). Tests to measure intelligence are numerous. One test that is frequently given to children and adolescents is the Stanford-Binet.

Intelligence in children is difficult to evaluate and is best tested on an individual basis. Personality tests such as picture story tests, inkblot tests, drawing tests, and sentence completion tests may also be administered. All such tests have their limitations, and of course their accuracy is subject to the abilities of the person interpreting them. Nonetheless, the tests are of value when used in conjunction with a thorough study of the child's physical, mental, emotional, and social development.

BOX 23–8

ELEMENTS INVOLVED IN MENTAL FUNCTIONING

- Level of consciousness
    Attention, short- and long-term memory, perceptions
- Thought processes
    Insight
    Judgments
    Affect
    Mood
- Expressive language
    Vocabulary, abstract thinking, intelligence

There are many causes of mental retardation. Some conditions that can develop during the neonatal period are phenylketonuria, hypothyroidism, fetal alcohol syndrome, Down syndrome, malformations of the brain (such as microcephaly, hydrocephalus, craniostenosis), and maternal infections such as cytomegalovirus (CMV; see Chapter 14). Birth injuries or anoxia during or shortly after delivery may also cause mental retardation. Conditions such as meningitis, lead poisoning, neoplasms, and encephalitis can cause mental retardation in a child or adult of any age. Heredity is a factor in mental retardation. It is also possible that living in a physically and emotionally deprived environment will cause the child to be mentally retarded.

The diagnosis is determined after a thorough study is made. The American Psychiatric Association provides a DSM-IV listing that defines diagnostic criteria for mental retardation. Conditions such as epilepsy, cerebral palsy, severe malnutrition, emotional disturbances, blindness, deafness, and speech disorders must be ruled out. In certain cases, early recognition and intervention can lessen or prevent mental retardation.

Other symptoms of mental retardation are associated with milestones of the growth process. Children who do not achieve milestones at the expected age may be cognitively impaired. Unusual clumsiness and failure to respond to stimuli are also early indications. Sometimes this disorder is not discovered until the child enters school. Each case must be frequently reevaluated according to the child's individual progress.

The Importance of Success in the Approach to the Mentally Retarded Child

We cannot all run at the same speed, sing (carry a tune) with the same ability, dance as gracefully, or draw as skillfully as some of our peers. Yet most of us get by. However, if one is not good in something, which, in our culture, is very important, such as reading, writing, and spelling, problems can develop. The problems usually relate to the consequences of chronic failure.

The pediatric nurse must assist the parents to understand that providing experiences that the child can be successful in and concentrating on strengths rather than weaknesses are the keys to dealing with children who are developmentally different. Children who experience consistent failure become angry. The anger causes behavior difficulties that can cloud the problem and the therapy.

Management and Nursing Goals. An individualized plan of care with goals and objectives is vital

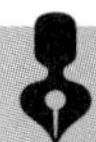

Nursing Tip

The retarded child needs to develop a sense of accomplishment. Do not "take over" projects because of your own need to assist or speed up the process.

Nursing Tip

Many retarded children have normal facial appearance. Many children with unusual faces are not retarded.

to managing mentally retarded children and helping their families. The initial step is to present the findings to the family and to provide the emotional support necessary to cope with a disabled child. The child's competence and adaptive behaviors should be discussed along with the deficiencies. Introduction to the multidisciplinary team for long-term management is important. Play therapy should be prescribed to nurture growth and development. The "Special Olympics" introduce healthy competition to the cognitively and physically impaired child. Receptive and expressive communication skills are developed with professional help.

Nurses must be familiar with the resources of the community so that they can direct the family to them. The local chapter of the National Association for Retarded Citizens may provide information and support. Summer camps, such as those run by the Easter Seal Society, provide stimulation and opportunities for socialization to children with mental and physical disabilities. The child guidance clinic or the psychological services of a nearby college or hospital may be utilized. Arrangements for proper dental care must be made because some children may be unable to cooperate with the necessary procedures.

The nurse caring for the retarded child in the hospital needs to know the child's stage of maturation and ability. A detailed history, including a habit and care sheet, is completed. Self-help activities are documented. Home routines are to be followed as closely as possible to avoid reversal of gains already made. Good communication between parents and nurse can help to make the transition from home to hospital as smooth as possible for the child. In obtaining information about the child from the parents, a positive approach is recommended. A request such as "Tell me about Carla's eating habits" is preferable to "Does she feed herself?" and is likely to yield more helpful information.

Prevention. The outlook is good for continued success in the prevention of mental retardation. Nurses can contribute to this by promoting genetic counseling, immunizations, newborn screening, and good prenatal care (Table 23–5). Comprehensive programs for early assessment and treatment of the mentally retarded must also be promoted. The nurse can serve as an advocate for the child and/or adolescent to help to ensure that their rights are upheld.

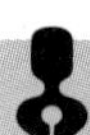

Nursing Tip

Nursing responsibilities to handicapped child

- Emphasize *strengths* present
- Maintain communication with family
- Avoid labels—use simple terms
- Contact school nurse—plan for school needs
- Provide daily experiences the child can succeed in
- Refer to local, state, and national support groups

Head Injuries

Head injuries are the major cause of death in children older than 1 year of age. More physical force is needed to produce brain trauma when the head is in a fixed position than when it is freely moving, a fact that supports the use of infant car seats. The incidence of head injury among children is high. A *concussion* is a temporary disturbance of the brain that is immediately followed by a period of unconsciousness. It jars the brain stem and is often accompanied by loss of memory of events that occurred immediately before (retrograde amnesia), during, and after the accident. A *skull fracture* indicates that the skull bone is broken or depressed. Bleeding may occur, resulting in pressure being exerted on the brain.

The response of the child to a head injury may differ from that of the adult. The location and type of skull fracture may not correlate with clinical

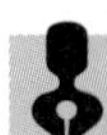

Nursing Tip

Retarded children have the same psychosocial needs as all other children but cannot express or respond as other children do.

Table 23–5
INTERVENTIONS CURRENTLY AVAILABLE TO PREVENT MENTAL RETARDATION

Factor	Intervention
Nearly total elimination	
Congenital rubella	Early immunization, antibody screening
Phenylketonuria, galactosemia, congenital hypothyroidism	Newborn screening, dietary management, replacement therapy
Kernicterus	Reduction of sensitization
Major reduction	
Tay-Sachs disease	Carrier screening, prenatal diagnosis in high-risk persons
Morbidity from prematurity	Newborn intensive care nurseries
Measles encephalitis	Early vaccination
Significant reduction	
Neural tube defects	Prenatal folic acid supplements
Lead intoxication	Screening for lead levels, improvement in environment, chelation when necessary
Fetal alcohol syndrome	Public education
Morbidity from head injury	Automobile child restraints, safety helmets and equipment
Child neglect and abuse	Parenting classes and family life education through the schools
Special assistance and relief	
Multiple handicaps, hearing, speech, Down syndrome	Early identification, support for families, genetic counseling of special risks

Adapted from Levine, M. D., Carey, W. B., & Crocker, A. C. (1992). *Developmental-behavioral pediatrics.* Philadelphia: Saunders.

findings. Careful clinical assessment is essential to determine the extent of brain injury. The surface area of a child's scalp is large and very vascular. Significant blood loss can result from scalp lacerations.

Pathophysiology. A skull fracture, brain concussion, contusion or intracranial hemorrhage may occur at the time of injury. Hypoxia, increased intracranial pressure, cerebral edema, and infection can occur within a few days. Hypoxia causes increased energy need of the brain that results in increased cerebral blood flow. This increased blood flow (hyperemia) increases cerebral edema. If the intracranial pressure rises too high, cerebral perfusion will diminish and brain damage or death will result. If the fontanels are open, the tolerance for increased ICP is higher in infants. Older children and adults do not have this advantage.

A child who sustains a mild bump to the head, retains consciousness, and does not vomit may have a covered ice pack applied to the site. During the first night following a bump on the head, parents are advised to be sure that they can arouse the child at least once, because intracranial bleeding occasionally occurs from a minor injury. If the child appears confused, has trouble seeing or speaking, or walks unsteadily, they should be advised to contact a physician. Confusion and amnesia following any head injury may indicate a concussion even if consciousness is not lost.

Infants who are roughly shaken *(shaken baby syndrome)* can sustain retinal, subarachnoid, and subdural hemorrhages in the brain and high-level cervical spine injuries resulting in permanent disability or death. Frequently, a child who has suffered a blow to the head is brought to the hospital for overnight observation to rule out or confirm the extent of injury. The child may experience all or some of the following symptoms: headache (manifested by fussiness in toddler), drowsiness, blurred vision, vomiting, and dyspnea. In severe cases, the child may be completely unconscious. Decerebrate or decorticate posturing may be evident (Fig. 23–14). In decerebrate rigidity, all four limbs are extended and the hands are pronated. In decorticate rigidity, the arms, wrists, and fingers are flexed. Plantar flexion occurs in the feet. Pathologic postures (posturing) are seen in severe brain injury. A careful history is obtained to determine any preexisting conditions and to ascertain the exact circumstances of the accident. Of particular importance is the child's state of consciousness immediately following the occurrence.

Children are handled gently and are inspected for injuries to other areas. They are placed in a crib or bed in accordance with their size. Side rails are raised, as seizures are not uncommon. The head of the bed is slightly elevated to decrease cerebral edema.

The nurse observes the child for signs of increasing ICP. Four components of a cranial or *neurologic*

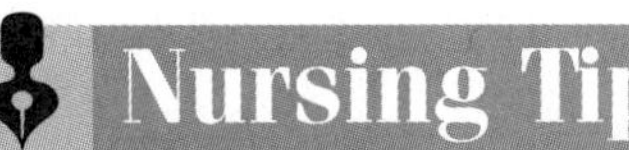

A positive glucose (dextrostix) test can determine if watery nasal discharge is cerebrospinal fluid (CSF) or a concurrent cold (rhinorrhea).

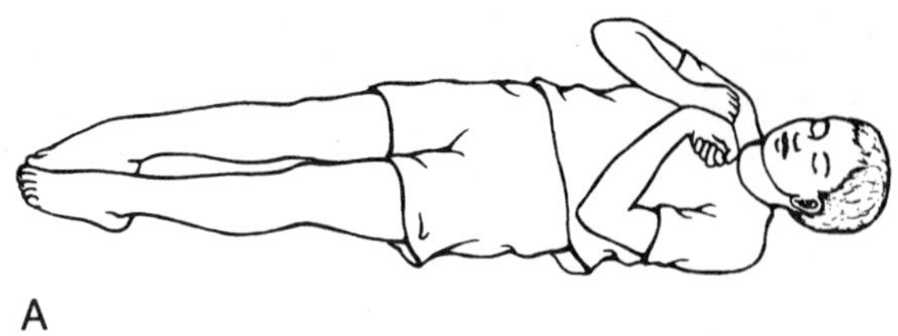

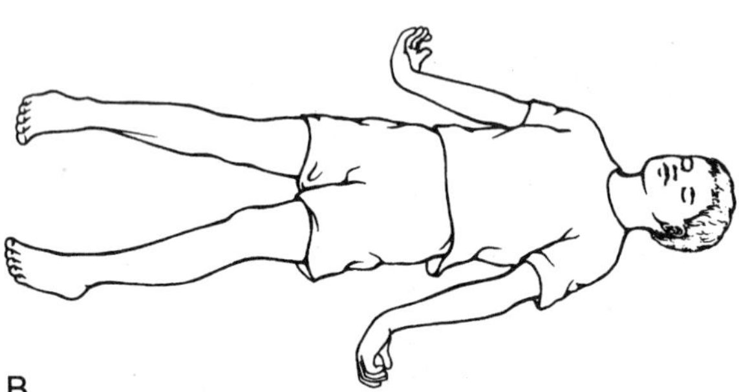

Figure 23–14. • Pathologic posturing that may occur in the patient with severe brain damage. **A,** Decorticate posturing. **B,** Decerebrate posturing.

check are (1) level of consciousness; (2) pupil and eye movement (Fig. 23–15); (3) vital signs; and (4) motor activity (see Table 23–6).

Level of Consciousness. Changes in level of consciousness are particularly meaningful and require immediate medical attention. The child's alertness on admission is recorded for use as baseline data. Response should be correlated with the developmental age of the child. Parents can be helpful in providing information about the child's usual capabilities. In general, children should be

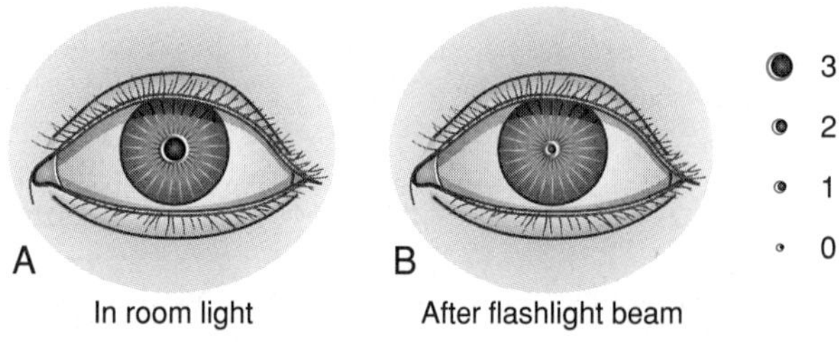

Figure 23–15. • The response of the pupil of the eye to a flashlight beam. **A,** The pupil of the eye is a "3" in room light. **B,** The pupil of the eye is a "1" after a flashlight beam is directed at the eye. The letters "B," "S," and "N" may be used to denote *B*risk, *S*low, or *N*on movement of the pupil response. This illustration would be recorded 3/1 B. The other eye should respond symmetrically. Sluggish movement, nonmovement, or asymmetrical response should be reported immediately.

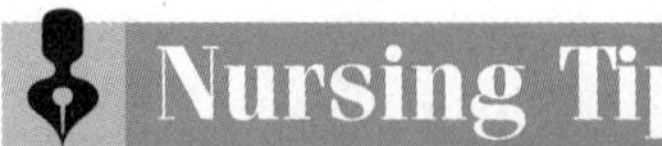

A concussion with resulting amnesia and confusion can be more serious than the presence of a fractured skull with no clinical symptoms.

oriented to person, time, and place (according to developmental capabilities). The nurse asks, "What is your name?" and "Where are you?" Older children may know the day of the week. The child should recognize parents. The nurse points to the mother and asks, "Who is this?" The child should be able to follow simple commands, such as "Turn over."

When the child does not respond to verbal stimuli, the upper arm is gently pinched and the response observed. The presence or absence of crying or speech are noted. It is not unusual for children to fall asleep, but they should be easily aroused. The nurse records changes in sleeping posture, movements of extremities, and any signs of tremors or restlessness. The bladder is observed for distention, which can contribute to irritability. Incontinence in the child who is toilet-trained is significant. The child's behavior is described in the nurse's notes. The Glasgow Coma Scale is valuable in determining various levels of consciousness. Table 23–7 shows a scale modified for infants.

Vital Signs. An increase in blood pressure and a decrease in pulse and respiration are evidence of ICP. Temperature elevations may be due to inflammation, systemic infection, or damage to the hypothalamus, which regulates body temperature. Mild elevations due to trauma are not uncommon during the first 2 days following a head injury.

Motor Activity. Because nerves energize the muscle tissue, any damage to the nervous system affects body movement. The quality and strength of muscle tone are observed in all four extremities. The child should be able to move the legs and push against the nurse's hands with both feet. The face should be symmetrical. The child can smile and frown. Drooping of the eyes *(ptosis),* inability to close the eyes tightly, and drooping of the corner of the mouth are considered pathological. The child

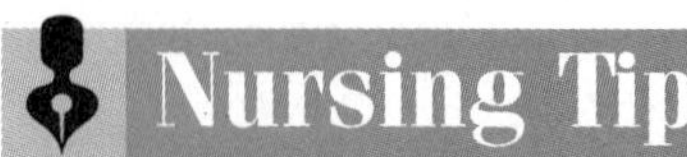

The presence of asymmetrical pupils following a head injury is a medical emergency.

Table 23–6
NEUROLOGIC ASSESSMENTS IN INFANTS AND CHILDREN

Many subtle clues to a change in neurologic status in infants and children can be missed unless the nurse aggressively assesses the child. The lack of the child's ability to communicate and cooperate poses a challenge in the neurological assessment of infants, but a knowledge of normal growth and development will aid the nurse in evaluating the status of his or her little client. For example, we know that by 6 months of age, an infant should turn his head toward the spoken word. However, assessing after a full feeding may cause a delayed response that may not be pathological.

Pain stimuli

There are two types of pain stimuli. *Central,* a response of the brain, and *peripheral,* a response of the spinal cord. Pain stimulus should continue for 30 s to assess optimal function response

Central pain stimulus

1. *Trapezius muscle.* Firmly pinch large muscle mass at the angle where the neck and shoulder meet
2. *Suborbital pressure.* Exert firm pressure on the "notch" that can be located under the center of the eyebrow

Level of consciousness

In children and adolescents we can asess the difference between arousal, awareness, orientation and memory. In infants, the Glasgow Coma Scale is used (see Table 23–7).

Arousal awareness

Child responds to his name, which is indicative basic cerebral function

Child can interact with environment indicating cerebral cortex functioning

A. *Orientation.* Assess awareness of person, place, or time. Use open-ended or multiple-choice question rather than a question that can be answered by yes or no
B. *Attention span.* Although attention span can differ with the age of child, the child would not normally fall off to sleep in the middle of response requiring rearousal stimuli. This should be recorded if it occurs
C. *Language.* Understanding the level of language development is essential in determining if language pattern is normal or abnormal. Speaking clearly and recognizing familiar objects is a skill that is age related in the pediatric setting
D. *Irritability, lethargy, and vomiting.* These are clinical symptoms of increased intracranial pressure in infants, in addition to signs such as a bulging fontanel
E. *Memory.* A child's ability to recognize family members or repeat what he had for breakfast is a valid assessment of memory

Cranial nerve assessment

Cranial nerve assessment is valuable in determining priority of need related to survival and safety

See Figure 23–8 and Table 23–1 (pp. 595–596)

A. *Cranial nerves 9 and 10* (glossopharyngeal and vagus). Control cough and gag reflex. Children under 6 years of age cannot voluntarily cough. Tongue blade stimulation of uvula should result in retching and gagging. Impaired responses can indicate need for nursing interventions to prevent aspiration
B. *Cranial nerves V and VII* (trigeminal and facial). Affect motor sensory responses in the face. Impaired functioning may require nursing interventions to protect the eye since the blink reflex will be lost
C. *Cranial nerves II and III* (optic and oculomotor). May alter pupillary response to light and will alter value of pupillary assessment
D. *Cranial nerve VIII* (acoustic). Alters hearing if injured
E. *Cranial nerve XII* (hypoglossal). Can be tested by asking child to stick out tongue. Loss of function will impair child's ability to suck
F. *Cranial nerve VI* (abducens) is most susceptible to increased intracranial pressure because of its long course. Inability to move eyes side to side and up or down would be an indication of impairment

Table continued on following page

Table 23–6
NEUROLOGIC ASSESSMENTS IN INFANTS AND CHILDREN *(Continued)*

Motor response
Symmetrical spontaneous body movements are an important observation to record. Asking child to follow a simple motor request is more accurate than a hand grasp, as in some age groups a hand grasp is a *reflex* rather than a *voluntary response.* A purposeful voluntary motor response is a more valuable assessment than a reflex response to remove irritants such as an attempt to pull out a nasogastric tube.

Posturing (see Fig. 23–14)
In children and adolescents, posturing can indicate a change in neurological status requiring immediate notification of the doctor
Decorticate. Flexion of arms to center to body and flexing of wrists indicate partial brain function (indicates injury to the cerebral cortex of the brain)
Decerebrate. Arms are extended along the side of the body and hands are pronated. This indicates brain stem function only (Fig. 23–14)
Opisthotonos position. Hyperextension of the neck and arching of the spine is a position assumed by infants with cerebral pathology (Fig. 23–9)

Eyes (see Fig. 23–15)
Pupils of the eyes should be observed for size, equality, and response to light. It may be best to evaluate the eye in a slightly darkened room so the pupils may be somewhat dilated and the response to sudden light from a flashlight can be readily assessed
Pupils that remain *pinpoint* can indicate damage to the pons or part of the brain stem or can indicate drug toxicity
Bilateral dilated pupils can be indicative of hypoxia or intoxication with atropinelike drugs
Pupils that are *unequal* in size can signal brain herniation; *immediate action is required*
Pupillary response to light can be brisk, sluggish, or absent. Recording should indicate size of pupil in normal light (e.g., 3), size of pupil after flashlight intervention (e.g., 1), and how fast the change occurred (B, brisk; S, sluggish/slow; A, absent). A normal recording for pupillary response would be: R 3/1 B; L 3/1 B. Keep in mind that infants and children who are blind will not have a meaningful light response test. When the pupil constricts in response to light be sure that constriction is maintained and that the eye does not redilate before light is removed.

Fontanel
A bulging anterior fontanel is indicative of increased intracranial pressure

Scalp vein distention
Scalp veins distend because of the obstruction of flow from the bridging veins of scalp to sagittal sinus

Ataxia; spasticity of lower extremities
Occur with damage to corticospinal pathways

Moro/tonic neck withdrawal reflexes
In infants absence of these reflexes can occur with increased intracranial pressure

Table 23–7
THE GLASGOW COMA SCALE MODIFIED FOR INFANTS

Age in Months	Response
1	1. None
	2. Crying to stimuli
	3. Crying spontaneously
	4. Blinks when eyelashes are touched
	5. Throaty noises
2	1. None
	2. Crying to stimuli
	3. Shuts eyes to light
	4. Smiles when caressed
	5. Babbles—single vowel sounds
3	1. None
	2. Crying to stimuli (moans)
	3. Stares to response and looks at environment
	4. Smiles to sound stimulation
	5. Coos, chuckles, *vowels* in a prolonged way
4	1. None
	2. Crying to stimuli (moans)
	3. Turns head to sound
	4. Smiles spontaneously or when stimulated, laughs when socially stimulated
	5. Modulating voice and perfect vocalization of vowels
5 and 6	1. None
	2. Crying to stimuli (moans)
	3. Localizes general direction of sound
	4. Discriminates family members
	5. Babbles to people, toys
7 and 8	1. None
	2. Crying to stimuli (moans)
	3. Recognizes familiar voices and family
	4. Babbles
	5. "Ba," "Ma," "Da"
9 and 10	1. None
	2. Crying to stimuli (moans)
	3. Recognizes (smiles or laughs)
	4. Babbles
	5. "Mama," "Dada"
11 and 12	1. None
	2. Crying to stimuli (moans)
	3. Recognizes—smiles
	4. Babbles
	5. Words (specifically "Mama" and "Dada")

From Zimmerman, S. S., & Gildea, J. H. (1985). *Critical care pediatrics.* Philadelphia: Saunders.

should be able to raise the arms and extend the palms upward and downward. Abnormal posturing is described and recorded.

Other Nursing Observations. Other factors include examination of wound swelling if a laceration of the head is present. The type and amount of drainage from the ears and nose are recorded. The nurse checks for *nuchal* (neck) rigidity, which might indicate infection. Occipital-frontal circumference of the head is monitored in infants, as are tension of the fontanels and presence of a high-pitched cry. Fluids are carefully monitored to control *cerebral edema.* Feeding difficulties should be noted as the child's diet is increased. The child is observed for signs of shock, which can also occur. Children whose condition has remained stable are discharged. Parents are instructed about any additional observations and follow-up care.

Near Drowning

Accidental drowning or near-drowning is the 4th leading cause of death for U.S. children under 19 years of age. Near drowning is defined as survival beyond 24 hours after submersion. Proper supervision and environmental safety precautions are the best measures to prevent drowning. In adolescents, the use of illicit drugs and alcohol during recreational swimming contributes to drowning incidents. The priorities include the immediate treatment of *hypoxia, aspiration,* and *hypothermia.*

With advances in emergency medical treatment by paramedics on site and the technology available in intensive care units in the hospital, cardiorespiratory survival has increased, but central nervous system injury remains the major cause of death or long-term disability.

Submersion of more than 10 minutes with failure to regain consciousness at the scene or within 24 hours is an ominous sign and indicates severe neurological deficits if the child survives. Respiratory and cardiovascular support, rewarming, and maintenance of adequate cerebral oxygenation are priorities of care. The parents need to be offered support, explanations of the therapy, and referral to social services, religious, or community agencies for follow-up.

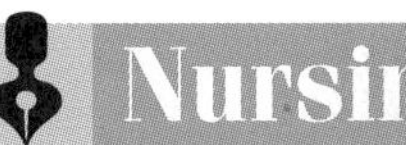

Nursing Tip

All children who experience near drowning should be admitted for a 24-hour observation period of close monitoring.

KEY POINTS

- Infants are more prone to ear infections than are older children because their eustachian tube is shorter, wider, and straighter.
- When instilling ear drops in infants, gently pull the pinna *down* and back. In children, the pinna is gently pulled *up* and back.
- In paralytic strabismus, the *unaffected* eye is patched.
- Level of consciousness is the most important indicator of neurologic health.
- Nursing care of the unconscious child includes assessing the child for increased intracranial pressure, maintaining an open airway, providing adequate nutrition and fluids, positioning, maintaining flexibility of joints, and preventing injury.
- Do not give aspirin or other salicylates to children with symptoms of influenza or chickenpox because the drug is linked to Reye's syndrome, a serious and life-threatening illness.
- Meningitis is an inflammation of the meninges that cover the brain and spinal cord.
- A high-pitched cry may be indicative of increased intracranial pressure (ICP).
- A seizure is a symptom of underlying pathology.
- Grand mal seizures have an aura, tonic and clonic phases, and post-ictal lethargy.
- Decerebrate, decorticate, or opisthotonos posturing indicates brain damage.
- The response of the pupils to light and level of consciousness are essential assessments to determine brain injury.
- The Glasgow Coma Scale is used to determine level of consciousness.
- The "shaken baby syndrome" can result in subdural hematoma and death.
- Confusion and amnesia after a head injury may indicate concussion even if consciousness is not lost.
- The four types of cerebral palsy are spastic, athetoid, ataxic, and mixed.
- Mental retardation involves three components: intelligence, adaptive behavior, and onset before 18 years of age.
- The priority of care for a child who has experienced near drowning is to prevent hypoxia, aspiration, and hypothermia.

MULTIPLE-CHOICE REVIEW QUESTIONS

Choose the most appropriate answer.

1. Symptoms of an earache in an infant include
   a. external drainage, pain, decrease in temperature.
   b. tugging at the ear, rolling head from side to side.
   c. crying, pointing to affected ear.
   d. redness of the cheeks, cyanosis of ear.
2. The medical term for crossed eyes is
   a. strabismus.
   b. amblyopia.
   c. myopia.
   d. PERRLA.
3. Reye's syndrome affects the
   a. stomach and intestine.
   b. islet of Langerhans.
   c. liver and brain.
   d. heart and blood vessels.
4. Mental retardation can be prevented by
   a. administering the Stanford-Binet test.
   b. a blood test at birth.
   c. careful preschool developmental screening.
   d. A urine test at 6 months of age.
5. The seizure in which the child cries out, falls to the floor, becomes rigid, and then has a convulsion is termed
   a. petit mal.
   b. Jacksonian.
   c. grand mal.
   d. atonic.

BIBLIOGRAPHY AND READER REFERENCE

Agency of Health Care Planning and Research (AHCPR). *Federal guidelines for treatment of OME in young children.* Publication #94-0620, 94-0623, and 94-0624, AHCPR Publication Clearing House. Silver Springs, MD: Author.

Alexander, K. (Ed.). (1995). *Lippincott manual of primary eye care.* Philadelphia: Lippincott.

Bacal, D., & Hertle, R. (1998). Don't be lazy about looking for amblyopia. *Contemporary Pediatrics, 15*(6), 99.

Behrman, R. E., Kleigman, R., & Arvin, A. (1996). *Nelson's textbook of pediatrics* (15th ed.). Philadelphia: Saunders.

Brown, T. P. (1994). Middle ear symptoms while flying: Ways to prevent severe outcome. *Postgraduate Medicine, 96,* 135.

Committee on Disabilities of the Group for Advancement of Psychiatry. (1997). Issues to consider in deaf and hard of hearing patients. *American Family Physician, 56*(8), 2057.

Cullen, P. M. (1995). Pharmacological supportive care of children with CNS tumors. *Journal of Pediatric Oncology Nursing, 12*(4), 230.

Dichter, M., & Brodie, M. (1996). New antiepileptic drugs. *New England Journal of Medicine, 334*(24), 1583.

Dodge, P. R. (1994). Neurological sequelae of acute bacterial meningitis. *Pediatric Annals, 23*(2), 101–106.

Epilepsy Foundation of America. (1989). *Seizure recognition and first aid.* Landover, MD: Author.

Farwell, J. R., et al. (1994). First febrile seizures characteristic of childhood seizure and illness. *Clinical Pediatrics, 33*(5), 2631.

Ferrie, C. D., et al. (1994). Video game epilepsy. *Lancet, 344*(8938), 1710.

Gregory, S., Sheldon, L. & Bishop J., (Ed.). (1995). *Deaf young people and their families: Developing an understanding.* Cambridge, MA: Harvard University Press.

Hamel, S., & Feldman, H. (1998). Focus on families caring for children with special needs. *Contemporary Pediatrics, 15*(4), 141.

Hilton, G. (1997). Seizure disorders in adults: Evaluation and management of new onset seizures. *The Nurse Practitioner, 22*(9), 42.

Kirkowski-Ziemba, S. (1995). Seizures. *American Journal of Nursing, 95*(2), 32.

MacDonald, D. (1998). Meeting special learning needs. *RN 61*(4), 33.

Mahan, L. K., & Escott-Stump, S. (1996). *Krause's food, nutrition & diet therapy* (9th ed.). Philadelphia: Saunders.

McNew, C., Hunt, S., & Warner, L. (1997). Helping your patient with epilepsy. *Nursing, 27*(9), 56.

Moore, J. M. (1995). CNS toxicity of cancer therapy in children. *Journal of Pediatric Oncology Nursing, 12*(4), 203.

Parell, G. S., & Becker, G. D. (1993). Inner ear barotrauma in scuba divers. *Archives of Otology, 119,* 455.

Prober, C. G. (1995). Commentary: The role of steroids in managing bacterial meningitis. *Pediatrics, 95,* 29.

Rhodes, W. M. (1997). Reye's syndrome, an update. *The Nurse Practitioner, 23*(12), 45–53.

Schein, J., & Stewart, D. (1995). *Language in motion: Exploring the nature of sign.* Washington, DC: Gallaudet University Press.

Shinnar, S., Amir, N., & Branski, D. (Ed.). (1995). *Childhood seizures.* New York: Krager.

Sy, W., & Shinnar, S. (1996). Managing adolescent seizure disorders. *Contemporary Pediatrics, 13*(10), 25–46.

Tennison, M. (1996). Discontinuing antiepileptics: When and how. *Contemporary Pediatrics, 13*(8), 49–60.

Thomas, R., & Taylor, K. (1997). *Journal of Maternal Child Nursing,* Assessing head injuries in children. *MCN 22*(4), 198–203.

Tully, S. B., Bar-Haim, Y., & Bradley, R. (1995). Abnormal tympanography after supine bottle feeding. *Journal of Pediatrics, 126,* 5105–5108.

Wilson, S., & Shinnar, S. (1996). Managing adolescent seizures. *Contemporary Pediatrics, 13*(10), 25.

Wolf, E. M. (1997). Communication with deaf surgical patients. *AORNJ, 26,* 39–47.

Wong, D. (1997). *Whaley & Wong's essentials of nursing care of children* (5th ed.). St. Louis, MO: Mosby.

Zamarchi, E., & Donati, M., et al. (1995). Fructose-1, 6-diphosphatase deficiency misdiagnosed as Reye's Syndrome. *Clinical Pediatrics, 34*(10), 561–564.

Zazove, P. (1997). Understanding deaf and hard of hearing patients. *American Family Physician, 56*(8), 1953.

chapter 24

The Child with a Musculoskeletal Condition

Outline

Objectives

On completion and mastery of Chapter 24, the student will be able to

- Define each vocabulary term listed.
- Demonstrate an understanding of age-specific changes that occur in the musculoskeletal system during growth and development.
- Discuss the types of fractures commonly seen in children and their effect on growth and development.
- List two symptoms of Duchenne's muscular dystrophy.
- Describe three types of child abuse.
- Identify symptoms of abuse and neglect in children.
- Differentiate between Buck extension and Russell traction.
- Describe two topics of discussion applicable at discharge for the child with juvenile rheumatoid arthritis.
- Describe the symptoms, treatment, and nursing care for the child with Legg–Calvé–Perthes disease.
- Compile a nursing care plan for the child who is immobilized by traction.
- Describe a neurovascular check.
- Describe the management of soft-tissue injuries.
- State two cultural or medical practices that may be misinterpreted as child abuse.
- Describe three nursing care measures required to maintain skin integrity in an adolescent child casted for scoliosis. Provide the rationale for each measure.

Vocabulary

arthroscopy
Bryant traction
Buck extension
compartment syndrome
compound fracture
contusion
Crutchfield tongs
epiphysis
gait
genu valgum
genu varum
greenstick fracture
hematoma
Milwaukee brace
neurovascular checks
retrograde amnesia
Russell traction
shin splint
spiral fracture
sprain

OVERVIEW

The musculoskeletal system supports the body and provides for movement. The muscular and skeletal systems work together to enable a person to sit, stand, walk, and remain upright. In addition, muscles move air into and out of the lungs, blood through vessels, and food through the digestive tract. They also produce heat, which aids in numerous body chemical reactions. Bones act as levers and provide support. Red blood cells are produced in the bone marrow, and minerals such as calcium and phosphorus are also stored there. Figure 24–1 describes some differences between the child's and adult's skeletal and muscular systems.

The musculoskeletal system arises from the mesoderm in the embryo. A great portion of skeletal growth occurs between the 4th and 8th weeks of fetal life. As the limbs elongate prior to birth, muscle masses form in the extremities. The Dubowitz scoring system (see Chapter 13, p. 331) is one measure of assessing neuromuscular maturity at birth. Testing various reflexes is another. Locomotion develops gradually and in an orderly manner in the growing child. A marked slowing down of growth is always a signal for investigation.

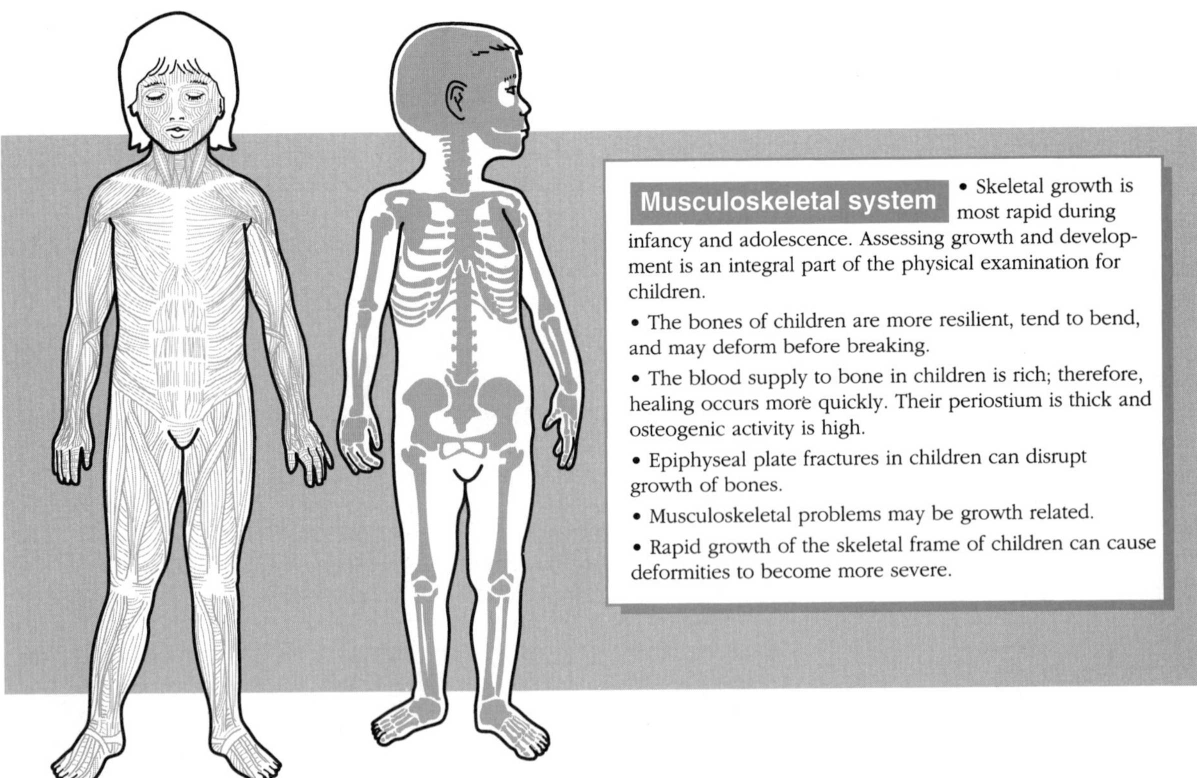

Figure 24–1. • Some musculoskeletal system differences between the child and the adult. The muscular system consists of the large skeletal muscles that enable us to move, as well as the cardiac muscle of the heart and the smooth muscle of the internal organs. The skeletal system consists of bones and cartilage. This system helps to support and protect the body.

ASSESSMENT OF THE MUSCULOSKELETAL SYSTEM IN THE GROWING CHILD

To assess the musculoskeletal system of the growing child and to identify deviations, the nurse must have a basic understanding of the effect of growth, neurologic development, and motor milestones at various ages. The newborn hip has limited internal rotation range of motion (ROM). The legs are maintained in a flexed position, and the lower leg has an internal rotation (internal tibial torsion) due to the effects of uterine positioning, which can last 4 to 6 months. The general curvature of the newborn spine is in a C shape from the thoracic to the pelvic level and changes with the mastery of motor skills to a double S curve in childhood. The newborn's feet normally turn inward *(varus)* or outward *(valgus),* but the turning-in self-corrects when the sole of the foot is stroked. The toddler's feet appear flat because of the presence of a fat pad at the arch. Any delay in neurologic development can cause a delay in the mastery of motor skills, which can result in altered skeletal growth.

Assessment of the musculoskeletal system includes observation, palpation, range of motion and gait assessment in children who can walk. Children who do not walk independently by 18 months of age have a serious delay and should be referred to a physician.

Assessment of Gait. The toddler who begins to walk has a wide, unstable *gait.* Arms do not swing with the walking motion. By 18 months, the wide base narrows and the walk is more stable. By 4 years of age, the child can hop on one foot and arm swings occur with walking. By age 6, the gait resembles the mature walk with equal stride lengths and associated arm swing. The trunk is centered over the legs and movement is symmetrical. When a child favors one side, pain may be present. Toe walking after 3 years of age can indicate a muscle problem.

In most cases, excessive in-toeing or pointing of the toe inward will clear by 4 years of age. These children trip and fall easily. Teaching proper sitting and body mechanics is the treatment of choice. Participation in ballet classes and ice skating will enhance hip flexibility. If the problem does not resolve, a brace may be prescribed. Failure to treat can result in hip, knee, or back problems in adulthood.

Young children appear "bow-legged" *(genu varum)* or knock-knee *(genu valgum)* with the knees turned inward until 5 years of age. Bowing is seldom pathologic. The ligaments that support the arch are not mature before 6 years of age, and so the child may appear to have flat feet. If the condition interferes with walking, an orthotic appliance can be prescribed for the child to wear inside the shoes. When the flat foot is painful, a referral for follow-up examination should be initiated. The role of the nurse is to reassure parents that unless there is associated pain or a problem with motor or nerve functions, many minor abnormal-appearing alignments will spontaneously resolve with activity.

Assessment of Muscle Tone. The nurse should assess symmetry of movement and the strength and contour of the body and extremities. The strength of the extremities can be tested by having the child push away the examiner's hand with his or her foot or hand.

Neurologic Examination. A neurologic assessment is a vital part of a comprehensive musculoskeletal examination. An assessment of reflexes, a sensory assessment, and the presence or absence of spasms should be noted.

X-Rays and Laboratory Tests

X-Rays. Routine radiographies are usually taken and the affected area is compared with the unaffected area.

Bone Scans. Are helpful in identifying pathology that may not clearly be seen on a routine x-ray, such as septic arthritis or tumors.

Computed Tomography (CT). Provides a cross-sectional picture of the bone and its relationship to other structures within the area of examination.

Magnetic Resonance Imaging (MRI). Does not involve harmful radiation; produces detailed pictures of the brain, spinal cord, and soft-tissue lesions, including a slipped femoral epiphysis.

Ultrasound. Does not involve harmful radiation or after effects. It is used to rule out foreign bodies in soft tissues, joint effusions, and developmental dysplasia of the hip.

Laboratory Studies. A complete blood count (CBC) and erythrocyte sedimentation rate (ESR) may rule out septic arthritis or osteomyelitis. Human leukocyte antigen (HLA) B-27 may help diagnose rheumatologic disorders.

A thorough history is necessary to determine the basis for musculoskeletal problems, which are often insidious in nature. The nurse determines the history of injury; location of pain; when symptoms started; any weakness, numbness, or loss of function in an extremity; and whether the problem is affecting the daily activities of the child. *Arthroscopies* are commonly done on adolescents with sports injuries. The physician is able to look inside the joint (usually the knee) to determine the extent of injury. The area is inspected, foreign particles removed, or repairs made to the torn menisci. A bone biopsy may reveal a malignancy. Muscle biopsy may detect muscular dystrophy.

Traction, casting, and splints are used in accordance with the patient's needs. Three types of skin traction are frequently used for the lower extremities of children. These are *Bryant traction, Buck extension,* and *Russell traction.* Children with musculoskeletal disorders may require lengthy hospitalization. Immobility causes a slowing down of body metabolism. Nursing interventions focus on maintaining body functions. Range-of-motion exercises and the use of a trapeze prevent muscle atrophy. Foods high in roughage stimulate the digestive tract and prevent constipation. Respiratory exercises prevent pneumonia. These and other measures can prevent complications that can lengthen hospitalization for the child. (Clubfoot and congenital hip dysplasia are discussed on pp. 356–357. Rickets is discussed in Chapter 27. General information on cast care is also found Chapter 14.)

Prevention of Pediatric Trauma

Accidents are common in childhood, but much can be done to prevent morbidity and mortality. Parents are responsible for maintaining a safe environment for their children. Nurses are responsible for educating parents and school teachers on how to prevent accidental injury and maintain a safe environment.

The proper use of pedestrian safety, car seat restraints, bicycle helmets, and other athletic protective gear, pool fences, window bars, deadbolt locks, and locks on cabinets can prevent unnecessary injury to children. Pediatric trauma can cause permanent disability or premature death. Nursing assessment and interventions can assist the injured child toward recovery. The nurse also has a community responsibility to support legislation that would maintain safe environments for children.

Differences between the Child and Adult. The pediatric skeletal system differs from the adult in that bone is not completely ossified, epiphysis are present, and the periosteum is thicker and produces callus more rapidly than the adult. The lower mineral content of the child's bone and greater porosity increases the strength of the bone. However, rotational or angular forces can stress ligaments that insert at the epiphyseal area of the bone and injury to the epiphysis can affect bone growth. Because of the presence of the epiphysis and hyperemia caused by the trauma, bone overgrowth is common in healing fractures of children under 10 years of age.

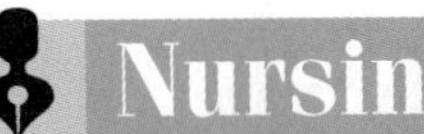

Nursing Tip

Principles of managing soft-tissue injuries:

- **R.** Rest
- **I.** Ice
- **C.** Compression
- **E.** Elevation

Pediatric Trauma

Soft-tissue injury usually accompanies traumatic fractures in the child at play or the adolescent involved in sports activities and include:

- *Contusions.* A tearing of subcutaneous tissue that results in hemorrhage, edema, and pain. Escape of blood into the soft tissue is referred to as a *hematoma,* or "black and blue mark."
- *Sprain.* When the ligament is torn or stretched away from the bone at the point of trauma, there may be resulting damage to the blood vessels, muscles, and nerves. Swelling, disability, and pain are major signs of a sprain.
- *Strain.* A microscopic tear to the muscle or tendon occurs over time and results in edema and pain.

Treatment of Soft-Tissue Injuries. Soft-tissue injuries should be treated immediately to limit damage from edema and bleeding. A cold pack and elastic wrap will reduce edema, bleeding, relieve pain, and should be applied at *alternating 30-minute intervals.* (After a 30-minute period ischemia can occur and that will impede the tissue perfusion.) Elevating the extremity above heart level reduces edema. When an elastic bandage is used for compression, a priority nursing responsibility is to perform neurovascular checks to ensure adequate tissue perfusion.

TRAUMATIC FRACTURES AND TRACTION

Definitions. A fracture is a break in a bone and is mainly caused by accidents. It is characterized by pain, tenderness on movement, and swelling. Discoloration, limited movement, and numbness may also occur. In a *simple fracture,* the bone is broken, but the skin over the area is not. In a *compound fracture,* a wound in the skin leads to the broken bone, and there is an added danger of infection. A *greenstick fracture* is an incomplete fracture in which one side of the bone is broken and the other is bent.

This type of fracture is common in children because their bones are soft, flexible, and more likely to splinter. In a complete fracture, the bone is entirely broken across its width. Figure 24–2 illustrates various types of fractures. When an x-ray reveals multiple fractures in various stages of healing, child abuse should be suspected.

Healing of a fracture in a child is more rapid than it is in an adult. The child's periosteum is stronger and thicker, and there is less stiffness on mobilization. Injury to the cartilaginous epiphyseal plate, found at the ends of long bones, is serious if it happens during childhood because it may interfere with longitudinal growth. Care of a patient in a cast is discussed on page 356. Casts may be made of plaster or fiberglass.

Fractures of the Femur in Early Childhood. The femur, the thigh bone, is the largest and strongest bone of the body. It is one of the most prevalent serious breaks that occur during early childhood. A *spiral fracture* of the femur is caused by a forceful twisting motion. When the history of an injury does not correlate with x-ray findings, child abuse should be suspected as spiral fractures can be the result of manual twisting of the extremity. The child complains of pain and tenderness when the leg is

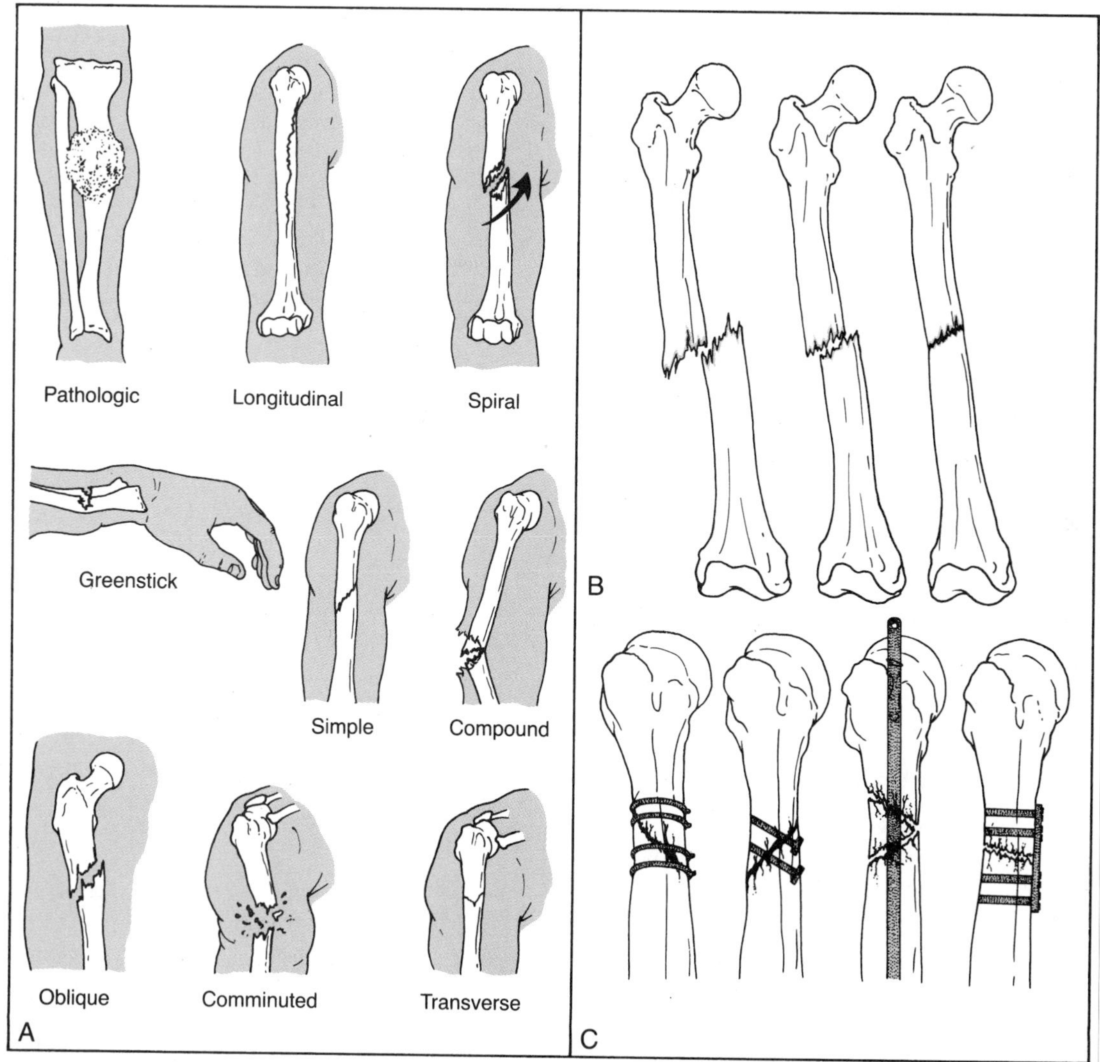

Figure 24–2. • **A,** Types of fractures. **B,** Reduction of a fractured bone. A gradual pull is exerted on the distal (lower) fragment of the bone until it is in alignment with the proximal fragment. **C,** Various methods of internal fixations, using plates, pins, nails, and screws to hold fragments of bone in place. (Redrawn from deWit, S. C. [1992]. *Keane's essentials of medical–surgical nursing* [3rd ed.]. Philadelphia: Saunders.)

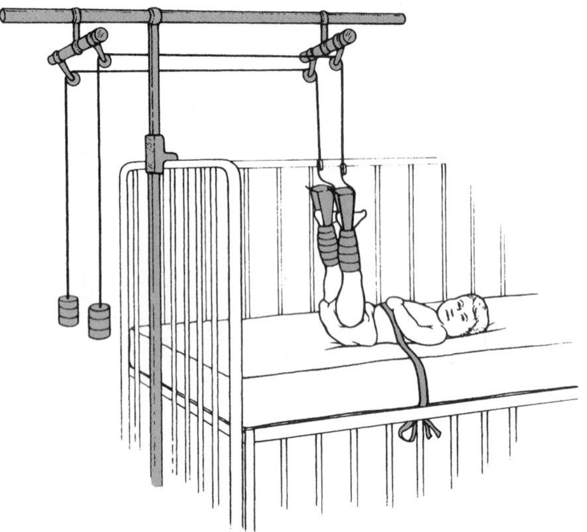

Figure 24–3. • Bryant traction is used for the young child who has a fractured femur.

moved and cannot bear weight on it. Clothes are gently removed, starting at the uninjured side and proceeding to the injured side. It may be necessary to cut the clothes. X-ray films confirm the diagnosis. Skin traction is used to reduce the fracture and keep the bones in proper alignment.

Bryant traction is used for treating fractures of the femur in children under 2 years or under 20 to 30 pounds. Weights and pulleys extend the limb as in the Buck extension; however, the legs are suspended vertically (Fig. 24–3). The weight of the child supplies the countertraction.

Nursing Assessment and Responsibilities. The nurse observes the traction ropes to be sure that they are intact, in the wheel grooves of the pulleys, and that the child's body is in good position. The legs should be at right angles to the body, and the buttocks raised sufficiently to clear the bed. Elastic bandages should be neither too loose nor too tight. A jacket restraint may be used to keep the child from turning from side to side. The weights are not removed once applied. *Continuous traction is necessary.* The weights must hang free, and the pull of the weights must not be obstructed by room furnishings, such as a chair. The weights are *not* lifted or supported when the bed is moved. The nurse performs a neurovascular check to the toes (see page 625) to see that they are warm and that their color is good (Fig. 24–4). Cyanosis, numbness, or irritation from attachments, tight bandages, severe pain, or absence of pulse in the extremities are reported immediately to the nurse in charge. A specific and serious complication of any traction is *Volkmann's ischemia* (*ischein,* "to hold back," and *haima,* "blood"), which occurs when the circulation is obstructed. Because the legs are elevated overhead, there is gravitational vascular drainage. Arterial occlusion can cause anoxia of the muscles and reflex vasospasm, which when unnoticed could result in contractures and paralysis.

The child is bathed and back and buttock care is given. A sheepskin padding may also be utilized. The sheets are pulled taut and are kept free of crumbs. The jacket restraint is changed when it is soiled. The child is encouraged to drink lots of fluids and to eat foods that are high in roughage to prevent constipation due to lack of exercise. Stool softeners may be necessary. A fracture pan is used for bowel movements, and a careful record is kept of eliminations. Deep-breathing exercises are encouraged to prevent collection of fluids in the lungs due to the child's immobility. These exercises may be done by blowing bubbles or blowing a pinwheel.

Diversional therapy is important, as hospitalization may be lengthy. Toys may be securely suspended over the child's head so that they are within easy reach. The child's crib is taken to the playroom when possible so that the child may experience the excitement of the activities there.

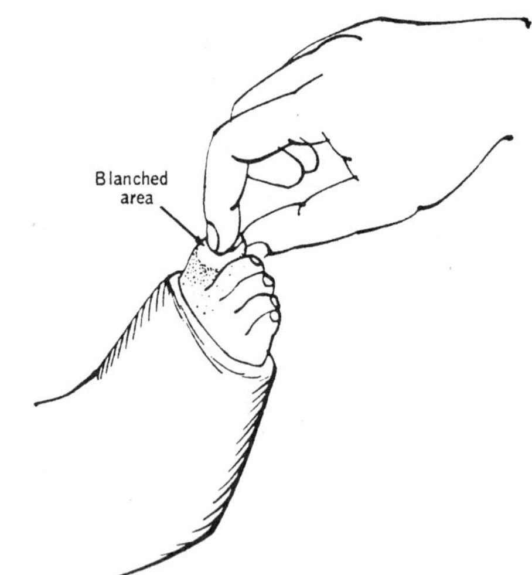

Figure 24–4. • Checking circulation to the toes or fingers. To check circulation (capillary refill), squeeze or press a toe or finger to blanch the skin. When the pressure is released the color should return quickly if the circulation is adequate. 1. If the toes do not blanch, congestion may be present and should be reported to the doctor. 2. If the blanching persists after pressure is released, the circulation is impaired. The doctor must be notified. 3. If extreme pain results from touching or moving the toes, report it to the doctor. (From Leifer, G. [1982]. *Principles and techniques in pediatric nursing.* Philadelphia: Saunders.)

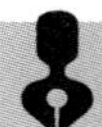

Nursing Tip

Checklist for traction apparatus:

- Weights are hanging freely
- Weights are out of reach of child
- Ropes are on the pulleys
- Knots are not resting against pulleys
- Bed linens are not *on* traction ropes
- Countertraction is in place
- Apparatus does not touch foot of bed

Tapes, CDs, stories, and other forms of entertainment are important aspects of a total nursing care plan. Pain control is essential. Parents are encouraged to visit the child as often as possible. With proper treatment, the prognosis for the child with this condition is good.

Neurovascular Assessment. A priority nursing responsibility in the care of a child with a fracture, who has a cast or ace bandage in place, is to perform neurovascular assessments or *neurovascular checks* at regular intervals. Aspects to check include:

- *Pain.* The location and quality of pain should be assessed and recorded. Pain control strategies and medication should be initiated as soon as possible. Pain at the trauma site that does not respond to medication may indicate a serious complication called *compartment syndrome.* Compartment syndrome is a term used to describe *ischemia* to an extremity due to pressure on the tissues caused by excessive edema. Surgery (fasciotomy) may be needed to reduce the pressure and increase tissue perfusion.
- *Pulse.* The quality of the pulse on the affected extremity should be compared to the unaffected extremity. A strong pulse indicates good blood flow necessary for healing.
- *Sensation.* Reduced sensation to touch (numbness or tingling) at a site distal to the fracture may indicate poor tissue perfusion and should be reported.
- *Color.* Pallor at the site distal to the fracture can indicate arterial insufficiency, whereas cyanosis of the site distal to the fracture can indicate venous stasis. Adequate blood supply and drainage are essential for optimum healing.
- *Capillary refill.* A compressed nailbed should return to its original color in less than 3 seconds. The findings should be compared with the unaffected extremity and the results recorded frequently (Fig. 24–4).
- *Movement.* The toes and fingers distal to the fracture site should be tested for movement. Since nerve injury can occur as a complication of skeletal fractures, the movement associated with specific nerve supply should be tested (Fig. 24–5).

Fractures and Traction in the Older Child. Traction is used when the cast does not maintain alignment of the two bone fragments. Skeletal muscles act as a splint for the fracture. Traction aligns the injured bone by the use of weights and countertraction. Immobilization is maintained until the bones fuse.

Buck skin traction (Buck extension) is a type of skin traction used in fractures of the femur and in hip and knee contractures. It pulls the hip and leg into extension. Countertraction is supplied by the child's body; therefore, it is *essential* that the child not slip down in bed and that the bed not be placed in high Fowler's position. Buck extension is sometimes used preoperatively, either unilaterally or bilaterally, to reduce pain and muscle spasm associated with a slipped capital femoral *epiphysis. Russell traction* is similar to Buck extension. However, in the former a sling is positioned under the knee, which suspends the distal thigh above the bed (Fig. 24–6). Skin traction is applied to the lower extremity. Pull is in two directions, vertically from the knee sling and longitudinally from the footplate (Fig. 24–7). This prevents posterior subluxation of the tibia on the femur, which can occur in children in traction. *Split Russell traction* uses two sets of weights, one suspending the thigh and the other exerting a pull on the leg, with weights at head and foot of the bed. In *skeletal traction,* a Steinmann pin

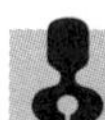

Nursing Tip

Checklist for patient in traction:

- Body in alignment
- Head of bed no higher than 20° (for countertraction)
- Heels of feet elevated from bed
- Range of movement (ROM) of unaffected parts checked at regular intervals
- Antiembolism stockings or foot pumps in place as ordered
- Neurovascular check performed regularly
- Skin integrity monitored regularly
- Pain unrelieved by medication reported
- Measures to prevent constipation
- Use of trapeze for change of position encouraged

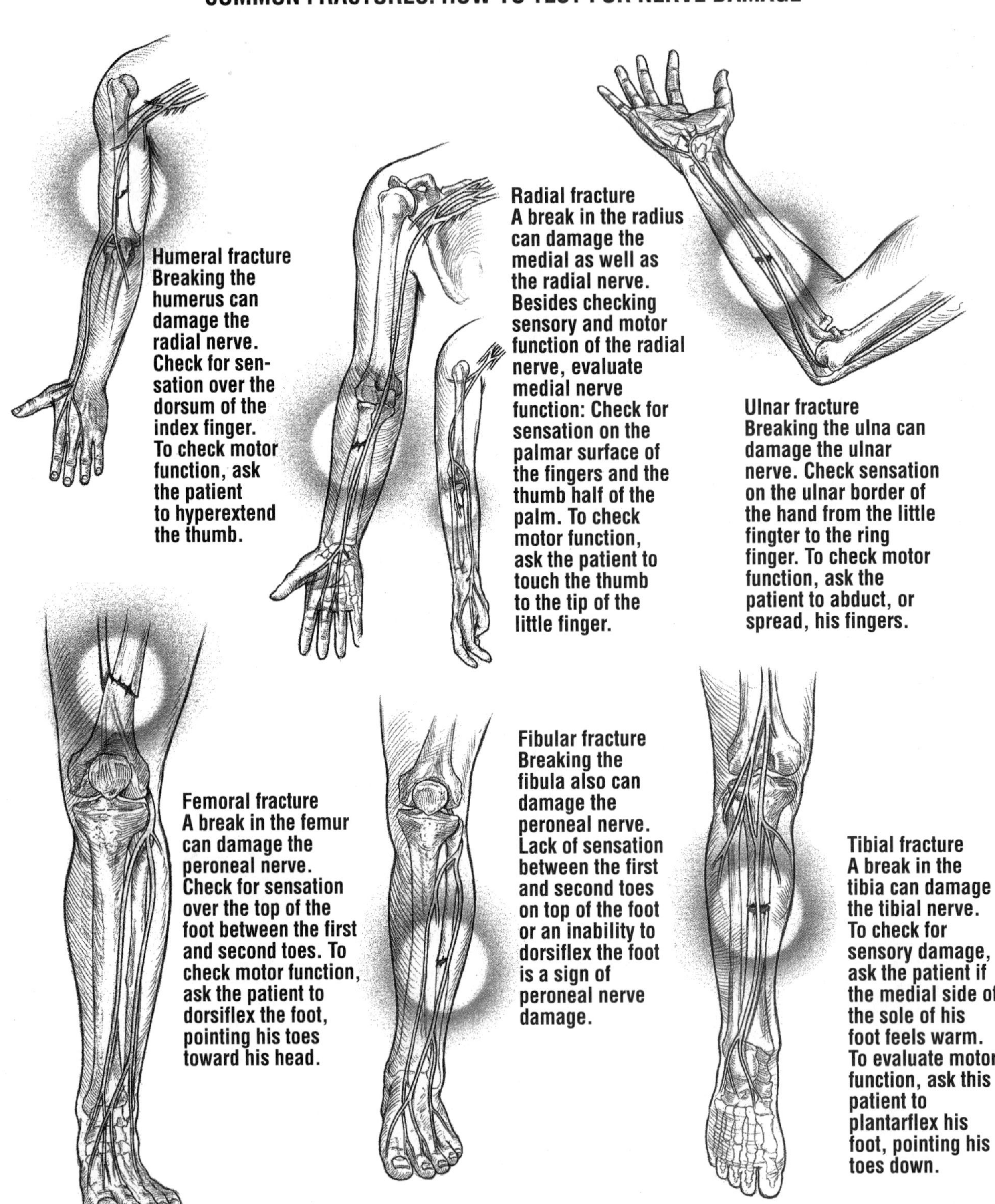

Figure 24–5. • Checking for nerve damage. Nerve damage can result from trauma and the motor sensory status of the extremity should be assessed and recorded. (Courtesy of Bert Oppenheim.)

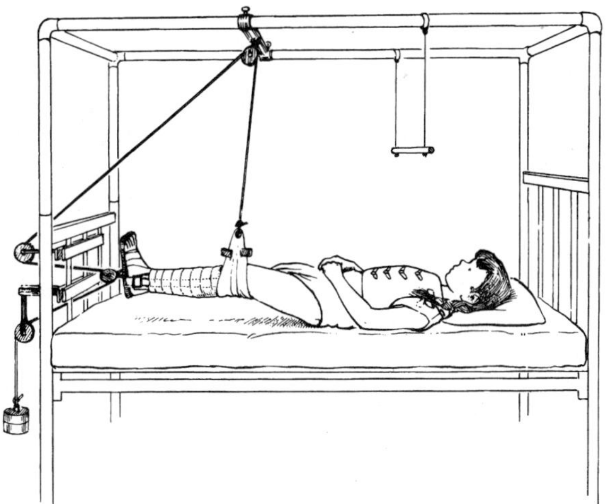

Figure 24–6. • Russell skin traction. (Modified from Tachdjian, M. [1972]. *Pediatric orthopedics.* Philadelphia: Saunders. Reprinted from Betz C., et al. [1994]. *Family-centered nursing care of children* [2nd ed., p. 1827]. Philadelphia: Saunders.)

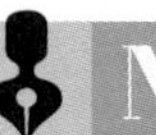

Nursing Tip

The "neurovascular check" for tissue perfusion is performed on the toes or fingers distal to an injury or cast and includes:

- Peripheral pulse
- Color
- Capillary refill time
- Warmth
- Movement and sensation

or Kirschner wire is inserted into the bone, and traction is applied to the pin. Daily care of the pin site is essential. Ninety–ninety traction with a boot cast or sling on the lower leg may be used (Fig. 24–8).

Crutchfield, or *Barton tongs* may be used in the skull to provide cervical traction (Fig. 24–9). Skeletal traction carries the added risk of infection from skin bacteria that may cause osteomyelitis. Balanced suspension, employing the *Thomas splint* and *Pearson attachments* is used to treat diseases of the hip as well as fractures in older children and adolescents. It may be used both before and after surgery. Nursing Care Plan 24–1 describes interventions for the child in traction. The child in traction experiences certain effects as a result of immobilization; these are illustrated in Figure 24–10. Visitors are important to the child in traction and a school tutor should be contacted so that the child will be able to return to class after healing occurs.

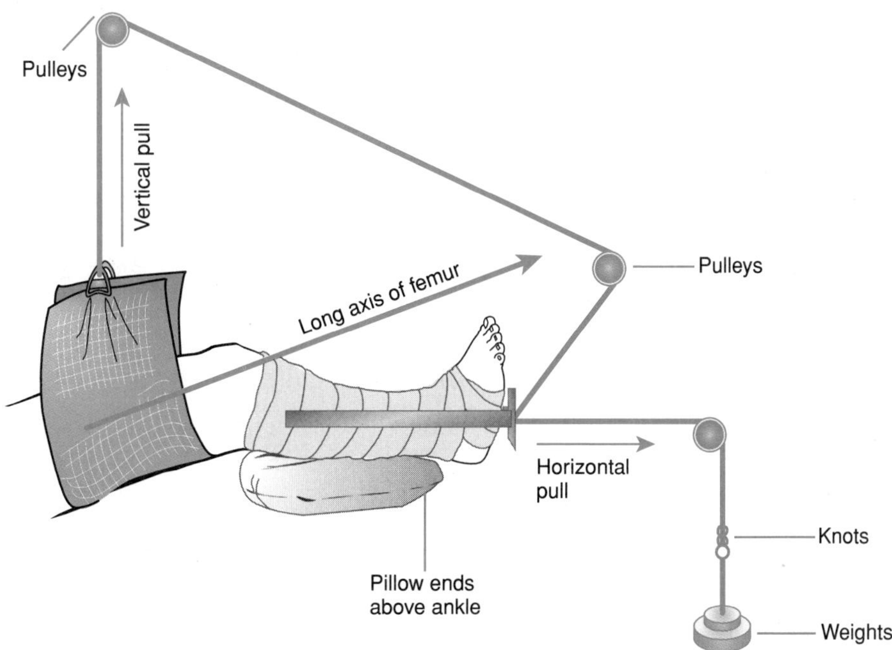

Figure 24–7. • Forces involved in traction. The placement of pulleys and angle of the joints determine the line of pull. In this case, the combined vertical and horizontal pull results in a pull on the long axis of the femur to reduce fracture displacement.

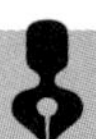

Nursing Tip

Compartment syndrome is a progressive loss of tissue perfusion due to an increase in pressure caused by edema or swelling that presses on the vessels and tissues. Circulation is compromised and the neurovascular check will be abnormal.

OSTEOMYELITIS

Description. *Osteomyelitis* is an infection of the bone that generally occurs in children younger than 1 year and in those between 5 and 14 years of age. It is more common in boys than in girls. *Staphylococcus aureus* is the organism responsible in 75% to 80% of cases in children over 5 years of age, and *Haemophilus Influenzae* is the most common cause in children under 3 years of age. This incidence may be reduced by the widening practice of routine infant immunization against this organism. Other organisms include group-A streptococci, and pneumococci. *Salmonella* and *Pseudomonas* are organisms often involved in adolescents who are intravenous (IV) drug users. Osteomyelitis may be preceded by a local injury to the bone, such as an open fracture, burn, or contamination during surgery. It may also follow a furuncle, impetigo, and abscessed teeth. In neonates a heel puncture or a scalp vein monitor can be the predisposing site of infection. The incidence of osteomyelitis has decreased as a result of antibiotics. Infective emboli may travel to the small arteries of the bone, setting up local destruction and abscess. For this reason, a careful search for infection in other bones and soft tissues is necessary.

Long bones contain few phagocytic cells (WBC) to fight bacteria that may come to the bone from another part of the body. The inflammation produces an exudate that collects under the marrow and cortex of the bone. The vessels in the area are compressed and thrombosis occurs that produces ischemia and resulting sensation of pain. The col-

Figure 24–8. • 90 degree–90 degree skeletal traction. A wire pin is inserted into the distal segment of the femur. The lower leg may be placed in a boot cast or is supported by a sling.

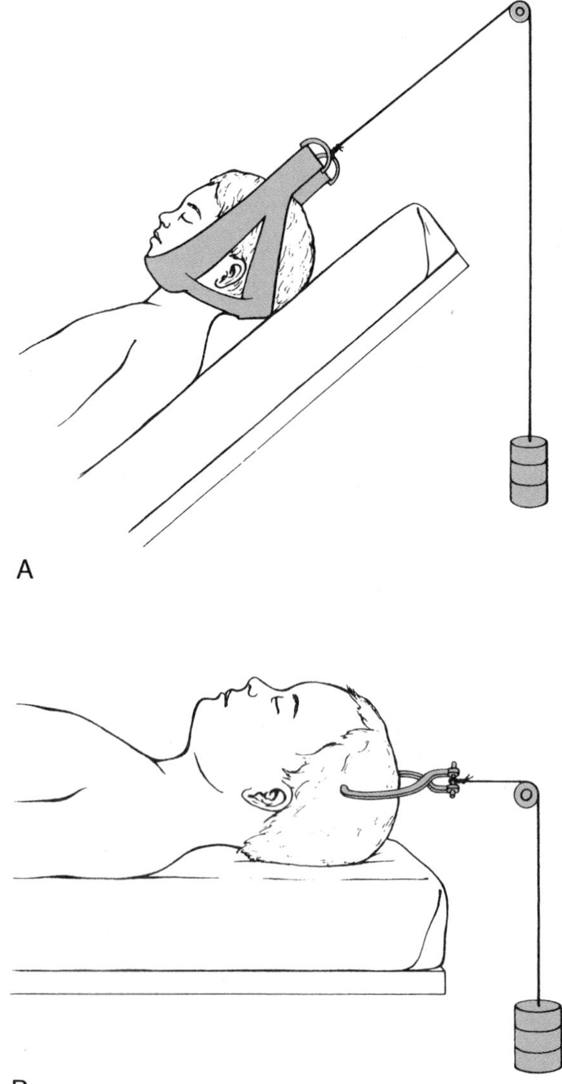

Figure 24–9. • **A,** Cervical traction. **B,** Crutchfield tong traction.

NURSING CARE PLAN 24–1

Selected Nursing Diagnoses for the Child in Traction

Nursing Diagnosis: Impaired physical mobility related to fixation devices

Goals	Nursing Interventions	Rationale
Child demonstrates how to obtain help via call bell Child will not develop complications of immobility as evidenced by intact skin, absence of respiratory and urinary infections Child will have a bowel movement on a regular basis	1. Draw picture of fracture for child and explain traction apparatus	1. An understanding of condition and of the type of traction used reduces anxiety and promotes compliance with treatment protocol
	2. Place call bell within easy reach of child	2. It is frightening to be immobilized; a call bell provides reassurance that help is at hand
	3. Change position as traction allows every 2 hours	3. Position changes every 2 hours helps to prevent skin breakdown
	4. Encourage exercise through play by doing pull-ups on trapeze apparatus	4. Exercise will help to prevent atrophy, joint contractures, and muscle weakness
	5. Institute range-of-motion exercises on unaffected extremities	5. Unaffected limbs need exercise to prevent stiffness, muscle atrophy, and deformities
	6. Encourage self-care	6. Promote self-directed wellness
	7. Encourage deep breathing with incentive spirometer or a toy	7. Deep-breathing exercises help to prevent pneumonia and atelectasis
	8. Observe for urinary tract infection	8. Kidney filtration slows down with immobilization; immobility causes minerals (e.g., calcium) to leave bones and pool in renal pelvis; stasis of urine is likely to occur, causing renal calculi
	9. Provide high-fiber diet and stool softeners	9. Bulk improves stool consistency and prevents constipation. Stool softeners prevent straining during defecation.
	10. Provide adequate fluids; monitor intake and output	10. Increased fluids are necessary to hydrate body, and decreases the risk of urine stasis and constipation.

Nursing Diagnosis: Pain due to tissue trauma

Goals	Nursing Interventions	Rationale
Child will be comfortable, as evidenced by a decrease in irritability, crying, body posturing, anorexia Older child verbalizes relief of pain	1. Administer pain medication prior to activity and before pain escalates	1. Child may be unable to verbalize pain. Premedication for pain allows for muscle relaxation and participation in activities
	2. Allow choice in method of pain relief, if possible	2. Allowing some choice, if there is one, to promote self-control
	3. Encourage child to hold favorite possession; provide pacifier for toddler	3. Favorite possessions and a pacifier are comforting, particularly to a small child
	4. Distract with music box or tapes, as age-appropriate	4. Distraction from a problem reduces stress and tension
	5. Listen and communicate with child	5. Listening to child gives nurse clues as to amount of pain; nonverbal cues are important in infants and toddlers
	6. Use touch as a comfort measure	6. Touch is particularly important in infants and toddlers but is comforting for all ages; proceed with caution if there is reason to suspect abuse
	7. Involve family in supporting child's ability to cope with pain	7. Child trusts family; family members may be able to suggest favorite types of comfort for child
	8. Consider cultural background in relation to pain expression	8. In some cultures, showing pain is considered cowardly

(Continued on following page)

NURSING CARE PLAN 24–1 *continued*

Selected Nursing Diagnoses for the Child in Traction

Nursing Diagnosis: Pain due to tissue trauma

Goals	Nursing Interventions	Rationale
	9. Monitor vital signs	9. A change in vital signs can indicate pain, infection, or poor tissue perfusion
	10. Provide support and education to family members	10. Family members who understand and participate in care can help the child to develop effective coping skills

Nursing Diagnosis: High risk for impaired skin integrity related to immobility, traction, poor circulation

Goals	Nursing Interventions	Rationale
Skin remains intact with no evidence of breakdown	1. Inspect skin regularly	1. Provides for early assessment of developing skin problems
Circulation of affected extremity is adequate as evidenced by normal capillary refill, equal and strong peripheral pulses, and sensation and motion in extremity	2. Check capillary refill of nailbeds in affected extremity	2. Impaired tissue perfusion will result in an increased capillary refill time
	3. Have child wiggle toes or fingers of affected extremity to determine sensation and motion	3. Wiggling toes and fingers determines mobility and sensation
	4. Assess restraining devices and elastic bandages for wrinkles or looseness	4. Excessive tightness or wrinkles in bandages can cause swelling and irritation of underlying tissue
	5. Utilize sheepskin underneath hips and back	5. Sheepskin may protect susceptible areas, such as bony prominences about sacrum
	6. Monitor traction device, including ropes, pulleys, and weights	6. To maintain effective traction, weights must be hanging freely, ropes must be securely on pulleys, and the traction device must be free of friction
	7. Maintain body alignment	7. Proper body alignment maintains a pull on the long axis of the bone
	8. Inspect pin sites for redness, swelling, or discharge; provide pin care according to protocol	8. Early intervention can prevent infection; pin care removes debris that can lead to infection or osteomyelitis

Nursing Diagnosis: Altered growth and development related to separation from family and friends

Goals	Nursing Interventions	Rationale
Child's developmental level is maintained	1. Allow child to choose age-appropriate games	1. Allowing child to choose activities increases active participation
	2. Encourage peer contact	2. Children, particularly those of school age and adolescents, must remain in contact with their peers to prevent feeling isolated
	3. Involve child-life specialist, or school teacher, to provide appropriate learning activities	3. Maintaining age-appropriate studies will allow the child to rejoin peers in school

lection of pus under the periosteum of the bone can elevate the periosteum, which can result in necrosis of that part of the bone. If the pus reaches the epiphysis of the bone in infants, infection can travel to the joint space, causing septic arthritis of that joint.

Local inflammation and increased pressure from the distended periosteum can cause pain. Older children can localize the pain and may limp. Younger children and infants will show decreased voluntary movement of that extremity. Associated muscle spasms can cause limited active ROM (Range of Motion). The child may refuse to stand or walk. Signs of local inflammation may be present. A detailed history may reveal possible sources of primary infection. Blood cultures to identify the organism may be valuable if the child has not been given antibiotics for the primary infection. A urine test for the presence of bacterial antigens and a tissue biopsy may be helpful to establish the diagnosis.

Manifestations. There is an elevation in white blood cell count and sedimentation rate. X-ray films fail to reveal infection until about 10 days later. A bone scan may be diagnostic.

Treatment and Nursing Care. Prompt and vigorous treatment are essential to ensure a favorable prognosis. Intravenous antibiotics are prescribed for a 4- to 6-week period. The high doses required indicate a nursing responsibility to monitor the infant or child for toxic responses and to ensure long-term compliance. The joint may be drained of pus arthroscopically or surgically to reduce pressure and avoid bone necrosis. The joint is immobilized in a functional position. If fever lasts beyond 5 days, a complication should be suspected. Early passive ROM exercises after the splint is removed may be advisable to reduce the occurrence of contracture. Gentle handling to minimize pain and use of appropriate pain relieving medications are essential. The child should be positioned comfortably with the limb supported by pillows or blanket rolls.

Routine cast or splint care, including frequent neurovascular checks (see p. 625), is a nursing responsibility. Bed rest is followed by wheelchair access, but weight bearing should be avoided. Diversional therapy, physical therapy, and tutorial assistance for school-age children should be provided so they can return to their class and classmates. Close interaction with home care providers is indicated.

DUCHENNE'S OR BECKER MUSCULAR DYSTROPHY (PSEUDOHYPERTROPHIC)

Description. The muscular dystrophies are a group of disorders in which progressive muscle degeneration occurs. The childhood form (Duchenne's muscular dystrophy) is the most common type. It has an incidence of about 0.14 in 3600 live born male infants of all races and ethnic groups. It is a sex-linked inherited disorder that occurs only in boys.

Manifestations. The onset is generally between 2 and 6 years of age; however, a history of delayed motor development during infancy may be evidenced. The calf muscles in particular become hypertrophied. The term *pseudohypertrophic* (*pseudo*, "false," and *hypertrophy*, "enlargement") refers to this characteristic. Other signs include progressive weakness involving frequent falling, clumsiness, contractures of the ankles and hips, and the Gower's maneuver (a characteristic way of rising from the floor) (Fig. 24–11). Intellectual impairment is common.

Laboratory findings show marked increases in blood creatine phosphokinase levels. Muscle biopsy reveals degeneration of muscle fibers and their replacement by fat and connective tissue. An *elec-*

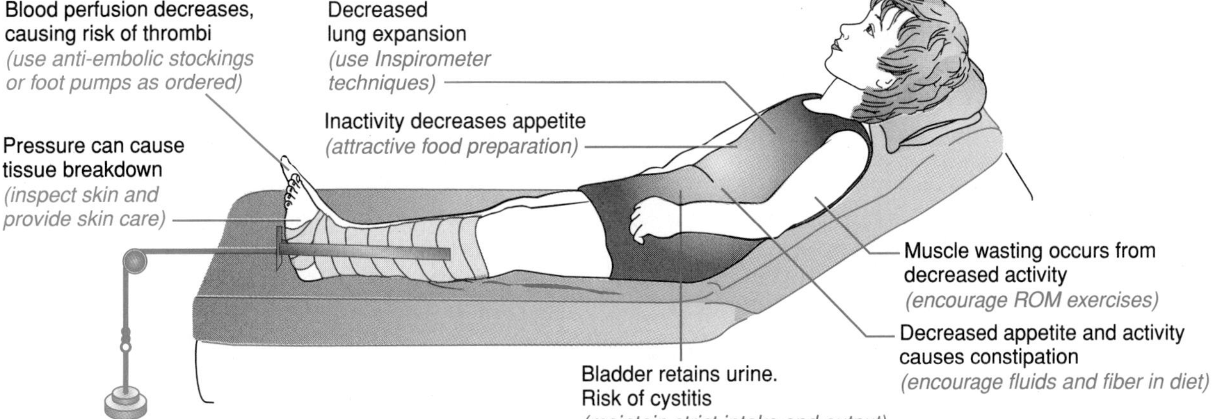

Figure 24–10. • Overcoming the effects of traction on a child.

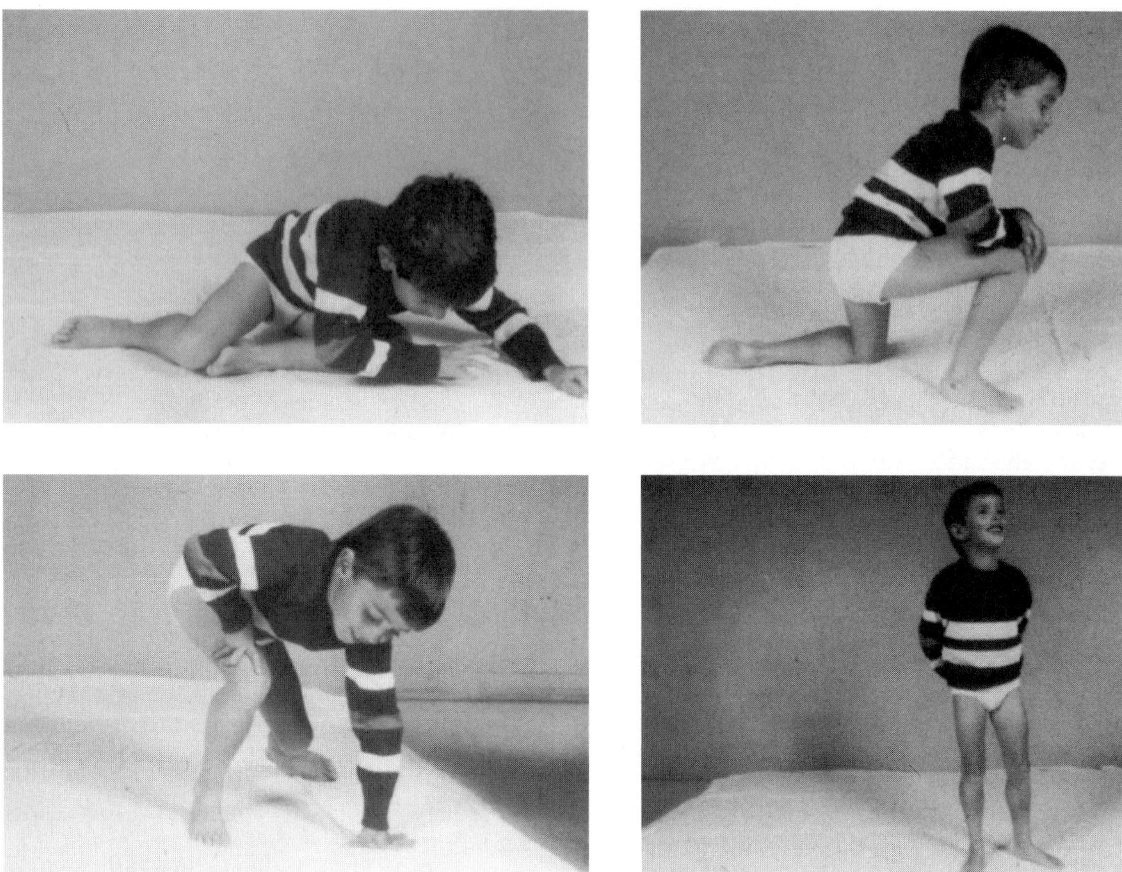

Figure 24–11. • Gowers' sign in a boy with hip girdle weakness from Duchenne-type muscular dystrophy. (From Behrman R. E., Kliegman, R. M., & Arvin, A. M. [1996]. *Nelson's textbook of pediatrics* [15th ed., p. 1478]. Philadelphia: Saunders.)

tromyogram (a graphic record of muscle contraction as a result of electrical stimulation) shows decreases in amplitude and duration of motor unit potentials. Electrocardiographic (EKG) abnormalities are also common. The disease becomes progressively worse, and wheelchair confinement occurs when the child is about 12 years old. Death is usually due to cardiac failure or respiratory infection. Mental retardation is not uncommon.

Treatment and Nursing Care. Treatment at this time is mainly supportive to prevent complications and maintain the quality of life. A multidisciplinary team should provide psychological support, nutritional support, physiotherapy, social/financial assistance, and, when necessary, respite and hospice care.

Compared with other children with disabilities, some children with muscular dystrophy may appear passive and withdrawn. Early on, depression may be seen because the child is unable to compete with peers. Social and emotional pressures on the child and family are great.

LEGG–CALVÉ–PERTHES DISEASE (COXA PLANA)

Description. Legg–Calvé–Perthes disease is one of a group of disorders called the *osteochondrosis* (*osteo,* "bone," *chondros,* "cartilage," and *osis,* "disease"), in which the blood supply to the epiphysis, or end of the bone, is disrupted. The tissue death that results from the inadequate blood supply is termed *avascular necrosis* (*a,* "without," *vasculum,* "vessels," and *nekros,* "death"). Legg–Calvé–Perthes disease affects the development of the head of the femur. Its cause and incidence are unknown. The disease is seen most commonly in boys between ages 5 and 12. It is more common in Caucasians. This disease is unilateral in about 85% of cases. Healing occurs spontaneously over 2 to 4 years; however, marked distortion of the head of the femur may lead to an imperfect joint or degenerative arthritis of the hip in later life. Symptoms include a painless limp and limitation of motion. X-ray films and bone scans confirm the diagnosis.

Treatment. Legg–Calvé–Perthes disease is a self-limiting disorder that heals spontaneously. The treatment involves keeping the femoral head deep in the hip socket while it heals and avoiding weight bearing. This is accomplished through the use of ambulation-abduction casts or braces that prevent subluxation (*sub,* "beneath," and *luxatio,* "dislocation") and enable the acetabulum to mold the healing head in such a way that it does not become deformed. This treatment may be preceded by bed rest and traction. The prognosis in Legg–Calvé–Perthes disease is fair. Some affected people may require hip joint replacement procedures as adults.

Nursing Care. Nursing considerations depend on the age of the patient and the type of treatment. When immobilization of the child is necessary, the general principles of traction, cast, and brace care are employed. Teaching and counseling are directed toward a holistic understanding of and interest in the individual child and family. Total immobility or partial mobility is particularly trying for children. The natural inclination to compete physically is thwarted. In some cases surgical immobilization is required. Pre- and postop care and care of a patient in a cast are discussed on pages 356 and 574.

OSTEOSARCOMA

Description. *Osteosarcoma* (*osteo,* "bone," *sarx,* "flesh," and *oma,* "tumor") is a primary malignant tumor of the long bones. The two most common types of bone tumors in children are osteosarcoma and Ewing's tumor. The mean age of onset of osteosarcoma is 10 to 15 years of age. Children who have had radiation therapy for other types of cancer and children with retinoblastoma have a higher incidence of this disease. Metastasis occurs quickly because of the high vascularity of bone tissue. The lungs are the primary site of metastasis; brain and other bone tissue are also sites of metastasis.

Manifestations. The patient experiences pain and swelling at the site. In adolescents this is often attributed to injury or "growing pains." The pain may be lessened by flexing the extremity. Later a pathologic fracture may occur. Diagnosis is confirmed by biopsy. A complete physical examination, including computed tomography (CT) and a bone scan, is done. Radiologic studies help to confirm the diagnosis.

Treatment and Nursing Care. Treatment of the patient with osteosarcoma consists of radical resection or amputation surgery. Internal prostheses are available for most sites. Long-term survival is possible with early diagnosis and treatment.

The nursing care is similar to that for other types of cancer. Problems of body image are particularly important to the self-conscious teenager. If amputation is necessary, the family and patient will need much support. The nurse anticipates anger, fear, and grief. Immediately following surgery, the stump dressing is observed frequently for bleeding. Vital signs are monitored. The child's position is as ordered by the surgeon. *Phantom limb pain* is likely to be experienced. This is the continued sensation of pain in the leg even though the leg is no longer there. It occurs because nerve tracts continue to report pain. This pain is very real and an analgesic may be necessary. Rehabilitation measures follow surgical recovery.

EWING'S SARCOMA

Description. Ewing's sarcoma was first described in 1921 by Dr. James Ewing. It is a malignant growth that occurs in the marrow of long bones. It occurs mainly in older school children and early adolescents. When metastasis is present on diagnosis, the prognosis is poor. Without metastasis there is a 60% survival rate. The primary sites for metastasis are the lungs and bones.

Treatment and Nursing Care. Amputation is not generally recommended for Ewing's sarcoma because the tumor is sensitive to radiation therapy and chemotherapy. This is a relief to the child and family. The child is warned against vigorous weight bearing on the involved bone during therapy to avoid pathologic fractures. Patients need to be prepared for the effects of radiation therapy and chemotherapy. The nurse supports the family members in their efforts to gain equilibrium following such a crisis.

JUVENILE RHEUMATOID ARTHRITIS

Description. Juvenile rheumatoid arthritis (JRA) is the most common arthritic condition of childhood. It is a systemic inflammatory disease that involve the joints, connective tissues, and viscera. It is not a rare disease, as an estimated quarter million children in the United States have the disorder (Behrman, Kliegman, & Arvin, 1996). The exact cause is unknown, but infection and an autoimmune response have been implicated.

Manifestations and Types. This disease has three distinct methods of onset: systemic (or acute febrile), polyarticular, and pauciarticular. The *systemic* form is manifested by fever above 103°F persisting for over 10 days, rash, abdominal pain, pleuritis, pericarditis, and enlarged liver and spleen. It occurs most frequently in children 1 to 3 and 8 to 10 years of age. Joint symptoms may be absent at onset but will develop in most patients. The *polyarticular* form can involve five or more joints often small joints of the hands and feet, which become swollen, warm, and tender. This form occurs throughout childhood and adolescence and predominantly affects girls. Approximately 40% of patients with JRA have the polyarticular type. The *pauciarticular* form is limited to four or fewer joints, generally the larger ones such as the hips, knees, ankles, and elbows. It occurs in children under age 3 years (mostly in girls) and in those over age 13 years (mostly in boys). Approximately 35% of patients with JRA have the pauciarticular form.

Children with pauciarticular disease are at risk for iridocyclitis (*irido,* "iris," *cycl,* "circle," and *itis,* "inflammation"), an inflammation of the iris and ciliary body of the eye also known as *uveitis.* Symptoms include redness, pain, photophobia, decreased visual acuity, and nonreactive pupils. All children with pauciarticular arthritis need slit-lamp eye examinations periodically. Distortion of the pupil and cataracts may occur. The long-term visual prognosis is uncertain. There are no specific tests or cures for JRA. The duration of the symptoms is important, particularly when they have lasted longer than 6 weeks. Diagnosis is determined by clinical manifestations, x-ray studies, laboratory results, and exclusion of other disorders. Aspirated joint fluid is yellow to green, cloudy, and has a low viscosity.

Treatment. The goals of therapy are to:

- Reduce pain and swelling.
- Promote mobility.
- Preserve joint function.
- Educate the patient and family.
- Help the child and family to adjust to living with a chronic disease.

Treatment is supportive. Drug therapy and exercise are the primary treatment. The three principal medications used in this condition are aspirin, corticosteroids, and nonsteroidal antiinflammatory (NSAIDs) agents, such as indomethacin or naproxen. Gold compounds are used when other measures prove ineffective. Regular monitoring of all medications is imperative.

Nursing Care. The nurse functions as a member of a multidisciplinary health care team that includes the pediatrician, rheumatologist, social worker, physical therapist, occupational therapist, psychologist, ophthalmologist, and school and community nurses. The child may be hospitalized during an acute episode or for an unrelated illness. Treatment consists of administering medications and providing warm tub baths, joint exercises, and rest. The physical therapist oversees the type and amount of exercise performed. Daily ROM exercises and play activities that incorporate specific routines help to preserve function, maintain muscle strength and to prevent deformities. One must be careful to avoid traumatizing an inflamed joint. Morning tub baths and the application of moist hot packs help to lessen stiffness. Resting splints may be ordered to prevent flexion contractures and preserve functional alignment. Proper body alignment with regular changes to the prone position (unless contraindicated) facilitates comfort. Either no pillow or a small flat pillow is advised for under the head. Measures to alleviate boredom are instituted.

Home Care. The patient is discharged with written instructions for home care. These are reviewed with family members to determine their level of understanding. A firm mattress or bed board is necessary to prevent joints from sagging. Age-appropriate tricycles and pedal cars promote mobility and exercise. Modifications in daily living, such as elevation of toilet seats, installation of hand rails, Velcro® fasteners, and so on, may be necessary. The importance of regular eye examinations is emphasized. Assist parents in planning nutritional meals. Weight gain is to be avoided as it places further stress on the joints. Unnecessary physical restrictions should be avoided, as these can lead to rebellion. Swimming is an excellent form of exercise.

School attendance is encouraged. Excessive absence from school, particularly for nonspecific complaints, may suggest that the child is depressed or overly preoccupied with the illness. In such cases, the meaning of the illness to the child and family and its effect on daily life need to be explored. Parents need assistance in establishing limits. Consistently negative behavior in social situations can present more problems than the actual disability. Overindulgence and preferential treatment often compromise the child's potential for happiness and independence. Siblings of chronically ill children may resent the special attention given to the patient. They may be torn by loyalty to the brother or sister and their own need to be with others. Parents need ongoing counseling and the services of various community resources. One resource is the Arthritis Foundation, which sponsors the American Juvenile Arthritis Organization. The child may benefit from socializing with other arthritic children.

This long-term disease is characterized by periods of remission and exacerbations. Nurses can serve as advocates for the child, that is, they can help alleviate stress by recognizing the impact of the disease and by openly communicating with the child, the family, and other members of the health-care team. Nurses support the child and family members and instill hope.

TORTICOLLIS (WRY NECK)

Description. *Torticollis* (*tortus,* "twisted," and *collium,* "neck") is a condition in which neck motion is limited because of shortening of the sternocleidomastoid muscle. It can be either congenital or acquired. It can also be either acute or chronic. The most common type is a congenital anomaly in which the sternocleidomastoid muscle is injured during birth. It is associated with breech and forceps delivery and may be seen in conjunction with other birth defects, such as congenital hip.

Manifestations. In congenital torticollis the symptoms are present at birth. The infant holds the head to the side of the muscle involved. The chin is tilted in the opposite direction. There is a hard palpable mass of dense fibrotic tissue (fibroma). This is not fixed to the skin and resolves by 2 to 6 months. Passive stretching and ROM exercises and physical therapy may be indicated. Feeding and playing with the infant can encourage turning to the desired side for correction. Operative correction is indicated if the condition persists beyond 2 years.

Acquired torticollis is seen in older children. It may be associated with injury, inflammation, neurologic disorders, and other causes. Nursing intervention is primarily that of detection. Infants who have limited head movements require further investigation.

SCOLIOSIS

Description. The most prevalent of the three skeletal abnormalities shown in Figure 24–12 is *scoliosis.* Scoliosis refers to an S-shaped curvature of the spine (Fig. 24–13). During adolescence, scoliosis is more common in girls. Many curvatures are not progressive and may require only periodic evaluation. Untreated progressive scoliosis may lead to back pain, fatigue, disability, and heart and lung complications. Skeletal deterioration does not stop with maturity and may be aggravated by pregnancy.

Causes. There are two types of scoliosis, functional and structural. *Functional* scoliosis is usually caused by poor posture, not by spinal disease. The curve is flexible and easily correctable. Structural or fixed scoliosis is due to changes in the shape of the vertebrae or thorax. It is usually accompanied by rotation of the spine. The hips and shoulders may appear uneven. The patient cannot correct the condition by standing in a straighter posture.

There are many causes of *structural* scoliosis. Some are congenital and develop in utero. These are noticeable at birth or during periods of rapid growth. *Neuromuscular* scoliosis is the result of muscle weakness or imbalance. It is seen in children with cerebral palsy, muscular dystrophy, and other conditions. The cause of *idiopathic* scoliosis is unknown; there may be a hereditary link.

Treatment. Treatment is aimed at correcting the curvature and preventing more severe scoliosis. Curves up to 20 degrees do not require treatment but are carefully followed. Curves between 20 and 40 degrees require daily exercise and the use of a *Milwaukee brace* (Fig. 24–14). This apparatus exerts

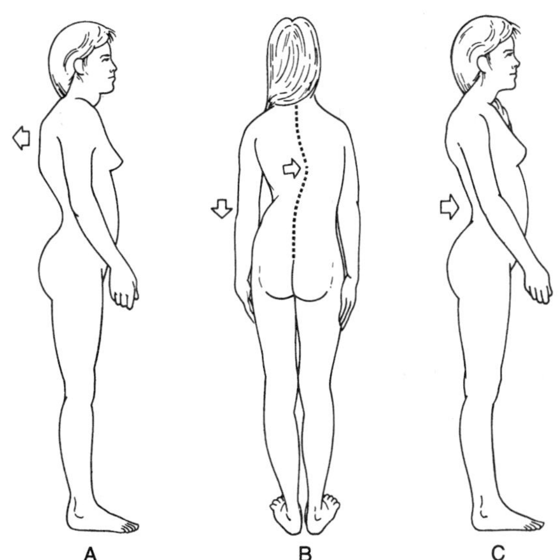

Figure 24–12. • **A,** Kyphosis involves a hunched back and outward curvature of the spine. **B,** In scoliosis, the spine has an S shape. **C,** In lordosis, the spine is curved in such a way that the pelvis tilts forward. (From Betz, C., et al. [1994]. *Family-centered nursing care of children* [2nd ed., p. 1853]. Philadelphia: Saunders.)

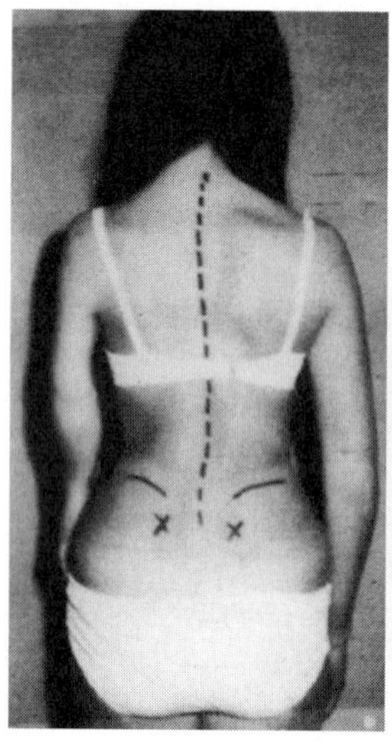

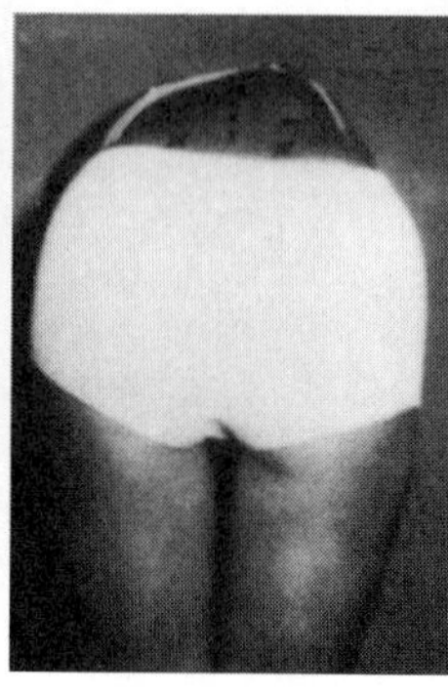

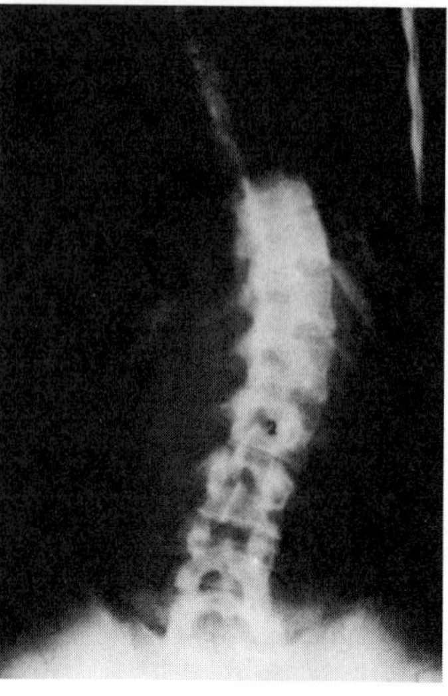

Figure 24–13. • Scoliosis. The spine rotates as it curves, with the spinous processes moving toward the concavity. The severe curve of 46 degrees seen by roentgenogram on the right is only partly recognizable when the patient stands upright. However, examination with the child's spine flexed shows the rotation on the right that indicates a structural scoliosis. (From Behrman R. E., Kliegman, R. M., & Arvin, A. M. [1996]. *Nelson's textbook of pediatrics* [15th ed., p. 1711]. Philadelphia: Saunders.)

pressure on the chin, pelvis, and convex (arched) side of the spine. It is worn approximately 23 hours a day and is worn *over* a T-shirt to protect the skin. An underarm modification of the brace (the Boston brace) is proving effective for patients with low curvatures. It is less cumbersome and more acceptable to the self-conscious young person. A transcutaneous electrical nerve stimulator (TENS) unit provides electrical stimulation to the muscles and is worn at night.

For curves of more than 40 degrees and for patients in whom conservative measures are not successful, hospitalization is required. A spinal fusion is performed. This is sometimes done in stages. A Harrington rod, Dwyer instrument or Luque wires may be inserted for immobilization during the time required for the fusion to become solid. Halo traction may be used when there is associated weakness or paralysis of the neck and trunk muscles (Fig. 24–15); it is also used in treating cervical fractures and fusions.

Figure 24–14. • The Milwaukee brace.

Nursing Care

Community Nursing. The management of scoliosis begins with screening. This is done before middle school. It should be a part of every yearly physical examination given to prepubescent youngsters. Camp nurses also need to be aware of symptoms. Early recognition is of utmost importance in detecting mild cases amenable to nonsurgical treatment.

The adolescent is prepared by explaining the purpose of the procedure and by being reassured that it merely entails observing the back while standing and bending forward. Adolescents need to know that it is simple, quick, and painless and that privacy will be afforded. They are instructed to wear clothing that is easy to remove, such as a pullover top. Boys disrobe to the waist, girls generally to the bra. No slip or undershirt should be worn.

Nursing Tip

Insertion of a Harrington rod or other metal device may delay a patient at an airport security scanner, as the metal could activate the alarm. The physician can supply a note to be used as clearance for air travel.

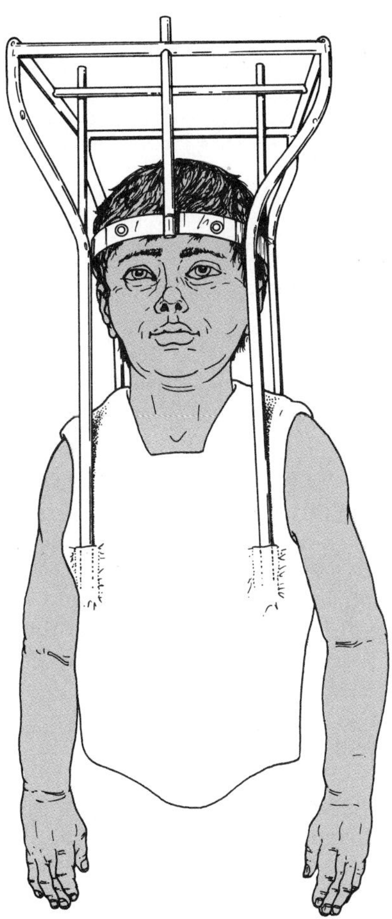

Figure 24–15. • Body jacket with halo apparatus.

The procedure consists of the nurse examining the spine from the front, side, and back while the adolescent stands erect and then observing the back as the adolescent bends forward. One looks initially for general body alignment and *asymmetry* (lack of proportion). In scoliosis, one shoulder may be higher than the other, a scapula may be prominent, the arm-to-body spaces may be unequal, or a hip may protrude; one arm may appear longer than the other when the person bends forward. Referrals are made as indicated to those who must obtain further treatment.

Nursing Care. The adolescent may be admitted overnight for a cast change or may require more extensive correction by spinal fusion. The nurse's knowledge of preadolescent and adolescent developmental tasks is imperative, because therapy often conflicts with these tasks.

Basic cast care is described on page 356. The adolescent in a body cast has many adjustments to make as a result of its weight and its restrictions on mobility. Ambulation is difficult, as is sleeping. Modifications must be made in bathing, shampooing, dressing, and eating. Teenagers are concerned about how they look in the cast, and clothes made especially for them boost their morale.

Routine preoperative nursing care of the adolescent is necessary for casting or spinal fusion. This includes instructing the adolescent and family about the purpose and extent of the cast or brace that may be prescribed. It is important that the nurse evaluate and document the adolescent's neuromuscular status at this time so that it may be used as a basis for comparison after the procedure is completed.

Much of the postoperative nursing care is directly related to combating the physical results of immobilization (see Fig. 24–10). The body systems become sluggish because of inactivity. This is evidenced in the gastrointestinal tract by anorexia, irregularity, and constipation. Allowing the adolescent to select foods with the aid of the dietitian is helpful in improving appetite. Increasing fluid intake reduces constipation. Cranberry juice helps to neutralize the alkaline content of urine and decreases the possibility of bladder infection.

The adolescent and parents are introduced to the multidisciplinary health care team and referral to the National Scoliosis Foundation and other agencies available within their community. Postoperative exercise, physical therapy, and promotion of adolescent school and developmental tasks are essential aspects of nursing care.

SPORTS INJURIES

A high percentage of adolescent males and females participate in athletic activities. The American Academy of Pediatrics recommends that a complete physical examination be given at least every other year during adolescence and that sports-specific examinations be given for those involved in strenuous activity on entry into junior or senior high school. Such examinations should be updated by an annual questionnaire. The family history and an orthopedic screening are important in identifying risk factors.

Prevention. Several factors help to prevent sports injuries. Some of these are adequate warm-up and cool-down periods; year-round conditioning; careful selection of activity according to physical maturity, size, and skill necessary; proper supervision by adults; safe, well-fitting equipment; and avoidance of participation when in pain or injured. Proper diet and fluids are also necessary. A few of the more common injuries are listed in

Table 24–1
SOME OF THE MORE COMMON SPORTS INJURIES

Type	Comment
Concussion	Any blow to the head followed by alterations in mental functioning should be treated as a possible concussion; observe carefully for sequelae
"Stingers" or "burners"	A common neck injury when a player hits another in the head in such sports as football or soccer; due to brachial plexus trauma; feels like an electrical jolt; usually mild, disappears suddenly; restrict sports activity until symptoms disappear; reassess protective gear
Injured knee	Usually a result of stress on the knee ligaments; potentially serious; should be evaluated by an experienced trainer or physician; may require arthroscopy
Sprain or strained ankle	May injure growth plate; x-ray films important in adolescent
Muscle cramps	Due to injury, alterations in blood flow, or electrolyte deficiencies. Important to warm up before activity; ensure fluid intake is adequate
Shin splints	Pain and discomfort in lower leg due to repeated running on a hard surface such as concrete; avoid such activity; use well-fitting shoes; decrease inflammation by rest

Table 24–1. The nurse has a major role in educating and directing parents to sources of accurate information to ensure that the physical, emotional, and maturational levels of the adolescent are appropriate for the activity (Table 24–2). Parents are encouraged to inquire as to the capabilities of personnel and availability of emergency services prior to the beginning of the competition.

FAMILY VIOLENCE

Violence has become a problem that affects children of all social classes across the nation. Family violence includes spousal abuse and child abuse, neglect, and maltreatment. Community violence is seen in neighborhoods where even non-gang–related adolescents "arm" themselves with guns and knives for "protection." Preschoolers who are allowed to repeatedly watch violent programs on television may be learning antisocial coping skills they will use as they grow and mature. The time spent watcing TV and the content of the programs should be controlled by parents so that TV exposure results in the acquisition of knowledge, skills, and information that will motivate learning. In homes where spousal and/or child abuse occurs, the child learns the behaviors that they will practice when

Table 24–2
SELECTED SPORTS ACTIVITIES AND THEIR RISKS

Sport	Risk
Gymnastics	Common problems associated with children engaging in gymnastics are delayed menstruation and eating disorders. Trauma and overuse injuries of the large joints and spine are common. Prevention includes muscle strengthening exercises, flexibility exercises, and wrist braces. Nutritional needs and education is essential
Ballet	Common problems associated with ballet often include delayed menarche and eating disorders. There is a high risk for stress fractures, strains, shin splints, and spinal deviations. Prevention includes nutrition planning and education and skilled coaching
Wrestling	Placement in a wrestling match is based upon weight. A binging and purging behavior is commonly found in athletes participating in wrestling. Concussions, neck strains and spinal injuries are common. Skin dermatitis and infection occurs from contact with floor mats. Skilled coaching, nutrition education, and planning are important
Football	Improvement in techniques, protective equipment and game exercises have decreased serious injuries in children participating on football teams
Hockey	A contact sport involving physical collisions and often puck and stick injuries as well. Proper protective equipment and sporting rules decrease the seriousness of injuries
Basketball, volleyball	Jumping sports that involve injury risk to ankles, knees, and fingers. Ankle sprain, tendinitis, stress fractures, and blisters are common complications of these sports
Running	Involves repeated poorly absorbed foot impact. Muscle fatigue, environmental temperature and running surface contribute to injuries. Preexercise, using good impact absorbing shoes, cross-training, and adequate rest are essential. *Shin splints* involves pain over the anterior tibia and results from tearing the collagenous fibers that connect muscle to bone. Shoe orthotics, running on a soft surface, cross-training, and rest are the priorities of management.
Skiing	Injuries are usually related to falls. Better equipment, controlled slope conditions, and separation of skill levels contribute to a decreased rate of injury.

BOX 24–1

FACTORS THAT MAY CONTRIBUTE TO OR TRIGGER CHILD ABUSE

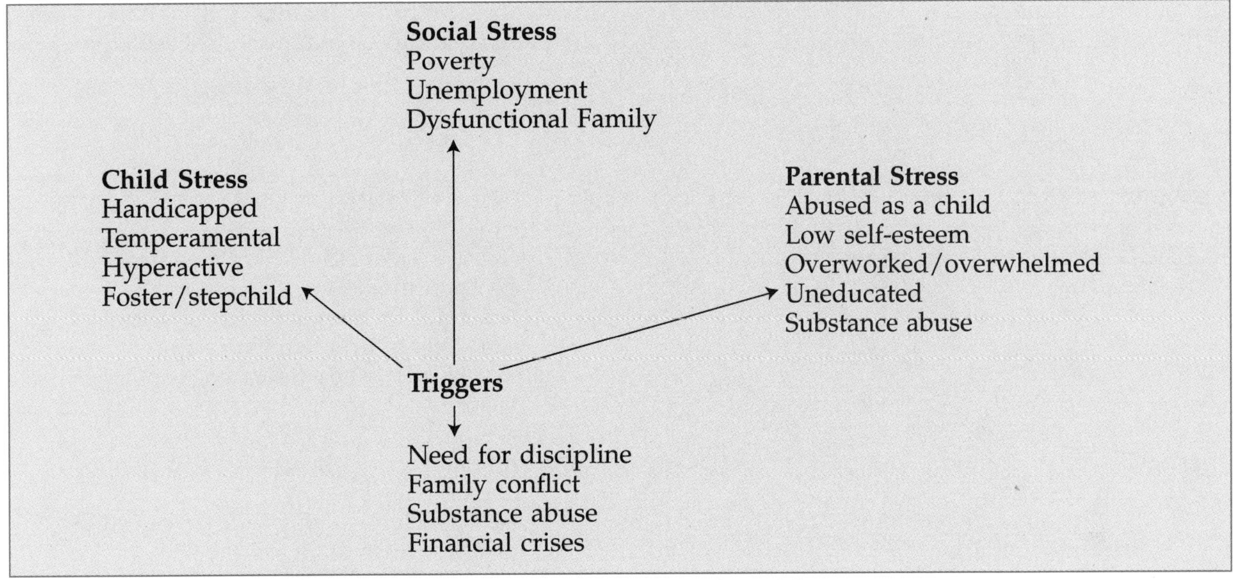

Abusive parents may love their child but respond to stress and triggers that provoke abusive behavior.

they become adults and the abuse cycle continues. Parents who are abusive are not usually psychotic or criminal. They may have a knowledge deficit about child care needs, as well as about child growth and development. Abusive parents are often without a support system, perhaps alone, angry, in crisis, or have unrealistic expectations (see Box 24–1).

CHILD ABUSE

Description. The term *battered child syndrome* was coined by Kempe in his landmark paper published in 1962 by the *Journal of the American Medical Association.* It refers to "a clinical condition in young children who have received serious physical abuse, generally from a parent or foster parent." The impact of Kempe's research was considerable and focused the attention of physicians on unexplained fractures and signs of physical abuse. Today, most authorities consider Kempe's definition narrow and have broadened it to include neglect and maltreatment.

According to the National Center on Child Abuse and Neglect, the incidence of the following aspects of child abuse has been increasing:

- *Emotional abuse.* Intentional verbal acts that result in a destruction of self-esteem in the child—can include rejection or threatening the child
- *Emotional Neglect.* An intentional omission of verbal or behavioral actions that are necessary for development of a healthy self-esteem. This can include social or emotional isolation of a child
- *Sexual Abuse.* Involves an act that is performed on a child for the sexual gratification of the adult
- *Physical Neglect.* The failure to provide for the basic physical needs of the child, including food, clothing, shelter, and basic cleanliness
- *Physical Abuse.* The deliberate infliction of injury on a child. It is suspected when an injury is not consistent with the history or developmental level of the child

The temperament of the child as well as that of the parent can be a causal factor in child abuse. Children who are different from others in any way are at particular risk. This includes preterm infants; sick, retarded, or disabled children; and merely unattractive children. Unwanted or illegitimate babies and stepchildren are especially vulnerable. It has been noted that people are often reluctant to report occurrences in middle- and upper-income families or when the incident involves friends or relatives.

Federal Laws and Agencies. By 1963 the United States Children's Bureau drafted a model mandatory state reporting law, which has been adopted in some form in all states. This law aids in establishing statistics and is based on the need to provide therapeutic help to both child and family. Immunity from liability is provided for persons reporting suspected cases. Most states have penalties for failure to report suspected child abuse. Referrals usually are made to the local Child Protective Services, and a case worker is assigned.

Nursing Care and Intervention. Nursing interventions for high-risk children is of utmost importance (Box 24–2). One approach currently taken is to identify high-risk infants and parents during the prenatal and perinatal periods. Predictive ques-

BOX 24–2

NURSING INTERVENTIONS FOR ABUSED AND NEGLECTED CHILDREN AND ADOLESCENTS

- Teach child anxiety-reducing techniques.
  - Gradual relaxation
  - Relaxation to music
  - Visual imagery
  - Exercise
  - Talking with safe, appropriate people about feelings
  - Choosing, building, and maintaining positive support systems
  - Ensuring personal safety
  - Setting boundaries
  - Establishing a safe, supportive relationship
  - Clarifying expectations and rules
  - Self-soothing techniques
- Assist child in managing his or her feelings.
  - Teach child to identify feelings.
  - Teach child to express feelings appropriately.
  - Teach child to modulate and control feelings.
  - Teach child to identify events that elicit strong positive and negative feelings.
  - Teach child to express feelings verbally instead of physically.
  - Teach child to normalize feelings resulting from abuse.
  - Teach child to share feelings appropriately with peer group.
  - Teach child to find commonality and support within group for feelings resulting from abuse.
- Teach child assertiveness skills.
  - Teach child to identify differences between assertiveness, passivity, and aggression.
  - Teach child to practice assertiveness skills.
  - Teach child to identify boundaries.
  - Teach child to understand when someone violates boundaries.
  - Teach child to practice responses when someone violates boundaries.
- Assist child in developing problem-solving skills.
  - Provide simple problem-solving model.
  - Increase awareness of child's control and decision-making.
  - Teach child to generate a list of possible solutions to problem situations.
  - Help child look at consequences of each solution.
  - Help child make best choice.
  - Help child give self positive and gentle negative feedback.
  - Coach problem-solving with actual situations as much as possible.
  - Teach good touch/bad touch.
  - Teach refusal skills.
  - Teach age-appropriate sexual expression.
  - Teach effects of substance abuse.
- Assist child in value building and clarification.
  - Define values.
  - Identify role of values.
  - Assist child in identifying and verbalizing values.
  - Help link child's values to child's actions.
  - Assist child in development of values.
  - Help child practice value-based decision-making.
- Assist child in enhancing his or her coping mechanisms.
  - Teach child to practice positive self-talk.
  - Help child set realistic expectations for self.
  - Assist child in learning to nurture self.
  - Teach child to practice relaxation.
  - Teach child to practice assertiveness and appropriate expression of feelings.
  - Assist child in learning to accept defeat and failure.
  - Help child identify and build skills, hobbies.
  - Encourage child to identify and focus on strengths.
  - Help child set and accomplish goals.
  - Assist child in developing organizational skills.

Bowden, V. R., Dickey, S. B., Greenberg, C. S. (1998). *Children and their families: The continuum of care.* Philadelphia: Saunders.

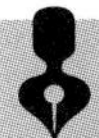

Nursing Tip

Reporting Suspected Abuse or Neglect

A citizen can report suspected child abuse or neglect by contacting the Children's Protective Services in the yellow pages of the telephone directory under "Social Service Organizations." This can be done anonymously. After obtaining the facts, the agency will inform the parents that a report is being filed and will check the condition of the child. A visit must be initiated within 72 hours. In most cases, this is accomplished within 48 hours or earlier if the situation is life-threatening. All persons who report suspected abuse or neglect are given immunity from criminal prosecution and civil liability if the report is made in good faith. Many professionals, such as physicians, nurses, and social workers, *must report child abuse.*

tionnaires are being used as screening tools in some clinics. Many hospitals also provide closer follow-up of mothers and newborns. Maternal–infant bonding and its significance to later parent–child relationships have been explored.

Nurses in obstetric clinics have the opportunity to observe parents and their abilities to cope. The history of the parent(s); desirability of the pregnancy; number of children already in the family; financial and personal stability of the family; types of support systems; and other factors may have a bearing on how the parents accept the new offspring. Pertinent observations include a description of parent–newborn interaction. Both verbal and nonverbal communications are important, as is the level of body and eye contact. Lack of interest, indifference, or negative comments about the sex, looks, or temperament of the baby could be significant.

In other areas, a cooperative team approach is necessary. This may include services, such as family planning, protective services, day care centers, homemakers, parenting classes, self-help groups, family counseling, child advocates, and a continued effort to reduce the incidence of preterm birth. Other related areas include financial assistance, employment services, transportation, emotional support and encouragement, and long-term follow-up care.

Individual nurses can help to detect child abuse by maintaining a vigilant approach in their work settings. Recordkeeping should be *factual* and *objective.* The pediatric nurse should make a point of reviewing old records of their patients, which may reveal repeated hospitalizations, x-ray films of multiple fractures, persistent feeding problems, history of failure to thrive, and a history of chronic absenteeism in school. Neglect or delay in seeking medical attention for a child or failure to obtain immunization and well-child care are sometimes significant findings. Children who seem overly upset about being discharged need to be brought to the attention of the physician. Runaway teenagers are frequently victims of abuse.

The abused child is approached quietly, and preparation for any treatment is carefully explained in advance. The number of caretakers should be kept to a minimum. The child may be able to express some hostility and fear through play or drawing. It is not unusual for these children to be either unresponsive or openly hostile or to show affection indiscriminately. Direct questioning is kept to a minimum. Praise is used when appropriate. Activities that promote physical and sensory development are encouraged. The nurse avoids speaking to the child about the parents in a negative manner. Other professionals are consulted about setting limits for poor behavior.

The nurse must acknowledge that in cases of child abuse there are always two victims: the child *and* the abuser. Because of personal problems, the abuser often leads an isolated life. Some have been battered or neglected children themselves. Many have unrealistic expectations about the child's intelligence and capabilities. There may be a role reversal in which the child becomes the comforter. Although removing the child from the home is one answer, many authorities believe that this can be more detrimental in the long run.

Being open to parents during this type of crisis is difficult but essential if the nurse wishes to be part of the solution rather than part of the problem. When placement in a foster home is necessary, parents experience grief, loss, and remorse. The child also mourns the loss of the family, even though there has been abuse. The nurse should be aware of the child's needs and facilitate expression of feelings of loss. The nurse who recognizes the

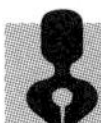

Nursing Tip

Bruises heal in various stages that are indicated according to color (1–2 days, swollen, tender; 0–5 days, red; 5–7 days, green; 7–10 days, yellow; 10–14 days, brown; 14–28 days, clear). Does the bruise match the caretaker's explanation of what happened?

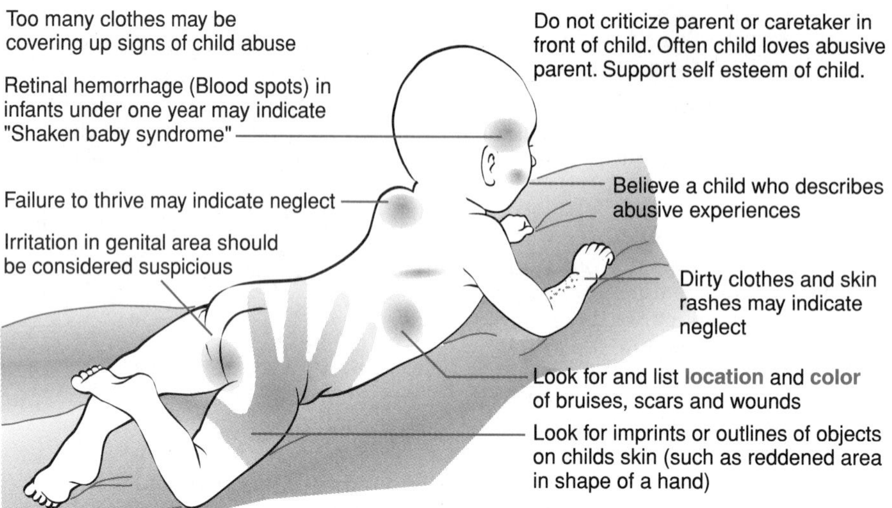

Figure 24–16. • Assessing for child abuse. The nurse should be alert for inconsistent statements about injuries; bruises at various stages of healing; delay in seeking care; history that is not compatible with injury or development.

potential for violence within us all is better able to respond to this complex problem.

Cultural and Medical Issues. Multiple factors should be considered when evaluating the child. A culturally sensitive history is essential. The nurse should be aware that what appears to be a cigarette burn could be a single lesion of impetigo. Mongolian spots can be mistaken for bruises. A severe diaper rash caused by a fungal infection can look like a scald burn. In some cases, loving parents can injure infants when shaking them to wake or feed them. They are not aware of the danger of "Shaken baby syndrome."

Some cultural practices can be interpreted as physical abuse if the nurse is not culturally aware of folk healing and ethnic practices. For example, "coining" of the body by the Vietnamese to allay disease can cause welts on the body. Burning small areas of the skin to treat enuresis is practiced by some Asian cultures. Forced kneeling is a common Carribean discipline technique. Yemenite Jews treat infections by placing garlic preparations on the wrists that can result in blisters. The Telugu people of Southern India touch the penis of a child to show respect.

The nurse should document all signs of abuse and interaction as well as verbal comments between the child and parents (Fig. 24–16). The child protective service should oversee any investigation that is warranted. Providing support to parents and child, an opportunity to talk in privacy and planning for follow-up care are basic nursing responsibilities. Parent education concerning growth and development is valuable.

KEY POINTS

- The age, neurologic development, and motor milestones achieved will influence the nursing assessment of the musculoskeletal system in a growing child.
- The normal gait of a toddler is wide and unstable. By age 6, the gait resembles a mature walk.
- Immobility causes a slowing down of body metabolism.
- Injury to the epiphyseal plate at the ends of long bones is serious during childhood because it may interfere with longitudinal growth.
- In a compound fracture, a wound in the skin leads to the broken bone, and there is added danger of infection.

- Any delay in neurologic development can cause a delay in mastery of motor skills, which can result in altered skeletal growth.
- Children who do not walk by 18 months of age should be referred for follow-up care.
- Rest, ice, compression, and elevation are the principles of managing soft-tissue injuries.
- Pain over a muscle area that does not respond to medication may indicate a complication known as *compartment syndrome.*
- A *neurovascular check* includes color, warmth, capillary refill time, movement, pulse, sensation, and pain.
- Tutorial assistance should be provided to school-age children who are hospitalized or immobilized for long periods of time.
- A complication of any traction is an arterial occlusion termed Volkmann's ischemia.
- Legg–Calvé–Perthes disease affects the development of the head of the femur.
- Juvenile rheumatoid arthritis is the most common arthritic condition of childhood.
- Medical treatment of scoliosis includes bracing, exercise, and the use of TENS electrical stimulation.
- Adolescents who participate in sports are subject to injuries, such as concussions and ligament injuries. Activities need to be selected carefully according to physical maturity, size, and skill required.
- A spiral fracture of the femur or humerus may be a sign of child abuse.
- Child abuse may be physical, emotional, sexual, or it may involve neglect.

MULTIPLE-CHOICE REVIEW QUESTIONS

Choose the most appropriate answer.

1. A disorder in which the blood supply to the epiphyses of the bone is disrupted is called
   a. muscular dystrophy.
   b. cerebral palsy.
   c. congenital hip dysplasia.
   d. Legg–Calvé–Perthes disease.
2. The term used when the circulation to a part of the body is obstructed is
   a. ischemia.
   b. ischesis.
   c. anemia.
   d. infarction.
3. Buck extension is an example of
   a. skin traction.
   b. skeletal traction.
   c. balanced traction.
   d. Bryant traction.
4. An *S*-shaped curvature of the spine seen in school-age children is
   a. sclerosis.
   b. sciatica.
   c. scabies.
   d. scoliosis.
5. A yellow bruise is approximately
   a. 2 days old.
   b. 5–7 days old.
   c. 7–10 days old.
   d. 10–14 days old.

BIBLIOGRAPHY AND READER REFERENCE

Ballock, T., & Richards, S. (1997). Hip dysplasia: Early diagnosis makes a difference. *Contemporary Pediatrics, 14*(7), 108.

Behrman, R. E., Kliegman, R. M., & Arvin, A. M. (1996). *Nelson's textbook of pediatrics* (15th ed.). Philadelphia: Saunders.

Benchot, R. (1996). The adolescent with slipped capital femoral epiphysis. *Journal of Pediatric Nursing, 11*(3), 175.

Betz, C., et al. (1994). *Family-centered nursing care of children* (2nd ed.). Philadelphia: Saunders.

Bowden, V., Dickey, S., & Greenberg, C. (1998). *Children and their families: A continuum of care.* Philadelphia: Saunders.

Bruce, R. N. (1996). Torsional and angular deformities. *Pediatric Clinics of North America, 43,* 867.

Chiocca, E. M. (1998). Action stat: Shaken baby syndrome. *Nursing 98, 28*(5), 33.

Chiocca, E. M. (1998). Child abuse and neglect: A status report. *Journal of Pediatric Nursing, 13*(2), 28.

Chiocca, E. M. (1998). The nurse's role in the prevention of child abuse and neglect. *Journal of Pediatric Nursing, 13*(3), 194.
Cookfair, J. M. (1996). *Nursing care in the community* (2nd ed.). St. Louis, MO: Mosby.
Curley, M. A., Smith, J. B., & Maloney-Harmon, P. (1996). *Critical care nursing of infants and children.* Philadelphia: Saunders.
Dubowitz, M., & King, H. (1995). Family violence: A child-centered family centered approach. *Pediatric Clinics of North America, 42,* 153.
Huston, C. J. (1998). Emergency! Cervical spine injury. *American Journal of Nursing, 98*(6), 33.
Ladebauche, P. (1997). Childhood trauma: When to suspect abuse. *RN, 60*(9), 38.
Mankin, K. P., & Zimbler, S. (11/97). Gait and leg alignment: What's normal and what's not. *Contemporary Pediatrics, 14*(11), 41.
Thomas R., & Taylor, K. (1997). Assessing head injuries in children. *MCN, 22*(4), 198.
Ulione, M. S. (1997). Health promotion and injury prevention in a child development center. *Journal of Pediatric Nursing, 12*(3), 148.
Unkila-Kallio, L., Kallio, M., et al. (1994). Serum-C reactive protein, ESR + WBC count in acute hematogenous osteomylites of children. *Pediatrics, 93,* 59.
Wong, D. (1997). *Whaley & Wong's essentials of pediatric nursing* (5th ed.). St. Louis, MO: Mosby.

chapter 25

The Child with a Respiratory or Cardiovascular Disorder

Outline

Objectives

On completion and mastery of Chapter 25, the student will be able to

- Define or identify each vocabulary term listed.
- Distinguish the differences between the respiratory tract of the infant and the adult.
- Describe the normal process of respiration.
- Identify three methods of preventing the spread of infection.
- Review the signs and symptoms of respiratory distress in infants and children.
- Discuss the nursing care of a child with pneumonia.
- Compare bedrest for a toddler with bedrest for an adult.
- Discuss the nursing care of a child with croup.
- Describe the treatment and nursing care of an infant with RSV.
- Recall the characteristic manifestations of allergic rhinitis.
- Recognize the precautions involved in the care of a child diagnosed with epiglottitis.
- Assess the control of environmental exposure to allergens in the home of a child with asthma.
- Express five goals of asthma therapy.
- Interpret the role of sports and physical exercise for the asthmatic child.
- Examine the prevention of SIDS.
- Recall four nursing goals in the care of a child with cystic fibrosis.
- Review the prevention of bronchopulmonary dysplasia.
- Discuss the postoperative care of a 5-year-old who has had a tonsillectomy.

(Continued)

Objectives (Continued)

- Devise a nursing care plan for the child with cystic fibrosis, including family interventions.
- List the general signs and symptoms of congenital heart disease.
- Differentiate among patent ductus arteriosus, coarctation of the aorta, atrial septal defect, ventricular septal defect, and tetralogy of Fallot.
- Discuss six nursing goals relevant to the child with heart disease.
- Discuss hypertension in childhood.
- Differentiate between primary and secondary hypertension.
- List the symptoms of rheumatic fever.
- Discuss the prevention of rheumatic fever.
- Describe a heart-healthy diet for a child over 2 years of age.
- Identify factors that can prevent hypertension.

Vocabulary

anastomosis	oxygen narcosis
carditis	polyarthritis
chorea	polycythemia
clubbing of fingers	pulse pressure
coryza	pursed-lip breathing
croupette	RAD (Reactive Airway Disease)
diaphragmatic hernia	shunt
dysphagia	status asthmaticus
heart defect	stenosis
heart failure	surfactant
hemodynamics	tachycardia
hyperlipidemia	tachypnea
hypothermia	"tet" spells
Jones criteria	tetralogy of Fallot
laryngeal spasm	thoracotomy
laryngomalacia	ventilation
meconium ileus	

RESPIRATORY SYSTEM

Development of the Respiratory Tract

Pulmonary structures differentiate in an orderly fashion during fetal life. This makes it possible to determine at what point a particular defect may have occurred. The laryngotracheal groove appears at 2 to 4 weeks of gestation. The trachea and the esophagus originate as one hollow tube and gradually, by the 4th week of fetal life, a septum forms to completely separate them. If the septum fails to form completely, a tracheoesophageal fistula occurs (see p. 723). By the 7th week of fetal life, the diaphragm forms and separates the chest from the abdominal cavity. If the diaphragm fails to close completely, a *diaphragmatic hernia* allows the abdominal contents (intestines, spleen, stomach) to enter the chest cavity and prevents the lungs from expanding fully. Alveoli and capillaries, necessary for gas exchange in the human body, are formed between the 24th and 28th weeks of fetal life. At the 24th week, the formed alveolar cells produce *surfactant.* (Surfactant prevents the alveoli from collapsing during respirations after birth.) A premature birth is therefore accompanied by problems with respiratory gas exchange. During fetal life, the lungs are filled with a fluid that has a low surface tension and viscosity and is rapidly absorbed after birth. Spontaneous respiratory movements occur in the fetus, although gas exchange occurs in the placenta. When surfactant is present in the lungs, the respiratory movements force some of the surfactant into the amniotic fluid. Surfactant is composed of *lecithin* and *sphingomyelin.* As the fetus matures, at about 35 weeks of fetal life, the lecithin component is twice that of the sphingomyelin. The analysis of the lecithin/sphingomyelin ratio (L/S ratio) by amniocentesis (see Chapter 5) is a method of determining fetal maturity and the ability of the fetus to survive outside the uterus.

Normal Respiration. The process of normal respiration is described in Figure 25–1.

Ventilation. *Ventilation,* the process of breathing air into and out of the lungs, is affected by several elements that interact:

- *Intercostal muscles, diaphragm, ribs.* These allow chest expansion and contraction. (Expansion of the chest lowers pressure in the chest cavity and air flows from higher pressure of the atmosphere into lower pressure of chest cavity. The opposite occurs during expiration.)
- *Brain.* The vagus nerve and the respiratory centers in the medulla of the brain regulate rhythmic respiratory movements. Signals sent to the respiratory center will increase or decrease respiratory rates.
- *Chemoreceptors.* These sensors respond to changes in the oxygen saturation in the blood by sending a signal to the pons, which is stimulated to increase respirations when the oxygen (O_2) saturation is low.

Note: A high carbon dioxide (CO_2) level in the blood and a low O_2 saturation stimulate the brain to increase the respiratory rate. However, in chronic lung disease, the receptors become tolerant to the high CO_2 and low O_2 concentration in the blood. Administration of supplemental oxygen increases the O_2 saturation level and may result in a decreased respiratory effort *(oxygen narcosis)* leading to respiratory failure. The differences between the respiratory tract of the growing child and that of the adult are shown in Table 25–1.

Procedures that may be performed on the child with a respiratory condition include throat and nasopharyngeal cultures, bronchoscopy, lung biopsy, arterial blood gas (Po_2, Pco_2) and pH analysis, pulse oximetry, transcutaneous monitoring, and various pulmonary function tests (PFTs). Chest x-ray films, computed tomography, radioisotope scan, bronchogram, and angiography may prove useful, depending on symptoms. The inspection, percussion, and auscultation procedures done by the nurse are of utmost value.

Nasopharyngitis

Description. A cold, also known as acute *coryza,* is the most common infection of the respiratory tract. It is caused by one or a number of viruses, principally the *rhinoviruses,* which are spread from one child to another by sneezing, coughing, and direct contact. The age, state of nutrition, and general health of the child contribute to the susceptibility level.

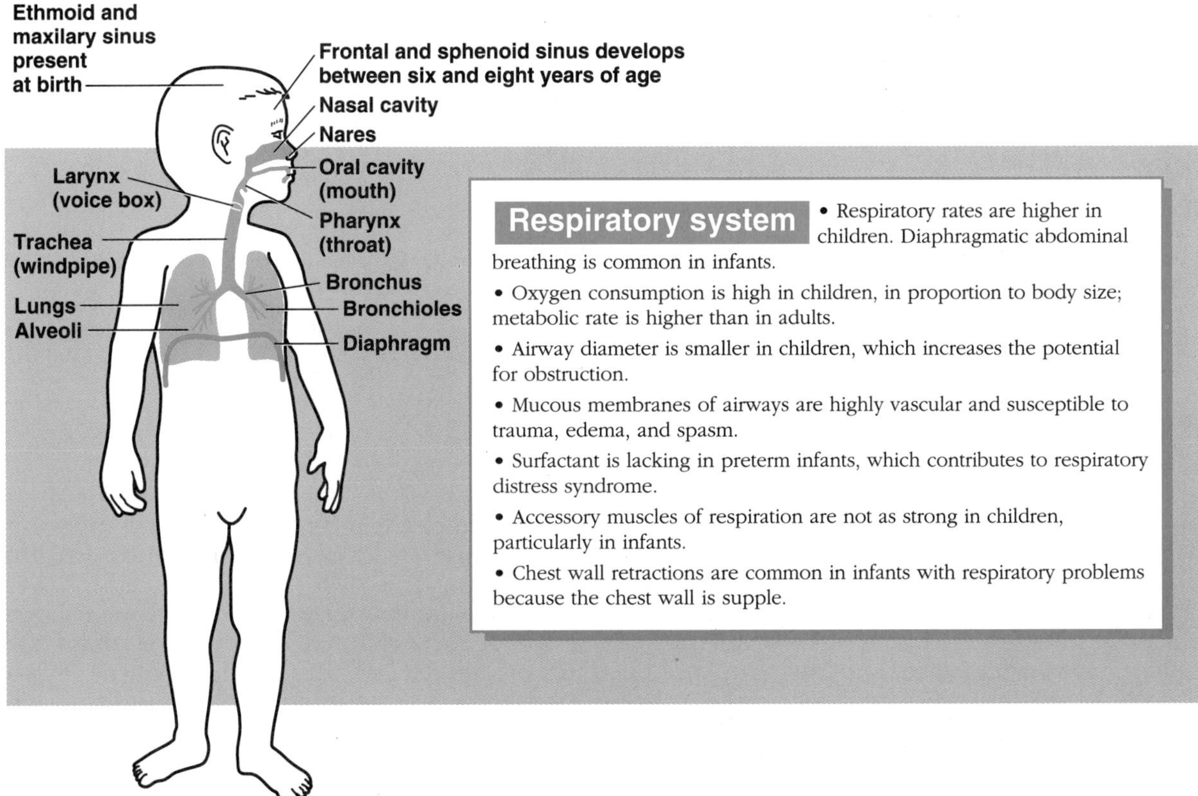

Figure 25–1. • Summary of respiratory features in children. The ribs and the diaphragm allow for inspiration of air. Air enters the body through the *nares,* or nostrils. The mucous membranes and cilia that line the respiratory tract warm, moisten, and filter the air as it passes to the *pharynx.* The pharynx contains the tonsils, which assist in infection control. The *larynx* at the upper end of the trachea contains the epiglottis, glottis and vocal cords, which prevent food and fluids from entering the trachea and allow voice sounds. The *trachea* is encircled by smooth muscle and cartilage to maintain patency and carries the air to the bronchi and then to the smaller bronchioles. The bronchioles continue to divide and lead to small, thin airsacs (alveoli) that are kept open on inspiration by the air contained in them. During expiration when the air sacs collapse, *surfactant* prevents the walls from sticking together, allowing for reinflation. Gas exchange occurs in the alveoli by diffusion to the bloodstream. The volume of air inhaled with each breath is related to body size.

Table 25–1
DIFFERENCES IN THE RESPIRATORY TRACT OF THE GROWING CHILD AND THAT OF THE ADULT

How Infant Differs from Adult	Significance
The infant relies primarily on abdominal muscles and the diaphragm for breathing. The intercostal muscles only stabilize the chest wall	Assessment of respiration is best accomplished by monitoring the rise and fall of the abdomen until 3 years of age when thoracic breathing begins. Adult-type breathing patterns are developed by 7 years of age Substernal retraction is a sign of respiratory distress in infants
In infants, the diaphragm is attached higher than in the adult and is stretched longer, limiting its ability to contract forcefully	Abdominal distention from formula or gas can interfere with movement of the diaphragm
The infant depends on the accessory muscles for respiratory efforts	Muscle fatigue can result in respiratory arrest
Infants are nose breathers and do not breathe through the mouth unless crying	Swelling of the nasal mucosa will interfere with sucking and cause irritability
In infants, tissue below the vocal cords is not firm and portions of the larynx are very narrow	Any edema or swelling can cause respiratory obstruction
The cartilage maintaining patency of the airway in infants is soft and not firm	Vagal nerve stimulation or muscle constriction can cause collapse of the airway and respiratory obstruction
The larynx and trachea are higher in the chest in infancy and descend slowly as the child grows	Positioning the infant or child for airway clearance and resuscitation is different than for adults. Excess flexion or extension of neck can cause respiratory obstruction
Alveoli in the lung divide and thin as the child grows and develops, resulting in increased surface area for gas exchange. The number of alveoli present at puberty is 9 times that of the infant	Less surface area in the alveoli is available for gas exchange, predisposing infants and young children to respiratory distress
Lung growth is inhibited by phenobarbital and excess insulin	Drugs and disease can inhibit lung development
Infants and young children have a small airway diameter	Edema or muscle spasm can rapidly cause respiratory obstruction
Newborns and infants produce less respiratory mucus (which serves as a cleansing agent)	Infants and children are more susceptible to respiratory infections
Infants have less developed smooth-muscle lining the airway than older children and adults	Bronchospasm may not occur in infants, and therefore wheezing may not be a presenting sign of a narrowed airway
In infants, the respiratory rate is higher and the breathing pattern is irregular	Meaningful assessment of respiration must be related to the age of the patient. Irregular respirations with short periods of apnea is normal for a young infant but abnormal in an adult

As the child becomes exposed to more children, the number of colds contracted increases. Parents may notice this, particularly during the child's first few years of day care or school because the child has had little opportunity to build up resistance. In temperate climates, the incidence of rhinoviral infection peaks in September and again in April or May, whereas in the tropics, peak occurrence occurs during the rainy season.

To prevent a cold the child's exposure to those with this virus is avoided to the extent possible. The rhinovirus is spread by contact with contaminated fingers touching the conjunctiva of the eyes or mucous membranes of the mouth. Routine handwashing practices, especially before rubbing the nose or sucking the fingers, can prevent the spread of the common cold.

The common cold differs from allergic rhinitis in that a child who has allergic rhinitis has no fever, purulent nasal discharge, or reddened mucous membranes. Sneezing, watery eyes, and itching are the primary manifestations of *allergic rhinitis.* In the older child or adolescent, persistent nasopharyngitis may be related to inhaled cocaine or other drug abuse.

Manifestations. The symptoms of a cold in an infant or small child are different from those in an adult. Children's air passages are smaller and more easily obstructed. The virus causes inflammation and edema of the membranes of the upper respiratory tract that damage cilia and prevent the drainage of mucous. Fever as high as 40° C (104° F) is not uncommon in children under 3 years of age. Nasal discharge, irritability, sore throat, cough, and general discomfort are present, and there may be vomiting and diarrhea. The diagnosis is complicated by the fact that many infectious diseases resemble the common cold during their onset. Complications of a cold include bronchitis, pneumonitis, and ear infections.

Treatment and Nursing Care. There is no cure for the common cold. When a cold is suspected, treatment should begin early. The treatment is designed to relieve the symptoms.

- *Rest.* Fatigue should be avoided. Confinement to bed for a child does not always result in physical rest. Bedrest in pediatrics means providing play therapy that promotes minimal activity. Watching TV on the couch, or playing quietly on a padded floor, may be more effective than jumping on the bed mattress. The nurse should consider the age and developmental level of the child and the activity level involved in the play when designing appropriate activities and guiding parents in the home care of their child.
- *Clean airways.* Congested nasal passages cause discomfort and prevent sucking of formula. Since fluid consumption is essential to prevent fever and dehydration, the airways need to be cleaned before feeding and before bedtime to provide a restful sleep. The nurse can teach the parents that instilling a few drops of saline into the nose and then suctioning with a bulb syringe (Chapter 12, Fig. 12–8) is the best way to clear the nostrils. Phenylephrine 0.125–0.25% may be instilled into the nose 15 to 20 minutes before bedtime. Stronger nosedrops or medicated nosedrops can be irritating to the mucosa of a young child's nasal passages. Nosedrops with an oily base should be avoided as they are readily aspirated and can cause problems. Rebound congestion will be avoided by limiting nose drop use to no more than 3 days.
- *Adequate fluid intake.* Anorexia is common in children with nasopharyngitis. Fluids should be encouraged to prevent dehydration. Cool, bland liquids are usually tolerated well in a child who has a sore throat.
- *Prevention of fever.* Ibuprofen (Motrin) or acetaminophen (Tylenol) can be administered when a high fever accompanies a cold. Parents should be cautioned to check the label of the medication for appropriate dosages. The safe dosage for Tylenol *elixir* differs from that of Tylenol *drops.*
- *Skin care.* A petroleum-based ointment can be applied to the nares and the upper lip to prevent skin irritation from a nasal discharge.

Moist air soothes the inflamed nose and throat. An electric cold air humidifier is safe and convenient. It must be cleaned and disinfected regularly. If a great deal of moisture is indicated, as in croup, the infant may be taken to a small room, such as the bathroom, and the hot water faucets or shower can be turned on to produce sufficient steam.

The older child is taught the proper way to remove nasal secretions from the nose. The mouth is opened slightly and secretions are gently blown through both nostrils at the same time. This method prevents infection from being forced into the eustachian tubes. Children must be taught to cover the mouth and nose when sneezing and to wash their hands afterward. Tissues must be properly discarded. Antibiotics are not effective against the common cold.

Acute Pharyngitis

Acute pharyngitis is an inflammation of the structures in the throat. This infection is common among children between ages 5 and 15. In 80% of cases the causative organism is a virus. Group-A beta-hemolytic streptococcus (strep throat) occurs in 20% of the cases. In children under age 3, the bacterium *Haemophilus influenzae* is common.

Manifestations, Treatment, and Nursing Care. Symptoms include fever, malaise, dysphagia (*dys,* "difficult," and *phagia,* "swallowing"), and anorexia. It is difficult to distinguish viral from bacterial types by symptoms only. Conjunctivitis, rhinitis, cough, and hoarseness with a gradual onset and persisting no longer than 5 days are characteristic of viral pharyngitis. In a child over 2 years of age, streptococcal pharyngitis characteristically includes high fever (104° F, or 40° C), difficulty in swallowing, and may last longer than 1 week. In children 6 months to 2 years of age, a postnasal discharge, fever, vomiting, anorexia, and enlarged tender cervical lymph nodes follows a course that may lead to complications. A strep throat is determined by throat culture. When the culture is positive, antimicrobial therapy (penicillin) is administered. It is prescribed orally for 10 days. Compliance is a problem; therefore, the nurse carefully explains to parents the need for the child to finish all of the medication. If the child is allergic to penicillin, erythromycin may be used. Acetaminophen (Tylenol) may be taken to relieve soreness of the throat. If the child is old enough to gargle, a solution of warm water and salt may be used.

Prompt treatment of strep throat is important to avoid serious complications, such as rheumatic fever, glomerulonephritis, peritonsillar abscess, otitis media, mastoiditis, meningitis, osteomyelitis, or pneumonia. The persistence of positive streptococcal culture after careful follow-up and therapy may indicate that the child is a group-A beta-hemolytic streptococcus carrier. However, it may also mean that the child did not complete the 10-day course of medication or that a penicillin-resistant organism has evolved. The child with strep throat is no longer infectious to others once penicillin therapy has begun.

Croup Syndromes

Description. *Croup* is a general term applied to a number of conditions whose chief symptom is a brassy (croupy) cough and varying degrees of inspiratory stridor (a harsh, high-pitched sound). When the larynx is involved, the clinical picture becomes more intense because of possible alterations in respiratory status, such as airway obstruction, acute respiratory failure, and hypoxia (Fig. 25–2). Acute spasmodic laryngitis is the milder form of the syndrome. Acute laryngotracheobronchitis is the most common. It is also referred to as subglottic croup, as edema occurs below the vocal cords. Croup can be benign or acute. Benign croup is frightening but rarely life threatening. Acute croup can develop into a respiratory emergency.

Benign Crouplike Conditions

Congenital Laryngeal Stridor (Laryngomalacia). Some infants are born with weakness of the airway walls and a floppy epiglottis that causes a stridor (crowlike noise) upon inspiration. There may be inspiratory retractions. The symptoms lessen when the infant is placed prone or propped in the side-lying position. Respiratory infection and crying may cause the symptoms to become frightening to the parents. The condition usually spontaneously clears, as the child grows and the muscles strengthen. The nurse should provide reassurance, suggest slow, small feedings, and a prone or side-lying position for the infant.

Spasmodic Laryngitis (Spasmodic Croup). Spasmodic croup usually occurs in children 1 to 3 years of age and is caused by a virus, allergy, or psychological triggers. Very often, gastroesophageal reflux (GER) will trigger an attack. Spasmodic croup has a sudden onset, usually at night and is characterized by a barking, brassy cough and respiratory distress. The child appears anxious and the parents become frightened. The attack lasts a few hours and by morning the child appears normal and in no distress. Increasing humidity and providing fluids are helpful measures.

Acute Croup

Laryngotracheobronchitis. This viral condition is manifested by edema, destruction of respiratory cilia and exudate, resulting in respiratory obstruction. Usually a mild upper respiratory infection precedes the development of a characteristic barking, or brassy cough. Stridor develops and classic symptoms of respiratory distress follow (see Fig. 25–2). The infant prefers to be held upright or sit up in bed *(orthopnea)*. Crying and agitation worsen the symptoms. Hypoxia can develop, accompanied by tachycardia and diminished breath sounds.

Treatment and Nursing Care. When the child is treated at home, parents are instructed to increase humidity levels around the child. This can be accomplished by using an electric cold water humidifier. The humidifier must be emptied, washed, and

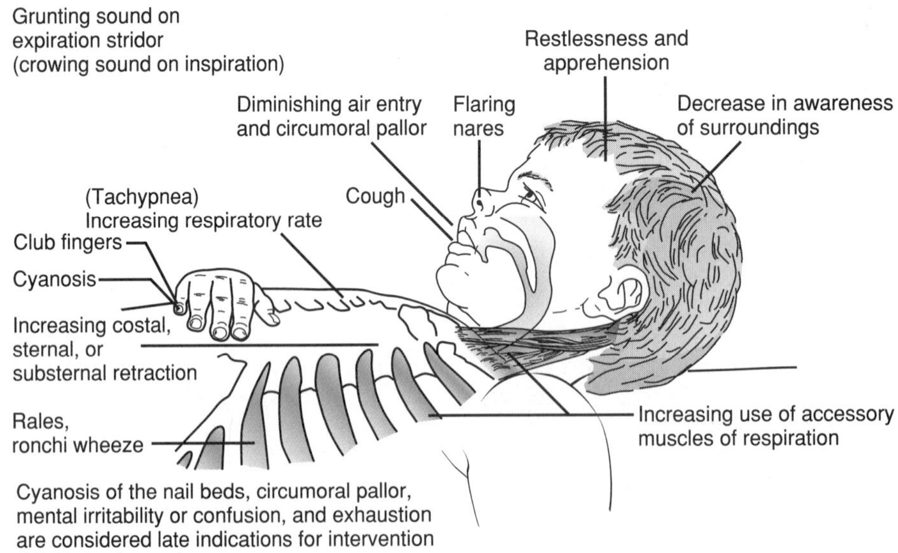

Figure 25–2. • Signs of respiratory distress in infants and children.

Nursing Tip

Respiratory illness is always potentially more serious in children than in adults.

disinfected each day to prevent the growth of microorganisms that occur in stagnant tap water. If parents are unable to obtain a vaporizer, the child can be taken into the bathroom where the hot water in the shower is turned on. The child inhales the moist air and the respiratory distress and laryngeal spasm are usually relieved. When continuing symptoms of respiratory distress require hospitalization the child is placed in a mist tent, or *croupette* (see p. 571). The cool air, well saturated in microdroplets that can enter the small airway of a child, cause mucosal cooling and vasoconstriction, and relieve the respiratory obstruction and distress. Intravenous fluids are prescribed to prevent dehydration and to decrease the risk of vomiting and aspiration that can occur after a coughing episode. Organization of care is essential to enable the child to have long periods of rest. The child will be placed on a cardiorespiratory monitor (CRM) and the vital signs observed closely. Oxygen is given to reduce hypoxia (see p. 571). Oxygen saturation is monitored and saturation levels are maintained above 90% (see Chapter 13, Fig. 13–6 for sensor application). Opiates are contraindicated because they depress respiration. Sedatives are contraindicated because increased restlessness is a primary sign of increased respiratory obstruction, and sedatives will mask signs of restlessness. Frequent racemic epinephrine inhalation therapy may relieve symptoms (Fig. 25–3). Corticosteroids may be prescribed to reduce the edema caused by inflammation and to prevent further destruction of ciliated epithelium. In some intensive care units, a helium-oxygen mixture is used to relieve dyspnea.

Epiglottitis

Epiglottitis is a swelling of the tissues *above* the vocal cords, that is, supraglottic swelling. This results in narrowing of the *airway inlet,* with the possibility of total obstruction. It is caused by *H. influenzae* type B and most often occurs in the child of age 3 to 6 years. It can occur in any season. The course is rapid and progressive. *Epiglottitis is a life-threatening medical emergency.* Blood gases fluctuate, and there is leukocytosis.

The onset is abrupt and the child presents with classic symptoms. The child insists on sitting up, leans forward, with the mouth open and drools saliva because of the difficulty in swallowing. The child appears wide-eyed and anxious, restless, and may emit a froglike croaking sound on inspiration. Cough is absent. Inspection of the throat would show an enlarged, reddened edematous epiglottis much like a "beefy-red thumb." However, the examining tongue blade may trigger a laryngo-spasm and result in sudden respiratory arrest. *Therefore it is a primary nursing responsibility to be sure there is a tracheotomy set at the bedside before any examination of the throat is attempted.*

Treatment. The treatment of choice is immediate tracheotomy or endotracheal intubation and oxygen to prevent hypoxia, brain damage, and sudden

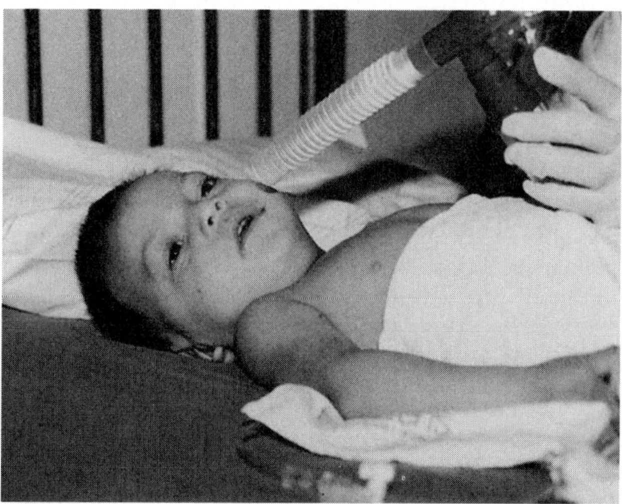

Figure 25–3. • A child receiving aerosol therapy (medicated nebulizer treatments). (From Ashwill, J., & Droske, S. [1997]. *Nursing care of children: Principles and practice.* Philadelphia: Saunders.)

death due to respiratory arrest. Parenteral antibiotic therapy usually results in a dramatic improvement within a few days.

Prevention. The American Academy of Pediatrics recommends that *H. influenzae* type B conjugate vaccines be administered beginning at 2 months of age as part of a regular immunization program for all children. This type of program will result in a decrease in the incidence of acute epiglottitis in children.

Bronchitis

Description. A study of the respiratory system reveals that the air tubes leading to the lungs resemble an upside-down tree. The trachea is the main trunk, with the bronchi, bronchioles, and alveoli as branches. These passages proceed from large to small and are lined with a continuous membrane. If there is an infection of the bronchial tree, it is seldom confined to one area but more often involves other structures.

Acute bronchitis is an infection of the bronchi. It seldom occurs as a primary infection, but is usually secondary to a cold or communicable disease. It is caused by a variety of organisms. Poor nutrition, allergy, and chronic infection of the respiratory tract may precipitate this condition. Most patients are under 4 years old.

Manifestations. A gradual onset of an unproductive "hacking" cough preceded by an upper respiratory infection, or "cold." The cough may become productive with purulent sputum. (Children under 7 years of age cannot voluntarily cough and usually swallow their sputum.)

Treatment. The use of cough suppressants before bedtime may be helpful to promote restful sleep. Antihistamines, cough expectorants, and antibiotics are usually not helpful. Most children recover uneventfully with symptomatic care at home.

Bronchiolitis

Acute bronchiolitis is a viral infection of the small airways (bronchioles) in the lower respiratory tract. It occurs in infants and children 6 months to 2 years of age, with a peak at 6 months of age. The small diameter of the small bronchiole in the infant is susceptible to obstruction when inflammation results in edema and excess mucous. The obstruction often leads to atelectasis. The gas exchange in the lungs becomes impaired and hypoxia occurs.

Manifestations. An upper respiratory infection, or cold, with a mild fever and serous (clear) nasal discharge is followed by the development of a wheezing cough and signs of respiratory distress (see Fig. 25–2). The increase in respiratory rate interferes with successful feeding and the infant becomes irritable and dehydrated. The respiratory syncytial virus (RSV) is the causative organism in 50% of cases. An apneic episode is usually the cause of hospitalization. Infants who have bronchiolitis may develop an hyperreactive airway or asthma later in life.

Treatment and Nursing Care. The treatment of an infant with bronchiolitis is symptomatic and similar to that of the child with croup (see p. 650). A semi-Fowler's position with a slightly hyperextended neck facilitates respirations. Oral feedings are often supplemented by IV fluids. Intake and output are recorded. Antibiotics and steroids have not shown to be effective. Bronchodilating aerosol therapy (Fig. 25–3) and high-humidity tents are prescribed. Frequent assessment of vital signs and monitoring of oxygen saturation levels are essential. If RSV is determined to be the causative agent, specific therapy is prescribed.

Respiratory Syncytial Virus

RSV is responsible for 50% of cases of bronchiolitis in infants and young children and is the most frequent cause of viral pneumonia. RSV is the single most important respiratory pathogen in infancy. RSV occurs worldwide and causes annual epidemics during winter months. Most children are infected with RSV before their fourth birthday, and reinfection is common, especially in children attending day care centers. Infants between 2 and 7 months of age can become seriously ill with this condition because their airways are so small and prone to obstruction by the thick mucus produced. Older children and adults are not as seriously ill and continue to go to work or school, becoming carriers and spreading the infection.

Transmission. RSV is spread by direct contact with respiratory secretions, usually by contaminated hand to mucous membrane (eyes, mouth, nose). RSV survives for more than 6 hours on countertops, tissues, and on a bar of soap. RSV is not spread via the airborne route. The incubation period is approximately 4 days.

Hospital cross infection is a major problem since caregivers may be carrying the organism. For this reason, an infant diagnosed with RSV infection is placed on standard (isolation) precaution to prevent the spread of RSV to other sick children.

RSV immunoglobulin has been used for preterm newborns with bronchopulmonary dysplasia who are at risk for infection. Smoking in the home, woodburning stoves, and kerosene heaters may increase the seriousness of symptoms of RSV bronchiolitis.

Diagnosis. An examination of nasopharyngeal washings for RSV antigens can be done while the child waits in the admitting unit so that the diagnosis is established before the infant is admitted to the pediatric unit.

Treatment and Nursing Care. The care of infants with RSV infection should be assigned to personnel who are not caring for patients at high risk for adverse response to RSV. Infection control techniques (see Appendix A) are employed to prevent the spread of infection to others on the unit. Mask, gown, and gloves are advisable during close contact with infants to prevent fomite spread. Frequent handwashing is essential. Liquid soap dispensers should be available at the sink as the organism survives on a dry bar of soap.

Support Infant and Families. Effective communication skills are necessary to provide support for parents of the infant who is seriously ill. The parent can be familiarized with the mist tent and encouraged to participate in the care and feeding of the infant.

Symptomatic Care. An ineffective breathing pattern is the priority nursing diagnosis for an infant hospitalized with RSV infection. Reporting *tachypnea* (increased respiration) and *tachycardia* (increased heart rate) is essential, as these vital sign changes may be indicative of hypoxemia. Auscultation of breath sounds and reporting wheezing, rales or ronchi are important. A child who has been wheezing and suddenly has a "quiet chest" on auscultation may be at risk of respiratory arrest. The higher pitched the wheeze, the more constricted is the airway. Signs of respiratory distress (Fig. 25–2) should be assessed and reported. Oxygen saturation levels are monitored and oxygen administered at levels needed to maintain a minimum of 90% to 95% saturation. Suctioning of mucus may be required to maintain a patent airway. Monitoring IV fluids and recording intake and output are essential to prevent dehydration. Urine output should be a minimum of 1–2 ml/kg/hr for infants and children. Pedialyte or Ricelyte are clear liquid electrolyte formulas prescribed for infants at risk of dehydration. The child should be weighed daily to detect early signs of dehydration. Inhaled bronchodilators or steroids are not helpful with RSV infections.

Antiviral Medication. Antiviral medication such as Ribovirin™ (virozole) is prescribed for use with severely ill infants or infants who have heart or lung problems that place them at high risk for serious complications. The medication has been found to be effective in the treatment of RSV infection but is rarely used prophylactically because of its serious side effects. Informed consent is usually required before treatment is initiated. The medication is administered by fine-droplet aerosol mist while the infant is in a mist tent. It is administered 18 to 24 hours a day for a minimum of 3 days. If the infant is on a ventilator, the nurse must monitor the ventilator tubes, which may be clogged by Ribovirin. Caregivers and visitors who are of childbearing age, pregnant, or breastfeeding should not care for infants receiving Ribovirin as teratogenic effects have been reported. The Ribovirin mist can cause precipitation on the surface of plastics and therefore caregivers with contact lenses may develop conjunctivitis because of the lens changes. Ribovirin may also act as an irritant to the upper respiratory tract of the caregiver, and therefore limited hours of contact and rotating assignments should be planned. When providing care to an infant receiving Ribovirin therapy, the nurse should turn off the nebulizer and allow the mist to settle before opening the mist tent and providing care. Linen removed from the bed should be slowly rolled and carefully folded to avoid releasing droplets of Ribovirin into the air.

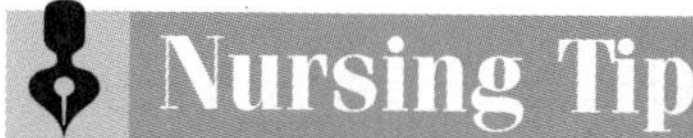

Nursing Tip

Caretakers who are pregnant or wear contact lenses should not give direct care to infants who are receiving Ribovirin aerosol therapy.

Complications. Infants who have a small airway size and are severely ill and hospitalized with RSV infection may be at risk for wheezing and hyperreactivity airway disease (RAD) later in life. Some studies (Martinez et al., 1995) have shown that the inflammation caused by RSV injures the respiratory epithelial cells, resulting in exposed sensory nerve fibers that respond easily to environmental irritants.

Pneumonia

Description. Pneumonia or pneumonitis is an inflammation of the lungs in which the *alveoli* (air sacs) become filled with exudate and surfactant may be reduced. The affected portion of the lung does not receive enough air. Breathing is shallow. As a result, the bloodstream is denied sufficient oxygen.

Pneumonia may occur as the initial or *primary* disease, or it may complicate another illness, in which case it is termed *secondary* pneumonia. Secondary pneumonia may accompany various communicable diseases or may follow surgery. It is more serious than primary pneumonia because the patient is already weak.

There are many types of pneumonia. Classification may be by causative organism (i.e., bacterial or viral) or by the part of the respiratory system involved (i.e., lobar or bronchial). Group B Streptococci is the most common cause of pneumonia in newborns, whereas chlamydia is the most common cause of pneumonia in infants 3 weeks to 3 months of age. The incidence of *H. influenzae* type B infection has been decreasing with current immunization programs. RSV, rhinovirus, adenovirus and pneumococcus are other organisms that are responsible for pneumonia in infants and children. Immunocompromised children may develop pneumonia caused by a gram-negative organism such as *Pneumocystis carinii* or fungi.

Toddlers frequently aspirate small objects such as peanuts or popcorn and develop pneumonia as a result; therefore, such foods are to be discouraged for this age group. *Lipoid* pneumonia occurs when the baby inhales an oil-based substance into the airways. It is less common today as children are seldom given cod liver or castor oil routinely, as they were in the past. Nose drops with an oil base are dangerous. The toddler who drinks kerosene may also develop a type of pneumonia. *Hypostatic* pneumonia may occur in patients who have poor circulation in their lungs and remain in one position too long. The child recovering from anesthesia needs to be turned frequently to stimulate circulation through the lungs. Early ambulation also accomplishes this.

Manifestations. The symptoms of pneumonia vary with the age of the patient and the causative organism. They may develop suddenly or may be preceded by an upper respiratory tract infection. The cough is dry at first, but it gradually becomes productive. Fever rises as high as 39.5° C to 40° C (103° F to 104° F) and may fluctuate widely during a 24-hour period. The respiratory rate may increase (tachypnea) to 40 to 80 breaths/min in infants and to 30 to 50 breaths/min in older children. Respirations are shallow in an attempt to reduce the amount of chest pain. The chest pain may be caused by a pleural irritation or a musculoskeletal irritation from frequent coughing. *Sternal retractions* may be seen when the assisting muscles of respiration are used. The nostrils may flare. The child is listless and has a poor appetite. The child tends to lie on the affected side. X-ray films confirm the diagnosis and determine whether there are complications. A differential white blood cell count is routinely done. Blood specimens show a marked increase in the number of white blood cells (16,000 to 40,000/mm^3). Cultures may be taken from the nose and throat.

Treatment. Treatment depends on the causative organism. Antipyretics are given to reduce fever. Oxygen is administered for dyspnea or cyanosis. When this treatment is begun early, the child is less restless and does not require as many sedatives or drugs to relieve pain. Since drug therapy has become so effective, many uncomplicated cases can be treated at home. Fluid intake should be increased, particularly clear fluids and "flattened" soft drinks. In infants younger than 6 months (Erythromycin Sulfisoxazole) Pediazole or Bactrim may be prescribed, but Amoxicillin is the drug of choice for children up to 5 years of age. Augmentin may be prescribed for *H. influenzae* type B (Hib) disease. Children who are allergic to penicillins will be treated with cephalosporins such as Suprax (cefixime). Rest, fluids, and a cough suppressant prior to bedtime are the basics of home care. Parent education concerning the need to complete all medication prescribed is essential. Tobacco use in the environment should be avoided and the need for Hib immunizations stressed. The use and disposal of tissues, covering the mouth during a cough, and modeling of proper handwashing techniques are preventative measures the nurse should teach the family.

Nursing Care. Nursing care in all types of pneumonia is basically the same. The age of the patient determines the nurse's approach and the type of equipment used. (The newborn receives oxygen in the isolette, whereas the older child requires a croupette or a larger tent.) Rest is an important part of the treatment. The nurse must be organized so that the child is not disturbed unnecessarily. Planned, quiet activities for the child are recommended (Fig. 25–4).

The nurse checks the vital signs at regular intervals. During the acute stages, the temperature may rise as high as 39.5° C to 40° C (103° F to 104° F). When a child is flushed with fever, *heavy clothing and blankets should be removed.* The nurse encourages the child to take fluids, flavored ice pops, or small sips of water frequently. If vomiting persists, parenteral fluids are given.

Tonsillitis and Adenoiditis

Description. The tonsils and adenoids, located in the pharynx (throat), are made of lymph tissue and are part of the body's defense mechanism against infection. The symptoms of tonsillitis includes difficulty in swallowing and breathing. Enlarged adenoids block the nasal passage, resulting

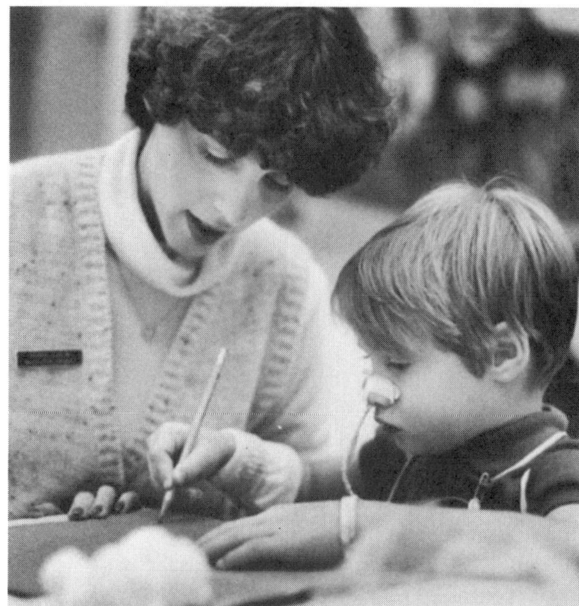

Figure 25–4. • Planned quiet activities help the hospitalized child to gain self-control following invasive procedures. (Courtesy of Blank Memorial Hospital for Children, Des Moines, IA.)

in mouth breathing. Other symptoms are similar to those of nasopharyngitis. Nursing care involves providing a cool mist vaporizer to keep the mucous membranes moist, salt water gargles, throat lozenges (if age appropriate), cool, liquid diet, and Tylenol® to promote comfort. Antibiotics are not usually prescribed unless a throat culture is positive for the streptococcal organism.

Treatment. The removal of the tonsils and adenoids, referred to as a "T&A," is usually not recommended for the child under 3 years of age. It is thought that if surgery is postponed, the condition may correct itself, since the tissues become smaller as the child grows. A *tonsillectomy* (removal of the palatine tonsils) is indicated only if persistent airway obstruction or difficulty in breathing occurs. The surgery is not performed during an acute infectious episode as inflamed tissue responds poorly to surgery.

Children are prepared for the surgery with age-appropriate explanations. Wording should be carefully selected, as young children may associate being "put to sleep" for the operation with their sick pet being "put to sleep" and never heard from again. Same-day surgery is the usual setting for tonsillectomy and the child returns home after a few hours. The presence of loose teeth should be reported to the anesthesiologist as there may be a danger of aspiration during the surgical procedure. Identification bands are applied and routine preop care initiated and documented.

Nursing Tip

After a tonsillectomy, milk and milk products may coat the throat and cause the child to clear his throat and further irritate the operative site.

Postoperative Care. Immediately following surgery, to facilitate drainage, the child is placed partly on the side and partly on the abdomen, with the knee of the uppermost leg flexed to hold the position. The child is watched carefully for evidence of bleeding, that is, an increase in pulse and respirations, restlessness, frequent swallowing (which may be from blood trickling down the back of the child's throat), and vomiting of bright red blood. An ice collar may be applied for comfort. The child's face and hands are wiped with a warm face cloth, and the hospital gown and linen are changed whenever necessary. Small amounts of clear liquids are given as tolerated. Synthetic fruit juices are used because they are not as irritating as natural juices. Red- or brown-colored juices are avoided as they make it difficult to evaluate the content of emesis and the presence of blood. A popsicle may appeal to the child. If these are well tolerated, progression to a soft diet is begun. The child is kept quiet for the remainder of the day. A small child may nestle on a parent's lap. Coughing, clearing the throat, and blowing the nose are avoided to decrease the risk of precipitating bleeding at the operative site. Appropriate pain relief is important and will minimize crying, which may further irritate the throat. Hemorrhage is the most common postoperative complication. The nurse should not assume that because surgery is minor it does not involve certain risks.

Written instructions are given to the parents when the child is discharged. The child should be kept quiet for a few days and should receive nourishing fluids and soft foods. After this, children may continue to take a nap or to have a rest period so that they have sufficient convalescent time. Acetaminophen (Tylenol) may be given to reduce throat discomfort. The child needs to be protected from exposure to infections. Gargling and highly seasoned food should be avoided during the first postoperative week.

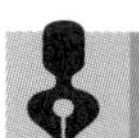

Nursing Tip

Frequent swallowing while the child is sleeping is an early sign of bleeding after a tonsillectomy.

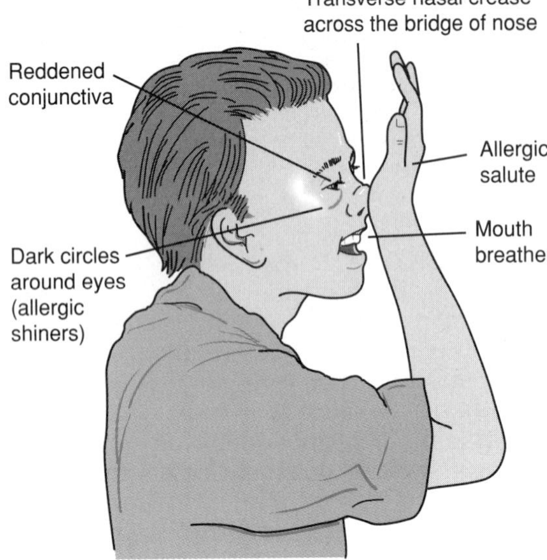

Figure 25–5. • The allergic salute. Signs of allergic rhinitis include a typical rubbing of the nose in response to nasal discharge *(allergic salute),* darkened circles under the eyes (allergic shiners) due to an obstruction of lymphatic and vein flow, and a *transverse crease* across the bridge of the nose resulting from the allergic salutes.

Allergic Rhinitis

Allergic rhinitis is an inflammation of the nasal mucosa caused by an allergic response. It often occurs during specific seasons and is referred to as *hay fever.* Allergic rhinitis is not a life-threatening condition and does not require hospitalization, but it occurs in 10% of children and accounts for many school absentee days.

Pathophysiology. The mast cells in the nasal mucosa respond to an antigen by releasing mediators such as histamine that cause edema and increased mucous secretion. A generalized parasympathetic response can follow. The child has a genetic predisposition to develop the allergy and exposure to the allergen triggers the response.

Manifestations. The characteristic signs of allergic rhinitis include nasal congestion, a clear watery nasal discharge, sneezing, and itching of the eyes (Fig. 25–5).

Diagnosis. Lab tests of the mucus membranes of the nose reveal presence of eosinophils, and skin testing may be positive for specific allergens (skin sensitization testing). The history shows a seasonal occurrence, a family history of allergy or asthma, typical appearance (Fig. 25–5), and absence of fever or purulent drainage.

Treatment. Symptomatic treatment revolves around the use of antihistamine (nonsedating) medications and decongestants to reduce edema of nasal mucous membranes. Topical medications should not be used because of a "rebound effect" that occurs with long-term use. Prophylactic therapy with cromolyn inhalants or glucocortioid nasal sprays may be prescribed if antihistamines are not effective, but this type of medication requires daily dosing and parent and child compliance. Immunotherapy for identified allergens may be prescribed. The main goals of the nurse are to help the parent to identify the difference between the allergy and a cold and provide referral for medical care and support during the long-term allergy testing and immunotherapy process. Teaching the family about controlling the environmental exposure to allergens is very important. Dust control, prevention of contact with animal dander, the use of air conditioners and high-efficiency particulate air (HEPA) filters in the home and the planning of vacation locales that

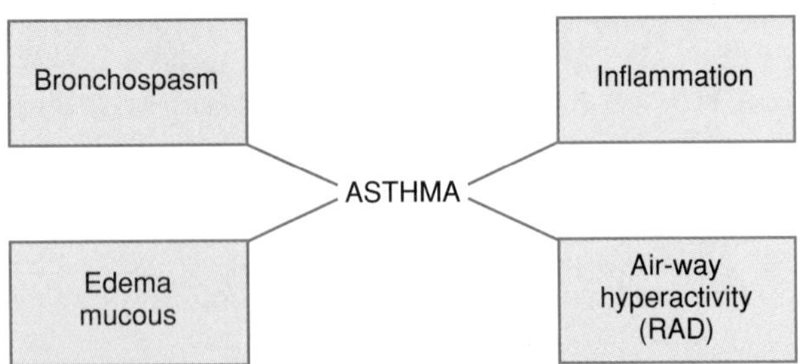

Figure 25–6. • There are four main components of asthma and the medication prescribed by the doctor is specifically designed to deal with the component manifested by the individual child. Inhaled corticosteroids may be prescribed for children with RAD, whereas inhaled bronchodilator is the treatment of choice for bronchospasm. A child with asthma can manifest one or more of the components of the asthma syndrome.

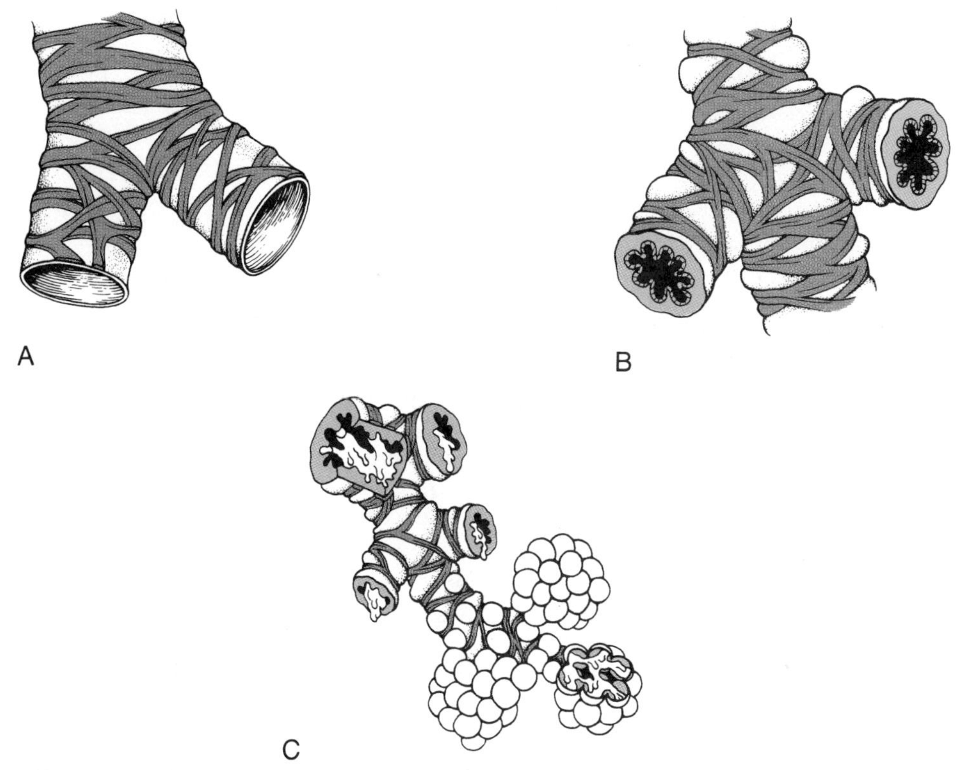

Figure 25–7. • Obstruction of bronchial asthma. **A,** Cross-section of normal bronchi. **B,** Asthmatic bronchi. **C,** Constriction, inflammation, and increased production of mucus.

do not present pollen challenges are some of the vital issues to discuss with the family.

Asthma

Description. Asthma is a *syndrome* (Fig. 25–6), caused by increased responsiveness of the tracheobronchial tree to various stimuli that results in reversible, *paroxysmal* (intermittent) constriction of the airways. The term *asthma* is a Greek word for panting or breathlessness. Asthma is the principal cause of chronic illness in children. It is the leading cause of school absenteeism, emergency room visits, and hospitalization. Although it may occur at any age, about 80% of asthma sufferers have their first symptoms before 5 years of age. Prior to puberty, about twice as many boys as girls are affected; thereafter, the sex incidence is equal.

Asthma is a recurrent and reversible obstruction of the airways in which bronchospasm, mucosal edema, and secretion and plugging of mucus contribute to significant narrowing of the airways and subsequent impaired gas exchange (Fig. 25–7). Both large and small airways may be involved. The onset of asthma may be triggered by house dust, animal dander, wool, feathers, pollen, mold, passive smoking, strong odors (as from wet paint, wood stoves, fireplaces), and certain foods. Vigorous physical activity, especially in cold weather, may precipitate an attack, as may rapid changes in temperature and humidity. Viral infections are also responsible. Emotional upsets, which affect smooth-muscle and vasomotor tone (*vas,* "vessel," and *motor,* "mover"), are closely intertwined with the condition. Whatever the precipitating cause, the response of the airways is similar. As the attack worsens, arterial blood gases change. P_{CO_2} rises and the blood pH falls, increasing respiratory acidosis and producing a strain on the heart. Children who are prone to allergies often develop asthma. Some children who suffer from infantile eczema (see p. 776) develop asthma as they grow older. A family history of allergies is often seen.

Diagnosis. A history, physical exam, and a response to bronchodilator therapy are the first diagnostic tools. An elevated eosinophil blood level is typical. Eosinophils in the sputum are also diagnostic. Allergy skin testing and a radioallergosorbent test (RAST) are measures that can identify sensitivity to allergens. Exercise testing and pulmonary function tests help to diagnose asthma and to assess progress of the syndrome.

Asthma is rarely diagnosed in infancy; the increased susceptibility of infants to respiratory obstruction and dyspnea in response to many different illnesses is due to:

- Decreased smooth muscle of an infant's airway
- Presence of increased mucous glands in the bronchi
- Normally narrow lumen of the normal airway
- Lack of muscle elasticity in the airway
- Fatigue prone and overworked diaphragmatic muscle on which infant respiration depends

The symptom of wheezing in infancy can be due to gastroesophageal reflux (GER), cystic fibrosis, or chronic aspiration often seen in developmentally delayed infants, or it may be a manifestation of a milk or food allergy.

Manifestations. The symptoms of asthma may begin slowly or abruptly. They may be mild, moderate, or severe. Obstruction is most severe during expiration as the airways become smaller during this phase of respiration (see Fig. 25–7). The trapped air in the lung causes hyperinflation and results in increased effort for breathing.

This can eventually put a strain on the heart. The hypoxia and resulting acidosis can then cause general pulmonary vasoconstriction that damages alveoli, decreases surfactant, and causes a chronic respiratory problem. In acute episodes, the patient coughs, wheezes, and has *difficulty breathing, particularly during expiration.* The child may complain that his or her chin, neck, or chest itches. Signs of air hunger, such as flaring of the nostrils, and use of the accessory muscles of respiration, that is, chest and abdominal muscles, may be evident. Orthopnea appears. The child is restless, perspires, and sometimes complains of abdominal pain. Pulse and respirations are increased, and rales, abnormal respiratory sounds, may be heard in the chest. Inflammation of the nose and sinuses may accompany asthma. The ability to participate in activities decreases.

These attacks often happen during the night and are frightening for both the child and parents. Repeated attacks over a long period may lead to emphysema. Chronic asthma is manifested by discoloration beneath the eyes (allergic shiners), slight eyelid eczema, and mouth breathing (Fig. 25–5).

Treatment and Long-Term Management. (See Box 25–1.) The main goals of asthma therapy are to:

- Maintain a near-normal pulmonary function
- Maintain a near-normal activity level
- Prevent chronic signs and symptoms
- Prevent exacerbations that require hospital treatment
- Prevent adverse responses to medication
- Promote self-care and monitoring consistent with developmental level

Medications. Bronchodilators or antiinflammatory agents may be prescribed.

Bronchodilators. Ventolin, Proventil (albuterol), Alupent (metaproterenol), and (Terbutaline) brethaire are examples of bronchodilators used for long-term management of asthma in children. The drug is inhaled with the aide of a metered dose inhaler (MDI). If a child has difficulty coordinating or inhaling the dose, a spacer device can be added. The nurse should teach the family how to use the devices and the precautions concerning frequency of doses. Theophylline is given orally, usually at night, in a liquid, tablet, or powder form that is sprinkled on a teaspoon of applesauce. The nurse should observe for signs of theophylline toxicity, which include restlessness, tremor, headache, tachycardia, abdominal pain, hypotension and diuresis and instruct the patient and family about drug–drug interactions (Table 25–2). Periodic serum levels must be taken to ensure safety. Toxicity can lead to convulsions and death. The family must be taught to tell the health care provider when the last dose of theophylline had been given when seeking medical care for asthma problems.

Antiinflammatory Drugs. *Cromolyn sodium* (Intal) is a nonsteroidal, antiinflammatory medication that is inhaled (Spinhaler). It's use is a *prophylactic,* or preventative. It cannot be used as a therapeutic drug for emergency care of respiratory distress. Intal is prescribed prior to exercise if a child has exercise-induced asthma to enable the child to participate in the activity. Daily doses are prescribed to ensure an adequate blood level. *Nedocromil* (Tilade), another *antiinflammatory,* may be prescribed. *Corticosteroids* are steroid, antiinflammatory medications that decrease inflammation. Inhaled preparations have less side effects than oral preparations and are used when bronchodilators are not effective. An increased appetite and euphoria are side effects of steroids.

Slow inhalation of an inhaled drug enables the drug to reach the lower airway. Rapid inhalation loses some of the dose, which is deposited on the sides of the pharynx. Nebulized inhalation therapy (med-nebs) is administered by the respiratory therapist in the hospital. Home care units are available (Fig. 25–3).

Nursing Care. The general control of environment is explained to the child and family. Avoiding

BOX 25–1
MANAGEMENT OF ASTHMA

Appropriate drug therapy Follow-up care Routine immunizations Influenza vaccine	Patient education	Measurement of lung function Environmental control of allergens and irritants

pet dander, mold, smoking, and dust is essential. Stuffed toys are not desirable. Humidity in living areas of the house should be controlled between 25% and 50%, as excess humidity (above 50%) promotes mold growth. Dust collectors, such as carpets, upholstery, or drapes should not be in the bedroom of an asthmatic child. Mattress covers, foam rubber pillows, and cotton blankets are preferred. Wool, down, and feather stuffed items should be avoided. Upholstery, drapes, and carpets can be sprayed every 3 months with 3% tannic acid or benzyl benzoate (acarasan) to kill dust mites, followed by cleaning and vacuuming. The use of HEPA filters in the bedroom and in the vacuum is advisable. Children can be taught to monitor their own lung function with the use of a peak flowmeter at home (Fig. 25–8). Involvement in self-care aids in compliance and results in better control of asthmatic symptoms.

Very often the parents and teachers exclude the child from physical activity in school because of the fear of triggering an asthmatic attack. School personnel must be taught by the school nurse the types of activities that are best tolerated by the asthmatic child. Swimming is best tolerated probably because of the high humidity in the air inhaled and the exhaling of air underwater is similar to "purse lip" exhaling. Sports such as baseball, short sprints, and gymnastics are well tolerated because the activity is intense but short. Intense activity that is prolonged, such as jogging, lap running, race running, or basketball is less tolerated by the asthmatic. Preexercise puffs of Intal and a warm-up before vigorous exercise can enable the child to participate more fully in age-appropriate school physical exercise. Many Olympic athletes have successfully managed their asthma symptoms. The promotion of normal growth and development is a basic goal in asthma care and participation with peers is important.

In more severe attacks the child is hospitalized.

Table 25–2
ASTHMA DRUG INTERACTIONS

Asthma Drug	Interacting Substance	Effect
Ephedrine	Antihypertensive drugs	Decrease antihypertensive effects
	Antidepressants (monoamine oxidase inhibitors [MAOIs] such as marplan, Nardil, Parnate	Can cause rise in blood pressure
	Antacids	Increases serum level of ephedrine
	Ammonium chloride expectorant	Reduces effectiveness of ephedrine
	Steroids	Lessen steroid effectiveness
Epinephrine	Antidepressants (tricyclic, e.g., Tofronil, Elavil) and MAOIs	Can cause tachycardia; high blood pressure, and cardiac arrhythmia
	B-adrenergic blockers such as Inderal (propranolol)	Can cause high blood pressure
	Digitalis	Can cause cardiac arrhythmia
Theophylline	Zyloprim (allopurinol)	Can cause tachycardia and zyloprim toxicity
	Antibiotics (Erythromycin)	Can cause theophylline toxicity
	Antibacterials (Cipro)	
	Rifampin	Decreases effectiveness of theophylline
	Tagamet (cimetidine)	Can cause theophylline toxicity
	Dilantin (phenytoin)	Can decrease effect of both drugs
	Phenobarbital	Decreases effect of theophylline
	Ephedrine	Can cause arrhythmia and nervousness
	Beta-blockers, e.g., propranolol (Inderal)	Decreases effect of theophylline
	Oral contraceptives	Can increase theophylline blood levels
	High-fat foods	Increase absorption of theophylline

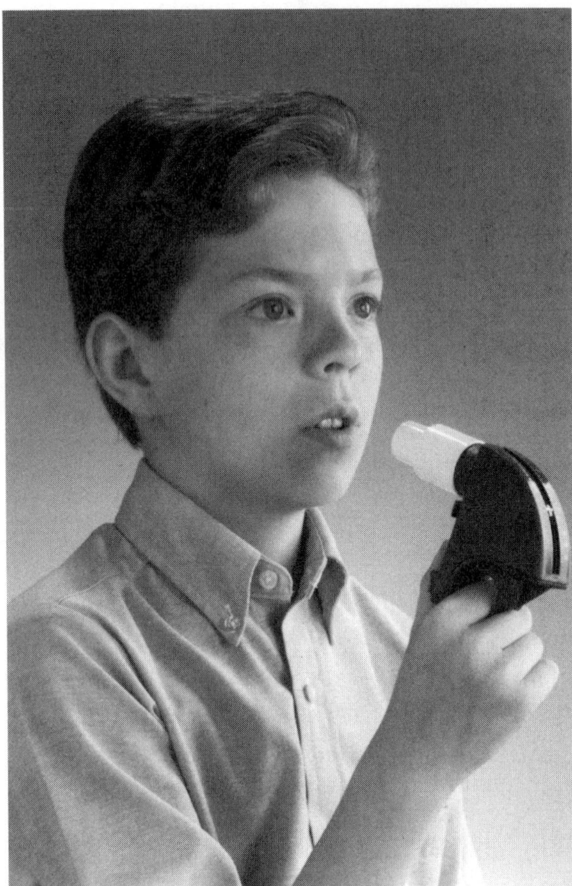

Figure 25–8. • Using the peak flow meter. Assessments should be done daily at home. The reading in the morning should be within 20% of the evening reading. (Courtesy of Ferraris Medical, Inc.)

The nurse limits conversation with the patient during the emergency period to questions that can be answered "yes" or "no." Oxygen will reduce hypoxia and improve the patient's color. It is administered by nasal prongs, hood, or mask.

If the child is in respiratory distress on admission, oxygen is administered per physician protocol and the child is positioned comfortably. One method is to place a pillow on the overbed table and have the patient extend the arms over it, elbows bent. This is comfortable and allows maximum utilization of the accessory muscles of breathing. Lung sounds are assessed for rhonchi, wheezing, or rales. Arterial blood gases and vital signs are monitored. The child is evaluated for clinical improvement (quieter, slower respirations, relaxed facial expression, cessation of retractions). Oral fluids are encouraged, as they help to liquefy secretions and are needed to compensate for fluid loss from dyspnea and diaphoresis. Carbonated beverages, such as ginger ale and colas, are avoided when the patient is wheezing. Beverages are served at room temperature because cold liquids can trigger reflex bronchospasm. Milk products are avoided because they tend to increase the production of mucus. Intake and output should be recorded. The patient is observed for cracked lips, absence of tears, poor skin turgor, and decrease in urinary output, all of which signal dehydration.

A well-balanced diet is necessary for the patient's general health. Ample time is allowed for meals, as respiratory distress may interfere with eating. The nurse organizes tasks so that the child obtains sufficient rest. The child is assisted with the use of the nebulizer if this is required. A sample clinical pathway for a child hospitalized with asthma is presented in page 661.

Self-Care. The child is gradually taught self-care. Patients are taught not to push themselves when they feel tightness in the chest, an early sign of difficulties. The importance of exercise to strengthen vulnerable lungs is emphasized. Yoga breathing exercises (Pranayama) can be effective when adolescents perform them in a warm, moist-air environment. *Purse-lip breathing* (blowing out as if blowing a kiss) and biofeedback are also helpful. The role of Vitamin B_6 in reducing asthma attacks is currently under study (Murphy & Kelly, 1996). Children are taught to observe "personal triggers" that are forewarnings of an attack. They are taught how to use the peak expiratory flowmeter. Other aspects of care include how to administer metered-dose inhalers and understanding medications and their possible side effects. Specific information about how often and when to use inhalers is paramount. The child is encouraged to discuss daily school routines. The physician is seen regularly to evaluate progress and readjust medications as needed. *The nurse reviews the signs of respiratory infection and where, when, and whom to call for help.* Early attention to symptoms may prevent escalation of the disease. The nurse listens to and supports parents and siblings. Asthma is a chronic disease, and the stresses associated with such conditions apply. Family lifestyle is evaluated and proper referrals initiated when needed. The family is encouraged to contact the American Lung Association or the Asthma and Allergy Foundation of America for information on existing programs that could be of benefit. Patients with severe asthma should wear a Medic-Alert bracelet and are educated and provided with injectable epinephrine (EpiPen or EpiPen Jr.) for emergency use.

Inhaler Therapy. Routine monitoring of airway obstruction should be part of comprehensive

ICD-9 Code: ______________________

ELOS: ______________________

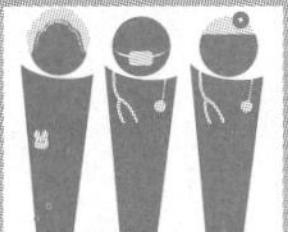

Clinical Pathway 25–1

An Interdisciplinary Plan of Care for the Child with Asthma

	Day 1	Day 2–3
Entrance Date/Time Initial	Date:________ Time:______ Initial:______	Date:________ Time:______ Initial:______
Goals	Establish initial degree of resp. distress Reverse airway obstruction Alleviate hypoxemia Identify asthma triggers Consider alternative explanations for wheezing R/O complicating factors: pneumothorax, pneumonia Patient/family verbalizes understanding of asthma	PL may be discharged when the following criteria are met: Peak flow > 80% of pts. baseline RA when sat. > 93% HR & RR normal for age Auscultation: minimal to no wheezing Albuterol nebs or MDI not more than q4h Tolerates PO well Family demonstrates knowledge of treatment plan Family demonstrates ability to provide care • use of nebulizer and/or MDI with spacer • use of peak flow meter for children 5 yr or > and documentation of readings, interpretation of readings • verbalize medication schedule • verbalize follow-up plan • have home nebulizer, if needed
Individualized Goals		
Labs	Consider: ABG—severe resp. distress Theophylline level (for pts on Theo) CBC if febrile	
Tests	Peak exp. flow > 5 yrs of age CXR: if not done PTA Spot check pulse oximetry for mild resp. distress Spot check SaO_2 for pts. on O_2 before resp. treatment	Peak exp. flow before & after resp. TX > 5 yrs of age (2 ×/day) → Monitor SaO_2 for pts receiving O_2 before TX (B.I.D.) →
Treatments	Adjust O_2 according to resp. status—keep SaO_2 > 93% → Monitor HR & RR Q 4″ → Routine I/O → Daily wts < 18 mo →	Wean O2 → room air Routine VS Encourage PO, decrease IVF
Individualized Treatments		

MC 3314 (front) (597)

Asthma MCF
Pads General
5/8/97

Continued on following page

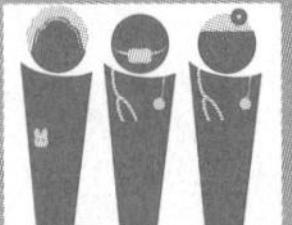

Clinical Pathway 25–1 *(Continued)*

An Interdisciplinary Plan of Care for the Child with Asthma

	Day 1	Day 2–3
Activity	As tolerated →	→
Diet	As tolerated →	→
Consults	Social Worker Case Manager Identify primary care provider Child Life, Respiratory Therapist Notify referring physician re; assessment & TX plan	Contact primary care provider
MEDS/I.V. Media/TV	Continue other maintenance meds Inhaled bronchodilator Q 2-4″ → IV fluids if not taking PO well or signs of dehydration Corticosteroids 2 mg/kg/day PO → Antibiotics if CXR + for pneumonia →	Decrease frequency to Q 4-6″ Consider: Inhaled steroids or cromolyn →
Equipment	Gemini IV pump MDI/spacer/compressed air nebulizer Suction/O_2 Peak flow meter > 5 yrs of age	Equipment and MEDS available prior to discharge
Teaching D/C Plan	Asthma education: → • pathophysiology of asthma/RAD • environmental control/triggers (esp. cigarette smoke) • medicine compliance, indications and side effects (highlight importance of corticosteroids in prevention of symptoms) • peak flow meter • home nebulizer/MDI with spacer use • s and sx of resp. distress • home treatment plan Hospital and unit policies	→ As for Day 1 Individualized TX plan Family verbalizes understanding of the plan: • phone call to PCP within 48″ • f/u office visit in one week
Individualized Teaching	Refer to Asthma Teaching Record → Refer to Discharge Plan of Care for individual discharge planning →	→

Signature	Initial	Signature	Initial	Signature	Initial	Signature	Initial

THIS DOCUMENT IS INTENDED AS A GUIDELINE AND SHOULD BE ADAPTED FOR INDIVIDUAL PATIENT NEEDS.

MC 3314 (back) (597)

Asthma MCF
Pads General
5/8/97

asthma management. A child of 6 years of age can self-test with adult supervision. A diary of peak flow readings (PFR) should be brought to the doctor during follow-up visits (Fig. 25–9). The nurse should be alert to the fact that compliance may be a problem with older children and adolescents who may cause false results by manipulating the unit.

Inhalers and spacers must be cleaned daily with water and weekly with vinegar and water as directed. A near-empty inhaler canister will float in a bowl of water. Measuring the cannister content level will enable the child to request a refill and avoid missing medication doses. Inhalers are designed to be used with an open-mouth technique, a closed-mouth technique, or a spacer or a mask for children under 3 years of age. Spacers are designed to help the child to coordinate inhalation with the release of the medication. A space is provided between the inhaler and the mouth for the puff of medication to float until the child breathes it in. The device will "whistle" if the breathing rate is too rapid. A mask that covers the nose and mouth of a child under 3 years of age who breathes through the nose contains a one-way valve that helps to deliver the inhaled medication. A Pulmo Aide nebulizer machine can be used in the home when inhalers are not appropriate for the individual child.

The nurse should help the child to see connections between triggers, medicines, and signs. For example, did the peak flow drop after contact with a cat or rabbit? Does the peak flow always change with a cold? Any time there is a change in peak flow, you should look for a trigger.

During every clinic visit, the nurse should have the child demonstrate the use of the inhaler or spacer and reinforce the principles involved. Inhaled antibiotic therapy for cystic fibrosis patients has recently been approved by the FDA. Inhaler therapy with specific "leucotriene modifiers" may be replacing corticosteroids inhalers for preventative therapy in asthma.

Nursing Tip

Principles of Asthma Treatment

- Daily monitoring
- Symptom diary
- Treatment plan with active participation of the child
- Identification and avoidance of triggers

Status Asthmaticus

When a child continues to have severe respiratory distress that is not responsive to drugs that may include epinephrine and aminophylline, the child has *status asthmaticus. This is a medical emergency.* The child requires immediate admission to the intensive care unit. Oxygen is administered via nasal cannula because mist in a mist tent can cause coughing or wheezing. Vital signs and the flow of IV medications are carefully monitored. Complying with the prescribed medical regimen, promptly seeking medical care when indicated, minimizing exposure to known allergens, wearing medical identification bracelets, and having a written crisis plan of management can minimize the life-threatening occurrence of status asthmaticus.

Cystic Fibrosis

Description. Cystic fibrosis (CF) is a major worldwide cause of serious chronic lung disease in children. It occurs in approximately 1 in 3000 live births of white infants and 1 in 17,000 births of black infants in the United States. It is most prevalent in Northern and Central Europeans. It is an inherited recessive trait with both parents carrying a gene for the disease. There is a defect in chromosome number 7. The defect in chromosome number 7 is thought to have developed many, many years ago as a self-protective response of the human body against cholera. As the body mutated chromosomes to develop a resistance to cholera, the change in the gene resulted in a defect that caused cystic fibrosis.

The basic defect in cystic fibrosis is an endocrine gland dysfunction that includes (1) increased viscosity (thickness) of mucous gland secretions; and (2) loss of electrolytes in sweat due to an abnormal chloride movement. Cystic fibrosis is considered a *multisystem* disease because the thick viscid secretions affect:

- *The respiratory system.* Small and large airways are obstructed by the thick secretions, resulting in difficulty in breathing. The accumulation and stasis of the thick secretions is a medium for growth of organisms that cause repeated respiratory infections. The thick secretions in the lungs and response of tissues to infections cause hypoxia that can result in heart failure. Emphysema, wheezes, and respiratory distress are common.
- *The digestive system.* The thickened secretions prevents the digestive enzymes from flowing to the gastrointestinal tract, resulting in poor absorption

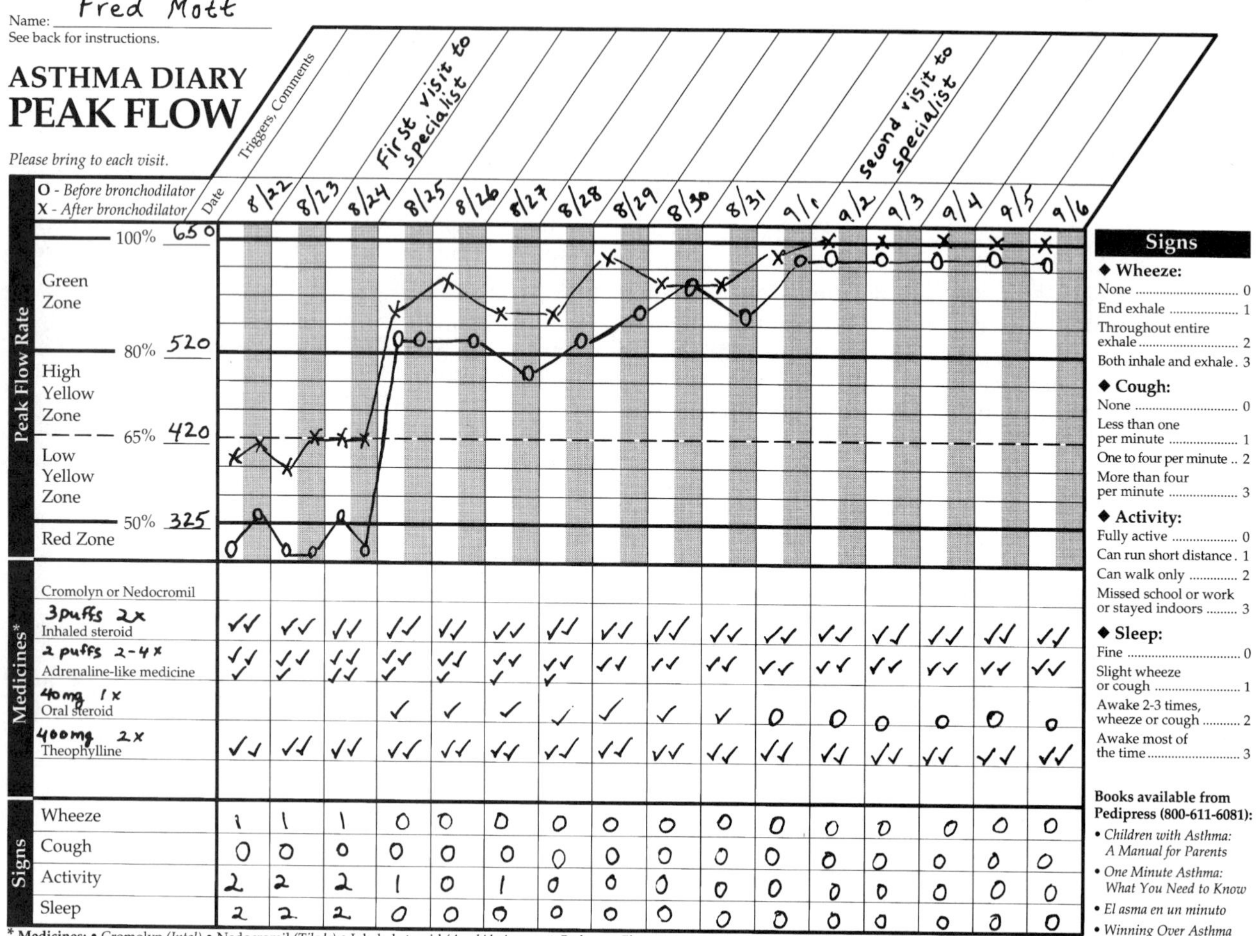

Figure 25–9. • The asthma diary. The clear column is for daytime PFR score and the shaded column is for nighttime peak flow scores. An x indicates PFR following inhaler therapy. An o indicates PFR without inhaler therapy. A check mark indicates medication taken. Asthma triggers/comments are recorded. The diary is brought to each follow-up clinic visit. (Courtesy of Pedipress, Inc., Amherst, MA.)

Peak Flow Diary. With the help of a peak flow diary, you and your doctor can work out a written plan that will help you to care for your (child's) asthma at home.

- *Date.* Fill in date above the grid.
- *Asthma care zones. Green zone:* Your current plan is effective. *Yellow zone:* Avoid triggers and change your medication routine (as directed by your doctor). *Red zone:* Take emergency medicine and see your doctor immediately.

Put your (child's) "personal best" peak flow score here: ________. This is the top of the Green Zone. On the table below, find the "personal best – 100%" score closest to your (child's) score. The top of the High Yellow Zone – 80%, the Low Yellow Zone – 65% and the Red Zone – 50% are listed below the personal best score. Place these numbers next to the 100%, 80%, 65%, and 50% on the diary.

If your (child's) personal best peak flow score has not yet been determined, discuss with your doctor. If your (child's) personal best peak flow rate reaches a higher level on two different days, change the scores using that number as the new personal best.

- *Day/night columns.* Use the clear column for daytime score (7 AM–7 PM) and the shaded column for nighttime score (7 PM–7 AM).
- *Plot peak flow score.* Use an "O" to plot scores blown before taking an inhaled *bronchodilator* and an "X" to plot scores blown after taking an inhaled bronchodilator. Estimate placement of mark between zone lines.
- *Peak flow trend.* Connect the O's with a line to illustrate a trend. Do the same thing for the X's.
- *Medicines.* Enter the name, dose, and number of doses per day for each medicine your doctor has instructed you to take. Put one check mark in the box for each dose given.
- *Signs.* Sign scores are listed on the right side of the diary. Enter each score by time of day. Cough is assessed during a 5-minute period.
- *Comments.* Enter comments above the date, such as "had cold," "rabbit in school," or "painting bedroom."

of food and growth failure. Bulky, foul-smelling stools that are frothy because of the undigested fat content are characteristic. Thick impacted feces can cause rectal prolapse. Pancreatic, liver, and biliary obstruction occurs.

- *Skin.* Loss of electrolytes (sodium and chloride) in the sweat causes a "salty" skin surface. Loss of electrolytes via the skin predisposes the child to electrolyte imbalances during hot weather.
- *Reproductive system.* Thick secretions can decrease sperm motility. Thick cervical mucous can inhibit sperm from reaching the fallopian tubes.

Manifestations. The manifestations of cystic fibrosis are illustrated in Figure 25–10.

Lung Involvement. The air passages of the lungs become clogged with mucus. There is a widespread obstruction of the bronchioles. It is difficult for the patient to breathe; expiration is especially difficult. More and more air becomes trapped in the lungs *(obstructive emphysema),* and small areas of collapse *(atelectasis)* may occur. Eventually, the chest assumes a barrel shape, with increased diameter across the front and back. The right ventricle of the heart, which supplies the lungs, may become strained and enlarged. *Clubbing of fingers and toes* (Fig. 25–11), a compensatory response indicating a chronic lack of oxygen, may be present. *Staphylococcus* and *Pseudomonas* infections can easily occur in the lungs and provide a suitable medium for the organisms' growth. This causes more thickening of the abnormal secretions, irritates and damages lung tissues, and further increases lung obstruction.

Dyspnea, wheezing, and cyanosis may occur. The child is irritable and tires easily. Gradually, there is a change in physical appearance. Evidence of obstructive emphysema, atelectasis, and fibrosis of lung tissue may also be present. The prognosis for survival depends on the extent of lung damage. However, this is only part of the picture, since cystic fibrosis also affects the pancreas and sweat glands.

Pancreatic Involvement. The pancreas lies behind the stomach. Some of its cells secrete pancreatic juice. This key digestive juice drains from the pancreatic duct into the duodenum at the same area in which bile enters. Changes occurring in the pancreas are due to obstruction by thickened secretions that block the flow of pancreatic digestive enzymes. As a result, foodstuffs, particularly fats and proteins, are not properly utilized by the body.

In infants, the stools may be loose. Gradually, because of impaired digestion and food absorption, the feces of the patient become large, fatty, and foul-smelling. They are usually light in color. The baby does not gain weight in spite of a good appetite and may look undernourished. The abdo-

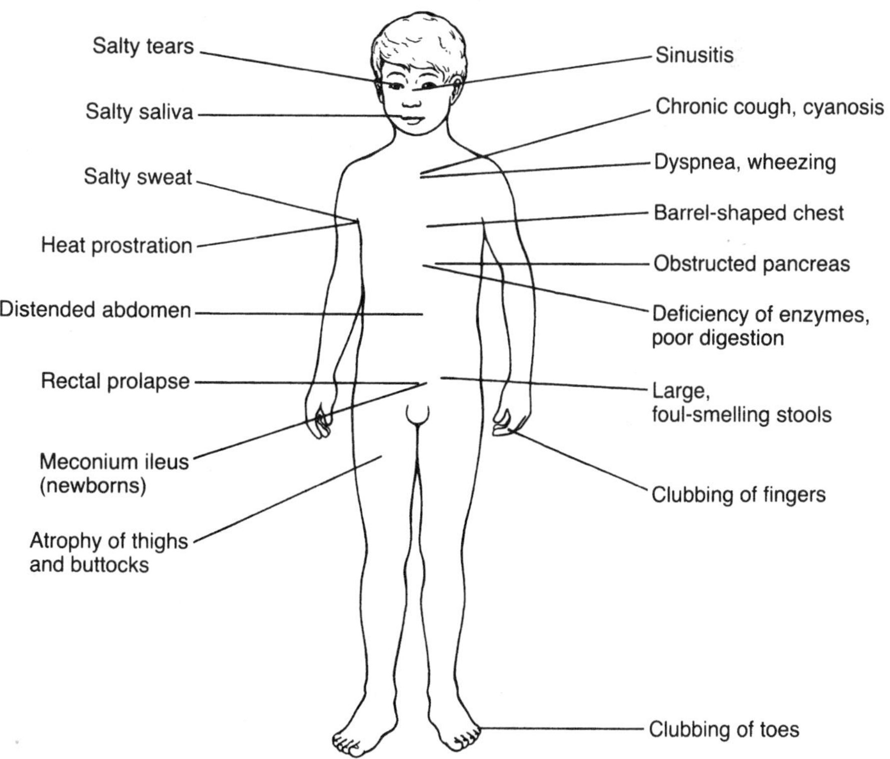

Figure 25–10. • Manifestations of cystic fibrosis.

men becomes distended, and the buttocks and thighs *atrophy* (waste away) as fat disappears from the main deposit sites.

A condition known as *meconium ileus* exists when the intestine of the newborn becomes obstructed with abnormally thick meconium while in utero. This condition is due to the absence of pancreatic enzymes that normally digest proteins in the meconium. The abnormal, puttylike stool sticks to the walls of the intestine, causing blockage. The presenting symptoms develop within hours after birth. The absence of stools and the presence of vomiting and of abdominal distention lead one to suspect intestinal obstruction. X-ray films confirm the diagnosis.

Sweat Glands. The sweat, tears, and saliva of the patient with cystic fibrosis become abnormally salty because of an increase in sodium chloride levels. Up to about 20 years of age, more than 60 mEq/l of sodium chloride in sweat is diagnostic of cystic fibrosis when one or more criteria are present. Levels of 40 to 60 mEq/l are highly suggestive. The analysis of sweat is a major aid in diagnosing the condition. The *sweat test* is the best diagnostic study. A dilute solution of pilocarpine is applied to the arm, and a weak electric current is used to stimulate sweating. A positive test should be repeated for confirmation. Because these patients lose large amounts of salt through perspiration, they must be watched for heat prostration. Liberal amounts of salt should be given with food, and extra fluids and salt should be provided during the hot weather.

Complications. Cystic fibrosis is often responsible for rectal prolapse in infants and children partly because of poor muscle tone in the rectal area and of the excessive leanness of the buttocks of the patient.

As the disease progresses, the liver may become hard, nodular, and enlarged. Cor pulmonale (*cor,* "heart," and *pulmon,* "lung"), heart strain due to improper lung function, is frequently a cause of death. There is a deficiency of vitamin A because the child is unable to absorb fats from which this vitamin is obtained. Sexual development may be delayed in these patients. Males are generally sterile; however, sexual function is unimpaired. Adolescent girls may experience secondary amenorrhea during exacerbations.

Treatment and Nursing Care

Respiratory Relief. (Oxygen therapy is discussed in page 570.) Antibiotics may be given as a preventive measure against respiratory infection; however, this treatment is controversial. Nursing Care Plan 25–1 summarizes interventions for the CF patient.

Intermittent aerosol therapy is administered to provide medication and water to the lower respiratory tract and to promote evacuation of secretions. Expectorants, especially the iodides, are also employed to thin secretions. Bronchodilators are used to increase the width of the bronchi, allowing free passage of air into the lungs.

Postural drainage and chest-clapping exercises are also of value (Fig. 25–12). These are performed by the physical or respiratory therapist during hospitalization. When postural drainage and chest clapping are done properly, the secretions in the chest are moved up and out. This should be explained to the parents so that they will continue this valuable procedure when the child comes home. Instructions may need to be frequently repeated to encourage full cooperation of the parents and child. These procedures are done following nebulization and at least 2 hours after eating. General exercise is good for the patient because it stimulates coughing. Somersaults, headstands, and wheelbarrow play within the child's endurance limits are therapeutic.

Breathing exercises may also be recommended for the older child. *Pursed-lip breathing* is one technique that is simple and effective. The patient is

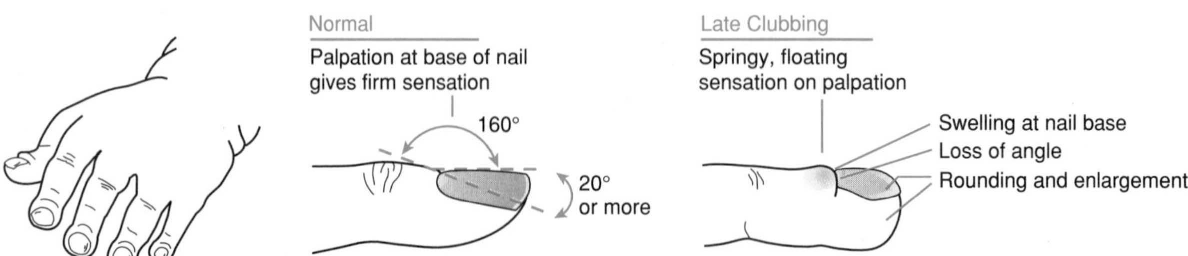

Figure 25–11. • Clubbing of the fingers. Clubbing of the fingers is a sign of chronic hypoxia.

NURSING CARE PLAN 25–1

Care of the Pediatric Patient with Cystic Fibrosis

Nursing Diagnosis: Potential for ineffective airway clearance related to inability to clear mucous from respiratory tract secondary to cystic fibrosis as evidenced by thick mucous production, unproductive/minimal cough, and adventitious breath sounds (wheezes, crackles, dyspnea, tachypnea, cyanosis)

Goals	Nursing Interventions	Rationale
Child will have an effective airway as demonstrated by effective cough, thin respiratory secretions, age-appropriate respiratory rate and effort, and O_2 saturation ≥ 92% on room air	1. Assess respiratory status (rate, depth, effort, breath sounds, oxygen saturation, and skin color) *at least* every 4 hr	1. Allows for early detection and intervention of changes in child's respiratory status
	2. Administer humidified oxygen as ordered by physician; monitor O_2 saturation frequently	2. Humidification helps to thin and loosen secretions. In chronic obstructive respiratory diseases, the respiratory center in the brain becomes tolerant of low O_2 saturation in the blood. Administering high concentrations of O_2 to patient with chronic lung disease can lead to oxygen narcosis
	3. Administer bronchodilators and expectorants as ordered by physician	3. These medications help the thinning, loosening, and expectoration of respiratory mucous
	4. Encourage age-appropriate oral intake of fluids	4. Helps to decrease the viscosity (thickness) of secretions
	5. Perform chest physiotherapy treatments (CPT) and postural drainage (PD) q4°/PRN. Perform CPT/PD 1 hour before or 2 hr after meals	5. CPT/PD help to mobilize secretions and to increase oxygenation. Performing 1 hr before or 2 hr after meals lessens the risk of vomiting and/or aspiration
	6. Teach the child how to do coughing and deep-breathing exercises. Use play therapy whenever possible. For example, using an inspirometer, "blowing up" the fingers of a clean glove	6. Children under the age of 7 cannot voluntarily produce an effective cough. Coughing and deep-breathing exercises helps with expanding the lungs and mobilizing secretions
	7. Teach parents/caregivers NOT to give over the counter (OTC) medications, especially cough suppressants, to the child with cystic fibrosis	7. Cough suppressant medication inhibits the cough reflex, leading to retained secretions and the possibility of respiratory infection

instructed to inhale through the nose, then to exhale through the mouth with the lips pursed as if whistling. Exhalation should be at least twice as long as inhalation. (If it takes 3 seconds to breathe in, 6 seconds are taken to allow all the air to escape.) The child is taught not to force the air out but to let it escape naturally.

Prevention of respiratory infections is essential. The child is isolated from patients and personnel who may harbor infections. The period of hospitalization is kept brief, if possible, to avoid cross-infection. This patient must be given the necessary immunizations against childhood diseases (see Chapter 31).

An oral pancreatic preparation, such as pancrelipase (Pancrease), is given to the child with each meal and snack to replace the pancreatic enzymes the child's body cannot produce. This medication is considered specific for the disease because it helps the child to digest and absorb food, thus improving the condition of the stools. If the child is ill and not eating, the medication is withheld. When meals are erratic, such as during vacations, medication is given when the largest amount of food will be consumed.

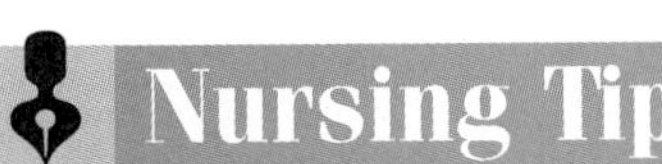

Chest physiotherapy should be done *between* meals.

NURSING CARE PLAN 25–1 *continued*

Care of the Pediatric Patient with Cystic Fibrosis

Nursing Diagnosis: Alteration in nutrition—less than body requirements related to decrease in the availability of pancreatic enzymes; poor intestinal absorption of nutritional intake; anorexia secondary to cystic fibrosis as evidenced by decreased oral intake, weight loss/failure to thrive, diarrhea, steatorrhea, or constipation

Goals	Nursing Interventions	Rationale
Child is able to ingest age-appropriate nutrition and maintain weight or gain height, weight according to the normal growth and development charts. Stools will be of normal color, consistency, and amount for age	1. Assess child's normal feeding patterns, dietary likes and dislikes and activity level	1. Knowing the child's preferences and activity level will aid in the plan of care in regards to the feeding of the child
	2. Administer pancreatic replacement enzymes and fat-soluble vitamin supplements as directed by physician before meals and snacks	2. Digestive and nutritional therapy consists of replacement of pancreatic enzymes and dietary adjustments. Administering supplemental fat-soluble vitamins is necessary because of the inability of the body to absorb fats
	3. Teach child (and parents) *not* to chew the capsules or "beads"; to swallow the medication whole; if powder form, sprinkle over a nonfat, nonprotein food, such as applesauce. Do not mix enzymes with hot (heat) foods, high-starch, or high-acid–containing foods. Wipe off any powder on oral mucosa of lips	3. Pancreatic enzymes are inactivated by heat, and acids are known to degrade the enzymes. Wipe the excess powder off mucosa to prevent excoriation or breakdown of mucosal membranes
	4. Note the color, consistency, amount, and frequency of stools. Notify physician of any changes, i.e., diarrhea, constipation, or steatorrhea	4. Pancreatic enzymes are known to cause constipation if taken in high doses or steatorrhea from malabsorption of fats and proteins due to low intake of the enzymes

Nursing Diagnosis: Alteration in family process related to chronicity of disease, need for outside support, and risk of life-threatening complications as evidenced by frequent physician office visits, hospitalizations, diminished focus on other siblings in home, and need for therapeutic interventions and compliance and home care routines

Goals	Nursing Interventions	Rationale
Family members verbalize their feelings about the impact cystic fibrosis has on them; are able to comply with therapeutic treatment plan; and utilize available resources within their community to assist in the care and treatment of their child	1. Assess educational level and amount of knowledge each family member has on cystic fibrosis *before* planning any family interventions or teaching sessions	1. Educational level will help to determine the type of teaching methods to be used, i.e., written, visual, hands-on, auditory. Having this information in advance helps the nurse to map out the plan of care and teaching. It also prevents the repetition of the same information or guides the nurse as to the amount of teaching/information required/or needed by the family.
	2. Assess level of impact disease has had on family	2. Guides the nurse in selecting appropriate referrals to community or support agencies needed by the family
	3. Teach and/or review with family the skills required in the daily care of the child with cystic fibrosis. For example, assessing respiratory rate and status; CPT/PD methods; monitoring stools; skin care; medication administration	3. Return demonstration enables the nurse to evaluate the ability of the family to provide effective home care

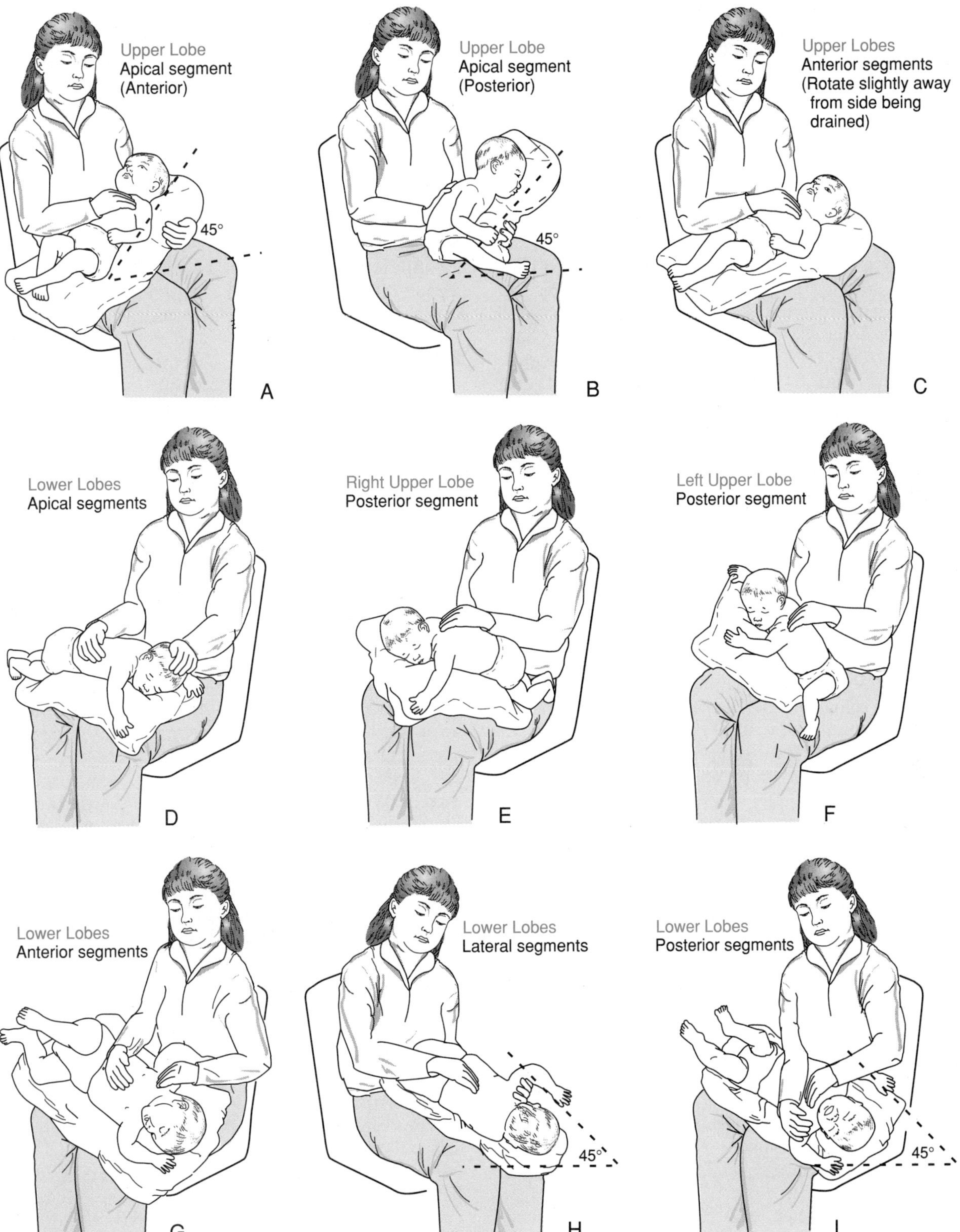

Figure 25–12. • Postural drainage. The positions for postural drainage are correlated with the segment being drained. In positions H and I, the child is shown on the right side; however, the child must also be turned to the left side to drain both lobes.

Nursing Tip

Pancreatic enzyme powder should be given with applesauce or other nonstarch, nonfat, nonprotein food.

Diet. The maintenance of adequate nutrition is essential. The diet is high in calories, as much as 50% above normal. There should be increased protein and moderate amounts of fat in conjunction with pancreatic extracts. Simple sugars are easy to digest, and banana products are particularly good. Fruits, cottage cheese, vegetables, and lean meats, which are high in protein and low in fat and starches, are recommended. Restrictions on ice cream, peanut butter, butter, french fries, and mayonnaise are advised. Extra salt may be provided by pretzels and salted bread sticks and crackers.

Supplements of vitamins A, D, and E in a water-miscible base are given each day in double the recommended dosage. Vitamin K may also be given when indicated. Salt tablets may be given to the older child during hot weather. Fluids may be encouraged because larger amounts of fluid are lost in the stools. The nurse may be asked to weigh the child daily.

The nurse feeding the infant with cystic fibrosis must be calm and unhurried. The baby needs careful burping to avoid abdominal distention. In general, the appetite is good. Older children need small amounts of food served attractively and frequently.

Because mealtime is a social time, the nurse remains with the child if the parents are not present. The nurse records the fluid intake at the end of the meal. The child's reaction to new foods and any variations in stools resulting from the foods are noted. The food refused and the type, character, and amount of vomiting, if any, are recorded.

General Hygiene. The nurse must pay special attention to the skin of the child with cystic fibrosis. The diaper area is cleansed following each bowel movement. An ointment to protect the skin is advisable because the character of the stool subjects the diaper area to irritation. The buttocks are exposed to air when a rash occurs. Because the patient has little fat and muscle, the position must be changed frequently, especially if the child is weak and cannot get out of bed. Frequent changes of position also prevent the development of pneumonia.

The child wears light clothing to avoid becoming overheated; it should be loose to allow freedom of movement. Good oral hygiene is necessary since the teeth may be in poor condition because of dietary deficiencies. Mouth care is given after postural drainage, as foul mucus may be raised, leaving an unpleasant taste in the patient's mouth.

Long-Term Care. The goals of care include minimizing pulmonary complications, ensuring adequate nutrition, promoting growth and development, and assisting the family to adjust to the chronic care required. Today the child with a lengthy illness spends most of the time at home. Hospitalization is mainly for diagnosis, relapses, and complications. This is extremely taxing financially, physically, and emotionally. The parents must distribute their time and energy within the family, yet give careful attention to their sick child or sometimes, children. How do they keep from spoiling the child? Do they limit the normal activities of the remaining children to spare the sick one? What about birthday parties, camping, Scouts, pets, epidemics at school? What does a trip to the shore or mountains entail? When do the husband and wife find time for themselves?

These seemingly overwhelming problems are faced daily by many people in every community. Parent groups are helpful in promoting exchange of ideas and in providing support. The National Cystic Fibrosis Research Foundation disseminates useful information. The nurse becomes familiar with the local chapter in the area so that parents are guided to reliable sources of information. Parents of these patients need encouragement and reassurance. Parents need explicit instructions regarding diet, medication, postural drainage, prevention of infection, rest, and continued medical supervision. Many families require the assistance of a social worker to secure funds for equipment and drugs. Genetic counseling is advised.

Emotional Support. The child who is chronically ill finds it hard to accept restricted activity. The amount and kinds of diversion required vary in cystic fibrosis because the disease affects children of all ages, and varies in severity.

It is thought that children benefit from simple, straightforward answers to questions about their illness. An uncomplicated diagram might be helpful. They should know why they must take medications with each meal, use the nebulizer, and have postural drainage. They should see and handle the unfamiliar equipment necessary for care.

The young child finds it more difficult to be separated from parents during hospitalization. Even when the prognosis is grave, a child's courage is sustained if parents are there. Visiting hours for parents must be flexible. Close contact by mail with school, church, and clubs is important for the school-age child. It is helpful for patients to develop an activity that they enjoy, such as piano or art. This increases feelings of worth and provides outlets for feelings. Consideration must be given to ways of fostering love, acceptance, trust, fair play, security, freedom of choice, creativity, and maintenance of self-identity.

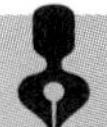

Nursing Tip

When oxygen is used in the home, the family should be taught safety precautions to prevent fire and injury.

Bronchopulmonary Dysplasia

Bronchopulmonary dysplasia is a fibrosis, or thickening, of the alveolar walls and the bronchiolar epithelium caused by oxygen concentrations above 40% or by the mechanical pressure ventilation given to newborns for a prolonged time. Swelling of the tissues causes edema, and the respiratory cilia are paralyzed by the high oxygen concentrations and lose their ability to clear mucous from the airways. Respiratory obstruction, mucous plugs, and atelectasis follow.

Prevention. Respiratory distress in the newborn is the major reason why oxygen and ventilators are used for prolonged periods. The main cause of respiratory distress in the newborn is prematurity. Therefore, prevention of preterm births is the best way of preventing bronchopulmonary dysplasia. The goal of treatment for respiratory distress in the newborn should be to administer only the amount of oxygen required to prevent hypoxia at the minimum ventilator pressures needed to prevent tissue trauma.

Symptoms. Symptoms of chronic respiratory distress (Fig. 25–2) include:

- Wheezing
- Retractions
- Cyanosis on exertion
- Use of accessory respiratory muscles
- Clubbing of the fingers
- Failure to thrive
- Irritability due to hypoxia

Treatment. Once bronchopulmonary dysplasia has developed, the goal of therapy is to reduce inflammation of the airway and to wean the infant from the mechanical ventilator. The infant may become oxygen dependent and develop reactive airway bronchoconstriction. Right-sided heart failure may develop. Fluid restriction, bronchodilators, and diuretics may be ordered. A tracheostomy may be also needed. Infants with bronchopulmonary dysplasia often develop respiratory stridor and retractions with even minor respiratory infections that result in repeated hospitalizations. Ongoing home care is required and respiratory problems persist through adulthood. Maintaining optimum growth and development is a challenge. Education and support of the family for a technology-dependent child at home are essential, and a multidisciplinary health care team approach is essential.

Sudden Infant Death Syndrome

Sudden infant death syndrome (SIDS) is clinically defined as the sudden, unexpected death of an apparently healthy infant between 2 weeks and 1 year, for which a routine autopsy fails to identify the cause. It is also referred to as "crib death" or "cot death." Although precise data are not available, it is estimated that in the United States SIDS kills about 6000 infants each year, or about 13 of every 10,000 live births. In industrialized countries, SIDS is one of the leading causes of death in early infancy; the peak incidence is between 2 and 4 months of age. Two clinical features of the disease remain constant: (1) death occurs during sleep; and (2) the infant does not cry or make other sounds of distress. It has occurred even when the parents were sleeping in the same room.

SIDS is thought to be caused by a brainstem abnormality of cardiorespiratory control. Increased risk factors for SIDS may include maternal smoking or cocaine use that causes hypoxia of the fetus, preterm birth, and poor postneonatal care. A face-down sleeping position may cause rebreathing of expired air or airway occlusion. Wrapping the infant who is placed face down may increase the risk for SIDS by preventing the infant from lifting and turning the face to the side. Infants who have apneic episodes are at risk of developing SIDS. Medications, such as caffeine and theophylline, have shown promise in selected groups of high-risk

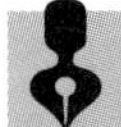

Nursing Tip

The American Academy of Pediatrics recommends that all healthy babies be placed on their back or side to help to prevent the occurrence of SIDS.

infants. Symptoms that may occur prior to the apneic episode include fever, fatigue during feedings, lethargy, and profuse sweating during sleep.

Prevention. For high-risk infants, home apnea monitors have been employed to warn parents of an impending problem and enable them to try to resuscitate the infant manually. All parents should have CPR education. The American Academy of Pediatrics in 1996 recommended that all healthy infants be placed in the supine (back-lying) position or the side-lying position on firm mattresses to prevent SIDS. The use of soft pillows or fluffy blankets for the infant to lie on is discouraged as it can prevent the infant from raising and turning his or her head. A national educational media campaign for this recommended positioning of infants may decrease the occurrence of SIDS.

Nursing Care. In talking with grieving parents after the death of their infant, the nurse must convey some important facts: that the baby died of a disease entity called sudden infant death syndrome, that currently the disease cannot be predicted or prevented, and that they are *not* responsible for the child's death. Grieving parents need time to say good-bye to their child. They are encouraged to hold and rock the infant, shed tears, and assist in burial preparations. This process, not common in the past, is conducive to the resolution of grief.

Parents experience much guilt and are catapulted into a totally unexpected bereavement that requires numerous explanations to relatives and friends. Often, needless blame has been placed on one parent by the other or by relatives. The family baby-sitter and physician may also be targets of attack. Emergency room personnel need to be especially sensitive and supportive during this crisis. There have been crib deaths for which parents have been charged with child abuse.

Nurses can recommend group therapy with other parents of SIDS victims. Two nationally supported organizations are The Compassionate Friends, Inc., and The National Sudden Infant Death Syndrome Foundation. These groups have local chapters in most states.

CARDIOVASCULAR SYSTEM

The cardiovascular system consists of the heart, the blood, and the blood vessels. As the heart beats, blood, oxygen, and nutrients are transported to all the tissues of the body, and waste products are removed. Because of anatomic and physiologic immaturity, the cardiovascular system of the child differs from that of the adult. Figure 25–13 summarizes some of these differences.

The cardiovascular system develops from the 3rd to 8th week of gestation. It is the first system to function in intrauterine life. When cardiovascular development is incomplete, heart defects occur. Fetal circulation is designed to serve the metabolic needs during intrauterine life and also to permit safe transition to life outside the womb.

Assessment for Suspected Cardiac Pathology. Although signs and symptoms of specific congenital heart defects relate to the specific pathology involved, several signs and symptoms are common to most infants with congenital cardiac problems. When the nurse assesses the child, the following observations should be reported:

- Failure to thrive, poor weight gain
- Cyanosis, pallor
- Visually observed pulsations in the neck veins
- Tachypnea, dyspnea
- Irregular pulse rate
- Clubbing of fingers
- Fatigue during feeding or activity
- Excessive perspiration, especially over forehead

Congenital Heart Disease

Congenital heart defects may be caused by genetic factors, maternal factors (such as drug intake or rubella illness), or environmental factors. Fetal echocardiography can detect cardiac malformations in high-risk cases. Acquired heart disease occurs *after* birth, as a result of a defect or illness.

Description. Congenital *heart defects* are not a problem for the fetus because fetal-maternal circulation compensates for all of its oxygen needs. However, at birth, the infant's circulatory system must provide for its own oxygen needs. Any heart defect or patent (open) fetal pathways in the cardiovascular system after birth will produce signs and symptoms that indicate an anatomic heart defect. Congenital heart disease occurs in approximately 8 out of 1000 births, and 50% of these infants evidence signs and symptoms before the 1st year of life. Some defects, such as mitral valve prolapse, may not be manifested until later in life.

Of the congenital anomalies, heart defects are the principal cause of death during the 1st year of life. Therefore, nurses must stress the need for good prenatal care and impress on parents the value of regular checkups at baby clinics. Many organic heart murmurs have been detected early in infancy at periodic checkups.

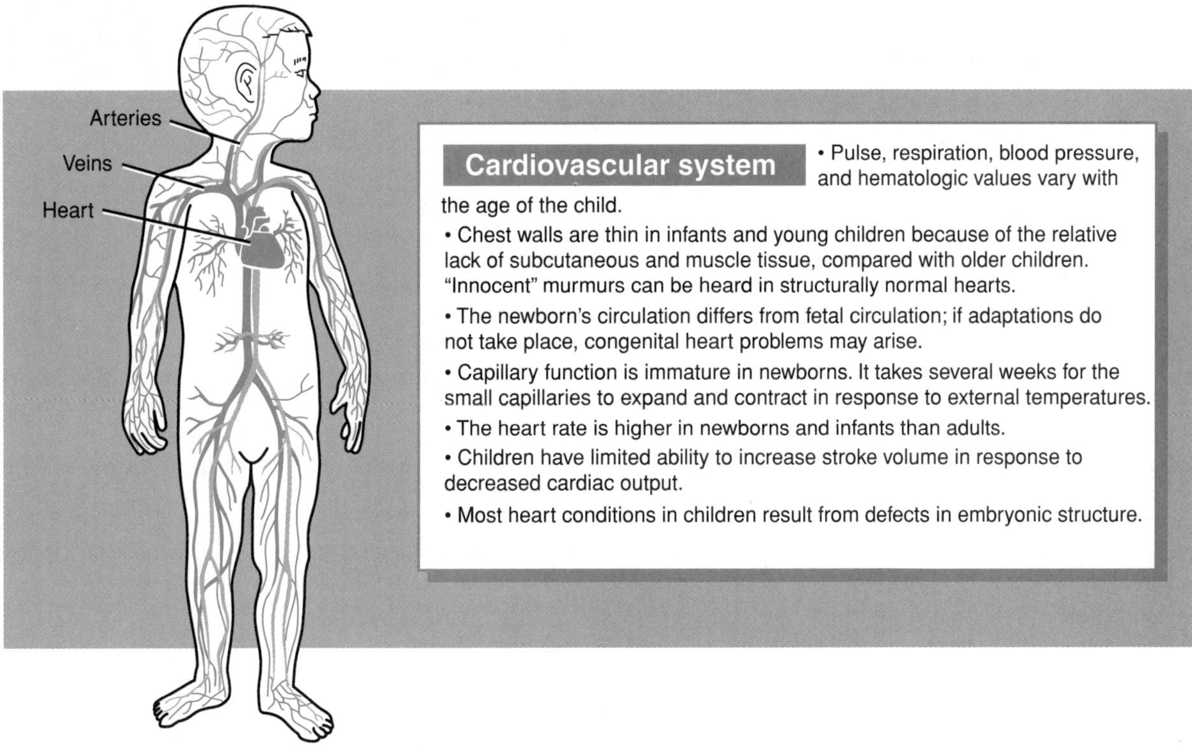

Figure 25–13. • Summary of some cardiovascular system differences between the child and the adult. The cardiovascular system consists of the heart, blood, and blood vessels. As the heart beats, blood, oxygen, and nutrients are transported to all the tissues of the body and waste products are removed.

Diagnosis and Treatment. The appearance of clinical symptoms and results of diagnostic tests aid in the diagnosis of congenital heart disease (Table 25–3). The treatment of most cardiac defects is surgical. A *thoracotomy* (chest incision) is performed and a cardiopulmonary bypass machine and *hypothermia* during the procedure minimize blood loss and enhance patient response. *Hypothermia* (*Hypo,* "under," and *thermal,* "heat") reduces the temperature of body tissues, resulting in a decreased need for oxygen. The cardiopulmonary bypass machine provides oxygenation of the body tissues while the surgeon stops the heart to perform surgery. Heart transplants may be the treatment of choice in cases such as a three-chambered heart.

Classification. Congenital heart defects can be divided into two categories: cyanotic and acyanotic. A more accurate classification is based on the effect of the defect on blood circulation. The study of blood circulation is termed *hemodynamics* (*hemo,* "blood," and *dynamics,* "power"). Blood always flows from an area of high pressure to an area of low pressure and takes the path of least resistance. Physiologically, defects can be organized into (1) lesions that increase pulmonary blood flow; (2) lesions that obstruct blood flow; and (3) lesions that decrease pulmonary blood flow. There are also mixed lesions. A *shunt* refers to the flow of blood through an abnormal opening between two vessels of the heart. Figure 25–14 compares the normal heart and the heart with various congenital defects.

Defects That Increase Pulmonary Blood Flow

Congenital heart defects that cause the blood to *return to the right ventricle and recirculate through the lungs* before exiting the left ventricle through the aorta, are known as defects that *increase pulmonary blood flow.* (For example, the defect in the atrial septum in the fetus allows blood to flow from the right atrium through the defect into the left atrium,

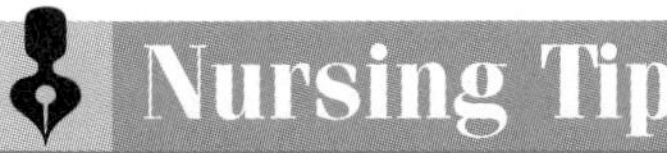

In congenital heart disease, cyanosis is *not always* a clinical sign.

providing a bypass of the lungs. After birth, the pressure is higher in the left atrium, and if the atrial opening persists, the blood flows *back* into the right atrium *(left-to-right shunt)* and then *recirculates* to the lungs, causing increased pulmonary flow. Some defects that increase pulmonary flow include: atrial septal defect; ventricular septal defect; and patent ductus arteriosus (see Fig. 25–14). In heart defects that result in increased pulmonary flow due to a left to right shunt, the oxygenated blood recirculates to the lungs and *cyanosis is rare.*

Atrial Septal Defect

In atrial septal defect (ASD), there is an abnormal opening between the right and the left atria. Blood that already contains oxygen is forced from the left atrium back to the right atrium. Most patients do not have symptoms. The defect may be recognized during a routine health examination, when a murmur is heard. Cardiac catheterization, electrocardiogram, and echocardiography may be performed to help to determine the diagnosis. The surgical repair involves a median *sternotomy* (*sternum,* and *otomy,* "cutting"). Closure is similar to that for ventricular septal defect (VSD; see the following discussion). Continued cardiology follow-up is necessary. Prognosis is excellent.

Ventricular Septal Defect

VSD is the most common heart anomaly. As the name suggests, there is an opening between the right and left ventricles of the heart. Increased pressure within the left ventricle forces blood back into the right ventricle (left-to-right shunt). A loud, harsh murmur combined with a systolic thrill is characteristic of this defect. The condition may be mild or severe. It is frequently associated with other defects. Many children with small defects may experience spontaneous closure during the 1st year of life as a result of growth.

Table 25–3

VALUE OF DIAGNOSTIC TESTS USED IN CONGENITAL HEART DEFECTS

Test	Definition	Value
Angiocardiography (selective)	Serial x-ray films of the heart and great vessels following injection of an opaque substance; a radiopaque catheter is moved into the heart chambers, and contrast medium is injected in specific areas	Abnormal communications in the heart can be observed; the course of the blood through the heart and great vessels can be traced
Aortography	X-ray films of the aorta after the injection of an opaque material	Useful in revealing patent ductus arteriosus
Radionuclide angiocardiography	Noninvasive nuclear procedure that permits visualization of the course of blood through the heart	May be used as a pre-cardiac catheterization screening study; provides assessment of congenital and acquired cardiovascular lesions and monitors the effects of therapy; an intravenous device is necessary to permit injection of the radionuclide
Barium swallow	Barium given by mouth	Shows indentation of the esophagus by the aorta or other vessels
Cardiac catheterization	A radiopaque catheter is passed through a cut-down site directly into the heart and large vessels	Reveals blood pressure within the heart; doctors can examine the heart closely with the tip of the catheter to detect abnormalities; blood samples can be obtained to determine oxygen content
Chest x-ray film	—	Provides a permanent record; shows abnormalities in shape and position of heart
Cineangiocardiography	Motion pictures of images recorded by fluoroscopy	Useful record and monitoring device
Echocardiography	The use of ultrasound to produce an image of sound waves of the heart; transducer placed directly on chest; sounds are analyzed on paper	Noninvasive procedure; localizes murmurs; determines if heart is structurally normal
Electrocardiogram	Tracing of heart action by electrocardiography	Detects variations in heart action and shows the condition of the heart muscle; may also be used as a monitoring device during cardiac catheterization
Magnetic resonance imaging	Noninvasive imaging technique that uses low-energy radio waves in combination with a magnetic field to generate signals that produce tomographic images	Very useful in diagnosing coarctation of the aorta

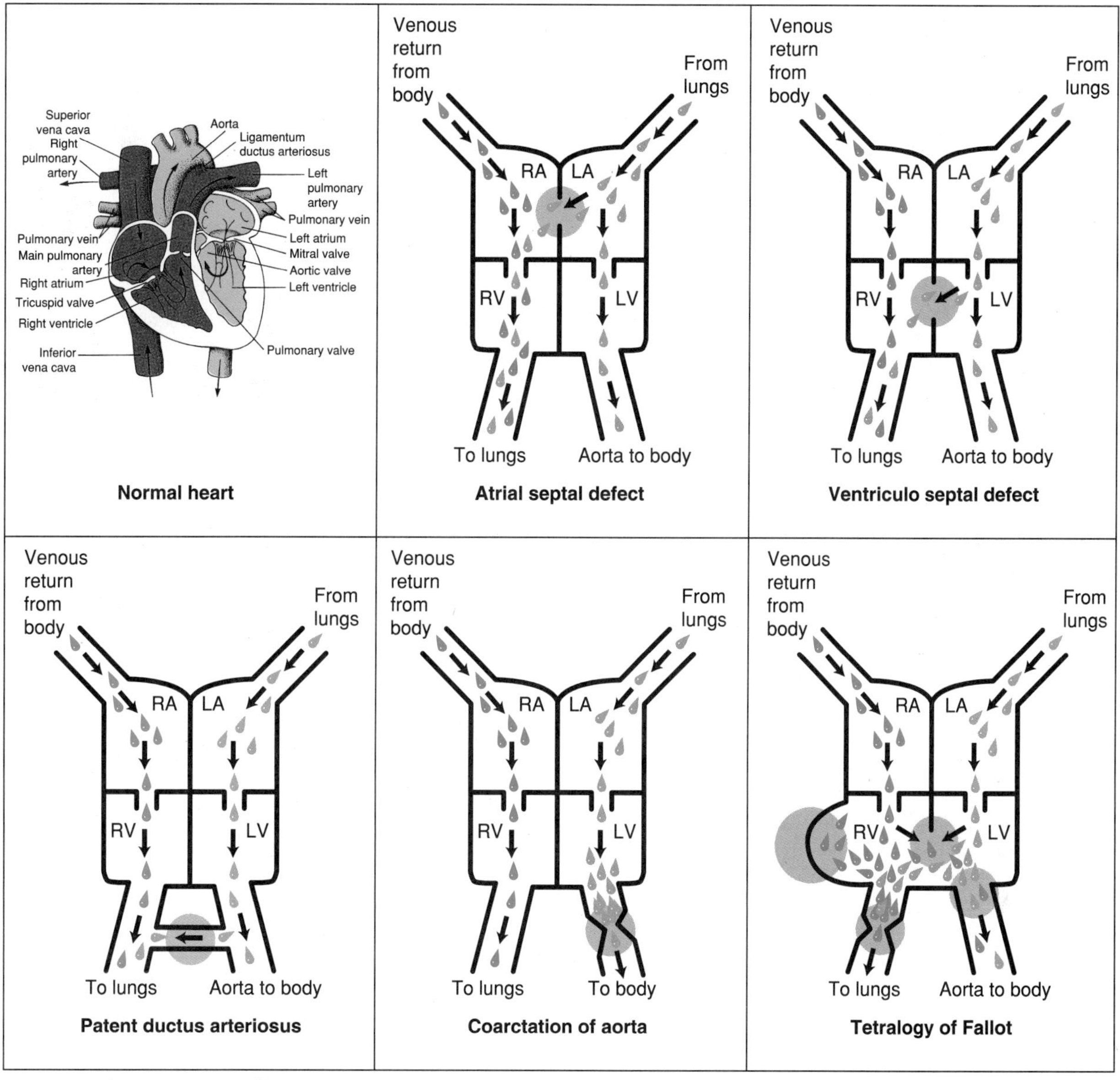

Figure 25–14. • The normal heart and various congenital heart defects.

Treatment includes close observation of the growing child. Antibiotic prophylaxis is necessary for dental care and minor surgical procedures to prevent bacterial endocarditis. The child is encouraged to live a normal life and undergoes frequent EKG and physical examinations to detect hypertrophy of the heart. If the septal defect is large, symptoms of pulmonary disease or heart failure may occur. Early surgical intervention has a low risk for most infants and prognosis is excellent. Normal growth and development are usually achieved within 1 or 2 years following surgery.

Open-heart surgery is performed under hypothermia. With the use of the heart-lung bypass machine, the condition can be corrected in a fairly dry or bloodless field. The hole is ligated with sutures or a synthetic patch. "The patch is not rejected because it is an inert substance and cardiac tissue completely covers the patch within 6 months after surgery" (Daberkow-Carson & Smith, 1994).

Patent Ductus Arteriosus

The circulation of the fetus differs from that of the newborn in that most of the fetal blood bypasses the lungs. The ductus arteriosus is the passageway (shunt) through which the blood crosses from the pulmonary artery to the aorta and avoids the deflated lungs. This vessel closes shortly after birth; however, when it does not close, blood continues to pass from the aorta, where the pressure is higher, into the pulmonary artery. This causes oxygenated blood to recycle through the lungs, overburdening the pulmonary circulation and making the heart pump harder.

The symptoms of patent ductus arteriosus (PDA) may go unnoticed during infancy. However as the child grows, dyspnea is experienced, the radial pulse becomes full and bounding on exertion, and there is an unusually wide range between systolic blood pressure and diastolic blood pressure. This is referred to as the *pulse pressure.* The *characteristic machinery-type murmur* may be heard. A two-dimensional echocardiogram is useful in visualizing and determining blood flow across the PDA.

PDA is one of the more common cardiac anomalies. It occurs twice as frequently in girls as in boys. Premature infants with hypoxia often respond to Indomethacin drug therapy that results in closure of the patent ductus arteriosus. Heart surgery is performed on all full-term newborns diagnosed with PDA to prevent congestive heart failure, emboli formation, and other complications. The ductus may be ligated via thoracotomy (incision into the chest) or via visually assisted thorascopic surgery (VATS) technique that eliminates the need for a large chest incision. The prognosis is excellent.

Obstructive Defect

Some congenital cardiac defects cause an obstruction to blood flow from the ventricles due to a *stenosis* (narrowing) of a vessel.

Coarctation of the Aorta

The word *coarctation* means "a tightening." In coarctation of the aorta, there is a constriction or narrowing of the aortic arch or of the descending aorta (the blood meets an obstruction) (see Fig. 25–14). Hemodynamics consists of increased pressure proximal to the defect and decreased pressure distally. The characteristic symptoms are a *marked difference in the blood pressure and pulses of the upper and lower extremities.* The patient may not develop symptoms until late childhood. Treatment depends on the type and severity of the defect. Infants who have associated congestive heart failure (CHF) are treated medically until the optimal time for surgery.

The surgeon resects the narrowed portion of the aorta and joins its ends. The joining is called an *anastomosis.* If the section removed is large, an end-to-end graft using tubes of synthetic polyester (Dacron) or similar material may be necessary. Because the graft will not grow, but the aorta will, the best time for surgery is between the ages of 2 and 4 years. Some children complain of leg pain after exercise. X-ray examination may reveal cardiac enlargement and "notching" of the ribs caused by vessels developed as collateral circulation. Pulses and blood pressure will differ in upper and lower extremities. A two-dimensional echocardiography can aid in diagnosis. If the condition is untreated, hypertension, congestive heart failure, and infective endocarditis may develop. As in PDA, closed-heart surgery is performed because the structures are outside the heart. The prognosis is good if there are no other defects and the child's physical condition is favorable at the time of surgery. If restenosis occurs after surgery for coarctation, a balloon angioplasty can relieve the obstruction. The nurse should observe the child with postcoarctation surgery for the development of hypertension and abdominal pain associated with nausea and vomiting, leukocytosis, and gastrointestinal bleeding or obstruction. Antihypertensive drugs, steroids, and nasogastric tube decompression are priority treatment of this postsurgical complication.

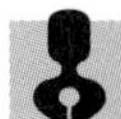

Nursing Tip

A difference in the blood pressure between the upper extremities and the lower extremities is a characteristic sign of coarctation of the aorta.

Defect That Decreases Pulmonary Blood Flow

When a congenital heart anomaly allows blood that has not passed through the lungs (unoxygenated blood) to enter the aorta and general circulation, a *decrease* in pulmonary blood flow occurs. Cyanosis due to the presence of unoxygenated blood in the circulation is a characteristic feature of this type of congenital heart anomaly.

Tetralogy of Fallot

Tetra means "four." In *tetralogy of Fallot* there are four defects: (1) stenosis or narrowing of the pulmonary artery, which decreases the blood flow to the lungs; (2) hypertrophy of the right ventricle, which enlarges because it has to work harder to pump blood through the narrow pulmonary artery;

Nursing Tip

Oxygen is a drug and administration should be correlated with monitoring of oxygen saturation levels. Too little oxygen can result in hypoxia; too much oxygen can result in lung damage.

(3) dextroposition (*dextro,* "right," and *position*) of the aorta, in which the aorta is displaced to the right and blood from both ventricles enters it; and (4) VSD (see Fig. 25–14).

When venous blood enters the aorta, the infant displays symptoms of cardiac problems. Cyanosis increases with age, and *clubbing of the fingers and toes* is seen. The child rests in a "squatting" position to breath more easily. This position increases systemic venous return. Feeding problems, growth retardation, frequent respiratory infections, and severe dyspnea on exercise are prevalent. The red blood cells (RBCs) of the body increase, causing *polycythemia* (*poly,* "many," *cyt,* "cells," and *hema,* "blood") to compensate for the lack of oxygen.

Narrowing of the pulmonary artery causes CHF due to the increased muscular force necessary to propel blood through the narrowed orifice. When unoxygenated blood enters the general circulation, *hypoxia* occurs, which may be manifested by cyanosis.

In response to chronic hypoxia, a *clubbing of the fingers* results (see Fig. 25–11). As a response to chronic hypoxia, the body produces more red blood cells, causing *polycythemia. Failure to thrive* results from decreasing energy and ability to eat and increased oxygen consumption. Multiple hospitalizations, cyanotic skin, and limited energy can impede growth and development both physically and socially.

Paroxysmal hypercyanotic, or *"tet" spells* occur during the first 2 years of life. Spontaneous cyanosis, respiratory distress, weakness, and syncope occur. They can last a few minutes to a few hours and are followed by lethargy and sleep. Parents and day care personnel need to be instructed to place the child in a knee–chest position when a "tet" spell occurs. Often, the child will pause and voluntarily *squat* in position until the attack abates. Recovery from the "tet" spell is usually rapid.

Diagnosis of tetralogy of Fallot is confirmed by chest x-ray that shows a typical *boot-shaped heart.* An EKG, two-dimensional echocardiography, and cardiac catheterization aid in the diagnosis.

Complications such as cerebral thrombosis due to polycythemia (thickened blood due to increased RBC) is a problem especially if dehydration occurs. Iron deficiency anemia develops because of decreased appetite and of the energy required to suck or eat. Bacterial endocarditis can occur and is prevented with prophylactic antibiotic therapy.

Treatment is designed to increase pulmonary blood flow to relieve hypoxia. A Blalock-Taussig surgical procedure can successfully be performed on newborns or premature infants. Open-heart surgery with total correction of all defects is usually done on the older, stable child with excellent results. In some cases, IV prostaglandin E therapy can open a constricted ductus arteriosus and allow for oxygenation of the body until surgery is performed.

General Treatment and Nursing Care of Children with Congenital Heart Defects. Some congenital heart defects are mild, perhaps causing a murmur, but requiring no specific treatment. Parents need to be guided to understand that the child should not be overprotected and restricted from normal activities related to optimum growth and development. Fear and anxiety can be transferred from the parents to the child. Education concerning general health, hygiene, dental care, balanced diet, and routine immunizations should be emphasized. In moderate heart anomalies, rough and competitive sports should be discouraged, but the child should not be excessively restricted in school PE activities. Some children will benefit from being transported to school so that energy can be consumed *during* school activities rather than by walking to school. Children who are active candidates for heart transplants should not receive live viral vaccinations. Prophylactic antibiotic therapy is indicated during routine dental care and infections are treated aggressively.

Nutritional guidance is aimed at preventing anemia and promoting optimal growth and development. In children with polycythemia, parents should be instructed in techniques of preventing dehydration. Family trips or vacations during the hot summer months require attention to the child's fluid needs to replace fluid loss from sweating. Vacations to high altitudes or very cold environments may cause adverse responses in a child who is already hypoxic or has cardiac problems.

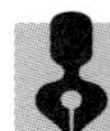

Nursing Tip

The four defects in tetralogy of Fallot are:

- Pulmonary artery stenosis
- Hypertrophy of right ventricle
- Dextra position of aorta
- Ventricular septal defect

Postoperative cardiac care usually takes place in an intensive care unit (ICU), where high-technology monitoring minimizes complications. The licensed vocational nurse will have contact with the child who is returning for postoperative checkups or is on a home care program following discharge. Providing routine supportive care, encouraging appropriate medical follow-up, and designing activities that promote optimal growth and development are primary goals of care. Currently, children with a history of congenital heart disease have difficulty obtaining independent health insurance. The problem may change with future legislation.

Defects That Cause Mixed Pathology

Hypoplastic Left Heart Syndrome

In hypoplastic heart syndrome, there is an underdevelopment of the left side of the heart, usually resulting in an absent or nonfunctional left ventricle and hypoplasia of the ascending aorta. The initial survival of the infant is dependent on a patent foramen ovale and ductus arteriosus to provide a pathway for oxygenated blood to the general body system. Other serious congenital anomalies may be present and the infant should be carefully assessed.

Symptoms include a grayish-blue color of the skin and mucous membranes, signs of congestive heart failure, including dyspnea, weak pulses, and a cardiac murmur. Survival beyond the first month of life without intervention is rare. With the advent of successful heart transplants, however, the prognosis of these infants is much brighter and emphasis is placed on maintaining life and hope until an appropriate heart is available for transplant. Following a transplant, immunosuppressive therapy to prevent organ rejection is essential.

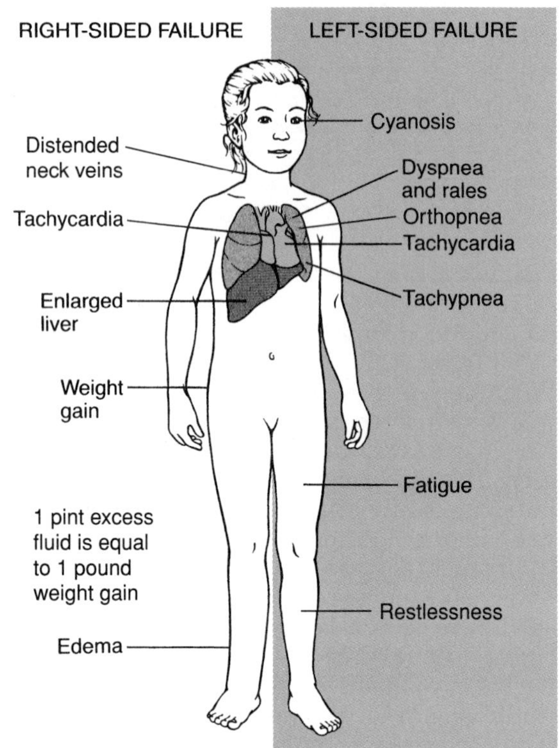

Figure 25–15. • Congestive heart failure. The *right* side of the heart moves unoxygenated blood to pulmonary circulation. A failure results in the backup of blood in the systemic venous system. The *left side* of the heart moves oxygenated blood from the pulmonary circulation to the systemic circulation. A failure results in backup into the lung. When the body tries to compensate for the problems, peripheral vasoconstriction occurs and results in cold, blue hands and feet, tachycardia, and tachypnea. Although heart failure may start as a right-sided or left-sided failure, eventually *both* sides become involved. (Redrawn from Pillitteri, A. [1992]. *Maternal and child health nursing: Care of the child bearing and child bearing family.* Philadelphia: Lippincott.)

Acquired Heart Disease

Acquired heart disease is a cardiac problem that occurs *after* birth. It may be a complication of a congenital heart disease, a response to respiratory infection, sepsis, hypertension, or severe anemia. *Heart failure* is defined as a decrease in cardiac output necessary to meet the metabolic needs of the body.

Congestive Heart Failure

Manifestations. Manifestations depend on the side of the heart affected (Fig. 25–15). Signs differ somewhat and are more subtle in infants. Some of these signs are cyanosis, pallor, rapid respiration, rapid pulse, feeding difficulties, fatigue, a weak cry, excessive perspiration (especially to the forehead), failure to gain weight, edema, and frequent respiratory infections.

Cyanosis. When observing color, the nurse notes whether the cyanosis is general or localized. If it is localized, the exact location is recorded in the nurse's notes, for example, hands, feet, lips, or around the mouth. Is the cyanosis deep or light? Is it constant or transient? Sometimes color improves during crying, and sometimes it gets worse; this is significant. If overt cyanosis is not apparent in the African-American infant, the palms of the hands and bottoms of the feet are observed. Clubbing of the fingers and toes (see Fig. 25–11, p. 666) as a result of blood pooling in the capillaries of the extremities in children with chronic hypoxia may be evident. The skin may be very pale or may be mottled. Sweating, particularly of the head, may be seen.

Rapid Respiration. Rapid respiration is called *tachypnea.* Over a rate of 60 breaths/min in a newborn at rest indicates distress. The amount of dyspnea does vary. In more acute cases, dyspnea is accompanied by flaring of the nostrils, mouth breathing, grunting, and sternal retractions (see Fig. 25–2, p. 650). The baby has more trouble breathing when flat in bed than when held upright. Air hunger is evidenced if the patient is irritable and restless. The cry is weak and hoarse.

Rapid Pulse. Rapid pulse is termed *tachycardia.* An increase in pulse rate is one of the first signs of CHF. The heart is pumping harder in an effort to increase its output and provide increased oxygen to all the tissues of the body. Cardiac output can be increased by one of two mechanisms, tachycardia or increased *stroke volume.* Stroke volume is the amount of blood ejected during one contraction. Because infants and small children have a limited ability to increase stroke volume, their heart rate increases. The heart is pumping harder to get sufficient oxygen to all parts of the body.

Feeding Difficulties. When the nurse tries to feed these infants, they tire easily. They may stop after sucking a few ounces. When placed in the crib, they cry and appear hungry. They may choke and gag during feedings; the pleasure of sucking is spoiled by their inability to breathe.

Poor Weight Gain. The patient fails to gain weight. A sudden increase in weight may indicate edema and the beginning of heart failure.

Edema. Blood flow to the kidneys is decreased, and the glomerular filtration rate slows. This causes both fluid and sodium to be retained. The nurse watches for puffiness about the eyes and, occasionally, in the legs, feet, and abdomen. Urine output may decrease.

Frequent Respiratory Tract Infections. Resistance is very low. Slight infections can be highly dangerous because the heart and lungs are already compromised. Immunizations are reviewed and updated as needed. The nurse prevents exposure to other children who have upper respiratory tract infections and other illnesses.

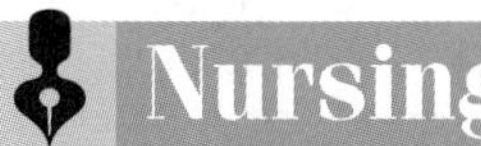

Nursing Tip

Early signs of congestive heart failure in infants that should be reported are:

- Tachycardia at rest
- Fatigue during feedings
- Sweating around scalp and forehead
- Dyspnea
- Sudden weight gain

Treatment and Nursing Care. The nursing goals significant to the care of children with heart defects are (1) to reduce the work of the heart; (2) to improve respiration; (3) to maintain proper nutrition; (4) to prevent infection; (5) to reduce the anxiety of the patient; and (6) to support and instruct the parents.

The nurse must organize care so that the baby is not unnecessarily disturbed. The patient needs a great deal of rest. A complete bath and linen change for an infant with a serious heart defect may not be a priority. The infant is fed early if crying and late if asleep. The physician orders the position in which the infant is placed. In some cases, the knee–chest position facilitates breathing; in other cases, a slanting position with the head elevated (Fowler's position) may be helpful. Older babies may be placed in infant seats.

Feedings are small and frequent. A soft nipple with holes large enough to prevent the infant from tiring is provided. Older children generally tolerate a "no-added-salt" diet. In some cases, nasogastric tube feedings are advantageous because they are less tiring for the patient. Oxygen is administered to relieve dyspnea. As breathing becomes easier, the baby begins to relax. A soft voice and gentle care soothe the patient. Whenever possible, the infant is held and shown love during feedings.

Digitoxin and digoxin (Lanoxin) are common oral digitalis preparations. In pediatric patients, Lanoxin is preferred because of its rapid action and shorter half-life. These agents slow and strengthen the heartbeat. The nurse counts the patient's pulse for 1 full minute before administering them. A resting apical pulse is most accurate. As a rule, *if the pulse rate of a newborn is below 100 beats/min the medication is withheld* and the physician is notified. In older children, the pulse rate should be above 70 beats/min. Because the pulse rate varies with the age of the child, it is ideal for the physician to specify in the written drug order at what heart rate the nurse should withhold the drug. When this is not done the nurse obtains clarification. The physician is notified when the drug is withheld.

If the patient vomits, the physician is contacted. Digitalis administration is not repeated until the physician confirms it is safe to do so. Tachycardia and irregularities in the rhythm of the pulse are significant and should be reported. Symptoms of toxicity include nausea, vomiting, anorexia, irregularity in rate and rhythm of the pulse, and a sudden change in pulse. If the baby is discharged while still receiving medication, the parents are taught how to take the pulse and what signs to be alert for when administering the drug.

Diuretics such as furosemide (Lasix) or chlorothiazide (Diuril) are useful in reducing edema. Careful monitoring of serum electrolyte levels prevents electrolyte imbalance, particularly potassium depletion. Parents of older patients are taught to recognize foods high in potassium, such as bananas, oranges, milk, potatoes, and prune juice. Diapers are weighed to determine urine output. Daily weighing of the baby also helps the physician to determine the effectiveness of the diuresis.

Complications other than cardiac decompensation (heart failure) may arise before or after surgery. Because of the increase in numbers of red blood cells circulating within the body (polycythemia), the blood becomes sluggish and prone to clots. When this is accompanied by dehydration, the threat of cerebral thrombosis may become a reality.

An accurate record of intake and output is essential. Signs of dehydration, such as thirst, fever, poor skin turgor, apathy, sunken eyes or fontanel, dry skin, dry tongue, dry mucous membranes, and decrease in urination, should be brought to the immediate attention of the nurse in charge. Pneumonia can occur rapidly. Fever, irritability, and increase in respiratory distress may indicate this condition. The patient's position is changed regularly to help prevent this setback.

The nurse working in a cardiac unit assesses the patient frequently for complications of cardiac and respiratory failure (Fig. 25–15) and should be competent in cardiopulmonary resuscitation techniques and the necessary modifications required for pediatric patients.

The parents of the child need support and understanding over a long time. A mother's fears and dependencies come to the surface when she gives birth to a baby with a defect. Because the heart is the body's major vital organ, this type of diagnosis causes much apprehension (Fig. 25–16). The physician has to reassure the parents without minimizing the danger involved. If the condition permits, the infant is sent home under medical supervision until the preferred age for surgery. The family must make every effort to provide the child with a normal environment within the necessary limits. It is easy for parents to become overpermissive because they do not wish the child to become unnecessarily excited. The child senses this and soon gains control of the home. This situation is difficult for everyone, but is especially exhausting and confining for the mother. Disciplining the child, such as with a time-out (chair time), is beneficial if done with consistency.

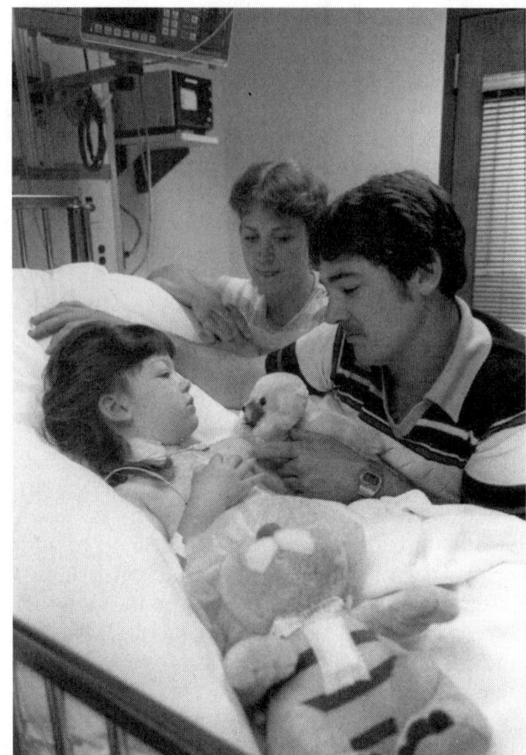

Figure 25–16. • Parents of children in cardiac intensive care units experience a great deal of anxiety because the heart is such a vital organ. (Courtesy of Mercy Hospital Medical Center, Des Moines, IA.)

The patterns formed during infancy can build the framework of a healthy personality for the patient. Children with heart conditions who are well integrated into family life have a decided advantage over children who are made to think they are invalids. Routine naps and early bedtime provide adequate rest for most patients. As children grow, they usually set their own limits on the amount of activity they can handle. Substitutions can be made for strenuous activities, such as bicycle riding, and for rigorous competitive games. The child receives the usual childhood immunizations. Prompt treatment of infections is important. A suitable diet with adequate fluids is necessary. Eating iron-rich foods is encouraged. Dental care should be regular. All-day attendance in school may be too tiring for the child; therefore, special provisions may be necessary. The child needs careful evaluation before any type of minor surgery is performed.

Some children will need occasional hospitalization for various tests or problems. They must be given simple explanations about their condition. They should be allowed to handle and to see hospital equipment before it is used whenever feasible.

Cardiac surgery is generally performed at a regional medical center where the necessary costly equipment is available. Chest tubes may be used postoperatively to remove secretions and air from the pleural cavity and to allow reexpansion of the lungs. These are attached to underwater-seal drainage bottles or a commercially manufactured disposable system, such as Pleur-Evac. Units for infants and older children are available. This system must be *airtight* to prevent collapse of the lung. Drainage bottles *are always kept below the level of the chest* to prevent backflow of secretions. This is especially important during transportation. *Two rubber-shod Kelly clamps must be available at all times* for emergency clamping of tubes. These are applied to the tubes as close as possible to the child's chest if a break in the system occurs.

Detailed discharge planning and coordination of community services are of value to the family. Over the years, the financial burden to the parents for medical and surgical necessities becomes phenomenal. All avenues for financial aid should be explored by qualified personnel. Nursing Care Plan 25–2 specifies interventions for the infant with a congenital heart defect complicated by CHF.

Rheumatic Fever

Description. Rheumatic fever (RF) is a systemic disease involving the joints, heart, central nervous system, skin, and subcutaneous tissues. It belongs to a group of disorders known as *collagen diseases.* Their common feature is the destruction of connective tissue. Rheumatic fever is particularly detrimental to the heart, causing scarring of the mitral valves. Its peak incidence is between the ages of 5 and 15. Rheumatic fever is common worldwide in lower-income groups and where overcrowded conditions exist. It is more prevalent during the winter and spring, and carrier rates among school children are believed to be higher during these seasons. Genetic factors have implicated an abnormal immune response.

Rheumatic fever is an autoimmune disease that occurs as a reaction to a group-A beta-hemolytic *Streptococcus* infection of the throat. The exact pathogenesis is unclear. The body becomes sensitized to the organism after repeated attacks and develops an allergic response to it. During the 1960s and 1970s, the disease almost disappeared; however in the late 1980s, a resurgence occurred in the United States. This has emphasized the need for a better understanding of its origin and transmission so that appropriate public health measures can be instituted.

Manifestations. Symptoms of rheumatic fever range from mild to severe and may not occur for 1 to 3 weeks after a strep throat infection (Fig. 25–17). The classic symptoms are *migratory polyarthritis* (wandering joint pains), *skin eruptions, chorea* (a nervous disorder), and *inflammation of the heart.* Subcutaneous nodules may appear beneath the skin, but are less common in children. Abdominal pain, often mistaken for appendicitis, sometimes occurs. Fever varies from slight to very high. Pallor, fatigue, anorexia, and unexplained nosebleeds may be seen. Rheumatic fever has a tendency to *recur,* and each attack carries the threat of further damage to the heart. The recurrences are most frequent during the first 5 years following the initial attack, and they decline rapidly thereafter.

Migratory Polyarthritis. The *polyarthritis* (*poly,* "many," *arthr,* "joint," and *itis,* "inflammation of") seen in rheumatic fever is distinctive in that it does not result in permanent deformity to the joint. It involves mainly the larger joints: knees, elbows, ankles, wrists, and shoulders. The joints become painful and tender and are difficult to move. *The symptoms last for a few days, disappear without treatment, and frequently return in another joint.* This pattern may continue for a few weeks. The symptoms tend to be more severe in older children. The joint may be visibly swollen and inflamed. On diagnosis salicylates are administered to relieve the pain.

Skin Eruptions. *Erythema marginatum,* the rash seen in rheumatic fever, consists of small red circles with red colored margins and a pale center, and wavy lines appearing on the trunk and abdomen. They appear and disappear rapidly and are significant in diagnosing the disease.

Sydenham's Chorea. Chorea is a disorder of the central nervous system characterized by involuntary, purposeless movements of the muscles. It may occur as an acute rheumatic involvement of the brain. Sydenham's chorea is primarily seen in prepubertal girls.

Attacks of chorea, which begin slowly, may be preceded by increased tension and behavioral problems. The child becomes "clumsy," may stumble and spill things, and may have difficulty buttoning clothes and writing. When the facial muscles are involved, grimaces occur. The child may laugh and cry inappropriately. In severe cases, the patient may

NURSING CARE PLAN 25–2

Selected Nursing Diagnoses for the Infant with a Congenital Heart Defect Complicated by Congestive Heart Failure

Nursing Diagnosis: High risk for altered cardiac output: decreased related to the heart's inability to pump enough blood to meet the metabolic needs of the body

Goals	Nursing Interventions	Rationale
Infant has adequate rest that is reflected by improved cardiac status (vital signs, laboratory results) Infant does not become chilled or overheated as evidenced by temperature evaluation of body and environment	1. Reduce workload on heart by maintaining a quiet environment; organize treatments so as to decrease disturbance; monitor vital signs carefully	1. Optimum rest will decrease demands on heart; pulse rate increases dramatically during congestive heart failure and may be one of the first signs of heart failure in the absence of fever
	2. Assess response to digoxin (if administered)	2. Digoxin is very effective in improving the workload of heart by increasing ventricular contractility and decreasing heart rate, but it is also lethal if levels become too high
	3. Use larger-holed nipples to minimize energy needed for sucking	3. Feeding difficulties are frequent because infants are subject to dyspnea, choking, and fatigue
	4. Avoid chilling by dressing infant appropriately for ambient temperature	4. Thermoregulation is important because extremes could increase the body's metabolic rate and oxygen requirements
	5. Report temperature increases	5. Could indicate infection

Nursing Diagnosis: High risk for impaired gas exchange related to excessive pulmonary congestion and anxiety

Goals	Nursing Interventions	Rationale
Infant balances energy demands with cardiac output as evidenced by stable vital signs and pink, warm skin Infant expends less effort and does not use accessory muscles to breathe	1. Monitor respiratory status frequently	1. Arterial blood gases or pulse oximetry provides important information as to respiratory status; pulmonary edema is manifested by tachypnea and decreased tidal volume
	2. Note color of extremities, lips, nail beds	2. Cyanosis of extremities, lips, and nail beds is a sign of decrease in peripheral tissue perfusion
	3. Note sternal retractions	3. Sternal retractions indicate a progression in respiratory distress; Cheyne-Stokes respirations indicate worsening heart failure
	4. Place in semi-Fowler position	4. Prevents abdominal organs from pressing on diaphragm (unless contraindicated because of other congenital defects)
	5. Assess for signs of respiratory infection, such as cough, increased dyspnea, fever, congestion, sneezing	5. Children with heart disease are subject to frequent respiratory infections; infection increases oxygen demand
	6. Avoid restrictive clothing	6. Restrictive clothing can inhibit breathing
	7. Administer oxygen to reduce stress on heart; monitor via pulse oximetry or arterial blood gases	7. Infants with congestive heart failure have decreased oxygenation of their tissues because of inadequate circulation; oxygen is given to increase the amount of O_2 in blood and to reduce hypoxia; suctioning and positioning can also improve tissue oxygenation

NURSING CARE PLAN 25-2 *continued*

Selected Nursing Diagnoses for the Infant with a Congenital Heart Defect Complicated by Congestive Heart Failure

Nursing Diagnosis: Altered nutrition—less than body requirements due to inadequate caloric intake related to fatigue, immature digestive tract, and poor sucking ability

Goals	Nursing Interventions	Rationale
Infant ingests adequate calories for growth by 24 hr Regurgitation decreases in frequency and amount Infant gradually ingests greater quantities of food Infant's weight begins to stabilize	1. Feed at first sign of hunger; crying wastes energy	1. Decrease energy expenditures
	2. Provide adequate rest before and after feeding	2. Infants tire easily; many babies are physically undeveloped (e.g., preterm infants); gavage feedings may be ordered to ensure adequate nutrients while decreasing energy requirements; avoiding procedures following feedings may prevent regurgitation
	3. Provide small, frequent feedings	3. Capacity of infant's stomach is small; frequent small feedings prevent regurgitation
	4. Weigh daily	4. Decreased renal perfusion results in salt and water retention, which leads to edema; daily weighings assist in determining effectiveness of treatment (many infants are on diuretics), nutritional status, and growth; also important in determining dosage of digoxin
	5. Administer potassium, if ordered, if infant is on diuretic or digoxin to prevent hypokalemia	5. Diuretics decrease salt and water retention related to decreased renal perfusion; since potassium may be lost during diuresis, hypokalemia may occur
	6. Monitor electrolytes	6. Diuretic agents may cause profound changes in electrolyte composition; therefore, frequent electrolyte evaluations are made; potassium depletion, especially in digitalized patient, is very dangerous; anatomic and physiologic makeup of infants and small children makes them vulnerable to imbalances in fluid and electrolytes, particularly during illness
	7. Administer vitamins	7. In severe heart failure, child is less likely to eat and may become malnourished from a decreased intake of nutrients; children in process of growth may require additional vitamins
	8. Keep accurate record of intake and output; weigh diapers	8. Diuretic therapy is used when edema and pulmonary congestion are associated with retention of sodium by kidneys; an accurate intake and output sheet determines necessity for hydration and reaction to medication and treatment protocol

(continued on following page)

become completely incapacitated, and deterioration in speech may be noticeable. Treatment of Sydenham's chorea is directed toward the relief of symptoms. The condition usually spontaneously disappears within weeks to months. Medication may also be required. The presence of Sydenham's chorea alone can support the diagnosis of rheumatic fever.

Rheumatic Carditis. *Carditis,* an inflammation of the heart, is a manifestation of rheumatic fever that can be fatal. It occurs more often in the young child.

NURSING CARE PLAN 25–2 *continued*

Selected Nursing Diagnoses for the Infant with a Congenital Heart Defect Complicated by Congestive Heart Failure

Nursing Diagnosis: High risk for altered family processes due to misunderstanding, feelings of helplessness, fatigue

Goals	Nursing Interventions	Rationale
Parents verbalize fears, ask questions Parents participate in the care of their infant if they wish and as feasible Parents verbalize the importance of managing their own stress	1. Assess parents' understanding of all treatments and procedures	1. Good teaching begins with exploring what person understands and building on the known
	2. Assess need for information	2. Pick opportune time to teach; if family is very stressed, little will be retained
	3. Encourage parents to participate in baby's care	3. Active participation by family helps to decrease anxiety
	4. Educate parents in procedures related to daily care, signs of congestive heart failure, conservation of baby's energy, feedings, medications (*Note:* Digoxin can be fatal if taken accidentally; inform parents not to leave drug where siblings could reach it)	4. Discharge planning begins on admission; hospitalization is often briefer, necessitating an early start; ensures uninterrupted care
	5. Allow siblings to visit	5. Sibling visits promote bonding, allay fears, and help children to feel a part of what is occurring
	6. Provide homelike atmosphere	6. Homelike atmosphere helps to reduce anxiety
	7. Educate as to local support groups	7. Because this disease is so frightening, support by others who have experienced similar crises is helpful
	8. Discuss necessity for parents to relieve their stress by exercise, meditation, communicating with one another, obtaining sufficient rest	8. Family's intactness is crucial for infant's health and happiness

The tissues that cover the heart and the heart valves are affected. The heart muscle, the myocardium, may be involved, as may the pericardium and endocardium. The *mitral valve,* between the left atrium and left ventricle, is frequently involved. Vegetations form that interfere with the proper closing of the valve and disturb its normal function. When this valve becomes narrowed, the condition is called *mitral stenosis.* Myocardial lesions called *Aschoff's bodies* are also characteristic of the disease. The burden on the heart is great because it has to pump harder to circulate the blood. As a result, it may become enlarged. Symptoms of poor circulation and heart failure may appear.

The patient has an irregular low-grade fever, is pale and listless, and has a poor appetite. Moderate anemia and weight loss are apparent. The child may experience dyspnea on exertion. *The pulse and respiration rates are out of proportion to the body temperature.* The physician may detect a soft murmur over the apex of the heart.

Diagnosis. The diagnosis of rheumatic fever is difficult to make, and for this reason the *Jones criteria* have been developed and modified over the years (Table 25–4). The presence of two major criteria or one major and two minor criteria, supported by evidence of recent streptococcal infection, indicates a high probability of rheumatic fever. A careful physical examination is done, and a complete history of the patient is taken. Certain blood tests are helpful. The erythrocyte sedimentation rate is elevated. Abnormal proteins, such as C-reactive protein may also be evident in the serum. Leukocytosis may occur but is not regularly present. Antibodies against the streptococci (measured by ASO titer) may also be detected. Additional studies may include chest x-ray films, throat culture, and lung tests. The electrocardiogram, a graphic record of the electrical changes caused by the beating of the heart, is very useful. Changes in conductivity, particularly a prolonged P-R interval (first-degree heart block), may indicate *carditis.*

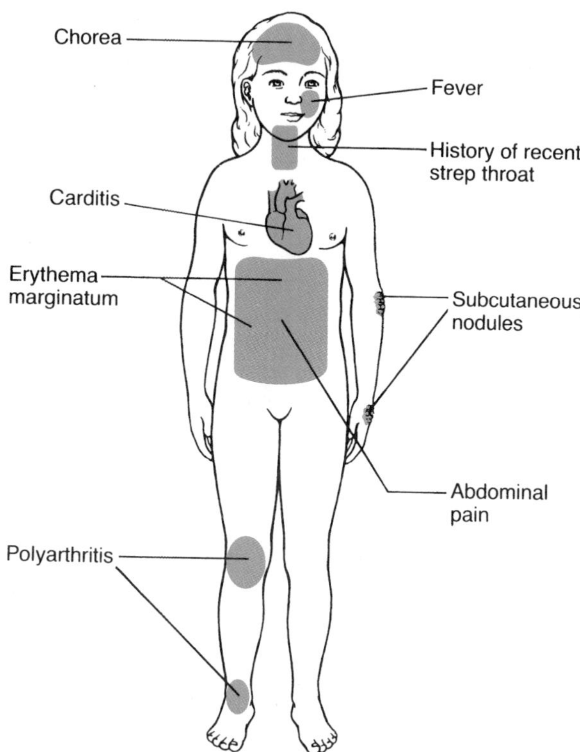

Figure 25–17. • Manifestations of rheumatic fever.

These tests are repeated throughout the course of the disease so that the doctor may determine when the active stage has subsided.

Treatment and Nursing Care. Treatment is aimed at preventing permanent damage to the heart. This is accomplished by antibacterial therapy, physical and mental rest, relief of pain and fever, and management of cardiac failure should it occur. Initial antibacterial therapy is directed toward eliminating the streptococcal infection. Penicillin is the drug of choice (given for a 10-day period) unless the patient is sensitive to it, in which case erythromycin is substituted.

Elimination of infection through medication is followed by long-term *chemoprophylaxis* (prevention of disease by drugs); intramuscular benzathine penicillin G is given monthly to patients with a history of rheumatic fever or evidence of rheumatic heart disease for a 5-year period or until 18 years of age. Oral administration is considered for patients with minimal involvement whose reliability about taking medications can be ascertained. Erythromycin is recommended for long-term therapy for patients who cannot tolerate penicillin. Financial assistance may be available to patients. Local heart associations, rehabilitation services, and state and municipal health departments are sources of such aid.

Antiinflammatory drugs are used to decrease fever and pain. Aspirin is the drug of choice for joint disease without evidence of carditis. The use of steroids is controversial. Concerns during therapy include aspirin toxicity and the effects of aspirin on blood clotting. Mild signs of Cushing's disease, such as moonface, acne, and hirsutism (increased hairiness), should be anticipated with the use of steroids. More severe reactions, such as gastric ulcer, hypertension, overwhelming infection, and toxic psychosis may occur. Phenobarbital is effective in reducing chorea. Padded side rails are used to protect the patient who experiences spasms. If CHF occurs, symptomatic treatment is given.

Bed rest during the initial attack is recommended, until the ESR returns to normal levels. The amount of work the heart has to do must be limited by resting the entire body. In this way, the circulation of the heart is slower, and the heart does not have to work as fast or as hard as when a patient is active. The nurse should teach parents and children the need for rest and the types of play activity appropriate during home care.

Nursing activities should be organized to ensure as few interruptions as possible to prevent tiring the patient. A bed cradle can be used to prevent pressure on painful extremities. Care includes special attention to the skin, especially over bony prominences; back care; good oral hygiene; and small frequent feedings of nourishing foods. Maintenance of healthy teeth and prevention of cavities are of special importance. The patient with rheumatic fever is particularly susceptible to *subacute bacterial endocarditis,* which can occur as a complication of dental or other procedures likely to cause bleeding or infection. Prophylactic antibiotic treatment is

Table 25–4
MODIFIED JONES CRITERIA

Major Criteria	Minor Criteria
Carditis	Fever
Polyarthritis	Arthralgia
Erythema marginatum	Previous history of rheumatic heart disease
Chorea	Elevated erythrocyte sedimentation rate
Subcutaneous nodules	Leukocytosis
	Altered P-R interval on electrocardiogram
	Positive C-reactive protein

A positive diagnosis of rheumatic fever cannot be made without the presence of two major criteria, or one major and two minor criteria, plus a history of streptococcal infection.

required before any dental procedure. Nutrition consists of small servings from the basic food groups. These are increased as the child's appetite improves. A record of fluid intake and output is kept, as overhydration may tax the heart. All efforts are made to provide emotional support for the child and family. Provisions should be made for the child to continue school studies.

Prevention. Prevention of infection and prompt treatment of group-A beta-hemolytic streptococcal infections can prevent the occurrence of RF. All throat infections should be cultured. Once a diagnosis of strep throat is established, the nurse stresses the need to complete antibiotic therapy even if symptoms disappear and the child "feels better." Close medical supervision and follow-up care are essential. The prognosis is favorable.

Systemic Hypertension

Description. Hypertension, or high blood pressure, is being seen more frequently during childhood and adolescence. Blood pressure is a product of peripheral vascular resistance and cardiac output. An increase in cardiac output or peripheral resistance results in an increase in blood pressure. Systemic blood pressure increases with age and is correlated with height and weight throughout childhood and adolescence (Table 25–5). *Significant hypertension* is considered when measurements are persistently between the 95th and 99th percentiles for the patient's age and sex. *Severe hypertension* is a blood pressure persistently at or above the 99th percentile for age and sex. When the cause of the increase in pressure can be explained by a disease process, the hypertension is referred to as *secondary.* Renal, congenital, vascular, and endocrine disorders represent the majority of illnesses that account for secondary hypertension. *Primary,* or *essential hypertension* implies that no known underlying disease is present. Nevertheless, heredity, obesity, stress, and salt intake can contribute to any type of hypertension.

Table 25–5
AVERAGE BLOOD PRESSURE MEASUREMENTS (90TH PERCENTILE LEVEL) IN CHILDHOOD

Weight (kg)	Systolic/Diastolic
4	86/68
6	106/65
14	106/68
25	111/70
35	114/72
45	117/75
60	124/80

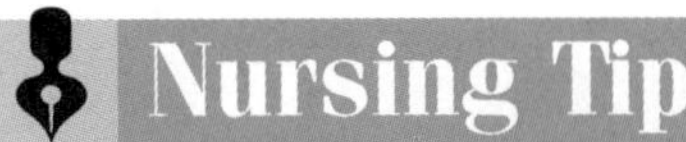

The blood pressure cuff should encircle two thirds of the length of the upper arm for an accurate blood pressure assessment.

There is increasing evidence that essential hypertension, although not generally seen until adolescence or adulthood, may have its roots in childhood. The prevention of this is significant in reducing stroke or myocardial infarction as a person ages. The assessment of blood pressure levels should be part of every physical examination during childhood. Hypertension is more prevalent in children whose parents have high blood pressure.

Manifestations. The child with high blood pressure rarely exhibits clinical symptoms. Frequent headaches, vision problems, or dizziness may or may not be related to hypertension but should be investigated. An elevated blood pressure is usually discovered during a routine physical exam.

Treatment and Nursing Care. The National Heart, Lung, and Blood Institute's Task Force on Blood Pressure Control in Children recommends that a blood pressure above the 95th percentile on three separate occasions be investigated further. Measuring blood pressure in young children requires careful attention to cuff size (see p. 544). The examination may cause stress, which also leads to inaccuracy. An adolescent who shows consistently high readings should be given a complete physical examination.

Treatment and nursing care involve nutritional counseling, reduction in sodium intake, weight reduction, and an age-appropriate program of aerobic exercise. Adolescents should be counseled concerning the adverse effects of drugs, alcohol, and tobacco on blood pressure. Drug therapy to reduce high blood pressure may not be effective in adolescents who are often noncompliant with long-term regimes.

For secondary hypertension, the underlying disease causing the high blood pressure is the focus of treatment. Diuretics, beta-blockers or ACE inhibitors, and calcium channel blockers are classifications of drugs that may be prescribed. Long-term therapy with diuretics may increase serum lipids and some beta-blocking–drugs (Propranolol) may reduce exercise tolerance and cause bronchospasms or sleep disturbances. The many side effects of long term anti-hypertensive drug therapy emphasizes

Table 25–6
AVERAGE PLASMA CHOLESTEROL AND TRIGLYCERIDE LEVELS IN CHILDHOOD

	Cholesterol	Triglycerides
Newborn	68	35
1–9 years	155–165	55–65
10–14 years	160	62–72
15–19 years	150–160	73–78

the need for aggressive prevention measures in childhood.

Prevention. The main focus of a hypertensive prevention program is patient education. The nurse can work with school personnel to promote awareness of the problem at PTA meetings. Community health fairs should offer blood pressure screening opportunities. Blood pressure measurement must be part of every routine physical examination. Risk factors, such as obesity, elevated serum cholesterol, high salt intake, sedentary lifestyle, and drug, alcohol or tobacco, use should be discussed. The effects of contraceptives on blood pressure and alternative options available for sexually active adolescents should be reviewed as appropriate.

Hyperlipidemia

Hyperlipidemia refers to excessive lipids (fat and fatlike substances) in the blood. Because there is evidence that the factors responsible for degenerative vascular disease may begin in childhood and that they may be somewhat controllable, considerable interest has developed in screening children for risk factors and in attempting to change these risks (Table 25–6).

Children with a parental history of cholesterol levels exceeding 240 mg/dl or a family history of early cardiac death (under age 55 years) should have their cholesterol levels tested. However, screening only those children who are identified as high risk may not reach all children who need follow-up care. Therefore, an active preventative program for all children and adolescents is essential. Lifelong healthy eating habits should be nurtured early and practiced by the entire family. A step-one dietary program involves no more than 300 mg of cholesterol per day and no more than 30% of total dietary calories from fat. Children under 2 years of age should not have a fat-restricted diet, as calories and fat are necessary for central nervous system growth and development. The AAP recommendations for heart-healthy guidelines are presented in Table 25–7.

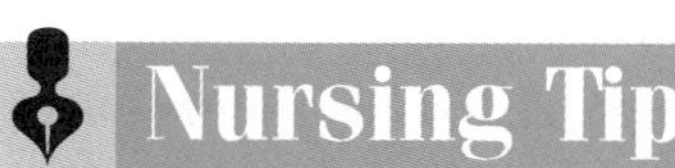

Children younger than 2 years of age should not be put on low-fat, high-fiber diets.

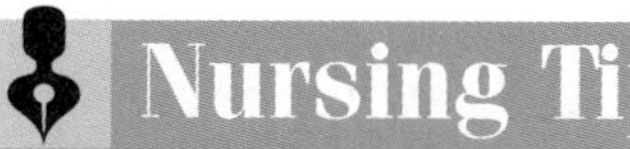

Hospitalization provides an excellent opportunity for the nurse to review heart-healthy information. Reviews of family history, lifestyle, and eating patterns are suitable interventions, even in the absence of high risk.

Kawasaki Disease

Kawasaki disease (KD) (Mucocutaneous Lymphnode Syndrome) occurs worldwide and is the leading cause of acquired cardiovascular disease in the United States. It usually affects children under 5 years of age. Studies have shown that KD may be a reaction to toxins produced by a previous infection with an organism such as the staphylococci. KD is not spread from person to person. The diagnosis is made by clinical signs and symptoms, since specific laboratory findings are not diagnostic. KD causes inflammation of the vessels in the cardiovascular system. The inflammation weakens the walls of the vessels and often results in an *aneurysm* (an abnormal dilation of the wall of a blood vessel). Aneurysms can cause thrombi (blood clots) to form, resulting in serious complications. About 40% of untreated children develop aneurysms of the coronary vessels, which can be life-threatening.

Manifestations. The onset is abrupt with a sustained fever, sometimes above 104° F, that does not respond to antipyretics or antibiotics. The fever lasts for more than 5 days. Conjunctivitis without discharge, fissured lips, a "strawberry tongue" (enlarged reddened papilla on the tongue), inflamed mouth and pharyngeal membranes, and enlarged nontender lymph nodes are seen. An erythematous skin rash develops, with swollen hands and desquamation (peeling) of the palms and soles. The child is very irritable and may develop signs of cardiac problems.

Treatment and Nursing Care. Intravenous gamma globulin given early in the illness can prevent the development of coronary artery pathology. Salicylate therapy (aspirin) is prescribed for its antithrombus properties. Warfarin (Coumadin)

Table 25–7
HEART-HEALTHY GUIDELINES FOR CHILDREN

Age	Guidelines
Infants	Breast milk or formula for 1 yr Rice or other single-grain cereal from 4–6 mo Balanced mixture of cereal, vegetables, fruits, and meats for second 6 mo of life Baby foods are labeled as to calories and nutrient composition; avoid foods with added sugar or salt; most baby foods with the exception of combined foods and desserts do not have these additives Babies do not need desserts to grow; infant fruits are more nutritious Fats do not need to be restricted in healthy infants
Toddlers and preschoolers	Avoid excessive fats, salt, and refined sugars Avoid salty snacks and sweet desserts Offer heart-healthy snacks of vegetables, fruits, finger foods Offer a variety of foods from the basic food groups Discourage the consumption of large amounts of milk, which can lead to nutritional imbalances
School-age children	Provide heart-healthy school lunches Role-model good daily exercise Screen children with family history of congenital heart disease (cholesterol, triglycerides, blood pressure)* Avoid obesity Discourage smoking
Adolescents	Emphasize importance of heart-healthy foods to improve endurance, good body image Avoid sedentary lifestyle Discourage excessive intake of dietary saturated fat, sodium, sugar, and excess calories Be a nonsmoking parent Assess stress management capabilities, counsel accordingly Screen periodically for serum cholesterol elevations, blood pressure Serial monitoring of adolescents deemed high risk (sustained high blood pressure readings on at least three separate occasions)

*Children over the age of 2 years with a family history of hyperlipidemia or early atherosclerotic heart disease should undergo routine screening for hyperlipidemia.

therapy may be prescribed if aneurysms are detected to prevent clot formation.

Nursing care is symptomatic and supportive. Parent teaching should be reinforced concerning the need to postpone active routine immunizations for several months following the administration of gamma globulin, which is an immunosuppressant. Low-dose aspirin therapy may be prescribed to prevent clot formation. Compliance may be a problem for any long-term regimen where medication must be taken when the child feels "well." The nurse should reinforce parent teaching concerning the recognition of cardiac problems and updating their CPR skills.

KEY POINTS

- Routine handwashing practices can prevent the spread of the common cold.
- Quiet play may be more restful than confinement to bed for toddlers and young children.
- Nosedrops with an oil base should be avoided.
- Laryngomalacia and acute spasmodic laryngitis are benign forms of croup. Laryngotracheo bronchitis and epiglottitis are acute types of croup.
- A croupette, or mist tent, provides moist air supersaturated with microdroplets that can enter the small airway of a child and relieve respiratory distress.
- A tongue blade examination of the throat can cause sudden respiratory arrest in a child with epiglottitis.
- Frequent swallowing while the child is sleeping is an early sign of bleeding immediately following a tonsillectomy.
- Coughing, clearing the throat, and blowing the nose should be avoided in the immediate postoperative period following a tonsillectomy.

- Swimming and sports activities that involve intermittent activity are well tolerated by asthmatic children.
- Cystic fibrosis is a multisystem disease characterized by an increased viscosity of mucous gland secretions.
- Signs and symptoms of congenital heart abnormalities in infants include dyspnea, difficulty with feedings, choking spells, recurrent respiratory infections, cyanosis, poor weight gain, clubbing of fingers and toes, and heart murmurs.
- The nursing goals significant to the care of children with heart defects are (1) to reduce the work of the heart; (2) to improve respiration; (3) to maintain proper nutrition; (4) to prevent infection; (5) to reduce the anxiety of the parent; and (6) to support growth and development.
- *Congenital heart defects* may be caused by genetic factors, maternal factors such as drug use or illness, or environmental factors. *Acquired heart disease* occurs *after* birth as a response to a defect or illness.
- Congenital heart defects that result in a recirculation of blood to the lungs do not usually produce cyanosis as a clinical sign.
- A congenital heart defect can cause an increase in pulmonary blood flow, a decrease in pulmonary blood flow, or an obstruction of blood flow.
- A difference in the blood pressure between the arms and the legs is characteristic of coarctation of the aorta.
- The defects in tetralogy of Fallot include pulmonary artery stenosis, hypertrophy of the right ventricle, dextro position of the aorta, and a ventricular septal defect.
- Hypercyanotic "tet" spells are relieved by placing the child in a knee–chest position.
- Signs of congestive heart failure in infants include tachycardia, at-rest fatigue during feedings, and perspiration around the forehead.
- The major Jones criteria that are diagnostic of rheumatic fever include polyarthritis, erythema marginatum, Sydenham's chorea, and rheumatic carditis.
- Chest tube drainage bottles must always be kept below the level of the chest.
- A child under 2 years of age should *not* have a fat-restricted diet.

MULTIPLE-CHOICE REVIEW QUESTIONS

Choose the most appropriate answer.

1. Which of the following is a priority nursing diagnosis in a child admitted with acute asthma?
   a. Risk for infection
   b. Altered nutrition
   c. Ineffective breathing pattern
   d. Body image disturbance
2. Which of the following signs or symptoms observed in a sleeping 2-year-old child following a tonsillectomy requires reporting and follow-up care?
   a. A pulse of 110
   b. A blood pressure of 96/64
   c. Nausea
   d. Frequent swallowing
3. The nurse is reinforcing teaching concerning the use of a cromolyn sodium inhaler for a 10-year-old with asthma. An accurate concept to emphasize would be:
   a. You should use the inhaler whenever you feel some difficulty in breathing.
   b. You should use the inhaler between meals.
   c. You should use the inhaler regularly every day even if you are symptom free.
   d. You can discontinue using the inhaler when you are feeling stronger.
4. When administering Lanoxin (Digoxin) to an infant, the medication should be withheld and the doctor notified if
   a. the pulse rate is below 60 beats/min.
   b. the infant is dyspneic.
   c. the pulse rate is below 100 beats/min.
   d. the respiratory rate is above 40/min.
5. An infant with tetralogy of Fallot is experiencing a "tet" attack involving cyanosis and dyspnea. Which position should the infant be placed in?
   a. Fowler's
   b. Knee–chest
   c. Trendelenburg's
   d. Prone

BIBLIOGRAPHY AND READER REFERENCE

American Academy of Pediatrics Committee on Infectious Diseases. (1996–1997). Reassessment of the Indications for Ribovirin Therapy in Respiratory Syncytial Virus Infection. *Pediatrics*, 137–140.

Ashwill, J., & Droske, S. (1997). *Nursing care of children: Principles and practice.* Philadelphia: Saunders.

Behrman, R. E., Kleigman, R., & Arvin, A. (1996). *Nelson's textbook of pediatrics* (15th ed.). Philadelphia: Saunders.

Berman, S. (Ed.) (1996). *Pediatric clinical decision making* (3rd ed., pp. 564–567). St. Louis, MO: Mosby.

Bing, M., Frishman, W., et al. (1997). Chronotherapy: Working with the body's rhythms. *Patient Care, 31*(15), 11.

Briening, E. (1998). Management of the pediatric patient in status asthmaticus. *Critical Care Nurse, 18*(1), 74.

Chiocca, E., & Russo, L. (1997). Action stat acute asthma attack. *Nursing 97, 27*(6), 57.

Coakley-Maller, E., & Shea, M. (1997). Respiratory infections in children. *Advance for Nurse Practitioners, 5*(9), 21–27.

Daberkow-Carson, E., & Smith, P. (1994). Altered cardiovascular junction. In Betz, C., Hunsberger, M., & Wrights, S. *Family centered nursing care of children*, 2nd ed. Philadelphia: Saunders.

Drazen, J. (1998). New directions in asthma drug therapy. *Hospital Practices, 33*(2), 25–27.

Fabius, D. (1994). Understanding heart sounds: Solving the mystery of heart murmurs. *Nursing 94, 24*(7), 39–44.

Groothuis, J. (1994). The role of antibody and use of RSV immunoglobulin in the prevention of RSV disease in preterm infants with and without BPD. *Pediatric Infectious Disease Journal, 13*, 454–458.

Gutgesell, H., Atkins, D., & Day, R. (1997). Common cardiovascular problems in the young: hypertension, hypercholesterolemia and preparticipation screening of athletes. *American Family Physician, 56*(8), 1993.

Hollingsworth, H. (1996). Allergic rhinoconjunctivitis current therapy. *Hospital Practice, 31*(6), 61–73.

Keddy, Gazarian P. (1997). Direct route for asthma therapy. *Nursing 97, 27*(10), 53.

Kemper, K. (1997). A practical approach to asthma management. *Contemporary Pediatrics 14*(8), 86.

Krishna, M., Chauhan, A. & Holgate, S. (1996). Molecular mediators of asthma: Current insights. *Hospital Practice, 31*(10), 115–130.

Lehr, M., & Simoes, E. (1998). A weapon against RSV for children at risk. *Contemporary Pediatrics, 15*(2), 78.

Martinez, F., Wright, A., Taussig, L., et al. (1995). Asthma and wheezing in the first six years of life. *New England Journal of Medicine, 332*, 133–138.

Mathews, P. (1997). Using a peak flow meter. *Nursing 97, 27*(6), 57–59.

Meert, K., Sarnaik, A., Gilmine, M., & Leek-Lai, M. (1994). Aerosolized Ribovirin in mechanically ventilated children with RSV lower respiratory tract disease. *Critical Care Medicine, 22,* 566–572.

Middleton, A. (1997). Managing asthma: It takes teamwork. *American Journal of Nursing, 97*(1), 39.

Miller, C., & Holden, P. (1998). Pediatric liquid ventilation. *RN, 61*(4), 57.

Moynihan, P., Naclerio, L., & Kiley, K. (1995). Parent participation. *Nursing Clinics of North American Nursing, 29*(2), 231–242.

Murphy, S., & Kelly, H. (1996). Advances in management of acute asthma in children. *Pediatric Review, 17,* 227.

National Asthma Education and Prevention Program: Expert Panel Report II. (1997). *Guidelines for the diagnosis and management of asthma.* Publication #97-4501. Bethesda, MD: US Department of Health and Human Services.

Norris, M. K. G., & Hill, C. S. (1994). Nutritional issues in infants and children with congenital heart disease. *Critical Care Nursing of North America, 9*(2), 153–164.

Reed, M. (Chair). (1997, December). RSV: Beyond the acute infection. Pediatric clinical pharmacy round table. New York: SCIENS Worldwide Medical Education.

Schidlow, D., & Callahan, C. (1996). Pneumonia. *Pediatrics in Review, 17*(9), 300–310.

Stinson, J., et al. (1995). Mothers' information needs related to caring for infants at home following cardiac surgery. *Journal of Pediatric Nursing, 10*(1), 48–57.

Toogood, J. (1994). Helping your patients make better use of MDIs and spacers. *Journal of Respiratory Disease, 15*(2), 151.

U.S. Department of Health and Human Services (1994, May). *Health technology assessment: Institutional and patient care criteria for heart-lung transplantation.* Washington, DC: Author.

Wagner, M., & Jacobs, J. (1997). Improving asthma management with peak flow meters. *Contemporary Pediatrics, 14*(8), 111.

Wang, E., Law, B., & Stephens, D. (1995). Pediatric Investigators Collaborative Network on Infections in Canada (PICNIC) prospective study of risk factors and outcomes in patients hospitalized with RSV lower respiratory tract infection. *Journal of Pediatrics, 126,* 212–219.

Wong, D. (1997). *Essentials of pediatric nursing* (5th ed.). St. Louis, MO: Mosby.

chapter 26

The Child with a Condition of the Blood, Blood-Forming Organs, or Lymphatic System

Outline

ANEMIAS
- Iron-Deficiency Anemia
- Sickle Cell Anemia
- Thalassemia

BLEEDING DISORDERS
- Hemophilia
- Idiopathic (Immunologic) Thrombocytopenic Purpura

DISORDERS OF WHITE BLOOD CELLS
- The Leukemias
- Hodgkin's Disease

NURSING CARE OF THE CHRONICALLY ILL CHILD

NURSING CARE OF THE DYING CHILD

Objectives

On completion and mastery of Chapter 26, the student will be able to

- Define each vocabulary term listed.
- Summarize the components of the blood.
- Recall normal blood values of infants and children.
- List two laboratory procedures commonly performed on children with blood disorders.
- Compare and contrast four manifestations of bleeding into the skin.
- List the symptoms, prevention, and treatment of iron-deficiency anemia.
- Recommend four food sources of iron for a child with iron-deficiency anemia.
- Recognize the effects on the bone marrow of increased RBC production due to thalassemia.
- Review the effects of severe anemia on the heart.
- Devise a nursing care plan for a child with sickle cell disease.
- Examine the pathology and signs and symptoms of sickle cell anemia.
- Describe four types of sickle cell crises.
- Discuss the nursing care of a child receiving a blood transfusion.
- Recall the pathology and signs and symptoms of hemophilia A and B.

(Continued)

Objectives (Continued)

- Identify the nursing interventions necessary to prevent hemarthrosis in a child with hemophilia.
- Discuss the effects of chronic illness on the growth and development of children.
- Plan the nursing care of a child with leukemia.
- Review the nursing care of a child receiving a transfusion.
- Contrast age-appropriate responses to a sibling's death and the nursing interventions required.
- Formulate techniques the nurse can use to facilitate the grieving process.
- Recall the stages of dying.
- Discuss the nurse's role in helping families to deal with the death of a child.

Vocabulary

alopecia	lymphadenopathy
Christmas disease	petechiae
ecchymosis	purpura
erythropoietin	respite care
hematoma	sickle cell crises
hemarthrosis	Sickledex
hematopoiesis	splenomegaly
hemosiderosis	thrombosis
icterus	

The blood and blood-forming organs make up the hematologic system. *Blood dyscrasias* or disorders occur when blood components fail to form correctly or when blood values exceed or fail to meet normal standards. Blood is vital to all body functions. Plasma and blood cells are formed at about the 2nd week of life in the embryo. Blood forms primarily in the liver at about the 5th week of development; later it forms in the spleen, thymus, lymph system, and bone marrow. In the fetus, blood is formed primarily in the liver until the last trimester of pregnancy.

During childhood the red blood cells are formed in the marrow of the long bones (such as the tibia and femur), and by adolescence, *hematopoiesis* (blood formation) takes place in the marrow of the ribs, sternum vertebrae, pelvis, skull, clavicle, and scapula. The rate of red blood cell (RBC) production is regulated by *erythropoietin.* This substance is produced by the liver of the fetus, but at birth the kidney takes over erythropoietin production. The lymph system includes lymphocytes, lymphatic vessels, lymph nodes, spleen, tonsils, adenoids, and the thymus gland. The lymphatic system drains regions of the body to lymph nodes where infectious organisms are destroyed and antibody production is stimulated. Lymph nodes are not palpable in the newborn, but cervical axillary and inguinal nodes are palpable by childhood. *Lymphadenopathy* is an enlargement of lymph nodes that is indicative of infection or disease. Figure 26–1 summarizes some of the differences between the child's and the adult's lymphatic system. Figure 26–2 depicts the main types of blood cells in the circulating blood.

Circulating blood consists of two portions: plasma and formed elements. The formed elements are erythrocytes (red blood cells), leukocytes (white blood cells), and thrombocytes (platelets). Erythrocytes primarily transport oxygen and carbon dioxide to and from the lungs and tissues. Leukocytes act as the body's defense against infections. Thrombocytes, along with portions of blood plasma, are involved with blood coagulation. In the young child, every available space in the bone marrow is involved with blood formation.

Lymphocytes, unlike other white blood cells, are produced in the lymphoid tissues of the body. They travel in the circulation but are more commonly found in the lymph tissue. They are released into the body to fight infection and provide immunity. Their numbers greatly increase in chronic inflammatory conditions. The spleen is the largest organ of the lymphatic system. One of the main functions of the spleen is to bring blood into contact with lymphocytes. Aside from trauma and rupture, the most frequently seen pathologic condition of the spleen is enlargement. This is termed *splenomegaly.* The spleen enlarges during infections, congenital and acquired hemolytic anemias, and liver malfunction.

Bone marrow aspiration is a procedure helpful in determining disorders of the blood. Numerous blood counts are utilized as well. Many are specific to a particular disease. The skin is sometimes an indicator of certain conditions of the blood. *Petechiae* (pinpoint hemorrhagic spots) and *purpura* (large petechiae) are often seen and should alert the nurse to the possibility of blood dyscrasia. The physician examines the liver and spleen by palpation and percussion to determine if they are enlarged.

ANEMIAS

Anemia can result from many different underlying causes. A reduction in the amount of circulating

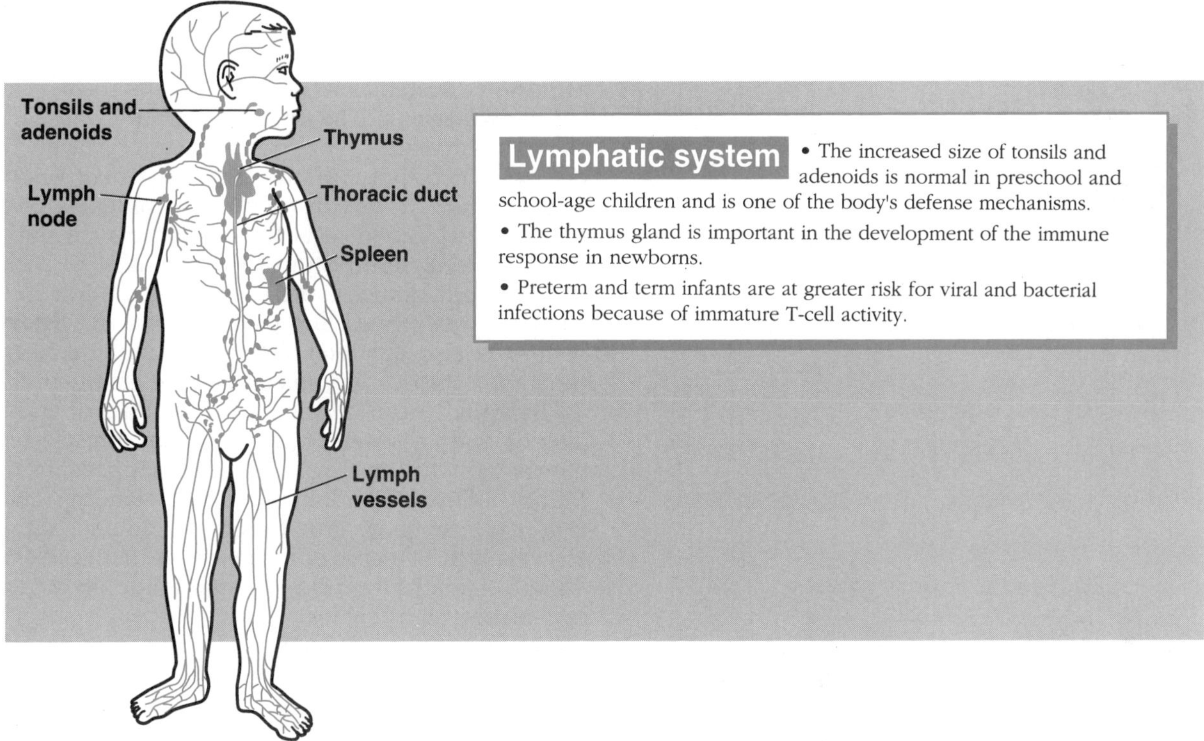

Figure 26–1. • Summary of lymphatic system differences between the child and the adult. The lymphatic system is a subsystem of the circulatory system. It returns excess tissue fluid to the blood and defends the body against disease.

hemoglobin reduces the oxygen-carrying ability of the blood. A hemoglobin level below 8 g/dl results in an increased cardiac output and a shunting of blood from the periphery of the body to the vital organs. Pallor, weakness, tachypnea, shortness of breath, and congestive heart failure can result. Table 26–1 reviews normal blood values in infants and children.

Iron-Deficiency Anemia

Description. The most common nutritional deficiency of children in the United States today is anemia due to insufficient amounts of iron in the body. The incidence is highest during infancy and adolescence, two rapid growth periods. Anemia (*an,* "without," and *emia,* "blood") is a condition in which there is a reduction in the amount and size of the red blood cells or in the amount of hemoglobin, or both. Iron-deficiency anemia may be caused by severe hemorrhage, the child's inability to absorb the iron received, excessive growth requirements, or an inadequate diet. Researchers have also found that feeding infants whole cow's milk can precipitate gastrointestinal bleeding resulting in anemia.

Prevention of iron-deficiency anemia begins with good prenatal care to ensure that the mother has a suitable intake of iron during pregnancy. During the first few months following birth the newborn relies on iron that was stored in the system during fetal life. Preterm infants may be deprived of a sufficient supply, since iron is obtained late in the prenatal period. Also, the iron stores of low-birth-weight babies and babies from multiple births are relatively small.

The highest incidence of this type of anemia occurs from the 9th month to the 24th month. During this rapid growth period, the baby outgrows the limited iron reserve that was in the body; in addition, iron-fortified formula and infant cereals may have been eliminated from the diet. Poorly planned meals or feeding problems also contribute to this deficiency. The mother may sometimes rely too heavily on bottle feedings to avoid conflict at meals. Unfortunately, milk contains very little iron. Instead, the amounts of solid food should be increased and the amount of milk decreased. Boiled egg yolk, liver, leafy green vegetables. Cream of Wheat, dried fruits (apricots, peaches, prunes, raisins), dry beans, crushed nuts, and whole-grain bread are good sources of iron. Iron-fortified cereals

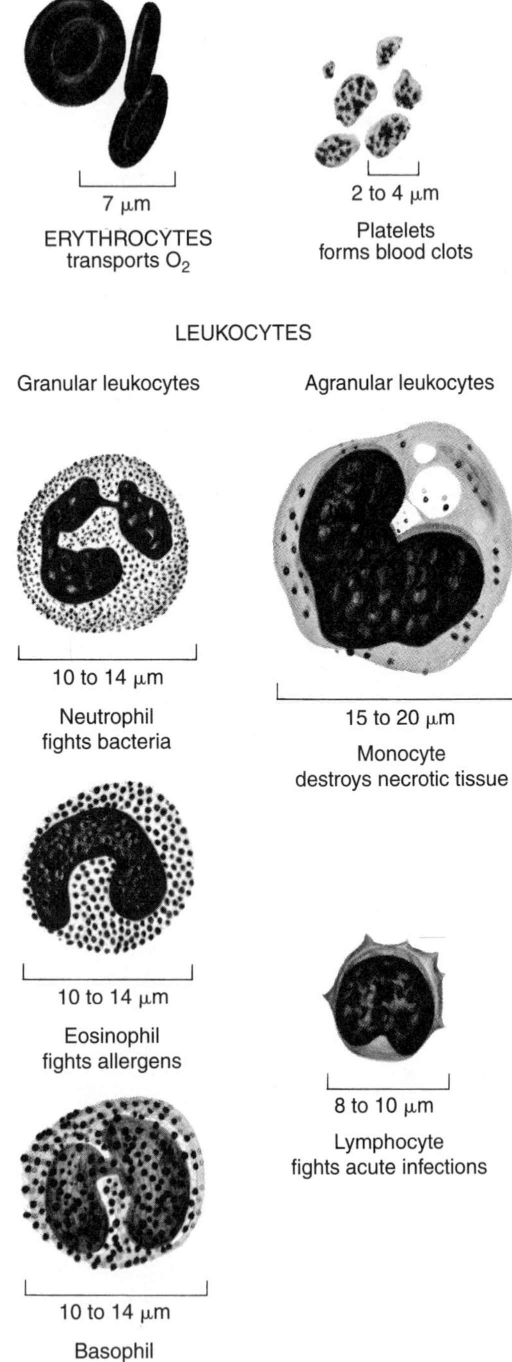

Figure 26–2. • Main types of blood cells in the circulating blood. (Adapted from Solomon, E. P., & Phillips, G. A. [1987]. *Understanding human anatomy and physiology* [p. 200]. Philadelphia: Saunders.)

eaten out of the box provide a nutritious snack. Unfortunately, not all the iron found in a food source is absorbed by the body. The bioavailability of iron in vegetables is less than that in meat.

Manifestations. The symptoms of iron-deficiency anemia are pallor, irritability, anorexia, and a decrease in activity. Many babies are overweight because of excessive consumption of milk (so called milk babies). Blood tests for anemia may include red blood cell count, hemoglobin, hematocrit, morphologic cell changes, and iron concentration. The stool may be tested for occult blood. A dietary history is also obtained. Sometimes a slight heart murmur is heard. The spleen may be enlarged.

Untreated iron-deficiency anemias progress slowly, and in severe cases the heart muscle becomes too weak to function. If this happens, heart failure follows. Children with long-standing anemia may also show growth retardation and cognitive changes. Screening procedures are suggested at 9 and 24 months for full-term infants and earlier for low-birth-weight babies.

Treatment. Iron-deficiency anemia responds well to treatment. Iron, usually ferrous sulfate, is given orally two or three times a day *between meals.* Vitamin C aids in the absorption of iron; therefore, giving juice when administering iron is suggested. Liquid preparations are taken through a straw to prevent temporary discoloration of the teeth. (Some available iron preparations do not have this disadvantage.) The toddler needs solid foods that are rich sources of iron. An iron-dextran mixture (Imferon) given intramuscularly is also highly effective. It must be injected deep in a large muscle using the Z-track technique to minimize staining and tissue irritation.

Parent Education. Parents need explicit instructions on proper foods for the infant. The nurse stresses the importance of breastfeeding for the first 6 months and the use of iron-fortified formula throughout the 1st year of life (the absorption of iron from human milk is much better than that from cow's milk). The amount of milk consumed during the day and night is determined. Solid food intake is reviewed and specific iron-enriched nutrients are suggested. The nurse considers financial, ethnic, and family preferences in discussions. Behavior

Nursing Tip

Avoid iron poisoning in children by keeping preparations well out of reach. Educate parents about this hazard.

Table 26–1

NORMAL BLOOD VALUES DURING INFANCY AND CHILDHOOD

Age	RBC (g/dL)	Hematocrit (%)	Leukocytes (WBC/mm³)	Neutrophils (%)	Lymphocytes (%)	Eosinophil (%)	Monocyte (%)
Neonate	16.5	50	12,000	40	63	3	9
3 Months	12	36	12,000	30	48	2	5
6 mo–6 yr	12	37	10,000	45	48	2	5
7–12 yr	13	38	8–10,000	55	38	2	5
Adult	14–16	42–47	8–10,000	55	35	3	7

concerns at mealtime may also need to be addressed.

The stools of babies placed on oral iron supplements are tarry green. Absence of this finding may indicate poor compliance with therapy by the parents. Oral iron preparations are not to be given with milk, which interferes with absorption. These preparations should be given between meals when digestive acid concentration is highest, in order to increase absorption. *It is important to emphasize that both dietary changes and supplemental iron therapy are necessary to eradicate iron-deficiency anemia.* Dietary changes must be lifelong to maintain good health and to prevent recurrence. Parents are encouraged to return for periodic evaluation of the child's blood status. Nursing Care Plan 26–1 specifies interventions for the child with iron-deficiency anemia.

Sickle Cell Anemia

Description. Sickle cell anemia is an inherited defect in the formation of hemoglobin. It occurs mainly in African-American populations, but it is also carried by some people of Arabian, Greek, Maltese, Sicilian, and other Mediterranean races. Many researchers believe that the gene for sickle cell anemia developed in these populations as protection against malaria. Sickling (clumping) due to decreases in blood oxygen may be triggered by dehydration, infection, physical or emotional stress, or exposure to cold. Laboratory examination of the affected child's blood shows that the red blood cell has changed its shape to resemble that of a sickle blade, from which the name of the disorder is derived (Fig. 26–3).

Sickle cells contain an abnormal form of hemoglobin termed *hemoglobin S* (the sickling type). The membranes of these cells are fragile and easily destroyed. Their crescent shape makes it difficult for them to pass through the capillaries, causing a pile-up of cells in the small vessels. This clumping together may lead to a *thrombosis* (clot) and cause an obstruction. *Infarcts,* or areas of dead tissue, may result when the tissue is denied proper blood supply. These generally develop in the spleen but may also be seen in other areas of the body, such as the brain, heart, lungs, gastrointestinal tract, kidneys, and bones. The patient feels acute pain in the affected area.

There are two types of sickle cell disorders: an asymptomatic (*a,* "without," and *symptoma,* "symptom") version, *sickle cell trait,* and a much more severe form requiring intermittent hospitalization, *sickle cell disease.*

Sickle Cell Trait. This form of the disease occurs in about 10% of the African-American population in the United States. The blood of the patient contains a mixture of normal (hemoglobin A) and sickle (hemoglobin S) hemoglobins. The proportions of hemoglobin S are low since the disease is inherited from only one parent. The doctor can distinguish sickle cell trait from the more severe disease by studying the patient's red blood cells and hemoglobin. Sickling is more rapid and extreme in the disease. In sickle cell trait, the hemoglobin and red blood cell counts are normal.

Sickle cell trait does not develop into sickle cell disease. Although there is no need for treating the patient with sickle cell trait, the patient *is* a carrier, and genetic counseling is important. Advice might be sought from a family physician, pediatrician, or genetic specialist. The nurse encourages and supports such efforts made by parents. The importance of regular visits to a well-child clinic or family-centered clinic is stressed. The nurse can also suggest organizations that help with transportation and baby-sitting problems that so often prevent parents from making maximum use of community facilities.

Sickle Cell Disease. This severe form of sickle cell disorder results when the abnormality is inherited from both parents (Fig. 26–4). *Each offspring* has one chance in four of inheriting the disease (not one of four children). The symptoms generally do not appear until the last part of the 1st year of life. There may be an unusual swelling of the fingers and toes. The symptoms of sickle cell ane-

NURSING CARE PLAN 26–1

Selected Nursing Diagnoses for the Child with Iron-Deficiency Anemia

Nursing Diagnosis: Knowledge deficit (parents) related to cause and treatment of anemia

Goals	Nursing Interventions	Rationale
Parents will verbalize understanding of the importance of dietary factors and iron supplements in the prevention and treatment of this condition Infant will ingest iron-rich formula plus two servings of iron-fortified cereal and iron supplement, if prescribed	1. Encourage breastfeeding	1. Absorption of iron from human milk is much better than that from cow's milk
	2. Encourage iron-rich formula for full 1st year	2. Cow's milk contains little iron
	3. Dispel myth that milk is a perfect food	3. Parents often rely too heavily on milk because it is easier than preparing solid foods, which baby may initially dislike; ingestion of large amounts of milk may interfere with absorption of iron supplements
	4. Give iron supplement between meals with juice	4. Vitamin C aids in absorption of iron

Nursing Diagnosis: Altered nutrition—less than body requirements related to iron-poor diet

Goals	Nursing Interventions	Rationale
Patient's hemoglobin level will improve with therapy; there will be no recurrence of anemia	1. Review 24-hr dietary history	1. Nurse can determine what foods are missing and quantities of food ingested; this information can be used as a baseline for teaching
	2. Review height and weight chart	2. Determines child's status in relation to norms; compares patient's present measurements with former rate of growth and progress
	3. Review solid food intake and suggest iron-rich foods as age appropriate	3. Solid foods high in iron need to be increased as age appropriate (egg yolk, liver, leafy green vegetables, Cream of Wheat, dried fruits, whole-grain bread, iron-fortified cereal)
	4. Educate parents as to how to administer iron supplement	4. Usually given orally two or three times a day between meals; supplements are easily forgotten because evidence of improvement is slow and signs of disease may not be noticeable; poisoning can result from overdose
	5. Stress importance of compliance with dietary regimen to prevent recurrence	5. Dietary changes must be lifelong to maintain good health

mia are caused by enlarging bone marrow sites that impair circulation to the bone and the abnormal sickle cell shape that causes clumping, obstruction in the vessel, and ischemia to the organ that vessel supplies.

There is chronic anemia. The hemoglobin level ranges from 6 to 9 gm/dl or lower. The child is pale, tires easily, and has little appetite. These manifestations of anemia are complicated by characteristic episodes of *sickle cell crises,* which are painful and can be fatal. Specific types of crises have been defined. They differ in pathology and may require somewhat different treatments (Table 26–2). Unfortunately, in some cases the sickle cell crisis is the first obvious manifestation of the condition. The patient appears acutely ill. There is severe abdominal pain. Muscle spasms, leg pains, or painful swollen joints may be seen. Fever, vomiting, hematuria, convulsions, stiff neck, coma, or paralysis can result, depending on the organs involved. The pa-

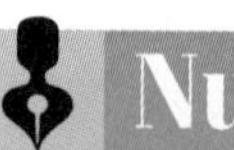

Nursing Tip

During sickle cell crises, anticipate the child's need for tissue oxygenation, hydration, rest, protection from infection, pain control, blood transfusions, and emotional support for life-threatening illness.

tient may be jaundiced. Cardiac enlargement and murmurs are not uncommon.

The sickle cell crises recur periodically throughout childhood; however, they tend to decrease with age. Between episodes, patients should be kept in good health. Immunizations of these children are particularly important, including *Haemophilus influenzae* and hepatitis B. Pneumococcal vaccine may be given to children over 5 years of age and should be administered to all children with sickle cell disease. Prophylactic penicillin G is highly effective in preventing serious pneumonia. Patients should refrain from becoming overly tired. They also should avoid situations such as flying in an unpressurized airplane or exercising at high altitude because oxygen concentrations are already reduced in their blood. Extra stress and exposure to cold may lower resistance, causing additional problems. Overheating, which can lead to dehydration, is also to be avoided. Oral intake of iron is of no value.

Diagnosis. The sickling test *(Sickledex)* is commonly used for screening. When the result is positive, hemoglobin electrophoresis ("fingerprinting") is employed. This procedure separates and records the various peptide patterns of the blood. It distinguishes between patients with the trait and those with the disease.

Treatment and Nursing Care. When the infant or child is hospitalized during a crisis, the treatment is supportive and symptomatic. The patient is confined to bed. Analgesics are given to relieve pain. Children in severe pain may need a continuous intravenous infusion containing a narcotic. If the patient has an infection, such as meningitis or pneumonia, antibiotics are given. Every effort is made to combat dehydration and acidosis. Small blood transfusions may be administered to increase the hemoglobin count, but the results are only temporary. Frequently, packed red blood cells are used for this purpose.

The nurse observes the overall appearance of the patient and assesses the developmental stage, body proportions, and relation of height and weight to age. Facial expressions, degree of restlessness, and areas of pain are noted and recorded. Elevated temperature; rapid, weak pulse; a sunken fontanel in infants younger than 18 months; weight loss; poor tissue turgor; dry skin, lips, and mucous membranes; and decrease in urination signal dehydration. If vomiting occurs, appropriate oral hygiene is given. The nurse observes and records infusions according to unit policy. An accurate record of intake and output is kept. Careful attention is given to the skin. Jaundice *(icterus)* can be

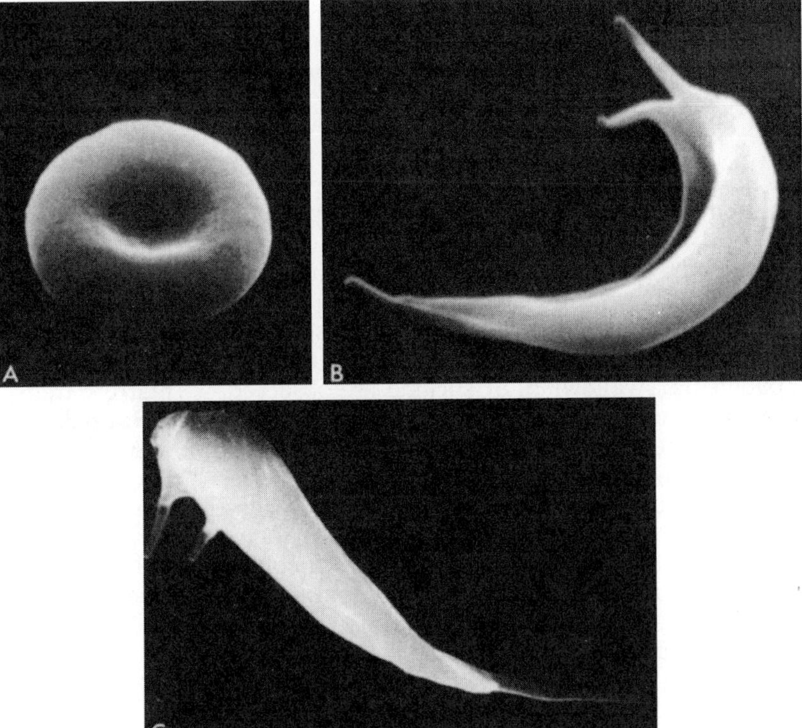

Figure 26–3. • Scanning electron micrograph of erythrocytes. Comparison of a normal cell **(A)** with deoxygenated sickled cells **(B, C)**. (Courtesy of Dr. James White. From Bunn, H. F., Forget, B. G., & Ranney, H. M. [1977]. *Human hemoglobins* [p. 240]. Philadelphia: Saunders.)

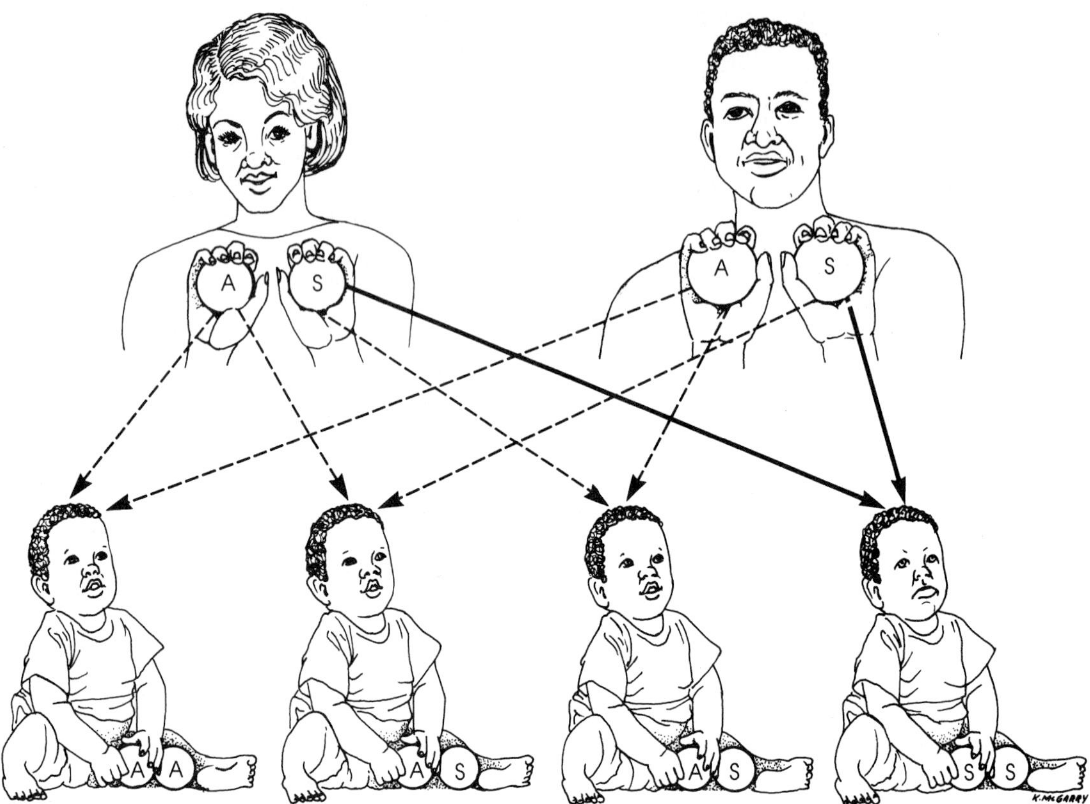

Figure 26–4. • How sickle cell disease is transmitted from parents to children. Parents who are carriers of the sickle cell trait do not show symptoms of the disease because hemoglobin A (the normal form of hemoglobin) in their red blood cells protects them from hemoglobin S (the sickling form). However, when two carriers become parents, the possibilities are as follows: One child in four will inherit all normal hemoglobin (AA) and thus be free of the disease; two children in four will inherit both hemoglobin A and hemoglobin S and thus become carriers (AS) of the trait, like their parents; and one child in four will inherit all sickling hemoglobin (SS) and thus be affected by sickle cell anemia.

detected by observing whether the skin (palms of the hands and soles of the feet) and the whites of the eyes have taken on a yellowish tinge. The patient's body position is changed gently.

Because sickle cell disease can affect muscle tone, any rigidity of muscles should be reported. Eye movements, swallowing, or sucking are observed. The nurse notes if the child is uncomfortable when flexing the neck to have a gown changed. The nurse watches for twitching about the face or elsewhere. Sickle cell disease may take a wide variety of courses. As always, the individual patient's progress is followed. Sometimes it is difficult to distinguish between a sickle cell crisis causing ischemia in the abdominal area from abdominal pain caused by appendicitis. The nurse must remember that pain experienced by a child with sickle cell disease may be caused by an unrelated condition.

Prevention of infection and dehydration are priority goals in the care of a child with sickle cell disease. Multiple transfusions of packed cells may be required to maintain adequate hemoglobin levels. The nurse should observe the child for reactions to the blood transfusion. *Hemosiderosis* (the deposit of iron into organs and tissues in the body) is a complication of this type of hemolytic disease. Bone marrow transplants have been successful.

Surgery. The approach to splenectomy in children with sickle cell disease has been conservative. Recurrence of acute splenic sequestration becomes less likely after 5 years of age. Routine splenectomy is not recommended, as the spleen generally atrophies on its own because of fibrotic changes that take place in patients with sickle cell disease.

Thalassemia

Description. The thalassemias are a group of hereditary blood disorders in which the patient's body cannot produce sufficient adult hemoglobin. The red blood cells are abnormal in size and shape and are rapidly destroyed. This abnormality results in a chronic anemia. The body attempts to compensate by producing large amounts of fetal hemoglobin. These disorders are caused by a deficiency in the normal synthesis of hemoglobin polypeptide chains. They are categorized according to the polypeptide chain affected as alpha-, beta-, gamma-, or delta-thalassemia.

The most common variety of thalassemia involves impaired production of beta chains and is known as *beta-thalassemia.* This variety consists of two forms, thalassemia minor and thalassemia major. Thalassemia major is also called Cooley's anemia. Thalassemia occurs mainly in persons of Mediterranean origin, for example, Greeks, Syrians, Italians, and their descendants elsewhere. The term is derived from the Greek *thalassa,* which means "sea." Thalassemia can also occur from spontaneous mutations.

Thalassemia Minor

Thalassemia minor, also termed *beta-thalassemia trait,* occurs when the child inherits a thalassemia gene from only one parent, that is, by heterozygous inheritance. It is associated with mild anemia. Hemoglobin concentration averages 2 to 3 gm/dl, lower than age-related values. These patients are often misdiagnosed as having an iron-deficiency anemia. Symptoms are minimal. The patient is pale, and the spleen may be enlarged. The patient may lead a normal life, with the illness going undetected. This condition is of genetic importance, particularly if both parents are carriers of the trait. Prenatal blood samples can detect thalassemia major in such cases.

Thalassemia Major (Cooley's Anemia)

When two thalassemia genes are inherited (homozygous inheritance), the child is born with a more serious form of the disease. A progressive, severe anemia becomes evident within the second 6 months of life.

The child is pale and hypoxic, has a poor appetite, and may have a fever. Jaundice, which at first is mild, progresses to a muddy bronze color due to *hemosiderosis,* a deposit of iron (released by blood cell destruction) into the tissues. The liver enlarges, and the spleen grows enormously. Abdominal distention is great, which causes pressure on the organs of the chest. Cardiac failure due to the profound anemia is a constant threat. Bone marrow space enlarges to compensate for an increased production of blood cells. Hematopoietic (*hema,* "blood," and *poiesis,* "to make") defects, a massive expansion of the bone marrow in the face and skull result in changes in the facial contour that give the child a characteristic appearance (Fig. 26–5). The teeth protrude because of an overgrowth of the upper jaw bone; the bone becomes thin and is subject to pathologic fracture.

The diagnosis is aided by the family history of thalassemia, radiographic bone growth studies, and blood tests. Hemoglobin electrophoresis is helpful in diagnosing the type and severity of the various thalassemias. The prognosis is poor. Death may be due to cardiac failure, severe anemia, or secondary infection.

Table 26–2

TYPES OF SICKLE CELL CRISES

Type	Comment
Vasoocclusive (painful crises)	Most common type, obstruction of blood flow by cells, infarctions, some degree of vasospasm Dactylitis, painful joints and extremities, abdominal pain (infarction or bleeding within liver, spleen, abdominal lymph node), central nervous system strokes, pulmonary disease, priapism
Splenic sequestration	Pooling of large amounts of blood in liver and spleen Spleen becomes massive Circulatory collapse, shock Children between 8 months and 5 years of age particularly susceptible Death may occur within hours of appearance of symptoms Minor episodes may resolve spontaneously Splenectomy may be indicated for children who have one or more severe crises
Aplastic crises	Bone marrow stops producing red blood cells, a number of infections may precipitate this (usually viral)
Severe anemia	Child may be transfused with fresh packed red cells
Hyperhemolytic	Rapid rate of hemolysis superimposed on already severe process, rare
Functional hyposplenism and overwhelming infection	Progressive fibrosis of spleen reduces its function, patient becomes more susceptible to infection

Data from Dickerman, J., & Lucey, J. (1985). *Smith's the critically ill child* (3rd ed.). Philadelphia: Saunders.

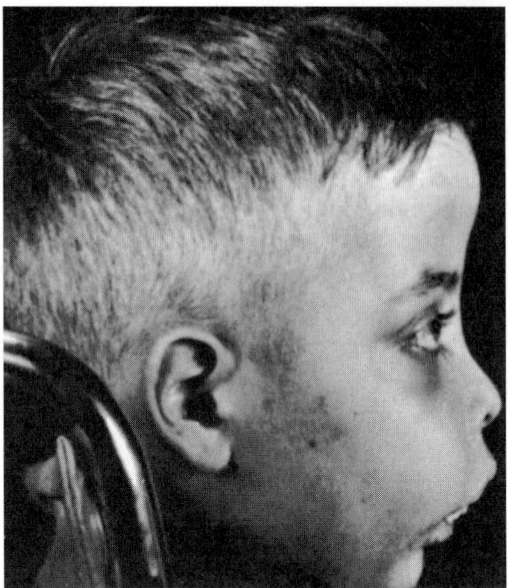

Figure 26–5. • Appearance of child with thalassemia major (Cooley's anemia). Note the overgrowth of the upper right jaw bone. (From Behrman, R. E., Kleigman, R. M., & Arvin, A. [1996]. *Nelson's textbook of pediatrics* [15th ed.]. Philadelphia: Saunders.)

Treatment and Nursing Care. The mainstay of treatment for thalassemia major is frequent blood transfusions to maintain the hemoglobin level above 10 gm/dl. As a result of repeated blood transfusions, excessive deposits of iron may be stored in the tissues. This is termed *hemosiderosis* and is seen especially in the spleen, liver, heart, pancreas, and lymph glands. Deferoxamine mesylate (Desferal Mesylate), an iron-chelating agent, is given to counteract hemosiderosis. Severe splenomegaly may occur in some children. Splenectomy may make the patient more comfortable, increase the ability to move about, and allow for more normal growth. After surgery these children are given prophylactic antibiotics to prevent infection. Bone marrow transplants are being performed with increasing success.

Nursing measures adhere to the principles of long-term care. The observation of the patient during a blood transfusion is discussed on pp. 707–708. Monitoring of vital signs is necessary to detect irregularities of the heart. Whenever possible, the same nurse cares for the patient during transfusions, blood tests, and other unpleasant procedures to provide security. Children are taught to regulate their activities according to their own tolerance.

The emotional health of the child and parents needs special consideration by the nurse. Every attempt to ease the strain of this prolonged illness must be made. Home care arrangements can be provided through community agencies. The family should be referred to the Cooley's Anemia Foundation for support and education. Older children need special support to accept changes in their body image caused by the disease. Suggestions applicable to the care of the chronically ill child are discussed throughout the text. Care of the dying child is discussed on pp. 713–717.

BLEEDING DISORDERS

Hemophilia

Description. Hemophilia is one of the oldest hereditary diseases known to humanity. In this disorder the blood does not clot normally, and even the slightest injury can cause severe bleeding. It has been called the disease of kings because it has occurred in children of several royal families in Russia and Europe. This congenital disorder is confined almost exclusively to males, but is transmitted by symptom-free females. Hemophilia is inherited as a sex-linked recessive trait. It is termed *sex-linked* because the defective gene is located on the X, or female, chromosome. Different combinations of genes account for the fact that some children inherit the disease, some become carriers, and others neither inherit nor carry the trait. New mutations do occur, and the reason for this is unclear. The sex of the fetus can be determined by amniocentesis. Fetal blood sampling detects hemophilia. Some carrier women can also be identified.

There are several types of hemophilia. There are more than 10 identified factors in the blood that are involved in the clotting mechanism. A deficiency in any one of the factors will interfere with normal blood clotting. The two most common types of hemophilia are *hemophilia B* or Christmas disease, which is a factor IX deficiency, and *hemophilia A*, which is a deficiency in factor VIII. For our purposes, this discussion is limited to classic hemophilia, or hemophilia A, which accounts for about 84% of cases.

Hemophilia A is due to a deficiency of coagulation Factor VIII, or antihemophilic globulin (AHG). The severity of the disease depends on the level of

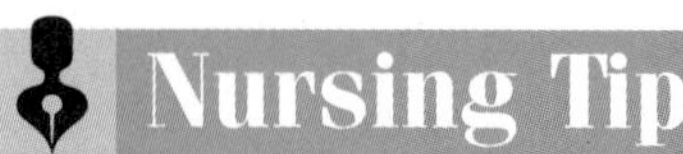

Nursing Tip

A classic symptom of hemophilia is bleeding into the joints (hemarthrosis).

Factor VIII in the plasma of the patient's blood. Some patients' lives are endangered by minor injury, whereas a child with a mild case of hemophilia might just bruise a little more easily than the normal person. The degree of severity tends to remain constant within a given family. The aim of therapy is to increase the level of Factor VIII to ensure clotting. It is possible to determine the level of Factor VIII in the blood by means of a test called the *partial thromboplastin time* (PTT), which can help to diagnose and assess the child's condition. Prenatal diagnosis by amniocentesis or fetoscopy is possible.

Manifestations. Hemophilia can be diagnosed at birth because maternal factor VIII cannot cross the placenta and be transferred to the fetus. It is usually not apparent in the newborn unless abnormal bleeding occurs at the umbilical cord or following circumcision. As the child grows older and becomes more subject to injury, it is found that the slightest bruise or cut can induce extensive bleeding. Normal blood clots in about 3 to 6 minutes. In a patient with severe hemophilia, the time required for clotting may be 1 hour or longer. Anemia, leukocytosis, and a moderate increase in platelets may be seen in the hemorrhaging child. There may also be signs of *shock.* Spontaneous hematuria is seen. Death can result from excessive bleeding anywhere in the body, but particularly when hemorrhage into the brain or neck occurs. Severe headache, vomiting, and disorientation may reflect cranial bleeds. Bleeding into the neck can cause airway obstruction. Bleeding into the ears and eyes can affect hearing and vision. Bleeding into the spinal column can instigate paralysis.

The circumstances leading to diagnosis may be the inability of a parent to stop a child's bleeding from a cut about the mouth or gums. A deciduous tooth loss may precipitate problems in a child who has a bleeding disorder. *Hematomas* may develop following immunization. An injured knee, elbow, or ankle presents particular problems. Hemorrhage into the joint cavity, or *hemarthrosis* (*hema,* "blood," *arthron,* "joint," and *osis,* "condition of"), is considered a classic symptom of hemophilia. The effusion (*ex,* "out," and *fundere,* "to pour") into the joint is very painful because of the pressure buildup. Repeated hemorrhages may cause permanent deformities that could incapacitate the child. This deformity is sometimes referred to as an ankylosis (*ankyle,* "stiff joint," and *osis,* "condition of").

Treatment and Nursing Care. The principal therapy for hemophilia is to prevent bleeding by replacing the missing factor. The development of recombinant antihemophilic factor, a synthetic product, has eliminated the need for repeated blood transfusions and its accompanying dangers (such as HIV and hepatitis infection). The missing factor is replaced by reconstituting the product with sterile water and administering it through an implanted intravenous port. Once the parents and child are taught how to administer the medication, treatment is carried out in the home. Diagnosed infants may receive prophylactic factor replacements at regular intervals to prevent hemarthrosis. Desmopressin acetate (DDAVP) is a nasal spray that can stop bleeding. It may be the treatment of choice for mild cases of hemophilia. Aminocaproic acid (Amicar) is an antifibrinolytic agent that can control bleeding that may occur due to dental care or other oral bleeding.

> **Nursing Tip**
>
> Drugs that contain salicylates are contraindicated for children with hemophilia.

Prophylactic factor replacement, combined with specific treatment prior to planned invasive procedures such as dental extraction or minor surgery, and education concerning the prevention of injuries that can cause bleeding, enable the hemophiliac child to live a normal life. Since young children often fall while playing, the joints of the knees, hips, and elbows can be protected by padding their play outfits. Appropriate sports activities should be selected to avoid undue injury and risk of bleeding episodes. When bleeding does occur, the traditional approach to care includes Rest, Ice, Compression, and Elevation (RICE). A medical alert identification band should be worn.

Home care programs are the treatment of choice. These greatly reduce the cost of treatment and decrease the risk of psychological trauma. A multidisciplinary approach to care assists families to develop healthy coping strategies to deal with a child who has a chronic illness.

It is difficult for parents not to be overprotective of these children. Children may resent being unable to participate in athletic activities with peers or may attempt to conceal their problem from others. Schooling should not be interrupted so that friendships are maintained with peers. The struggle to protect these children and still foster independence and a sense of autonomy may seem monumental to parents who work away from home. Allowing children to participate in decision making about their care and focusing on their strengths are helpful.

Parent groups and professional counseling may provide support to enable children and parents to develop a healthy attitude toward the condition. Organizations that may be helpful are the National Hemophiliac Foundation and the American Red Cross. Genetic counseling and family planning services should be offered to the family and the adolescent.

Platelet Disorders

The reduction or destruction of platelets in the body interferes with the clotting mechanism. Skin lesions that are common to these disorders include *petechiae,* a bluish nonblanching pinpoint size lesion; *purpura,* groups of adjoining petechiae; *ecchymosis,* an isolated bluish lesion larger than a petechiae; and a *hematoma,* which is a raised ecchymosis.

Idiopathic (Immunologic) Thrombocytopenic Purpura

Description. Idiopathic (immunologic) thrombocytopenic purpura (ITP) is an acquired platelet disorder that occurs in childhood. It is the most common of the purpuras, a group of disorders affecting the numbers of platelets or their function. The cause is unknown, but it is thought to be an autoimmune system reaction to a virus. Platelets become coated with antiplatelet antibody, are "perceived" as foreign material, and are eventually destroyed by the spleen. ITP occurs in all age groups, with the main incidence seen between 2 and 4 years.

Manifestations. The classic symptoms of this disease include being easily bruised, which results in petechiae (pinpoint hemorrhagic spots beneath the skin) and purpura (hemorrhage into the skin). About 30% of the patients also have nosebleeds. There may have been a recent history of rubella, rubeola, or viral respiratory infection. The interval between infection and onset is about 2 weeks. The platelet count is below 20,000/mm^3 (normals range between 150,000 and 400,000/mm^3). Diagnosis is confirmed by bone marrow aspiration to rule out leukemia. The bruises of ITP must be distinguished from those of child abuse.

Treatment and Nursing Care. When platelets are low, the greatest danger is spontaneous intracranial bleeding. Neurologic assessments are therefore a priority of care. Treatment is not indicated in most cases of ITP. Spontaneous remission occurs in about 6 weeks to 4 months. A few children go on to have chronic ITP. Drugs that interfere with platelet function should be avoided to prevent bleeding. These include aspirin, phenylbutazone (Butazolidin), and phenacetin, an ingredient of acetylsalicylic acid, phenacetin, and caffeine (APC). Activity is limited during the acute stage to avoid bruises from falls and trauma. Nursing considerations for the more acutely ill child focus on observing the patient for signs of bleeding. The child should use soft toothbrushes for oral hygiene to minimize tissue trauma. When there has been a large amount of blood loss, packed red blood cells may be administered. Platelets are usually not given because they are destroyed by the disease process. Steroids such as prednisone may be prescribed. Intravenous gamma globulin may be used to elevate platelet counts. In cases of chronic ITP a splenectomy may be indicated to minimize the release of antiplatelet antibody. Complications of ITP include bleeding from the gastrointestinal tract, hemarthrosis, and intracranial hemorrhage. Mortality in childhood ITP is less than 1%. All children need to be immunized against the viral diseases of childhood to prevent this complication.

DISORDERS OF WHITE BLOOD CELLS

The Leukemias

Description. Leukemia (*leuko,* "white," and *emia,* "blood") is a malignant disease of the blood-forming organs of the body that results in an uncontrolled growth of immature white blood cells. The immature cells are termed *blasts,* or stem cells. This term comes from the Greek *blastos,* meaning "germ" or "formative cell." The nurse may see the terms lymphoblasts or myeloblasts referred to in descriptive histories. Leukemia is the most common form of childhood cancer. In the past it was considered fatal. However, the prognosis has improved greatly with modern treatments and medication. About 2,000 new cases of childhood leukemia are diagnosed in the United States every year. About 40 children per million under the age of 15 years are affected.

The leukemias involve a disruption of bone marrow function due to the overproduction of immature white blood cells (WBCs) in the marrow. Although the WBC count can be as high as 50,000 to 100,000, the cells are immature and do not function as healthy WBCs do to fight infection. *Increased susceptibility to infection results.* The WBC "take over" the centers that are designed to form red blood cells and *anemia* results. When the WBC infiltrate and "take over" the centers that form platelets, the reduced platelets cause *bleeding tendencies*. The invasion of the bone marrow causes weakening of the bone and pathologic *fractures* can occur.

Leukemia cells can infiltrate the spleen, liver, and lymph glands, causing fibrosis and diminishing their function. The cancerous cells invade the central nervous system and other organs, draining these organs of their nutrients and finally causing metabolic starvation of the body. Leukemias are classified according to the type of white blood cell affected: (1) acute lymphocytic (ALL); (2) acute nonlymphocytic (ANLL); or (3) acute myelocytic (AML). The discussion focuses on the most common childhood leukemia, ALL.

Manifestations. The most common symptoms during the initial phase of the illness are low-grade fever, pallor, tendency to bruise, leg and joint pain, listlessness, abdominal pain, and enlargement of lymph nodes. These symptoms may develop gradually or may be sudden in onset. As the disease progresses, the liver and spleen become enlarged. The skin may be an unusual lemon-yellow. *Petechiae* and *purpura* may be early objective symptoms. Anorexia, vomiting, weight loss, and dyspnea are also common. The kidneys and testicles may enlarge, and the patient may develop hematuria.

Because the white blood cells are not functioning normally, bacteria easily invade the body. Ulcerations develop about the mucous membranes of the mouth and anal regions and have a tendency to bleed (Fig. 26–6). Anemia becomes severe despite transfusions. The child may die as a direct result of the disease or from secondary infection. The symptoms are the same regardless of the type of white blood cell affected, and they vary widely with each patient, depending on the parts of the body involved.

Diagnosis. The diagnosis of leukemia is based on the history and symptoms of the patient and the results of extensive blood tests that demonstrate the presence of leukemic blast cells in the blood, bone marrow, or other tissues. Because the bone marrow is where many white and red blood cells are formed, a bone marrow aspiration is commonly performed. A piece of the marrow of the bone is removed from the sternum or, more often in children, the iliac crest. A special needle is used and the marrow is studied in the laboratory (Fig. 26–7). X-ray films of the long bones show changes in the bones. After the diagnosis has been confirmed, a spinal tap determines central nervous system (CNS) involvement. Kidney and liver function studies are also performed because normal function of these organs is absolutely necessary for chemotherapy to be used in treating the disease.

Treatment and Nursing Care. The treatment of a child with cancer involves the multidisciplinary health care team (pediatrician, pathologist, oncologist, nurse, radiotherapist, nutritionist, psychologist, and school personnel). As with any diagnosis of cancer, the leukemic child is usually referred to a specialized center where facilities for required care are available. School tutoring and counseling should be continuous in the hospital setting and in the home during home care to provide optimum growth and development. Chemotherapy is carried out in specialized units with specially trained personnel. Although therapy may be effective in reducing leukemic cells, the side effects of treatments need to be addressed. Bone marrow suppression requires that the family be taught about infection prevention. Adequate hydration should be emphasized to minimize kidney damage. Active routine immunizations need to be delayed while the child is receiving immunosuppressive drugs as the body will not be able to manufacture antigens as expected. Parents should report any exposure to infections such as chickenpox so that immunoglobin can be administered. Chickenpox can be life-threatening to a child who is immunosuppressed.

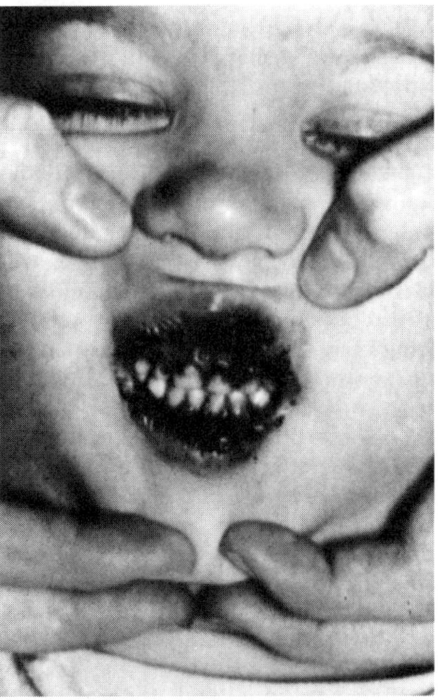

Figure 26–6. • The mouth lesions of leukemia. (From Blake, F., Wright, F., & Waechter, E. [1970]. *Nursing care of children* [8th ed.]. Philadelphia: Lippincott.)

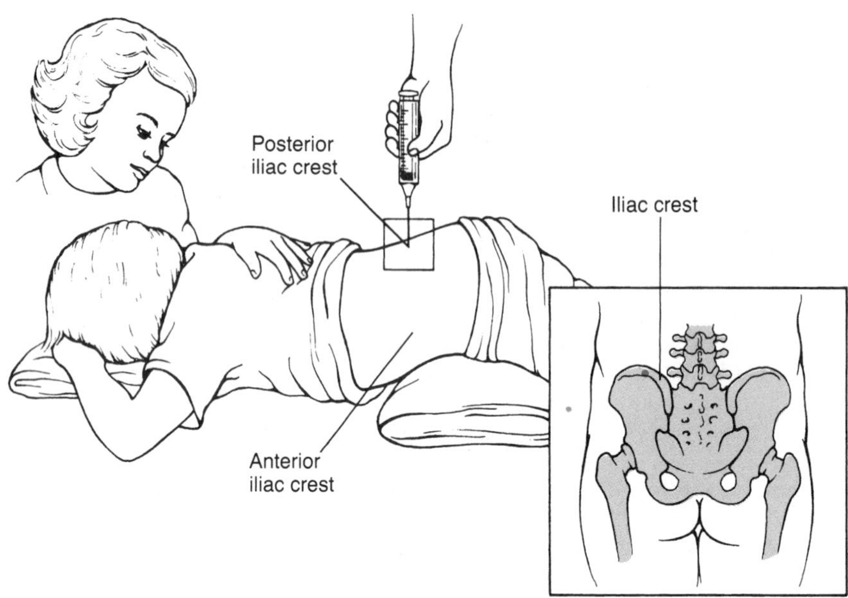

Figure 26–7. • Bone marrow aspiration. Because many white and red blood cells are formed in the bone marrow, a bone marrow aspiration can determine the type and quantity of cells present and help to rule out or to confirm a serious disease.

Nausea and vomiting are common complications of chemotherapy and result in decreased appetite, weight loss, and generalized weakness. Presenting the child's favorite foods in an attractive manner is essential. Total parenteral nutrition (TPN) may be indicated to support nutritional needs. A bone marrow transplant may be useful. An autologous transplant uses the child's own bone marrow that has been purged of malignant cells. An allogeneic bone marrow transplant is taken from a donor who matches the child. Transplanted marrow rejection is a risk. When the child is hospitalized "reverse isolation" precautions may prevent nosocomial infections. The nurse should refer parents to available support groups. The Ronald McDonald house and hospice programs help parents and families to cope with this illness. Since hair loss *(alopecia)* is a side effect of chemotherapy, the child can be offered a hat or a wig to help to preserve a positive body image. An intake and output record is maintained and meticulous oral hygiene is given.

The development of specific chemotherapeutic agents for acute leukemia has significantly changed the survival time. In most cases of ALL, it is now possible to induce remissions that may be maintained for prolonged periods (longer than 3 years). There is mounting optimism that some patients may never relapse and that the chemotherapy may thus represent a complete cure. Other acute varieties show a less predictable response to therapy. Untreated leukemia results in death from infection or hemorrhage in about 6 months. Components of chemotherapy include (1) an induction period; (2) CNS prophylaxis for high-risk patients; (3) maintenance; (4) reinduction therapy (if relapse occurs); and (5) extramedullary disease therapy.

The list of medications for treatment of this disease is growing (Box 26–1). A combination of drugs used to induce remissions includes prednisone, vincristine sulfate, and daunorubicin or L-asparaginase. They work within 4 to 6 weeks in about 95% of children with ALL. The therapeutic effects of these drugs are of short duration, however, so it is necessary to use additional drugs that help to maintain the remissions. The steroid-prednisone has the side effects of masking the symptoms of infection, increasing fluid retention, inducing personality changes, and causing the child's face to appear moon-shaped. Methotrexate and 6-mercaptopurine are useful in maintaining remissions because they act against chemicals vital to the life of the white blood cell. These powerful medications produce side effects of varying degrees, such as nausea, diarrhea, rash, hair loss *(alopecia),* fever, anuria, anemia, and bone marrow depression. Peripheral neuropathy may be signaled by severe constipation due to decreased nerve sensations to the bowel. The nurse should consult a pharmacology text for information about the particular drugs used for the patient to anticipate potential problems.

Children's anxiety often centers on their symptoms. They fear that the treatments necessary to correct their problems may be painful, as indeed some are, for example, venipunctures, bone marrow aspirations, and blood transfusions. Their trust in others is in a precarious balance. Nurses must inform children of what they are about to do and why it is necessary. The explanation is given in terms the child will understand.

The child may ask the nurse the inevitable question, "Am I going to die?" One suggestion is to reply with a question, such as "Why do you ask that? Do you feel sick today?" This may encourage the child to verbalize feelings. The pediatric nurse who gives patients permission to discuss their concerns will find opportunities to clear up misconceptions and to decrease children's feelings of isolation. Hope is conveyed because it is indispensable to continued functioning, although the nature of hope may change from that of cure to additional time to live.

The patient is frequently observed for signs of infection. Particular attention is paid to potential infected sites, such as the patient's mucous membranes and puncture breaks in the skin from laboratory or therapeutic procedures. Pierced ears are observed for inflammation. Vital signs are observed for subtle variances, as steroid therapy may mask these indicators. The patient is turned often and observed for skin breakdown, particularly in the perianal area. Nutritious meals and supplemental feedings that are high in protein and calories are offered. Parents and the child are taught what to look for and report.

Thrombocytopenic bleeding is a frequent complication of leukemia. The nurse observes the patient's skin for petechiae and ecchymosis. Nosebleeds are common and are treated by application of cold and pressure.

The mouth is inspected daily for ulcerations and hemorrhage from the gums. It may be rinsed with a prescribed solution of one part hydrogen peroxide to four parts saline solution. Commercial mouthwashes are used with caution because they may alter normal flora and may cause fungal overgrowth. A Water-Pik is helpful in massaging and toughening the gums. If the child is comatose, mouth care supplies are kept at the bedside. A soft sponge toothbrush is helpful. The nurse may also clean food particles from the patient's teeth with a piece of gauze wrapped around the finger. Petroleum jelly or cold cream is applied to dry, cracked lips.

The nurse observes the patient for gastrointestinal bleeding, evidenced by hematemesis (*hema,* "blood," and *emesis,* "vomiting") and bloody or tarry stools. Hemarthrosis (*hema,* "blood," *arthron,* "joint," and *osis,* "condition of") may develop. This makes moving about painful; therefore, nursing intervention is necessary to make the patient more comfortable in or out of bed. The nurse manipulates catheters and suction drainage gently to avoid irritation of the sensitive mucosa. Scanning the patient's unit for environmental hazards is also important. Emergency procedures for control of bleeding should be reviewed.

Care of a Child Receiving a Transfusion. Platelets and packed red blood cells may be given to the

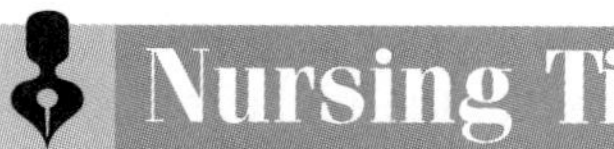

Nursing Tip

Bleeding from the nose or mouth may be evidenced by a soiled pillowcase or sheet.

BOX 26–1

AN EFFECTIVE TREATMENT REGIMEN FOR LOW-RISK ACUTE LYMPHOBLASTIC LEUKEMIA

Remission Induction (4–6 Weeks)
Vincristine 1.5 mg/m^2 (max 2 mg) IV/wk
Prednisone 40 mg/m^2 (max 60 mg)/day PO
L-Asparaginase *(Escherichia coli)* 10,000 U/m^2/day biweekly IM

Intrathecal Treatment
Triple therapy: methotrexate,* hydrocortisone,* and cytosine arabinoside* weekly × 6 during induction, and then every 8 wk for 2 yr

Systemic Continuation Treatment
6-Mercaptopurine 50 mg/m^2/day PO
Methotrexate 20 mg/m^2/wk PO

With Reinforcement
Vincristine 1.5 mg/m^2 (max 2 mg) IV every 8 wk
Prednisone 40 mg/m^2/day by mouth × 7 days every 4 wk

*The dose of intrathecal medication is age-adjusted.
From Behrman, R. E. (1996). *Nelson's textbook of pediatrics* (15th ed.). Philadelphia: Saunders.

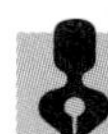

Nursing Tip

If a blood transfusion reaction occurs, stop the infusion, keep the vein open with normal saline solution, and notify the charge nurse. Take the patient's vital signs and observe closely.

child. Hemolytic reactions caused by mismatched blood are rare. Nevertheless, the registered nurse should positively identify donor and recipient blood types and groups on labels and the patient's chart with another professional. Blood is infused through a blood filter to avoid impurities. Medications are *never* added to blood. Blood is administered *slowly.* The intravenous site is frequently checked for infiltration. The patient is observed for *signs of transfusion reaction,* which include chills, itching, rash, fever, headache, and pain in the back. If such a reaction occurs, the tubing should be clamped off immediately, the line kept open with normal saline solution, and the nurse in charge notified.

Transfusions with piggyback setups are common. Blood and normal saline or other suitable intravenous solutions are connected by a stopcock. When blood must be stopped, tube patency can be maintained by opening the saline line. Necessary emergency medications can thus be administered and the site preserved for future infusions. An *autosyringe* may be used to administer small amounts of blood. The line is flushed with normal saline before and after instillation.

Circulatory overload is always a danger with children. *An infusion pump is routinely used to regulate blood flow.* Dyspnea, precordial pain, rales, cyanosis, dry cough, and distended neck veins are indicative of circulatory overload. Apprehension can also be a warning signal of air emboli or electrolyte disturbance. The nurse must maintain a high level of alertness for such signs, particularly in children whose conditions warrant repeated transfusions. If a reaction occurs, the blood bag and tubing are saved and returned to the blood bank. Most transfusion reactions occur within the first 10 minutes of administration; nevertheless, the patient is carefully monitored throughout this treatment. Diphenhydramine (Benadryl) may be ordered for allergic reactions. Aminophylline may be ordered for wheezing. Oxygen may be necessary to relieve dyspnea and cyanosis. Blood transfusions administered through central lines must be warmed to prevent cardiac arrhythmias. Establish baseline data (temperature, pulse, respiration, and blood pressure) before transfusion and monitor for changes. It is helpful if the parents remain with the child during this time. Suitable diversions minimize boredom.

Hodgkin's Disease

Description. Hodgkin's disease is a malignancy of the lymph system that primarily involves the lymph nodes. It may metastasize to the spleen, liver, bone marrow, lungs, or other parts of the body. The presence of giant multinucleated cells called *Reed-Sternberg cells* is diagnostic of the disease. Hodgkin's disease is rarely seen before 5 years of age, but the incidence increases during adolescence and early adulthood. It is twice as common in boys as in girls.

Table 26–3
CRITERIA FOR STAGING OF HODGKIN'S DISEASE

Stage	Criteria
I	Disease restricted to single site or localized in a group of lymph nodes; asymptomatic
II	Two or more lymph nodes in the area or on the same side of the diaphragm
III	Involves lymph node regions on both sides of the diaphragm, involves adjacent organ or spleen
IV	Diffuse disease, least favorable prognosis

Manifestations. The presenting symptom of Hodgkin's disease is generally a painless lump along the neck. Characteristically, there are few other manifestations. Generally the swelling is first noted by the patient or parents. In more advanced cases, there may be unexplained low-grade fever, anorexia, unexplained weight loss, night sweats, general malaise, rash, and itching. Diagnosis is confirmed by x-ray films, body scan, lymphangiogram, and a biopsy of the node. Stages of Hodgkin's disease are defined in Table 26–3.

Treatment. Well-established treatment regimens are now being utilized to combat this illness. Both radiation therapy and chemotherapy are used in accordance with the clinical stage of the disease. The combination of nitrogen mustard, vincristine sulfate (Oncovin), procarbazine hydrochloride, and prednisone is a common protocol. It is referred to as the MOPP regimen. Another drug combination currently being used is Adriamycin (doxorubicin hydrochloride), bleomycin, vinblastine sulfate, and dacarbazine (ABVD). The prognosis for remission is favorable. Cure is primarily related to the stage of the disease at diagnosis.

Nursing Care. Nursing care is mainly directed toward the symptomatic relief of the side effects of radiation therapy and chemotherapy. Education of the patient and family is paramount, as most patients are cared for in the home. The nurse should explain the myriad of diagnostic tests to be performed and prepare the child for the typical procedures and aftereffects.

Following a lymphangiogram, the skin and urine may take on a bluish color. The child and parents should be prepared to deal with the impact on the child's self-image. The school nurse should be contacted to implement a schedule that will promote growth and development while preventing overfatigue. Adolescents may be interested in sperm banking before immunosuppressive therapy is initiated. A common side effect of radiation is malaise. The teenager tires easily and may be irritable and anorectic. The skin in the treated area may be sensitive and needs to be protected against exposure to sunlight and irritation. After treatment a sun-blocking agent containing paraaminobenzoic acid (PABA) should be used to prevent burning. The attending physician may prescribe an ointment to relieve itching. Nothing should be applied to the treatment area without the recommendation of the physician. There may be diarrhea after abdominal irradiation. The patient *does not* become radioactive during or after therapy.

Following splenectomy, the patient faces the long-term risk of serious infection. This risk is explained to the parents and teenager. Elevations of temperature need to be monitored carefully. There may also be infection with little or no fever as a result of masking by certain medications. In such cases, cultures of blood, urine, sputum, or stool may need to be taken. Parents or the adolescent are instructed to feel free to call the clinic, particularly if there is a change in the condition or apprehension or confusion about symptoms. Medication readjustments should not be attempted unless specifically advised by the physician. Emotional support of the teenager is age appropriate. Nurses must particularly be prepared for periods of anger, which may be directed at them. Suitable outlets, such as the use of a punching bag, allows for safe direction of anger. Routine use helps to prevent a buildup of tension. Activity in general is regulated by the patient. The physician advises the patient if special precautions are necessary.

The appearance of secondary sexual characteristics and menstruation may be delayed in pubescent patients. This can be a source of anxiety. The nurse respects the patient concerns and can be most effective by listening empathetically (Nursing Care Plan 26–2).

NURSING CARE OF THE CHRONICALLY ILL CHILD

Chronic Illness. Chronic illness during childhood often impacts growth and development (Table 26–4). Specific programs that foster feelings of security and independence within the limits of the situation are essential. Behavior problems are lessened when patients can verbalize specific concerns with persons sensitive to their problems. If they feel rejected by and different from their peers, they may be prone to depression. To be in school and to be considered one of the group is very important to children. Hospital school programs provide familiarity and enable patients to keep pace with their classmates. The recreational therapist may also be helpful in combating boredom and providing outlets for tension.

Nurses need to help patients to accept their body with all its strengths and imperfections. They must develop an awareness of the teenager's particular fears of forced dependence, bodily invasion, mutilation, rejection, and loss of face, especially within peer groups. The nurse anticipates a certain amount of reluctance to adhere to hospital regulations, which reflects the adolescent's need for self-determination. Recognizing this as an asset rather than a liability enables the nurse to respond creatively.

Developmental Disabilities. Children who have a developmental disability that affects their intellect or ability to cope face some unique difficulties. They may often be overprotected, unable to break away from supervision, and deprived of necessary peer relationships. The pubertal process with its emerging sexuality concerns parents and may precipitate a family crisis.

Home Care. Most children with acute and chronic conditions are being cared for in the home. Home health care and other community agencies work together to provide holistic care. *Respite care* provides trained workers who come into the home for brief periods to relieve parents of the responsibility of caring for the child. This enables the parents to shop, do business transactions, or simply take a much-needed vacation. The school systems also share in the responsibility of care, which is crucial if a family is to be successful in home care. One mother, whose 13-year-old daughter has a severe developmental disability (cerebral palsy, blindness, scoliosis, mental retardation), offered these suggestions for the health care worker assisting in the home:

- Observe how the parents interact with the child.
- Do not wait for the child to cry out for attention, as the youngster may be unable to communicate in this way.
- Watch for facial expression and body language.
- Post signs above the bed denoting special considerations, such as "Never position on left side" and "Do not feed with plastic spoon."
- Listen to the parents and observe how they attend to the physical needs of the youngster.

(Text continued on page 713.)

NURSING CARE PLAN 26–2

Selected Nursing Diagnoses for the Adolescent Receiving Cancer Chemotherapy

Nursing Diagnosis: Knowledge deficit concerning prevention of infection due to myelosuppression

Goals	Nursing Interventions	Rationale
Patient will remain free of infection as evidenced by temperature of 36.5–37.6° C (99.7–99.6° F); skin and mucous membranes will show no signs of irritation or inflammation Patient's hemoglobin level will improve with therapy; there will be no recurrence of anemia	1. Instruct patient about body's immune system and immunotherapy as age appropriate; use visual aids	1. A malignant process depresses the immune system at onset of disease; chemotherapy further suppresses it and causes some physical changes that increase chances of infection
	2. Monitor white blood cell count and interpret blood values at patient's level of understanding	2. Leukopenia (decreased white blood cells), which predisposes patient to infection, and thrombocytopenia (decreased platelets), which predisposes patient to bruising and bleeding, are the most serious side effects; anemia due to decreased erythrocyte count is also a side effect but is more easily treated
	3. Place patient in private room, avoid crowds, practice proper handwashing and good personal hygiene, monitor temperature	3. Bone marrow suppression as a side effect of chemotherapy or radiation predisposes child to anemia, infection, and bleeding; in addition to treatment effects, patients with leukemia are particularly vulnerable because their bone marrow is depressed as a result of disease; neutropenia may result; infection can be life-threatening
	4. Observe mouth and perianal area for infection	4. Ulcerations of mouth and anus are common; meticulous rectal care will prevent natural microbial flora (*Escherichia coli*) from being introduced by a break in mucosa; enemas and rectal temperatures are avoided because of this; stomatitis is a frequent side effect of chemotherapy
	5. Use soft toothbrush, Water-pik, soothing mouthwashes	5. Protecting membranes decreases the likelihood of capillary damage and of mucous membrane breakdown
	6. Limit exposure to direct sunlight	6. Photosensitivity is a side effect of some chemotherapeutic drugs

Nursing Diagnosis: High risk for hemorrhage due to platelet deficit from bone marrow suppression

Goals	Nursing Interventions	Rationale
Patient shows no signs of bleeding, as evidenced by stable vital signs and absence of hematuria, petechiae, and ecchymosis	1. Observe for hematuria, hematemesis melena, epistaxis, petechiae, and ecchymosis	1. Bleeding from these sites can occur because of myelosuppression
	2. Increase fluid intake	2. Patient may be febrile; a liberal fluid intake also prevents hemorrhagic cystitis; vomiting from chemotherapy may deplete fluid volume, and patient may become dehydrated
	3. Use local measures if necessary to control bleeding	3. Direct pressure reduces small bleeds; avoid puncture wounds whenever possible; bandages and old blood are promptly removed, since they provide media for infection
	4. Monitor platelet counts and assist patient in types of safe activity when count is low	4. Children with low platelet counts are advised to avoid temporarily activities that might cause bleeding or injury (skateboarding, contact sports, and so on); aspirin is avoided, because it destroys platelets

NURSING CARE PLAN 26–2 *continued*

Selected Nursing Diagnoses for the Adolescent Receiving Cancer Chemotherapy

Nursing Diagnosis: Altered nutrition due to stomatitis, nausea, and vomiting

Goals	Nursing Interventions	Rationale
Patient is able to eat frequent small meals; caloric intake is adequate for age Nausea and vomiting will decrease; patient's weight will stabilize	1. Inspect mouth daily for ulcerations	1. Mouth lesions may lead to anorexia; early treatment is necessary
	2. Serve bland, moist, soft diet	2. Prevents trauma to mouth and lesions of the esophagus
	3. Apply local anesthetics to ulcerated areas before meals	3. Protects lesions and makes eating easier
	4. Monitor weight	4. Malnutrition may be present; weight loss is common owing to nature of treatments and side effects of medication, such as nausea and vomiting
	5. Alert patient to expected reactions to treatment protocol	5. Preparing patient in advance reduces anxiety
	6. Give antiemetic prior to onset of nausea and vomiting	6. Regularly scheduled antiemetics reduce discomfort of nausea and vomiting
	7. Suggest appropriate relaxation techniques	7. Symptoms can be controlled or lessened by relaxation techniques

Nursing Diagnosis: Disturbance in body image due to moon face, hair loss; patient may have amputation

Goals	Nursing Interventions	Rationale
Patient verbalizes some satisfaction with appearance	1. Allow teenager to ventilate feelings about body	1. Accept all feelings
	2. Provide continuity of care	2. Teenagers need persons they can trust; continuity of care provides this
	3. Utilize wigs, scarfs, eyebrow pencil, false eyelashes; stress that hair loss is temporary; suggest clothing that minimizes body changes and enhances appearance	3. Looking and feeling attractive are morale boosters
	4. Have patient draw "How it feels to be sick," "How it feels to be well"; discuss	4. Indirect communication is helpful for self-conscious teenager; drawing provides an outlet for expression of feelings

Nursing Diagnosis: Disturbance in self-esteem and independence/dependence tasks

Goals	Nursing Interventions	Rationale
Patient will participate in self-care and daily hygiene	1. Involve patient in decision making as age appropriate	1. Patients are less anxious if they can gain a measure of control over their lives; denial of this increases noncompliance
	2. Set appropriate limits on disruptive behavior	2. Limit setting denotes caring; providing structure promotes security, particularly in a strange setting
	3. Avoid overprotection, overattention, overanxiety; foster independence	3. These behaviors may make patient feel different and not in control

Nursing Diagnosis: Fear of sexual dysfunction due to treatment modalities

Goals	Nursing Interventions	Rationale
Patient expresses understanding of information	1. Address sexuality issues and concerns	1. A teenager is a teenager first and a cancer patient second; all normal longings and fears concerning sexuality, enticing the opposite sex, and so on remain imprisoned unless someone is willing to listen and, more often than not, bring up the subject

(continued on following page)

NURSING CARE PLAN 26–2 *continued*

Selected Nursing Diagnoses for the Adolescent Receiving Cancer Chemotherapy

Nursing Diagnosis: Social isolation related to interrupted schooling, rejection by peers

Goals	Nursing Interventions	Rationale
Patient remains in contact with peers	1. Provide opportunity for group discussions with peers; encourage letter writing, telephone calls; suggest cancer camp; respect privacy with adolescent visitors; contact spiritual advisor, church youth groups, and the like	1. Immersion into a peer group is one of the tasks of adolescence; long-term disease may disrupt this task and isolate the patient

Nursing Diagnosis: Fear of death due to treatment or nature of disease

Goals	Nursing Interventions	Rationale
Patient expresses two concerns regarding life expectancy Patient expresses hope, although this may be changed from "hope" of cure to prolonged life	1. Convey empathic understanding of patient's and family's worries, fears, and doubts	1. Fear of death is like an elephant in a living room that everyone pretends does not exist; by refusing to discuss it, family can pretend that it will not happen; because no feelings are shared, each member suffers in isolation; sharing a threat lessens burden and brings members closer; nevertheless, sharing cannot be forced on persons who are not ready for it
	2. Determine patient's perception of diagnosis, for example, "What are your concerns?"; "How can I help?"	2. Misconceptions abound in life-threatening illness as patient is in crisis
	3. Support "hope" by clarifying and by educating patient about disease and side effects	3. Hope is important to patient and family members; it may be hope of celebrating a birthday or seeing a special friend; it may be hope that suffering will end
	4. Avoid discounting patient by making statements such as "I know exactly how you feel" or "You shouldn't feel that way" or by changing the subject	4. Expression of feelings is basis for identifying effective coping methods
	5. Draw and discuss "strongest feeling I've had today"	5. Patient can distance himself or herself from feelings through drawings. This makes the feelings less threatening

Table 26–4

THE EFFECTS OF CHRONIC ILLNESS ON GROWTH AND DEVELOPMENT*

Age	Feature	Effect
Infancy	Trust	A visible defect can retard bonding. Prolonged illness may separate child from family. Irritability promotes parental negativity
Toddler	Autonomy	Physical restrictions impede development of motor and language skills. Toilet training may be delayed. Actual fear may erode self-confidence. Separation anxiety occurs
Preschooler	Initiative	Impaired ability to experience the world outside of the family impedes social skills. Overprotective parents delay learning self-discipline. May develop negative body image. Develops sense of guilt at inability to master tasks
School Age	Industry	Loss of grade level in school due to illness and inability to participate or compete can lead to sense of inferiority. Sense of independence and accomplishment can be lost. Being different from peers may impede sense of belonging
Adolescent	Identity	Feels loss of control and inability to conform with peers. Developing self-concept may become negative. May grieve for a lost ability. Enforced dependence may impair plans for future goals. Rebellion results in decreased compliance

*Chronic illness can impede growth and development. The nurse should reinforce teaching concerning the developmental needs of chronically ill children at different age levels to promote self-acceptance and a positive self-esteem.

- Do not be afraid to ask questions or discuss apprehensions you may feel about your ability to care for the child.
- Be attuned to the needs of other children in the home.
- Be creative in exploring avenues for socialization, as these teenagers are seldom invited to birthday or slumber parties.
- Explore community facilities or support groups that might benefit the family.

The Care of the Chronically Ill Child. The chronically ill child needs to be a contributing member to the family unit. Often when health care activities inhibit development and prevent peer socialization opportunities, both the child and the parent will discard the health care practice. The child needs to be treated normally, avoiding overprotection and overrestriction. Focusing on what the child *can* do and providing experiences that are *successful* is more effective than focusing on the disability.

Involvement of the entire family with the care of the chronically ill child aids in normal family interaction. Respite care opportunities are needed to provide parents with a normal spousal relationship. The child should be integrated into the community and the society rather than isolated from them. Nurses can assist the child and the family to develop strategies to cope with chronic illness and to promote optimum growth and development. The wellness of the child should be the center of the child's life, rather than the disability.

NURSING CARE OF THE DYING CHILD

Facing Death

Facing death is often a difficult personal issue for the nurse. The nurse needs to understand the grieving process; personal and cultural views concerning that process; the views of a parent losing a child; and the perceptions of the child facing death. Integrating these understandings and helping all involved to cope successfully involves a multidisciplinary approach. The response to a child's death is influenced by whether there was a long period of uncertainty prior to the death or whether it was a sudden unexpected event. The nurse must show compassion, but function in a clinically competent, professional manner. Demonstrating a nonjudgmental approach when the personal or cultural practices of the family conflict with the nurse's own values presents a challenge. Sensitive effective care can be provided only if the nurse is aware of these needs of the family. The nurse can facilitate the grief process by anticipating psychological and somatic responses and maintaining open communication. The family's efforts to cope, adapt, and grieve must be supported.

The response of family to the death of the child may initially be manifested by somatic distress, such as weakness, anguish, or shortness of breath. A family member may feel detached from the world and have a sense of unreality or disbelief. A sense of guilt and blame may follow ("I should have" or "I could have"). Hostility is a normal response and may drive away those that do not understand its normalcy in the acute grieving process. A restlessness and general irritability or inability to function may follow. Assistance in the care of other children or household responsibilities may be necessary. Nursing priorities include being a patient and family advocate, providing support, and facilitating the grieving process.

Self-Exploration

One important, if not the most important, task to prepare for working with the dying patient is self-exploration. Our own attitudes about life and death affect our nursing practice. Emotions buried deep within us can form barriers to effective communication unless they are recognized and released. How we have or have not dealt with our own losses affects our present lives and our ability to relate to patients. Nurses must recognize that *coping is an active and ongoing process.* At times we need loving detachment from patients and their families to become revitalized. We must find constructive outlets, such as exercise and music, to maintain our equilibrium. An active support system consisting of nonjudgmental people who are not threatened by natural expressions of feelings is crucial. Proper channeling of these emotions can be a valuable part of our empathetic response to others. *It is vital that nurses support one another in the work environment.*

The Child's Reaction to Death

Each child, like each adult, approaches death in an individual way, drawing on limited experience. Nurses must become well acquainted with patients and view them within the context of the family and social culture. Their anxiety often centers on symp-

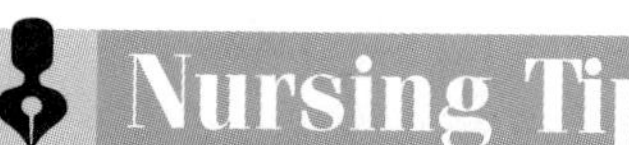

Brothers and sisters often feel neglected and lonely. They are frustrated because they are unable to comfort their parents and loved ones.

toms. They fear that treatments may be painful. Nurses must be honest and inform patients about the upcoming procedures in terms that the child will understand. Expressing feelings is encouraged: "You seem angry." Sufficient time for a response is allowed. Children should be allowed to have as much control over what happens to them as possible. This is fostered by including them in decisions that concern their welfare. However, the child should not be offered a choice when there is none. Children often communicate symbolically. The nurse *listens* to what they say to adults, to their toys, and to other children. Crayons and paper are provided.

Although age is a factor, the child's level of cognitive development, rather than chronologic age, affects the response to death (Table 26–5). Children younger than 5 years are mainly concerned with separation from their parents and abandonment. (Even adults are threatened by thoughts of dying alone.) Preschool children respond to questions about death by relying on their experience and by turning to fantasy. They may believe death is reversible or that they are in some way responsible. Children do not develop a realistic concept of death as a permanent biologic process until the age of 9 or 10.

Dying adolescents face conflicts between their treatment regimens and their need to establish independence from their parents and conformity with their peers. This leads to anger and resentment, which are frequently displaced on to hospital staff members. An atmosphere of acceptance and nonjudgmental listening allow patients freedom to ventilate their hostility in a nonthreatening environment. Nursing Care Plan 26–3 specifies nursing interventions for the dying child.

The Child's Awareness of His or Her Condition

Surprising as it may seem, many investigators have shown that terminally ill children are generally aware of their condition, even when it is carefully concealed. This is reflected in their drawings and play and can be detected through psychological testing. Failure to be honest with children leaves them to suffer alone, unable to express their fears and sadness or even to say good-bye.

Physical Changes of Impending Death

Physical changes that take place when death is impending include cool, mottled, cyanotic skin and the slowing down of all body processes. There may be loss of consciousness, although hearing is intact. Rales in the chest may be heard, which result from increased secretions pooling in the lungs. Movement and neurologic signs lessen. If thrashing or groaning occurs, the patient is assessed for pain and pain relief should be provided.

Stages of Dying

The stages of dying as detailed by Kübler-Ross (1975)—denial, anger, bargaining, depression, acceptance, and then reaching out to help others—can be applied to parents and siblings as well as to the sick child. (Nurses may also respond with similar feelings.) It is important to accept and to support each participant at whatever stage has been reached and not to try to direct progress. Nurses should be available and make their availability known (Table 26–6).

Parents are encouraged to assist in the care of their child (Fig. 26–8). This is facilitated by hospice and the movement toward supervised home care. It is therapeutic for children to be in their own surroundings whenever possible. Siblings involved in the patient's care feel less neglected, and the sacrifices they must make become more meaningful. Discussions before death allow them to make amends for their hostilities toward the sick child. The family's religious and spiritual philosophy can

Table 26–5
A CHILD'S RESPONSE TO A SIBLING'S DEATH

Age	Response/Understanding	Parent Guidance
Infant	Does not understand concept of death. Reacts on emotional level to anxiety of parents	Maintain normal routine Utilize support network to assist in care
Preschooler	Think death is temporary. May blame self for sibling's death	Use accurate terms and simple explanations Reassure child and *listen*
School Age	Realizes death is final. May be interested in details of death. May fear parents will die. May try to "take care" of parents	Respond to child's need for reassurance and security Refer to death using accurate terms Allow child to participate in funeral and feel useful
Adolescent	Can understand abstract concept of death but has feelings of own immortality. May express anger at death of sibling	Accept behavior Encourage communication and discussion

NURSING CARE PLAN 26–3

Selected Nursing Diagnoses for the Dying Child

Nursing Diagnosis: Anxiety, anticipatory (family members) due to potential death of child

Goals	Nursing Interventions	Rationale
Parents will express two anxieties to nurse Communications among parents, other children, patient, and nurse remain open	1. Remain available to family as child grows weaker	1. Nurse's presence provides support
	2. Give parents permission to talk and grieve about upcoming death and to think about funeral arrangements if they choose	2. Helps to prepare family for the inevitable; sorts out and identifies actual sources of feelings
	3. Involve siblings in plans and progress of brother or sister	3. Siblings will feel less isolated
	4. Provide permission for laughter, play, friends (make every day count)	4. Laughter and play reduce tension
	5. Suggest that overprotection and attention, even when provided out of love, can be detrimental to dying child	5. Child will feel more in control if not overprotected
	6. Encourage family to maintain as normal a lifestyle as possible, and each member to take time for own needs (continue to go to hairdresser, a movie—whatever they previously enjoyed)	6. When all members are taking care of themselves, they will have more energy to cope with crises
	7. Facilitate honesty about child's imminent death among family members and patient	7. Information helps to relieve anxiety
	8. Explain that family members often cannot support one another, as each grieves in his or her own way	8. Explanation of this to family helps to relieve the guilt stemming from irritability or anger
	9. Recognize that grief is often expressed as anger	9. Anger is a natural emotion; it is not fearsome in itself, although its expression may be; family has a right to all feelings
	10. Provide for ventilation of guilt ("If only I had taken her to the doctor sooner" and the like)	10. Prevents accumulation or repression of guilt
	11. Suggest meditation, progressive relaxation, guided imagery	11. Helps to reduce stress

(continued on following page)

be a source of strength and support, as can caring neighbors and friends.

Statistics show a high correlation between the death of a child and divorce. Nurses must observe signs of tension between parents so that suitable intervention may be established. Each parent grieves in an individual time and way, often making it difficult for spouses to be supportive of each other. The suppression of strong feelings of guilt, helplessness, and outrage can be devastating. Feelings left unexpressed can cause depression and/or physical illness.

Kübler-Ross (1969) reminds us that dying is the easy part. Helping our patients to live until they die

Table 26–6

THE NURSE'S ROLE IN HELPING THE FAMILY COPE WITH THE DYING CHILD

Listen	Giving advice is a reflection of the nurse's need to "solve the problem"
Provide privacy	Family needs to express their emotions and comfort each other without being embarrassed
Therapeutic intervention	Assess coping behaviors and work with clergy and social workers to meet immediate needs for patient comfort and family coping
Provide information	Avoid the tenseness of waiting for test results. Be truthful to the child and family
Use appropriate phrases and open-ended statements	When speaking with a sibling of a child that has died, avoid using terms such as "he isn't hurting anymore," "he is living with God or a deceased relative," "he has passed away." These terms are confusing to children. Explanations should be short, direct, and truthful.

NURSING CARE PLAN 26–3 *continued*

Selected Nursing Diagnoses for the Dying Child

Nursing Diagnosis: Anxiety (dying child) due to pain, isolation, lack of information

Goals	Nursing Interventions	Rationale
Child verbalizes feelings of comfort; if nonverbal, child rests comfortably, no crying Child is not isolated Child verbalizes understanding of treatment, procedures, outcome as age appropriate	1. Administer pain relievers as necessary	1. Child may deny pain because of fear of treatment
	2. Encourage parents to hold, cuddle, touch child as condition permits	2. Reduces anxiety, thereby reducing pain
	3. Encourage visits from friends and siblings as age appropriate	3. Provides emotional support and distraction from disease
	4. Decorate hospital room with cards, pictures, mementos; provide telephone as age appropriate	4. Attractive environment promotes mental health
	5. Investigate possibility of home or hospice care	5. Familiar and stable environment may facilitate child's emotional healing
	6. Explain all procedures	6. Information relieves anxiety
	7. Assess child's knowledge about impending death	7. Nurse can determine level of understanding as age appropriate; this assists in communication
	8. Answer all questions about death honestly, use open-ended questions to assist patient in expression of feelings	8. Conveys that all feelings are acceptable
	9. Listen to what child says in play	9. Children work through many fears in play
	10. Assist child in drawing "a wish," "yesterday, today, tomorrow"	10. Drawings promote the release of feelings and a means of communication
	11. Allow child to grieve (behavior may be sulky, cranky, withdrawn)	11. Therapeutic grieving prevents depression

Nursing Diagnosis: Grieving, actual: related to death of child

Goals	Nursing Interventions	Rationale
Family members have an opportunity to say good-bye Family members express feelings of grief, fear, anger, loss, guilt	1. Provide time for family to be alone with dead child as desired	1. Family needs to say good-bye
	2. Remain available, express your own loss and grief	2. Parents derive comfort from knowing others loved their child
	3. Assist parents in making decisions	3. Even a simple decision such as when to telephone relatives becomes monumental at this stage
	4. Offer a beverage	4. Denotes concern
	5. Assess spiritual need; refer to pastoral counseling if desired	5. A belief in God provides strength for many persons; pastoral counselors are effective
	6. Respect family's beliefs, worldview, philosophy	6. Many beliefs may be unconventional
	7. Listen to expressions of grief	7. Family needs to repeat story to work through grief

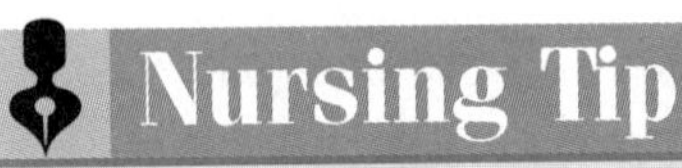

Grandparents, teachers, and friends are also grieving. Be alert for all significant others.

is the real challenge. She discusses this beautifully in *A Letter to a Child with Cancer,* which she wrote in response to a child's request, "What is life, what is death, and why do little children have to die?" Consult a librarian to locate this classic book and others published especially to help children and parents with dying and grief. There are several hospices in the United States that limit their services to children. St. Mary's Hospice in Bay Side, New York, is credited with being the first.

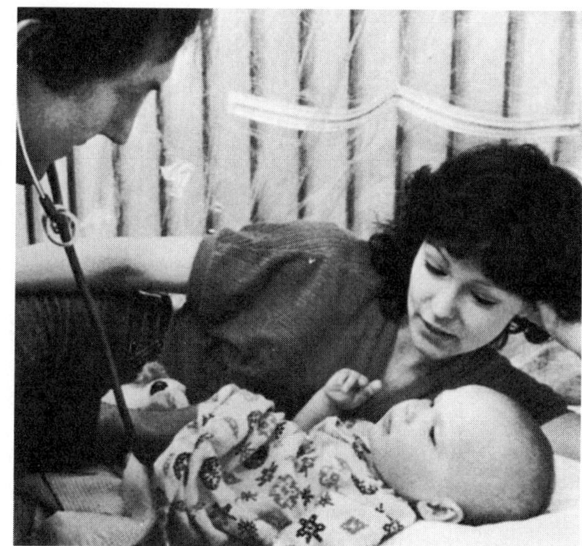

Figure 26–8. • Close contact between caregivers and family is of great importance for a child who has a potentially life-threatening disease. (Courtesy of Blank Memorial Hospital for Children, Des Moines, IA.)

KEY POINTS

- Circulating blood consists of two portions: plasma and formed elements.
- Bone marrow aspiration is one procedure that is helpful in determining disorders of the blood.
- The most common nutritional deficiency of children in the United States is iron-deficiency anemia.
- Sickle cell disease is an inherited defect in the formation of hemoglobin. The cells become crescent-shaped and clump together.
- Massive expansion of the bone marrow in thalassemia causes changes in the contour of the child's skull and face.
- Hemophilia A is due to a deficiency in coagulation factor VIII and hemophilia B (Christmas disease) involves a deficiency of factor IX.
- Hemarthrosis (bleeding into the joints) is a characteristic sign of hemophilia A.
- Hemosiderosis (deposits of iron in the organs and tissues) is a complication of multiple transfusions in hemolytic blood disorders.
- Signs of transfusion reactions include chills, itching rash, fever, and headache.
- *Petechiae* are bluish pinpoint lesions on the skin. *Purpura* are groups of adjoining petechiae; *ecchymosis* is an isolated bluish lesion larger than petechiae, and a *hematoma* is a raised ecchymosis.
- Leukemia is the most common form of childhood cancer.
- Diagnostic procedures for patients with blood disorders are often invasive or painful. The nurse prepares and supports the patient and family during these procedures.
- Maintenance of schooling, adequate hydration and nutrition, prevention of infection, promotion of a positive self-image, and meticulous oral hygiene are essential components of nursing care of a leukemic child.
- Reed-Sternberg cells are diagnostic for Hodgkin's disease.
- Children who are chronically ill need to be aided in mastering developmental tasks.
- The stages of dying according to Kübler-Ross includes denial, anger, bargaining, depression, acceptance, and reaching out to help others.
- The nurse can help the family of a dying child by listening and assessing their needs; reinforcing information; providing privacy; and using appropriate phrases and open-ended statements.

MULTIPLE-CHOICE REVIEW QUESTIONS

Choose the most appropriate answer.

1. When the patient experiences apprehension and urticaria while receiving a blood transfusion, the nurse
   a. slows the transfusion and takes the patient's vital signs.
   b. observes the child for further transfusion reactions.
   c. stops the transfusion, lets normal saline run slowly, and notifies the charge nurse.
   d. stops what he or she is doing and takes the patient's history.
2. The role of platelets in the blood is to
   a. carry oxygen to the tissues.
   b. fight germs and overcome infection.
   c. help the body to stop bleeding.
   d. provide nutrition to the body.
3. Which of the following principles should the nurse teach the parent concerning administering liquid iron preparations to her child with iron-deficiency anemia?
   a. Allow preparation to mix with saliva and bathe the teeth before swallowing.
   b. Warm the medication before administering.
   c. Administer between meals.
   d. Administer in the bottle of formula.
4. Thalassemia major (Cooley's anemia) is treated primarily with
   a. a diet high in iron.
   b. multiple blood transfusions.
   c. bed rest until the sedimentation rate is normal.
   d. oxygen therapy.
5. Which of the following is a characteristic manifestation of Hodgkin's disease?
   a. Petechiae
   b. Erythematous rash
   c. Enlarged lymph nodes
   d. Pallor

BIBLIOGRAPHY AND READER REFERENCE

American Academy of Pediatrics. (1996). Health supervision for children with sickle cell disease and their families. *Pediatrics, 98,* 467.

American Cancer Society. (1986). *What will I tell the children?* Omaha, NE: Eppley Cancer Institute.

Behrman, R. E., Kleigman, R., & Alvin, A. (1996). *Nelson's textbook of pediatrics* (15th ed.). Philadelphia: Saunders.

Behrman, R., & Kleigman, R. (1998). *Essentials of pediatrics* (3rd ed.). Philadelphia: Saunders.

Bunting, E. (1996). *Sunflower house: The process of life.* Philadelphia: Saunders.

Charachi, S., Terrin, M., Moore, R., et al. (1995). Effect of hydrooxurea on frequency of painful crises in sickle cell anemia. *New England Journal of Medicine, 32,* 1317.

Chiocca, E. (1996). Sickle cell crises. *American Journal of Nursing, 96*(9), 49.

Diaz, M. (1995). When a baby dies. *American Journal of Nursing, 95*(11), 54.

Faulkner, K. (1997). Talking about death with a dying child. *American Journal of Nursing, 97*(6), 64.

Friebert, S., & Shurin, S. (1998). ALL: Diagnosis and outlook. *Contemporary Pediatrics, 15*(2), 118.

Friebert, S., & Shurin, S. (1998). ALL: Treatment and beyond. *Contemporary Pediatrics, 15*(3), 39.

Gutgesell, H., Barst, R., Humes, R., et al. (1997). Common cardiovascular problems in the young. *American Family Physician, 56*(7), 1825–1830.

Hoole, A., Pickard, C. G., Jr., Ovimette, R., et al. (1995). *Disorders of the hematopoietic system.* In *Patient care guidelines for the nurse practitioner* (4th ed.). Philadelphia: Lippincott.

Joffrion, L., & Douglas, D. (1994). Grief resolution. *Journal of Psychosocial Nursing, 32*(3), 13.

Keffer, J., & Keffer, H. (1994). The DNR order. *AORN, 59*(3), 641.

Knafl, K., & Breitmayer, B. (1996). Family response to childhood chronic illness: Description of management styles. *Journal of Pediatric Nursing, 11*(5), 315.

Kubler-Ross, E. (1982). *On child and death.* New York: Macmillen

Kubler-Ross, E. (1975). *Death, the final stage of growth.* Englewood Cliffs, NJ: Prentice-Hall.

Leifer, R. (1997). *The happiness project: Transforming the three poisons that cause suffering we inflict on ourselves and others.* Ithaca, NY: Snow Lion Publishers.

Levi, R. (1995). Childhood ilness through a child's eyes. *The ACCH Advocate,* 2(1), 43–45.

Mahan, C., & Escott-Stump, S. (1996). *Krause's food, nutrition, and diet therapy* (9th ed.). Philadelphia: Saunders.

McIntier, T., Sr. (1995). Nursing the family when a child dies. *RN, 58*(2), 50.

Neville, K. (1996). Psychological distress in adolescents with cancer. *Journal of Pediatric Nursing, 11*(4), 243–251.

Oleske, J., & Boland, M. (1997). When a child with a chronic condition needs hospitalization. *Hospital Practice, 32*(6), 167.

Orto, C. (1995). *Joint bleeding in hemophilia: The hemophilic nursing handbook.* National Hemophilic Foundation.

Perrett, R. (1996). Buddhism, euthanasia, and the sanctity of life. *Journal of Medical Ethics, 22,* 309–313.

Smith-Stoner, M., & Frost, A. (1998). Coping with grief and loss. *Nursing 98, 28*(2), 49.

Snyder, C. *Oncology nursing.* Boston: Little Brown.

Wong, D. (1997). *Whaley & Wong essentials of pediatric nursing.* St. Louis, MO: Mosby.

Zimmerman, S., Ware, R., & Kinney, T. (1997). Gaining ground in the fight against sickle cell disease. *Contemporary Pediatrics, 14*(10), 154.

chapter 27

The Child with a Gastrointestinal Condition

Outline

Objectives

On completion and mastery of Chapter 27, the student will be able to

- Define each vocabulary term listed.
- Discuss three common gastrointestinal anomalies in infants.
- Interpret the nursing management of an infant with gastroesophageal reflux.
- Discuss the postoperative nursing care of an infant with pyloric stenosis.
- Explain why infants and young children become dehydrated more easily than adults do.
- Differentiate between three types of dehydration.
- Trace the route of the pinworm cycle and describe how reinfection takes place.
- Review the prevention of the spread of thrush in infants and children.
- Prepare a teaching plan for the prevention of poisoning in children.
- List two measures to reduce acetaminophen poisoning in children.
- Indicate the primary source of lead poisoning.

Vocabulary

antihelmintics	overnutrition
colitis	parenteral fluids
colonoscopy	pica
dehydration	poisoning
endoscopy	polyhydramnios
enterocolitis	projectile vomiting
gastroenteritis	pruritus
homeostasis	reflux
incarcerated	sigmoidoscopy
isotonic	stenosis

OVERVIEW

The gastrointestinal (GI) tract transports and metabolizes nutrients necessary for the life of the cell. It extends from the mouth to the anus. Nutrients are broken down into absorbable products by enzymes from various digestive organs. The anatomy of the digestive tract, with some of the differences between the child and adult, is depicted in Figure 27–1. The primitive digestive tube is formed by the yolk sac and is divided into the foregut, midgut, and hindgut. The foregut evolves into the pharynx, lower respiratory tract, esophagus, stomach, duodenum, and beginning of the common bile duct. The midgut elongates in the 5th fetal week to form the primary intestinal loop. The remainder of the large colon is derived from the primitive hindgut. The liver, pancreas, and biliary tree evolve from the foregut. At 8 weeks gestation, the anal membrane ruptures, forming the anal canal and opening.

A number of procedures are available to determine GI disorders. Laboratory work, such as a complete blood count (CBC) with differential will reveal anemia, infections, and chronic illness. An elevated erythrocyte sedimentation rate (ESR) is indicative of inflammation. A sequential multiple analysis (SMA 12) will reveal electrolyte and chemical imbalances. X-ray films include GI series, barium enema, and flat plates of the abdomen. *Endoscopy* allows direct visualization of the GI tract through a flexible lighted tube. Upper endoscopy permits visualization and biopsy of the esophagus, stomach, and duodenum. It is also valuable to remove foreign objects and cauterize bleeding ves-

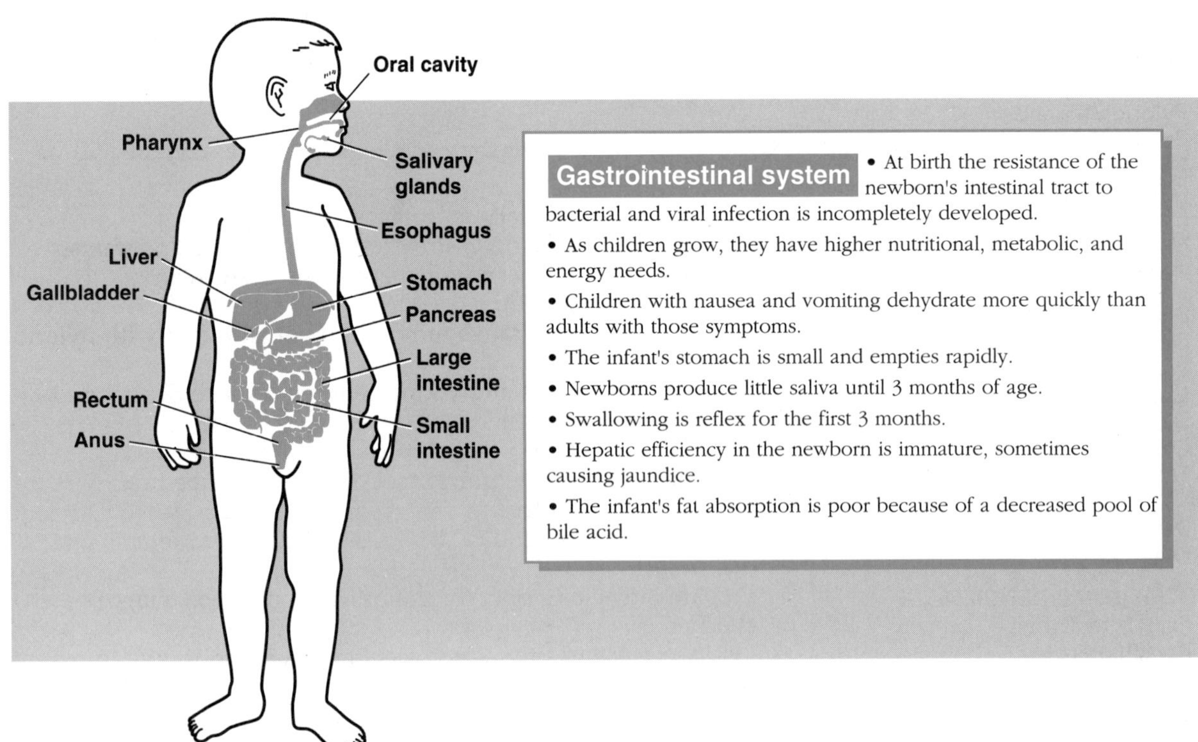

Figure 27–1. • Some of the gastrointestinal system differences between the child and adult. The digestive system consists of the digestive tract and the glands that secrete digestive juices into the digestive tract. This system mechanically and chemically breaks down food and eliminates wastes.

sels. Visualization of the bile and pancreatic ducts is also possible through endoscopy. The lower colon is inspected by *sigmoidoscopy. Colonoscopy* provides visualization of the entire colon to the ileocecal valve. Stool cultures and rectal biopsy are also important diagnostic tools. Ultrasonography is a noninvasive procedure useful in visualizing intestinal organs and masses, particularly of the liver and pancreas. Liver blood tests include serum glutamic-pyruvic transaminase (SGPT), serum glutamic oxaloacetic transaminase (SGOT), prothrombin time (PT), and partial thromboplastin time (PTT). Liver biopsy may also be indicated. Overall malabsorption tests, such as the 72-hour fecal fat test and the Schilling test, which can determine the absorption capacity of the lower ileum, are also useful.

Symptoms of GI disorders may be manifested by systemic signs such as *failure to thrive* (FTT; failure to develop according to established growth parameters such as height, weight, and head circumference) or jaundice. *Pruritus* (itching) in the absence of allergy may indicate liver dysfunction. Local manifestations of a GI disorder include pain, vomiting, diarrhea, constipation, rectal bleeding, and hematemesis.

Nursing intervention focuses on providing adequate nutrition and freedom from infection, which can result from malnutrition or depressed immune function. Developmental delays in children should be investigated to determine whether they are related to the GI system. Skin problems in these patients may be related to pruritus from liver disease, to irritation from frequent bowel movements, or to other disorders. Pain and discomfort may occur during acute episodes, but they may also be due to medication side effects, or they may be referred pain. Cleft lip and cleft palate are discussed in Chapter 14. Anorexia is discussed in Chapter 32, and necrotizing entercolitis is discussed in Chapter 13.

CONGENITAL DISORDERS

Esophageal Atresia

Tracheoesophageal Fistula (TEF)

Description. Atresia of the esophagus is due to a failure of the tissues of the GI tract to separate properly from the respiratory tract early in prenatal life. There are four types of atresia:

- The upper esophagus and the lower esophagus (leading from the stomach) end in a blind pouch.
- The upper esophagus ends in a blind pouch; the lower esophagus (leading from the stomach) connects to the trachea.
- The upper esophagus is attached to the trachea and the lower esophagus (leading from the stomach) is also attached to the trachea.
- The upper esophagus connects to the trachea and the lower esophagus (leading from the stomach) ends in a blind pouch.

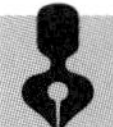

Nursing Tip

Drooling in the newborn is pathologic because salivary glands do not develop for several months.

The diagnosis of this condition is based on clinical manifestations and confirmed by x-ray.

Manifestations. The earliest sign of TEF occurs prenatally when the mother develops *polyhydramnios.* When the upper esophagus ends in a blind pouch, the fetus cannot swallow the amniotic fluid, resulting in an accumulation of fluid in the amniotic sac (polyhydramnios). At birth, the infant will *vomit* and *choke* when the first feeding is introduced. Because the upper end of the esophagus ends in a blind pouch, the newborn cannot swallow accumulated secretions and will appear to be drooling. Although drooling after 3 months of age is related to teething, drooling in a newborn is pathologic and related to atresia. When the upper esophagus enters the trachea, the first feeding will enter the trachea and result in *coughing, choking, cyanosis,* and *apnea.* If the lower end of the esophagus (from the stomach) enters the trachea, air will enter the stomach each time the infant breathes, causing abdominal distention.

Treatment and Nursing Care. The nursing goals involve preventing pneumonia, choking, and apnea in the newborn. Assessment of every newborn during the first feeding is essential. The first feeding usually consists of clear water or colostrum (if breastfed) to minimize the seriousness of aspiration should it occur. If symptoms are noted, the infant is placed on nothing by mouth (NPO), suctioned to clear the airway and positioned to drain mucous from the nose and throat. Surgical repair is essential for survival (see Preoperative Care, Chapter 22).

Imperforate Anus

Description. Imperforate anus occurs in about 1 in 5,000 live births. The lower GI tract and the anus

Nursing Tip

Newborn infants should not be discharged before a meconium stool is observed and recorded.

arise from two different tissues. Early in fetal life the two tissues meet and join, and then a perforation of tissue separating them occurs, allowing for a passageway between the lower GI tract and the anus. When this perforation does not take place, the lower end of the GI tract and the anus end in blind pouches. This is called *imperforate anus.* There are four types of imperforate anus, ranging from a stenosis to complete separation or failure of the anus to form.

Manifestations. A routine part of the newborn assessment is to determine the patency of the anus. Often the first temperature of the newborn is taken rectally to ascertain patency. (All subsequent and routine temperature readings are usually take via the axillary route.) Failure to pass meconium in the first 24 hours must be reported. Infants should not be discharged to the home before a meconium stool is passed.

Treatment and Nursing Care. Once the diagnosis is established, the infant is placed on nothing by mouth and prepared for surgery. Diagnosis is confirmed by x-ray or MRI. The initial surgical procedure may be a colostomy. Subsequent surgery can reestablish the patency of the anal canal.

Pyloric Stenosis

Description. Pyloric stenosis (narrowing) is an obstruction at the lower end of the stomach (pylorus) caused by an overgrowth (hypertrophy) of the circular muscles of the pylorus or by spasms of the sphincter. This condition is commonly classified as a congenital anomaly; however, its symptoms do not appear until the baby is 2 or 3 weeks old. Pyloric stenosis is the most common surgical condition of the digestive tract in infancy (Fig. 27–2). Its incidence is higher in boys than in girls, and it has a tendency to be inherited.

Manifestations. Vomiting is the outstanding symptom of this disorder. The force progresses until most of the food is ejected a considerable distance from the mouth. This is termed *projectile vomiting,* and it occurs immediately after feeding. The vomitus contains mucus and ingested milk. The baby is constantly hungry and will eat again immediately after vomiting. Dehydration, as evidenced by sunken fontanel, inelastic skin, and decreased urination, and malnutrition can develop. An olive-shaped mass may be felt in the right upper quadrant of the abdomen. Ultrasonography or scintiscans are commonly used today for diagnostic purposes, as it is noninvasive and accurate. In severe cases, the outline of the distended stomach and peristaltic waves are visible during feeding.

Treatment. The operation performed for pyloric stenosis is called a *pyloromyotomy* (*pylorus, myo,* "muscle," and *tomy,* "incision of"). The surgeon incises the pyloric muscle to enlarge the opening so that food may easily pass through it again. This is done as soon as possible if the infant is not dehydrated.

Nursing Care. The dehydrated infant is given intravenous fluids preoperatively to restore fluid and electrolyte balance. If this is not done, shock may occur during surgery. Thickened feedings may be given until the time of operation in hopes that some nutrients will be retained. The physician prescribes the degree of thickness of the formula, which is given by teaspoon or through a nipple with a large hole. The infant is bubbled *before* as well as *during* feedings to remove any gas accumulated in the stomach. The feeding is done slowly, and the baby is handled gently and as little as possible. The infant is placed on the right side following feedings. The pylorus is on the right side

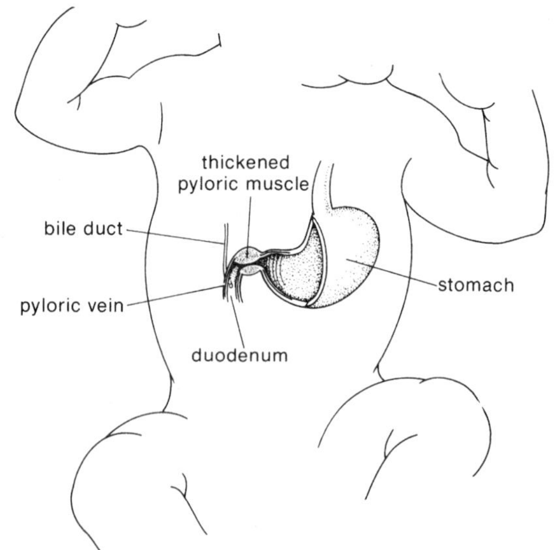

Figure 27–2. • Pyloric stenosis. Hypertrophy or thickening of the pyloric sphincter blocks the stomach contents, causing the infant to regurgitate forcefully. Serious electrolyte imbalances ultimately occur, and surgery is necessary to correct the condition. (From Betz, C., Hunsberger, M., & Wright, S. [1994]. *Family-centered nursing care of children* [2nd ed.]. Philadelphia, Saunders.)

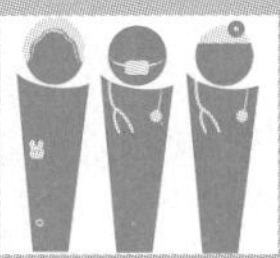

Clinical Pathway 27–1

An Interdisciplinary Plan of Care for the Infant with Pyloric Stenosis

	Patient/Family Intermediate Outcomes		
Nursing Diagnosis	Day: Admission	Day: Postop 1	Day: Postop 2
Fluid Volume Deficit: related to effects of persistent vomiting	Child shows improved fluid and electrolyte balance.	Child demonstrates normal fluid and electrolyte balance, as evidenced by normal urine output (1 mL/kg/hr), moist mucous membranes, good skin turgor, laboratory values within normal limits.	→
Altered Nutrition: less than body requirements related to persistent vomiting	Child stops vomiting.	Child ingests and retains small amounts of formula.	Child ingests and retains sufficient nutrients to meet dietary needs.
Pain: related to incision, muscle cutting and manipulation during surgery		Child has signs of pain recognized and interventions promptly implemented. Child experiences minimal levels of pain.	→
Knowledge Deficit: related to treatments, surgery, postoperative care	Parents verbalize understanding of treatments and surgery.	Parents verbalize understanding of postoperative pain management, feeding, and incision care.	Parents verbalize understanding of home care and follow-up needs.

(continued on following page)

of the abdomen; thus, drainage into the intestine is facilitated. Fowler's position is preferred to aid gravity in passing milk through the stomach (see Fowler's sling, Fig. 27–7). If vomiting occurs, the nurse may be instructed to *refeed* the infant. Charting of the feeding includes time, type, and amount offered; amount taken and retained; and type and amount of vomiting. The nurse also notes whether the baby appeared hungry after the feeding or vomiting.

The nurse obtains and records a baseline weight and weighs the infant at about the same time each morning. Other factors to be charted include the type and number of stools and the color of urine and frequency of voiding (intake and output). Position is changed frequently because the infant is weak and vulnerable to pneumonia. All procedures designed to protect from infection must be strictly carried out.

The care of the infant following surgery includes a careful observation of vital signs and administration of intravenous fluids. The wound site is inspected frequently (see Chapter 22 for postoperative care). Since the surgery involves cutting into the hypertrophied muscle, but *not through the mucous membrane of the bowel,* the infant will not need nasogastric decompression postoperatively and will be able to resume oral feedings shortly after responding from anesthesia. The doctor prescribes oral feedings of small amounts of sugar and water that gradually increase until a regular formula can be taken and retained. Overfeeding is avoided and the nurse reviews feeding techniques with parents. The diaper is placed low over the abdomen to prevent contamination of the wound site. See Clinical Pathway 27–1 for Pyloromyotomy.

Celiac Disease

Description. Celiac disease is also known as *gluten enteropathy* and *sprue* and is the leading malabsorption problem in children. The cause is thought to be an inherited disposition with environmental triggers.

Manifestations. Symptoms are not evident until

Clinical Pathway 27–1 *(Continued)*

An Interdisciplinary Plan of Care for the Infant with Pyloric Stenosis

Care Intervention Categories	Day: Admission	Day: Postop 1	Day: Postop 2
Consults	Surgical consult		
Labs	CBC, electrolytes Repeat electrolytes prn to monitor Cl^- and CO_2 values		
Medications and IVs	IV fluids: maintenance and replacement Give acetaminophen with codeine or acetaminophen p.r.n. for pain	Heparin lock IV when tolerating PO fluids	Discontinue IV if tolerating PO fluids
Nutrition	NPO	Give 10 mL oral electrolyte solution after recovered from anesthesia; start pyloric refeeding protocol (increasing feeding volumes from clear fluids to dilute to full-strength formula); repeat previous step if emesis × 1, notify surgeon if emesis × 2.	Give full-strength formula at normal feeding volumes.
Pain management	Give acetaminophen with codeine or plain (see medications above) Flex knees; position to avoid stretching abdominal muscles. Burp frequently to avoid abdominal distention.	→	→
Procedures	NG tube to gravity drainage	Discontinue NG tube before starting feedings	
Radiology	Sonogram of abdomen and barium study p.r.n. to confirm diagnosis		

(continued)

6 months to 2 years of age when foods containing gluten are introduced to the infant. Gluten is found in wheat, barley, oats, and rye. Repeated exposure to the gluten causes damage to the villi in the mucous membranes of the intestine resulting in malabsorption of food. The infant presents with failure to thrive. *Stools are large, bulky, and frothy* because of undigested contents. The infant is irritable. Diagnosis is confirmed by serum IgA test and small-bowel biopsy.

Treatment and Nursing Care. The treatment involves a lifelong diet restricted in wheat, barley, oats, and rye. It is a nursing challenge to teach the family the importance of dietary compliance. A professional nutritionist or dietician can aid in identifying foods that are gluten free. Long-term bowel pathology can occur if dietary compliance is not lifelong.

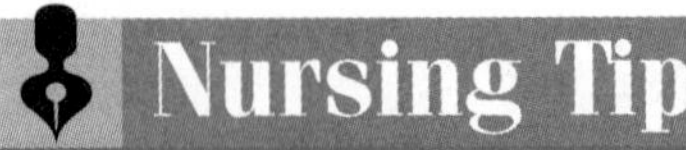

Nursing Tip

A bulky, frothy, stool may indicate a malabsorption is present.

Clinical Pathway 27–1 *(Continued)*

An Interdisciplinary Plan of Care for the Infant with Pyloric Stenosis

Care Intervention Categories	Day: Admission	Day: Postop 1	Day: Postop 2
Teaching/discharge planning	Teach parents about preoperative care routines. Teach parents about surgical routines; review postoperative care.	Teach parents methods of pain assessment and management; reintroduce feedings; provide incision care. Assess what supplies will be needed at home (medications, dressings) and ability of parents to obtain them.	Evaluate parent's ability to manage pain, feed, and care for incision; review techniques p.r.n. Discharge child when full oral feedings are tolerated.
Vital signs/baseline parameters	Vital signs with blood pressure on admission and q 4 hr	→	→
	Daily weight	→	→
	Urine specific gravity each shift	→	
	Intake and output	→	→

Adapted from Bowden, V., Dickey, S., & Greenberg, C. (1998). *Children and their families: The continuum of care.* Philadelphia: Saunders.

Hirschsprung's Disease (Aganglionic Megacolon)

Description. Hirschsprung's disease occurs when there is an *absence of ganglionic innervation to the muscle of a segment of the bowel.* This usually happens in the lower portion of the sigmoid colon. Because of the absence of nerve cells, there is a lack of normal peristalsis. This results in chronic constipation. Ribbonlike stools are seen as feces pass through the narrow segment. The portion of the bowel nearest to the obstruction dilates, causing abdominal distention (Fig. 27–3). It is seen more often in boys than girls and has familial tendencies. The incidence is approximately 1 in 5000 live births. There is a higher incidence in children with Down syndrome. The condition may be acute or chronic.

Manifestations. In the newborn, failure to pass meconium stools within 24 to 48 hours may be a symptom. In the infant, constipation, ribbonlike stools, abdominal distention, anorexia, vomiting, and failure to thrive may be evident. Often the parent brings the young child to the clinic after trying several over-the-counter laxatives to treat the constipation without success. If the child is untreated, other signs of intestinal obstruction and shock may be seen. The development of *enterocolitis* (inflammation of the small bowel and colon) is a serious complication. It may be signaled by fever, explosive stools, and depletion of strength. Diagnostic evaluation usually includes a barium enema and rectal biopsy, which shows a lack of innervation. Anorectal manometry tests the strength of the internal rectal sphincter. In this procedure, a balloon catheter is placed into the rectum, and the pressure exerted against it is measured.

Treatment and Nursing Care. Megacolon is treated by surgery. The impaired part of the colon is removed, and an anastomosis of the intestine is performed. In newborns a temporary colostomy may be necessary, and more extensive repair may follow at about 12 to 18 months. Closure of the colostomy follows in a few months.

Nursing care is age-dependent. In the newborn, detection is a high priority. As the child grows older, careful attention to a history of constipation and diarrhea is important. Signs of undernutrition, abdominal distention, and poor feedings are suspect.

Because the distended bowel in a child with megacolon provides a larger mucous membrane surface area that will come in contact with fluid inserted during an enema, an increased absorption

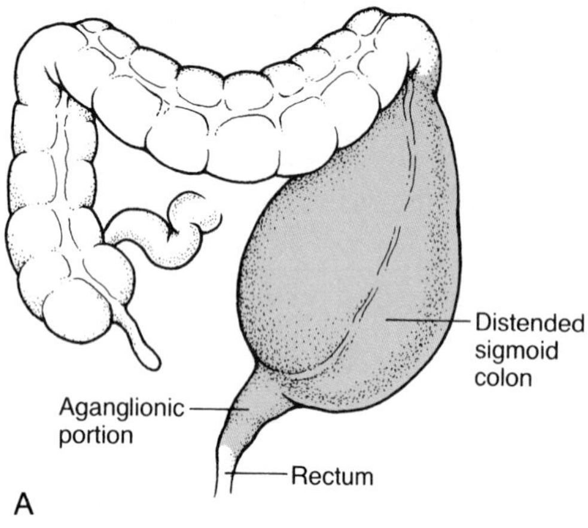

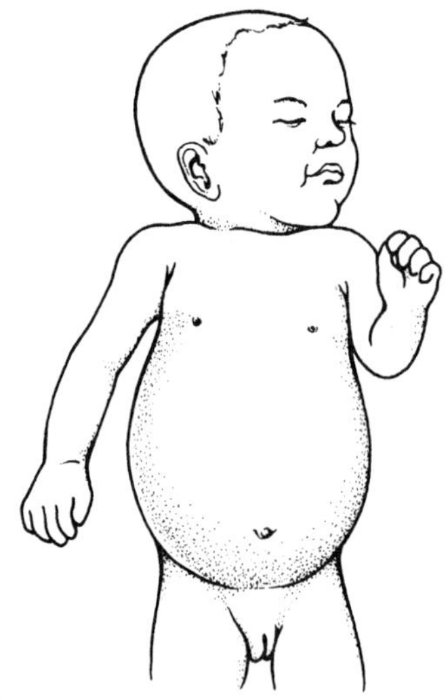

Figure 27–3. • Hirschsprung's disease (megacolon). **A,** There is no ganglionic nerve innervation or peristalsis in the narrowed section. **B,** The adjacent bowel becomes enlarged, causing distention of the abdomen.

of the fluid can be anticipated. For this reason, when a child is given an enema at home, normal saline, not tap water, is used. Tap water enemas in infants and small children can lead to water intoxication and death. Parents can obtain normal saline solution from the pharmacy without prescription, or they can make it at home by using one half of a teaspoon of noniodized salt to 1 cup of lukewarm tap water. The amount of fluid administered should be determined by the health care provider. The nurse stresses to parents the importance of adding salt to water. Postoperative care of children is discussed in Chapter 22.

Intussusception

Description. Intussusception (*intus,* "within," and *suscipere,* "to receive") is a slipping of one part of the intestine into another part just below it (Fig. 27–4). It is frequently seen at the ileocecal valve, where the small intestine opens into the ascending colon. The *mesentery,* a double fan-shaped fold of peritoneum that covers most of the intestine and is filled with blood vessels and nerves, is also pulled along. Edema occurs. At first this telescoping of the bowel causes intestinal obstruction, but as peristalsis forces the structures more tightly, strangulation takes place. This portion may burst, causing peritonitis.

Intussusception generally occurs in boys between 3 months and 6 years of age who are otherwise healthy. Its frequency decreases after 36 months of age. Occasionally the condition corrects itself without treatment. This is termed a spontaneous reduction. However, because the patient's life is in danger, the doctor does not waste time waiting for this to occur. The prognosis is good when the patient is treated within 24 hours.

Manifestations. In typical cases, the onset is sudden. The infant feels severe pain in the abdomen, evidenced by loud cries, straining efforts, and kicking and drawing of the legs toward the abdomen. At first there is comfort between pains, but the intervals shorten and the condition becomes worse. The child vomits. The stomach contents are green or greenish-yellow; this is due to bile stain, and the contents are described as bilious. Bowel movements diminish, and little flatus is passed. Movements of blood and mucus that contain no feces are common about 12 hours after the onset of the obstruction; these are termed *currant jelly stools.* The child's fever may run as high as 106°F (41.1°C), and signs of shock, such as sweating, weak pulse, and shallow, granting respirations are evident. The abdomen is rigid.

Treatment and Nursing Care. Intussusception is an *emergency,* and because of the severity of symptoms, most parents contact a doctor promptly. The diagnosis is determined by the history and physical findings. The doctor may feel a sausage-shaped mass in the right upper portion of the abdomen during bimanual rectal and abdominal palpation. Abdominal films also may indicate the mass. A barium enema is the treatment of choice, with surgery scheduled if reduction is not achieved. The recurrence rate following barium enema reduction is about 10%.

During the operation, a small incision is made into the abdomen, and the wayward intestine is "milked" back into position. The intestine is inspected for gangrene, and if all is well, the abdomen is sutured. Barring complications, recovery is straightforward. If the intestine cannot be reduced or if gangrene has set in, a resection is done and the affected bowel is removed. The cut end of the ileum is joined to the cut end of the colon; this is called an *anastomosis.* Routine pre- and postoperative care is discussed in Chapter 22.

Meckel's Diverticulum

Description. During fetal life the intestine is attached to the yolk sac by the vitelline duct. If this duct fails to disappear completely, a small blind pouch may form. This condition is termed Meckel's diverticulum (Fig. 27–5). It usually occurs near the ileocecal valve. It may be connected to the umbilicus by a cord. A fistula may also form. This sac is subject to inflammation, much like the appendix. This disorder is the most common congenital malformation of the gastrointestinal tract. It is seen more frequently in boys.

Manifestations. Symptoms may occur at any age but appear most often before age 2. Painless bleeding from the rectum is the most common sign. Bright-red or dark-red blood is more usual than tarry stools. Abdominal pain may or may not be present. In some persons it may exist without causing symptoms. Barium enema and radionuclide scintigraphy are useful in diagnosing Meckel's diverticulum. X-ray films are not helpful because the pouch is so small that it may not appear on the screen.

Treatment and Nursing Care. The diverticulum is removed by surgery. Nursing care is the same as for the patient undergoing exploration of the abdomen. Because this condition appears suddenly and bleeding causes parental anxiety, emotional support is of particular importance.

Hernias

Description. An *inguinal* hernia is a protrusion of part of the abdominal contents through the inguinal canal in the groin. It is more common in boys than in girls. It is also seen frequently in preterm infants. An *umbilical* hernia is a protrusion of a portion of intestine through the umbilical ring (an opening in the muscular area of the abdomen through which the umbilical vessels pass, Fig. 27–6). This type of hernia appears as a soft swelling covered by skin, which protrudes when the infant cries or strains. Hernias may be present at birth (congenital) or may be acquired, and they can vary in size. A hernia is termed reducible if it can be put back into place by gentle pressure; if this cannot be done, it is called an irreducible or an *incarcerated* (constricted) hernia. Incarceration occurs more often in infants under 10 months of age. Hernias may be bilateral.

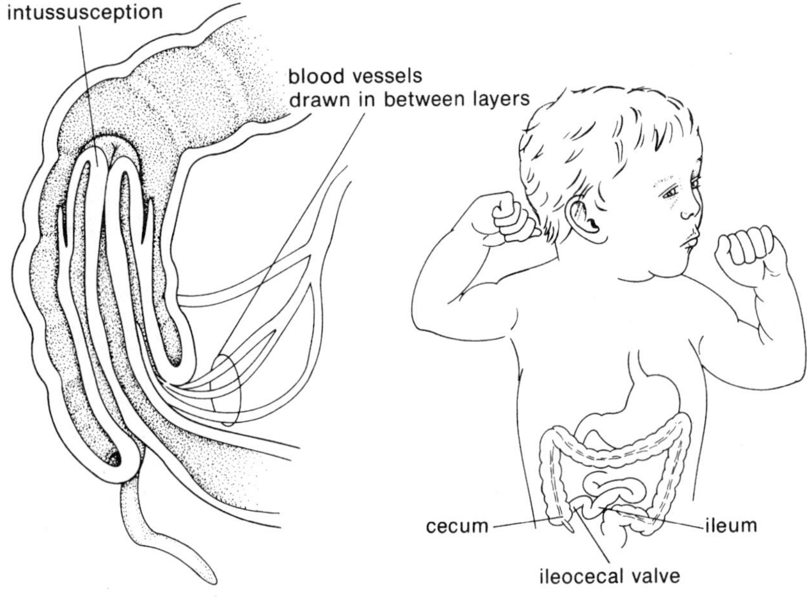

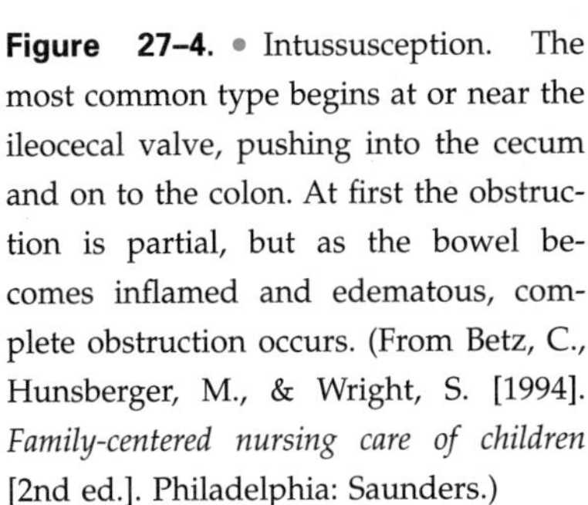

Figure 27–4. • Intussusception. The most common type begins at or near the ileocecal valve, pushing into the cecum and on to the colon. At first the obstruction is partial, but as the bowel becomes inflamed and edematous, complete obstruction occurs. (From Betz, C., Hunsberger, M., & Wright, S. [1994]. *Family-centered nursing care of children* [2nd ed.]. Philadelphia: Saunders.)

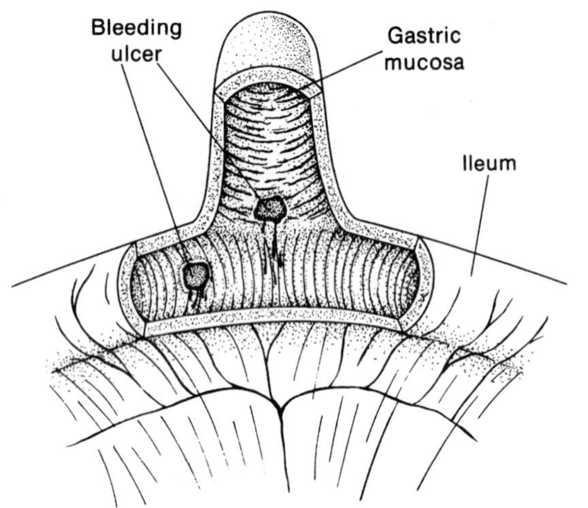

Figure 27–5. • Meckel's diverticulum is a congenital anomaly characterized by an outpouching of the ileum. (From Betz, C., Hunsberger, M., & Wright, S. [1994]. *Family-centered nursing care of children* [2nd ed.]. Philadelphia: Saunders.)

Manifestations. The infant with a hernia may be relatively free of symptoms. Irritability, fretfulness, and constipation are sometimes evident. The diagnosis is made when physical examination shows a mass in the area that reappears from time to time, particularly when the child cries or strains. A *strangulated* hernia occurs when the intestine becomes caught in the passage and the blood supply is diminished. This happens more frequently during the first 6 months of life. Vomiting and severe abdominal pain are present. Emergency surgery is necessary if strangulation occurs, and in some cases a bowel resection is performed.

Treatment and Nursing Care. Hernias are successfully repaired by the surgical operation called a herniorrhaphy. This is a relatively simple procedure that is tolerated well by the child. Most children are scheduled for same-day surgery units. The benefits of this method are both economic and psychological. Parents are instructed to bring the fasting child to the hospital about 1 hour before surgery. Parents remain with the child during the entire time except

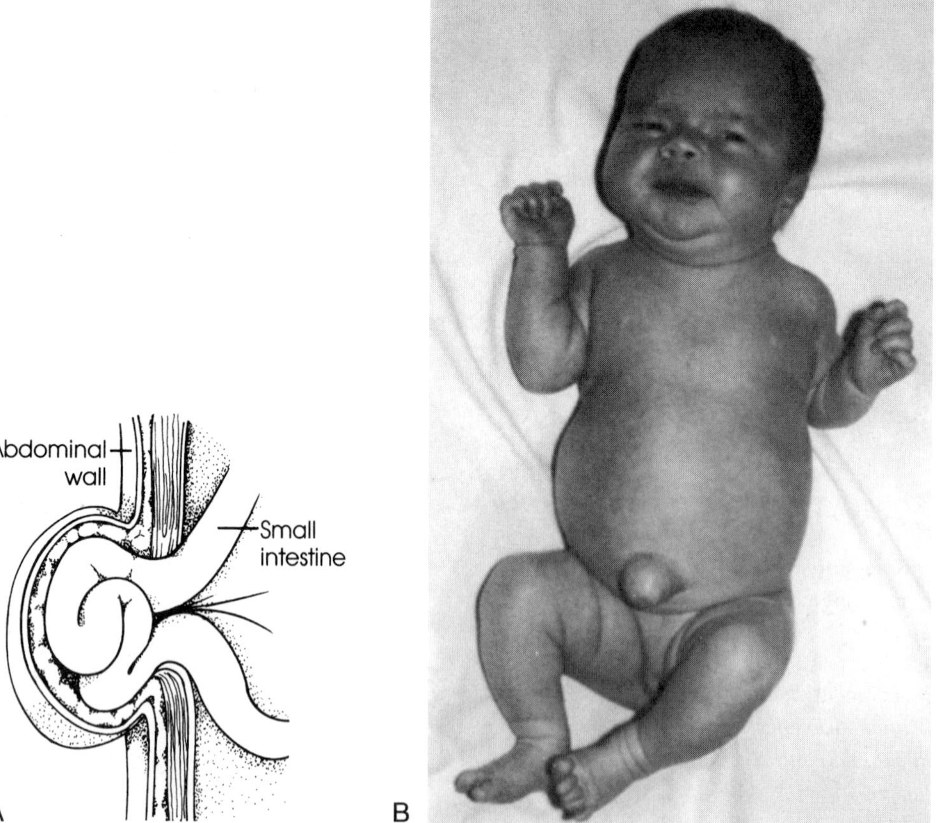

Figure 27–6. • **A,** Umbilical hernia. **B,** Infant with an umbilical hernia. (From Marlow, D. R., & Redding, B. A. [1988]. *Textbook of pediatric nursing* [6th ed.]. Philadelphia: Saunders.)

during the actual procedure. They are encouraged to assist in routine postoperative care.

Often no dressing is applied to the wound. Sometimes a waterproof collodion dressing, which looks like clear nail polish, is applied. Postoperative care is directed toward keeping the wound clean. Diapers are left open for this purpose. Wet diapers are changed frequently.

DISORDERS OF MOTILITY

Gastroenteritis

Description. *Gastroenteritis* involves an inflammation of the stomach and the intestines; *colitis* involves an inflammation of the colon; *enterocolitis* involves an inflammation of the colon and the intestine. The most common noninfectious causes of diarrhea involve food intolerance, overfeeding, improper formula preparation, or ingestion of high amounts of sorbitol, a substance found in sweetened "sugar-free" products. The priority problem in diarrhea is fluid and electrolyte imbalance and failure to thrive.

Treatment and Nursing Care. Treatment is focused on identifying and eradicating the cause. Nursing responsibilities include teaching parents and caregivers proper diet and feeding techniques that are age appropriate. The priority goal of care includes preventing fluid and electrolyte imbalance.

Oral dehydrating solutions (ORT), such as Pedialyte, Lytren, Ricelyte, and Resol are used for infants in small frequent feedings. Although formula feeding is withheld, breastfeeding can accompany ORT treatment, because of its osmolarity, antimicrobial properties, and enzyme content.

The nursing care includes maintaining intake and output records and providing skin care and frequent diaper changes to prevent excoriation from the frequent stools. Parents should be taught good handwashing techniques, principles of food handling, and principles of cleanliness and of infection prevention. The infant should be weighed daily, observed for dehydration or overhydration, and kept warm. Enteric precautions and standard precautions should be employed to prevent the spread of infection (see Appendix A).

Vomiting

Description. Vomiting, a common symptom during infancy and childhood results from sudden contractions of the diaphragm and muscles of the stomach. It must be evaluated in relation to the child's overall health status. Persistent vomiting requires investigation because it results in dehydration and electrolyte imbalance. The continuous loss of hydrochloric acid and sodium chloride from the stomach can cause *alkalosis.* In this condition, the acid–base balance of the body becomes disturbed because of a loss of chlorides and potassium. This can result in death if the patient is left untreated.

Manifestations. The child may vomit from various causes. Some stem from improper feeding techniques that should be assessed by the nurse. Sometimes the difficulty lies with formula intolerance. The introduction of foods of a different consistency may also precipitate this symptom.

Other causes of vomiting are systemic illness such as increased intracranial pressure or infection. Aspiration and aspiration pneumonia are serious complications of vomiting. In aspiration, vomitus is drawn into the air passages on inspiration, causing immediate death in extreme cases. Health professionals and laypersons should become familiar with life-saving procedures such as CPR for use in such emergencies.

Treatment and Nursing Care. To prevent vomiting, the nurse must carefully feed and bubble the baby. Treatments are avoided immediately following feedings. The baby is handled as little as possible following feedings. To prevent aspiration of vomitus, the nurse places the infant on the right side following feedings. When an older child begins to vomit, the head is turned to one side, and an emesis basin and tissues are provided.

Factors to be charted include time, amount, color (bloody, bile-stained), consistency, force, frequency, and whether or not vomiting was preceded by nausea or by feedings. Intravenous fluids may be given (Chapter 22). Oral fluids are withheld for a short time to allow the stomach to rest. Gradually, sips of water are given according to the infant's tolerance and condition. The patient's intake and output are carefully recorded so that the physician is able to compare the kidney output with the total fluid intake.

When vomiting is persistent, drugs such as trimethobenzamide (Tigan) or promethazine (Phenergan) may be prescribed. They are available in rectal suppository form. The nurse lubricates the suppository and inserts it well into the rectum, where it dissolves. Slight pressure is exerted over the anus for a short time to ensure the suppository is not expelled. Charting includes the time administered and whether or not vomiting subsided.

Gastroesophageal Reflux

Description. Gastroesophageal reflux (GER, or chalasia) results when the lower esophageal sphincter is relaxed or not competent, which allows stomach contents to be easily regurgitated into the esophagus.

The term *chalasia* is derived from the Greek word *chalasis,* which means "relaxation." Although many infants have this condition to a small degree, about 1 in 300 to 1 in 1000 have significant reflux and associated complications. The condition is associated with neuromuscular delay and is seen frequently in preterm infants and children with neuromuscular disorders, such as cerebral palsy and Down syndrome. In many infants, the symptoms decrease around 12 months, when the child stands upright and eats more solid foods.

Manifestations. The symptoms include vomiting, weight loss, and failure to thrive. The vomiting occurs within the 1st and 2nd week of life. The baby is fussy and hungry. Respiratory problems can occur when vomiting stimulates the closure of the epiglottis and the infant presents with apnea. Aspiration of vomitus can also occur.

Treatment and Nursing Care. A careful history is taken. Of particular interest are when the vomiting started, type of formula, type of vomiting, feeding techniques, and the baby's eating in general. Tests used to determine the presence of GER include a barium swallow under fluoroscopy or esophagoscopy. Esophageal sphincter pressure may also be measured. Prolonged esophageal pH monitoring is one of the most definitive diagnostic tests and helps to determine the acuity of the disease and the course of treatment.

Therapy depends on the severity of symptoms. Some parents need only reassurance and education about feeding the baby. The routine includes careful burping, avoiding overfeeding (which distends the stomach), and proper positioning. In infants with more complicated GER, medication and surgical intervention may be required. Parents are instructed to burp the baby well. Feedings are thickened with cereal. After being fed, the baby is placed in an upright position or propped on the right side. The body is inclined about 30 to 40 degrees, and the baby is held in place by a Fowler's sling (Fig. 27–7). Sitting upright in an infant seat is not recommended because it increases intraabdominal pressure. Medications that relax the pyloric sphincter and promote stomach emptying may be utilized. Metoclopramide (Reglan) or bethanechol chloride (Urecholine) are two such medications. They are administered before meals.

Diarrhea

Description. Diarrhea in the infant cannot be defined in the same way as diarrhea in the adult. The number of stools per day is not often significant in the infant. Diarrhea in infancy is a sudden increase in stools from the infant's normal pattern, with a *fluid consistency,* with a *color* that is green, or containing mucous or blood. *Acute* sudden diarrhea is most often due to an inflammation or infection or a response to a medication, food, or poisoning. *Chronic diarrhea* lasts for more than 2 weeks and may be indicative of a malabsorption problem, long-term inflammatory disease, or allergic responses. *Infectious diarrhea* is caused by viral, bacterial, or parasitic infection and usually involves gastroenteritis.

Manifestations. The symptoms of diarrhea may be mild or extremely severe. The stools are watery and are expelled with force (explosive stools). They may be yellowish-green. The baby becomes listless, refuses to eat, and loses weight. The temperature may be elevated and the infant may vomit. Dehydration is evidenced by sunken eyes and fontanel and by dry skin, tongue, and mucous mem-

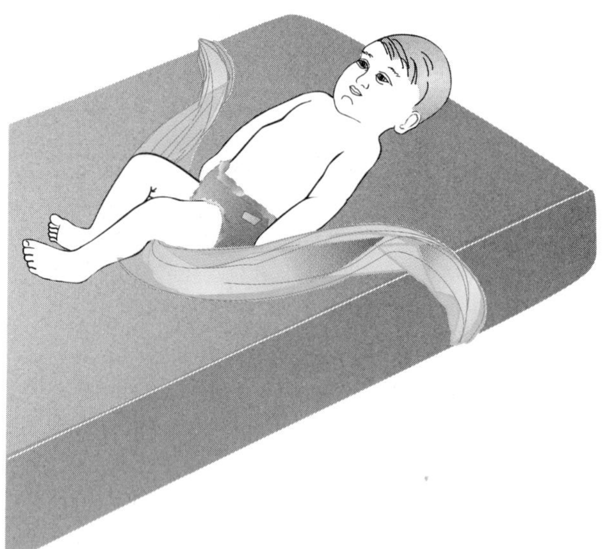

Figure 27–7. • The Fowler's sling. The Fowler's sling is used to maintain Fowler's position and to prevent the infant from sliding down to the foot of the bed. The bed is in Fowler's position; the rolled blanket is tucked under the mattress on each side at armpit level; when the infant is in side-lying position or prone, the legs *straddle* the sling to maintain positioning. (From Leifer, G. [1982]. *Principles and techniques in pediatric nursing,* 4th ed. [p. 82.] Philadelphia: Saunders.)

Nursing Tip

Green, watery stools may indicate diarrhea in infants.

branes. Urination may become less frequent. In severe cases, the excessive loss of bicarbonate from the gastrointestinal tract results in acidosis.

Infectious diarrhea in infants is commonly caused by the rotavirus that occurs often in day care centers; by *Escherichia coli,* which is caused by lack of hygiene or poorly cooked foods; *Salmonella* from contaminated food or pet (especially turtles) contact; by *Shigella;* and by other organisms. *Clostridium difficile* often follows antibiotic therapy. *Giardia lamblia* is an intestinal protozoan that causes diarrhea. It is spread by contaminated water, unsanitary conditions, and fecal contamination by animals. Prevention is important and centers around teaching the basics of hygienic practices, handwashing, and the use of disinfectants.

Mild diarrhea in older children may be treated at home under a doctor's direction, provided that there is a suitable caregiver. Treatment is essentially the same. The intestine is rested by reducing intake of solid foods. Clear fluids, such as flat ginger ale, gelatin desserts, tea, and popsicles, are usually well tolerated. High-sodium broths are avoided to prevent electrolyte imbalance. Other foods are added to the diet gradually. A soft diet (sometimes called a BRAT diet, for *b*ananas, *r*ice cereal, *a*pplesauce, and *t*oast with jelly) may be resumed when liquids are well tolerated. Creamed soups are avoided. Crackers and pretzels are gradually added. A regular intake is usually resumed within 2 to 3 days. Milk and butter are cautiously added as the patient's condition improves. Nursing Care Plan 27–1 provides nursing interventions for the care of a child with diarrhea.

Constipation

Description. Constipation is difficult or infrequent defecation with passage of hard, dry fecal material. There may be associated symptoms, such as abdominal discomfort or blood-streaked stools.

Manifestations. The frequency of bowel movements varies widely in children. There may be periods of diarrhea or *encopresis* (constipation with fecal soiling). Constipation may be a symptom of other disorders, particularly obstructive conditions. Diet, culture, and social, psychological, and familial patterns may also influence its occurrence. The use of laxatives and enemas should be discouraged. Most children use the bathroom every day, but they may be hurried and have an incomplete bowel movement. Some children are embarrassed or even afraid to use school or public bathrooms.

Treatment and Nursing Care. Evaluation begins with a thorough history of dietary and bowel habits. Some infants respond to formula with a high iron content by developing constipation. Changing to a low-iron formula may be helpful. The frequency, color, and consistency of the stool are noted. The nurse inquires about any medication the child may be taking. The parents are asked to define what they mean by constipation. Parent teaching concerning prevention of constipation is essential.

Dietary modifications include adding more roughage in the diet. Foods high in fiber include whole-grain breads and cereals, raw vegetables and fruits, bran, and popcorn for older children. Increasing fluid intake is also important. A stool softener such as docusate sodium (Colace) may be prescribed. The child is encouraged to try to move the bowels at the same time each day to establish a routine. The child should not be hurried. Increased exercise may help sedentary children.

Fluid and Electrolyte Imbalance

Principles of Fluid Balance in Children. Infants and small children have different *proportions of body water and body fat,* from those of adults (Fig. 27–8), and the water needs and water losses of the infant, per unit of body weight, are greater. In children under 2 years of age, *surface area* is particularly important in fluid and electrolyte balance because more water is lost through the skin than through the kidneys. The surface area of the infant is from two to three times greater than that of the adult in proportion to body volume or body weight. *Metabolic rate* and *heat production* are also two to three times greater in infants per kilogram of body weight. This produces more *waste products,* which must be diluted to be excreted. It also stimulates respiration, which causes greater evaporation through the lungs. Compared with adults, a greater percentage of body water in children under age 2 is contained in the *extracellular compartment.*

Fluid turnover is rapid, and dehydration occurs more quickly in infants than in adults (Table 27–1 and Box 27–1). The infant cannot survive as long as the adult in the presence of continued water depletion. A sick infant does not adapt as rapidly to shifts in intake and output because the kidneys lack maturity. They

NURSING CARE PLAN 27–1

Gastroenteritis (Diarrhea/Vomiting)

Nursing Diagnosis: Fluid volume deficit related to diarrhea and/or vomiting as evidenced by weight loss, output greater than intake, emesis, liquid stools, decreased urine output, abdominal distension/rebound tenderness, excoriation of perianal mucosa, hypotensive, increased pulse rate, change in skin turgor, lethargy, irritability

Goals	Nursing Interventions	Rationale
Infant/child's weight is within 5% of normal baseline Bowel movements will be reduced in number within 24 hours (of nursing intervention) Urine output is above 1 cc/kg/hr Infant/child is free from fluid/electrolyte imbalance	1. Weigh infant/child daily	1. Daily *accurate* weights are necessary to ascertain the amount of fluids lost through liquid stools and/or vomiting
	2. Monitor vital signs, e.g., temperature, pulse, respirations, blood pressure, and skin turgor.	2. Helps determine if the infant/child is responding appropriately to medical and nursing interventions.
	3. Record intake and output accurately, including ice chips, intravenous fluids, gelatins, or other food products that become waterlike at room temperature	3. Accurate recording of intake and output is necessary to determine the amount of fluid replacement required
	4. Observe/monitor intravenous fluid administration	4. Fluid depletion occurs very rapidly in infants and small children as they have different proportions of both body water and fat from an adult. IV fluids may be needed to prevent dehydration, electrolyte imbalance, shock, and death
	5. Notify health care provider of decreased number of stools, ability to drink liquids without emesis; increased urine output, and improvement in vital signs and skin turgor	5. Prevents overhydration of infant/child
	6. Obtain fresh stool specimen, if ordered, and send to laboratory for analysis	6. A fresh sample is required to determine if there are any ova (eggs) or parasites in the stool that could be the cause of the gastroenteritis
	7. Resume oral liquids/foods gradually, starting with ordered rehydration fluids	7. Rehydration fluids help to decrease the mobility of colon, rests intestinal tract, and decreases the risk of water toxicity

Nursing Diagnosis: High risk for altered skin integrity related to frequency of stools as evidenced by excoriation of skin/tissue in perianal area, erythema, depending on age of child, pain with each stooling; complaint of burning/pain in perianal area

Goals	Nursing Interventions	Rationale
Infant/child shows improvement or resolution of erythema and exhibit tissue intact and free from secondary infection	1. Change diapers/underwear as soon as a stooling occurs; cleanse perianal area with warm water using a soft cloth free of any alcohol	1. Liquid stools generally contain high amounts of acids. The longer the stool is in contact with the infant/child's skin, the greater the risk of excoriated tissue. Alcohol can be very painful on impaired tissue
	2. Leave buttocks exposed to air whenever possible (usually *after* the diarrhea slows down or stops)	2. Air helps to keep the skin dry and free from any irritation such as diapers or underwear rubbing on the skin
	3. Apply soothing balm or ointment to affected area, *after* thorough cleansing, sparingly	3. The balm or ointment is a protective barrier on the infant/child's skin. If the ointment is placed on uncleansed skin, the infant/child is at increased risk of excoriation
	4. If medicated powders are prescribed and/or used, teach parent to put powder in their hand and then apply on the infant/child's buttocks and to keep powder container away from infant/child	4. If powder is "sprayed" on to buttocks, the infant/child is at risk of inhaling the powder

(continued)

NURSING CARE PLAN 27-1 *continued*

Gastroenteritis (Diarrhea/Vomiting)

Nursing Diagnosis: Parental knowledge deficit related to diarrhea in infants/children as evidenced by lack of previous experience

Goals	Nursing Interventions	Rationale
Parents will verbalize understanding of the dietary restrictions, potential complications, and method of treatment for gastroenteritis/diarrhea	1. Instruct parents on proper methods of making, reconstituting, and storing of formulas, oral fluid replacements, and foods	1. Ensure that parents understand that improper handling or storing of food products can increase the risk of further gastroenteritis
	2. Teach/reinforce proper handwashing techniques, especially after handling soiled diapers and clothing and before preparing and/or eating a meal	2. Handwashing is the first in the line of defense in preventing the spread of infection
	3. Explain that dehydration occurs rapidly in infants and small children. Because of this fact, the parents need to seek help from their health care provider early so as to prevent potential hospitalization and/or further complications	3. Early detection and interventions prevent more severe complications from the dehydration that occurs with gastroenteritis
	4. Teach parents that some over-the-counter remedies for vomiting and diarrhea can be harmful to infants and small children	4. Absorbents such as kaolin and pectin may alter the consistency and appearance of stools, decreasing the frequency of evacuation; but may mask actual fluid loss

are less able to concentrate urine and require more water than an adult's kidneys to excrete a given amount of solute. Disturbances of the gastrointestinal tract frequently lead to vomiting and diarrhea. Electrolyte balance depends on fluid balance and cardiovascular, renal, adrenal, pituitary, parathyroid and pulmonary regulatory mechanisms. Many of these mechanisms are maturing in the developing child and are unable to react to full capacity under the stress of illness such as diarrhea and vomiting.

Oral Fluids

Whenever possible, fluids are given by mouth. It is the most natural and satisfactory method. Nurses must use their ingenuity to coax sick children to take enough fluids because they may refuse food and water and do not understand their importance for recovery. Toddlers and infants are not capable of drinking by themselves. The busy nurse must find time to offer fluids and must be patient and gently persistent. Liquids are offered frequently and in small amounts. Brightly colored containers and drinking straws may help. Frozen fruit flavored ice sticks may be more readily accepted than juice in a cup. The nurse keeps an accurate record of the patient's intake and output.

Nursing Tip

All children with vomiting or diarrhea must have an accurate intake and output recorded.

Parenteral Fluids

Parenteral (*para,* "beside or apart from," and *enteron,* "intestine") *fluids* are those given by some route other than the digestive tract. They are necessary when sickness is accompanied by vomiting or loss of consciousness or when the gastrointestinal system requires rest. Parenteral fluids are needed in severe cases of vomiting and diarrhea in which the loss of excessive water and electrolytes will lead to death if untreated. It also provides a means for the safe and effective administration of selective parenteral medications. Solutions given parenterally must be sterile to prevent a general or local infection. The nurse must be aware of the importance of parenteral therapy and assessments required.

The infant or child receiving parenteral fluids needs the nurse's warmth and affection. A pacifier should be used whenever infants are NPO. Parents should be encouraged to pick up and hold or rock their children who are receiving IV therapy. Arm boards prevent the child from pulling out the IV and protect the tubing. Parenteral therapy is discussed in Chapter 22.

Dehydration

Description. When a person is in good health, the intake and output of fluids are balanced and *homeostasis* (a uniform state) exists. This is accomplished by appropriate shifts of fluids and electrolytes across cellular membranes and by elimination of products of metabolism that are no longer needed or are in excess. The volume of blood plasma and interstitial and intracellular fluids remains relatively constant. Dehydration occurs whenever fluid output exceeds fluid intake, regardless of the cause.

Manifestations. Disorders of fluids and electrolytes—sodium (Na), potassium (K), calcium (Ca), and magnesium (Mg)—are more complex in growing children. A newborn's total weight is approximately 77% water, compared with 60% in adults (see Fig. 27–8). This varies with the amount of fat. Also, the daily turnover of water in infants is equal to almost 24% of total body water, compared with about 6% in adults. A baby's body surface in comparison with weight is three times that of the older child; therefore, the baby is subject to greater evaporation of water from the skin. The younger the patient, the higher the metabolic rate and the more unstable the heat-regulating mechanisms. (Elevations in temperature also increase the rate of water loss.) Rapid respirations speed up this process, and when diarrhea is present, additional fluid is lost in the stools. Immaturity of the kidneys impairs the infant's ability to conserve water. The average urine output in infants and children is seen in Table 27–2. Preterm and newborn infants are also more susceptible to dehydration from variations in room temperature and humidity. When this is

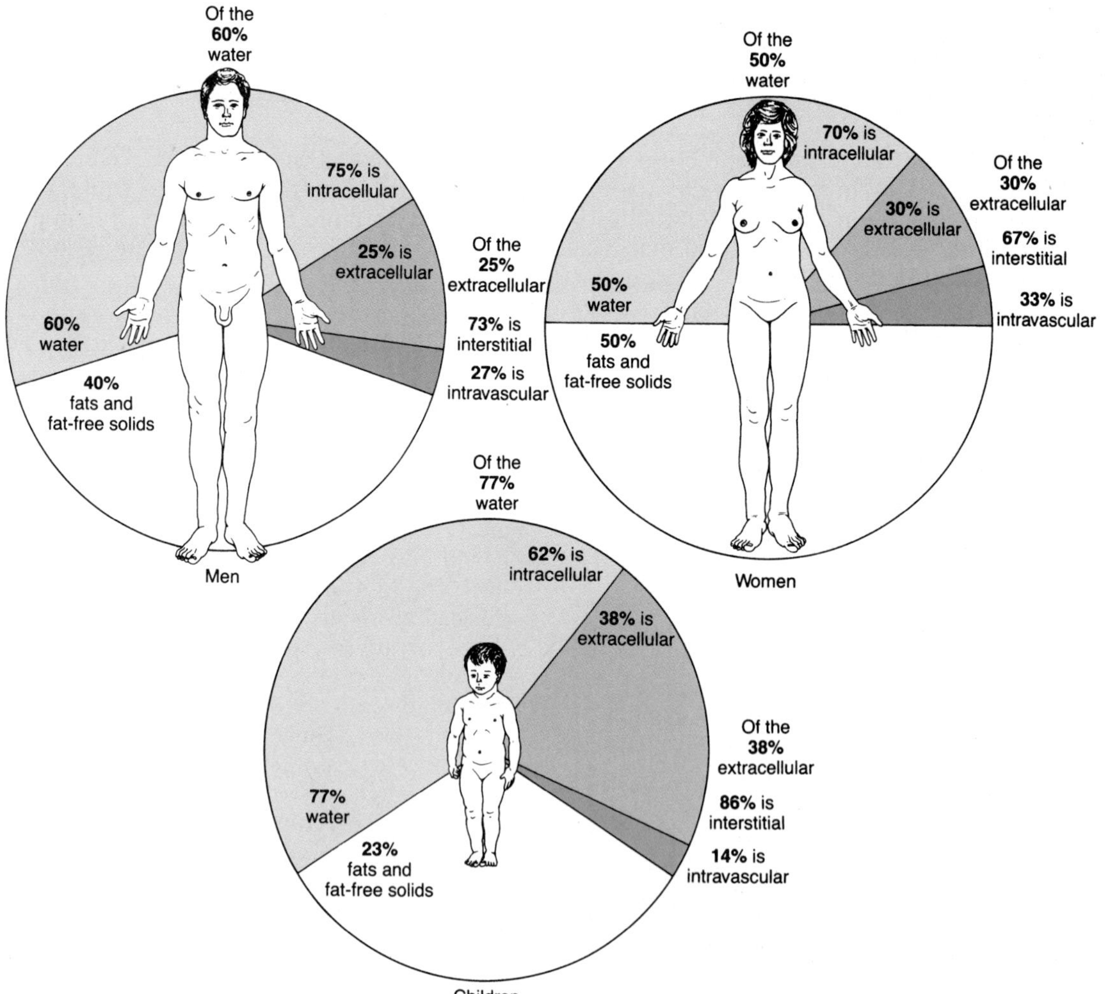

Figure 27–8. • Relationship of body water and body solids to the body weight of the adult man and woman and the child.

Table 27–1
SIGNS OF ISOTONIC, HYPERTONIC, AND HYPOTONIC DEHYDRATION

Area of Assessment	Signs of Dehydration: Isotonic	Hypertonic	Hypotonic
Weight loss	Mild dehydration—up to 5% weight loss Moderate dehydration—5% to 10% weight loss Severe dehydration—over 10% weight loss		
Behavior	Irritable and lethargic	Irritable when disturbed; lethargic	Lethargic to delirious; coma
Skin turgor	Dead elasticity	Good turgor; "foam rubber" feel	Very poor turgor; clammy
Mucous membranes	Dry	Parched	Clammy
Eyeballs and fontanel	Sunken and soft	Sunken	Sunken and soft
Tearing and salivation	Absent or decreased	Absent or decreased	Absent or decreased
Thirst	Present	Marked	Present
Urine	Decreased output; serum globulin (SG) elevated	Normal to decreased output; SG elevated or decreased	Decreased output; SG elevated
Body temperature	Subnormal to elevated	Elevated	Subnormal
Respiration	Rapid	Rapid	Rapid
Blood pressure	Normal to low	Normal to low	Very low
Pulse	Rapid	Rapid	Rapid
Blood chemistry	Blood urea nitrogen (BUN) increased	BUN increased	BUN increased
	Na decreased	Na increased	Na decreased
	K normal or increased	K decreased	K varies or increased
	Cl decreased	Cl low during correction	Cl decreased
	pH usually decreased	Ca decreased	

Courtesy of P. Chinn.

coupled with higher fluid losses, life-threatening deficits can ensue within a few hours.

Problems of fluid and electrolyte disturbance require evaluation of the type and severity of dehydration, clinical observation of the patient, and chemical analysis of the blood. The types of dehydration are classified according to the level of serum sodium, which depends on the relative losses of water and electrolytes. These types are usually termed *isotonic* (the patient has lost equal amounts of fluids and electrolytes), *hypotonic* (the child has lost more electrolytes than fluid), and *hypertonic* (more fluids are lost than electrolytes; Table 27–3).

These classifications are important because each form of dehydration is associated with different relative losses from intracellular fluid (ICF) and extracellular fluid (ECF) compartments, and each requires certain modifications in treatment. *Maintenance* fluid therapy replaces normal water and electrolyte losses, and *deficit* therapy restores preexisting body fluid and electrolyte deficiencies. The

BOX 27–1

ASSESSMENT OF THE DEHYDRATED CHILD

History
Weight change, history of illness contacts, stool and vomiting frequency

Clinical Examination
Daily weight, skin turgor, mucous membrane moisture, fontanel fullness, and mental state

Laboratory Studies
Complete blood count, electrolytes, blood urea nitrogen, creatinine, osmolarity, glucose, calcium

Urinalysis
Specific gravity, pH, glucose, ketones, amino acids, other appropriate cultures

Table 27–2
AVERAGE DAILY EXCRETION OF URINE

Age	Fluid Ounces	Milliliters
1st and 2nd days	1–2	30–60
3rd to 10th days	3–10	100–300
10th day to 2 mo	9–15	250–450
2 mo to 1 yr	14–17	400–500
1–3 yr	17–20	500–600
3–5 yr	20–24	600–700
5–8 yr	22–34	650–1000
8–14 yr	27–47	800–1400

Table 27–3
ESTIMATION OF DEHYDRATION

Clinical Sign	Degree: Mild	Moderate	Severe
Weight loss (%)	5	10	15
Behavior	Normal	Irritable	Hyperirritable to lethargic
Thirst	Slight	Moderate	Intense
Mucous membrane	May be normal	Dry	Parched
Tears	Present	+/−	Absent
Anterior fontanel	Flat	+/−	Sunken
Skin turgor	Normal	+/−	Increased

From Graef, J., & Cone, T. (1988). *Manual of pediatric therapeutics* (4th ed.). Boston: Little, Brown. With permission.

composition of intravenous fluids and the amount and rate of flow are important in preventing complications.

Shock (hypovolemia) is the greatest threat to life in isotonic dehydration. The electrolyte content of oral fluids is particularly significant in the care of infants and small children suffering from disorders of fluid balance and receiving infusions. Commercially prepared electrolyte solutions are available and are called oral rehydrating solutions. Children with hypotonic dehydration, that is, excess water with sodium electrolyte depletion, are at risk for water intoxication. This can also occur if tap water enemas are given to small children. Potassium is lost in almost all states of dehydration. *Replacement potassium is administered only after normal urinary excretion is established.*

Overhydration

Description. Overhydration results when the body receives more fluid than it can excrete. This can occur in patients with normal kidneys who receive intravenous fluids too rapidly. It also can occur in a patient receiving acceptable rates of fluid, especially when the patient's illness is related to disorders of fluid mechanism.

Manifestations. Edema is the presence of excess fluid in the interstitial (*interstitium,* "a thing standing between") spaces. Interstitial fluid is similar to plasma, but it contains little protein. In healthy persons, it responds well to shifts in fluid balance. *Any factor causing sodium retention can cause edema.* The flow of blood out of the interstitial compartments also depends on adequate circulation of blood and lymph. Low protein levels can also disturb osmotic cellular pressure, causing edema. This is seen in patients with nephrosis, in which large amounts of albumin are lost.

Trauma to or infections of the head can cause cerebral edema, which can be life-threatening. Constrictive dressing may obstruct venous return, causing swelling, particularly in dependent areas. *Anasarca* (*ana,* "throughout," and *sarx,* "flesh") is a severe generalized edema. Early detection and management of edema are essential. Taking accurate daily weights is indispensable, as is close attention to body weight changes. Vital signs, physical appearance, and changes in urine character or output are noted. Edema in infants may first be seen about the eyes and in the presacral, occipital, or genital areas. In pitting edema, after exerting gentle pressure with the finger, the nurse notices an impression in the skin that lasts for several seconds.

Infants receiving IV therapy have an IV and oral intake recorded. If the oral intake falls below prescribed rates, then the IV rate is increased. If the oral intake exceeds prescribed levels, the IV rate is decreased or the IV is hep-locked to maintain patency and avoid overhydration.

Electrolyte Imbalance. The nurse must be able to assess the electrolyte needs of the child (Table 27–4). When fluid snacks or nourishment are ordered, the selection of fluid can influence the treatment given for dehydration. For example, if the child has a hypertonic type of dehydration (which means there is excess sodium) and the nurse offers the child tomato juice, the high sodium content of tomato juice will negatively impact the child's prescribed treatment. If the child has hypotonic dehydration (which means the child has deficient electrolytes) and the nurse offers plain water, she will also impact the child's care negatively. It is a nursing responsibility therefore to correlate laboratory findings of the individual child with fluids and foods offered to the child.

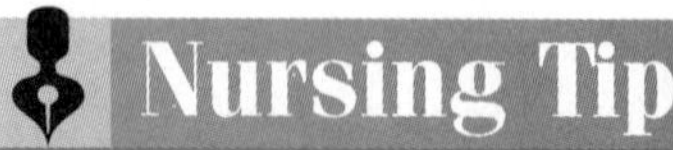

The nurse must document at least one void has occurred before IV potassium is administered.

NUTRITIONAL DEFICIENCIES

Because infancy is a period of rapid growth, poor nutrition is particularly dangerous at this time. Severe vitamin deficiencies are rare in prosperous countries; those that do occur are caused by poverty, ignorance, or neglect. Figure 27–9 shows a

Table 27–4
INTERPRETING ABG VALUES

	Acid	Normal	Alkaline
pH	<7.35	7.35–7.45	>7.45
(Respiratory parameter) $PACO_2$	>45	35–45	<35
(Metabolic parameter) HCO_3	<22	22–26	>26

- Where the patient's pH falls will indicate acidosis or alkalosis
- If the pH falls in the same line as the HCO_3, the problem is *metabolic.*
- If the pH falls in the same box as $PACO_2$, the problem is *respiratory.*

Interpreting a sample patient's lab values

pH $PACO_2$ HCO_3	pH HCO_3	$PACO_2$	

Interpretation:
- The column the pH is in tells you *acidosis* is the problem.
- The HCO_3 (the metabolic parameter) is in the same line as the Ph, therefore, the problem is *metabolic acidosis.*

Interpreting a sample patient's lab values

pH $PACO_2$ HCO_3		HCO_3	Ph $PACO_2$

Interpretation: Place the patient's lab values in the appropriate columns.
- The column the pH is in tells you *alkalosis* is the problem.
- The $PACO_2$ (the respiratory parameter) is in the same line as the pH, therefore, the problem is *respiratory alkalosis.*

Adapted from Mays, D. (1995). Turn ABG's into child's play. *RN, 58*(1), 37–38. Reprinted with permission copyright 1995 Medical Economics.

child, from the United States, with general, moderate malnutrition. Severe malnutrition is still rampant in many underdeveloped countries. Every person must be concerned with the plight of the starving child. Sometimes the baby's body is unable to utilize food even though the diet is adequate. An example of this is celiac disease, in which the intestines are unable to handle fats and starches. Severe malnutrition may also be seen in failure to thrive.

Failure to Thrive

Description. Failure to thrive (FTT) describes infants and children who, without an obvious cause, fail to gain and often lose weight. Although this condition can be caused by organic abnormalities, this discussion is limited to environmental etiologies. Infants who fail to thrive are frequently admitted to the hospital for evaluation with presenting symptoms of weight loss or failure to gain, irritability, and disturbances of food intake, such as anorexia or pica (abnormal consumption of nonfood materials). Vomiting, diarrhea, and general neuromuscular spasticity sometimes accompany the condition. The child has a complete work-up to identify organic reasons for failure to thrive and the cause is treated. FTT can be caused by environmental stresses. Children fall below the 3rd percentile (some authorities suggest the 5th) in weight and height on standard growth charts. Their development is delayed. Children who fail to thrive seem apathetic. Some have a "ragdoll limpness" (hypotonia), and often they appear wary of their caretakers. Others appear stiff and unresponsive to cuddling. The personality of the baby may not foster maternal attachment. Failure to thrive with malabsorption has been reported with frequency among autistic children and among institutionalized retarded children.

Manifestations. There can be a disturbance in the mother–child or caretaker–child relationship. The situation is complex and often associated with marital discord, economic pressures, parental immaturity, low stress tolerance, and single parenthood. Alcohol and drug abuse can be present. Many

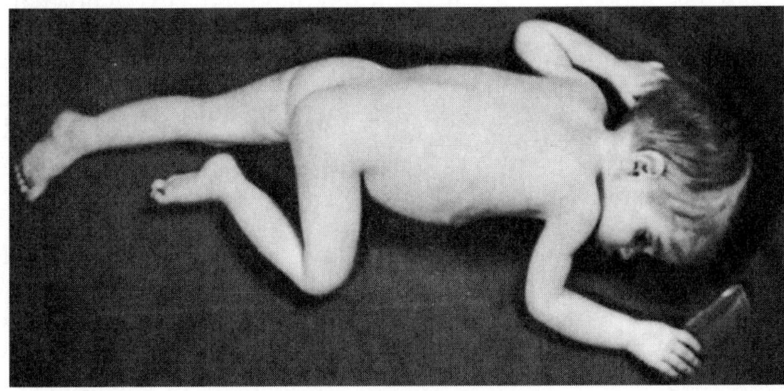

Figure 27–9. • This child has general malnutrition of moderate degree, frequently seen in the United States. (Courtesy of University of Rochester, Rochester, NY.)

mothers feel deprived and unloved and have conflicting needs. Infants suffer from the inability to establish a sense of trust in their caretakers. Their coping abilities are affected by a lack of nurturing. Outward neglect and physical abuse are not uncommon.

Prevention of environmental failure to thrive consists chiefly of social measures, such as parenting classes, family planning, and early recognition and support of families at risk. All children should receive routine health assessments. The pregnancy history may detect circumstances that may contribute to lack of bonding, such as an unplanned pregnancy or desertion by the child's father. Planning interventions that will enhance parent–infant interaction is an important nursing responsibility.

Treatment and Nursing Care. Treatment involves a multidisciplinary approach in accordance with the circumstance; that is, physician, nurse, social worker, family agency, and counselor may all participate. If no progress can be made, temporary or permanent placement of the child or children in a foster home may be required. During hospitalization one nurse per shift is selected to increase nurturing and interaction with the infant and parent.

Treatment of the child who fails to thrive requires maturity on the part of the nurse. It is vital to support rather than reject the mother. Maternal attachment can be facilitated by listening and helping the mother to understand her feelings and frustrations and to explore her choices. The nurse encourages her to assist with the daily care of her child. The child's uniqueness and responses to mother are stressed. The nurse points out developmental patterns and provides anticipatory guidance in this area. Frequently the mother's "lack of interest" stems from her own insecurities. Parents Anonymous and parent aides are other resources.

The prognosis of this condition is uncertain. Emotional starvation, particularly in the early years, can be psychologically traumatic. Inadequacies in intelligence, language, and social behavior have been documented in children who fail to thrive.

Kwashiorkor

Description. Kwashiorkor is a protein deficiency. In many parts of the world, children still starve to death. There are no well-planned maternal and child health programs to elevate health standards in these localities. In some areas, superstition and ignorance prevent children from utilizing nutritious foods found in their environment. In kwashiorkor, there is a severe deficiency of protein in the diet in spite of the fact that the number of calories consumed may be nearly adequate. It belongs to a class of disorders termed protein-energy malnutrition.

Manifestations. Kwashiorkor occurs in children 1 to 4 years of age who have been weaned from the breast. Kwashiorkor means, in native dialect, "the disease of the deposed baby when the next one is born," indicating that the child no longer breastfeeds because a sibling is born and takes over the breast of the mother. Oral intake then is deficient in protein. The child fails to grow normally. Muscles become weak and wasted. There is edema of the abdomen that may become generalized. Diarrhea, skin infections, irritability, anorexia, and vomiting may be present. The hair becomes thin and dry. Because protein is the basis of melanin, a substance that provides color to hair, melanin becomes deficient. This is the reason the earliest sign of this protein malnutrition is a white streak in the hair of the child (depigmentation). The child looks apathetic and weak.

Treatment and Nursing Care. Treatment for kwashiorkor is mainly preventive. Although hunger may never be completely erased in the world, many private, public, and world health agencies sponsor programs in an effort to alleviate such suffering. Simple protein powder sprinkled on the culturally prepared meal will alleviate the problem. Early dietary treatment in established cases may prevent more serious growth retardation.

Rickets

Description. Rickets is a disease of infancy and childhood caused by deficient amounts of vitamin D. Vitamin D and exposure to sunshine are necessary for the proper absorption and metabolism of calcium and phosphorus, which are needed for normal growth of bones.

Manifestations. The classic symptoms of rickets are bowlegs; knock-knees; beading of the ribs, called the *rachitic rosary;* and improper formation of the teeth.

Treatment and Nursing Care. The widespread use of vitamin supplements and fortification of foods have largely eliminated the problem of rickets in North America. The nurse should guide parents concerning the need for an optimum, well-balanced diet, exercise, and exposure to outdoor sunlight.

Scurvy

Scurvy is a disease caused by insufficient fruits and vegetables that contain vitamin C in the diet. The symptoms of scurvy include joint pains, bleeding gums, loose teeth, and lack of energy. Good sources of vitamin C are citrus fruits and raw, leafy vegetables. Vitamin C is easily destroyed by heat and exposure to air. Small amounts of water should be used for cooking vegetables to prevent vitamin C from being destroyed, since it is also water-soluble. It may be given to infants in the form of orange juice, which should not be boiled. Vitamin supplements prescribed for infants and children contain vitamin C. The vitamin is not stored in the body and requires a daily intake from food sources.

INFECTIONS

Thrush (Oral Candidiasis)

Description. Thrush is an infection of the mucous membranes of the mouth caused by the fungus *Candida.* This organism is normally present in the mother's vagina and is nonpathogenic. However, the altered conditions in the vagina produced by pregnancy may lead to the development of monilial vaginitis. The mucous membranes of the baby's mouth may become infected by direct contact with this infection during delivery or by contact with the mother's or nurse's contaminated hands. Cross-infection of other newborns may result.

Manifestations. White patches that resemble milk curds appear on the tongue, inner lips, gums, and oral mucosa. They are painless but cannot be wiped away. Anorexia may be present. The systemic symptoms are mild if the infection remains in the mouth; however, it can pass along the mucous membranes into the gastrointestinal tract, causing inflammation of the esophagus and stomach. Pneumonitis may also develop. *Epstein's pearls,* which are small, white, epithelial cysts that appear along both sides of the midline of the hard palate, are sometimes mistaken for thrush. These are harmless and gradually disappear.

Nursing Tip

In the home, parents are taught to drop nystatin or other medication slowly into the side of the baby's mouth. Medication needs to remain in contact with "patches" as long as possible. Instruct parents to watch for dehydration (e.g., decrease in number of wet diapers due to the baby's refusal to take fluids because of mouth discomfort.

Treatment and Nursing Care. This infection responds well to the local application of an antibiotic suspension, such as nystatin (Mycostatin). The mouth is swabbed three or four times a day between feedings with a sterile applicator moistened with the prescribed solution. With proper care, the condition disappears within a few days following its onset.

Newborns suspected of having thrush are cared for using isolation (standard) precautions. Individual feeding equipment is necessary, and the equipment should be sterile. Disposable bottles or prefilled formula bottles are used. Disposable nipples, pacifiers, and bottles, are preferred.

Candida infection of the diaper area presents as a bright red, sharply demarcated diaper rash. Nystatin cream is often prescribed.

Worms

Enterobiasis (Pinworms)

Description. Of the several varieties of worms that affect humans, the most common is the pinworm, *Enterobius vermicularis* (*enteron,* "intestine," *bios,* "life," and *vermis,* "wormlike"). It is seen more often in toddlers but can develop in older children and adults. The pinworm looks like a white thread about ⅓ inch. It lives in the lower intestine, but comes out of the anus to lay its eggs, generally during the night. These eggs become infective a few hours after they have been deposited. This type of parasite spreads from one person to another, particularly where there are large groups of children in close contact with one another. The child becomes infected by ingesting the eggs. The route of entry is the mouth. Reinfection takes place by way of the rectum to the fingers to the mouth or by way of the rectum to the clothing to the fingers to the mouth.

Manifestations. The nurse or parent may notice that the child scratches the anal area and may complain of itching. There may be associated irritability and restlessness. Weight loss, poor appetite, and fretfulness during the night may develop. The rectal area may become irritated from scratching. A special pinworm diagnostic tape or paddle or a tongue blade covered with cellophane tape, sticky side out, may be placed against the anal region to obtain pinworm eggs (the scotch tape test). This is done early in the morning, before the child has a bowel movement, bathes, or scratches the anal area with the fingers. The tape is put on a glass slide and examined under a microscope. The eggs are typical of pinworms.

Treatment and Nursing Care. Several effective *anthelmintics* (*anti,* "against," and *helminth,* "worms") are available. Mebendazole (Vermox) is a single-dose, chewable tablet and is the drug of choice for children over age 2. Pyrantel pamoate (Antiminth) also controls the infestation. Pyrvinium pamoate (Povan) suspension, a one-dose treatment, is an alternative drug; nurses advise parents that Povan stains and turns the stools red.

The child must be taught to wash the hands well following bowel movements. The child's fingernails are kept short. A soothing ointment is applied to the rectal area. The patient should wear clean underwear that fits snugly to avoid scratching with the fingers.

All symptomatic members of the family should be treated for this condition to prevent reinfection. Pregnant women should not take Vermox and should consult a physician before taking any alternative drug. In the home, the toilet seat is scrubbed daily. Cloth diapers and bed linens are washed in hot water.

Ascariasis (Roundworms)

Ascaris lumbricoides is a roundworm infestation that can be asymptomatic or can cause abdominal pain. The infestation is estimated to affect 1 billion persons worldwide. It thrives in warm climates and among the impoverished. In the United States, it is seen more often in the southern states and among immigrants and migratory workers living below poverty levels. It is caused by the unsanitary disposal of human feces and poor hygiene practices. An egg from an infected person can survive for weeks in the soil. The child ingests eggs from contaminated soil. The eggs develop into larvae in the intestine, penetrate the intestinal wall, and enter the liver, from which they circulate to the lungs and heart. The patient is generally without symptoms until the larvae reach the glottis, are coughed up, swallowed, and enter the small intestine. There they develop into adult male and female species. They survive on undigested food in the canal and produce eggs that are expelled in the child's feces. A chronic cough without fever is characteristic of this condition. Diagnosis is made by confirmation of the eggs in the patient's stool. The treatment of ascariasis is the same as that for enterobiasis (pinworms). Nursing considerations are outlined in Nursing Care Plan 27–2.

POISONING

Goals in the treatment of poisoning are to

- Remove the poison
- Prevent further absorption
- Administer antidote/call Poison Control Center
- Provide supportive care—seek medical help

Volume of a Swallow. The volume of a swallow has been estimated to be 0.21 ml per kg. Thus a child 2 to 3 years of age who takes one swallow may have ingested about 3 ml of poison.

Principles of Care. Education of parents and children is the best way to prevent poisoning. The school and the clinic are the best resources that should be used in an active accident prevention program. Table 27–5 lists common poisonous plants.

Poison Control Centers. The telephone number of the poison control center is listed in the telephone directory and should be posted near the phone.

Ipecac Syrup. Ipecac can be kept in the home out of reach of children. Doses up to 15 ml may be given to children over 1 year of age with 200 ml of water to induce vomiting. Ipecac should *not* be used with corrosive, alkali, gasoline, and cleaning fluid ingestion or if child is not fully conscious. Table 27–6 indicates how to assess the type of toxic substance ingested according to the smell of the vomitus.

Activated Charcoal. Activated charcoal will absorb poisons such as strychnine, atropine, Malathion, and arsenic compounds. However, activated charcoal if given together with ipecac, will neutralize each other, rendering both ineffective in the treatment of poisoning.

Tannic Acid. Tannic acid precipitates alkaloid and metallic poisons preventing absorption into the body. *Gastric lavage* and *dialysis* are used in the hospital setting to clear poisons from the stomach and the blood.

Drugs

Acetaminophen Poisoning

Acetaminophen overdose is listed along with other poisons commonly encountered in pediatrics in Box 27–2.

NURSING CARE PLAN 27–2

Selected Nursing Diagnoses for the Preschool Child with Ascariasis (Roundworm Infestation)

Nursing Diagnosis: High risk for altered nutrition—less than body requirements related to anorexia, nausea, deprivation of host nutrients by parasites

Goals	Nursing Interventions	Rationale
Child maintains adequate growth and development parameters for age as evidenced by weight and growth charts	1. Administer appropriate antiparasitic medication as prescribed: mebendazole (Vermox) single-dose, chewable tablet; pyrantel pamoate (Antiminth)	1. Several drugs are effective against ascariasis; none is useful during the pulmonary phase of the infection
	2. Offer light diet until digestive symptoms subside	2. Child may experience anorexia, stomach pain
	3. Observe child for nausea, diarrhea, regurgitation, or passage of adult worms in stool	3. Larvae rise to the oropharynx and are swallowed; obstruction of the intestine by adult worms can occur
	4. Observe for signs of associated anemia	4. Children with few resources may have poor eating habits; anorexia may accompany disorder
	5. Monitor child's growth with growth grid	5. To ascertain growth and development parameters for comparison
	6. Assess child's behavior—is it age appropriate?	6. Child may come from dysfunctional family; pica may be present

Nursing Diagnosis: Knowledge deficit (parents) regarding mode of transmission

Goals	Nursing Interventions	Rationale
Parents verbalize knowledge of transmission of roundworm	1. Draw picture for parents showing the roundworm life cycle	1. Visual aids to promote understanding; disease is caused by soil contaminated by human feces or subsequently by eating raw fruits and vegetables contaminated by flies
	2. Point out that these worms have high egg outputs	2. Eggs also remain infective in soil for weeks
	3. Explain roundworms only live in human hosts	3. Dispelling misinformation is of importance in education
	4. Emphasize strict handwashing practices; preschool child is taught to wash hands before meals and is supervised	4. Handwashing removes eggs and other organisms
	5. Emphasize washing of all raw fruits and vegetables before eating	5. These foods may be contaminated by flies and infested soil
	6. Stress necessity of laundering towels, sheets, underwear, and night clothing	6. Eggs may be found on articles contaminated by soil; disease is perpetuated by poor sanitary facilities and poor hygiene practices
	7. Advise of necessity of treating all family members	7. This will prevent transmission and reinfection
	8. Suggest services of public health nurse if this appears warranted	8. Proper referrals will ensure follow-through

(continued on following page)

Description. Acetaminophen (Tylenol) has now replaced aspirin as the most commonly ingested drug that causes toxicity. This is because it is so widely used and because aspirin associated with Reye's syndrome is no longer recommended for fever in children with flulike symptoms. Acetaminophen poisoning occurs most often from acute overdose rather than from the cumulative effects seen with aspirin. Because acetaminophen is metabolized in the liver, overdose results in hepatic destruction. With early treatment most children recover without complications. Tylenol drops and Tylenol Elixer each have a different potency. When "1 teaspoon of Tylenol" is advised, the nurse must be sure the parent understands which preparation to purchase or a massive overdose can occur.

Manifestations. Manifestations and treatment modalities that the nurse might anticipate in patients with acute poisoning are shown in Box 27–3.

Treatment and Nursing Care. The stomach is emptied by lavage or induced emesis from syrup of ipecac. Depending on the serum acetaminophen

NURSING CARE PLAN 27–2 *continued*

Selected Nursing Diagnoses for the Preschool Child with Ascariasis (Roundworm Infestation)

Nursing Diagnosis: Knowledge deficit (parents) regarding growth and development parameters of preschooler that predispose child to infestation from parasites

Goals	Nursing Interventions	Rationale
Parents verbalize knowledge of growth and development of preschool child Parents verbalize necessity for hygienic practices to prevent parasitic infection from various sources	1. Review growth and development of preschooler	1. Many parents have little knowledge of growth and development
	2. Emphasize need for all members of family to use frequent and thorough handwashing	2. Handwashing is most effective method of preventing disease transmission; remind small child
	3. Stress need for child to wear shoes when outdoors	3. Going barefoot is discouraged because of danger of hookworm, which penetrates bare feet
	4. Explain necessity for keeping dogs and cats away from sandboxes	4. Sandboxes contaminated by dog or cat feces may lead to *Toxocara canis* or *Toxocara cati*
	5. Advise periodic cleansing of toys to avoid pinworms and other parasites	5. Children often play with community toys; they are chewed on, dropped on ground, and so on
	6. Remind parents to teach preschool child not to put dirt and other contaminated objects into mouth	6. Prevention of parasitic and other diseases may be accomplished by these simple measures
	7. Suggest that child's fingernails be trimmed frequently	7. This prevents larvae from accumulating under nails
	8. Suggest parents wash hands well before and after handling raw meats	8. Raw meats often contain disease organisms, which can cause food poisoning and other conditions
	9. Emphasize need to cook beef and pork adequately	9. This prevents tapeworm infestation

level, this may be followed by the N-acetylcysteine (Mucomyst) antidote. In small children, it may be administered directly into the nasogastric tube following lavage. Otherwise it is generally given orally every 4 hours for 72 hours. This medicine has a bad smell and taste and the patient needs coaxing and support to assist with compliance. The medicine may be mixed with a soft drink or juice. Liver enzymes (SGOT and SGPT) are monitored. Prevention of overdose is of utmost importance. Even in uncomplicated cases, the child is subject to unpleasant, stressful procedures. Because parents are often

Table 27–5
COMMON HOUSEHOLD PLANTS THAT ARE POISONOUS

Plant	Action
Azalia Buttercup Marigold	Cause symptoms of aconitine poisoning
Lantana Jimsonweed	Cause symptoms of atropine poisoning
Sweetpea Black mountain laurel	Cause symptoms of curare poisoning
Apricot pits Peach pits Elderberry	Cause symptoms of cyanide poisoning
Camellia seeds Foxglove Oleander	Cause symptoms similar to digitalis poisoning
Goldenrod Nightshades Poinsettia	Cause symptoms of nitrate poisoning
Laurel Maryvana Water hemlock	Cause symptoms of resin poisoning
Camellia Marigold Tulips Violets	Cause symptoms of salicylates poisoning

Note: These plants should not be used to landscape the backyard of homes with young children.

Table 27–6
ASSESSING FOR POISONING BY SPECIFIC ODOR OF VOMITUS

Odor of Vomitus	Probable Content
Sweet	Chloroform, acetone
Bitter almond	Cyanide
Pear	Chloral hydrate
Garlic	Phosphorous, arsenic
Shoepolish	Nitrobenzene
Violet	Turpentine

Note: The nurse should report and document the specific odor of vomitus, which can be helpful in determining the specific poison contained in the substance ingested.

informed that acetaminophen is "safer" than aspirin, they may be more careless in storing it.

Salicylate Poisoning

Description. Aspirin (acetylsalicylic acid) poisoning is seen less frequently than in the past because of safety packaging and the increase in use of acetaminophen. Nevertheless, aspirin is often used in most homes and may be stored carelessly on bedside stands or in a mother's purse. Oil of wintergreen (methyl salicylate) is also extremely hazardous when mistakenly administered as cough medicine or swallowed by the curious child. It is

BOX 27–2

POISONS COMMONLY ENCOUNTERED IN PEDIATRICS

Acids
Toilet bowl cleaners
Swimming pool pH adjustment solutions
Concentrated acids in hardware and paint stores

Alkalines
Clinitest tablets
Drain-cleaning crystals
Dishwasher soaps
Industrial cleaners (brought home in unlabeled containers)

Medications
Diet pills
Sleeping pills
Sedatives
Cold remedies
Birth control pills
Vitamin supplements, iron
Diarrhea remedies (Lomotil)
Menstrual pain relievers
Antipyretics (aspirin, acetaminophen)
Oil of wintergreen

Cyanide
Pesticides
Metal polishes
Photographic solutions
Fumigating products

Ethanol
Alcoholic beverages
Cold remedies
Perfumes
Mouthwashes
Aftershave lotions

Petroleum Distillates
Heavy greases, oils
Turpentine
Furniture polishes
Gasoline, kerosene
Lighter fluid

Insecticides
Home gardening products
Recently sprayed lawns

Carbon Monoxide
Accidental
Suicidal

Lead
Paint
Air
Food
Ant poison
Unglazed pottery
Colored newsprint
Curtain weights
Fishing sinkers
Lead water pipes
Acid juices in leaded pottery

Athropods, Insect Stings
Spiders (brown recluse, black widow)
Certain scorpions
Insects (bees, wasps, hornets)

Snakes
Rattlesnakes
Moccasins
Copperheads
Others

Poisonous Plants
Boston ivy
Split-leaf philodendron
Umbrella plant
Azalea
Daffodil
Foxglove
Mistletoe
Tulip
Others

sometimes used as a home remedy for arthritic pain. Even a dose as small as 1 teaspoon can cause a child's death.

Manifestations. This drug acts rapidly but is excreted slowly. Ingestion of 150 mg/kg causes symptoms. Although most cases of aspirin poisoning are emergencies, a child may unknowingly be poisoned by aspirin's cumulative effect. The use of several aspirin-containing products at once, for example, over-the-counter cold remedies and aspirin, can be hazardous. Time-release aspirin is especially dangerous, because the symptoms of poisoning are delayed and aspiration of the stomach is of little avail. It is wise, therefore, to read labels carefully and to administer aspirin sparingly. It is even better to use it only under a physician's direction.

Treatment and Nursing Care. Vitamin K is administered to control bleeding. Peritoneal dialysis (*peritoneum* and *dialysis,* "passing of a solute through a membrane") is a therapeutic measure used in acute renal failure. The therapy utilizes the principles of osmosis and diffusion through the semipermeable peritoneal membrane, with the purpose of removing toxic substances from the blood. Hemodialysis is another method used for essentially the same purpose.

The nurse must realize the danger of drug poisoning and must constantly practice and teach safety measures to prevent tragedies. Treatment, utility rooms, and drug baskets are scrutinized to ensure that nothing harmful is within reach of ambulatory children.

BOX 27-3

ANTICIPATED CARE FOR POISONING

Anticipate

Emptying. (Lavage, ipecac, activated charcoal)
Central nervous system. Restlessness, agitation, seizures, coma
Respiratory. Airway obstruction, hypoventilation, hypoxia, oxygen therapy, respiratory arrest, cardiopulmonary resuscitation (keep artificial airway handy), chemical pneumonitis
Cardiovascular. Difficulties with electrolytes, blood urea nitrogen, creatinine, glucose; need for electrocardiogram monitor
Gastrointestinal. Difficulty swallowing, abdominal pain, possible gastrostomy
Kidneys. Urine specific gravity, intake and output, intravenous tubes
Methods to increase elimination. Cathartic, forced diuresis, dialysis, hemoperfusion
Hypo- or hyperthermia. Sponge baths, cooling blanket
Child. Physical and psychological crises
Parents. Guilt, anger, family dysfunction

Lead Poisoning (Plumbism)

Description. Lead poisoning results when a child repeatedly ingests or absorbs substances containing lead. The primary source is paint from old, deteriorating buildings. The lead contents of food, water, and air have decreased substantially since 1990. Lead poisoning is most common in children between the ages of 1½ and 3 years. The incidence is increased in tenement areas of large cities. Although the incidence is highest among the poor, lead poisoning is also found among suburban and middle-class children.

The children chew on windowsills and stair rails. They ingest flakes of paint, putty, or crumbled plaster. Eating nonfood items is called *pica.* Food, particularly fruit juices consumed from improperly glazed earthenware, is another source. Lead poisoning among Mexican Americans may be due to azarcon, a bright-orange powder containing approximately 93.5% lead. Azarcon is used as a folk remedy to treat empacho and other digestive problems in infants. Lead poisoning among Hmong Laotian refugees may be due to Paylooah, a bright orange-red powder, which may be used for fever or rash. Unwashed fresh fruit sprayed with insecticides and dust from enclosed shooting galleries are also culprits. Another source is dust in homes near lead-processing plants. "Spitballs" made from the colored section of newspaper comics is also a source of lead poisoning.

Lead can have a lasting effect on the nervous system, especially the brain. The incidence is high among siblings of an affected child and recurrence is common. Mental retardation may occur in severe cases. In much of the United States, lead poisoning is a reportable disease. The Agency for Toxic Substances and Diseases Registry (ATSDR) provides information on this condition.

Manifestations. The symptoms occur gradually and range from mild to severe. Because the infant's or young child's central nervous system is extremely vulnerable, acute symptoms of encephalitis may follow a relatively short period of exposure. The lead settles in the soft tissues and bones and is excreted in the urine. In the beginning, weakness, weight loss, anorexia, pallor, irritability, vomiting, abdominal pain, and constipation may be seen. In the later stages, signs of anemia and nervous sys-

NURSING CARE PLAN 27–3

Selected Nursing Diagnoses for the Child with Lead Poisoning

Nursing Diagnosis: Pain related to multiple injections

Goals	Nursing Interventions	Rationale
Child experiences minimal pain as evidenced by vocalization, facial expression, and body language Child engages in play and sleeps well	1. Prepare child for injection through needle play; anticipate frustration and anger 2. Rotate sites of injection; when an intravenous route cannot be used chelation therapy is given intramuscularly into a large muscle mass. Move painful areas slowly and gently	1. Preparation reduces anxiety levels, helps patient to feel more in control 2. Rotation of sites prevents formation of painful fibrotic areas; EDTA is so painful that physician may order combining local anesthetic procaine with the drug; it is drawn into syringe last so that it enters child first

Nursing Diagnosis: Knowledge deficit (parents) related to the dangers of lead ingestion

Goals	Nursing Interventions	Rationale
Parents can list the environmental sources of lead Parents verbalize early symptoms of poisoning	1. Obtain a careful history concentrating on possible exposure to lead 2. Discuss common environmental sources of lead: peeling paint from dilapidated housing, and other areas such as day care, folk remedies, occupations of household adults 3. Assess child's nutritional status 4. Review early signs and symptoms of disease for detection 5. Enlist services of public health nurse and social services	1. A careful history will provide a course of direction 2. Information increases understanding and compliance 3. These children may be malnourished or may have a history of pica 4. Patients may experience behavior changes of irritability, hyperactivity, distractibility 5. Environment must be modified before child returns; child must have lead blood levels regularly monitored

tem involvement, such as muscular incoordination, neuritis, convulsions, and encephalitis, are seen.

Treatment and Nursing Care. Blood and urine tests are performed to determine the amount of lead in the system. Lead is especially toxic to *the synthesis of heme* in the blood; heme is necessary for hemoglobin formation and for functioning of renal tubules. Blood lead levels are the primary screening test. X-ray films of the bones show further deposits of lead. The history of the patient may reveal *pica.* This is a condition in which the child has a distorted appetite and eats a variety of things that most persons consider unpalatable, such as sand, grass, wool, glass, plaster, coal, animal droppings, and paint from furniture.

Treatment is aimed at reducing the concentration of lead in the tissues and blood. Chelating agents that render the lead nontoxic and increase its excretion in the urine are given in more severe cases. Calcium disodium edetate (CaEDTA) and dimercaprol are commonly used. CaEDTA may be given intravenously or as a deep intramuscular injection. Mild symptomatic lead poisoning may be treated with meso-2,3,-dimercaptosuccinic acid (DMSA). It can be given orally, has not been associated with serious side effects, and does not cause zinc depletion, as does CaEDTA. Complete deleading takes several months, and retreatment may be necessary when the child has an acute infection or other metabolic disturbance. The prognosis depends on the extent of poisoning. All children with elevated lead blood levels need to be followed to evaluate developmental and intellectual milestone achievement.

Prevention of this condition is foremost. Lead paint should not be used on children's toys or furniture. Instead, one should use paint marked for indoor use. Nursing Care Plan 27–3 presents a summary of interventions for the child experiencing lead poisoning. Nursing care is mainly symptomatic.

FOREIGN BODIES

About 80% of all foreign body ingestion occurs in children between 6 months and 3 years of age. About 80% of the foreign bodies ingested will pass through the GI tract, but others require surgical removal. The high curiosity of the young child and the tendency to place objects in the mouth increase the susceptibility to accidental ingestion of a non-food object. Unless the object is sharp or large, passage through the GI tract can take up to 4 to 6 days. The child is cared for at home and the nurse should emphasize the importance of cutting and examining each stool until the object is passed successfully. The nurse should caution parents not to use laxatives and to maintain a normal diet to avoid intestinal spasms that may precipitate an obstruction. Parents should be instructed to notify the doctor if abdominal pain or vomiting occurs. Follow-up care and teaching concerning safety in the environment and prevention of ingested or inhaled foreign bodies are priority nursing responsibilities.

KEY POINTS

- The newborn should be closely observed for signs of tracheoesophageal fistula, which includes coughing, choking, cyanosis, and apnea during feedings.
- Drooling in the newborn may be a sign of an obstructed esophagus (TEF).
- The first stool of the newborn should be documented to record patency of the anus.
- Pyloric stenosis is caused by a hypertrophy of the pyloric muscles and is manifested by projectile vomiting.
- Nursing care for the child with pyloric stenosis involves frequent assessment, careful feeding, positioning on the right side following feedings, and education and support of the parents.
- Large, bulky, frothy stools are characteristic of malabsorption syndromes.
- Celiac disease is caused by an intolerance to gluten in the diet.
- Tap water should not be used for enemas in children with megacolon, to avoid development of water intoxication.
- Intussusception is characterized by "currant jelly stools."
- Hirschsprung's disease occurs when there is an absence of ganglionic innervation of the muscle of a segment of the bowel.
- The treatment of gastroesophageal reflux includes thickened feedings, burping, and maintaining Fowler's position.
- In an infant, a diarrhea stool is manifested by a watery consistency and a greenish color that may contain mucus or blood. Frequency of bowel movements, by itself, is not an indication of diarrhea in infants.
- Teaching parents basic hygienic practices, handwashing, and animal handling can prevent outbreaks of diarrhea.
- The functions of the GI tract have a great influence on the fluid and electrolyte balance in infants and children.
- The higher daily exchange of water that occurs in infants leaves them less volume reserve when they are dehydrated.
- Oral rehydrating solutions are commercially prepared electrolyte solutions
- Isotonic dehydration is the loss of equal amounts of water and electrolytes. Hypertonic dehydration is the loss of more water than electrolytes. Hypotonic dehydration is the loss of more electrolytes than water.
- Infants who are fed by the intravenous route should be picked up and held and allowed to suck on a pacifier.
- Kwashiorkor is a protein deficiency characterized by a depigmented (white) streak of hair.
- Disposable nipples, pacifiers and bottles should be used for infants with thrush.
- Pinworm is diagnosed by a "scotch tape test." Preventing the child from scratching the anal area is an essential part of breaking the cycle of worm re-infestation.
- A chronic productive cough without fever is part of the roundworm life cycle in children.
- The nurse should teach parents not to store poisonous substances in food containers.
- Prevention of accidental poisoning should be part of every parent teaching plan.
- Pica, the eating of non-food items, is characteristic of children with lead poisoning.
- Lead poisoning (plumbism) can cause neurological damage.

MULTIPLE-CHOICE REVIEW QUESTIONS

Choose the most appropriate answer.

1. The pathology of pyloric stenosis is due to
   a. edema of the pyloric muscle.
   b. ischemia of the pyloric muscle.
   c. hypertrophy of the pyloric muscle.
   d. neoplastic obstruction.
2. Which of the following menu selections is best for a child diagnosed with celiac disease?
   a. Pizza and chocolate cake.
   b. Spaghetti and blueberry muffin.
   c. Chicken sandwich on whole-wheat bread.
   d. Corn tortilla and fresh fruit.
3. Following surgery for pyloric stenosis, the nurse could anticipate that the infant
   a. will have nasogastric suction for 24 hours.
   b. will be fed clear liquids within 6 hours.
   c. will remain NPO for 24 to 48 hours.
   d. will be fed formula within 4 hours.
4. Pinworms are diagnosed by
   a. seeing the worm in the stool.
   b. a blood antigen level.
   c. a "scotch-tape" test in early morning.
   d. a stool laboratory exam taken at hour of sleep.
5. Priority teaching for a parent of a child who ingested a foreign body includes
   a. encouraging the use of mild laxatives every night.
   b. slicing each stool passed to observe for the foreign body.
   c. encouraging a daily enema until the foreign body is passed.
   d. keeping the child NPO until the foreign body is passed.

BIBLIOGRAPHY AND READER REFERENCE

Ashwill, J., & Droske, S. (1997). *Nursing care of children.* Philadelphia: Saunders.

Behrman, R. E., Kleigman, R., & Arvin, A. (1996). *Nelson's textbook of pediatrics* (15th ed.). Philadelphia: Saunders.

Ellenhorn, M. J. (1997). *Ellenhorn's medical toxicology* (2nd ed.). Baltimore: Williams & Wilkins.

Erickson, T. B., Goldfrank, L. R., & Kulig, K. (1997). How to treat the poisoned patient. *Patient Care, 31*(13), 161–183.

Litovitz, T., Felberg, L., White, S., et al. (1996). 1995 Report on the American Association of Poison Control Center's toxic exposure surveillance system. *American Journal of Emergency Medicine,* 14(5), 487.

Lovejoy, F. H. (1992). Childhood poisonings: What role for ipecac and charcoal. *Contemporary Pediatrics, 9*(12), 99–108.

Mack, R. B. (1998). "Some-die-wholly in half a breath"—gun blueing poisoning. *Contemporary Pediatrics,* 15(2), 95.

Mack, R. B. (1996). Don Giovanni and hellfire: Turpentine poisoning. *Contemporary Pediatrics, 13*(7), 67–79.

Mahan, L. K., & Escott-Stump, M. (1996). *Krause's food, nutrition, & diet therapy* (9th ed.). Philadelphia: Saunders.

Mays, D. A. (1995). Turn ABGs into child's play. *RN, 58*(1), 36–39.

Rice, K. H. (1994). Oral rehydration therapy: A simple, effective solution. *Journal of Pediatric Nursing, 9*(6), 349–356.

Stifler, J., & Shanahan, N. (1994). The IV bubbles and boards system. *Journal of Pediatric Nursing,* 9(6), 417–419.

Wong, D. (1997). *Whaley's & Wong's essentials of pediatric nursing.* St. Louis, MO: Mosby.

Wood, R. A. (1997). Anaphylaxis in children. *Patient Care, 31*(13), 161–183.

chapter 28

The Child with a Genitourinary Condition

Outline

Objectives

On completion and mastery of Chapter 28, the student will be able to

- Define each vocabulary term listed.
- Differentiate between nephrosis and acute glomerulonephritis.
- Name the functional unit of the kidney.
- List four urologic diagnostic procedures.
- Discuss the skin care pertinent to the child with nephrosis.
- Explain any alterations in diet applicable to the child with nephrosis.
- Outline the nursing care for a child who is diagnosed as having Wilms' tumor.
- Discuss the impact of genitourinary surgery on the growth and development of children at various ages.
- Discuss the impact of undescended testes on fertility.

Vocabulary

ascites
chordee
cryptorchidism
cystitis
cystometrogram
dysuria
encopresis
enuresis
epispadias
frequency
glomeruli
gonad
hydrocele
hydronephrosis
hyperkalemia
hyperlipidemia
hypoalbuminemia
hypospadias
nephron
neutropenia
nocturia
oliguria
orchiopexy
phimosis
polyuria
pyelonephritis
urethritis
urgency
vesicoureteral reflux

DEVELOPMENT OF THE URINARY TRACT

The urinary system consists of two kidneys, two ureters, the urinary bladder, and the urethra. Figure 28-1 depicts these structures and how they differ in the developing child and in the adult. The function of the kidneys is to rid the body of waste products and to maintain body fluid homeostasis (Fig. 28–2). The kidneys also produce substances (e.g., erythropoietin-stimulating factor, ESF) that stimulate red blood cell formation in the bone marrow, and renin that regulates blood pressure. Microscopically, the functional unit of the kidneys is the nephron. Each kidney contains over 1 million nephrons. Although the newborn's kidneys are immature, they function quite effectively. Nevertheless, the functional limitations must be considered carefully when the newborn is premature or ill. This applies especially to the administration of medications, formula, and parenteral fluids.

Soon after implantation, the embryonic mass differentiates into three distinct layers of cells. These layers are called the *ectoderm, mesoderm,* and *endo-*

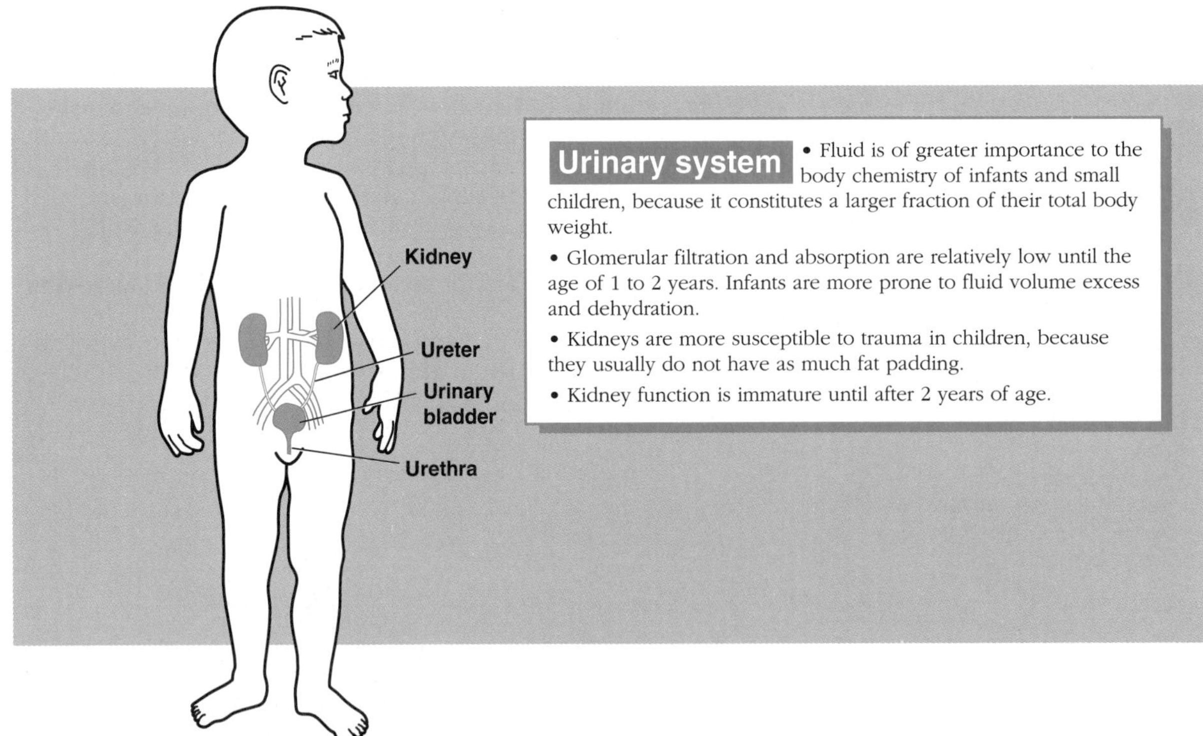

Figure 28-1. • Summary of some urinary system differences between the child and the adult. The urinary system is the main excretory system. The kidneys remove wastes and excess materials from the blood and produce urine. This system helps to regulate blood chemistry.

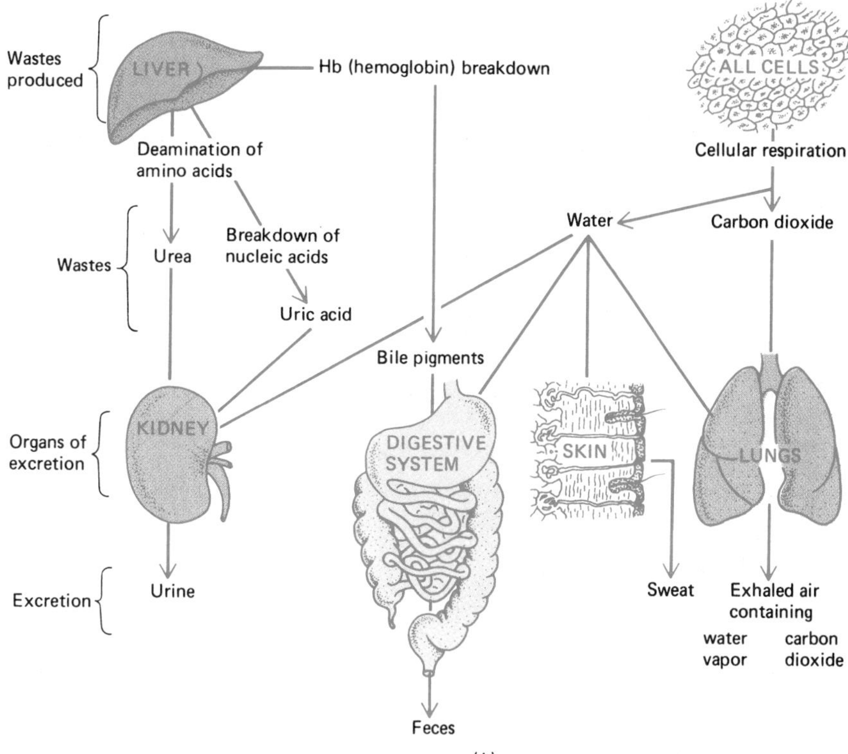

Figure 28-2. • The kidneys, lungs, skin, and digestive system participate in the disposal of metabolic wastes. Nitrogenous wastes are produced by the liver and transported to the kidneys. The kidneys excrete these wastes in the urine. All cells produce carbon dioxide and some water during cellular respiration. (From Solomon, E. P., & Phillips, G. A. [1987]. *Understanding human anatomy and physiology* [p. 310]. Philadelphia: Saunders.)

derm. The urinary and reproductive organs originate from the mesoderm. At about the 3rd month of gestation, the fetal kidney begins to secrete urine. The amount gradually increases as the fetus matures, and it contains an increased portion of amniotic fluid volume. An absence or small amount of amniotic fluid may indicate genitourinary difficulties.

The kidney and urinary tract develop about the same time as the ears form during fetal life. There is an unexplained relationship between low-set ears in the newborn and urinary tract anomalies. When assessing the newborn, an imaginary line should be drawn between the outer canthus of the eye and the occiput. The line should cross the tip of the earlobe. If the tip of the earlobe falls below this line, the assessment should be recorded and reported.

DEVELOPMENT OF THE REPRODUCTIVE SYSTEMS

Figure 28–3 shows the female and male reproductive systems and lists some of the differences between children and adults. The reproductive system provides for perpetuation of the species. Each sex is equipped with a gonad, which provides a reproductive cell, and a set of accessory organs. The gonads (ovaries in the female and testes in the male) produce sex cells and hormones that affect the reproductive organs and other body systems.

Sex is genetically determined at the time of fertilization. The presence of a Y chromosome is essential for the development of the testes and their hormones. Sex differentiation occurs early in the embryo. The organs specific to the male or female child develop. Before this, the embryo has neither male nor female characteristics. The development of the ovaries occurs later than that of the testes. By the 12th week, the external genitals of the fetus are recognizably male or female.

Several tests are helpful in diagnosing conditions of the reproductive tract. These include a Papanicolaou (Pap) smear, serologic blood tests, cultures, ultrasound procedures, pregnancy tests, and routine blood and urine tests. Sexual abuse in children may be manifested by such behaviors as urinary frequency, excessive masturbation, encopresis (fecal soiling beyond 4 years), severe nightmares, bedwetting, irritation or pain in the genital area, and a decrease in physical or emotional development. Suggestive posturing by young children or explicit knowledge of sex acts shown by children under 8

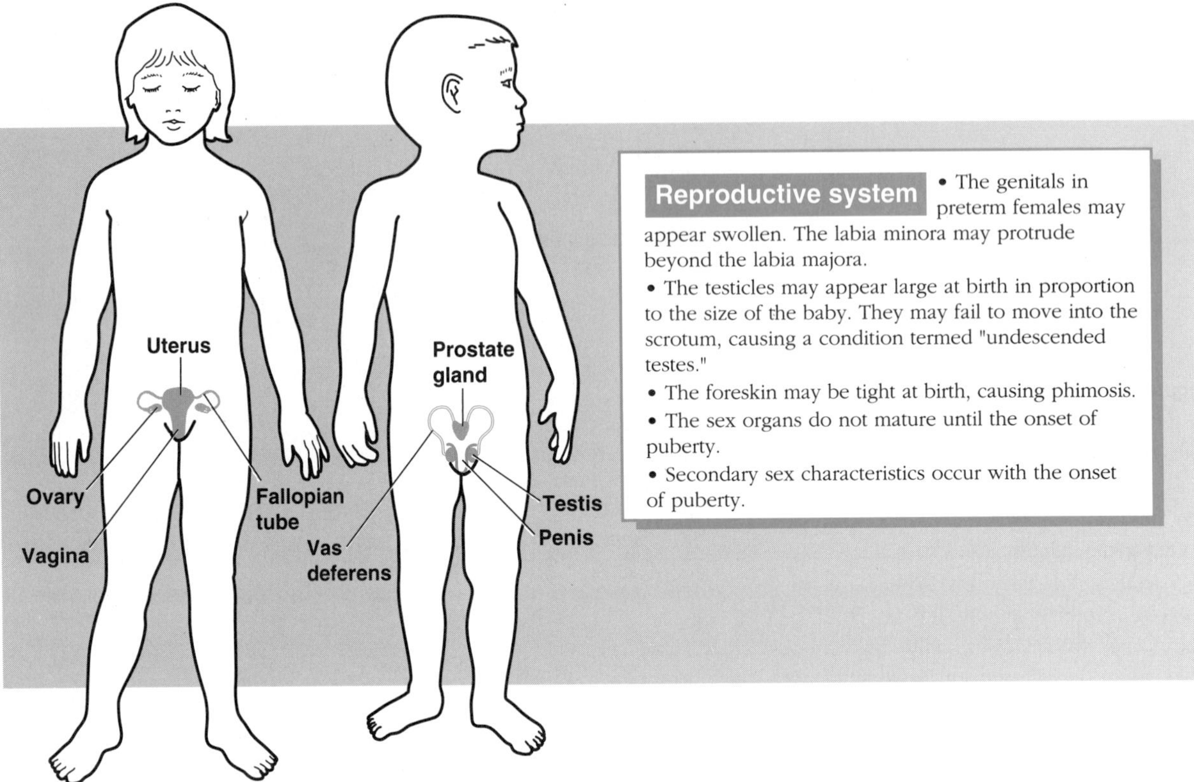

Figure 28-3. • Summary of some reproductive system differences between the child and the adult male and female. Each reproductive system consists of gonads and associated structures. The reproductive system maintains sexual characteristics and perpetuates the species.

years old needs further investigation. Menstrual disorders and premenstrual syndrome are discussed in Chapter 11. Sexually transmitted diseases are discussed in Chapter 11.

Assessment of Urinary Function

Urologic diagnostic procedures include urinalysis, ultrasonography, intravenous pyelogram, and computed tomographic (CT) scan of the kidneys. Renal biopsy is used to diagnose the extent of kidney disease. A uroflow is an assessment procedure used to determine the rate of urine flow. The child voids into a receptacle, and a uroflowmeter graphs the volume. This is useful in diagnosing stricture or scarring. Cytoscopy is useful for investigating congenital abnormalities or acquired lesions in the bladder and lower urinary tract or for catheterization. X-ray examination of the bladder and urethra before and during micturition is called voiding cystourethrography. The *cystometrogram* and urethral pressure profile assess bladder capacity and function. Both tests require catheterization and infusion of sterile water. Common lab tests are reviewed in Table 28–1.

Terms commonly used to describe urinary dysfunction include:

- *Dysuria.* Difficulty in urination
- *Frequency.* Abnormal number of voidings in a short period
- *Urgency.* Urge to void but inability to do so
- *Nocturia.* Awakening during the night to void
- *Enuresis.* Uncontrolled voiding after bladder control had been established
- *Polyuria.* Increased urinary output
- *Oliguria.* Decreased urinary output

Anomalies of the Urinary Tract

Phimosis

Description. *Phimosis* is a narrowing of the preputial opening of the foreskin, which prevents

Table 28–1
COMMON LAB TESTS FOR URINARY TRACT FUNCTION

Test	Normal Levels*	Significance of Deviation
Blood		
Blood urea nitrogen (BUN)	Newborn: 4–18 Child: 5–18	High BUN indicates renal disease, dehydration, steroid therapy
Uric acid	Child: 2–5	Renal disease
Creatinine	Infant: 0.2–0.4 Child: 0.3–0.7 Adolescent: 0.5–1.0	Severe renal disease
Urine		
Red blood cells	<2	Trauma, infection, stones
Bacteria	Few	Infection
Casts	Occasional	Glomerular disease, pyelonephritis
White blood cells	<2	Infection
Ketones	0	Stress; diabetes mellitus
Glucose	0	Diabetes mellitus
Protein	0	Glomerular kidney disease
pH	Newborn: 5–7 Child: 4.8–7.8	Potassium deficiency, electrolyte imbalance
Specific gravity	Newborn: 1.001–1.020 Child: 1.001–1.030	Dehydration Overhydration, renal disease, pituitary malfunction

*Values for different age groups are indicated only when relevant.

the foreskin from being retracted over the penis (Fig. 28–4). This is normal in newborns and usually disappears by three years of age. In some children this narrowing may obstruct the stream of urine, causing dribbling or irritation. The condition can be corrected by circumcision.

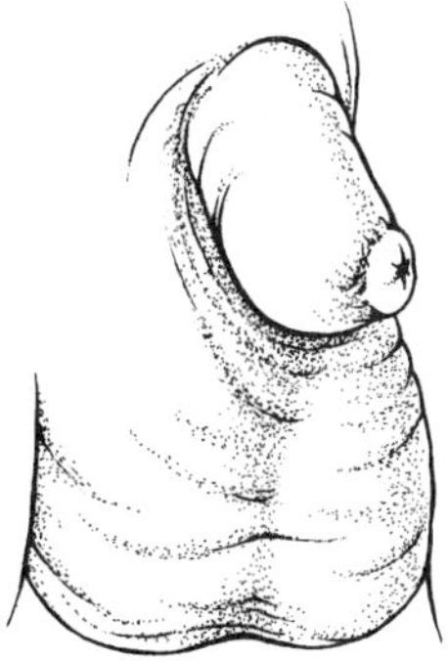

Figure 28-4. • Phimosis. The foreskin is advanced and fixed; it cannot be retracted over the glans.

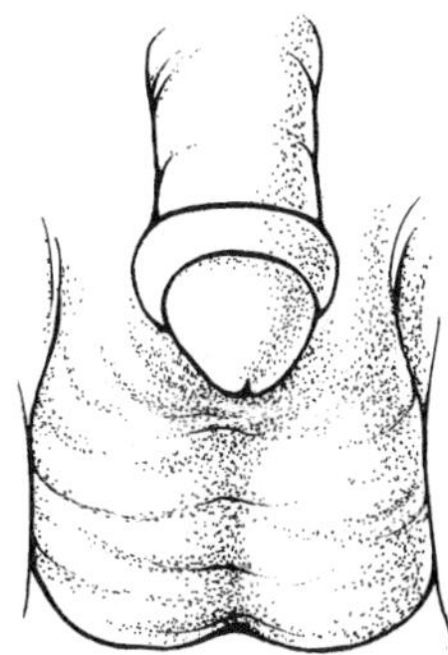

Figure 28-5. • Paraphimosis. The foreskin is retracted and fixed; it cannot be returned to its original position. Constriction impedes circulation.

When circumcision is performed on an older boy, careful explanations and reassurance are provided. The nurse is sensitive to the child's embarrassment and fear. Postoperatively the penis is covered with a petroleum gauze. It is tender and may burn on urination.

Cleansing of the uncircumcised penis and retraction of the foreskin are discussed in Chapter 12. Forcible retraction of a tight foreskin is avoided because it can lead to *paraphimosis* (Fig. 28–5). When this occurs, the foreskin cannot be returned to its normal condition. There may be swelling due to the constriction. This condition requires immediate evaluation by a physician.

Hypospadias and Epispadias

Description. *Hypospadias* is a congenital defect in which the urinary meatus is not at the end of the penis but on the lower shaft. In mild cases it is just below the tip of the penis, but it may be found at the midshaft or near the penal-scrotal junction. This deformity, unlike epispadias, is fairly common, occurring in 1 out of 250 to 500 newborn boys. In *epispadias* the opening of the urinary meatus is on the upper surface of the penis (Fig. 28–6). Hypospadias may be accompanied by *chordee,* a downward curvature of the penis caused by a fibrotic band of tissue.

Treatment and Nursing Care. The alert nurse may discover hypospadias or epispadias in the nursery during neonatal assessment. In many mild cases, surgery is not necessary for either condition unless the location and extent of the defect are such that the child will not be able to stand to void or the defect would cause psychological problems or difficulties in future sexual relations. Treatment consists of surgical repair, usually performed before 18 months of age. It is sometimes done in stages, depending on associated defects. Most techniques

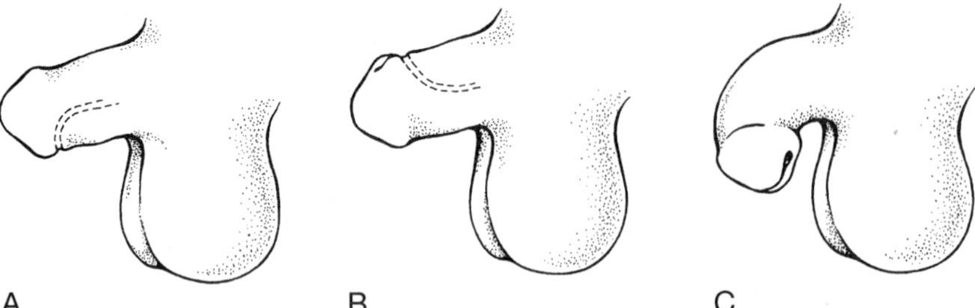

Figure 28-6. • **A,** Hypospadias. **B,** Epispadias. **C,** Chordee.

can be performed during same-day surgery. Routine circumcision of the newborn is avoided in these children, as the foreskin may be useful in the repair. Postoperatively a urinary catheter may be required. Parents are instructed in the home care of the catheter. Medication for bladder spasms may be required.

As this condition is corrected at a time in childhood when fears of separation and mutilation are great, attention is directed to psychological considerations. In the older child, questions about virility and reproduction may surface and need to be addressed.

Exstrophy of the Bladder

Description. In exstrophy of the bladder, the lower portion of the abdominal wall and anterior wall of the bladder are missing. As a result, the bladder lies open and exposed on the abdomen (Fig. 28–7). Exstrophy is due to a failure of the midline to close during embryonic development. Other congenital anomalies may also be present. This anomaly occurs in 1:40,000 live births and more often in boys than in girls.

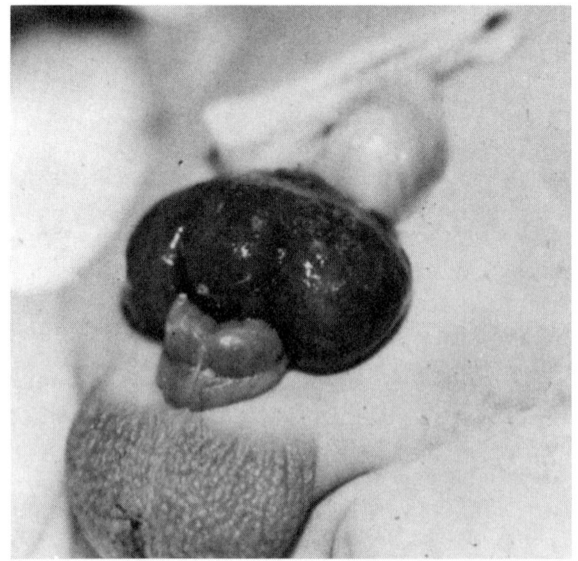

Figure 28-7. • Bladder exstrophy. (From Behrman, R. [1992]. *Nelson's textbook of pediatrics* [14th ed., p. 1373]. Philadelphia: Saunders.)

Manifestations. This disorder is noticeable by fetal sonogram. The defect may range from a small cutaneous fistula in the abdominal wall to complete exstrophy (the turning inside out of an organ). Urine leaks continually from the bladder. The skin around the bladder becomes excoriated. Other anomalies are common.

Treatment and Nursing Care. The bladder is covered with a plastic shield or appropriate dressing to protect its mucosa but allow for urinary drainage. This also protects the bladder from irritation by bedclothes or diapers. The skin is protected by a suitable ointment. Diapers are generally placed under rather than around the infant. The baby is positioned so that urine drains freely. Antibiotics are given to prevent infection. Surgical closure is ideally performed during the first 48 hours of life.

Obstructive Uropathy

Description. Many conditions, such as calculi (stones), tumors, strictures, and scarring may cause an obstruction of the normal flow of urine (Fig. 28–8). These conditions may be congenital or ac-

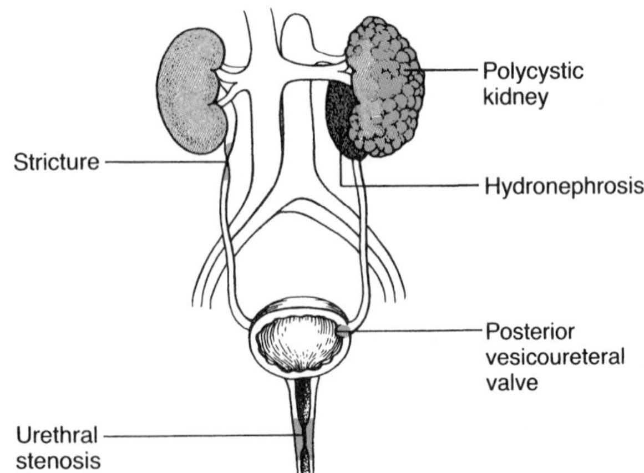

Figure 28-8. • Frequent sites of urinary obstruction.

quired. Blockage may be either partial or complete. One or both kidneys may be affected. The pathologic changes depend on the nature and location of the problem. *Hydronephrosis* (*hydro,* "water," and *nephro,* "kidney") is the distention of the renal pelvis due to an obstruction. The pelvis of the kidney becomes enlarged and cysts form. This may eventually damage renal nephrons, resulting in deterioration of the kidneys. *Polycystic kidney* refers to a condition in which large, fluid-filled cysts form in place of healthy kidney tissue in the fetus. This is inherited as an autosomal recessive trait. Kidney damage can result in inability of the kidney to concentrate urine, resulting in metabolic acidosis. Urine that is not excreted promptly can promote the growth of organisms that cause urinary tract infection.

Treatment and Nursing Care. Urinary diversion is necessary in certain conditions, and it may be accomplished by several procedures (Table 28–2). This type of surgery is a source of great apprehension for parents. The physical care of the child with a urinary stoma (artificially created opening or passage) presents hygiene problems, skin problems, and difficulties in leaving the infant in the care of others. Frequent trips to the clinic add to the strain of everyday life.

Stress from the urinary diversion is age related. The toddler may be unable to attain independence in toilet training. The school-age child suffers from being different and may have a distorted body image. The adolescent may have lowered self-esteem and is concerned about sexuality. Parents with affected newborns grieve for the loss of a perfect child and experience concerns about the length and quality of the infant's life. The nurse anticipates the impact of this type of diagnosis and incorporates suitable psychological interventions into daily care. Providing emotional support and teaching parents how to prevent infection are priorities of care.

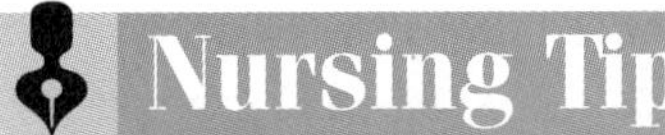

Most newborns urinate within the first 24 hours of life. Recording and reporting the presence or absence of urination is very important.

Assessing for a Distended Bladder. To assess for a distended bladder palpate below the umbilicus, moving toward the symphysis until a smooth round firm bladder rim is felt. The normal bladder is not palpable as it lies behind the symphysis pubis.

Acute Urinary Tract Infection

Description. Urinary tract infections are common in children. They are more common in girls (except during the neonatal period) than in boys and occur predominantly in the 7 to 11 age group. Of all infections, 75% to 90% are caused by *Escherichia coli,* followed by *Klebsiella* and *Proteus* (Behrman, Kleigman, & Arvin, 1996). The nurse will see the following terms used to describe the location and problem of urinary tract disturbances:

- *Urethritis.* Infection of the urethra
- *Cystitis.* Inflammation of the bladder
- *Bacteriuria.* Bacteria in the urine
- *Pyelonephritis.* Infection of the kidney and renal pelvis
- *Ureteritis.* Infection of the ureters
- *Vesicoureteral reflux.* Backward flow of urine into the ureters.

Several factors account for the preponderance in girls. These include a shorter urethra, the location of the urethra closer to the anus, wearing of nylon

Table 28–2
SURGICAL PROCEDURES USED IN URINARY DIVERSION

Procedure	Definition
Ureterostomy	Surgical implantation of ureters to outside abdominal wall; allows urine to drain into collection device
Ileal or colon conduit (artificial channel)	Diverts urine at ureter, bypassing bladder and urethra; ureters are removed from bladder and attached to ileum or colon, which then acts as a bladder without voluntary control of voiding; patient has stoma, which is larger and not as prone to stenosis as ureterostomy; child wears ileostomy appliance (*Note:* Urine from a conduit may appear cloudy from the secretions of the bowel conduit; this is not a sign of urinary tract infection)
Nephrostomy	Tube passes through flank into pelvis of kidney, allowing urine to be drained from pelvis (bypassing ureter, bladder, and urethra; drains into ostomy bag)
Suprapubic tube placement	Suprapubic tube is placed above pubis into bladder to provide urinary drainage
Vesicostomy (*vesico,* "bladder," *stoma,* "passage")	Surgical opening into bladder between umbilicus and pubis; bladder wall brought to surface of abdomen

underwear, use of bubble bath, retention of urine, and vaginitis. In young girls with repeated infections, incest or other sexual abuse should be considered.

Certain chemical and physical factors are important. Normal urine is acidic. Alkaline urine favor pathogens. Urine that remains in the bladder for a period of time serves as an excellent medium for bacterial growth. In certain conditions, such as *vesicoureteral reflux,* the urine is forced backward from the bladder into the ureters during urination (Fig. 28–9).

Manifestations. Signs and symptoms of urinary infection are age dependent. Infants frequently present with fever, weight loss, failure to thrive, nausea, vomiting, and frequent urination. Foul-smelling urine and persistent diaper rash may also be indicators. In the older child, urinary frequency, pain during micturition, onset of bedwetting in a previously "dry" child, abdominal pain, and hematuria may be present. When the kidney is involved, there may be fever, chills, and flank pain.

The diagnosis depends on the culture of bacteria from the urine. In toilet-trained children, a midstream urine specimen is obtained after cleansing the urethral meatus and rinsing with sterile water. Catheterization may be necessary to obtain a sterile specimen. An intravenous pyelogram, cystogram, or sonogram may be indicated.

Treatment and Nursing Care. Acute cystitis is treated promptly to avoid pyelonephritis. Sulfonamides or broad-spectrum antibiotics are usually prescribed. If anatomic defects are present, surgical correction may be suggested. Methods of preventing urinary tract infections are taught to parents and to the patient, as age appropriate. The nurse stresses the need for proper amounts of fluid to maintain sterility and flushing of the bladder. Nursing Care Plan 28–1 presents the nursing considerations appropriate for these patients. The prognosis is excellent with prompt treatment. Some patients develop chronic pyelonephritis and experience recurring infections. More seriously ill children may require hospitalization. Blood pressure, weight, and fever are important parameters to observe in detecting early complications in such children. Anticipatory guidance by explaining procedures helps decrease the child's and the parents' stress levels.

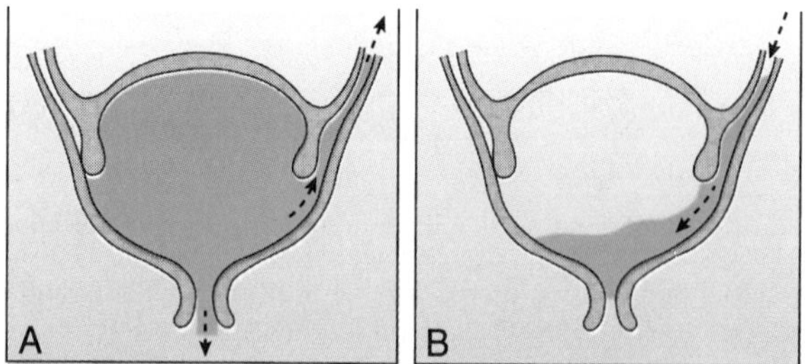

Figure 28-9. • Vesicoureteral reflux. Congenital abnormalities of the junction between the bladder and the ureters can force urine to flow backward into the ureters during voiding **(A).** After voiding, residual urine from the ureter remains in the bladder **(B).**

Nephrotic Syndrome (Nephrosis)

Description. Nephrotic syndrome refers to a number of different types of kidney conditions that are distinguished by the presence of marked amounts of protein in the urine. Minimal change nephrotic syndrome (MCNS), found in approximately 85% of cases, is discussed here.

Nephrosis is more common in boys than in girls and is seen most often in children 2 to 7 years of age. The specific cause is unknown but may be related to a thymus T-cell dysfunction. The prognosis is good in steroid-responsive patients. Most children have periods of relapse until the disease resolves itself.

Manifestations. The characteristic symptom of nephrosis is *edema.* This occurs slowly; the child does not appear to be sick. It is first noticed about the eyes and ankles and later becomes generalized. The edema shifts with the position of the child during sleep. The patient gains weight because of the accumulation of fluid. The abdomen may become distended *(ascites).* The child is pale, irritable, and listless and has a poor appetite. Blood pressure is usually normal.

Urine examination reveals albumin (protein). The *glomeruli,* the working units of the kidneys that filter the blood, become damaged and allow albumin and blood cells to enter the urine. The level of protein in the blood falls; this is termed *hypoalbuminemia* (*hypo,* "below," *albumin,* and *emia,* "blood"), and the cholesterol content rises; this is termed *hyperlipidemia* (*hyper,* "above," *lipos,* "fat," and *emia,* "blood"). Vomiting and diarrhea may also be present. Renal biopsy and examination of the tissue under light and electron microscopes provide valuable information.

Treatment

Control of Edema. The child with nephrosis is given medications designed to reduce proteinuria and consequently edema. Steroid therapy is currently used for this purpose. Oral prednisone is initially given. The dosage is reduced for mainte-

NURSING CARE PLAN 28–1

Selected Nursing Diagnoses for the Child with a Urinary Tract Infection

Nursing Diagnosis: Altered patterns of urinary elimination related to dysuria, incontinence

Goals	Nursing Interventions	Rationale
Child does not complain of frequency, urgency, or pain on urination Infant does not strain or fret before voiding Child verbalizes reasons for frequent bladder emptying	1. Administer antibiotics as prescribed	1. Antibiotics are chosen according to urine culture and sensitivity; Pyridium may be given to decrease dysuria
	2. Encourage complete bladder emptying; explain necessity for this, as age appropriate	2. Standing urine in the bladder is very susceptible to the growth of organisms
	3. Remind child to void frequently; anticipate incontinence	3. Under normal conditions the bladder flushes away organisms by regularly ridding itself of urine; this prevents organisms from accumulating and invading nearby structures; the convalescent bladder is less resistant to invasion than is a healthy bladder
	4. Encourage fluids	4. Child may be febrile; increasing fluids decreases the concentration of solutes and alleviates urinary stasis
	5. Keep accurate intake and output records	5. This is essential to determine the progress of treatment since the kidneys and bladder play an important part in fluid balance
	6. Teach child how to collect urine specimens, if age appropriate	6. Education ensures that specimen will be correctly obtained without contamination
	7. Provide privacy	7. Children must be given same courtesy as adults, as they are sensitive and embarrassed by body exposure

Nursing Diagnosis: Knowledge deficit concerning hygiene measures useful in prevention of urinary tract infection

Goals	Nursing Interventions	Rationale
Girl demonstrates on doll how to wipe herself after voiding Child verbalizes methods to accomplish this	1. Instruct girl in importance of wiping self from front to back	1. Good perineal hygiene avoids fecal contamination of urethra
	2. Emphasize need to avoid bubble baths, water softeners	2. Oils in these products are known to irritate urethra
	3. Encourage use of showers	3. These hygienic measures are helpful in preventing infection
	4. Explain need for cotton underwear	4. Cotton underwear is more absorbent
	5. Suggest juices such as apple or cranberry to maintain acidity of urine	5. Acidifying urine decreases rate of bacterial multiplication; an acid-ash diet of meats, cheese, prunes, cranberries, plums, and whole grains is also beneficial
	6. Recommend frequent pad change for menstruating girls and proper genital cleansing during period	6. Old pooled blood fosters growth of organisms; proper cleansing helps to prevent irritation

(Continued)

nance therapy, which continues for 1 to 2 months. Because steroids mask signs of infection, the patient must be watched closely for more subtle symptoms of illness. Children are prone to infection when absolute granulocyte counts fall below 1000 cells mm ^{3}. This is called *neutropenia.*

The child's skin is examined at sites of punctures, wounds, pierced ears, and catheters. The nurse watches for temperature variations and changes in behavior. Suspicions are promptly reported, as septicemia is life-threatening. Prompt antibacterial therapy is begun when an acute infection is recognized. Diuretics have not generally been effective in reducing nephrotic edema. Immunosuppressive therapy (i.e., cyclophosphamide [Cytoxan] and chlorambucil) has shown promise for some steroid-resistant children.

Diet. A well-balanced diet high in protein is desirable because protein is constantly being lost in the urine. The carbohydrate and fat content of the

NURSING CARE PLAN 28–1 *continued*

Selected Nursing Diagnoses for the Child with a Urinary Tract Infection

Nursing Diagnosis: Knowledge deficit (parents) concerning follow-up care

Goals	Nursing Interventions	Rationale
Parents verbalize necessity for continued supervision and medication	1. Instruct parents to administer medication as prescribed and to continue for length of time recommended by the physician	1. Typical course of antibiotic treatment is 7–10 days; emphasize need to complete prescribed dosage
	2. Suggest patient avoid hot tubs or whirlpool baths	2. May be potential sources of infection
	3. Remind parents of necessity of adequate hydration for child	3. Children dehydrate very quickly
	4. Instruct parents that recurrence is most likely within 3–12 mo following infection, often asymptomatic	4. Emphasize the need for routine office visits to pick up asymptomatic infections
	5. Explain necessity for periodic follow-up urine cultures	5. Recurrence is common; a urine culture obtained approximately 1 wk after medicine is discontinued will determine if medication has eradicated bacteria

diet should be high enough to prevent protein from being used for energy. If either dietary protein or body protein is used for energy, the waste product urea is excreted through the kidneys, which increases their workload. Parents are instructed to avoid adding salt to foods served whenever edema is present. Fluids are not restricted.

Care of Ascites. *Ascites,* an abnormal collection of fluid in the peritoneal cavity, is seen in advanced cases of nephrosis. This fluid can also cause pressure on the heart and the organs of respiration. The doctor can remove some of this fluid by a procedure known as an *abdominal paracentesis* (*para,* "beside," and *kentesis,* "puncture"). Fluid may also accumulate in the chest. This is termed *hydrothorax* (*hydro,* "water," and *thorax,* "chest"). The procedure used to remove fluid from the chest is called thoracentesis (*thorax,* "chest," and *kentesis*). Corticosteroid and medical diuresis have greatly reduced the need for these procedures.

Mental Hygiene. The nurse provides supportive care to the parents and child through the course of this disease. Whenever possible the child is treated at home and brought to the hospital for special therapy only. Parents are instructed to keep a daily record of the child's weight, urinary proteins, and medications. Signs of infection, abnormal weight gain, and increased protein in the urine must be reported promptly. The child is allowed up and about after the acute stage of the illness subsides to participate in normal childhood activities.

Nursing Care. The nursing care of the child with nephrosis is of the greatest significance because the disease requires long-term therapy. The child is periodically hospitalized and becomes a familiar personality to hospital personnel. The following factors are important in creating nursing care plans for each child.

Skin Care. Good skin care is especially important during periods of marked edema. The skin is bathed daily and whenever necessary. Special attention is given to the neck, underarms, groin, and other moist areas of the body. The patient is handled gently to prevent injury to the skin. The male genitals may become edematous; they are bathed and a scrotal support is applied. Cotton is used to separate the skin surfaces to prevent the formation of a rash. Children who are not toilet trained require meticulous care of the diaper area because urine acidity predisposes to skin breakdown.

Positioning. The patient is turned frequently to prevent respiratory infection. A pillow placed between the knees when the patient is lying on the side prevents pressure on edematous organs. The child's head is elevated from time to time during the day to reduce edema of the eyelids and to make the patient more comfortable. Swelling impairs the circulation of the lacrimal secretions. It may therefore be necessary to bathe the eyes to prevent the accumulation of exudate.

Diet. The appetite of the patient is poor. Small quantities of food are attractively arranged and served on brightly colored dishes. The child's favorite foods are served if they are nutritious. Colored straws may also be used. If the parents are available, the child can enjoy their company during meals.

Nursing Tip

Remember to measure and record urine specimens sent to the laboratory.

The child's intake and output are strictly charted. This is the responsibility of the nurse, regardless of who feeds the patient. Parents are instructed to inform the nurse of how much fluid has been taken. The importance of keeping *proper fluid balance sheets* (i.e., intake and output records) for patients with diseases of the kidneys cannot be overemphasized.

Urine Assessment. As stated, the patient's urine must be carefully measured. Diapers may be weighed on a gram scale before application and after removal (1 gm = 1 ml). The weights are marked on the diaper. A careful check of the number of voidings is of particular value. The character, odor, and color of the urine are also important. If a 24-hour urine collection is ordered, *every* voided specimen within that time must be saved or the test will not be valid. The specimens are collected in a large bottle or container that is correctly labeled. Some tests require that certain preservatives be added to the container; this matter is clarified before the procedure begins.

Weight, Protection from Infection. The patient is weighed two or three times a week to determine changes in the degree of edema. The child is weighed on the same scale each time, and at about the same time of day. Abdominal girth (circumference) should also be measured every day.

Nurses make every effort to protect the child from exposure to upper respiratory tract infections. Children who are up and about must not be allowed to wander into areas where they would be in danger of contracting an infection. *No vaccinations or immunizations should be administered while the the disease is active and during immunosuppressive therapy.*

The vital signs of a patient with nephrosis are taken regularly. Ordinarily there is no elevation of temperature unless an infection is present. Blood pressure remains normal. Parental guidance and support are given by all members of the nursing team. The child with nephrosis is kept under close medical supervision over an extended period. Prognosis is considered favorable.

Acute Glomerulonephritis

Description. Acute glomerulonephritis (AGN), formerly called *Bright's disease,* is an allergic reaction (antigen–antibody) to a group-A beta-hemolytic streptococci infection. It may appear after the patient has had scarlet fever or skin infections. The body's immune mechanisms appear to be important in its development. Antibodies produced to fight the invading organisms also react against the glomerular tissue. Glomerulonephritis is the most common form of nephritis in children, and it occurs most frequently in boys 3 to 7 years of age. Both kidneys are usually affected.

The nephron is the working unit of the kidneys. Nephrons number in the millions. Within the bulb of each nephron lies a cluster of capillaries called the glomerulus. It is these structures that are affected, as the name implies. They become inflamed and sometimes blocked, permitting red blood cells and protein, which are normally retained, to enter the urine. The kidneys become pale and slightly enlarged. Table 28–3 compares nephrosis with AGN.

The prognosis is excellent. Patients with mild cases of the disease may recover within 10 to 14 days. Patients with protracted cases may show urinary changes for as long as 1 year but have complete recovery. Observation for complications that involve hypertensive changes to the blood supply of the brain necessitate careful assessment and care of each patient.

Table 28–3
COMPARISON OF NEPHROSIS WITH ACUTE GLOMERULONEPHRITIS

	Nephrosis	Acute Glomerulonephritis
Cause	Unknown, may be a thymus T-cell dysfunction	Response to infection with group-A beta-hemolytic streptococci
Edema	Massive edema Anasarca: whole-body edema Ascites: fluid in abdominal cavity	Periorbital edema (puffiness of eyes)
Blood pressure	Usually normal	Usually moderately elevated
Urine tests	Proteinuria Trace of blood	Trace of protein Hematuria (resolves within 1 mo, but urinary symptoms may persist for 1 yr)
Pallor	Pallor in excess of anemia (appearance due to edematous tissue)	Pallor related to anemia

Note: The signs and symptoms of nephrosis and acute glomerulonephritis are similar. Careful analysis and comparisons reveal significant differences. Either condition can lead to renal failure and its consequences.

Manifestations. From 1 to 3 weeks after a streptococcal infection has occurred, the parent may notice that the child's urine is smoky brown or bloody. This is frightening to the parent and child, and most parents immediately seek medical advice. Periorbital edema (mild swelling about the eyes) may also be present, with fever (high at first but gradually leveling off to about 37.8°C [100°F]), headache, diarrhea, and vomiting. Urinary output is decreased. The urine specific gravity is high, and albumin, red and white blood cells, and casts may be found on examination. The blood urea nitrogen level is elevated, as are the serum creatinine and sedimentation rate. The serum complement level is usually reduced. *Hyperkalemia* (excessive potassium in the blood) may produce cardiac toxicity. Hypertension may occur.

Treatment and Nursing Care. Although children may feel well, activity is limited until gross hematuria subsides. The urine is regularly examined. Every effort is made to prevent children from becoming overtired, chilled, or exposed to infection. As renal function is impaired, there is danger of accumulation of nitrogenous wastes and sodium in the body. Penicillin is given during the acute phase and may be continued orally for some time to prevent renewed infection.

Nursing care is supportive. Prevention of infection, fatigue, maintenance of accurate intake and output records, and frequent assessment of vital signs are essential.

Although glomerulonephritis is generally benign, it can be a source of anguish for the parents and child. If the patient is treated at home, the parents must plan activities to keep the child occupied with quiet activity. They must understand the importance of continued medical supervision, as follow-up urine and blood tests are necessary to assess progress. All children with hypertension should be monitored for signs of increased intracranial pressure.

Wilms' Tumor

Description. Wilms' tumor, or *nephroblastoma* (*nephro,* "kidney," *blasto,* "bud," and *oma,* "tumor"), is one of the most common malignancies of early life. It is an embryonal adenosarcoma (*adeno,* "glandular," and *sarcoma,* "cancer of connective tissue") that is now known to be associated with certain congenital anomalies, particularly of the genitourinary tract. It is thought to have a genetic basis.

About two thirds of these growths are discovered before the child is 3 years old. During the early stages of growth, as with some other malignancies, there are few or no symptoms. A mass in the abdomen is discovered generally by a parent or by the physician during a routine checkup. X-rays of the kidneys (most importantly, intravenous pyelograms) reveal a growth and verify the fact that the remaining kidney is normal. The tumor compresses kidney tissue and is usually encapsulated. Renal damage may cause hypertension. Chest x-ray films, ultrasound, bone surveys, liver scan, and CT may also be indicated. Wilms' tumor seldom affects both kidneys.

Treatment and Nursing Care. Treatment of the Wilms' tumor patient consists of a combination of surgery, radiation therapy, and chemotherapy. The kidney and tumor are removed as soon as possible after the diagnosis has been confirmed. It is important to prepare the parents and the child for the extent of the incision, which is considerable. The National Wilms' Tumor Study (NWTS) lists several categories of effective treatment. Five stages of tumor activity are cited, and appropriate refinements in radiation therapy and chemotherapy are suggested. Children with localized tumors (stage I and stage II) have a 90% chance of cure. Patients younger than 2 years of age have a higher rate of response to therapy.

General nursing measures for the comfort of the patient are carried out. One factor pertinent to this condition is that all unnecessary handling of the abdomen is to be avoided, as it can cause the tumor to spread. The doctor explains this to the parents, and in the hospital a sign is placed on the crib or child: "Do not palpate abdomen." Abdominal palpation, as part of the daily assessment, is omitted. Nursing Care Plan 28–2 outlines care for a child undergoing surgery of the renal system. Chemotherapy and radiation following surgery are usually completed at a cancer center.

Hydrocele

Description. A *hydrocele* (*hydro,* "water," and *cele,* "tumor") is an excessive amount of fluid in the sac that surrounds the testicle, which causes the scrotum to swell (Fig. 28–10). When the testes descend into the scrotum in utero, the *processus vaginalis,* a fold of tissue, precedes them. This tissue ordinarily fuses, separating the peritoneal cavity from the scrotum. When this fusion does not take place, peritoneal fluid may enter the inguinal canal. Its appearance in the newborn is not uncommon, and in many cases the condition corrects itself by 1 year of age.

Treatment. If a chronic hydrocele persists beyond 1 year, it is corrected by surgery. Routine

NURSING CARE PLAN 28-2

Selected Nursing Diagnoses for the Child Undergoing Surgery of the Renal System

Nursing Diagnosis: Anxiety related to surgical experience

Goals	Nursing Interventions	Rationale
Parents state two ways they are coping with the stress of this surgery Child verbalizes understanding of procedure, as age appropriate	1. Provide surgical tour, include wake-up room	1. Explanations and familiarity with physical surroundings may decrease apprehension
	2. Encourage parents to remain with child, as appropriate	2. Child is more secure when parents are close by
	3. Explain mask and anesthesia equipment	3. It is frightening to have something placed over face; equipment is intimidating
	4. Determine small child's words for penis, urination	4. This will promote understanding postoperatively
	5. Provide support and reassurance	5. Urinary surgery may raise anxiety about sexual function, which parents or patients are often unable to express

Nursing Diagnosis: High risk for ineffective airway clearance related to poor cough effort associated with postanesthesia, postoperative immobility, pain

Goals	Nursing Interventions	Rationale
Patient maintains airway patency as evidenced by clear lung sounds, vital signs within normal range	1. Assist child to turn, cough, deep-breathe; reposition infants	1. Prolonged postoperative immobility leads to decreased chest expansion, pooling of mucus in bronchi, and hypostatic pneumonia; in nephrectomy patients, incision is close to diaphragm, making breathing painful; allow infants to cry for a few seconds to ensure deep breathing; if secretions are present, coughing will generally follow; ambulate as ordered
	2. Monitor vital signs frequently	2. Monitoring vital signs will assess cardiovascular function and tissue perfusion
	3. Teach splinting of incision preoperatively	3. Splinting incision lessens pain
	4. Teach incentive spirometry preoperatively	4. Spirometry promotes alveolar inflation, restores and maintains lung capacity, and strengthens respiratory muscles; it also provides immediate feedback about the effectiveness of deep breathing
	5. Assess and medicate for bladder spasm and incisional pain	5. Postoperative pain and discomfort may make patients reluctant to turn, cough, and deep-breathe

(Continued)

postoperative nursing care is given. This is outlined in Chapter 22. Same-day surgery may be arranged.

Cryptorchidism

Description. The testes are the male sex glands. These two oval bodies begin their development in the abdominal cavity below the kidneys in the embryo. Their function is to produce spermatozoa (male sex cells) and male hormones, particularly testosterone. Toward the end of the 7th fetal month, the testes begin to descend along a pathway into the scrotum. If this descent does not take place normally, the testes may remain in the abdomen or inguinal canal. This condition is common in about 30% of low-birth-weight infants. When one or both testes fail to lower into the scrotum, the condition is termed *cryptorchidism* (*kryptos,* "hidden," and *orchi,* "testis"). The unilateral form is more frequently seen.

NURSING CARE PLAN 28–2 *continued*

Selected Nursing Diagnoses for the Child Undergoing Surgery of the Renal System

Nursing Diagnosis: High risk for fluid volume deficit related to patient's age, surgery, catheters, refusal to drink

Goals	Nursing Interventions	Rationale
Vital signs remain within normal limits Patient's hydration and acid–base balance remain stable as evidenced by laboratory reports	1. Regulate intravenous fluids	1. Child will probably take nothing by mouth for a brief period prior to and following surgery; intravenous fluids maintain hydration and replace lost electrolytes
	2. Keep accurate intake and output records	2. Careful monitoring of fluid intake and output will identify early renal complications
	3. Weigh infants daily	3. Daily weights in infants will assist in monitoring under- or overhydration; comparison with preoperative weight will assess infant's nutritional progress
	4. Record separate output for each drainage tube	4. An unexpected reduction in urine flow requires prompt intervention; each catheter drains into its own collection bag, so that source of reduced flow will be immediately noticed
	5. Observe fontanels of infants for depression	5. Depressed fontanels, sunken eyeballs, lack of tears, dark circles around eyes, and poor skin turgor denote dehydration, which can occur quickly in infants and children
	6. Begin clear oral fluids gradually	6. Replacement of fluids and electrolytes by mouth is generally considered to be the safest method; clarify ambiguous orders, such as "force fluids," "restrict fluids," particularly in infants and small children with urologic disorders, cardiac conditions, and so on
Child's temperature will remain at or below 38° C (100.4° F); incision site will not be erythematous or foul-smelling	1. Assess for signs of infection	1. Fever, incisional tenderness, redness, drainage from incisions, lethargy indicate infection
	2. Observe and record patency, color, amount, and consistency of drainage	2. Catheters can become plugged by mucous shreds, blood clots, and chemical sediment; plugging of conduits can lead to infection of urinary tract, urine stasis, and if obstruction persists, hydronephrosis
	3. Obtain urine cultures as indicated	3. Pathogens in urine are most specifically determined by culture; goal is to obtain urine that is uncontaminated by organisms outside urinary tract
	4. Maintain aseptic closed drainage system	4. Maintaining a closed drainage system aids in preventing infection; careful handwashing before and after handling of catheter or drainage system is also of importance

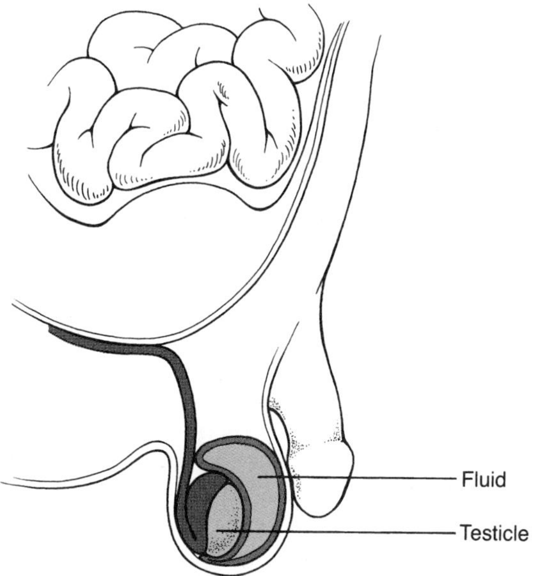

Figure 28-10. • Hydrocele.

Because the testes are warmer in the abdomen than in the scrotum, the sperm cells begin to deteriorate. If both testes are affected, sterility results. *Inguinal hernia* often accompanies this condition. Secondary sex characteristics, such as voice change and growth of facial hair, are not affected, since the testes continue to secrete hormones directly into the bloodstream. Acute scrotal pain may indicate a *testicular torsion* (twisting), which requires immediate surgery to preserve testicular function.

Treatment and Nursing Care. Occasionally, a testis or the testes spontaneously descend during the 1st year of life. Hormonal management before surgery consists of the administration of human chorionic gonadotropin (HCG). This hormone is useful as a diagnostic aid, and it may also precipitate the descent of the testes. If this does not occur, an operation called an *orchiopexy* (*orchio,* "testicle," and *pexy,* "fixation") is performed.

Although an orchiopexy improves the condition, the fertility rate among these patients, even when only one testis is undescended, may be reduced. In addition, the incidence of testicular tumors is increased in these patients during adulthood. Parents are told to teach the growing child the importance of self-examination of the testes. When the child returns from surgery, care is taken to prevent contamination of the suture line and scrotal support is maintained.

The psychological approach of the nurse to the patient and his family is important because of the embarrassment they may feel. People may ask the child why he is being operated on when there is no visible evidence of trauma. This problem is frequently compounded by the fact that the older child may have been told not to discuss his condition; in addition, his understanding of his problem and just what is going to happen in surgery may be vague. Therefore, the nurse caring for the child should know what he has been told and how he feels about his operation to give emotional support. Terminology is clarified. The nurse assures the child that his penis will not be involved in the surgery.

The parents, too, may have anxieties that they cannot verbalize. It is difficult for many of them to communicate with their child about such matters. They may also fear that the child will become homosexual or less virile. A thoughtful, sensitive nurse who tries to anticipate these and other related feelings and fears promotes the child's adjustment.

Impact of Urinary or Genital Surgery on Growth and Development

Surgery of the urinary or genital tract impacts growth and development. Preschoolers may perceive the treatment as punishment. Separation anxiety during hospitalizations peak and preventive strategies should be explained to the parents. The body image of the child needs to be assertively maintained whenever surgery is delayed beyond infancy. Between 3 and 6 years of age, the child becomes curious about sexual differences and may masturbate. Surgical interventions during this stage of development require guidance and preparation to minimize the negative impact on growth and development.

During home care, tub baths may be contraindicated, dressings to "private parts" of the body need to be inspected daily and restriction on play activities that involve straddle toys (tricycles, rocking horses, etc.) are necessary. Adolescents may be concerned about effects of surgery on appearance and sexual abilities.

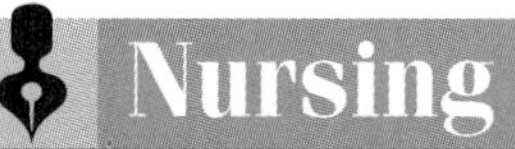

The bladder capacity of a child can be approximated by the formula: age in years + 2 = ounces of bladder volume or capacity.

KEY POINTS

- The functional unit of the kidney is the nephron.
- Children with hypospadias are born with the urethral opening located on the undersurface of the penis.
- Bladder exstrophy is a serious congenital defect in which the bladder lies exposed on the lower portion of the abdominal wall. Surgical correction of this defect is lifesaving.
- Obstruction of the urinary tract may lead to hydronephrosis, a distention of the kidney pelvis. This is a serious condition because it could eventually lead to kidney failure if untreated.
- To avoid fecal contamination of the urinary tract, girls are taught to wipe the perineal area from front to back after urination.
- Ascites is an abnormal collection of fluid in the peritoneal cavity. It is seen in advanced cases of nephrosis and other conditions.
- The accurate charting of intake and output on patients with kidney problems is absolutely essential to their treatment and recovery. This includes ostomy and urinary drainage.
- Accurate blood pressure measurements will detect hypertension, a condition frequently associated with kidney problems.
- Normally urine flows from the ureters into the bladder, and almost no flow reenters the ureters. Repeated urinary tract infections or improper position of the ureters or sphincters in the bladder at birth may result in reflux of urine into the ureters.
- Good health habits include assessing one's own body including the genitals.
- Early treatment of cryptorchidism is necessary to preserve testicular function.
- A hydrocele is an excessive amount of fluid in the sac that surrounds the testicle. It causes the scrotum to swell.
- Undescended testes *(cryptorchidism)* refers to a condition in which the testes do not lower into the scrotum during the fetal period but remain in the abdomen or inguinal canal after birth.

MULTIPLE-CHOICE REVIEW QUESTIONS

Choose the most appropriate answer.

1. The nurse understands that genitourinary surgery impacts growth and development. When caring for a 4-year-old child postoperatively, a priority nursing responsibility would include:
   a. Strategies to preserve child's body image
   b. Assurances that appearance and sexual function will not be affected
   c. Providing age-appropriate toys such as tricycles
   d. Preventing embarrassment by limiting family and friends visiting
2. The administration of prednisone to children with nephrosis creates the problem of
   a. intolerance of foods.
   b. increased risk of infection.
   c. increased periorbital edema.
   d. weight loss.
3. The reason for daily weights in children with nephrosis is to monitor
   a. weight loss from low-protein diet
   b. accuracy of fluid balance sheets
   c. changes in the amount of edema
   d. percentile on growth grid
4. A *priority* nursing responsibility in the care of a child with Wilms' tumor is to
   a. maintain accurate intake and output records.
   b. omit abdominal palpation during daily assessments.
   c. maintain strict bedrest.
   d. assess neurologic function.
5. Accurate fluid intake and output records are particularly important in patients with kidney disease because
   a. they aid in assessing kidney damage.
   b. they help to determine nutritional adequacy.
   c. they are important in assessing hypertension.
   d. they provide a reliable method of determining infection.

BIBLIOGRAPHY AND READER REFERENCE

Baker, A., & Davis, A. (eds.). (1997). *Pediatric parenteral nutrition.* New York: Chapman and Hall.

Behrman, R. E., Kleigman, R., & Arvin, A. (1996). *Nelson's textbook of pediatrics* (15th ed.). Philadelphia: Saunders.

Bowden, V., Dickey, S., & Greenberg, C. (1998). *Children and their families: The continuum of care.* Philadelphia: Saunders.

Green, D. M., D'Angio, G., Beckwith, J., et al. (1996). Wilms' tumor. *CA: A Cancer Journal for Clinicians, 46*(1), 46–63.

Hagerman, R. J. (1997). Meeting the challenge of fragile X syndrome. *Patient Care, 31*(4), 146–162.

Kirton, C. (1997). Assessing for bladder distention. *Nursing 97, 27*(4), 64.

Mahan, L., & Escott-Stumps, S. (1996). *Krause's food, nutrition & diet therapy* (9th ed.). Philadelphia: Saunders.

Reynolds, E., & Haberman, A. (1995). Diagnosis and management of pyelonephritis in infants. *MCN, 20*(2), 78–84.

Stevens-Simon, C. (1997). Reproductive health care for your adolescent female. *Contemporary Pediatrics, 14*(2), 35–69.

Vogt, B. (1997). Identifying kidney disease. *Contemporary Pediatrics, 14*(3), 115–127.

Wong, D. (1997). *Whaley & Wong's essentials of pediatric nursing.* St. Louis, MO: Mosby.

Zook, R. (1997). Handling inappropriate sexual behavior with confidence. *Nursing 97, 27*(4), 65.

chapter 29

The Child with a Skin Condition

Outline

Objectives

On completion and mastery of Chapter 29, the student will be able to

- Define each vocabulary term listed.
- Recall the differences between the skin of the infant and that of the adult.
- Describe two topical agents used to treat acne.
- Summarize the nursing care for a child who has infantile eczema. State the rationale for each nursing measure.
- Discuss the symptoms and treatment of pediculosis.
- Differentiate among first-, second-, and third-degree burns in anatomic structures involved, appearance, level of sensation, and first aid required.
- List five objectives of the nurse caring for the burned child.
- Describe how the response of the child with burns differs from the adult.
- Identify the principles of topical therapy.
- Examine the emergency treatment of three types of burns.
- Differentiate four types of topical medication.
- Discuss the prevention and treatment of frostbite.

Vocabulary

allergens
alopecia
autograft
chilblain
comedones
crust
curling ulcer
débridement
dermabrasion
ecchymosis
emollient
eschar
exanthem
frostbite
heterografts
hives
homografts
ileus
isograft
macule
MRSA
papule
pediculosis
pruritus
pustule
sebum
TBSA
vesicle
xenograft

SKIN DEVELOPMENT AND FUNCTIONS

The main function of the skin is *protection.* It acts as the body's first line of defense against disease. It prevents the passage of harmful physical and chemical agents and *prevents the loss of water and electrolytes.* It also has a great capacity to regenerate and repair itself.The skin and the structures derived from it, such as hair and fingernails, are known as the *integumentary system.* Figure 29–1 depicts these structures and how they differ in the developing child and in the adult.

Maintaining skin integrity is important to self-esteem and therefore has a psychological as well as a physiologic component. This is particularly evident in patients with facial disfiguration. Four basic skin sensations—pain, temperature, touch, and pressure—are felt by the skin in conjunction with the nervous system. The skin also secretes sebum, which helps to protect and maintain its texture. The outer surface of the skin is acidic, with a pH of 4.5 to 6.5 to protect the skin from pathologic bacteria, which thrive in an alkaline environment.

The skin is composed of two layers: the epidermis, derived from the ectoderm, and the dermis, derived from the mesoderm. Vernix caseosa, a

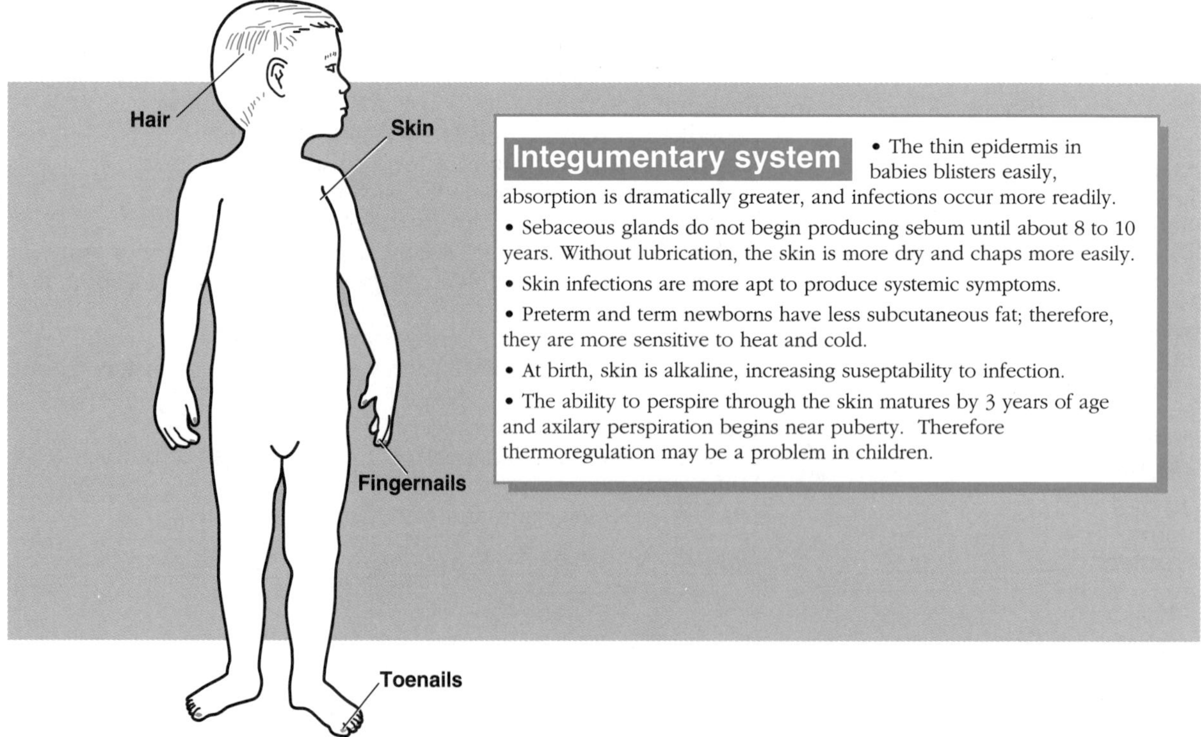

Figure 29–1. • Summary of some integumentary system differences between the child and the adult. The integumentary system consists of the skin and the structures derived from it. This system protects the body, helps to regulate body temperature, and receives stimuli such as pressure, pain, and temperature.

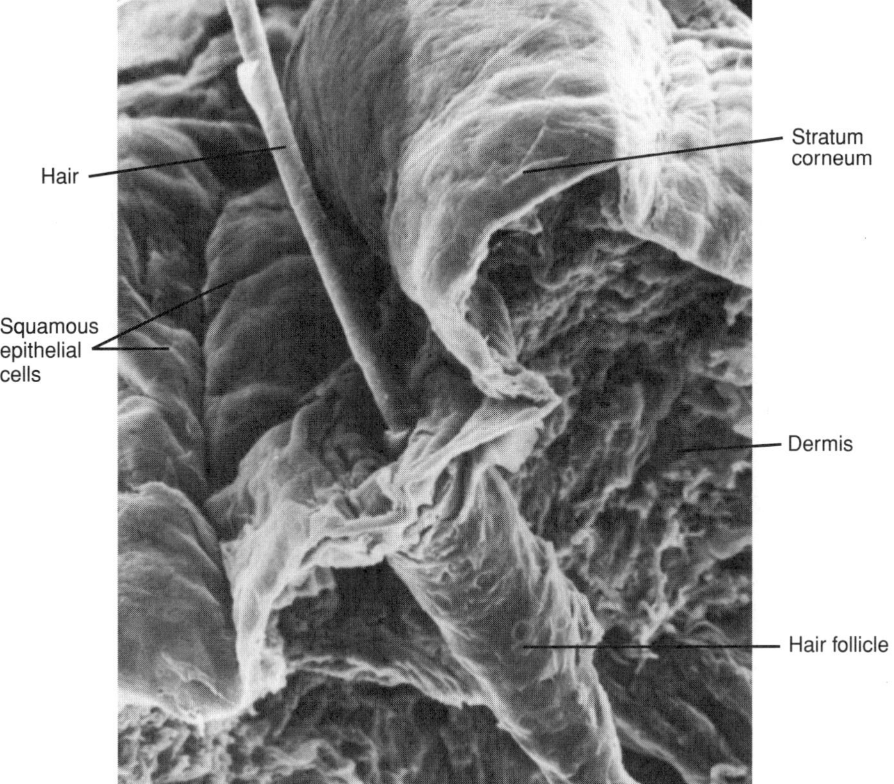

Figure 29–2. • Scanning electron micrograph of human skin showing hair follicle, approximately 250 times life size. (Courtesy of Dr. Karen A. Holbrook. From Solomon, E. P., & Phillips, G. A. [1987]. *Understanding human anatomy and physiology* [p. 62]. Philadelphia: Saunders.)

cheeselike substance, covers the fetus until birth. This protects the fetal skin from maceration as it floats in its watery home. The fetal skin is at first so transparent that blood vessels are clearly visible. Downy lanugo hair begins to develop at about 13 to 16 weeks, especially on the head. At 21 to 24 weeks, the skin is reddish and wrinkled, with little subcutaneous fat. Adipose tissue forms during later weeks. At birth, the subcutaneous glands are well developed, and the skin is pink and smooth with a polished look. It is thinner than the skin of an adult. Figure 29–2 is an electron micrograph of human skin with a hair follicle.

Certain skin conditions in children may be associated with age, as in the case of milia in babies and acne in adolescents. A skin condition may be a manifestation of a systemic disease, such as chickenpox. Some lesions, such as strawberry nevi and mongolian spots, are congenital. Other skin lesions, such as those seen in rubella and fifth disease, are self-limited and do not require treatment.

There are great individual differences in skin texture, color, pH, and moisture. Skin color is an important diagnostic criterion in cases of liver disease, heart conditions, and child abuse and for overall assessment. Complete blood counts and serum electrolyte levels are helpful in diagnosing skin conditions. Skin tests are used in diagnosing allergies. The tine test is useful in screening for tuberculosis. Skin scrapings are used for microscopic examination. The Wood light is an instrument used to diagnose certain skin conditions. It reflects a particular color according to the organism present.

Hair condition is important to observe. Hair is inspected for color, texture, quality, distribution, and elasticity. Hair may become dry and brittle and may lack luster owing to inadequate nutrition. Hair may begin to fall out or even change color during illness or the ingestion of certain medications.

Skin conditions may be acute or chronic. The nurse should describe the lesions with regard to size, color, configuration (e.g., butterfly rash), presence of pain or itching, distribution (e.g., arms, legs, behind ears), and whether the rash is general or local. *Hives,* a general rash that appears abruptly, is frequently an allergic or medication reaction. The condition of the skin around the lesions is also significant, as is the skin turgor. Managing itching is a key component in preventing secondary infection from scratching. Dressings and ointments are applied as prescribed. Preventing tetanus is a consideration in open wounds. Mongolian spots and physiologic jaundice are covered in

BOX 29–1
TERMS USED TO DESCRIBE SKIN CONDITIONS

Ecchymosis: black and blue-purple mark (bruise)

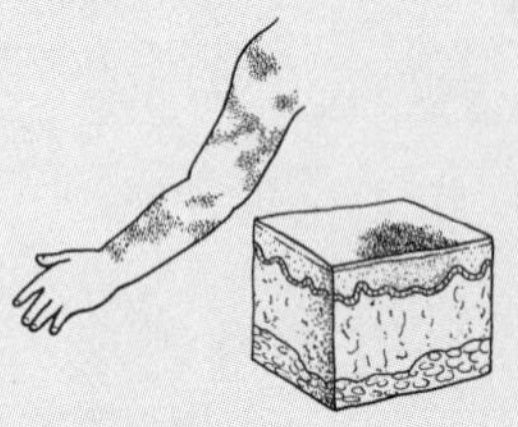

Crust: scab

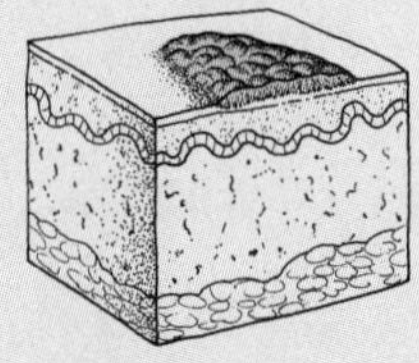

Macule: flat rash (freckles)

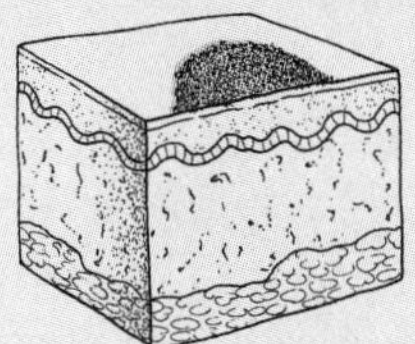

Papule: elevated area (pimple)

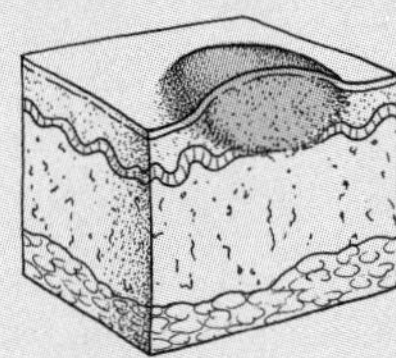

Pustules: elevated, pus filled (impetigo, acne)

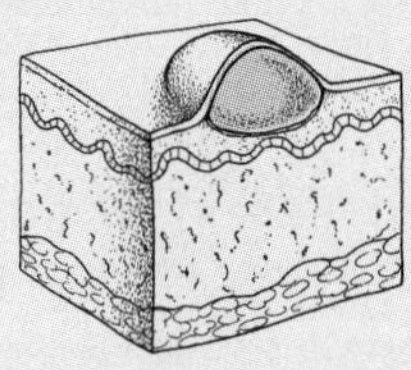

Stye: infection of eyelash follicle

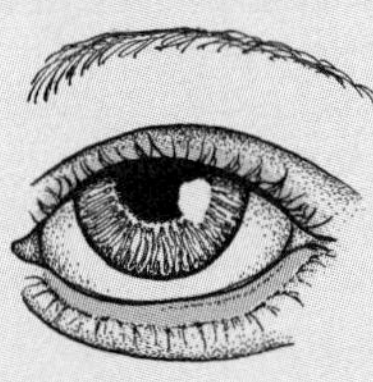

Vesicle: elevated fluid-filled blister (cold sore, chickenpox)

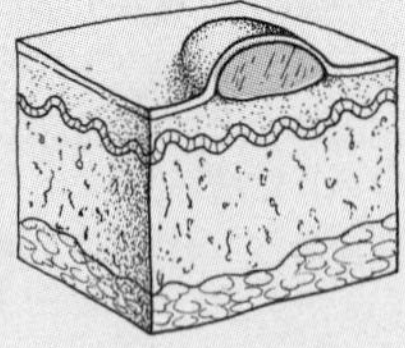

Wheal: raised red, irregular (mosquito bite, allergic reactions)

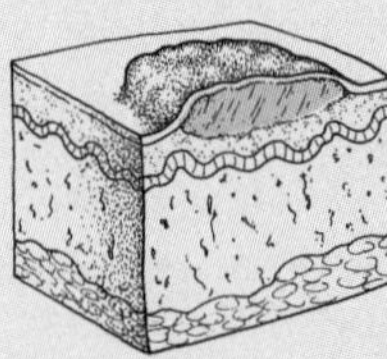

Chapter 12. The communicable diseases are discussed in Chapter 31.

Skin Lesions. Many childhood infectious diseases, such as measles (see Color Plate Fig. 3), German measles (see Color Plate Fig. 4), and chickenpox (see Color Plate Fig. 5), involve the presence of an *exanthem* (a skin rash). Box 29–1 identifies terms used to describe some conditions of the skin that the nurse may witness. Some rashes begin as one lesion and evolve into others. For example, the pattern of chickenpox rash is macule, papule, vesicle, and crust.

CONGENITAL LESIONS

Strawberry Nevus

The strawberry nevus is a common *hemangioma,* which may not become apparent for a few weeks after birth. Although it is harmless and disappears without treatment, it is disturbing to parents, especially when it appears on the head or face (Fig. 29–3). At first it is flat, but it gradually becomes raised. The lesion is bright red, elevated, and sharply demarcated. The lesions gradually blanch, and 60% disappear spontaneously by 5 years of age; 90% by 9 years of age. Laser treatment or excision may be considered if the area becomes ulcerated. Parents are frequently quizzed about the growth by insensitive persons and may be advised of various unorthodox treatments. The nurse offers support and reassurance to parents and corrects misinformation.

Port Wine Nevus

Port wine nevi are present at birth and are due to dilated dermal capillaries. The lesions are flat, sharply demarcated, and purple to pink. The lesion darkens as the child gets older. If the area is small, cosmetics may disguise the lesion. If the area is large, laser surgery may be indicated.

INFECTIONS

Miliaria

Description. Miliaria (prickly heat) refers to a rash caused by excess body heat and moisture. There is retention of sweat in the sweat glands, which have become blocked or inflamed. Rupture or leakage into the skin causes the inflamed response. It appears suddenly as tiny pinhead-sized reddened papules with occasional clear vesicles. It may be accompanied by *pruritus* (itching). It is seen in infants during hot weather or in newborns who sleep in overheated rooms. It often occurs in the diaper area or in the folds of the skin where moisture accumulates. Plastic enclosures on diapers

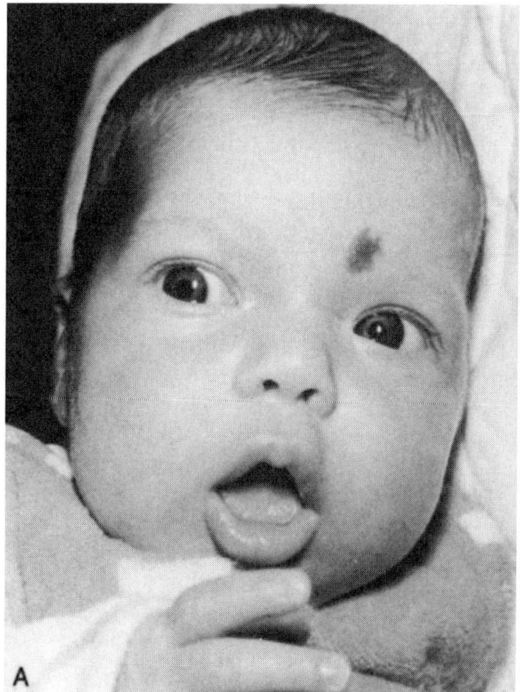

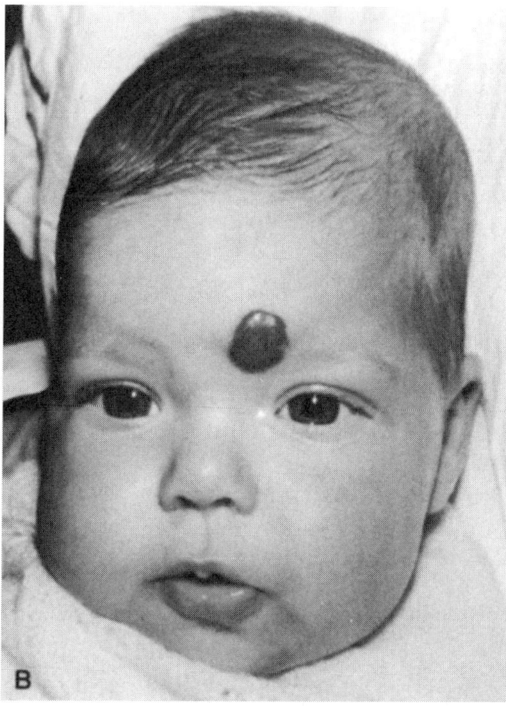

Figure 29–3. • Strawberry nevus. **A,** Appearance 4 days after birth. **B,** Appearance 6 weeks later; the nevus has enlarged and become raised above the skin. This minor lesion can result in major psychological problems. (From Beischer, N. A., & MacKay, E. B. [1986]. *Obstetrics and the newborn* [2nd ed., p. 637]. Philadelphia: Saunders/Bailliere Tindall.)

hold in body warmth that results in a rash. This harmless condition may be reversed by removing extra clothing, bathing, skin care, and frequent diaper changes.

Intertrigo

Description. Intertrigo (*in,* "into," and *terere,* "to rub") is the medical term for chafing (see Color Plate Fig. 6). It is a dermatitis that occurs in the folds of the skin. The patches are red and moist and are usually along the neck and in the inguinal and gluteal folds. This condition is aggravated by urine, feces, heat, and moisture. Prevention consists of keeping the affected areas clean and *dry.* The child is allowed to be out of diapers to expose the area to air and light (Fig. 29–4). Maceration of the skin can lead to secondary infections.

Seborrheic Dermatitis

Description. Seborrheic dermatitis (cradle cap) is an inflammation of the skin that involves the sebaceous glands (see Color Plate Fig. 7). It is characterized by thick, yellow, oily, adherent, crustlike scales on the scalp and forehead. The skin beneath the patches may be red. Less often it may involve the eyelids, external ear, and inguinal area. Secondary bacterial and yeast infections may occur. It is seen in newborns, in infants, and at puberty. In newborns it is commonly known as "cradle cap." It is seen in babies with sensitive skin, even when the head and hair are washed frequently. Seborrhea resembles eczema; however, it usually does not itch and there is a negative family history. In adolescence it is more localized, usually confined to the scalp. A condition resembling seborrheic dermatitis is common in human immunodeficiency virus (HIV)–infected children and adolescents.

Treatment. Treatment consists of shampooing the hair on a regular basis. In newborns if the scales are particularly stubborn, they may be softened by applying baby oil to the head the evening before and shampooing the hair in the morning. The scalp is rinsed well. A soft brush is helpful in removing loose particles from the hair. The nurse teaches the parent how to shampoo an infant's head using the football hold (see Chapter 22, Fig. 22-4). In adolescents a dandruff-control shampoo is used. Medications such as sulfur, salicylic acid, or hydrocortisone may be prescribed. Topical antifungal agents effective against *Pityrosporum* have also been suggested. Response is usually rapid.

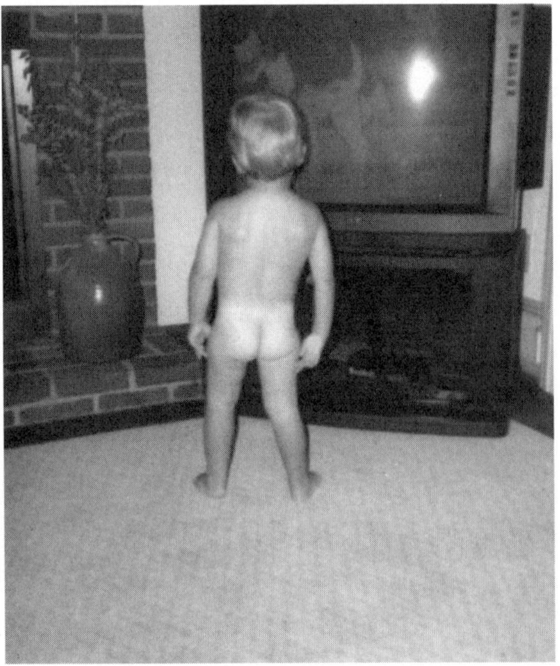

Figure 29–4. • The child with chafing or a rash in the diaper area benefits from periods of exposure to air and/or sunlight.

Diaper Dermatitis

Description. Diaper dermatitis (diaper rash) is a frequently seen condition that results when the skin becomes irritated by prolonged contact with urine, feces, retained laundry soaps, and friction. It may be seen in response to the addition of solid foods or with a change in breast or bottle feedings. Changes in detergent, water softeners, the use of wipes that contain fragrance or chemicals, or other household substances may precipitate the irritation. The rash may appear as a simple erythema (redness) (see Color Plate Fig. 8) or may be evidenced by scales, blisters, and ulcerations. Perianal involvement may be apparent if the baby has loose stools. A beefy red rash in the diaper area may be indicative of a *Candida* (thrush) infection.

Treatment and Nursing Care. It is easier to prevent diaper rash than to cure it. This is accomplished by frequent diaper changes to limit the exposure to moisture. The diaper is periodically removed to expose the skin to light and air. With each diaper change, the perineal area is thoroughly cleansed (preferably with warm water) and gently dried. Plastic pants are avoided. After bowel movements, the area is cleansed with mild soap and water. *The skin folds are thoroughly washed, rinsed, and dried.* If a rash is persistent, the pediatrician may prescribe a light application of a mild hydrocortisone ointment. Superabsorbent disposable diapers reduce the occurrence of diaper rash, but frequent diaper changes and skin care remain essential. Petrolatum, A and D ointment, or zinc oxide ointment are protective ointments that can be applied between diaper changes and removed with mineral oil before reapplying after a diaper change.

Acne Vulgaris

Description. Acne is an inflammation of the sebaceous glands and hair follicles in the skin (see Color Plate Fig. 9). At puberty, because of hormonal influence, the sebaceous follicles enlarge and secrete increased amounts of a fatty substance called *sebum.* Genetic factors and stress are also thought to play a part. The course of acne may be brief or prolonged (lasting 10 years or longer). Premenstrual acne in girls is not uncommon. The principal lesions include comedones, papules, and nodulocystic growths.

A *comedo* (plural, *comedones*) is a plug of keratin, sebum, and bacteria. Keratin is a protein substance that is the main constituent of epidermis and hair. There are two types of comedones, open and closed. In the open comedo, or blackhead, the surface is darkened by melanin. Closed comedones, or whiteheads, are responsible for the inflammatory process of acne. With continued buildup, the walls of the follicle rupture, releasing their irritating contents into the surrounding skin. A pustule may appear when this develops near the exterior. This process occurs no matter how carefully the teenager washes because surface bacteria are not involved in the pathogenesis. Acne is usually seen on the chin, cheeks, and forehead. It can also develop on the chest, upper back, and shoulders. It usually is more severe in winter.

Treatment. The basic treatment of acne has changed considerably over the past few years. It is no longer thought that certain foods trigger the condition: therefore, restriction of chocolate, peanuts, and cola drinks is unwarranted. A regular, well-balanced diet is encouraged. Patients who are not taking tetracycline or vitamin A benefit from sunshine. General hygienic measures of cleanliness, rest, and avoidance of emotional stress may help to prevent exacerbations.

Routine skin cleansing is indicated, and greasy hair and cosmetic preparations should be avoided. Excessive cleansing of the skin can be harmful, however, since it irritates and chaps the tissues. Squeezing pimples ruptures intact lesions and causes local inflammation. The topical preparations recommended include benzoyl peroxide gels, such as Benzagel, Panoxyl, or Desquam-X, which dry and peel the skin and suppress fatty acid growth. Vitamin A acid (Retin-A) help to eliminate keratinous plugs. Vitamin A acid can increase sensitivity to the sun, so precautions should be taken when it is used. Tetracycline or erythromycin may be given in conjunction with topical medications in more serious cases. Monilial vaginitis is a secondary complication sometimes seen when these drugs are used, and this should be explained to the unsuspecting teenage girl. Topical antibiotics such as clindamycin (Cleocin T) or erythromycin (T-Stat, A/T/S) are also available.

> **Nursing Tip**
>
> Topical Benzoyl Peroxide and Retin-A neutralize each other when applied together.

Isotretinoin (Accutane) is given to patients with severe pustulocystic acne who have been unable to benefit from other types of treatment. It has many side effects; thus the patient must be carefully monitored. *It is not prescribed during pregnancy or to those at risk for pregnancy because of the possibilities of fetal deformity.* Planing of the skin to minimize scarring *(dermabrasion)* is done selectively, as it is not always successful.

Acne is distressing to the adolescent, particularly when the face is extensively involved. Sometimes even a minimum problem is seen as disastrous when it happens before an important event. The self-conscious young person feels different and embarrassed. The nurse who is attuned to the feelings of individuals can provide understanding support. Although the teenager is educated to assume responsibility for the regimen, including the parents helps to prevent conflict surrounding it. Drug-induced acne can be a problem for children on long-term steroids, phenobarbital, phenytoin, lithium, vitamin B_{12}, or medications containing iodides or bromides.

Herpes Simplex Type I

Description. Herpes simplex type I, a viral infection, is commonly known as a cold sore or fever blister. It may begin by a feeling of tingling, itching, or burning on the lip. Vesicles and crusts form (see Color Plate Fig. 10). Spontaneous healing occurs in about 8 to 10 days. Communicability is highest early in the formation and is spread by direct contact. Recurrence is common because the virus lies dormant in the body until it is activated by stress, sun exposure, menstruation, fever, and other causes. Patients need to become familiar with their own personal triggers. Herpes can be serious in newborns and in patients who are immunocompromised.

Treatment and Nursing Care. Topical acyclovir may reduce viral shedding and hasten healing. In the hospital, ointments are applied with gloved hands. Contact (standard) precautions should be followed (see Appendix A). Patients are instructed not to pick at lesions, as this may cause spreading to other sites. They should not share lipstick and should avoid kissing while lesions are active. Sensitivity to the self-conscious teenager who has a cold sore is important. Genital herpes caused by the herpes virus type II and spread by sexual intimacy is discussed in Chapter 11, Table 11–1. The distinction between the two types has become less clear because of an increase in the practice of oral-genital sex.

Infantile Eczema

Description. Infantile eczema, or atopic dermatitis, is an inflammation of genetically hypersensitive skin. The pathophysiology is characterized by local vasodilatation in affected areas. This progresses to *spongiosis,* or the breakdown of dermal cells and the formation of intradermal vesicles. Chronic scratching produces weeping and results in lichenification, or coarsening, of the skin folds. The exact cause of this condition is difficult to pinpoint, as it is believed to be mainly due to allergy. Infantile eczema is rarely seen in breastfed babies until they begin to eat additional food. It seems to follow a definite familial history of allergies; emotional factors are often involved.

Eczema actually is a symptom rather than a disorder. It indicates that the infant is oversensitive to certain substances called *allergens,* which enter the body via the digestive tract (food), by inhalation (dust, pollen), by direct contact (wool, soap, strong sunlight), and by injections (insect bites, vaccines). Some children develop the triad of atopic dermatitis, asthma, and hay fever.

Manifestations. Although infantile eczema can occur at any age, it is more common during the first 2 years. The pruritic lesions form vesicles that weep and develop a dry crust. They are more severe on the face, but may occur on the entire body, particularly in the skin folds (see Color Plate Fig. 11). Eczema is worse in the winter than in the summer and has periods of temporary remission.

The baby scratches because the itching is constant, and he or she is irritable and unable to sleep. The lesions become easily infected by bacterial or viral agents. Infants and children with eczema should not be exposed to adults with "cold sores" because they may develop a systemic reaction with high fever and multiple vesicles on the eczematous skin. Eczema may flare up following immunization. Laboratory studies may show an increase in immunoglobulin E and eosinophil levels.

Treatment and Nursing Care. Treatment of the child with infantile eczema is aimed at promoting comfort by relieving symptoms. An emollient bath is sometimes ordered for its soothing effect on the skin. Oatmeal and a mixture of cornstarch and baking soda are examples of substances prescribed. The baby's hair is washed with a soap substitute rather than a shampoo. Some dermatologists believe that bathing should be kept to a minimum. The physician may suggest that a bath oil such as Alpha-Keri be used as the lesions begin to heal. This prevents the skin from becoming too dry. To be correctly used, bath oils should be added after the patient has soaked for a while and the skin is hydrated. In this way, moisture is sealed rather than excluded, as it is when oil is added before the patient gets into the tub. Whenever possible, patients are treated at home because of the danger of infection in the hospital.

Corticosteroids may be administered systemically or locally. Antibiotics are needed if infection is present. Medication to help to relieve itching is ordered for the patient. A child who is uncomfortable and unable to sleep should receive sedation.

The nurse plays a vital role in the treatment of patients with skin problems (Nursing Care Plan 29–1). The nurse should assess the ability of the family to cope with care of this child at home. Techniques of home bathing or application of soaks combined with quiet playtime enhances family coping. Control of itching is essential. Ointments are applied with a gloved hand to minimize contact with the skin. The fingernails of the child are cut short and cotton gloves or socks can be used to prevent scratching. Appropriate dress is advised, as are using cotton fabric and avoiding wool and stuffed animals due to their allergy potential. Clothes should be laundered using mild soaps and avoiding products that contain fragrances or harsh chemicals. Parents should be taught the principles of general hygiene to avoid secondary infection of the open skin lesions. A hypoallergenic formula and a plan to identify possible food allergens are explained to parents. The types of topical medications are listed in Table 29–1.

Parent Teaching Concerning Topical Therapy. Skin lesions can be pruritic (itchy) scaling, weeping,

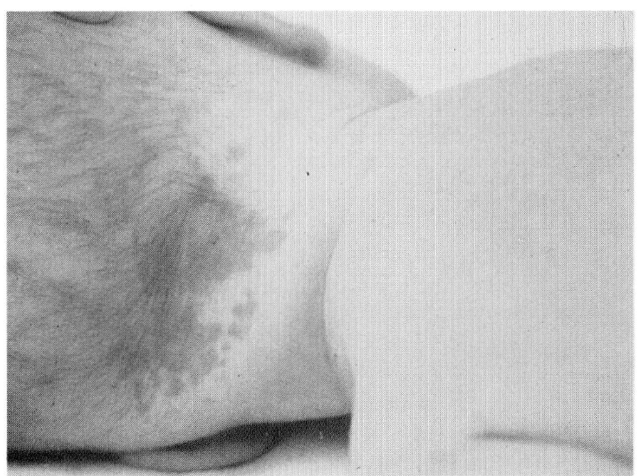

Figure 1. Stork bites (telangiectatic nevi). These flat, red areas are seen on the nape of the neck and on the eyelids. They result from the dilation of small vessels. (Courtesy of Jane Deacon, MS, RN, NNP, The Children's Hospital, Denver, CO.)

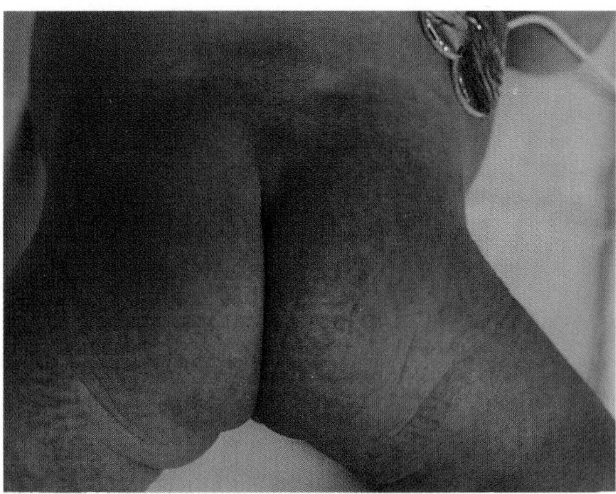

Figure 2. Mongolian spots (hyperpigmentation) are bluish discolorations of the skin, found mainly in newborns with dark skin tones. The sacral and gluteal areas are the usual sites. (From Gorrie, T. S., McKinney, E. S., Murray, S. S. [1994]. *Foundations of maternal newborn nursing.* Philadelphia: W. B. Saunders.)

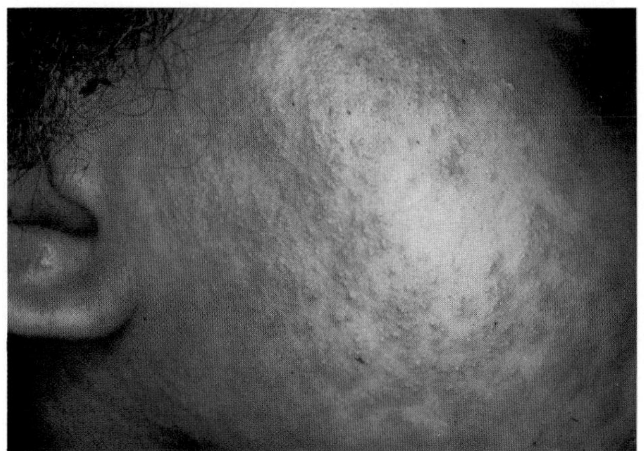

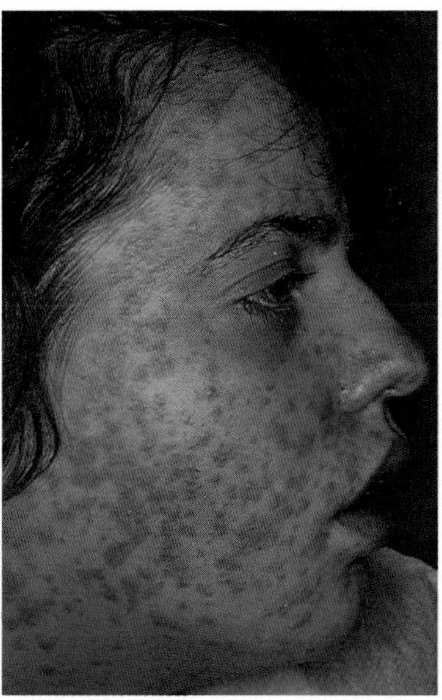

Figure 3. Measles (rubeola). Red-purple maculopapular blotchy rash in dark skin (*A*) and in light skin (*B*) appears on third or fourth day of illness. Rash appears first behind ears and spreads over face, then over neck, trunk, arms and legs; looks "coppery" and does not blanch. Also characterized by Koplik's spots in mouth—bluish white, red-based elevations of 1 to 3 mm. (*A*, From Feigin, R. D., & Cherry, J. D. [1987]. *Textbook of pediatric infectious diseases* [2nd ed.]. Philadelphia: W. B. Saunders, p. 807. *B*, From Hurwitz, S. [1981]. *Clinical pediatric dermatology: A textbook of skin disorders of childhood and adolescence*. Philadelphia: W. B. Saunders, p. 350.)

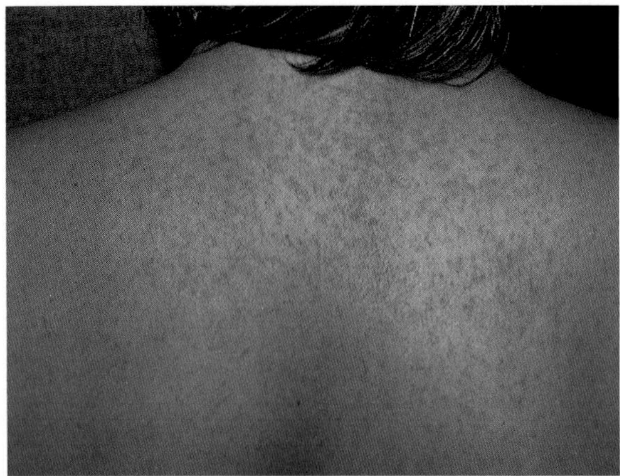

Figure 4. German measles (rubella). Pink papular rash (similar to measles but paler) first appears on face, then spreads. Distinguished from measles by presence of neck lymphadenopathy and absence of Koplik's spots. (From Hurwitz, S. [1993]. *Clinical pediatric dermatology: A textbook of skin disorders of childhood and adolescence* [2nd ed.]. Philadelphia: W. B. Saunders, p. 356.)

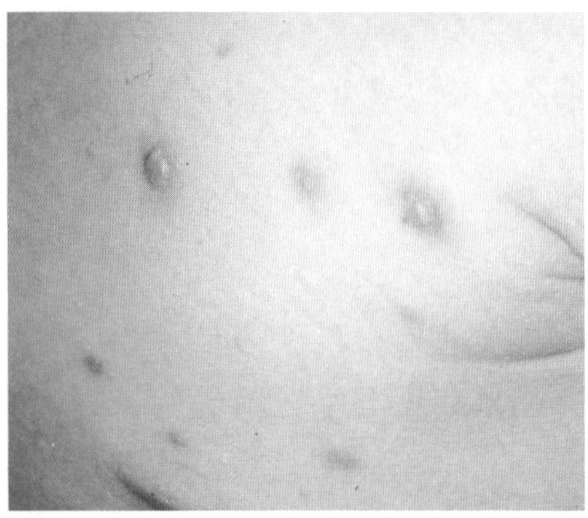

Figure 5. Chicken pox (varicella). Small tight vesicles first appear on trunk, then spread to face, arms, and legs (not palms or soles). Vesicles erupt in succeeding crops over several days, then become pustules, and then crusts. Intensely pruritic. (From Feigin, R. D., & Cherry, J. D. [1987]. *Textbook of pediatric infectious diseases* [2nd ed.]. Philadelphia: W. B. Saunders, p. 807.)

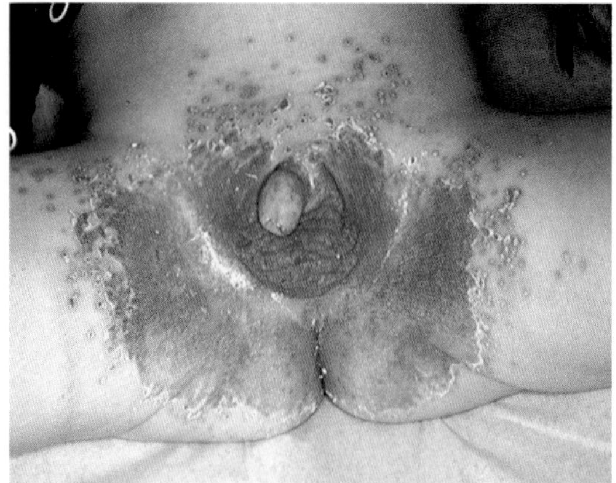

Figure 6. Intertrigo (candidiasis). Red, moist patches with sharply demarcated borders, some loose scales. Usually in genital area extending along inguinal and gluteal folds. Infectious disease aggravated by urine, feces, heat, moisture. (From Hurwitz, S. [1993]. *Clinical pediatric dermatology: A textbook of skin disorders of childhood and adolescence* [2nd ed.]. Philadelphia: W. B. Saunders, p. 36.)

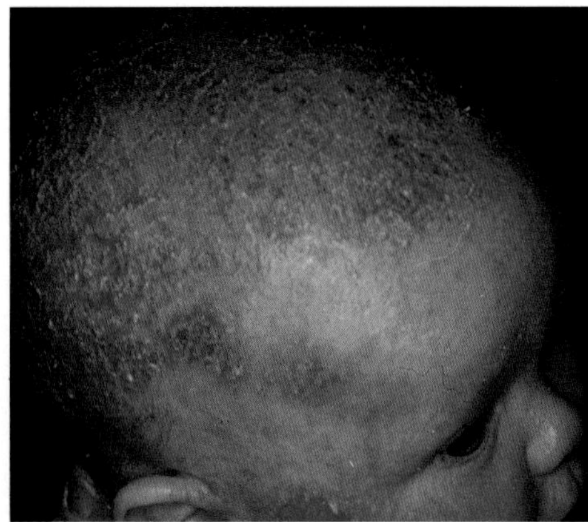

Figure 7. Seborrheic dermatitis (cradle cap). Thick, yellow, greasy, adherent scales on scalp and forehead; very common in early infancy. Resembles eczema lesions except cradle cap is distinguished by absence of pruritus, "greasy" yellow-pink lesions, and negative family history of allergy. (From Hurwitz, S. [1993]. *Clinical pediatric dermatology: A textbook of skin disorders of childhood and adolescence* [2nd ed.]. Philadelphia: W. B. Saunders, p. 17.)

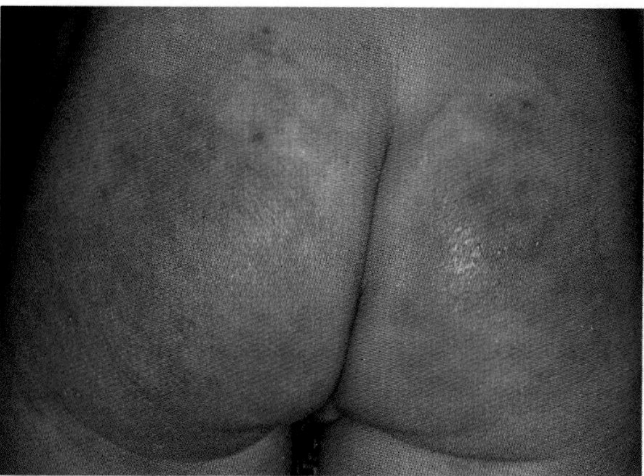

Figure 8. Diaper dermatitis. Red moist maculopapular patch with poorly defined borders in diaper area, extending along inguinal and gluteal folds. History of infrequent diaper changes or occlusive coverings. Inflammatory disease due to skin irritation from ammonia, heat, moisture, occlusive diapers. (From Hurwitz, S. [1993]. *Clinical pediatric dermatology: A textbook of skin disorders of childhood and adolescence* [2nd ed.]. Philadelphia: W. B. Saunders, p. 37.)

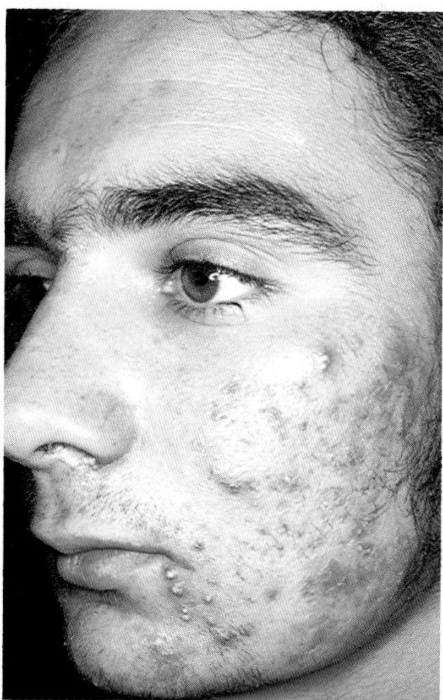

Figure 9. Acne. Acne is the most common skin problem of adolescence. An increase in sebaceous gland activity creates increased oiliness. Almost all teens have some acne, even if it is the milder form of open comedones (blackheads) and closed comedones (whiteheads). Severe acne includes papules, pustules, and nodules. The lesions usually appear on the face and sometimes on the chest, back, and shoulders. (From Hurwitz, S. [1993]. *Clinical pediatric dermatology: A textbook of skin disorders of childhood and adolescence* [2nd ed.]. Philadelphia: W. B. Saunders, p. 137.)

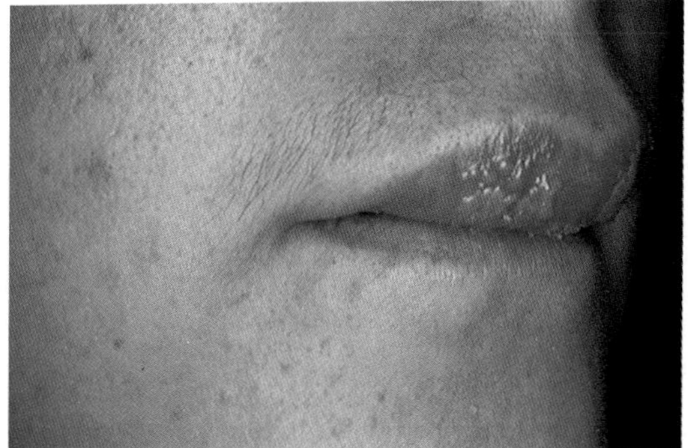

Figure 10. Herpes simplex (cold sores). Begins with skin tingling and sensitivity. Erupts with tight vesicles, then pustules, then crust. Common location is upper lip; also appears in genitalia. (From Hurwitz, S. [1993]. *Clinical pediatric dermatology: A textbook of skin disorders of childhood and adolescence* [2nd ed.]. Philadelphia: W. B. Saunders, p. 321.)

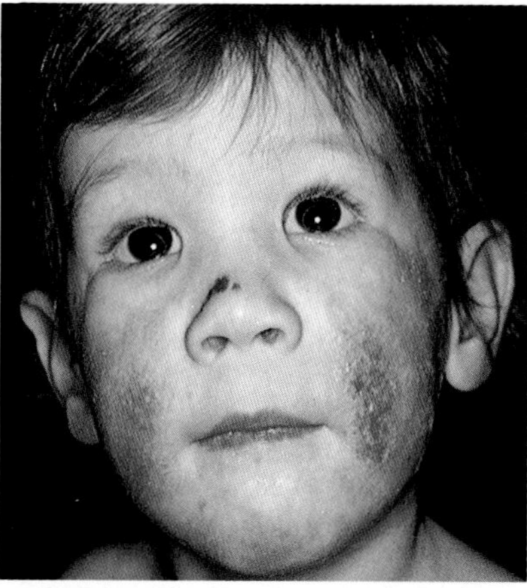

Figure 11. Infantile eczema (atopic dermatitis). Erythematous papules and vesicles, with weeping, oozing, and crusts. Lesions usually on scalp, forehead, cheeks, forearms and wrists, elbows, backs of knees. Paroxysmal and severe pruritus. Family history of allergies. (From Hurwitz, S. [1993]. *Clinical pediatric dermatology: A textbook of skin disorders of childhood and adolescence* [2nd ed.]. Philadelphia: W. B. Saunders, p. 280.)

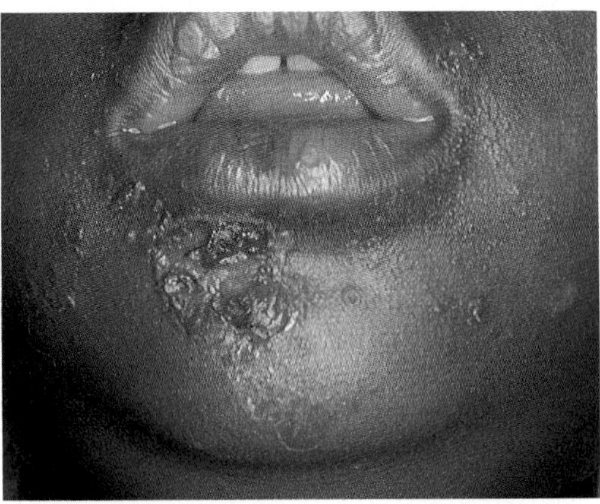

Figure 12. Impetigo. Moist, thin-roofed vesicles with thin erythematous base. Rupture to form thick honey-colored crusts. Contagious bacterial infection of skin; most common in infants and children. (From Hurwitz, S. [1993]. *Clinical pediatric dermatology: A textbook of skin disorders of childhood and adolescence* [2nd ed.]. Philadelphia: W. B. Saunders, p. 280.)

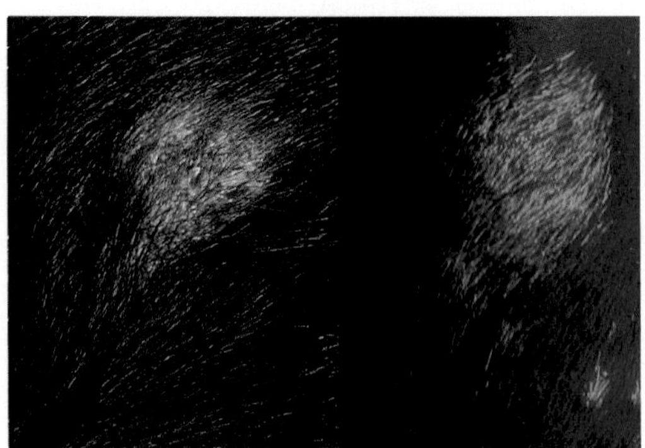

Figure 13. Tinea capitis (scalp ringworm). Rounded patchy hair loss on scalp, leaving broken off hairs, pustules, and scales on skin. Due to fungal infection; lesions fluoresce under Wood's light. Usually seen in children and farmers; highly contagious. (From Lookingbill, D. P., & Marks, J. G. [1993]. *Principles of dermatology* [2nd ed.]. Philadelphia: W. B. Saunders, p. 282.)

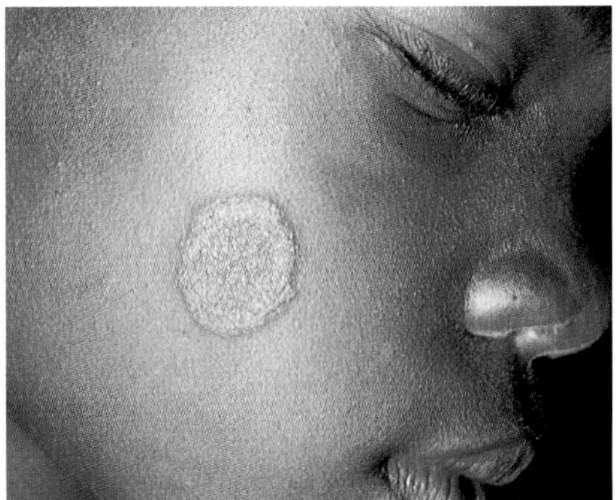

Figure 14. Tinea corporis (ringworm of the body). Scales—hyperpigmented in whites, depigmented in dark-skinned persons—on chest, abdomen, back of arms, forming multiple circular lesions with clear centers. (From Hurwitz, S. [1993]. *Clinical pediatric dermatology: A textbook of skin disorders of childhood and adolescence* [2nd ed.]. Philadelphia: W. B. Saunders, p. 380.)

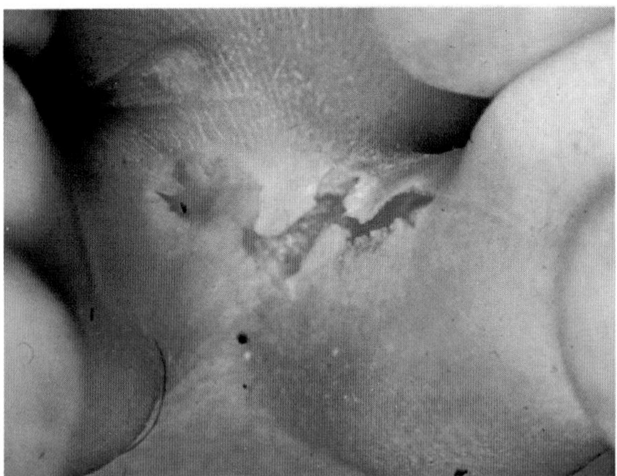

Figure 15. Tinea pedis (ringworm of the foot). "Athlete's foot," a fungal infection, first appears as small vesicles between toes, sides of feet, soles. Then grows scaly and hard. Found in chronically warm moist feet: children after gymnasium activities, athletes, aging adults who cannot dry their feet well. (From Feigin, R. D., & Cherry, J. D. [1987]. *Textbook of pediatric infectious diseases* [2nd ed.]. Philadelphia: W. B. Saunders, p. 813.)

NURSING CARE PLAN 29–1

Selected Nursing Diagnoses for the Child with Eczema

Nursing Diagnosis: Skin integrity impaired related to inflammation

Goals	Nursing Interventions	Rationale
Child's skin does not show signs of irritation or infection	1. Describe types of lesions, configuration, and location	1. Eczema has a typical pattern of distribution; vesicles, oozing, and crusting may denote infection
	2. Provide supervision rather than restraints whenever possible	2. Elbow restraints may assist in avoiding self-inflicted skin damage due to scratching and picking; restriction of movement to infants has been related to learning difficulties and other problems, therefore, judicious application of any restraint is necessary
	3. Keep fingernails short	3. Trimming fingernails and covering hands with "sock mittens" will reduce excoriation from scratching
	4. Administer medicated baths such as Aveeno	4. Medicated baths soothe and rehydrate the skin
	5. Apply wet dressings	5. Wet dressings promote cooling of the skin, which decreases inflammation and itching (pruritus)
	6. Adminsiter oral antibiotics and sedatives as prescribed	6. Systemic antibiotics such as erythromycin may be prescribed if there is an infection; sedatives reduce itching
	7. Apply steroid ointments as prescribed	7. Steroid creams reduce inflammation

Nursing Diagnosis: High risk for altered nutrition—less than body requirements, related to irritability, sensitivity to certain foods

Goals	Nursing Interventions	Rationale
Child will eat portions of each meal and maintain weight Child receives adequate nutrition as evidenced by growth charts and other parameters	1. Serve hypoallergenic diet if prescribed	1. This is a basic diet in which only one new food is added at a time to determine whether the infant is allergic to it
	2. Determine specific food sensitivities from parents if child is not on diet	2. Parents have the most knowledge from experience with their child
	3. Observe child for food sensitivities	3. Any food can produce allergic symptoms, but some are thought to be highly allergenic; certain antigens (foreign protein) may enter the bloodstream and activate antibody formation of immune system; one reason this takes place during infancy is that a baby's gastrointestinal tract is immature; allergy may be outgrown as body systems mature
	4. Administer vitamins and mineral supplements as prescribed	4. Child may be deficient in nutrients owing to irritability and food restrictions; adequate intake of vitamins and minerals is essential to the maintenance of healthy skin (particularly vitamins A, B, and C)
	5. Provide adequate fluids	5. Adequate hydration prevents drying of the skin and pruritus, and it makes the skin less prone to breaks, which can become infected

(Continued)

NURSING CARE PLAN 29–1 *continued*

Selected Nursing Diagnoses for the Child with Eczema

Nursing Diagnosis: Knowledge deficit (parents) related to nature of disorder

Goals	Nursing Interventions	Rationale
Parents verbalize understanding of potential allergens Parents state that they have an understanding of disease process	1. Advise parents to remove articles that irritate skin, for example, wool, and to provide loose cotton clothing	1. Clothing with rough and tightly woven fibers will prevent natural evaporation from skin; wool may cause an allergic reaction; sweating increases itching
	2. Encourage parents to use mild detergents, rinse clothes thoroughly	2. Avoiding strong detergents and rinsing clothing thoroughly will prevent skin flareups
	3. Expose infant to sunlight, but monitor carefully	3. Although sunlight is beneficial, overexposure to ultraviolet rays can seriously damage the skin; infants and young children require special protection from the sun because their epidermis is thin; exposure time should be brief, even on hazy days
	4. Help parents to identify products in which wheat, milk, eggs may not be readily apparent	4. Food labels are read carefully to determine content
	5. Advise parents to expect exacerbations and remissions	5. Eczema is a chronic disease that takes time and energy to control

or crusted. Most skin lesions cause psychological stress, which should be addressed for both the parents and the child with the skin lesion. Prevention of secondary infection is essential and the nurse should help the parent to understand the signs of inflammation or infection. When topical medication is applied, the lesions may change in form or color as they heal. Parents should be advised of changes to expect and when to seek follow-up advice. The nurse should teach parents the principles and techniques of applying topical medication, which includes:

Table 29–1

TYPES OF TOPICAL MEDICATIONS

Type	Definition
Cream	A water-based emulsion of oil in water that is nongreasy for use on weeping lesions
Ointment	An oil-based emulsion of water in oil that is clear and greasy. Used on dry skin; does not rub off easily
Lotion	A suspension of powder in water that sould be shaken well before using. It may be drying. Often used on scalp lesions
Aerosol spray	Suspension of medication in an alcohol base. Alcohol evaporates, leaving medication on the skin. Effective for hairy areas
Gel	A clear, semisolid emulsion. Liquefies when applied to skin
Bath oils	Bath oils are not used in pediatrics because they lubricate the sides of the tub, causing falls and injuries. The value of the treatment must be weighed with the risks involved. Colloidal oatmeal baths may be soothing

- Absorption is best when an ointment is applied following a warm bath.
- Medication should be applied by stroking in the direction of hair growth. (Circular or rubbing motions can inflame hair follicles).
- The use of elbow restraints can prevent an infant from scratching while allowing freedom of movement.

Over-the-Counter Skin Products. Parents should be guided in the use of over-the-counter products that affect skin health. Simple ointments such as petrolatum, A & D, and zinc oxide are helpful only if they are washed off completely between diaper changes. Cornstarch can support *Candida* infection and should be avoided. Frequent diaper changes are essential. High-absorbency disposable diapers decrease wetness of the skin and commercially laundered cloth diapers kill organisms on the diaper. Both help to prevent diaper dermatitis. Home-laundered diapers are not subject to high temperatures and soaps often contain fragrances that may be irritating. Commercially pre-

Nursing Tip

Parents should be taught that "kissing a wound to make it better" can introduce organisms that can cause infection.

pared wipes can leave the skin moist; warm water and a mild soap are less irritating. If paper towels are used, prints should be avoided as the color dyes can be irritating to the skin. Cortisone creams should be avoided, because it may temporarily clear the rash but does not resolve the underlying cause that will prevent recurrence.

Staphylococcal Infection

Description. The genus of bacteria called *Staphylococcus* comprises common bacteria that are found in dust and on the skin. Under normal conditions, they do not present a problem to the healthy body's defenses. If the number of organisms increases in preterm and newborns, whose general resistance is low, skin infections may occur. An abscess may form, and infection may enter the bloodstream. This condition is called *septicemia.* Pneumonia, osteomyelitis, or meningitis may result. Primary infection of the newborn may develop in the umbilicus or circumcision wound. It may occur while the newborn is in the hospital or after discharge. This infection spreads readily from one infant to another. Small pustules on the newborn must immediately be reported.

Treatment and Nursing Care. Antibiotics effective against the appropriate strain of *Staphylococcus* are administered. Ointments may be locally applied. In past years, the staphylococci that invaded the body developed resistance to the drugs in current use. Methicillin-resistant *Staphylococcus aureus* (MRSA) infections are resistant to antibiotics and are handled under strict isolation (standard) precautions. The use of disposable individual equipment for patients and aseptic techniques can decrease nosocomial spread.

Scalded skin syndrome is caused by *S. aureus.* The lesions begin with a mild erythema with sandpaper texture, vesicles appear, rupture and peeling occurs, leaving a bright red surface exposed. The skin looks as if it had been scalded and often child abuse is suspected. Intravenous antibiotics, strict isolation, and prevention of secondary infection are priorities. Maintenance of warmth and of fluid–electrolyte balance are also important in the plan of care. Healing usually takes place without scarring.

Impetigo

Description. Impetigo is an infectious disease of the skin caused by staphylococci or by group A beta-hemolytic streptococci. It results when the organism comes in contact with a break in the skin, such as an insect bite. The bullous form seen primarily in infants is usually staphylococcal, whereas nonbullous types are more commonly seen in children and young adults. Both organisms can usually be cultivated in the latter. The newborn is susceptible to this infection because resistance to skin bacteria is low. Impetigo tends to spread from one area of skin to another and is contagious.

Manifestations. The first symptoms of a bullous lesion are red papules (pimples) (see Color Plate Fig. 12). These eventually become small vesicles or pustules surrounded by a reddened area. When the blister breaks, the surface beneath is raw and weeping. The lesions may occur anywhere, but are most often found around the nose and mouth and in moist areas of the body, such as the creases of the neck, axilla, and groin. In older children, a crust may form, and scratching may cause further infection.

Treatment and Nursing Care. Systemic antibiotics are administered either orally or parenterally. Parents are instructed to wash the lesions three or four times a day to remove crusts. Ointments such as mupirocin (Bactroban) may be prescribed for topical application. Prevention of the disease by treating small cuts promptly is important.

The prognosis with proper treatment is good. The nursing care consists primarily of preventing this disease. Education of parents includes reminding them of the necessity for prompt attention to minor cuts and bites. In diagnosed cases, compliance with the treatment regimen is needed to prevent the spread of infection to other children and family members. If the diagnosis is made in the newborn nursery, the baby is isolated to prevent other newborns from becoming infected. Nephritis may occur as a complication of beta-hemolytic streptococcal infections.

Fungal Infections

Description. Fungal infections are caused by closely related fungi that have a preference for invading the stratum corneum, hair, and nails. The word *tinea* comes from the Latin "worm." The common name for this infection is *ringworm.* Fungi are larger than bacteria. Some fungi may be transmitted from person to person and others from animal to person. The name denotes the part of the body involved.

Tinea Capitis. Tinea capitis ("ringworm of the scalp") is seen in school children. It is characterized by patches of *alopecia* (hair loss). The hair loses pigment and may break off. The papules become pustules, which progress to red scales. There are areas of circular balding (see Color Plate Fig. 13).

Diagnosis is made by history and appearance. Some strains of tinea capitis glow green under a *Wood light.* This condition is treated with griseofulvin (Fulvicin, Grisactin), which is administered by mouth. It is given with or after meals to avoid gastrointestinal irritation and increase absorption. Suspensions should be well shaken. Parents are instructed to continue therapy as long as ordered and not to miss a dose. Exposure to the sun is avoided. Treatment may be necessary for 8 to 12 weeks. Children may go to school but are warned not to exchange hats, combs, or other personal items. This infection can be stubborn and may take several weeks to clear.

Tinea Corporis. Tinea corporis ("ringworm of the skin") is evident as an oval scaly inflamed ring with a clear center. It is seen on the face, neck, arms, and hands (see Color Plate Fig. 14). It can be transmitted by infected pets. Treatment consists of local application of an antifungal preparation such as clotrimazole or haloprogin twice daily for 2 to 4 weeks. More severe cases may require oral griseofulvin treatment.

Tinea Pedis. Tinea pedis refers to *athlete's foot.* Lesions are located between the toes, on the instep, and on the soles (see Color Plate Fig. 15). There is accompanying pruritus. It occurs more often in preadolescents and adolescents. It is diagnosed by direct microscopic scrapings of the lesions. Treatment consists of topical therapy with an antifungal preparation. Oral griseofulvin therapy may also be given. Adolescents are cautioned to avoid alcohol when taking this medicine, as it may cause tachycardia and flushing.

Because this condition is aggravated by heat and moisture, feet need to be carefully dried, especially between the toes. Clean socks are worn. Shoes need to be well ventilated. Plastic shoes that retain heat are avoided. Recurrences are common.

Tinea Crurus. Tinea crurus ("thigh") affects the groin area and is commonly referred to as "jock itch." It occurs on the inner aspects of the thighs and scrotum. The initial lesion is small, raised, and scaly. It spreads, and tiny vesicles occur at the margins of the rash. Local application of tolnaftate liquid (Tinactin, Aftate) or powder is effective. Stinging may occur when a spray solution is applied. General hygiene should be stressed.

Pediculosis

The infestation of humans by lice is termed *pediculosis.* There are three types: pediculosis capitis, head lice; pediculosis corporis, body lice; and pediculosis pubis, crabs or pubic lice. The various types usually remain in the part of the body designated by their name. They are transmitted from person to person or by contact with contaminated articles. Their survival depends on the blood they extract from the infected person. Severe itching in the affected area is the main symptom. Treatment in all cases is aimed at ridding the patient of the parasite, treating the excoriated skin, and preventing the infestation of others. The most common form seen in children is head lice.

Pediculosis Capitis

Description. Pediculosis capitis, known commonly as head lice, affects the scalp and hair. The louse lays eggs, called nits, which attach to the hair, and hatch within 3 or 4 days (Fig. 29–5). Head lice are more common in girls than in boys because of hair length and the tendency to share combs and hair ornaments. The parasite may be acquired from hats, combs, or hairbrushes. It is easily transferred from one child to another and is seen most frequently in the school-age child and in preschool children who attend day care centers.

Manifestations. Children with pediculosis capitis suffer from severe itching of the scalp. They scratch their heads frequently and often cause further irritation. The hair becomes matted. Pustules and excoriations may be seen about the face. Nurses admitting patients to pediatric units should be on the alert for head lice. In particular, the nurse inspects the hairline at the back of the neck and about the ears. Crusts, pediculi, nits, and dirt may cause matting of the hair and a foul odor. When the condition is discovered, it is handled with discretion so as not to embarrass the child or parents.

Treatment and Nursing Care. Treatment is directed toward killing the lice, getting rid of the nits, and managing any infections of the face and scalp. Family members and playmates of the child should be examined and treated as necessary. Prescription shampoos, such as pyrethrin, are commonly used. Retreatment may be necessary in 1 week to 10 days. Lindane (Kwell) has also been used; however, it has more reported side effects (consult circular).

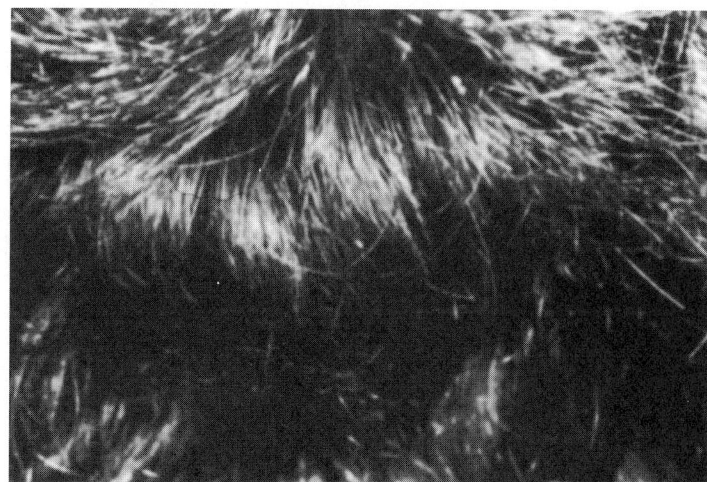

Figure 29–5. • Pediculosis. White nits or eggs of head lice attached to hair. (From Levy, M. [1991]. Disorders of the hair and scalp in children. *Pediatric Clinics of North America, 38,* 917.)

If the eyebrows and eyelashes are involved, a thick coating of petroleum jelly (Vaseline) may be applied, followed by removal of remaining nits. Nits on the head are removed by combing the hair with a fine-tooth comb dipped in a 1:1 solution of white vinegar and water. The hair is then washed. In some cases, recovery is hastened by cutting the hair. Contact (standard) precautions should be followed.

Children should be cautioned against swapping caps, head scarves, and combs. Parents are instructed to inspect the child's head regularly. Parents are encouraged to report infestations to the school nurse, as widespread outbreaks are periodically encountered.

Scabies

Description. Scabies is a parasitic infection caused by the itch mite. *Sarcoptes scabiei.* It is seen worldwide. It is caused by the adult female mite, who burrows under the skin and lays eggs. The mite has a round body and four pairs of legs and is visible by microscopic examination. A characteristic burrow is sometimes seen under the skin, particularly between the fingers. Burrows contain eggs and feces of the mite. Itching is intense, especially at night. A vesiculopustular lesion can occur in children.

Scabies may occur anywhere on the body but is seldom seen on the face. It thrives in moist body folds, but in young children the lesions may appear on the head, palms, and soles of the feet. It is spread by close personal contact, including sexual relations. It is rarely transmitted by fomites because the isolated mite dies within 2 to 3 days.

Treatment and Nursing Care. Treatment consists of the application of permethrin (Elimite). It can be used for children older than 2 months of age. Parents are instructed to follow the directions carefully. All family members, baby-sitters, and close associates require treatment. Contact standard precautions are followed (Appendix A).

INJURIES

Burns

Description. Burns occur frequently during childhood. They are the leading cause of accidental death in the home for children between the ages of 1 and 4 years. Sometimes burns are a result of child abuse and neglect. The two times of day in which burns are most likely to occur are the early morning hours before parents awaken and after school.

Types of burns include:

- *Thermal.* Due to fire or a scalding vapor or liquid
- *Chemical.* Due to a corrosive powder or liquid
- *Electrical.* Due to electrical current passing through the body
- *Radiation.* Due to x-rays or radioactive substances

Burns can involve the skin or the mucous membranes. When a child is burned by fire near the face, the flames may be *inhaled,* causing a burn of the mucous membrane lining the airway. Assessing for resulting edema and respiratory distress is a priority. When a formula or food is heated in the microwave oven, "hot-spots" occur that can cause burns to the mucous membranes lining the mouth.

Differences in responses of children to a burn:

- The child's skin is thinner than the adult, lending to a more serious depth of burn with lower temperatures and shorter exposure than adults.
- The large body surface area of the child results in greater fluid, electrolyte, and heat loss.
- Immature response systems in young children can cause shock and heart failure.
- The increased metabolism rate (BMR) of a child results in increased protein and calorie needs.
- Smaller muscle and fat content in the body results in protein and caloric deficiencies when oral intake is limited.
- The skin is more elastic in children, causing pulling on the scarring areas, resulting in formation of a larger scar.
- The immature immune system predisposes the child to developing infections that complicate burn treatment.
- The prolonged immobilization and treatment required for burns adversely affects growth and development.

Classification. The severity of a burn depends on the area, *extent,* and *depth* of involvement. The size of the burn is calculated as a percentage of total body surface (TBSA) (Fig. 29–6). In children, age-related charts are used because their body proportions differ from those of adults and a standard (rule of nines) cannot be applied. The extent of destruction of the skin is described as partial-thickness or full-thickness. In partial-thickness burns, only part of the skin is damaged. Full-thickness burns are more extensive and may require skin grafting. The classification of and first aid treatment for burns are summarized in Table 29–2. One can survive a rather extensive superficial burn, whereas a deep burn involving a smaller surface area can threaten the patient's life. Table 29–3 discusses children's response to burn injuries.

Burns can also be complicated by fractures, soft-tissue injury, or preexisting conditions such as diabetes, obesity, epilepsy, and heart or renal disease. Moderate burns are considered to be: (1) partial-thickness burns involving 15% to 30% of body surface; or (2) full-thickness burns involving less than 10% of body surface. Major burns are (1) partial-thickness types involving 30% or more of body surface; or (2) full-thickness burns involving 10% or more of body surface. Second- and third-degree burns must be regarded as open wounds that have the added danger of infection.

Care of Electrical Burns. When electricity is the cause of the injury, the child should be assessed for entry and exit lesions that may appear as a small erythematous area. The location of the entry and exit wounds indicate the path of electricity through the body. Muscle damage can occur, and if the electric current passed through the heart, cardiac muscle damage can result. Deep-muscle damage can cause renal impairment from myoglobinuria. The child should be observed closely for responses with EKG monitors and vital signs recorded, and cardiac enzymes assessed before discharge.

Nursing Tip

Electrical burns of the mouth are common in small children who put everything into their mouths. Biting into electrical cords is not unusual. Such wounds are usually deep and leave an entrance and exit burn. They are subject to bleeding for several weeks.

Emergency Care. Community education programs emphasize the response to a child with a burn injury. The school nurse plays a major role in the education process.

- *Stop the burning process.* Stop, drop, and roll is the sequence of care. Rolling the child in a blanket smothers the flames. A caustic powder should be brushed off before water is used to wash the area, to avoid spreading contact with the caustic substance. Electricity should be turned off before touching a child who has been electrocuted.
- *Assess the injury.* ABC = Airway Breathing Circulation of the victim. CPR is initiated if appropriate. Minor burns can be treated, major burns should be assessed by a physician.
- *Cover the burn.* The burned area should be covered with a clean cloth to minimize contact with air, to reduce pain, to minimize hypothermia, and to prevent contamination of the wound. Burned clothing and jewelry should be removed as metal retains heat and continues the burn injury.
- *Transport to a hospital.* Do not give any fluids by mouth because peristalsis may have diminished in response to the burn injury. If available, IV fluids and oxygen should be administered and the child comforted and reassured.

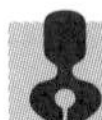

Nursing Tip

The small child is taught to stop, drop, and roll, should the clothes become ignited.

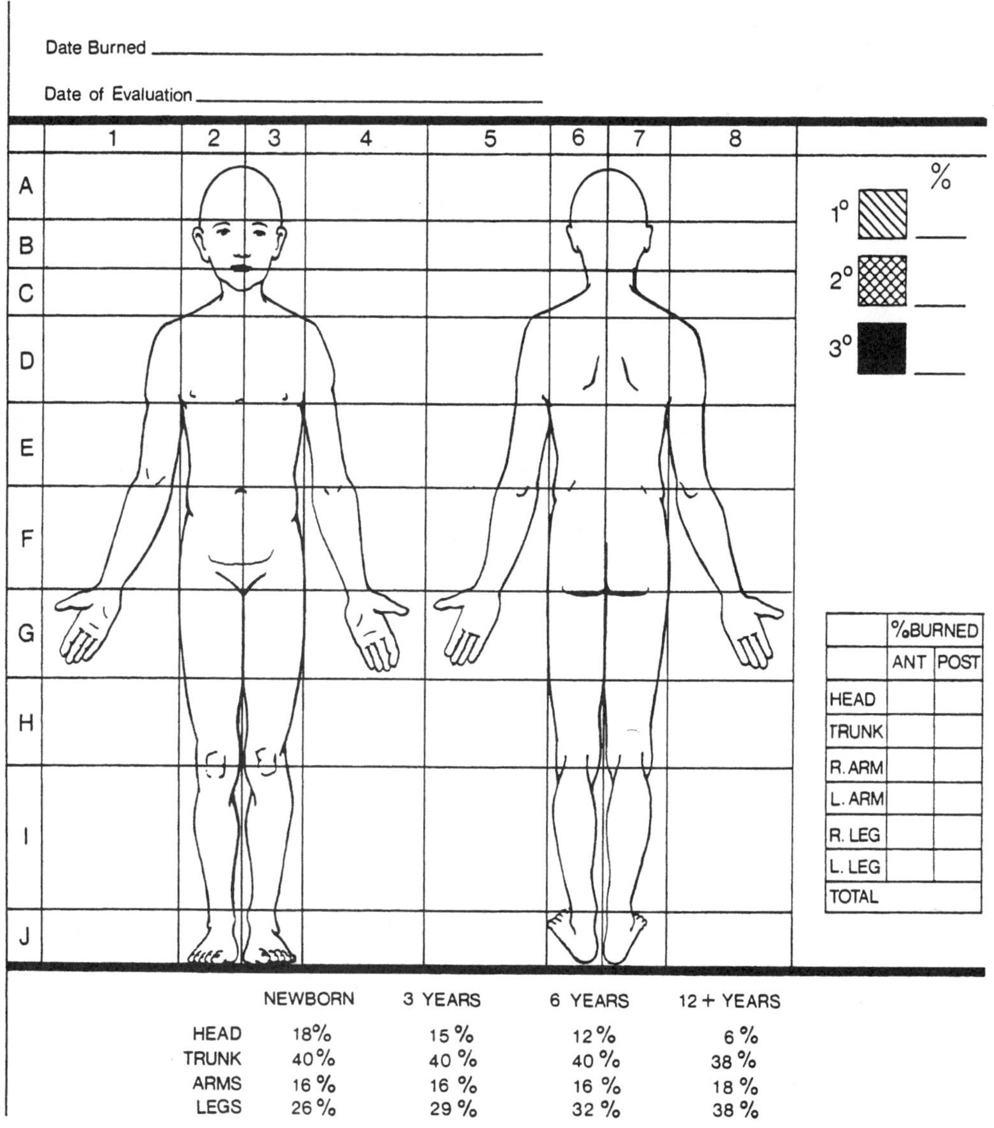

Figure 29–6. • A chart used to determine developmentally related percent body burn surface area (BSA). The percent of BSA involved is the basis for determining the fluid and nutritional needs of the burned child. In children younger than 3 years of age, some hospitals use the "rule of nines" which assigns the infant's head as 18% of TBSA and the lower extremities 14% of TBSA with 9% assigned to each arm and 1% to the hands or palms. (Courtesy of Shriners Hospital for Crippled Children, Burn Institute, Boston, MA.)

Care of Minor Thermal Burns. Minor burns are treated at home and followed with clinic visits until healing is complete. The wound is cleansed, and an antimicrobial ointment applied with a loose dressing. Blisters are not disturbed. Dressings are changed as prescribed and the parent is advised to report any sign of infection. The status of tetanus immunization is reviewed and updated as needed. Pain relief is administered as needed. The wound of a minor burn is usually completely healed within 20 days. Evaluation of scarring and effect on range of motion (ROM) will determine future follow-up needs.

Care of Major Burns. The immediate treatment of shock in cases of severe burns is handled by the physician, nurse, and respiratory therapist and other specialists in the emergency room or in some instances the operating room. Priorities include establishing an airway in patients with facial burns or smoke inhalation, instituting intravenous life-

Table 29–2
CLASSIFICATION AND FIRST-AID TREATMENT OF BURNS

Degree	Anatomy and Depth	Appearance and Sensation	First-Aid Treatment
First	Epidermis only	Skin red but blanches easily on pressure and refills quickly; painful, indicating tissue viability	Immerse in cold water to halt burning process; apply an antimicrobial ointment
Second			
Superficial	Epidermis and much of dermis; partial thickness	Blistered, moist, pink, or red; painful, indicating tissue viability	If area is small, treat as for first-degree burn, apply antimicrobial ointment; otherwise treat as for deep dermal burn
Deep dermal	Extends deep into dermis; partial thickness but can become full thickness with infection, trauma, or poor blood supply	Mottled; red, tan, or dull white; blisters; painful, indicating tissue viability	Immerse in cold water to halt burning process; cover with sterile dressing or clean cloth to prevent contamination and decrease pain from contact with air; avoid breaking blisters; seek medical attention immediately
Third	Subdermal; involves entire skin and all its structures; full thickness	Tough, leathery, dry; does not blanch or refill; dull brown, tan, black, or pearly white; painless to touch, indicating death of tissue	Halt burning process by immersing in cold water or rolling in blanket or rug; wrap in clean sheet or other sterile dressing; provide blanket for warmth; have victim lie down; DO NOT apply ointment or any other substance to burned area; take patient to nearest emergency treatment center immediately

lines, and assessing burn wounds and other, perhaps initially unrecognized, injuries. At times, some of these procedures are carried out simultaneously.

Establishing an Airway. Cyanosis, singed nasal hairs, charred lips, and stridor are indications that flames may have been inhaled. An endotracheal tube is inserted to maintain an adequate airway, although this is not required for all patients. This permits delivery of humidified air with oxygen, easy removal of secretions from respiratory passages, and use of a pressure ventilator if needed. Sedation is administered with caution to avoid further respiratory embarrassment.

If *eschar* (*eschara,* "scab") from burns on the trunk inhibits respirations, an incision called an *escharotomy* is made to prevent restriction of chest movement. Blood gas levels, including level of carbon monoxide, are ascertained. The child is placed on sterile sheets. Attendants wear face masks, sterile gown, and gloves.

Intravenous infusions are begun to prevent intravascular dehydration and electrolyte imbalance.

Table 29–3
RESPONSE TO BURN INJURY IN CHILDREN*

Response	Effect
Increased capillary permeability; hypovolemia	Loss of plasma, proteins, and fluids; shock
Increased blood flow to vital organs and decreased blood flow to periphery of body and nonvital organs	Peristalsis ceases (ileus)
	Curling's ulcer forms in stomach
Increase in body metabolism to maintain heat	Increased BMR can strain the heart by causing increased cardiac output
Damage to red blood cells and hemolysis resulting in anemia	Anemia causes increased cardiac output to maintain perfusion
Open wounds of burn can predispose to infection	Immature immune system can be overwhelmed and sepsis can result
Dead tissue provides a media for bacterial growth	
Waste products accumulate in blood due to anemia and slow perfusion of nonvital organs	Renal failure, cardiac failure, and pulmonary edema can complicate toxicity from burn injury

*Thermal injuries produce both local and systemic effects.

Ringer's lactate solution is often used initially. Within 24 to 48 hours, when capillary permeability is restored, albumin or plasma may be used.

Laboratory studies include hematocrit and sodium chloride, potassium, carbon dioxide, blood urea nitrogen, creatinine, and serum protein levels. Blood typing and cross-matching are performed. Fluid therapy requires close monitoring throughout hospitalization. To determine urine volume and characteristics, a urinary catheter is inserted and an intake and output record is maintained.

The loss of fluid causes renal vasoconstriction, leading to depressed glomerular filtration and oliguria. Without adequate therapy, acute renal failure can develop. Urine output is observed hourly. It varies considerably, but on the average 20 to 30 ml/hr for patients older than 2 years is considered adequate during the resuscitative stage. The patient's present weight is recorded and is used as baseline data for determining adequacy of treatment.

A nasogastric tube is inserted and is attached to low Gomco suction. This empties the stomach and prevents complications such as gastric dilatation, vomiting, and paralytic ileus. The patient has nothing by mouth for the first 24 hours. Sporadic bleeding as a result of *Curling's* or stress ulcer is not uncommon in patients with severe burns; the administration of antacids, such as magnesium hydroxide (Maalox), has helped to reduce its incidence.

Wound Care. Immediate care of the wound itself includes cleansing and *débridement* (removal of dried crusts) of necrotic tissue. The loss of skin increases the threat of infection, and fluid loss due to evaporation can be significant. The immune system is depressed. Strict asepsis is maintained, and the wound site is treated in accordance with the physician's instruction. A tetanus immunization history is obtained, and tetanus prophylaxis is administered as required. Low doses of penicillin may be prescribed to prevent streptococcal infection.

A semiopen method of burn dressing may be used, although exposure methods may be useful on accessible areas such as the face. The wound is covered by a few layers of sterile gauze that has been saturated with antibacterial ointment or cream. The gauze is held in place by elastic netting (Fig. 29–7). When the wound is being dressed, *no two burn surfaces should touch.* A sterile blanket may be used to prevent chilling. The wound is cleansed by tub baths, or in many cases, whirlpool baths are utilized to soften necrotic areas and débride the wound. Débridement is done when needed to cleanse the wound and prepare the new granulation tissue for grafting. The use of enzymes such as Travase may be prescribed. The burn area is closed and resurfaced by grafting.

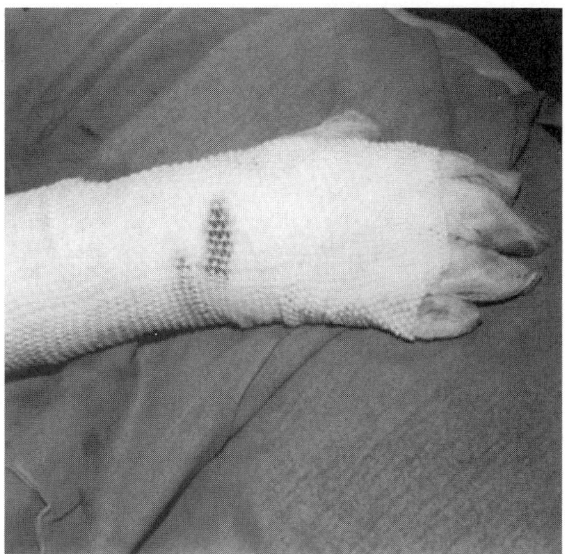

Figure 29–7. • Occlusive dressing applied to a burned hand. (Courtesy of the Burn Center at St. Agnes Medical Center, Philadelphia, PA. From deWitt, S. C. [1992]. *Essentials of medical–surgical nursing* [2nd ed., p. 641]. Philadelphia: Saunders.)

Skin Grafts. Temporary grafts are used during the acute stage of recovery. They protect the wound from infection and reduce fluid loss but are eventually rejected by the body. Temporary grafts include *homografts,* usually tissue from cadavers free from disease, and *heterografts,* tissues obtained from different species. Heterografts are also referred to as *xenografts* (*xeno,* "foreign," and *graft,* "slice of skin").

Many grafts are derived from pigskin, which is available commercially either fresh or frozen; these biologic dressings are frequently used in children and are called porcine *xenografts* (Fig. 29–8). They are particularly useful in partial-thickness or deep dermal burns and have greatly improved burn management. Deep dermal wounds may be preceded by tangential (merely touching) excision, which is a surgical technique of removing burned

Nursing Tip

A severe burn can cause loss of function in two of the most important properties of the skin: the ability to protect against infection and the ability to prevent loss of body fluid.

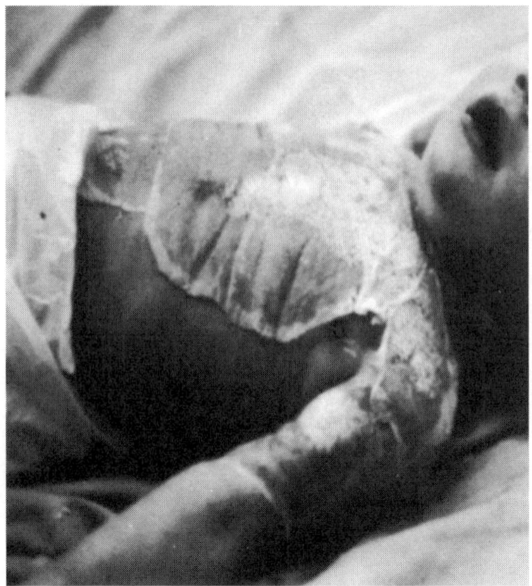

Figure 29–8. • Porcine dressing. (Courtesy of St. Agnes Medical Center Photography Department, Philadelphia. From Marlow, D. R., & Redding, B. A. [1988]. *Textbook of pediatric nursing* [6th ed., p. 801]. Philadelphia: Saunders.)

eschar with a dermatome. Thin layers are shaved down to the live tissues, and temporary porcine grafts are applied.

There are two types of permanent grafts, *autografts* and *isografts.* An autograft (*auto,* "self") is healthy tissue obtained from another part of the patient's body. An *isograft* (*iso,* "equal") is obtained from the patient's identical twin. Permanent grafts are done during the rehabilitative stage of the patient's illness to improve appearance and function. The site from which the tissue has been removed is called the *donor area.*

Advances in grafting techniques have improved the overall prognosis in burn patients and have helped to minimize scarring. A split-thickness skin graft can be prepared with the use of a dermatome. In extensive burns, it is sometimes difficult to find enough intact skin for use. Special methods such as the Tanner mesh graft may be used. In this method, a strip of split-thickness skin is run through a special cutting machine that makes multiple slits to expand the skin to provide more coverage, in some cases as much as nine times the original area of the skin. The graft is sutured in place to maintain tension.

The "postage-stamp" graft consists of small pieces of donor skin placed on the granulation tissue. Spaces between grafts allow for drainage and healing. Full-cover grafts are sheets of skin placed intact over the wound. These are cosmetically more effective than patch and mesh grafts but are not always available. The donor site is covered with xenograft or fine mesh gauze; it heals in about 2 weeks. Newly grafted areas are covered with sterile dressings. Every effort is made to prevent *bleeding* and *infection.* The areas surrounding the wound are observed for edema and impaired circulation.

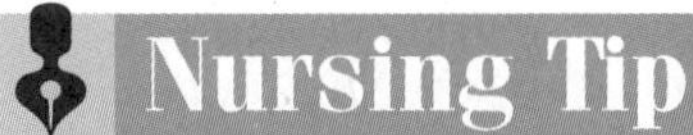

Nursing Tip

In cases of car, house, or airplane fires, patients may face additional crises, such as loss of relatives, pets, and possessions.

Nursing Care. Children who have suffered extensive burns and survive the early dangers face a long period of hospitalization and require specialized care. The various aspects of nursing care differ with the age of the patient, the area of the burn, and the type of treatment used. Nursing Care Plan 29–2 lists some interventions for children with burns. Table 29–4 lists topical agents used in treating burn patients.

Protective isolation (standard precautions) is instituted. All instruments that come in contact with the wound must be sterile. Ointments are applied with a gloved hand or a sterile tongue depressor. Care must be taken to avoid injury to granulation tissue. If the wound is to be covered, a layer of fine mesh gauze is secured with sterile fluffs, followed by Kling bandages and a stockinette or elastic tubular netting. With young children, restraints may be required to keep their fingers away from the wound.

The nurse reports signs of infection immediately. These are elevation of temperature, pulse, and respiration; restlessness and confusion; pain; purulent drainage; and odor of wound dressing. A careful description of the wound in nurse's notes facilitates daily comparison and determination of progress. All infection must be cleared before skin grafting can be performed.

The nurse remains alert for signs of fluid overload, in particular, behavioral changes and altered sensorium. Oral fluids, although initially restricted to prevent nausea and vomiting, are necessary during the convalescent stages, to prevent kidney damage and to maintain body fluid requirements. The nurse must use ingenuity to persuade the child to take sufficient amounts of fluids. An accurate record of intake and output of fluids is kept.

There is an increase in demands on the metabolism as it deals with this trauma, and more calories are spent as water evaporates from the wound site. Frequent feedings of foods high in calories, protein,

NURSING CARE PLAN 29–2

Selected Nursing Diagnoses for the Child With Burns (Subacute Phase)

Nursing Diagnosis: High risk for infection related to loss of protective layer of skin secondary to burn

Goals	Nursing Interventions	Rationale
The child's rectal temperature will not be elevated Skin around wound remains intact and is not red or warm to touch	1. Wash hands for 1 full minute before touching patient	1. Handwashing is essential to prevent introducing pathogens; the immune system of a child is immature, which results in an increased susceptibility to infection and organ failure
	2. Wear sterile gown, gloves, and mask when handling burn wound	2. Necrotic tissue serves as an excellent breeding ground for microorganisms, which multiply rapidly in a burn wound
	3. Use sterile bed linens if exposure method is utilized	3. When wound is exposed to air, nurse must constantly observe patient for signs of infection; serous fluid that exudes from wound hardens and forms a covering, but bacteria may enter through breaks in dried exudate
	4. Cleanse wound as ordered	4. Hydrotherapy is often used to cleanse burned area; children lose heat more rapidly than adults do; therefore, nurse must maintain warmth of water and room temperature
	5. Apply prescribed antibacterial ointments	5. Antibacterial ointments reduce number of organisms in wound; after 18–24 hours, if left untreated, a wound becomes colonized with pathogenic bacteria
	6. Obtain wound cultures as ordered	6. Cultures provide baseline data; antibiotics are prescribed to treat specific organisms
	7. Screen visitors for infections	7. Child needs to be protected from infected persons
	8. Check vital signs, especially temperature	8. Decrease excessive metabolic expenditures (child should not become overheated or chilled); temperature readings can determine early signs of general sepsis, wound infection, or bacterial pneumonia
	9. Observe wound for purulent, foul drainage	9. Purulent, foul drainage indicates wound infection
	10. Handle child gently	10. Gentle handling will prevent injury to wound or donor site

(Continued)

and iron are therefore necessary. A high-protein diet, a normal diet with added amounts of meat, milk, eggs, fish, or poultry, is usually prescribed. Iron therapy may be initiated if anemia begins to develop. Eggnogs are nourishing between-meal drinks for burn patients with such needs. Small amounts are offered frequently. Vitamins A, B, and C and zinc sulfate are given to hasten healing and to stimulate the appetite. Gavage feedings may be necessary. Accurate daily records of foods consumed, calorie count, and patient's weight will help to determine the nutritional status.

The nurse bears in mind that other parts of the body that are not affected need exercise and proper positioning to prevent painful contractures. The child's position is changed every 2 to 4 hours unless

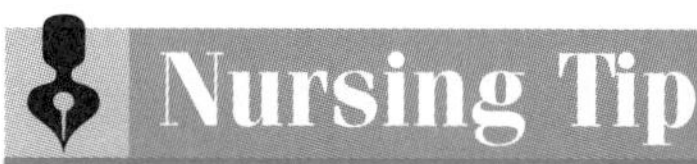

Disorientation, fever, and diminished bowel sounds may be early signs of sepsis.

NURSING CARE PLAN 29–2 *continued*

Selected Nursing Diagnoses for the Child With Burns (Subacute Phase)

Nursing Diagnosis: Altered nutrition—less than body requirements, related to hypermetabolism as the body attempts to restore tissue

Goals	Nursing Interventions	Rationale
Child ingests sufficient calories to compensate for catabolism as evidenced by normal healing and stable body weight	1. Provide high-calorie, high-protein meals and snacks	1. Although edema usually accompanies a severe burn, a gradual weight loss follows because of increased energy and protein requirements
	2. Avoid painful procedures around mealtime	2. Discomfort decreases child's appetite
	3. Cater to child's food preferences as feasible	3. Children frequently lack appetite; poor nutritional status impairs wound healing, compromises immune response, and increases chance of infection
	4. Provide nourishing between-meal feedings	4. Child's metabolic demands may require two to three times normal calorie intake for age
	5. Administer supplementary vitamins and minerals	5. Anorexia may lead to vitamin deficiencies
	6. Anticipate total parenteral nutrition	6. If caloric requirements cannot be met, supplemental feedings may be required
	7. Provide companionship at meals	7. Parents understand child's food preferences; they may bring food from home if feasible; presence of nurse may distract child from discomfort and promote socialization

Nursing Diagnosis: High risk for altered skin integrity, pressure ulcers related to immobility

Goals	Nursing Interventions	Rationale
Child's skin is not erythematous and shows no signs of breakdown	1. Turn patient frequently	1. Frequent repositioning prevents pressure necrosis
	2. Check peripheral areas for color, capillary refill, pulse, sensation, motion	2. Burns that encompass whole circumference of extremities (circumferential burns), such as fingers and toes, and chest require careful attention, particularly in first few hours following injury; edema puts pressure on underlying blood vessels and nerves; children's fingers and toes are very small and thin, and circulation can be cut off very easily
	3. Keep child from picking and scratching; restrain if necessary	3. Itching is common with burns; scratching can cause infection

Nursing Diagnosis: High risk for impaired physical mobility related to burn

Goals	Nursing Interventions	Rationale
Child demonstrates full range of motion Child does not develop contractures	1. Explain and perform range-of-motion exercises	1. Contractions that limit function can develop from scar formation and immobility of unaffected limbs
	2. Encourage water play	2. Water soothes the stressed child; other games that encourage use of limbs are also beneficial
	3. Observe for constricting eschar, particularly over joints	3. Early intervention prevents or minimizes contractures

contraindicated. A footboard is used to prevent footdrop. Support should be given by means of pillows, sandbags, and rolled towels as necessary.

The physical therapist attends the child regularly to exercise and keep the joints limber and healthy. The child begins to ambulate as soon as possible. Self-help activities and mobility are encouraged. Pressure splints or elasticized garments help to

NURSING CARE PLAN 29–2 *continued*

Selected Nursing Diagnoses for the Child With Burns (Subacute Phase)

Nursing Diagnosis: High risk for fluid volume deficit related to loss of fluids via open wound

Goals	Nursing Interventions	Rationale
Fluids and electrolytes are maintained as evidenced by laboratory data and clinical signs Skin turgor and urinary output are adequate	1. Monitor electrolyte levels 2. Encourage fluid intake 3. Observe urinary output 4. Monitor IV fluids 5. Keep *accurate* intake and output records 6. Observe patient for evidence of fluid overload, such as altered behavior or sensorium 7. Test tissue turgor	1 to 7. Throughout recovery process, fluid and electrolyte balance fluctuates with surgical procedures, sepsis, and evaporative losses; careful monitoring is needed until wound is healed; errors in fluid therapy in children can be life-threatening, as infants, in particular, have high rates of heat exchange relative to size and weight, high rates of water exchange in relation to total body water, and significant differences in muscle, water, and electrolyte composition; they also require relatively larger volumes of urine for excretion of waste products than do adults, and insensible water losses when expressed in terms of body weight are significantly greater in children than in adults

Nursing Diagnosis: Pain related to burn, nature of treatment

Goals	Nursing Interventions	Rationale
Patient is comfortable as evidenced by nonirritable behavior and absence of crying	1. Avoid drafts or overheating by adjusting room temperature	1. Body responds to a large burn area by increasing metabolic rate; oxygen comsumption increases as temperature, respirations, and heart rate rise; controlled environment reduces water evaporation and heat losses from the wound; increases comfort of patient
	2. Administer pain relievers before dressing changes	2. Adjust time of dressing change to coincide with peak action of pain reliever
	3. Observe for hostility, irritability, depression, guarding of body parts, which may indicate pain in nonverbal child	3. Children do not understand necessity for treatments; they protest loudly and are afraid; dressing changes are painful and difficult for nurse and child; determining child's level of pain tolerance during a procedure is helpful in assisting child to stay in control; allowing pauses when tension escalates is of importance
	4. Allow child to express feelings	4. Expression of feelings is necessary for a healthy personality
	5. Use distraction techniques	5. Distraction may take child's mind off pain
	6. Provide tactile contact	6. Appropriate touch is an important aspect of human communication, especially with nonverbal child

(Continued)

NURSING CARE PLAN 29–2 *continued*

Selected Nursing Diagnoses for the Child With Burns (Subacute Phase)

Nursing Diagnosis: High risk for disturbance of self-concept related to scars, disfigurement, isolation

Goals	Nursing Interventions	Rationale
Child maintains healthy self-concept during rehabilitation period as evidenced by a sense of humor, absence of depression, and increased acceptance of body disfigurement	1. Reassure child and parents	1. A calm and straighforward manner promotes confidence
	2. Help to alleviate guilt	2. Acknowledging guilt feelings validates reality and facilitates problem solving
	3. Explore feelings concerning physical appearance by having patients draw themselves before and after burn	3. Patient may gain insight from drawing; aids in expression of feelings; a series of drawings provide more information than does one drawing
	4. Discuss ways to camouflage disfigurement	4. Often families have false hope about plastic repair; plastic surgery may restore function, but evidence of burn may still need to be camouflaged
	5. Anticipate regressive behavior	5. Regression often occurs in patients in crisis as patient tries to return to a safer time of life
	6. Incorporate developmental aspects into nursing care plans	6. Incorporating developmental aspects is particularly relevant for accident prevention and nursing intervention
	7. Encourage contact with peers	7. Reentry into social life can be problematic, particularly with disfigurement of face and neck; child may need to "test the waters" gradually; burn camps are available at major treatment centers

Nursing Diagnosis: High risk for dysfunctional grieving related to appearance

Goals	Nursing Interventions	Rationale
Child is able to observe burn wound and feels free to express negative as well as positive feelings to nurse	1. Support patient in expressing grief concerning "imperfect appearance"	1. Verbalization of grief reduces its impact
	2. Anticipate grief reflected as anger and fear as well as sadness	2. Anger, fear, and grief are normal responses to loss

Nursing Diagnosis: Knowledge deficit in child and family regarding accident prevention

Goals	Nursing Interventions	Rationale
Family verbalizes understanding of the importance of installing smoke detectors and sheltering children from strong sunlight, hot liquids, electrical outlets, etc.	1. Assess knowledge of accident prevention in this and other areas	1. Accidents and injuries are major cause of death in children over 1 yr of age
	2. Provide ongoing education as required	2. Ongoing education is necesary, as child is constantly developing new motor and cognitive skills that may carry risks
	3. Assess parenting skills, suggest classes if needed	3. Many adults have not had good role models for parenting; they may under- or overestimate child's capabilities

reduce scar tissue and are sometimes worn for months following discharge (Fig. 29–9).

Emotional Support. A burn injury is taxing to the child and parents. It requires long periods of hospitalization and frequent readmissions. The accident itself is terrifying for the child, but it is made even worse if it was caused by disobedience. Nurses encourage children to express their feelings. Analgesics are administered *prior* to painful procedures. The long-term patient requires diversions of various types. School tutors are requested and contact is maintained with peers through cards or e-mail.

Nurses give constant support to the parents, who usually feel guilty if their child was injured in an accident. Nurses indicate by their manner that they

Table 29–4
TOPICAL AGENTS USED IN TREATING BURN PATIENTS

Agent	Comment
Silver sulfadiazine cream 1% (Silvadene)	Effective against gram-negative and gram-positive bacteria and yeast (*Candida albicans*) Do not use if patient is allergic to sulfa drugs Cream does not sting, softens eschar Do not waste (expensive) Gently remove old cream before reapplying
Mafenide acetate 10% (Sulfamylon)	Effective against gram-positive and gram-negative organisms Painful because it draws water out of the tissues; pain may last 15–30 min or longer Remain with child after application for comfort and diversion Allergic rash common Tendency to cake, best used with hydrotherapy Potential for metabolic acidosis
Silver nitrate 0.5% ($AgNO_3$)	Effective against gram-negative organisms Dressing must be kept *wet* and changed frequently Stains unburned skin, linen, and most surfaces a dark brown or black Eschar becomes light brown

do not blame the parents for what has happened. Preparation for discharge begins early. The multidisciplinary health care team includes the doctor, nurse, school nurse, schoolteacher, physiotherapist, and psychologist. Instructions are given about wound care, diet, exercise, and rest. Return appointments are made, and referral agencies are contacted. Methods to improve the physical appearance of the patient are discussed. The importance of burn prevention cannot be overemphasized.

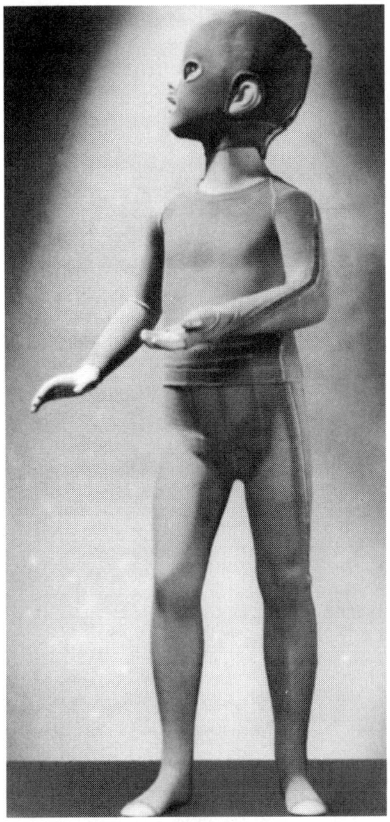

Figure 29–9. • Pressure garments for various body parts. (Courtesy of Jobst Institute, Inc., Toledo, OH.)

Frostbite

Frostbite is the result of freezing of a body part. *Chilblain* is a cold injury with erythema, vesicles, and ulcerative lesions occurring as a result of vasoconstriction. Education to prevent cold injury is essential for those living or visiting cold climates. School nurses play a vital role in educating parents and children. Adequate layered clothing including hats and gloves (wool over cotton) is preferred. In exposure to extreme cold, warmth is lost in the periphery of the body before the core temperature drops. Therefore, in extreme cases of exposure to freezing temperatures, the head and torso should be warmed before the extremities, to ensure survival with minimal consequences. Frostbitten extremities appear pale, hard and are without sensation. Dry clothing should be applied and muscle activity should be encouraged. Blankets or sleeping bags are initially used to start rewarming. Warm moist oxygen, warming blankets, and warming baths are used. A deep purple flush appears with the return of sensation, which is accompanied by extreme pain. Pain relief and monitoring of vital signs are essential. Blistering and ulcers can occur and are treated with whirlpool soaks. Skin damage is similar to that incurred with burns. Frostbite can result in *necrosis* (death) of tissue and require amputation.

KEY POINTS

- The skin is the body's first line of defense against disease.
- Certain skin conditions are symptoms of systemic disease.
- Common skin problems in infants are diaper dermatitis, seborrheic dermatitis, and atopic dermatitis (eczema).
- A strawberry nevus is an example of a hemangioma.
- Pediculosis is the term for lice. Lice may occur on the head, body, or pubic area.
- Tinea pedis, or athlete's foot, is prevented by drying the feet well, particularly between the toes, and wearing well-ventilated footwear.
- A severe burn can cause loss of function in two of the most important properties of the skin: the ability to protect against infection and the ability to prevent the loss of body fluid.
- Electrical burns carry the risk of thrombosis and tissue damage in other parts of the body.
- The severity of a burn depends on the area, extent, and depth of involvement.
- Preventing infection is an important nursing intervention for patients with burns or any skin lesion.
- Frostbite can cause tissue damage similar to burns.
- Absorption of topical hydrating medication is best when applied following a warm bath.
- Types of burns include thermal; electrical; chemical; and radiation.

MULTIPLE-CHOICE REVIEW QUESTIONS

Choose the most appropriate answer.

1. Pain relief is important in the burn patient because
   a. it prevents discomfort.
   b. the child must be kept from crying.
   c. parents become upset.
   d. pain contributes to shock.
2. Which of the following would be contraindicated in a patient with infantile eczema?
   a. Wrapping the baby in a wool blanket
   b. Covering hands with cotton mittens
   c. Using elbow restraints to prevent scratching
   d. Using open, wet dressings
3. A characteristic of third-degree burns not present in second-degree burns is
   a. lack of pain.
   b. blisters, warmth.
   c. redness.
   d. severe pain.
4. Which of the following is contained in a colloid bath often prescribed for children with dermatitis?
   a. Bath oil
   b. Glycerine soap
   c. Oatmeal
   d. Salt, or saline solution
5. The cause of infantile eczema may be the basis of a teaching plan for the child's parent. Infantile eczema is most likely caused by
   a. an infection with *Staphylococcus aureus.*
   b. a parasitic skin disease.
   c. poor hygiene.
   d. an allergic response.

BIBLIOGRAPHY AND READER REFERENCE

Behrman, R., & Kleigman, R. (1998). *Nelson's essentials of pediatrics.* Philadelphia: Saunders.

Behrman, R. E., Kleigman, R., & Arvin, A. (1996). *Nelson's textbook of pediatrics* (15th ed.). Philadelphia: Saunders.

Betz, C., Hunsberger, M., & Wright, S. (1994). *Family-centered nursing care of children* (2nd ed.). Philadelphia: Saunders.

Blawat, D., & Banks, P. (May 1977). Comforting touch: Using topical skin preparations. *Nursing 97, 27*(5), 46.

Bowden, V., Dickey, S., & Greenberg, C. (1998). *Children and their families: The continuum of care.* Philadelphia: Saunders.

Cohen, B. (1997). Warts and children: Can they be separated. *Contemporary Pediatrics, 14*(2), 128.

Eckler, J. (1997). Pediculosis Do's and Don'ts. *Nursing 97, 5,* 63.

Heymann, P., Rakes, G., Loach, T., & Murphy, D. (1997). Recognizing the young atopic child. *Contemporary Pediatrics, 14*(4), 131.

Kaiser, H. B., Kaliner, M. A., et al. (1997). Who needs allergy testing? *Patient Care, 31*(14), 169–183.

Mimouni, K., Mimouni, M., Zeharia, A., & Mukamel, M. (1995). Prognosis of infantile seborrheic dermatitis. *Journal of Pediatrics, 127*(5), 744–745.

Peters, S. (1997). Treating dermatitis in children: The role of topical corticosteroids. *Advance for Nurse Practitioners, 52*(2), 50–51.

Romeo, S. (1995). *Atopic dermatitis: The itch that rashes. Pediatric Nursing, 21*(2), 157–161.

Schmitt, B. D. (1996). When your child has impetigo. *Contemporary Pediatrics, 13*(6), 71–72.

Singleton, J. (June 1997). Pediatric dermatoses: Three common skin disruptions in infancy. *Nurse Practitioner, 22*(6), 32.

Usatine, R., Quan, M., & Strick, R. (1998). Acne vulgaris: A treatment update. *Hospital Practice, 33*(2), 111.

Whaley, D. (1997). *Whaley & Wong's essentials of pediatric nursing.* St. Louis, MO: Mosby.

chapter 30

The Child with a Metabolic Condition

Outline

OVERVIEW

INBORN ERRORS OF METABOLISM
- Tay-Sachs Disease

ENDOCRINE DISORDERS
- Hypothyroidism
- Diabetes Insipidus
- Diabetes Mellitus

DIET THERAPY FOR CHILDREN WITH DIABETES AND OTHER METABOLIC DISORDERS

Objectives

On completion and mastery of Chapter 30, the student will be able to

- Define each vocabulary term listed.
- Relate why growth parameters are of importance to patients with a family history of endocrine disease.
- Compare the signs and symptoms of hyperglycemia and hypoglycemia.
- Differentiate between type I and type II diabetes.
- List a predictable stress that the disease of diabetes has on children and families during the following periods of life: infancy, toddlerhood, preschool age, elementary school age, puberty, and adolescence.
- Outline the educational needs of the diabetic child and parents in the following areas: nutrition and meal planning, exercise, blood tests, administration of insulin, and skin care.
- List three precipitating events that might cause diabetic ketoacidosis.
- List three possible causes of insulin shock.
- Explain the Somogyi phenomenon.
- Discuss the preparation and administration of insulin to a child, highlighting any differences between pediatric and adult administration.
- List two benefits of exercise for the diabetic teenager.
- List the symptoms of hypothyroidism in infants.
- Discuss the dietary adjustment required for a child with diabetes insipidus.

Vocabulary

antidiuretic
gestational
glucagon
glycosuria
glycosylated hemoglobin test
hormone
hyperglycemia
hypoglycemia
hypotonia
ketoacidosis
lipoatrophy
polydipsia
polyphagia
polyuria
Somogyi phenomenon
target organ
vasopressin

OVERVIEW

The two major control systems that monitor the functions of the body are the nervous system and the endocrine system. These systems are interdependent. The endocrine, or ductless, glands regulate the body's metabolic processes. They are primarily responsible for growth, maturation, reproduction, and response of the body to stress. Figure 30–1 depicts the organs of the endocrine system and outlines how this system in children differs from that in adults. *Hormones* are chemical substances produced by the glands. They pour their secretions directly into the blood that flows through them. An organ specifically influenced by a certain hormone is called a *target organ.* Too much or too little of a given hormone may result in a disease state. Most of the glands and structures of the endocrine system develop during the 1st trimester of fetal development.

Maternal endocrine dysfunction may affect the fetus; therefore, an in-depth maternal history is a valuable tool in nursing assessment. The absence or deficiency of an enzyme that has a role in metabolism causes a defect in the metabolism process that can result in illness. Most inborn errors of metabolism can be detected by clinical signs or screening tests that can be performed in utero. Lethargy, poor feeding, failure to thrive, vomiting, and enlarged liver may be early signs of an inborn error of metabolism in the newborn. When clinical signs are not manifested in the neonatal period, an infection or body stress can precipitate symptoms of a latent defect in the older child. Unexplained mental retar-

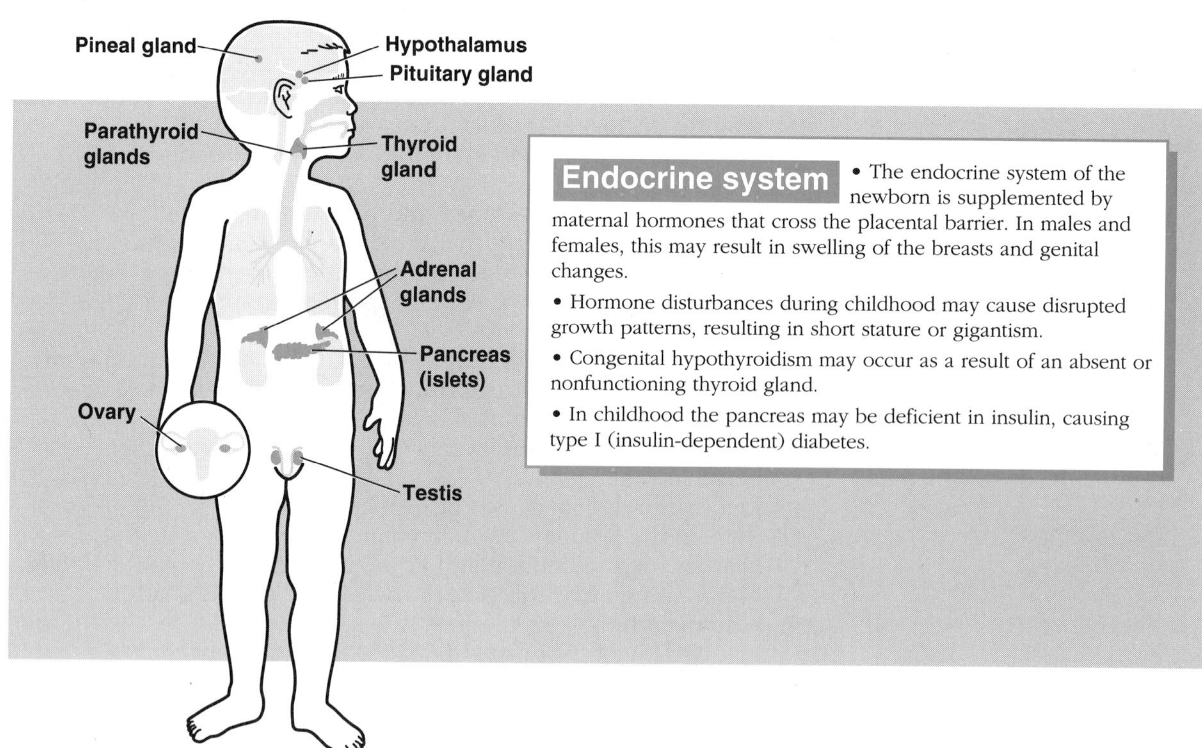

Figure 30–1. • Summary of some endocrine system differences between the child and the adult. The endocrine system consists of the ductless glands that release hormones. It works with the nervous system to regulate metabolic activities.

dation, developmental delay, convulsions, an odor to body or urine, or episodes of vomiting may be subtle signs of a metabolic dysfunction. Phenylketonuria (PKU), galactosemia, and maple syrup urine disease are discussed in Chapter 14. Cystic fibrosis is discussed in Chapter 25.

Radiographic studies to determine bone age are valuable diagnostic tools. Serum electrolytes and glucose, hormonal, and calcium level tests may be required. Phenylketonuria testing of newborns is an important screening device for identifying an enzyme deficiency. Chromosomal studies and tissue biopsy are other diagnostic tools. Sexual maturation and skin texture, pigment, and temperature may be indicators of specific disorders. Thyroid function tests may be required. Ultrasound is helpful in determining the size and character of the adrenal glands and ovaries as well as other organs. A 24-hour urine specimen may reveal important data. The glucose tolerance test is commonly performed to detect and monitor diabetes. Genetic counseling can help to prevent some disorders.

INBORN ERRORS OF METABOLISM

The term *inborn errors of metabolism* was coined at the turn of the century by Garrod. There are literally hundreds of these hereditary biochemical disorders that affect body metabolism. The pattern of inheritance is generally autosomal recessive. These conditions range from mild to severe.

Tay-Sachs Disease

Description. In Tay-Sachs disease, there is a deficiency of *hexosaminidase*, an enzyme necessary for the metabolism of fats. Lipid deposits accumulate on nerve cells, causing both physical and mental deterioration. This is a disease that is found primarily in the Ashkenazic Jewish population. It is an autosomal recessive trait carried by 1 in 30 Ashkenazic Jewish population, resulting in a birthrate occurrence of 1 in 4000 live births.

Manifestations. The infant with Tay-Sachs disease is normal until about 5 to 6 months of age, when physical development begins to slow. There may be head lag or inability to sit. The disease progresses, and when deposits occur on the optic nerve, blindness may result. Mental retardation eventually develops, as the brain cells become damaged. Most children die before the age of 5 from secondary infection or malnutrition.

Treatment and Nursing Care. There is no treatment for this devastating disease. The nursing care is mainly palliative. Mos
with periodic hospitali
such as pneumonia. Cha
of the dying child. Carr
screening tests. Genetic
have markedly decrease
Sachs disease.

ENDOCRINE DISORDERS

Hypothyroidism

Description. Hypothyroidism occurs when there is a deficiency in the secretions of the thyroid gland. It may be congenital or acquired. It is one of the more common disorders of the endocrine system in children. The thyroid gland controls the rate of metabolism in the body by the production of thyroxine (T_4) and triiodothyronine (T_3). In congenital hypothyroidism, the gland is absent or not functioning. The symptoms of hypothyroidism may not be apparent for several months.

Juvenile hypothyroidism is acquired by the older child. It may be caused by a number of conditions, the most common being lymphocytic thyroiditis. Often it appears during periods of rapid growth. Infectious disease, irradiation for cancer, certain medications containing iodine, and lack of dietary iodine (uncommon in the United States) may predispose one. Symptoms, diagnosis, and treatment are similar to those mentioned for congenital hypothyroidism. Because brain growth is nearly complete by 2 to 3 years of age, mental retardation and neurologic complications are not seen in the older child.

Manifestations. The baby is very sluggish and sleeps a lot. The tongue becomes enlarged, causing noisy respiration (Fig. 30–2). The skin is dry, there is no perspiration, and the hands and feet are cold. The infant feels floppy when handled. This *hypotonia* also affects the intestinal tract, causing chronic constipation. The hair eventually becomes dry and brittle. If left untreated, irreversible mental retardation and physical disabilities result.

Treatment and Nursing Care. Early recognition and diagnosis are essential to prevent the developing sequelae. A screening test for hypothyroidism may be performed at birth. It consists of T_4 measurement and a thyroid-stimulating hormone measurement when T_4 is low. This is generally part of an overall screen for other metabolic defects. Treatment involves administration of the synthetic hormone sodium levothyroxine (Synthroid or Levothroid). Hormone levels are monitored regularly.

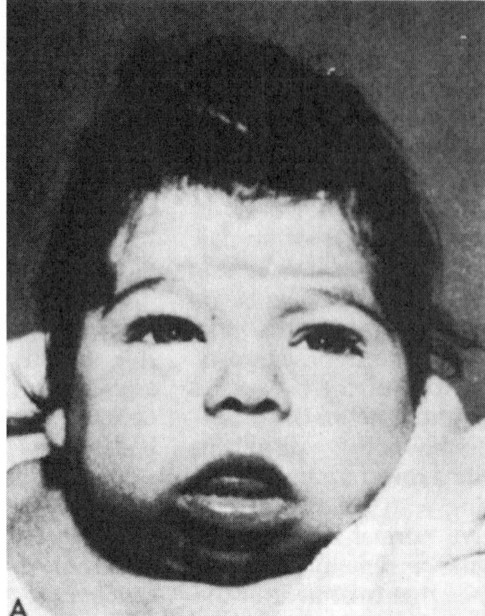

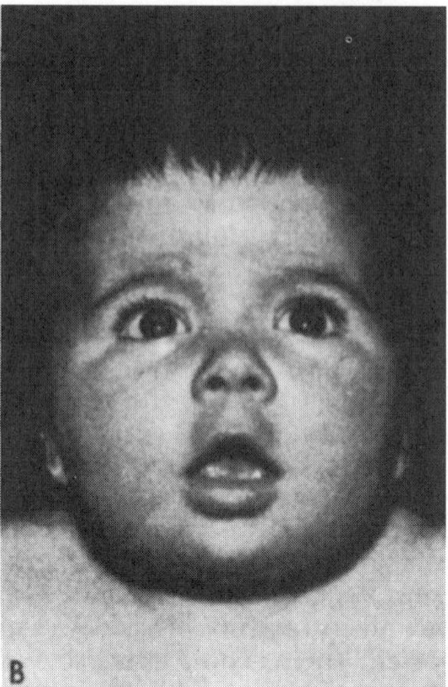

Figure 30–2. • **A,** Congenital hypothyroidism in a 6-month-old infant. The infant fed poorly and was constipated. She had a large tongue, poor head control, puffy face, and persistent nasal discharge. **B,** Same infant 4 months after treatment. Note the decreased facial puffiness and the alert expression. (From Behrman, R., Kleigman, R., & Arvin, A. [1996]. *Nelson's textbook of pediatrics* [15th ed.]. Philadelphia: Saunders.)

Therapy reverses the symptoms and prevents further mental retardation but does not reverse existing retardation. This is why early detection of congenital hypothyroidism is so important. Medication is taken at the same time each day, preferably in the morning. Parents are cautioned not to interchange brands. Children may have reversible hair loss, insomnia, and aggressiveness, and their school work may decline during the first few months of therapy. This is temporary. Full therapeutic effect may take 1 to 3 weeks. Medication is not to be discontinued because replacement for hypothyroidism is lifelong. Parents are instructed about these measures and advised to consult their physician before giving other medications. Table 30–1 describes common metabolic dysfunctions.

Diabetes Insipidus

Diabetes Insipidus can be hereditary (autosomal dominant) or acquired as the result of a head injury or tumor. It is the result of posterior pituitary *hypofunction* that results in a decreased secretion of *vasopressin,* the *antidiuretic hormone.* A lack of antidiuretic hormone results in uncontrolled diuresis. The kidney does not concentrate the urine during dehydration episodes.

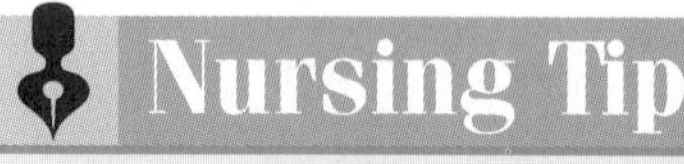

Nursing Tip

Growth hormone is administered at bedtime to simulate natural timing of hormone release.

Manifestations. *Polydipsia* and *polyuria* are the initial signs. The infant cries and prefers water to milk formula. Loss of weight, growth failure, and dehydration occur rapidly. As the child grows older, enuresis may be a problem. Excessive thirst and the search for water overshadow the desire to play, explore, eat, learn, or sleep. Perspiration is deficient and skin is dry.

Treatment and Nursing Care. Treatment involves hormone replacement of vasopressin in the form of Desmopressin by subcutaneous injection or DDAVP nasal spray. Parents should be taught to monitor for signs of overdosage, which include symptoms of water intoxication (edema, lethargy, nausea, CNS signs). Children with diabetes insipidus who are admitted to the hospital in an unconscious state and are unable to express thirst, are at great risk. A medical identification bracelet should be worn. School personnel should be advised of the needs of the child. Often school protocol limits children's access to bathrooms and water fountains even during or after physical activity. These restrictions could be life-threatening to a child with diabetes insipidus. The nurse should contact the school nurse and PE instructors and educate parents concerning the child's needs and the lifelong administration of the medication. Home care instructions should include recognizing signs of water intoxication.

Diabetes Mellitus

Description. Diabetes mellitus (DM) is a chronic metabolic condition in which the body is unable to utilize carbohydrates properly because of a deficiency of insulin, an internal secretion of the beta-cells of the pancreas. Insulin deficiency leads to impairment of glucose transport (sugar cannot pass into the cells). The body is also unable to store and utilize fats properly. There is a decrease in protein synthesis. When the blood glucose level becomes dangerously high, glucose spills into the urine and diuresis occurs. Incomplete fat metabolism produces ketone bodies that accumulate in the blood. This is termed *ketonemia.* Untreated diabetes can lead to coma and death.

Etiology. Diabetes mellitus is considered to be an autoimmune disease that may involve a defect in chromosome number six. A trigger, or stressor, such as a virus, causes destruction of the beta-cells in the Isles of Langerhans of the pancreas resulting in the manifestation of illness. It is the most common endocrine disorder of childhood, and it has a number of physical, emotional, and developmental consequences. Constant attention to dietary intake and daily administration of medication place a stress on the growing child. Long-term complications relating to kidney disease, blindness, circulatory problems, and neuropathy loom in the future for these children. Treatment is designed to optimize growth and development and to minimize complications.

Classification. Diabetes is not a single entity but rather a syndrome. To help to eliminate confusion in terminology, the National Institutes of Health appointed an international committee, the National Diabetes Data Group, to classify the carbohydrate intolerance syndromes. As more is learned about diabetes, further refinements in classification will be necessary. Three of the categories pertinent to this discussion of pediatric diabetes are described here:

- *Type I, insulin-dependent diabetes mellitus (IDDM).* This was formerly termed juvenile-onset diabe-

Table 30–1
METABOLIC DYSFUNCTIONS

Gland	Problem	Involved Hormone	Manifestation	Rx
Pituitary—anterior	Decreased hypopituitarism	Growth hormone	Short stature, dwarfism	Synthetic growth hormone replacement
	Increased hyperpituitarism	Growth hormone	Before epiphyseal closure, gigantism After epiphyseal closure, acromegaly Sexual precocity (puberty before 8–9 yr)	Surgery, irradiation Radioactive implants Monthly hormone injection to control secretions until puberty
Pituitary—posterior	Decreased hypopituitarism	Decreased antidiuretic hormone	Diabetes insipidus (see p. 798)	Vasopressin by injection or nasal spray
	Increased hyperpituitarism	Increased antidiuretic hormone	Syndrome of inappropriate antidiuretic hormone secretion (SIADH)	Fluid restriction and hormone antagonists
Parathyroid	Decreased hypoparathyroidism	Decreased parahormone	Decreased blood calcium and increased phosphorus causing tetany and laryngospasm	Calcium gluconate, vitamin D supplements
	Increased hyperparathyroidism	Increased parathromone	Elevated blood calcium and lowered phosphorus levels causing spontaneous fractures and CNS problems	Restore calcium balance, excise tumor
Adrenal	Decreased adrenal cortical insufficiency (Addison's disease)	Decreased steroids, sex steroids, epinephrine	Craving for salt, seizures, neurologic and circulatory changes, decreased sexual development	Replace cortisol and body fluids, genetic sexual assessment
	Increased hyperadrenalism	Increased cortisol	Cushing syndrome, hyperglycemia, electrolyte problems, pheochromocytoma	Depends on cause, tumor removal

tes. It is characterized by absolute or complete insulin deficiency. Childhood diabetes is usually of this type. Although there may be some insulin production during certain phases of the disease, patients eventually become insulin deficient. They are prone to ketosis.

- *Type II, non-insulin dependent diabetes mellitus (NIDDM).* This was formerly called adult-onset diabetes. These persons are not usually dependent on insulin and rarely develop ketosis. Although NIDDM may occur at any age, it generally develops after the age of 40. When type II diabetes is seen in young adults, it is sometimes called maturity-onset diabetes of youth. Table 30–2 lists clinical features of type I and type II.
- *Secondary diabetes.* Secondary diabetes may be caused by diseases that involve the pancreas, such as cystic fibrosis or cancer; hormonal causes; drug-induced causes; or other syndromes. Secondary diabetes is often reversed by treating the underlying cause. *Gestational diabetes* is the appearance of symptoms for the first time during pregnancy (see Chapter 5).

Type I IDDM Diabetes

Incidence. Approximately 12 million Americans have diabetes. In the United States, the annual incidence is about 10 to 12 new cases per 100,000 children (Behrman & Kleigman, 1998). The frequency is increasing. Some factors contributing to this are (1) patients with diabetes are living into their reproductive years and having children; (2) feeding cows milk to children under 2 years of age; (3) obesity has increased; and (4) good prenatal care has decreased the mortality rates of mothers and babies. Specific viral infections can also trigger IDDM.

Symptoms of IDDM may occur at any time in childhood, but the rate of occurrence of new cases is highest among 5- and 7-year-old children and pubescent children 11 to 13 years of age. In the former group, the stress of school and the increased exposure to infectious diseases may be responsible. During puberty, increased growth, increased emotional stress, and insulin antagonism of sex hormones may be implicated. It occurs in both sexes with equal frequency. The disease is more difficult to manage in childhood because the patients are growing, they expend a great deal of energy, their nutritional needs vary, and they have to face a lifetime of diabetic management. Young children with IDDM often do not demonstrate the typical "textbook" picture of the disorder. The initial diagnosis may be determined when the child presents with ketoacidosis. Therefore, the nurse must be particularly astute in subjective and objective observations.

Manifestations. Children with diabetes present a classic triad of symptoms: polydipsia, polyuria, and polyphagia. The symptoms appear more rapidly in children. The patient complains of excessive thirst *(polydipsia),* excretes large amounts of urine frequently *(polyuria),* and is constantly hungry *(polyphagia).* An insidious onset with lethargy, weakness, and weight loss is also common. Anorexia may be seen. The child who is toilet-trained may begin wetting the bed or have frequent "accidents" during play periods, may lose weight, and is irritable. The skin becomes dry. Vaginal yeast infections may be seen in the adolescent girl. Abdominal cramps are common. There may be a history of recurrent infections. The symptoms may go unrecognized until an infection becomes apparent or coma results. Laboratory findings indicate glucose in the urine (glycosuria or glucosuria). *Hyperglycemia* (*hyper,* "above," *gly,* "sugar," and *emia,* "blood") is also apparent.

The Honeymoon Period. When IDDM is initially diagnosed and the child is stabilized on insulin dosage, the condition may appear to improve. Insulin requirements decrease and the child feels well. This phenomenon supports the parent's phase of "denial" in accepting the long-term diagnosis of DM for their child. The "honeymoon period" lasts a short time (a few months), and parents must be encouraged to closely monitor blood sugar levels to avoid complications.

Table 30–2
CLINICAL FEATURES OF TYPE I AND TYPE II DIABETES

Feature	Type I (IDDM)	Type II (NIDDM)
Onset	Abrupt, frequently can date week of onset	Insidious, often found by screening tests
Body size	Normal or thin	Frequently obese
Blood glucose	Fluctuates widely with exercise and infection	Fluctuations are less marked
Ketoacidosis	Common	Infrequent
Sulfonylurea-responsiveness	Rare	Greater than 50%
Insulin required	Almost all	Less than 25%
Insulin dosage	Increases until stable glucose control	May remain stable

IDDM, insulin-dependent diabetes mellitus; NIDDM, non-insulin-dependent diabetes mellitus.

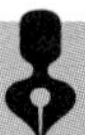

Nursing Tip

A period of remission, or the "honeymoon" phase of the disease, may occur within a few weeks of beginning insulin administration. There is a decline in insulin need and improved metabolic control. This, however, is temporary.

Diagnostic Blood Tests

Blood Glucose. A random blood glucose may be drawn at any time and requires no preparation of the client. The results should be within normal limits for both nondiabetics and diabetics in good control.

Fasting Blood Glucose. Fasting blood glucose is a standard and reliable test for diabetes. The blood glucose level is measured in the fasting patient, usually first thing in the morning. If the patient has a dextrose intravenous solution running, the results of the test will not be accurate. If the child is known to have diabetes, food and insulin are withheld until after the test. If a person's blood glucose is greater than 140 mg/dl on two separate occasions and the history is positive, the patient is considered to have diabetes and requires treatment. In nondiabetics the results are usually less than 115 mg/dl. A high blood glucose level before eating is a clear sign of diabetes.

Glucose Tolerance Test. Another test to determine the amount of sugar in the blood is the glucose tolerance test. Results are plotted on a graph (Fig. 30–3). An intravenous glucose tolerance test is preferred in children, as oral glucose tolerance tests have had low detection rates. Glucose is administered intravenously over several minutes to the fasting child. Blood samples are taken at 30, 60, 90, 120, and 180 minutes. Generally, small amounts of water are allowed. Parents and teenagers are advised to bring reading material, homework, headsets, and so on to the physician's office or laboratory, as the procedure is time-consuming. A blood glucose concentration greater than 200 mg/dl is considered positive. Normal values may not return for over 3 hours.

Glycosylated Hemoglobin Test. The *glycosylated hemoglobin test* (GHb) reflects glycemic levels over a period of months. Values are found to be elevated in virtually all children with newly diagnosed diabetes. This study also helps to confirm the results of blood and urine tests done either at home or by the doctor. Glucose in the bloodstream is constantly entering red blood cells and linking with, or glycosylating, molecules of hemoglobin. The more glucose is in the blood, the more hemoglobin becomes coated with glucose. The red blood cells carry this glucose until they are replaced by cells with fresh hemoglobin. This process takes about 3 to 4 months. Values vary according to measurement used. Values of 6% to 9% represent very good metabolic control. Values above 12% indicate poor control. One clinic awards an "under 9" badge to their patients who achieve this value and reports that a low glycosylated hemoglobin test can be a tremendous psychological boost.

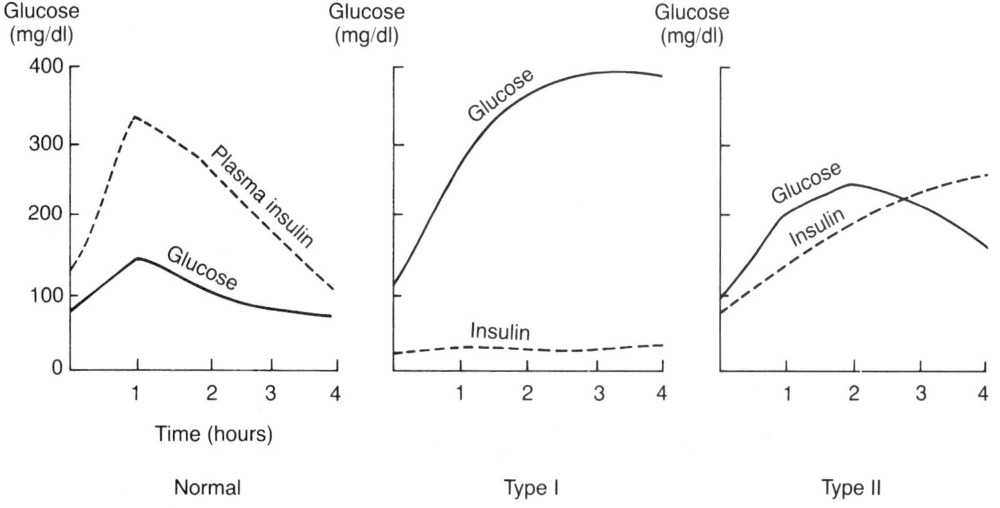

Figure 30–3. • The glucose tolerance test: *Left,* normal; *center,* type I diabetes; *right,* type II diabetes. The graphs show the relationship between the ingestion of glucose and the level of plasma insulin over 4 hours in a normal person and in persons with type I and type II diabetes. (Adapted from Waechter, E. H., & Blake, F. G. [1976]. *Nursing care of children* [9th ed.]. Philadelphia: Lippincott.)

Table 30–3
HYPERGLYCEMIA AND HYPOGLYCEMIA

Hyperglycemia (ketoacidosis)	Hypoglycemia
Cause	
Insulin underdose	Excess exercise
Food overdose	Too little food
	Insulin overdose
Signs and symptoms	
Polyuria, polydipsia, polyphagia	Fatigue
Fruity odor to breath	Hunger
Fatigue	Pale, clammy
Abdominal pain	Diaphoresis
Red lips, flushed face	Tremors
Dehydration	Lethargy
Disorientation	Headache
Drowsiness progressing to coma	
Deep, rapid (Kussmaul) respirations	
Treatment	
Regular insulin	Administer glucogon or orange juice or CHO orally

Glycosylated albumin (fructosamine) is a test used to measure blood glucose control over the preceding 7 to 10 days. C-peptide (connecting chains of insulin peptides) may also be measured to determine how much insulin the body is producing (endogenous). This is of particular value during the "honeymoon" period of the disease.

Diabetic Ketoacidosis (DKA). Diabetic *ketoacidosis* is also referred to as *diabetic coma,* although a person may have diabetic ketoacidosis with or without being in a coma. It may result if a diabetic patient contracts a secondary infection and does not follow proper self-care. It may also result, as occurs fairly often in diabetic children, if the disease proceeds unrecognized. Even minor infections, such as a cold, increase the body's metabolic rate and thereby change the body's demand for insulin and the severity of diabetes.

Symptoms of ketoacidosis are compared to those of hypoglycemia in Table 30–3. Diabetic teaching should include this information. The symptoms range from mild to severe and occur within hours to days.

Treatment and Nursing Care. The aims of treatment in type I diabetes are (1) to ensure normal growth and development through metabolic control, (2) to enable the child to cope with a chronic illness, have a happy and active childhood, and be well integrated into the family, and (3) to prevent complications. Complications can be minimized by maintaining blood glucose at consistently normal levels. Teaching ideally begins when the diagnosis is confirmed. A planned educational program is necessary to provide a consistent body of information, which can then be individualized. The patient's age and financial, educational, cultural, and religious background must be considered. Many hospitals hold group clinics for diabetic patients and their relatives. These sessions are conducted by the multidisciplinary health care team and include the diabetes nurse educator, dietitian, and pharmacist. Patients who are living with the disease provide encouragement and help by sharing concerns. Health professionals become directly involved with the patient's progress and can offer necessary feedback and support. Continuous follow-up is essential.

Because diabetic children are growing, additional dimensions of the disorder and its treatment become evident. Growth is not steady but occurs in spurts and plateaus that affect treatment. Infants and toddlers may have hydration problems, especially during illness. Preschool children have irregular activity and eating patterns. School-age children may grieve over the diagnosis and ask, "Why me?" They may use their illness to gain attention or to avoid responsibilities. The onset of puberty may require adjustments in insulin as a result of growth and the antagonistic effect of the sex hormones on insulin. Adolescents often resent this condition, which deviates from their concept of the "body ideal." They have more difficulty in resolving their conflict between dependence and independence. This may lead to rebellion against parents and treatment regimens.

The impact of the disease on the rest of the family must also be considered. Parents may also feel guilty for having passed on the disease. Siblings may feel jealous of the attention the patient receives. The sharing of responsibility by parents is ideal but not necessarily a reality. Some may have difficulty accepting the diagnosis and the more regimented lifestyle it imposes. Family members must cope with their individual reactions to the stress of the illness.

Children must assume responsibility for their own care gradually and with a minimum of pressure. Overprotection can be as detrimental as neglect. Parents who have received satisfaction from their child's dependence on them may need help "letting go." Diabetic camp experience is helpful in this respect. A medical identification bracelet should be worn.

The nursing management of childhood diabetes requires knowledge of growth and development, pathophysiology, blood glucose self-monitoring, nutritional management, insulin management, in-

NURSING CARE PLAN 30–1

Selected Nursing Diagnoses for the Child with Diabetes Mellitus

Nursing Diagnosis: High risk for injury related to hypoglycemia or diabetic ketoacidosis (hyperglycemia)

Goals	Nursing Interventions	Rationale
Child is able to measure blood glucose with glucometer, as age appropriate Child is adequately hydrated as evidenced by good tissue turgor and intake and output records Child is asymptomatic of hypoglycemia or hyperglycemia	1. Teach child home glucose monitoring	1. Self-care increases feelings of control
	2. Record vital signs regularly	2. Vital signs detect infection and illness, which affect diabetes; in ketoacidosis, Kussmaul respirations may be seen until blood pH and serum bicarbonate normalize
	3. Monitor fluid intake and output	3. Dehydration may occur as a result of vomiting, polyuria, and hyperglycemia
	4. Serve meals and snacks on time	4. Serving meals on time prevents hypoglycemia and minimizes hyperglycemia
	5. Administer or have patient administer insulin as ordered	5. Insulin is individualized to meet the response of patients. It cannot be taken by mouth, as stomach juices would destroy it before it could be used
	6. Assess level of consciousness	6. Both hypoglycemia and hyperglycemia affect sensorium, depending on stage of reaction
	7. Carefully observe patient for signs of hypoglycemia or hyperglycemia	7. Many factors such as diet, increased exercise, or illness can contribute to the body's balance of insulin and glucose; changes in hormone levels that accompany menstruation can cause swings of high or low blood sugar

Nursing Diagnosis: Knowledge deficit regarding exercise

Goals	Nursing Interventions	Rationale
Child describes physical exercise program Child is prepared for hypoglycemia, should it occur	1. Assess child's activity level as age appropriate	1. Exercise increases glucose utilization
	2. Explain that exercise lowers the blood sugar and in this respect acts like more insulin	2. Patient may need to adjust insulin for days when involved in high-impact exercise
	3. Instruct as to symptoms of hypoglycemia such as irritability, shakiness, hunger, headache, altered levels of consciousness	3. Early recognition and prompt treatment will prevent injury
	4. Teach child importance of carrying extra sugar when exercising or playing sports	4. Taking sugar reverses symptoms of hypoglycemia
	5. Teach child dangers of swimming alone	5. Child could drown if symptoms occur

Nursing Diagnosis: Knowledge deficit regarding identification

Goals	Nursing Interventions	Rationale
Child states understanding of importance of wearing proper identification bracelet Family acquires identification bracelet	1. Child demonstrates proper identification	1. Diabetes symptoms may be mistaken for other conditions, such as flu
	2. Encourage purchase of means of identification	2. Child may be unconscious or too young to inform others of condition

sulin shock, exercise, skin and foot care, infections, effects of emotional upsets, and long-term care. Nursing Care Plan 30–1 lists interventions for the child with diabetes mellitus.

Teaching Plan for Children with Diabetes. The patient and family are instructed about the location of the pancreas and its normal function. The nurse explains the relationship of insulin to the pancreas,

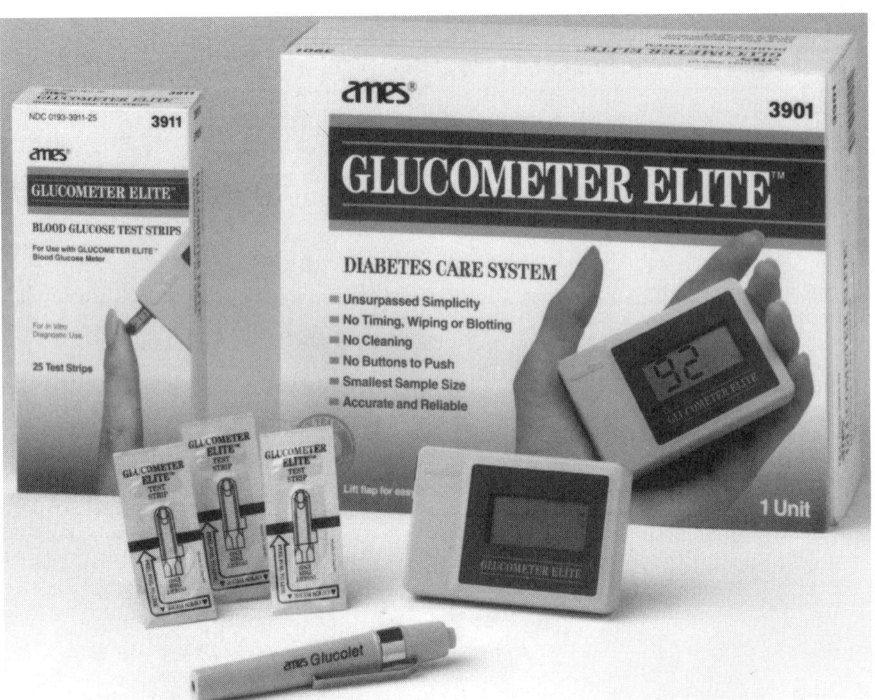

Figure 30–4. • Glucometer used to determine blood glucose values. (Courtesy of Miles, Inc., Diagnostics Division, Tarrytown, NY.)

differentiating between type I and type II diabetes. All information is given gradually and at the level of understanding of the child and family. Audiovisual aids and pamphlets are incorporated into the session. If the patient is newly diagnosed, hospitalization offers opportunities for instruction.

Blood Glucose Self-Monitoring. Patients can test their own blood glucose in the home. While still being supervised by and consulting with the physician, the patient can make rational changes in insulin dosage (sliding scale dosage) based on home blood glucose tests, nutritional requirements, and daily exercise. This is of great psychological value to the child, teenager, and parents, as it reduces feelings of helplessness and complete dependence on medical personnel. Home glucose monitoring should be taught to all young patients or their caretakers. The patient must not only be skilled in the techniques but also understand the results and how to incorporate them into daily regimens. This means involving the entire health care team in ongoing supervision, demonstrations, and support. Although instructions come with the various products, patients need individual training.

Glucometer systems provide readouts and automatically store data by time and date. Some also keep track of diet and the amount of exercise for the day. This can be connected to a computer or computer printer for review. Records can be transmitted over the telephone to the physician.

Obtaining blood specimens have been simplified by the use of capillary blood-letting devices, such as the Glucolet. This device automatically controls the depth of penetration of the lancet into the skin. Other brands include the Hamalet, Autoclix, Monoject, and Autolet. The sides of the fingertips are recommended testing sites, as there are fewer nerve endings and more capillary beds in these areas. The best finger to use is the middle, ring, or little finger on either hand. If the child washes the hands in warm water for about 30 seconds, the finger will bleed more easily. To perform the test, a drop of blood is put on a chemically treated reagent strip. The test strip with a drop of blood is inserted into the glucometer, and the blood glucose reading appears (Fig. 30–4).

Cost, convenience, and portability are factors to consider when selecting devices. Most products can be obtained at the local pharmacy. Newer and more precise instruments are being developed constantly. Frequency of use is determined by the amount of diabetes control required by the particular child.

DIET THERAPY FOR CHILDREN WITH DIABETES AND OTHER METABOLIC DISORDERS

Nutritional Management. The triad of management of diabetes comprises a well-balanced diet, insulin, and regular exercise. The importance of glycemic control in decreasing the incidence of symptoms and complications of the disease has been established. The advent of blood glucose self-monitoring is affecting food intake, in that diets can be fine-tuned and more flexible while the cornerstone of *consistency* (in amount of food and time of feeding) is maintained. Contrary to popular belief, there is no scientific evidence that persons with diabetes require special foods. In fact, if it is good for the diabetic, it is good for the entire family. The nutritional needs of diabetic children are essentially no different from those of nondiabetic children, with the exception of the elimination of concentrated carbohydrates (simple sugars). These cause a marked increase in blood glucose and should generally be avoided.

The goals of nutritional management in children are to ensure normal growth and development, to distribute food intake so that it aids metabolic control, and to individualize the diet in accordance with the child's ethnic background, age, sex, weight, activity, family economics, and food preferences. Once a diet prescription is received from the physician, the dietitian assists the family in designing an individualized diet plan. The dietitian also explains the use of exchange lists.

Education of the patient is ongoing. Too much information given at one time may overwhelm the parents and discourage the child. Well-informed nurses can offer much reinforcement and support. They can clarify such terms as dietetic, sugar-free, juice-packed, water-packed, and unsweetened. Meal trays in the hospital provide an excellent opportunity for teaching. Children should bring their lunch to school. Teenagers need to be advised that alcohol lowers the blood sugar. It suppresses gluconeogenesis and is high in calories. Most cocktail mixes contain sugar; however, water, sugar-free pop, club soda, and tomato juice do not. Although the consumption of alcohol is discouraged, the young person who wishes to drink should do so after dinner or should consume the beverage with some type of food. Respecting cultural patterns and personal preferences is important. The content of foods commonly found in fast-food chain restaurants is available through the American Diabetes Association.

The importance of fiber in diets is well documented. In the diabetic patient, soluble fiber has been shown to reduce blood sugar levels, lower serum cholesterol values, and sometimes reduce insulin requirements. Fiber appears to slow the rate of absorption of sugar by the digestive tract. Raw fruits and vegetables, bran cereals, wheat germ, beans, peas, and lentils are good sources of soluble fiber.

Glycemic Index, Cholesterol, Artificial Sweeteners. The glycemic index for selected foods has an impact on the manipulation of dietary needs. Because persons with diabetes have an increased risk for atherosclerosis, the reduction of serum cholesterol is another concern. These persons (like most of the general public) need to reduce their intake of animal fats or substitute vegetable fat for animal fat. This is accomplished by consuming less beef and pork and more lean meat, chicken, turkey, fish, low-fat milk (depending on age of patient), and vegetable proteins. The form of food is also significant. An apple, apple juice, and applesauce may precipitate different blood sugar responses. Portions, the type of processing, cooking, and combinations of foods have also been shown to have a bearing on these responses.

Aspartame (NutraSweet) was approved by the Food and Drug Administration in 1981. It is used in items that do not require cooking. Aspartame is made of two amino acids. Both contain insignificant amounts of carbohydrate. One granulation form is called Equal. Sorbitol, mannitol, and xylitol are sugars commonly found in foods called "sugar-free." These substances are absorbed more slowly into the bloodstream. Large amounts of sorbitol can cause diarrhea and overuse should be avoided.

Insulin Management. Insulin is used principally as a specific drug for the control of diabetes mellitus. When injected into the diabetic patient, it enables the body to burn and store sugar. Current data emphasize the importance of blood glucose control in the prevention of microvascular disease. Insulin pumps are used in certain patients (Fig. 30–5). More highly purified insulins are being developed to reduce complications. *Human insulin,* which is not made from humans but is produced biosynthetically in bacteria using recombinant DNA technology, is widely used. It is reported to be very similar to the body's natural insulin. One example is Humulin, manufactured by the Eli Lilly Company.

The dose of insulin is measured in units, and special syringes are used in its administration. U-100 (100-unit) insulin is the standard form. Each marking on the 1-ml (100-unit) syringe represents 2 units of insulin. The 50-unit disposable syringe is

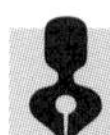

Nursing Tip

Instruct the patient and family to read food labels carefully. The word *dietetic* does not mean *diabetic.* Dietetic merely means something has been changed or replaced; for example, the food may have less salt or less sugar.

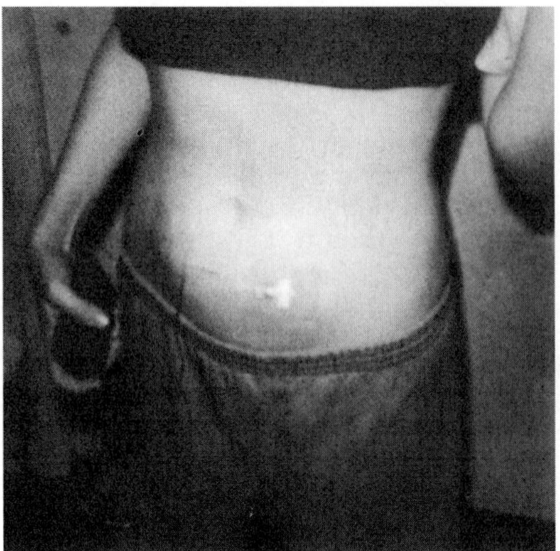
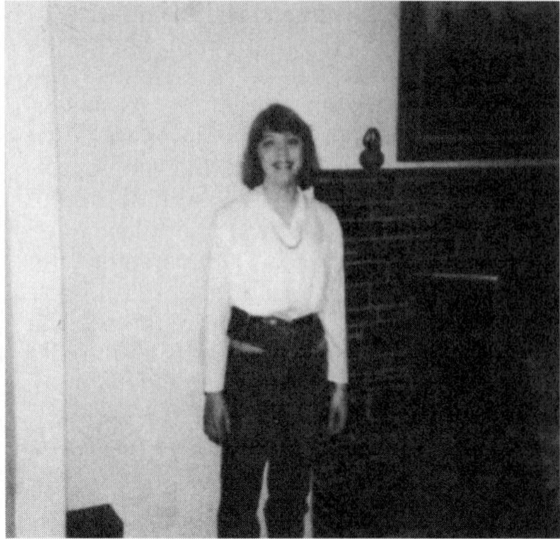

Figure 30–5. • The insulin pump offers continuous subcutaneous insulin infusion without the need for frequent injections.

intended for small doses. All vials of U-100 insulin have color-coded caps, and all labels bear black printing on a white background. Bold letters indicate type: "R" for regular, "P" for protamine zinc insulin (PZI), "N" for neutral protamine Hagedorn (NPH) insulin, "L" for lente, "U" for ultralente, and "S" for semilente.

It is important to teach the parents and child about the administration of insulin. Insulin cannot be taken orally because it is a protein and would be broken down by the gastric juices. The usual method of administration is *subcutaneously* (Fig. 30–6). When injected at a 90-degree angle, the short needle enters the subcutaneous space. This technique may be easier for the child to learn because it takes less coordination to administer than a 45-degree-angle technique. Automatic injection devices (Fig. 30–7), the insulin pump, and needle-free injectors such as Medi-Jector, EZ, or Tendertouch are fairly easy to use and promote independence in the child. A child can generally be taught to perform self-injection after the age of 7. The doctor prescribes the type and amount of insulin and specifies the time of administration.

The site of the injection is rotated to prevent poor absorption and injury to tissues (Fig. 30–8). Injection model forms made from construction paper and site rotation patterns are useful. One suggested site rotation pattern is to use one area for 1 week. For each injection, a different site within that area is used. Injections should be about 1 inch apart. The young child can use a doll to practice self-injection.

Insulin should not be injected into an area that has a temporarily increased circulation. A more rapid than expected effect can trigger hypoglycemia. For example, a more rapid circulation to the legs can be expected in a child who is riding a tricycle, therefore the thigh should not be selected as a site for injection. If a teen returns from playing

Nursing Tip

Take snacks seriously—they are an important part of the day's food supply.

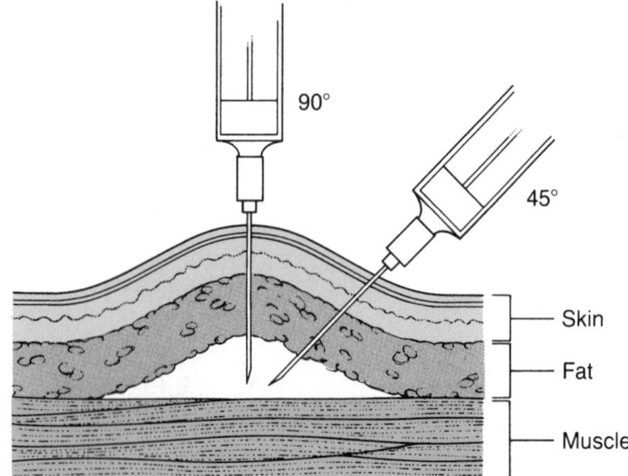

Figure 30–6. • Subcutaneous injection of insulin. (From Betz, C., Hunsberger, M., & Wright, S. [1994]. *Family-centered nursing care of children* [2nd ed.]. Philadelphia: Saunders.)

Nursing Tip

When mixing insulin, always withdraw the regular insulin first and then add the long-acting insulin into the syringe.

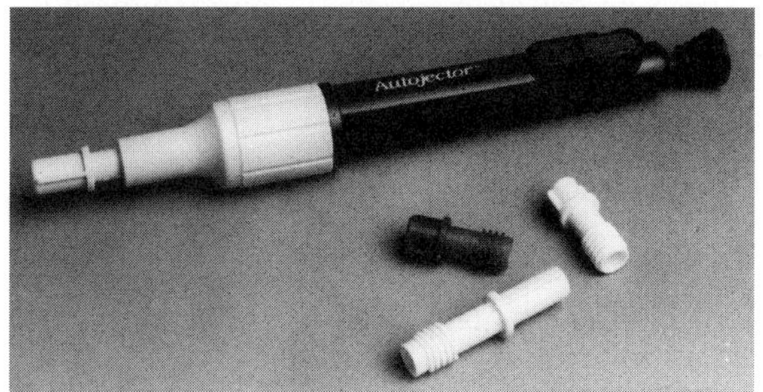

Figure 30–7. • The Autojector delivers the predrawn dosage at the preset depth by a button control. It has four depth adjusters. (Courtesy of Ulster Scientific, New Paltz, NY.)

tennis, the upper arm is avoided as an injection site following that type of activity.

Lipoatrophy (*lipo,* "fat," and *atrophy,* "loss of") and *lipohypertrophy* (*lipo,* and *hypertrophy,* "increase of") refer to changes that can occur in the subcutaneous tissue at the injection site. Proper rotation of sites and the availability of the newer purified insulins have helped to eliminate this condition. The child is taught to "feel for lumps" every week and to avoid using any sites that are suspicious.

The various types of insulin and their action are

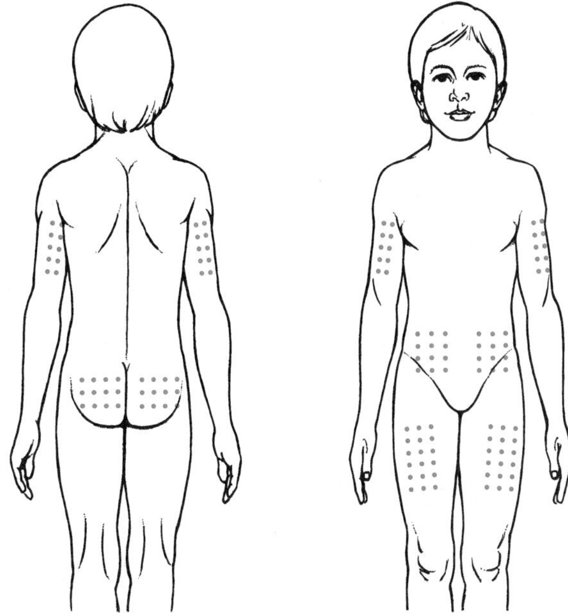

Figure 30–8. • Sites of injection of insulin. (From Betz, C., Hunsberger, M., & Wright, S. [1994]. *Family-centered nursing care of children* [2nd ed.]. Philadelphia: Saunders.)

listed in Table 30–4. The main difference is in the amount of time required for it to take effect and the length of protection time. The values listed in Table 30–4 are only *guidelines.* The response of each diabetic child to any given insulin dose is highly individual and depends on many factors, such as site of injection, local destruction of insulin by tissue enzymes, and insulin antibodies.

Regular or crystalline insulin is a purified form of

Table 30–4
HYPOGLYCEMICS: INSULIN

		Hypoglycemic Effect		
	Brand Name(s)	***Onset (hr)***	***Peak (hr)***	***Duration (hr)***
Rapid-acting				
Lispro	Lispro	15–30 min	30–90 min	2–4
Regular insulin	Humulin R Novolin R Velosulin	0.5–1	2–4	6–8
Semilente insulin	Semilente	1–1.5	5–10	12–16
Intermediate-acting				
Lente insulin	Humulin L Novolin L	1–2.5	7–15	24
Neutral protamine Hagedorn (NPH) insulin	Humulin N Insulintard Novolin N	1–1.5	4–12	24
Long-acting				
Protamine zinc insulin (PZI)	PZI	4–8	8–24	24–36
Ultralente insulin	Humulin U Ultralente	4–8	10–30	>36

From Hodgson, B. B., Kizior, R. J., & Kingdon, R. T. (1993). *Nurse's drug handbook.* Philadelphia: Saunders; and Behrman, R., & Kleigman, R. (1998). *Nelson's essentials of pediatrics.* Philadelphia: Saunders.

regular insulin and is less likely to cause allergic reactions. Both NPH, an intermediate type, and PZI, a long-lasting insulin, have had small amounts of chemicals added to prolong their action and to make them more stable. They offer protection over a period of hours, enabling the patient to do without repeated injections of unmodified insulin. They are cloudy and require mixing before being withdrawn from the vials. This is done by gently rolling the bottle between the palms of the hands. Insulin is not used if it is discolored.

Frequently the physician orders a combination of a short-acting insulin and an intermediate-acting one; for example, "Give 10 units of NPH insulin and 5 units of regular insulin at 7:30 A.M." This offers the patient immediate and longer-lasting protection. NPH or Lente insulin may be given in the same syringe as regular or crystalline insulin (Fig. 30–9). Long-acting types of insulin are seldom given to children because of the danger of *hypoglycemia* during sleep. Stable premixed insulins are now available.

Insulin Shock. Insulin shock, also known as *hypoglycemia* (*hypo*, "below," *glyco*, "sugar," and *emia*, "blood"), occurs when the blood sugar level becomes abnormally low. This condition is caused by too much insulin. Factors that may account for this imbalance include poorly planned exercise, reduction of diet, and errors made because of improper knowledge of insulin and the insulin syringe.

Children are more prone to insulin reactions than adults because (1) the condition itself is more unstable in young people, (2) they are growing, and (3) their activities are more irregular. Poorly planned exercise is frequently the cause of insulin shock during childhood. Hospitalized patients who are being regulated must be observed frequently during naptime and at night. The nurse becomes suspicious of problems if unable to arouse the patient or if the child is perspiring heavily.

The symptoms of an insulin reaction, which range from mild to severe, are generally noticed and treated in the early stages. They appear suddenly in the otherwise well person. Examination of the blood would reveal a lowered blood sugar level. The child becomes irritable and may behave poorly, is pale, and may complain of feeling hungry and weak. Sweating occurs. Symptoms related to disorders of the nervous system arise because glucose is vital to the proper functioning of nerves. The child may become mentally confused and giddy, and muscular coordination is affected. If insulin shock is left untreated, coma and convulsions can occur.

The immediate treatment consists of administering sugar in some form, such as orange juice, hard candy, or a commercial product such as Glutose. The patient begins to feel better within a few minutes and at that time may eat a small amount of protein or starch (sandwich, milk, cheese) to prevent another reaction. *Glucagon* is recommended for the treatment of severe hypoglycemia. It quickly restores the child to consciousness in an emergency; the child can then consume some form of sugar or a planned meal.

The *Somogyi phenomenon* (rebound hyperglycemia) occurs when blood glucose levels are lowered to a point at which the body's counterregulatory hormones (epinephrine, cortisol, glucagon) are released. Glucose is released from muscle and liver cells, which precipitates a rapid rise in blood glucose. It is generally the result of chronic insulin use, especially in patients who require fairly large doses of insulin to regulate their blood sugar. Hypoglycemia during the night and high glucose levels in the morning are suggestive of the phenomenon. The child may awaken at night or have frequent nightmares and experience early morning sweating and headaches. The child actually needs *less* insulin, not more, to rectify the problem.

The Somogyi phenomenon differs from the *dawn phenomenon,* in which early morning elevations of blood glucose occur *without* preceding hypoglycemia but may be a response to growth hormone secretion that occurs in the early morning hours. Together the Somogyi and dawn phenomena are the most common causes of instability in diabetic children. Testing blood glucose around 3 AM helps to differentiate the two conditions and assists in regulating insulin dosage.

Exercise. Exercise is important for the patient with diabetes because it causes the body to use sugar and promotes good circulation. It lowers the blood glucose, and in this respect it acts like more insulin. The diabetic patient who has planned vigorous exercise should carry extra sugar to avoid insulin reactions. The patient should also carry money for candy or a drink or to use a telephone. The blood glucose level is high directly after meals, so the child can participate in active sports at such times. Games enjoyed directly before meals should be less active. The diabetic child is able to participate in almost all active sports. Poorly planned exercise, however, can lead to difficulties.

Skin Care. The patient is instructed to bathe daily and dry well. Cleansing of the inguinal area, axillae, perineum, and inframammary areas is especially important, as yeast and fungal infections tend to occur there. Skin is inspected for cuts, rashes, abrasions, bruises, cysts, or boils. These lesions are managed promptly. If skin is very dry, an oil such as Alpha-Keri may be used in the bath water. Adolescents are taught to use electric razors.

1. Wash your hands.
2. Gently rotate the intermediate insulin bottle.
3. Wipe off the tops of the insulin vials with an alcohol sponge.
4. Draw back an amount of air into the syringe equal to the total dose.
5. Inject air equal to the NPH dose into the NPH vial. Remove the syringe from the vial.

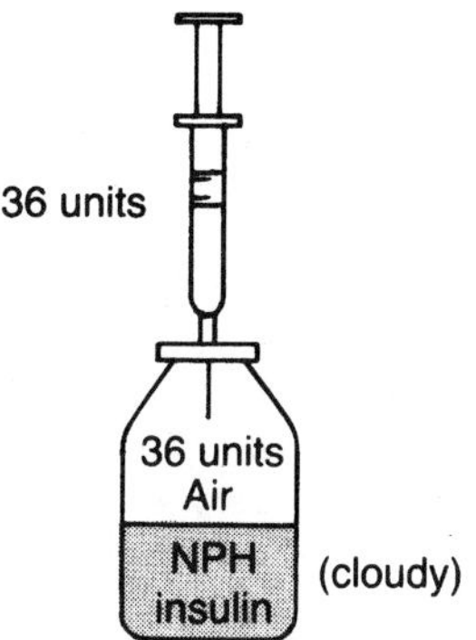

6. Inject air equal to the regular dose into the regular vial.

12 units

12 units
Air

Regular
insulin

(clear)

7. Invert the regular insulin bottle and withdraw the regular insulin dose.

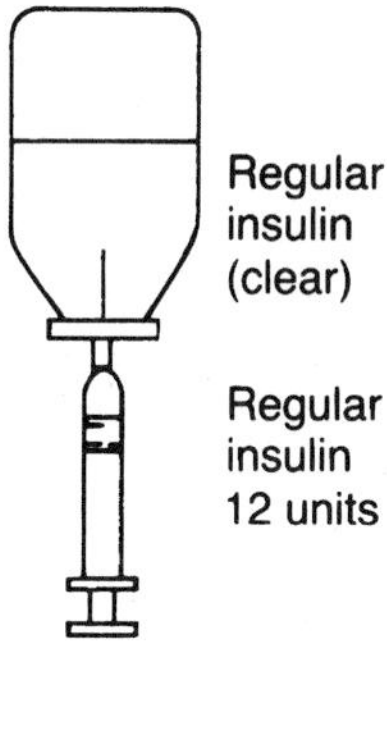

8. Without adding more air to the NPH vial, carefully withdraw the NPH dose.

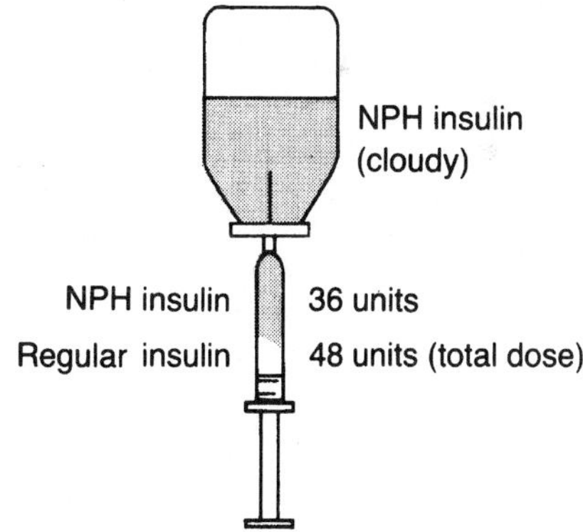

Figure 30–9. • Mixing insulin. This step-order process avoids the problem of contaminating the regular insulin with the intermediate insulin. If contamination of the regular insulin does occur, the rapid-acting effect of this drug would be dampened, and it would be unreliable as a quick-acting insulin in an acute situation such as diabetic ketoacidosis. (From Price, M. J. [1983]. Insulin and oral hypoglycemic agents. *Nursing Clinics of North America, 18,* 687–706.)

Exposing the skin to extremes in temperatures is avoided. Injection sites are inspected for lumps.

Foot Care. Although circulatory problems of the feet are less common in children, proper habits of foot hygiene need to be established. Patients are instructed to wash and dry their feet well each day. The feet are inspected for interdigital cracking, and the condition of the toenails is checked. Nails are trimmed straight across. Corn remedies, iodine, or alcohol should not be used. Socks are changed daily, and tight socks or large ones that bunch up are avoided. Shoes are replaced often as the child grows. The child should not go barefoot.

Infections. Immunizations against communicable diseases are essential.

Emotional Upsets. Emotional upsets can be as disturbing to the patient as an infection and may require food or insulin adjustments, or both. Table 30–5 lists nursing interventions for stress on child and family related to type I diabetes.

Urine Checks. Routine urine checks for sugar are being replaced by the more accurate glucose blood monitoring. However, this procedure does not test for acetone, which the patient may need to determine, particularly when the blood glucose level is high and during illness. Daily urine checks may be advocated for some patients. Saying urine "check" rather than "test" is less confusing to young children.

Glucose-Insulin Imbalances. The patient is taught to recognize the signs of insulin shock and ketoacidosis (see Table 30–3). Early attention to change and daily recordkeeping are stressed. Many excellent teaching films and brochures are available. The child should wear an identification bracelet. Wallet cards are also available. Teachers, athletic coaches, and guidance personnel are informed about the disease and should have the telephone numbers of the patient's parents and physician.

Travel. With planning, children can enjoy travel with their families, and older adolescents can travel alone. Before leaving, the child should be seen by the physician for a checkup and prescriptions for supplies. A written statement and a card identifying the child as diabetic should be carried. Time changes may affect meals. Additional supplies of insulin, sugar, and food are kept with the child. These are never checked with luggage, especially on an airplane, as they may be lost. If foreign travel is planned, parents need to become familiar with the food in the area so that dietary requirements can be met. Local chapters of the American Diabetes Association or the Juvenile Diabetes Foundation can help vacationing families in an emergency.

Follow-up Care. The child needs to see the physician regularly. The patient should also be taught to visit the dentist regularly for cleaning of teeth and gums. Brushing and flossing daily are essential. Eyes should be examined regularly; blurry vision must not be disregarded. Magazines such as *Diabetes Forecast* and *Diabetes in the News* offer excellent suggestions and guidance.

Surgery. The diabetic usually tolerates surgery well. Insulin may be given before or after the operation. If the patient is restricted to nothing by mouth, calories may be supplied by intravenous glucose. Details vary according to the procedure and the patient's treatment for diabetes. Careful review of the patient's history helps in formulating nursing care plans and provides a basis for teaching.

Prospects for the Future. Diabetic research is being conducted on many fronts. Geneticists are helping to determine how diabetes is inherited so that one day they will be able to predict who will inherit the disease. Pancreas transplantation has been performed, and the success rate is improving. Beta-cell transplantation in animals has resulted in their cure. An artificial pancreas is another possibility; its precursors might be the insulin pumps used today. The laser beam has aided the treatment for complicated eye conditions. Such advances hold promise for resolving or eradicating the dilemma of diabetes. Diet therapy for various types of endocrine disorders is reviewed in Table 30–6.

Table 30–5

NURSING INTERVENTIONS FOR PREDICTABLE TYPES OF STRESS ON A CHILD WITH TYPE I DIABETES AND ON THE FAMILY

Age	Issue	Nursing Interventions
Infant	Trust versus mistrust Onset and diagnosis particularly difficult during infancy; anxiety can be transmitted to baby	Stress consistency in fulfilling needs Involve both parents in education Avoid information overload Instill hope and confidence Focus on child rather than disease Review normal growth and development of infancy Assist in problem-solving (baby-sitters, difficulty in obtaining specimens, baby food exchange lists, and so on)
Toddler	Autonomy versus shame and doubt	Prepare child for procedures or separations Encourage exploration of environment Stress limit setting as a form of love
	Is this a temper tantrum or high or low blood sugar?	Admit it is difficult to distinguish temper tantrums from symptoms If behavior worsens or is prolonged or if physical symptoms appear, check blood sugar Provide 24-hr telephone number
Preschool	Initiative versus guilt	Foster sense of competence
	May view injections as punishment	Educate parents to provide consistent warmth, reassurance, and love
	May view denial of sweets as lack of love	Discuss feelings about child's life and diabetes Avoid negative connotation by words, for example, "bad blood test," "cheating" Help parents sort out child's fantasies
	"Picky eater"	Plan favorite party dishes on occasion Invite a playmate for lunch Suggest alternative nutritious snacks
Elementary school	Industry versus inferiority	Assist child in how to respond to teasing from peers ("Yecch, needles")
	Patients may feel they will be cured by hospitalization	Explain "honeymoon" stage of disease
	Grief over lack of cure	Accept child's disappointment
	Rebellion over treatment regimen	Gradually assume self-management of insulin and specimen tests; this increases feelings of mastery and control
	Rebellion over food plan	Provide lists of fast-food exchanges
	Anxiety about disclosure of condition to friends	Group-related education with diabetic peers
	Embarrassed about reactions in school, missed days	Promote open dialogue among health personnel and teachers, school nurse, fellow students
	Unpredictable effects of exercise	Continually reinforce treatment principles with specific regard to hypoglycemia or hyperglycemia and emergencies
Puberty	"Bouncing" blood sugars may make child feel out of control	Explain that growth and sex hormones affect blood sugars Girls, in particular, experience difficulties about the time of menstruation Adjustments in insulin and food are common for most diabetics at this stage
	Anger at the disease: "Why must I be different?"	Assist patient in acceptable ways of expressing anger; discuss anger with parents, as they are often its target
	More frequent hospitalizations	Provide encouragement and support; be alert to marital stress and sibling deprivation

Table 30–6
DIET THERAPY IN PEDIATRIC METABOLIC DISORDERS

Disorder	Major Signs and Symptoms	Dietary Regime
Phenylketonuria (PKU)	Mental retardation	Low phenylalanine diet, Lofenalac formula for infants
Celiac disease	Chronic diarrhea, irritability, distention, failure to thrive	Eliminate gluten, use corn flour and vitamin B supplements
Cystic fibrosis	Thick mucus causes obstruction of pancreatic enzymes and poor absorption of nutrients, flatulence and foul-smelling stools	Pancreatic enzyme replacement with normal meals
Lactose intolerance	Abdominal distension, cramps, diarrhea, failure to thrive	Lactose-free diet. Use Prosobee, soy formulas, avoid milk/milk products
Galactose intolerance	Jaundice, vomiting, convulsions, lethargy, blindness	No galactose or lactose in diet, use milk substitutes
Fructose intolerance	Vomiting, diarrhea, failure to thrive	Fructose-free diet, avoid honey, fruit, sorbitol, and sucrose. Offer vitamin C and vegetables.
Maple syrup urine disease	Acidosis, convulsions	Low-leucine and low-valine diet
Urea cycle defect	Lethargy	Low-protein diet
Acidemia	Seizures, elevated ammonia levels	
Diabetes insipidus	Inability to concentrate urine, diuresis	Unrestricted water intake
Diabetes mellitus	Inability to produce insulin to metabolize sugar, protein, and fat	Controlled sugar intake regulated with insulin administration; high-fiber, balanced diet

KEY POINTS

- The two major systems that control and monitor the functions of the body are the nervous system and the endocrine system.
- The term *inborn error of metabolism* refers to a group of inherited biochemical disorders that affect body metabolism.
- Screening programs for early detection of inborn errors are important because some conditions can cause irreversible neurologic damage.
- Diabetes mellitus type I (IDDM) is the most common endocrine disorder of children. The body is unable to utilize carbohydrates properly because of a deficiency of insulin, an internal secretion of the pancreas.
- The symptoms of diabetes appear more rapidly in children. Three symptoms are polydipsia, polyuria, and polyphagia.
- The mainstays of the management of diabetes are insulin replacement, diet, and exercise.
- Diabetic ketoacidosis is a serious complication that may become life-threatening.
- Self-management to maintain glucose control and to prevent complications is a major goal of education of the child with diabetes.
- A deficiency in the secretion of the thyroid gland is termed hypothyroidism. It may be congenital or acquired and requires lifelong treatment by oral administration of a synthetic thyroid hormone.
- The glycosylated hemoglobin test reflects glucose control over a period of months.
- Excess intake of sugar substitutes such as sorbitol can cause diarrhea.
- A child with diabetes insipidus requires unlimited access to water.
- Growth hormone is administered at bedtime to stimulate the natural time of hormone release.

MULTIPLE-CHOICE REVIEW QUESTIONS

Choose the most appropriate answer.

1. Which of the following is an important aspect of a teaching plan for the parent of a child with hypopituitarism?
   a. The child should be enrolled in a special education program at school.
   b. The routine administration of growth hormone should be administered at bedtime.
   c. All family members should have an endocrine work-up.
   d. The routine medication should be administered before the school day starts.
2. A child who has diabetes asks why he cannot take insulin orally instead of by subcutaneous injection. The best response of the nurse would be:
   a. Pills are only for adults.
   b. Insulin is destroyed by digestive enzymes.
   c. Insulin can cause a stomach ulcer.
   d. Insulin interacts with food in the stomach.
3. Which of the following may indicate a need for insulin in a diabetic child?
   a. Diaphoresis and tremors
   b. Red lips and fruity odor to the breath
   c. Confusion and lethargy
   d. Headache and pallor
4. The nurse teaches the diabetic child to rotate sites of insulin injection in order to:
   a. prevent subcutaneous deposit of the drug.
   b. prevent lipoatrophy of subcutaneous fat.
   c. decrease the pain of injection.
   d. increase absorption of insulin.
5. Kussmaul respirations are seen in diabetic children with
   a. neuropathy.
   b. ketoacidosis.
   c. hypoglycemia.
   d. retinopathy.

BIBLIOGRAPHY AND READER REFERENCE

Behrman, R., & Kleigman, R. (1998). *Nelson's essentials of pediatrics.* Philadelphia: Saunders.

Behrman, R., Kleigman, R., & Arvin, A. (1996). *Nelson's textbook of pediatrics* (15th ed.). Philadelphia: Saunders.

Betz, C., Hunsberger, M., & Wright, S. (1994). *Family-centered nursing care of children* (2nd ed.). Philadelphia: Saunders.

Bowden, V., Dickey, S., & Greenberg, C. (1998). *Children and their families: The continuum of care.* Philadelphia: Saunders.

Cookfair, J. (1996). *Nursing care in the community.* St. Louis, MO: Mosby.

Davies, R. (1996). Caring for patients with diabetes insipidus. *Nursing 96,* 5, 62–63.

Faulkner, M. (1996). Family responses to children with diabetes and their influence on self-care. *Journal of Pediatric Nursing, 11*(20), 82–93.

Maffeo, R. (1997). Helping families cope with type I diabetes. *American Journal of Nursing, 6* 36–39.

Mahan, L., & Escott-Stump, S. (1997). *Krause's food, nutrition & diet therapy* (9th ed.). Philadelphia: Saunders.

McConnell, E. (1997). Monitoring blood glucose levels at the bedside. *Nursing, 27*(4), 28.

Oleske, J., & Boland, M. (1997). When a child with a chronic condition needs hospitalization. *Hospital Practice, 32*(6), 167.

Robertson, C. (1998). When your patient is on an insulin pump. *RN, 61*(3), 30.

Wong, D. (1997). *Whaley & Wong's essentials of pediatric nursing.* St. Louis, MO: Mosby.

chapter 31

The Child with a Communicable Disease

Outline

Objectives

On completion and mastery of Chapter 31, the student will be able to

- Define vocabulary terms listed.
- Discuss three principles involved in standard precautions used to prevent the transmission of communicable diseases in children.
- Discuss national and international immunization programs.
- Describe the nurse's role in the immunization of children.
- Interpret the detection and prevention of common childhood communicable diseases.
- Discuss the characteristics of common childhood communicable diseases.
- Formulate a nursing care plan for a child with AIDS.
- Demonstrate a teaching plan for preventing STDs in an adolescent.

Vocabulary

acquired immunity	papule
active immunity	passive immunity
body substance	pathogens
endemic	pathonomonic
epidemic	portal of entry
erythema	portal of exit
fomite	prodromal
incubation period	pustule
macule	reservoir for infection
natural immunity	STD
nosocomial infection	standard precautions
opportunistic infection	vector
pandemic	vesicle

COMMUNICABLE DISEASE

There have been only a few brief periods in history when infectious disease did not dominate the attention of health care professionals. In spite of immunization, sanitation, antibiotics, and other controls, the world continues to face infectious agents such as human immunodeficiency virus (HIV), hepatitis, tuberculosis, and sexually transmitted diseases (STDs). In spite of our knowledge of immunizations, some children still suffer from common communicable diseases (Table 31–1). Antibiotic-resistant organisms increase, and immunocompromised patients are threatened by nonpathogenic organisms. Prevention and control are key factors in managing infectious disease.

Common Childhood Communicable Diseases

The incidence of common childhood communicable diseases has dramatically decreased as immunological agents have been developed. Diseases such as smallpox have declined to a point worldwide that routine immunizations are no longer recommended. (A brief review of smallpox is presented in this chapter because the nurse must be able to identify a smallpox lesion and refer for follow-up care to avoid an outbreak of this deadly illness.) Providing all children with the appropriate immunizations is the health care challenge of today. Airplane travel is commonplace and rapid transmission of contagious diseases from around the world requires alert assessment by the nurse and all health care workers.

REVIEW OF TERMS

A *communicable disease* is one that can be transmitted, directly or indirectly, from one person to another. Organisms that cause disease are called *pathogens.*

The *incubation* period is the time between the invasion by the pathogen and the onset of clinical symptoms. The *prodromal* period refers to the initial stage of a disease: the interval between the earliest symptoms and the appearance of a typical rash or fever. Children are frequently contagious during this time, but because the symptoms are not specific they may attend preschool or another group program and spread the disease. A *fomite* is any inanimate material that absorbs and transmits infection. A *vector* is an insect or animal that carries and spreads a disease. A *pandemic* is a worldwide high incidence of a communicable disease. An *epidemic* is a *sudden* increase of a communicable disease in a localized area. An *endemic* is an expected *continuous* incidence of a communicable disease in a localized area. *Body substance* refers to moist secretions or parts of the body that can contain microorganisms. Emesis, saliva, sputum, semen, urine, feces, and blood are examples of body substances. Body substance precautions indicate the need to wear disposable protective gloves and/or garments when coming in contact with these body substances. A *portal of entry* is a route by which the organisms enter the body (for example, a cut in the skin). A *portal of exit* is the route by which the organisms exit the body (for example, feces or urine). A *reservoir for infection* is a place that supports the growth of organisms (for example, standing, stagnant water). The *chain of infection* refers to the way in which organisms spread and infect the individual (Fig. 31–1). Standard precautions are found in Appendix A. Careful handwashing is basic and essential to contain infection.

HOST RESISTANCE

Many factors contribute to the virulence of an infectious disease. The age, sex, and genetic makeup of the child have a bearing. The nutritional status of the person, as well as physical and emotional health, is also important. The efficiency of the blood-forming organs and of the immune systems

Table 31–1
COMMUNICABLE DISEASES OF CHILDHOOD

Disease	Causative Organism	Signs and Symptoms	Incubation Period	Prevention/ Treatment	How Long Contagious	Nursing Interventions
Chicken pox (varicella)	Varicella zoster virus	Prodromal signs include mild fever followed by macules, papules, vesicles, pustules, and scabs. All stages of lesion are present on the body at the same time	2–3 weeks (13–17 days average)	Vaccine available; acyclovir (zovirax) or immune globulin given to immunosuppressed children who are exposed	6 days after appearance of rash	Trim fingernails to prevent scratching. (Removal of scabs may cause scars). Calamine lotion may reduce itching. Isolate from others
Smallpox (variola)	Virus	Child appears toxic. Macules, papules, vesicles, pustules, and scabs appear. Only one stage of the lesion at a time is present on the body.	6–18 days (12 days average)	Routine smallpox vaccination is no longer recommended unless patient is traveling into high-risk country	Highly contagious; CDC notification required	A toxic illness with a high mortality rate. Strict isolation required preferably in a negative pressure room and restricted caregivers
German measles (rubella)	Rubella virus	Mild fever and cold symptoms precede a rose-colored maculopapular rash. Enlarged glands at back of neck and ears	2–3 weeks (18 day average)	All infants should receive vaccine, with boosters at preschool age	Until rash fades (5 days)	Symptomatic treatment and comfort measures. Avoid exposing any woman who might be in early months of pregnancy as rubella can cause fetal anomalies
Measles (rubeola)	Virus	Fever, cough, conjunctivitis followed by small white (koplik spots) on inner cheeks (exanthem), then maculopapular rash erupts (exanthem)	1–2 weeks (10 days average)	All infants should receive vaccine at 15 months and boosters at preschool age. Gamma globulin may be given after exposure. Vitamin A is recommended to reduce morbidity	From 4 days before to 5 days after rash appears	Symptomatic care. Isolate, provide quiet activities. Utilize measures to reduce eyestrain caused by photophobia. Detailed oral care
Fifth disease (erythema infectiosum)	Human parvovirus B19 (HPV)	Child has "slapped cheek" appearance. Generalized rash appears, subsides, and reappears if skin is irritated by sun or heat	4–14 days	None	During incubation period	This is a benign condition unless child is immunocompromised. Isolation not required. May last 1–3 weeks.

Table continued on following page

Table 31–1 *(Continued)*

COMMUNICABLE DISEASES OF CHILDHOOD

Disease	Causative Organism	Signs and Symptoms	Incubation Period	Prevention/ Treatment	How Long Contagious	Nursing Interventions
Roseola (exanthem subitum) (sixth disease)	Herpes virus 6 (HHV 6)	Persistent high (103°F–105°F) fever that drops rapidly as the rash appears. The maculopapular rash is nonpruritic and blanches easily	2 weeks	None; high fever may precipitate convulsions	Until rash fades	Rest and quiet should be provided. Teach parents temperature-reducing techniques and prevention of seizures
Mumps (parotitis)	Paramyxovirus	Fever, headache, glands near ear and toward jaw line ache and develop painful swelling. Enlarged parotid gland. May be bilateral	14–21 days (18 days average)	Vaccine after 15 mo of age (MMR)	Until swelling subsides	Encourage fluids, ice compresses to neck for comfort. Isolate
Whooping cough (pertussis)	*Bordetella pertussis*	Fever, cold, cough. Spells of coughing accompanied by a noisy gasp for air that creates a "whoop"	5–21 days (10 days average)	Vaccinate all infants with series (DPT). Exposed unvaccinated child may be given erythromycin. Cool mist tent, antibiotics used for treatment	Several weeks	Isolate, bed rest, provide abdominal support during coughing spell. Refeed if vomits. Observe for airway obstruction
Polio (infantile paralysis; poliomyelitis)	Enterovirus	Fever, headache, stiff neck and stiff back, paralysis	1–2 weeks	Start complete series of polio vaccines in infancy. May require respirator care	1 week for throat secretions; 4 weeks for feces	Isolate, bed rest, observe for respiratory distress. Position, physiotherapy, and range of movement exercises
Infectious mononucleosis (glandular fever)	Epstein-Barr virus (EBV)	Low-grade fever, malaise, jaundice, enlarged spleen	2–6 weeks	Limit contact with saliva. Do not share eating utensils	(Spread by direct contact only)	Rest and supportive treatment. Isolation not required. Provide school tutoring to maintain grade level
Hepatitis A	Enterovirus 72	Fever, anorexia, headache, abdominal pain, malaise, jaundice, dark urine, and chalklike stools	15–45 days	Hepatitis A vaccine recommended for children traveling to endemic areas. Gamma globulin if child is exposed	Virus may be shed for 6 months in neonates	Educate family and community concerning ingestion of contaminated water or shellfish from contaminated water or swimming in contaminated water. Proper handwashing essential. Standard precautions essential

Table continued on following page

Table 31–1 *(Continued)*
COMMUNICABLE DISEASES OF CHILDHOOD

Disease	Causative Organism	Signs and Symptoms	Incubation Period	Prevention/ Treatment	How Long Contagious	Nursing Interventions
Hepatitis B	HBV virus	Symptoms same as type A. Can manifest liver pathology	30–180 days	Hepatitis B vaccine (HBV) series during newborn period or for health care workers or travelers. Interferon or reverse transcriptase inhibitors may be effective treatment. Liver transplant may be necessary. Immune globulin may be indicated for exposed susceptible children	May persist in carrier state	Prevent contact with blood or blood products. Identify high-risk mothers and newborns. Educate concerning need for vaccination
Lyme disease	*Borrelia Burgdorferi*	Skin lesions at site of tick bite. Macule with raised border and clear center. May "burn." Fever, arthralgia. May lead to heart and neurologic involvement	3–32 days	Wear protective clothing in wooded area. Inspect for ticks following play when camping. Light-colored clothing makes tick more noticeable. Remove tick with tweezer. Inspect pets. Treat with amoxicillin or doxycycline	Spread by infected tick	Educate concerning prevention of exposure
Tuberculosis	*Mycobacterium tuberculosis*	Low-grade fever, malaise, anorexia, weight loss, cough, night sweats. Children often asymptomatic. Adenopathy, pneumonia and positive tuberculin skin test	2–10 weeks airborne droplet infection	Early detection by routine PPD skin test. Examine contacts. Exposed children may receive isoniazid (INH) and rifampin, which inhibits growth of organism	After treatment when cough subsides	Isolate newborn from infected mother. Identify contacts. Isolate, using special mask (see Appendix A)
Diphtheria	*Corneybacterium diptheriai*	Common cold with purulent nasal discharge. Malaise, sore throat. White or gray membrane forms in throat, causing respiratory distress	2–5 days	DPT vaccine to all infants. Intravenous antibiotics and antitoxin, tracheotomy required. Oxygen and suction as needed		Observe for respiratory, cardiac, and CNS involvement. Isolate. Identify contacts for treatment

affects resistance. Important factors in host resistance to disease include:

- *Intact skin and mucous membranes.* A break in the skin can be a portal of entry for an organism that can cause illness.
- *Phagocytes* in the blood attack and destroy organisms.
- The functioning *immune system* in the body responds to fight infection. Some factors in this immune response include interferon, T-cells, B-cells, and antibodies. Vaccinations assist the

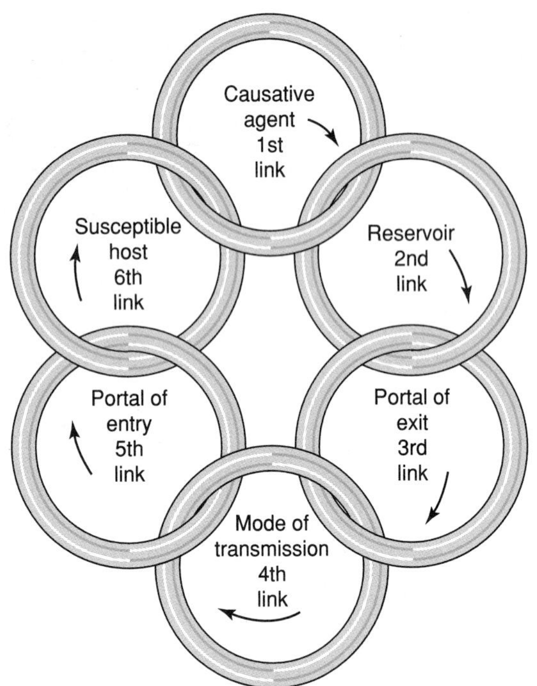

Figure 31–1. • The chain of infection. The process by which pathogens are transmitted from the environment to a host, invade the host, and cause infection. (From Leahy, J., & Kizilay, P. [1998]. *Foundations of nursing practice. A nursing process approach.* Philadelphia: Saunders.)

body to manufacture antibodies that can help the child to resist infections.

The child who has an underlying condition, such as diabetes, cystic fibrosis, burns, or sickle cell disease, may be more susceptible to certain organisms.

Children with acquired immunodeficiency syndrome (AIDS), cancer, or children receiving steroid or immunosuppressive drugs often have depressed immune systems. This makes them very susceptible to *opportunistic infections* as well as to pathogens (an *opportunistic infection* is caused by organisms *normally* found in the environment that the immune-suppressed individual cannot resist or fight). An infection acquired in a health care facility during hospitalization is termed a *nosocomial infection.*

Types of Immunity. Immunity is *natural* or *acquired* resistance to infection. In *natural immunity,* resistance is inborn. Some races apparently have a greater natural immunity to certain diseases than others. Immunity also varies from person to person. If two persons are exposed to the same disease, one may become very ill and the other may have no evidence of the disease.

Acquired immunity is not due to inherited factors but is acquired as a result of having the disease or is artificially acquired by receiving vaccines or immune serums. Vaccines contain live weakened or dead organisms that are not strong enough to cause the disease, but stimulate the body to develop an immune reaction and antibodies. When the person produces their own immunity, it is called *active immunity.*

If a person needs immediate protection from a disease, *antibodies* can be obtained in immune serums; most are from animals, but some are from humans. For example, tetanus serum, used to prevent lockjaw, is procured from the horse, but gamma globulin, which is rich in antibodies, is obtained from human blood. This type of immunity, known as *passive immunity,* acts immediately but does not last as long as immunity that the body actively produces. Passive immunity *provides* the antibody. It does not stimulate the system to produce its own antibodies.

A *carrier* is a person who is capable of spreading a disease but does not show evidence of it. Typhoid is an example of a disease spread by a carrier.

Transmission of Infection. Infection can be transmitted from one person to another by *direct* or *indirect* means. *Direct transmission* involves contact with the person who is infected (the body fluids of that person, such as nasal discharge or an open lesion). *Indirect transmission* involves contact with objects that have been contaminated by the infected person. These objects are called *fomites.* Doorknobs, used tissues, countertops, and toys are examples of fomites. For example, the respiratory syncytial virus (RSV) lives on dry soap for several hours. Therefore picking up soap used by a person infected with the RSV virus transmits the organism. This is one of the reasons why liquid soap is advocated. The chain of infection transmission is shown in Figure 31–1. Preventing the spread of infection depends on breaking the chain.

Various tests are available to determine whether an individual is susceptible to a particular disease. Examples are the *Schick test* for diphtheria, the *Dick test* for scarlet fever, and the *tuberculin test* for tuberculosis (the tine test or the Mantoux intradermal skin test are also tests for tuberculosis).

MEDICAL ASEPSIS AND STANDARD PRECAUTIONS

The purpose of medical aseptic techniques used with *all* patients is to prevent the spread of infection from one child to another or from the child to the nurse. A person or object is considered *contaminated* if it has touched the infected patient or any equipment or fomite that has come in contact with the patient. People or articles that have had no contact with the patient are considered *clean.*

Articles that have come in direct contact with the patient must be disinfected before they can be used by others. When something is disinfected, microorganisms in or on it are killed by physical or chemical means. The autoclave, which uses steam under pressure, is considered effective in killing most germs when the article is adequately exposed and sterilized for the proper length of time.

All children suspected of having a communicable disease who are admitted to the hospital are placed on isolation *(standard)* precautions until a definite diagnosis is established. A private room or negative-pressure room is assigned. (See Appendix A for specific precautions and practices involved.)

Disposable items are used whenever possible; they include diapers, tissues, needles, suction catheters, thermometers, suture sets, dishes, nursing bottles, and utensils. They are double-bagged and disposed of according to hospital procedure.

The nurse must understand the importance of protecting himself or herself and others from the contagious patient. This is accomplished by specific precautions, called *standard precautions,* or *universal precautions.* The Centers for Disease Control (CDC) recommends *standard* precautions for *all* patients; that involves handwashing, the use of disposable gloves, mask and eye protection, and gowns to protect the nurse's clothing from becoming soiled (Fig. 31–2). In addition to these precautions, *trans-*

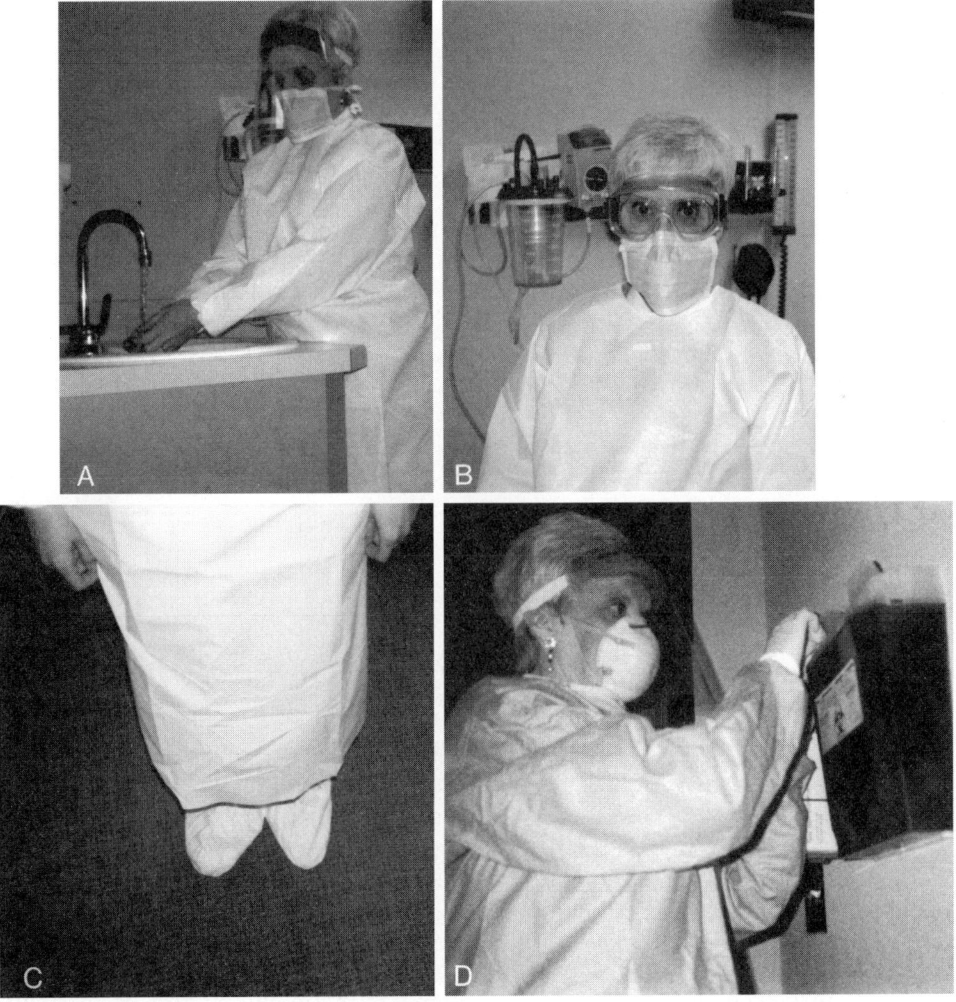

Figure 31–2. • Health care workers should routinely use appropriate barrier precautions to prevent skin and mucous membrane exposure when contact with a patient's blood or other body fluids is anticipated. **A,** Nurse wearing a face shield, disposable mask, and covergown and *washing hands thoroughly.* **B,** Protective goggles. **C,** Paper disposable boots to cover shoes in areas such as the delivery and operating rooms. **D,** Nurse wearing a mask, splash mask, and gloves. All sharp items are placed in puncture-resistant containers. (Courtesy, Columbia/HCA Portsmouth Regional Hospital.)

mission-based precautions are designed according to the method of spread of infection, such as large droplet, airborne droplet, or contact with a wound or drainage.

Large droplet infection precautions are used with diseases such as pertussis and influenza. The patient coughs or sneezes and the droplets can contaminate an area 3 feet around the patient. Beyond 3 feet, a mask and gown are not necessary.

Airborne infection precautions are used for patients with conditions such as tuberculosis, varicella (chickenpox), and rubeola (measles). Small airborne particles caught on floating dust in the room can be inhaled any place in the room. The use of negative-pressure rooms and of masks and gowns when entering the room is recommended.

Contact precautions are used when the condition transmits organisms via skin-to-skin contact or indirect touch of a contaminated fomite. Gloves and a gown are worn for close contact with RSV; hepatitis A patients who are incontinent, contagious skin diseases such as impetigo, or wound infections. Some diseases may have more than one mode of spread and therefore require more than one precaution technique.

Because isolation procedures vary from hospital to hospital and from hospital to home, a minimum of specific procedures are presented. Standard precautions are discussed in Appendix A and describe the protocols for use of gowns, masks, and other protective clothing. Disposable gloves should be worn whenever touching any body substance. You should be wearing gloves if you are touching something that is moist and not yours.

Protective Isolation. Protective isolation (also called *reverse isolation* or barrier technique) is used for patients who are *not* communicable, but have a lowered resistance and are highly susceptible to infection. This simple procedure reduces the incidence of nosocomial (hospital) infections. The patient is placed in a private room with the door closed. It is recommended that all persons wear gown, mask, and gloves when attending the child in reverse isolation. Protective isolation units, such as life islands, are also available. Both the child and family need adequate explanations.

Handwashing. The nurse must wash hands between patients and after removing gloves. Antibacterial soaps may be used in some units, but overuse can irritate skin. Paper disposable gowns are used. The gown is used once and discarded in a plastic isolation laundry bag held by a ringstand.

Family Education. Education of family members must be ongoing. Factors to be emphasized include the necessity for immunization of children, proper storage of food (particularly perishables), use of pasteurized milk, proper cooking of meats, cleanliness in food preparation, and proper handwashing. Review the ways in which infectious diseases are spread. Children need to be taught to avoid using community hand towels. Other modes of transmission, such as crowded living conditions, insects, rodents, and sandbox, may also be discussed.

> **Nursing Tip**
>
> Apply lotions to open lesions sparingly to avoid absorption that could lead to drug toxicity.

RASHES

Many infectious diseases begin with a rash (see Color Plate Figs. 3 to 5). Rashes tend to be itchy (pruritic) and uncomfortable. Symptomatic care is provided by prescribing Tylenol and Benedryl or topical lotions. Rashes can be described as:

- *Erythema.* A diffused reddened area on the skin
- *Macule.* A circular reddened area on the skin
- *Papule.* A circular reddened area on the skin that is elevated.
- *Vesicle.* A circular reddened area on the skin that is elevated and contains fluid
- *Pustule.* A circular reddened area on the skin that is elevated and contains pus
- *Scab.* A dried pustule that is covered with a crust
- *Pathognomonic.* Term used to describe a lesion or symptom that is *characteristic* of a specific illness. For example, koplik spots are pathognomonic for measles.

WORLDWIDE IMMUNIZATION PROGRAMS

Healthy People 2000

The United States Public Health Service has made immunization against childhood communicable diseases of 95% of all children in the United States a goal to achieve by the year 2000. Some reasons for the current low vaccination rate include: knowledge deficit of parents; lack of accessibility to vaccination clinics; cost of vaccinating children; fear of adverse reactions; misunderstandings about contraindications; and failure to track or follow-up on immunization records. Federally funded programs to provide the vaccine and to educate are needed. The effort of the World Health Organization (WHO) and United Nations Children's Fund (UNICEF) have resulted in dramatic declines in vaccine-preventable illnesses worldwide, especially in Third World countries. New vaccines are developed and assessed for routine use in endemic areas. The influenza vaccine, the pneumococcal vaccine, varicella vaccine, and RSV immune globulin are available for children. Vaccines for cholera and yellow fever are available for families traveling to endemic areas. The Centers for Disease Control (CDC) provide advice concerning vaccinations needed for persons traveling to various parts of the world.

The Nurse's Role

Worldwide immunization practices have eliminated smallpox as a threat. Measles is rarely seen in developed countries. Current vaccinations against varicella, hepatitis, influenza (for high-risk children), and pneumonia (for children over 2 years) are available, and the challenge is to make them accessible. The nurse is a vital link in educating parents about the need for immunizations.

The Vaccine. Correct *storage* of vaccines is essential to ensure potency. The nurse should check the label to determine if refrigeration is needed. The correct *route of administration* is important to achieve immunization. The oral, subcutaneous, and intramuscular routes are used for various vaccines. Series of dosage and administration to achieve desired antibody levels and appropriate boosters to maintain immunity are needed. The nurse can educate parents and school personnel about immunization schedules and should assess the immunization status of each child at every clinic visit.

Immunization Schedule for Children

Informed consent concerning the potential risks and documentation of immunization is essential. Parents should have copies of their child's immunization records. The immunization program for children in the United States is described in Figure 31–3.

Contraindications to live virus vaccine administration include

- Immunocompromised state
- Pregnancy
- Bacteremia or meningitis
- Immunocompromised caregiver in the home (OPV)

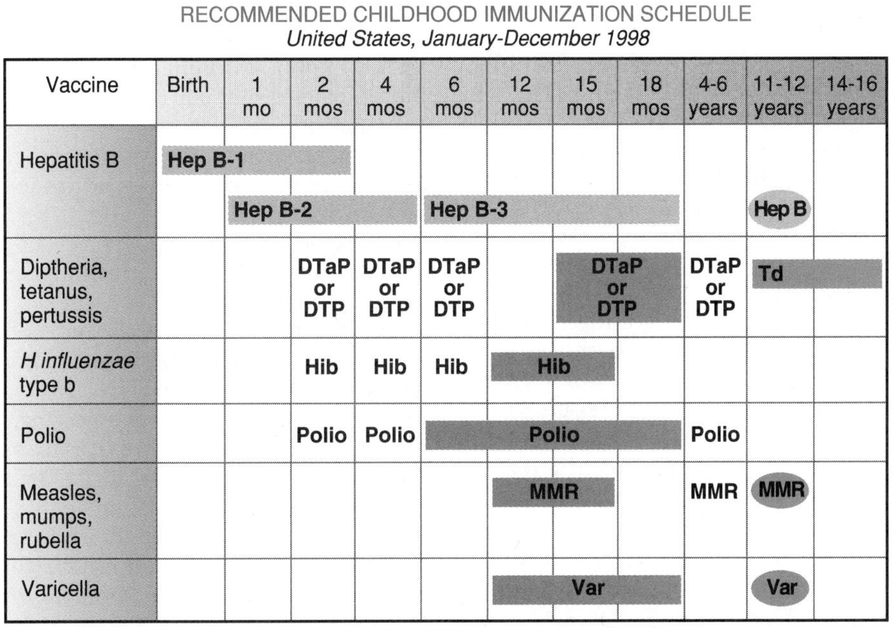

RECOMMENDED CHILDHOOD IMMUNIZATION SCHEDULE
United States, January-December 1998

Vaccine	Birth	1 mo	2 mos	4 mos	6 mos	12 mos	15 mos	18 mos	4-6 years	11-12 years	14-16 years
Hepatitis B	Hep B-1										
		Hep B-2			Hep B-3					Hep B	
Diptheria, tetanus, pertussis			DTaP or DTP	DTaP or DTP	DTaP or DTP		DTaP or DTP		DTaP or DTP	Td	
H influenzae type b			Hib	Hib	Hib	Hib					
Polio			Polio	Polio	Polio				Polio		
Measles, mumps, rubella						MMR			MMR	MMR	
Varicella						Var				Var	

Figure 31-3. • Immunization schedule. *Bars,* range of age for appropriate administration of vaccines to infants and children; *oval,* assessment for need at that age. DPT; HBV; Hib are given IM. MMR and IPV are given SC. OPV is given orally. Var, varicella vaccine; Hep, hepatitis; DPT or DtaP, diphtheria and tetanus toxoids and acellular pertussis vaccine; HBV, hepatitis B vaccine; Hib, *Haemophilus influenzae* B vaccine.

Nursing Tip

The pertussis vaccine is not given to children older than 7 years of age.

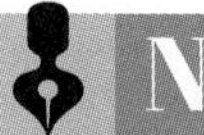

Nursing Tip

An interrupted vaccination series can continue without restarting the entire series.

- Corticosteroid therapy (requires individual evaluation)
- History of high fever (105°F) following previous vaccinations

SEXUALLY TRANSMITTED DISEASES

Overview. *Sexually transmitted disease (STD)* is the general name given to infections that are spread through direct sexual activity. This term replaces venereal disease. Two common types of STDs are gonorrhea and syphilis; however, over 20 other diseases are now considered prevalent. Some of these are scabies, pediculosis pubis, herpes progenitalis, genital warts, chlamydial infection, cytomegalovirus, and AIDS. Gonorrhea occurs far more frequently than does syphilis, but the effects of untreated syphilis are more debilitating. One may contract both diseases at the same time. Each can be transmitted by a pregnant woman to her unborn child, causing serious problems in the fetus, such as blindness, birth defects, and death.

The earliest record of STDs appears in the Bible and was written about 1500 BC. It was thought that with the advent of penicillin, STDs would be eradicated, but there has been a widespread resurgence, particularly among teenagers. The United States Public Health Service is calling it "an epidemic" and a "national health emergency." The incidence of STDs surpasses that of all other communicable diseases combined, except the common cold.

The reasons for this resurgence are many. They involve cultural, economic, social, and moral factors that are intertwined. Specific reasons cited include changing values and lifestyles of society; an increase in sexual contacts; the increase in the mobility of society and surges in population; the reluctance of many persons to seek medical help (particularly adolescents); inadequate education about STD's; and changes in common methods of contraception. The occurrence of an STD in a prepubertal patient should always prompt investigation into the possibility of sexual abuse.

Nursing Tip

The earliest age a vaccine can be administered is the youngest age the infant can respond by developing antibodies to that illness.

Nursing Care and Responsibilities

Regardless of the medical professional's feelings about the changes in society and sexual permissiveness, the consequences of these changes must be recognized and managed (Nursing Care Plan 31–1). Nurses who wish to help teenagers with STDs must create an environment in which the teenage patients will feel safe and at ease. What adolescents need at this point is ego support, which the nurse is able to provide through listening and through a nonjudgmental attitude.

The nurse approaches the patient with sensitivity and recognizes that the teenager is embarrassed and in need of privacy, especially during examinations. Girls are often afraid and always nervous about a pelvic examination. This is true even when their outward manner may seem otherwise. Careful explanations are needed. The patient is draped appropriately, and the nurse remains during the examination to provide reassurance. The findings are discussed with the patient, and questions are encouraged. Most teenagers need to be drawn out and do not readily ask questions, even when they do not understand.

The requirement to report sexual contacts is an emotionally charged topic that often prevents patients from seeking help. The person who is assured of confidentiality and who has been treated in a dignified manner is more apt to cooperate. Girls who are sexually active must be taught to take responsibility for their own health. Young people need to be made aware of the fact that sex with only one partner does not eliminate the risk, as this person may have had contact with others; the partner needs only one sexual experience with one infected person to transmit the disease.

Changes in methods of contraception have been cited as one reason for the increased incidence of STDs. As more women used birth control pills and

NURSING CARE PLAN 31-1

Selected Nursing Diagnoses for the Adolescent With a Sexually Transmitted Disease

Nursing Diagnosis: Knowledge deficit regarding genital hygiene

Goals	Nursing Interventions	Rationale
Adolescent verbalizes understanding of general hygiene measures related to the genitals	1. Assess patient's knowledge of cleansing genitals	1. Patient education is an ongoing responsibility of entire health care team; it communicates interest and concern for adolescent's welfare; both formal and informal teaching are necessary
	2. Educate as to effective genital care	2. Adolescent girls need to wipe themselves from front to back to avoid spreading bacteria from the anus to the vagina
	3. Stress importance of drinking lots of fluids and voiding regularly to avoid cystitis and other infections	3. Good fluid intake prevents stagnation of urine in the bladder; frequent voiding cleanses urethra
	4. Suggest that teenage girls wear loose-fitting cotton underwear	4. Cotton underwear is absorbent; tight-fitting garments restrict perineal ventilation and may contribute to vaginitis
	5. Recommend that bubble baths, hygiene sprays, and douching be avoided	5. These products and procedures may cause irritation; douching is unnecessary, and some believe it is detrimental, as it washes away normal protective mucus and bacterial flora of vagina and may introduce bacteria; tampons need to be changed at least three to four times a day during menses; wash hands before and after changing
	6. Uncircumcised boys need to retract foreskin and cleanse penis regularly	6. This prevents smegma from collecting under foreskin and causing irritation
	7. Suggest importance of daily baths and showers with particular attention to cleansing of genital area	7. Soap and water are all that are necessary for keeping perineal and perianal areas clean; thorough drying of genitals prevents irritation
	8. Educate as to normal secretions of genital area	8. All adolescent girls have normal, nonbloody, asymptomatic vaginal discharge called leukorrhea; this discharge is secreted by endocervical glands; this keeps mucous membranes of vagina moist and clean; the urethra in a boy should show no signs of discharge, infection, or abnormal tissue growth
	9. Suggest that adolescents become aware of their personal anatomy and seek health care for any deviations or abnormal secretions	9. Patients who are familiar with their own anatomy can identify abnormal changes

(Continued)

intrauterine devices (IUDs), fewer men used condoms ("rubbers"), which helped to reduce the spread of infection by protecting the partner from direct contact with the organisms. This trend is changing because of AIDs. The proper use of male and female condoms is described in Chapter 11, Box 11–4. The use of foam and other local agents prior to intercourse lowers the pH of the vagina and decreases (but does not eliminate) the risk of infection. The pill actually raises the pH of the vagina, increasing the susceptibility to infection. Disease organisms may also travel along the wick of an intrauterine device. Douching is not an effective means of birth control and may force disease organisms into the uterus. Some means of reducing the risk of STDs include bathing the external genitals

NURSING CARE PLAN 31–1 *continued*

Selected Nursing Diagnoses for the Adolescent With a Sexually Transmitted Disease

Nursing Diagnosis: Knowledge deficit regarding transmission of STDs

Goals	Nursing Interventions	Rationale
Patient verbalizes understanding of transmission of STDs Patient does not evidence symptoms of rash, pain, itching, odor, or discharge Patient verbalizes knowledge that some infections may have no symptoms	1. Encourage limitation of partners, preferably limiting sex to one partner	1. Limiting partners reduces exposure to STDs
	2. Discourage sex with strangers (a pickup or prostitute)	2. These persons are more apt to be infected; there is little way of knowing their health history
	3. Instruct adolescents that use of oral contraceptive does not protect against STDs	3. The pill actually raises the pH of the vagina, increasing the susceptibility to infection
	4. Emphasize importance of using latex condoms when having intercourse	4. Lambskin and natural-membrane condoms are not as effective against virus that leads to AIDS (human immunodeficiency virus [HIV]) because of pores in material; on package look for words *latex* and *5% nonoxynol 9* (a spermicide)
	5. Suggest that vaginal sprays, douches, and lubricants that lower vaginal pH may protect against some STDs but are *not* effective against HIV	5. HIV is carried in body secretions of infected person, particularly in blood and semen; mixing of body secretions is to be avoided
	6. Educate as to importance of avoiding anal intercourse, particularly with a person who injects drugs	6. Drug users are a very high-risk group for AIDS and other STDs; rectal intercourse is particularly contraindicated because even small breaks in the rectal mucosa provide a direct route to the blood stream
	7. Dispel misinformation	7. There is a great deal of misinformation concerning STDs
	8. Stress importance of keeping clinic appointments and taking all medications prescribed should one become infected	8. Follow-up care is essential for the health and welfare of patient and patient's contacts

and perianal area with soap and water and urinating before and after intercourse. There is no immunity to STDs; one can be infected repeatedly. The best way to prevent these disorders is to avoid sexual contact with infected persons. The percentage of patients hospitalized with STDs is small because of adequate outpatient treatment measures. The nurse must be familiar with the requirements and techniques of standard precautions (see Appendix A).

The nurse assesses the person's level of knowledge and provides information at an understandable level. Many young people have little knowledge of their body and their developing sexuality. Others have mild to deep-seated emotional problems that need to be addressed. They may be using sex to escape from reality, to express hostility or rebellion, or to call attention to themselves. They may be involved in relationships they no longer desire, so they need help in formulating positive attitudes toward themselves. They also need help understanding their behavior and that of others. In

Nursing Tip

The use of condoms to prevent STDs, although recommended, is not considered 100% effective because condoms are apt to slip or break during intercourse and can be damaged by oil-based lubricants.

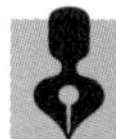

Nursing Tip

Sex education is not limited to the mechanics of intercourse, but rather includes the feelings involved in a sexual experience: expectations, fantasies, fulfillments, and disappointments.

particular, adolescents need to learn that they are responsible for their own actions if they choose to be sexually active.

Prevention

The prevention of STDs is everyone's concern and demands individual initiative and responsibility. Table 31–2 describes age-appropriate interventions. Nurses must keep themselves informed about the latest techniques in diagnosis and treatment. Education of the public, particularly young people, is paramount. Nurses who work in settings frequented by teenagers can distribute some of the many excellent health pamphlets available. Structured courses in sex education should include presentations on STDs (there are also excellent audiovisual aids) and discussion of how one establishes healthy sexual behavior patterns. The community health or school nurse is involved in case finding and referral. Delays due to fear of disclosure have tragic results. Legislation in all 50 states permits physicians to treat infected minors without first obtaining parental consent. Individual sexually transmitted diseases are discussed in Chapter 11.

Acquired Immunodeficiency Syndrome (AIDS) in Children

Pediatric AIDS is a worldwide public health problem with a devastating outcome. It is the 5th leading cause of death in the United States of children under 15 years of age. In 1996, 540,000 cases of AIDS in adults and 7,296 cases of AIDS in children under 13 years of age were reported. Eighteen percent of the nation's AIDS cases are adolescents. These numbers do not count those who may be exposed or who test positive but do not exhibit signs and symptoms of AIDS. Children usually acquire the AIDS infection by:

- Contact with an infected mother at birth (approximately 90% of cases in infants)
- Sexual contact with an infected person
- Use of contaminated needles or contact with infected blood

Table 31–2

NURSING CARE TO PREVENT AND TREAT STDS

Nursing goals

To provide anticipatory guidance concerning sexuality at a level that the child or young person can comprehend throughout developmental cycle
To prevent infection
To identify early symptoms and provide prompt treatment if infection occurs
To prevent sequelae

Assessment	Nursing Interventions
Children under age 12	Provide age-appropriate instruction concerning sexuality; also explore expected patterns that might occur before next visit
Puberty and adolescence	Review structure and function of reproductive systems; review personal hygiene; discuss values and decision-making, possible sexual behavior and consequences, prevention of pregnancy and STDs
Self-concept: anticipate evidence of fear, embarrassment, anger, and decreased self-esteem upon suspicion of infection	Create nonjudgmental atmosphere, listen, assess level of knowledge, observe nonverbal behavior, establish confidentiality; provide privacy when assisting with pelvic or genital examination; provide appropriate draping of patient; realize anger is often a mask for depression, grief—do not take personally
Skin and hair	It is not uncommon to see skin rashes, "crabs" (pubic lice), or scabies (mites) Clothing is disinfected by washing in hot water
Sexual partners	Determine sexual preference; investigate and direct to treatment; persons with multiple sexual partners, homosexuals, persons with new partners, and those with history of prior STD are at particular risk
Sexual intercourse	Abstain during treatment; use condom to prevent reinfection
Medication	Take all of prescribed medication; if on tetracycline, advise to take 1 hr before or 2 hr after meals (on empty stomach); avoid dairy products, antacids, iron, and sunlight
Compliance with treatment	Stress importance of follow-up, routine Pap smears
Sequelae	Discuss possible complications of specific disorders such as birth defects, infertility

Educating the public about the role of unprotected sex and IV drug abuse in increasing the risk of AIDS infection is a public health challenge.

AIDS is caused by a retrovirus known as the human immunodeficiency virus type 1 (HIV-1) that attacks lymphocytes (the white blood cells that protect one from disease). It appears to cause an imbalance between the helper T-cells ($CD4^+$) that support the immune system and the suppressor T-cells that shut it down. In a person not infected with HIV, the number of $CD4^+$ cells remains constant over time. In an HIV-infected person, as months and years go by, the number of $CD4^+$ cells drops. The $CD4^+$ cell count is a measure of the damage to the immune system caused by HIV and of the body's ability to fight infection. A physician uses the $CD4^+$ cell count to help to decide what medical treatments are best for the individual.

A series of terms for this disorder have been developed, but the disease is now classified along a continuum by the Centers for Disease Control. The categories include:

- *Asymptomatic infection.* This refers to a latent period. Individuals in this category have positive antibody tests, indicating exposure to the virus, but are not ill.
- *Symptomatic HIV infection.* Many individuals have this earlier and milder condition (compared with AIDS). This has formerly been referred to as AIDS-related complex, or ARC.
- *AIDS.* This refers to the most advanced involvement, which includes the finding of HIV antibodies in the patient's blood, the presence of complicating opportunistic infections, and other criteria.

Children do not get AIDS from casual relationships at schools and medical facilities or through family living. The virus is infectious but not highly contagious, and the circumstances for acquiring it are specific, as indicated. Improved attention to hygiene practices in response to this disease can only be applauded.

Because passive transmission of antibodies from the mother occurs, babies are born with antibodies that crossed the placenta. Some babies' systems become clear of antibodies in about 15 months, whereas other babies eventually experience the infection. Because of the transference of antibodies, the standard enzyme-linked immunosorbent assay (ELISA) and Western blot tests used to diagnose HIV infection in older children and adults are less reliable until after 15 months of age.

Manifestations. Criteria for the disease in children have been outlined by the Centers for Disease Control in Atlanta. Initial symptoms in infancy are vague and include failure to thrive, lymphadenopathy (enlarged lymph glands), chronic sinusitis, and nonresponse to treatment of infections. The patient becomes subject to overwhelming infection. Opportunistic infections, such as oral thrush, *Pneumocystis carinii* pneumonia, herpes viruses, and cytomegalovirus take advantage of the body's depressed immune system. Kaposi's sarcoma, a rare type of skin cancer, appears to be less common in children than in adults. Serious bacterial infections, such as meningitis, impetigo, and urinary tract problems, are reported in children. The symptoms of HIV infection generally develop more rapidly in infants, and this may be attributed to the infant's immature immune system.

Treatment and Nursing Care. Treatment and nursing care are supportive because there is no cure for AIDS at this time. Assessment and care of the child with HIV or AIDS are critically important. Education concerning long-term compliance with prescribed medication and supportive care to promote growth and development are essential. Nursing Care Plan 31–2 provides selected nursing diagnoses and interventions for the patient with AIDS.

Psychological support for these children is paramount. Sensory stimulation and touching are especially important for infants. The effects of isolation can be physically and emotionally devastating to the developing child. Many babies are abandoned, outlive their mothers, or must live in foster care. Unique programs such as Children's AIDS Program (CAP) provide homelike respite care environment and day care. The goal of the program is to help families living with HIV infection to stay together.

The nurse anticipates interventions related to the care of the child with a life-threatening disease. Efforts to support families in crisis are particularly pertinent. Often the extended family must take over. Many families have few financial resources and are exhausted from the child's frequent hospitalizations and physical care. They need to be introduced to such agencies as social service, financial aid, AIDS and grief support groups, home health, nutritional programs such as Women, Infants, and Children (WIC), and hospice.

Several medications are used to manage AIDS in children. Zidovudine (ZDV) significantly prevents transmission from mother to fetus when given after the first trimester of pregnancy. Didanosine (DDI), Nevirapine (a reverse transcriptase inhibitor), and protease inhibitors such as Invirase or Ritonavir (norvir) are sometimes used in combination therapy for children who test positive for the AIDS virus. Some current drugs used in the treatment of AIDS include Zidovudine, Videx, Hivid (zalcitabine), Stavudine (zerit), and Lamivudine (epivir). The drugs are very expensive. A fungal infection

NURSING CARE PLAN 31–2

Selected Nursing Diagnoses for the Newborn/Infant with AIDS

Nursing Diagnosis: High risk for infection related to HIV attack on T-lymphocytes and the suppression of antibody function

Goals	Nursing Interventions	Rationale
Patient remains free from infection as evidenced by intact skin, absence of respiratory distress, and normal laboratory findings	1. Anticipate opportunistic infections, as patient's immune system is depressed	1. Opportunistic infections are those that occur due to opportunity afforded by poor health of patient; newborns and preterms have immature immune systems, and so are particularly susceptible; once infected, they have few reserves
	2. Monitor respiratory status closely; watch for restlessness, apprehension	2. Lungs are a target for infection; patients are subject to pneumonia, particularly *Pneumocystis carinii*
	3. Examine patient regularly for infection (puncture sites, mouth, rectum, pierced ears)	3. Thrush and herpes simplex are common in children; perianal region is in danger of secondary infection from feces
	4. Reposition frequently	4. Frequent repositioning reduces pooling of secretions in lungs
	5. Administer antipyretics and antibiotics as prescribed	5. These will increase patient comfort; may help to ward off infection; pneumonia requires aggressive efforts to identify pathogen; fever is common

Nursing Diagnosis: Nutritional alterations—less than body requirements related to anorexia, anemia, thrush

Goals	Nursing Interventions	Rationale
Nutrition maintained as evidenced by normal healing, muscle tone, and body weight	1. Offer small portions of high-calorie, bland foods often	1. Child has poor appetite; may have mouth sores
	2. Provide oral formula to infants as prescribed	2. Must have sufficient nutrients to meet growth and development and to maintain body expenditures
	3. Administer nasogastric tube feedings if ordered	3. Preterms and weakened infants may require nasogastric feedings
	4. Provide hyperalimentation therapy if ordered	4. Nutritional supplements may be necessary as disease progresses; prognosis is poor, despite aggressive management
	5. Provide for mobility to ensure muscle strength	5. Immobility contributes to wasted muscles; toddlers need to be up and around as condition permits
	6. Chart intake and output, daily weights	6. These patients become easily dehydrated. Daily weights will determine nutritional progress

Nursing Diagnosis: High risk for injury related to changes in central nervous system and from decreased blood components

Goals	Nursing Interventions	Rationale
Parents become aware of potential sources of injury; parents recognize signs of bleeding Child will not show signs of injury as evidenced by absence of petechiae	1. Provide developmentally safe environment	1. Children are accident prone; normal cuts and abrasions become easily infected; impetigo can be very dangerous for this child
	2. Observe skin for petechiae and bruising, explain to parents	2. Thrombocytopenia is common; Kaposi's sarcoma, a form of skin cancer, is rare in children, but may be seen in adolescents; looks like bruise in early stages
	3. Monitor laboratory reports (prothrombin times, hematocrit, and so on)	3. Cultures of blood, urine, throat, and stool may be ordered; child may be unable to generate a white cell response great enough to be detected in laboratories; may also be abnormal response of cells

(Continued)

NURSING CARE PLAN 31–2 *continued*

Selected Nursing Diagnoses for the Newborn/Infant with AIDS

Nursing Diagnosis: Skin integrity: impaired integrity related to immunosuppression

Goals	Nursing Interventions	Rationale
Skin remains intact; patient is able to eat without discomfort	1. Inspect mouth often for lesions (*Candida albicans*) 2. Apply nystatin suspension if ordered 3. Observe frequently for diaper rash; apply prescribed ointment; maintain skin intactness by thorough, gentle cleansing	1. Mouth sores may prevent child from eating 2. Nystatin may soothe and promote healing 3. Skin is subject to breakdown and infection

Nursing Diagnosis: Infection: high risk for transmission related to disease organism

Goals	Nursing Interventions	Rationale
Infection is contained through the use of universal blood and body fluid precautions	1. Observe isolation technique; use universal precautions for blood and body fluids; maintain enteric and needle precautions similar to those for hepatitis B; wear gloves for diaper change, specimen collections (especially blood); handle secretions and excretions with care; utilize good handwashing techniques	1. Centers for Disease Control and Prevention regulations request standard precautions to prevent body secretions, especially blood, from infecting caregivers (see Appendix A)

Nursing Diagnosis: Knowledge deficit of family

Goals	Nursing Interventions	Rationale
Family verbalizes understanding of disease process, transmission, and necessary precautions	1. Clarify misconceptions about the disease 2. Help to prepare parents for possible poor prognosis 3. Prepare parents adequately for discharge from hospital 4. Encourage parents to stay abreast of current, unfolding information 5. Provide ongoing support services	1. Misconceptions create anxiety; there are a lot of misconceptions about acquired immunodeficiency syndrome (AIDS) 2. Prognosis is generally death; zidovudine (AZT) is showing promise for delaying onset of AIDS if used after positive serologic testing; much controversy about testing exists 3. Children should remain with their families and, if possible, be managed out of the hospital with medical and social supports 4. Newer developments may change picture of disease; instills some hope in family 5. Because of the stigma, possible length, and prognosis of this disease, families require much support

Nursing Diagnosis: Fear (parents and patient)

Goals	Nursing Interventions	Rationale
Parents verbalize fears; family develops coping skills that assist them in managing stress related to life-threatening disease	1. Encourage family to support one another and keep lines of communication open 2. Alert parents to self-help groups 3. Acquire accurate knowledge about disease 4. Dispel inordinate fears of general public	1. Fear is reduced if it can be shared 2. AIDS support groups, hospice; discuss value of life support measures; families may be faced with such difficult decisions 3. There is much inaccurate information about how AIDS is acquired and transmitted 4. It is important that pediatric nurses be well informed about the disease

called *Pneumocystis carinii* is the first opportunistic infection to affect the pediatric patient. Prophylactic medications are available. The nurse should be alert for central nervous system involvement such as failure to achieve developmental milestones, or motor deficits. Respiratory syncinctial virus (RSV), pneumonia, renal failure, and gastrointestinal malfunction often plague the pediatric AIDS patient.

Children should be assessed for the need for updating routine immunizations. The major difference in the childhood immunization of affected children is that live polio-virus vaccine is omitted. Instead, inactivated polio virus vaccine is substituted. Tuberculosis testing is done routinely and as needed. Several antiviral drugs are being tested in children. Early diagnosis and treatment can improve the quality and length of life for many children.

KEY POINTS

- *Standard precautions* are techniques recommended by the CDC to prevent the transmission of communicable diseases.
- *Body substance* refers to moist secretions of the body that can contain microorganisms.
- An *opportunistic infection* is caused by organisms normally found in the environment that the immunosuppressed child cannot fight.
- Immunization programs in the United States provide *active* immunity for children.
- Proper handwashing is the basic essential factor to prevent the transmission of infection.
- Proper storage of vaccines and appropriate routes of administration are essential to ensure the potency of the vaccine.
- Education of parents about the need for immunizations against common childhood communicable diseases is a primary nursing responsibility.
- Koplik spots are white spots on the mucous membrane of the oral cavity that occur prior to a skin rash and are indicative of measles (Rubeola) infection.
- In chickenpox (varicella) all stages of the skin lesions are present on the skin at the same time.
- A child with German measles (rubella) should not be cared for by a woman in early months of pregnancy as the virus can cause fetal anomalies.
- In children with roseola, a persistently high fever *suddenly* drops as the rash erupts.
- Gamma globulin offers *passive* immunity for exposed children who are immunosuppressed.
- Listening skills and a nonjudgmental attitude is essential when caring for adolescents with STDs.
- Children acquire the AIDS infection by contact with an infected mother at birth, sexual contact with an infected person, or use of contaminated needles during drug use.
- The long-term nursing goals in the care for a child with AIDS are to promote compliance for long-term drug therapy and to provide support to maintain optimum growth and development.

MULTIPLE-CHOICE REVIEW QUESTIONS

Choose the most appropriate answer.

1. The nurse is caring for a newborn with AIDS. Which of the following is a priority goal?
   a. Encourage breastfeeding.
   b. Prevent infections.
   c. Provide initial immunizations.
   d. Notify Social Services.
2. An adolescent diagnosed with AIDS asks about the mode of transmission for the illness. An accurate response is that it was most likely:
   a. a casual contact with a friend who is HIV positive.
   b. a latent response to an inherited predisposition.
   c. use of a contaminated toilet seat.
   d. contact with contaminated body substance through sex or IV needle use.
3. When providing play therapy for a child with a communicable disease who is in an isolation room, a priority principle or rationale for selection would include:
   a. The toy should be appropriate for a child on bed rest with minimal activity.
   b. Most children love books.
   c. It is best to bring the child's favorite toy from home.
   d. The toy should be washable.
4. A parent brings a 2-month-old infant to the clinic for the second in the immunization series. The nurse should prepare for administration of which of the following immunizations?
   a. DPT; Hib; polio
   b. DPT; polio; MMR
   c. DPT; polio; varicella
   d. td; hepatitis; MMR
5. The DPT immunization is administered
   a. orally.
   b. subcutaneously.
   c. intramuscularly.
   d. intravenously.

BIBLIOGRAPHY AND READER REFERENCE

American Academy of Pediatrics. (1997). HIV infection. In Peter, G. (Ed.), *1997 Redbook Report of Committee on Infectious Diseases.* Elk Grove Village, IL: Author.

Behrman, R., & Kleigman, R. (1998). *Nelson's essentials of pediatrics.* Philadelphia: Saunders.

Berkowitz, C. (1996). *Pediatrics, a primary care approach.* Philadelphia: Saunders.

Bonny, A., & Biro, F. (1998). Recognizing and treating STD's in adolescent girls. *Contemporary Pediatrics, 15*(3), 119.

Borton, D. (1997). Isolation precautions: Clearing up the confusion. *Nursing 97, 27*(1), 49.

Coles, B., & Hipp, S. (1996). Syphilis among adolescents: The hidden epidemic. *Contemporary Pediatrics, 13*(6), 5.

Denny, F., & Henderson, F. (1996). Renegade streptococci. *Contemporary Pediatrics, 13*(9), 104.

Finan, S. (1997). Promoting healthy sexuality guidelines for school age child and adolescent. *Nurse Practitioner, 22*(11), 62.

Finberg, L. (1998). *Saunders manual of pediatric practice.* Philadelphia: Saunders.

Flasker, V. D. J., & Unguarski, P. (1995). *HIV/AIDS, A guide to nursing care* (3rd ed.). Philadelphia: Saunders.

Frankenburg, W. (1996). The "Partners" program: A prescription for preventative care. *Contemporary Pediatrics, 13*(6), 65.

Goldgeier, M. (1996). Fungal infections. *Contemporary Pediatrics, 13*(9), 21.

Greenfield, L., Marcuse, E., & Bibus, D. (1998). Calling the shots: A guide to immunization resources. *Contemporary Pediatrics, 15*(4), 125.

Grubman, S., & Oleske, J. (1998). *HIV infection in infants, children and adolescents in AIDS* (3rd ed). Wormser, G. (ed.). Philadelphia: Lippincott.

Healthy People 2000. (1991). National Health Promotion and Disease Prevention DHHS Publication #9150212, USDHHS, Washington, DC.

Heitman, B., Irizarry, A. (1997). Recognition and management of toxoplasmosis. *Nurse Practitioner, 22*(9), 75.

Lederman, H. (1996). IVIG therapy (Intravenous Immune Globulin). *Contemporary Pediatrics, 13*(6), 75.

Lehman, D., & Lieberman, J. (1998). Polio vaccines: Time for change. *Contemporary Pediatrics, 15*(1), 58.

Scott, P., Clark, J., & Miser, W. (1997). Update on primary prevention and outbreak. *American Family Physician, 56*(4), 1121.

Sparks, L., & Russell, C. (1998). The new varicella vaccine: Efficacy, safety and administration. *Journal of Pediatric Nursing, 13*(2), 85.

Stiehm, R., Yamauchu, T., & Maher, C. (1997). Infections in children: How many are too many. *Patient Care,* June 15, 156.

Tarantala, D., & Mann, J. (1996). Global expansion of HIV infection and AIDS. *Hospital Practice, 31*(10), 63.

Unguarski, P. (1997). Update on HIV infection. *American Journal of Nursing, 97*(1), 44.

U.S. Department of Health and Human Services, Public Health Service, Center for Disease Control, Atlanta, Georgia. (1997). USPHS/IDSA Guidelines for prevention of opportunistic infections in persons infected with HIV. *American Family Physician, 56*(4), 1131.

Volberding, P. (1998). An aggressive approach to HIV antiretroviral therapy. *Hospital Practice, 33*(1), 81.

Weyer, D. (1997). Skin: A window to the immune system. *Advice for Nurse Practitioners, 5*(10), 22.

Wong, D. (1997). *Whaley and Wong's essentials of pediatric nursing.* St. Louis, MO: Mosby.

chapter 32

The Child with an Emotional or Behavioral Condition

Outline

Objectives

On completion and mastery of Chapter 32, the student will be able to

- Define each vocabulary term listed.
- Discuss the impact of early childhood experience on a person's adult life.
- List symptoms of potential suicide in children and adolescents.
- Discuss immediate and long-range plans for the suicidal client.
- Differentiate among the following terms: psychiatrist, psychoanalyst, clinical psychologist, and counselor.
- List five criteria for referring a child to a mental health counselor or agency.
- List four behaviors that may indicate substance abuse.
- Name two programs for members of families of alcoholics.
- Discuss problems facing children of alcoholics.
- List four symptoms of attention deficit hyperactivity disorder.
- Describe techniques of helping children with attention deficit hyperactivity disorder to adjust to the school setting.
- Compare and contrast characteristics of bulemia and anorexia nervosa.

Vocabulary

art therapy
behavior modification
bibliotherapy
DSM-IV
dysfunctional
family therapy
intervention
milieu therapy
play therapy
polypharmacy
psychosomatic
recreation therapy

THE NURSE'S ROLE

The nurse is often the person who has the greatest amount of contact with the family. Assessing child–parent relations is an important and ongoing aspect of care. To work effectively with the disturbed child, nurses first must understand the types of behavior considered within normal range. Nurses are valuable members of the multidisciplinary health care team in that they work closely with hospitalized acutely ill children, long-term chronically ill children, and children in school. Nurses should keep a careful record of behavior and note relationships with members of the family. Such notations are meaningful to the physician and other staff members who are as concerned with preventing problems from arising as they are with treating them. Is 4-year-old Janice wetting the bed? What about Bobby who continually bangs his head against the crib during naptime? What does Manuel do in the playroom? Is he sitting alone in a corner? Does he hit the other children? Is he constantly in motion? Does Eric seem indifferent to attempts to establish rapport? Is there a physical cause for his behavior? An action in itself might be considered within the normal limits of behavior, but carried to extremes it may interfere with the child's experience of and reaction to reality and requires further investigation.

Everyday, everywhere, children are trying to cope with stress. Many succeed and grow stronger; some do not. Early childhood intervention programs are helpful in preventing major problems that impact growth and development. Parenting classes teach what to expect at various ages and stages. They also stress the importance of age-appropriate discipline and guidance. Parent groups provide education, socialization, and support. Other agencies provide a variety of services. Some services include the National Alliance for the Mentally Ill (NAMI), Family Service Association of America, Inc., Toughlove, and the Youth Suicide National Center. Nurses need to be aware of such resources to guide parents appropriately (see Appendix B).

Nursing Tip

Parents provide important assessment data about the child that the young child cannot provide. They are also important in bringing the child to therapy. Discrediting parents threatens the child and is not therapeutic.

When parents request guidance, the nurse encourages them to seek help from their family physician or pediatrician or from a community mental health center. In the hospital, a psychiatric clinical nurse specialist (CNS) is an excellent resource. If the child is in school, the services of the school psychologist or guidance counselor may prove valuable. Some churches employ counselors who are available free of charge to parishioners. Families who lack adequate financial resources can be directed to appropriate agencies. Some agencies not only provide emergency funds, but can also set up a budgeting system for those receiving meager wages. This is particularly helpful when parents are young teenagers.

No matter how dysfunctional the parent–child relationship, most children consciously and unconsciously identify with parental values. Discrediting parents threatens the child's security and creates anxiety. The nurse reassures parents and helps them regain or maintain confidence in their parenting role. In addition, because children do not seek treatment on their own, the nurse should assist parents in becoming invested in the treatment modality. Finally, as a professional, the nurse supports organizations concerned with mental health, votes on issues that are pertinent to the welfare of children in the community, and offers services when they are needed.

TYPES AND SETTINGS OF TREATMENT

The first psychiatric clinic for children in the United States was established in Chicago in 1909 to serve delinquents. The basic staff of the modern child guidance clinic is composed of a psychiatrist, a psychologist, a social worker, a pediatrician, and the nurse. Usually the child guidance clinic provides diagnostic and treatment services. It may be part of a hospital, a school, a court, or a public health or welfare service, or it may be an independent agency.

The *psychiatrist* is a medical doctor who specialized in mental disorders. The *psychoanalyst* is usually a psychiatrist but may be a psychologist; all psychoanalysts have advanced training in psychoanalytic theory and practice. The *clinical psychologist* has an advanced degree in clinical psychology from a recognized university. Many of these specialists work in the school system with children, teachers, and families to prevent or resolve problems. A *counselor* is a professional with a master's degree from an accredited institution. Many counselors specialize in a specific area, such as substance abuse or counseling of children. In most states, counselors have to be licensed.

Children who do not respond well to individual outpatient therapy may require the type of care provided in residential treatment centers. Their home situations may be so disruptive that they might benefit from a change of environment. This alternative also provides a cooling-down period for the family. *Family therapy* is begun. The length of stay varies from 1 to 3 weeks. Partial hospitalization programs in which the child attends therapy during the day and returns home at night are popular.

Intervention may involve individual, family, or group therapy; behavior modification; or milieu therapy; or it may involve a combination of these. *Behavior modification* focuses on modifying specific behaviors by means of stimulus and response conditioning. *Milieu therapy* refers to the physical and social environment provided for the child. *Art therapy,* music therapy, and *play therapy* are particularly helpful in dealing with younger children who have difficulties expressing themselves. *Recreation therapy* is also valuable. *Bibliotherapy,* the reading of stories about children in a situation similar to the child's, is also therapeutic. Creating an *emotionally safe environment* is basic to all forms of therapy.

ORIGINS OF EMOTIONAL AND BEHAVIORAL CONDITIONS

Early childhood experiences are critical to personality formation. Situations that disrupt family patterns can have a lasting impact on the child. Children who come from dysfunctional families may suffer from any of the following: failure to develop a sense of trust (in their caretakers and environment), excessive fears, misdirected anger manifested as behavior problems, depression, low self-esteem, lack of confidence, and feelings of lack of control over themselves and their environment. These and other manifestations may make children feel negative about themselves and the world. They experience guilt and may blame themselves when confronted with disappointment and failure.

Growing up can be painful even under the best circumstances. It is difficult for the child in the early school years to live up to so many rapidly developing standards. Guilt and anxiety develop. Finger-sucking, nail-biting, excessive fears, stuttering, and conduct problems are reflections of nervous tension.

The current trend toward prevention by identifying risk factors and advocating early *intervention* is a major goal of children's mental health services. The term *psychosomatic* has come to refer to the bodily dysfunctions that seem to have emotional or mental bases. Each person has a different potential for coping with life. Truancy, lying, stealing, failure in school, and a crisis such as death or divorce of parents are but a few of the difficulties that may require intervention. Box 32–1 summarizes some of the disorders that can affect behavior and appear during infancy, childhood, and adolescence. Some behavioral disorders are caused by genetic factors;

BOX 32–1

SUMMARY OF DISORDERS USUALLY FIRST EVIDENT IN INFANCY, CHILDHOOD, AND ADOLESCENCE

- Adjustment disorders
- Anxiety disorders (separation, obsessive-compulsive)
- Attention deficit hyperactivity disorder
- Autistic disorder
- Bipolar depression
- Conduct disorder
- Developmental disorders (e.g., language, math)
- Eating disorders (anorexia, bulemia, pica)
- Encopresis
- Enuresis
- Major depression
- Mental retardation
- Oppositional disorder
- Schizophrenia
- Sleep disorders
- Stereotyped movement disorders (tics, Tourette's syndrome)
- Stuttering
- Substance abuse

Data adapted from American Psychiatric Association. (1994). *Diagnostic and statistical manual of disorders—DSM-IV* (4th ed.). Washington DC: Author.

for example, autism is thought to have autosomal recessive inheritance.

ORGANIC BEHAVIOR DISORDERS

Childhood Autism

Autism is a developmental disorder manifested by motor sensory, cognitive, and behavioral dysfunctions. It involves impaired social interaction, communication, and interests. It may be caused by a defect in neurogenesis in the early weeks of fetal life (Courchesne). It may also involve an abnormal neurochemical status with some abnormalities in catecholamine pathways and increased serotonin levels. It occurs in 3–4 of 10,000 children and is more common in males.

Autism is usually diagnosed by 4 years of age although symptoms appear earlier. Failure to use eye contact and look at others, poor attention behavior, and poor orienting to one's name are significant signs of dysfunction by 1 year of age. Research has shown that cognitive delays, if present, do not always occur early. Peer-related social behavior normally develops early in the preschool period. Symbolic play normally emerges by 2 years of age. Autistic children do not show interest in other children. Autistic children also have difficulty engaging in pretend play. Parallel play is the preference for the autistic child. Early identification and intervention may help the autistic child. The nurse who is alert to identify dysfunctions in the social behavior of young children can facilitate early referral that may result in more meaningful social advances for the autistic child. Treatment of autism involves providing well-structured home and school environments, behavioral modification, and in some cases the use of specific drugs.

Drug therapy in autism is not curative. The goal of drug therapy is to reduce behavioral symptoms that interfere with cognitive development and family interactions. Haloperidol calms the child without sedating, but offers no help with learning abilities.

Stimulants such as amphetamines decrease hyperactivity, but impair cognition and may increase self-injurious behavior. Popranolol, buspirone, and valproic acid have been helpful in reducing aggressive behavior in autistic children. High-dose vitamin B therapy has been used to treat autistic children; however, research has shown that high doses deplete magnesium and other B complex vitamins and may cause sensory neuropathy. Fenfluramine, an appetite suppressant, and Naltrexone, an opioid antagonist, have been experimentally used to increase attention span and improve IQ. A multidisciplinary approach to care is essential. The nurse's role is to identify abnormal behavior as early as possible, refer for follow-up care, and monitor side effects of medications prescribed.

During hospitalization, the nurse should provide a highly structured environment with few distractions. A normal homelike routine should be maintained whenever possible, with safety a priority. Communication should be at the child's developmental level, using one request at a time in a slow and friendly manner.

A high intelligence and development of meaningful language by 5 years of age is a favorable prognosis, although most autistic children require long-term care.

Obsessive-Compulsive Disorders in Children

Obsessive compulsive disorder (OCD) is a disorder in which a recurrent, persistent, repetitive thought invades the conscious mind *(obsession)* or a ritual movement or activity that is not related to adapting to the environment assumes inordinate importance *(compulsion)*. The rituals or movements may involve touching an object, saying a certain word, or washing the hands repetitively. OCD in children differ from OCD in adults in that the symptoms are not usually part of an obsessive personality. The behavior may start as early as age 4, but may not be noticed as interfering with daily functioning until 10 years of age or older. Children usually are aware of their compulsive behavior and may voluntarily control themselves while in school with peers. Untreated, the problem grows to interfere with total functioning. OCD is related to depression and other psychiatric disorders such as Tourette's syndrome, and suicidal behavior is a high risk for adolescents with OCD.

OCD does not involve impairment of cognitive function or interpersonal relationships. OCD is of genetic origin. Some research studies show involvement of the basal ganglia of the frontal lobe and a problem with neurohormonal system. Children often become withdrawn and isolated from peers and family. Poor school performance is related to compulsive repetitive behavior, rather than a deficit in intelligence. Family conflicts arise to compound the problem. Clomipramine is one medication used to control behavior. Fluoxetine and Fluvoxamine alter serotonin and are effective for OCD problems.

Behavior therapy combined with medication provides the best results. The treatment involves "exposure and response prevention." However, the child must be motivated and capable of following directions for behavior therapy to be successful. Parent and sibling involvement and support is essential. The nurse's role is to assess normal growth and development and understand that ritualistic behavior, that is normal at 3 years of age is normally replaced by hobbies of collecting and special interests by 8 years of age. Prolonged ritualistic behavior should be referred for follow-up care. Assessing response to and side effects of medications is an important nursing role.

ENVIRONMENTAL OR BIOCHEMICAL BEHAVIOR DISORDERS

Depression

Depression in a child is not as easy to identify as depression in the adult. Many children have difficulty expressing their feelings and often "act out" their concerns. Depression is an emotion common to childhood. Sadness over grades, moving to a new community, or the loss of a pet may trigger a depressive mood that results in either a dependent-type behavior or a disruptive-type behavior. These manifestations are resolved in a short time and are considered perfectly normal. A major depressive or mood disorder is usually characterized by a prolonged behavioral change from baseline that interferes with schooling, family life, and/or age-specific activities. Symptoms can include loss of appetite, sleep problems, lethargy, social withdrawal, and sudden decrease in grades. In young children head banging, truancy, lying, and stealing can occur. Depressive behavior, left untreated, can lead to substance abuse and/or suicide. Major depression occurs in about 1% of children younger than school age, 2% of school age children, and 5% of adolescents. Inheritance factors, organic factors, and environmental factors all contribute to major depressive disorders in children. Treatment of depressive disorders is usually on an outpatient basis and may include prescribed drugs.

Nursing responsibilities include recognizing signs of depression and initiating appropriate and prompt referral (Nursing Care Plan 32–1). Educating parents and school personnel concerning the identification of children at risk is an important nursing function in the community as well as the hospital setting.

Suicide

Suicide is the third leading cause of death in adolescents after accidents and homicide. Completed suicides are more common in boys than in girls, but girls make more attempts. Many adolescent suicides are not intended to end in death, but are a cry for help that may end tragically. The risk for successful suicide increases when there is a plan of action, a means to carry out the plan, and an absence of obvious resources to turn to for help. The breakdown of family ties, pressure to succeed, or foiled relationships may trigger a low self-esteem or frustration that results in the turning of feelings of hostility or hopelessness inward.

Suicidal behaviors can be identified as *suicidal ideation*, which involves thoughts about suicide; *suicidal gestures*, which is an attempt at a suicidal action that does not result in injury; and a *suicidal attempt*, which is an action that is seriously intended to cause death (although it may be unsuccessful). Some adolescents may exhibit rage behavior or an emotional outburst that results in an *impulsive act* that can result in accidental death. Some adolescents display a chronic type of high-risk behavior that can lead to serious injury or death. The nurse's role lies in education, prevention, and identification of those children at risk and prompt referral for follow-up care.

Some manifestations of suicidal behavior include a flat affect or "fixed" facial expression; deterioration in school performance; isolation from friends and family; changes in physical appearance; giving away of cherished possessions; and talk of death. The nurse is a vital link in working with school personnel to develop peer support groups and educate families concerning community resources available. Mental health associations, hotlines, drop-in centers, runaway houses, and free clinics are community resources that can be called upon.

Substance Abuse

Substance abuse is the illegal use of drugs, alcohol, or tobacco for the purpose of producing an altered state of consciousness. Substances may be ingested, injected, or inhaled to produce the desired effect. Four levels of substance abuse have been established: *experimentation, controlled use, abuse,* and *dependence.* Although there is often a fine line between controlled use and abuse, frequency may be a major signal. This is especially true when accompanied by inappropriateness, for example,

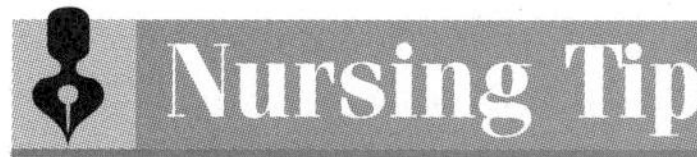

Every threat of suicide must be taken seriously.

NURSING CARE PLAN 32–1

Selected Nursing Diagnoses for the Depressed Adolescent

Nursing Diagnosis: High risk for violence: self-directed, related to depression and stress

Goals	Nursing Interventions	Rationale
Adolescent states whether suicide is contemplated Adolescent does not harm self and states two healthy coping measures Adolescent verbalizes acceptance of protective measures Family verbalizes seriousness of suicidal threats	1. Ask adolescent if suicidal thoughts are present	1. This information is important to know, as it will determine intervention; most depressed teenagers are filled with contradictory feelings; talking honestly about them helps to clarify them
	2. Inquire as to precipitating event: broken romance, poor grades, and so on	2. Suicidal reactions are associated with feelings of hopelessness often related to loss of a significant or valued relationship or a disappointment
	3. Determine if adolescent has specific suicidal plan	3. How person plans to take life is one of most significant criteria of assessing suicidal potential; more specific plans are a more dangerous threat
	4. Determine if person has a history of suicidal attempts	4. If patient has made serious attempts in past, situation is considered more critical
	5. Determine if person has history of emotional instability	5. History of emotional instability is more dangerous
	6. Determine if adolescent has means available	6. If the means to commit suicide are available (i.e., pills, gun), threat is imminent and more serious
	7. Provide supervision as outlined by physician or institution	7. Surveillance and support by staff and family are important
	8. Determine if safe contract has been signed	8. This is a written agreement that person will contact a nurse, counselor, or crisis line or go to an emergency room before harming self
	9. Attend team conferences	9. It is wise to have available as many persons as possible to support one another and share stress of situation
	10. Administer antidepressants if ordered	10. Antidepressants elevate the mood of the client; unfortunately, most antidepressants must be taken for 3–4 wk before a therapeutic response is evident; some require monitoring of blood values
	11. Monitor room for potentially dangerous articles	11. Belts, glasses, rope, and other materials may be used to self-destruct
	12. Explain precautions to adolescent and family members	12. Explanations will lessen fear and increase compliance
	13. Reinforce the seriousness of adolescent's suicidal threat to parents	13. *All* suicidal threats need to be taken seriously

(Continued)

"getting stoned" at the weekend party versus on the way to school. There are two kinds of dependence, *psychological* and *physical.* Psychological dependence includes craving for and a compulsive need to use a substance. Physical dependence occurs with drugs such as heroin and alcohol. People become "hooked on the drug," and in addition to psychological dependence they experience physical

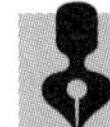

Nursing Tip

When a teenager feels hopeless and talks about feeling useless or worthless, do not contradict what the youngster has to say. Instead listen, indicate your understanding, and encourage the expression of feelings.

NURSING CARE PLAN 32–1 *continued*

Selected Nursing Diagnoses for the Depressed Adolescent

Nursing Diagnosis: Ineffective individual coping related to poor self-esteem, isolation, inability to deal with painful feelings

Goals	Nursing Interventions	Rationale
Adolescent makes positive statement about self Adolescent accepts positive statements from others Adolescent accepts presence of nurse, peers, or significant others Adolescent gradually deals with painful feelings by sharing and expressing them either verbally or nonverbally Adolescent speaks in future terms	1. Have client list two positive things about self	1. Determines adolescent's strengths so that nurse can build on them
	2. Instruct adolescent to draw "how I see myself" and "how others see me"	2. Provides valuable information about person's self-esteem; self-destructive behavior reflects underlying depression related to low self-esteem and anger directed inward; drawing offers a release from feelings, helps to clarify emotions, and is a vehicle for discussion between client and nurse
	3. Build extra time into visits so that adolescent does not feel rushed; give your undivided attention	3. This indicates that you are truly interested; ringing telephone and personal interruptions devalue visit
	4. Instruct adolescent to draw a box and put things that bring happy feelings in the box; then instruct to draw another box and place things that cause sadness in that box; encourage adolescent to verbalize feelings about drawings; respect adolescent's wish not to talk should this occur	4. Drawings help clients to distance themselves from problem and see it more clearly
	5. Review methods of coping	5. Discovering how the patient coped in the past when he or she was less distressed is of importance so that these methods can be reinforced
	6. Suggest healthy methods of coping such as exercise, relaxation tapes, talking things out with parents or peers	6. Many teenagers are not aware of healthy coping methods

withdrawal symptoms. *Tolerance* develops when a user's body becomes accustomed to certain drugs. The person must then increase the dose each time to maintain its effect. Table 32–1 summarizes the characteristics of some of the more commonly abused drugs and the adolescent's reactions to them. Table 32–2 lists street names for some of these drugs.

Alcohol. Experimentation with alcohol has traditionally been accepted as a normal part of growing up. All states have legal drinking age laws that are well defined and implemented. However, studies have shown that one in seven (14.5%) of eighth graders have experimented with beverages containing alcohol. Nurses need to educate the public that alcoholism is a disease with established criteria that is both treatable and preventable. The devastating physical consequences of alcohol abuse as well as the increased risk of accidents and injury should be discussed with children starting as early as elementary school age. School nurses and parent teachers associations can work together to prevent alcohol abuse and identify alcohol abusers who can be referred for follow-up care. Al-Anon, Alateen, AA (Alcoholics Anonymous) are programs listed in most local telephone directories in the United States that welcome the young adolescent seeking help with an alcohol problem. Alcoholism is often a family disease. Adults often serve alcohol freely at social events in the home and therefore offer mixed messages about alcohol use to their children.

Cocaine. The easy availability of cocaine and the affordability of "crack" cocaine are the causes of increased experimentation by children. The drug can be "snorted," smoked, or used intravenously. The drug can cause life-threatening systemic responses as well as aggressive, antisocial behavior.

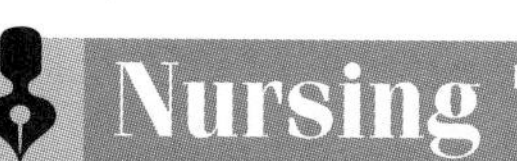

It has been estimated that over 2 million people are using cocaine on a regular basis. "Crack" is a popular form that can be extremely addictive.

Acute overdose can result in death. Treatment usually requires in-patient residential care.

Gateway substances are common household products that can be abused to achieve an altered state of consciousness, or "high." A feeling of euphoria can be followed by central nervous system depression, seizures, and cardiac arrest. These substances include cleaning fluid, glue, lighter fluid, paints, shoe polish, various aerosols, and gasolines that are inhaled in various ways. They are called

Table 32–1
CHARACTERISTICS OF ABUSED DRUGS AND THEIR ACUTE REACTIONS IN ADOLESCENTS

Class	Example	Route	Behavioral Signs	Physical Signs	Medical Complications
Opiates	Heroin, methadone, morphine	Subcutaneous, intranasal, intravenous	Euphoria, lethargy to coma	Constricted pupils, respiratory depression, cyanosis, rales, needle marks	Injection site infection, hepatitis, bacterial endocarditis, amenorrhea, peptic ulcer, pulmonary edema, tetanus
Hypnotics sedatives	Barbiturates, glutethimide	Oral, intravenous	Slurred speech, ataxia, short attention span, drowsiness, combativeness, violence	Constricted pupils (barbiturates), dilated pupils (glutethimide), needle marks	Injection site infection, hepatitis, endocarditis
	Alcohol	Oral	As above		Gastritis, central nervous system infection, depression
Stimulants	Amphetamines	Oral, subcutaneous, intravenous	Hyperactivity, insomnia, anorexia, paranoia, personality change, irritability	Hypertension, weight loss, dilated pupils	Injection site infection, hepatitis, endocarditis, psychosis, depression
	Cocaine	Intravenous, intranasal	Restlessness, hyperactivity, occasional depression or paranoia	Hypertension, tachycardia	Nausea, vomiting, inflammation or perforation of nasal septum
Hallucinogens	LSD, THC, PCP, STP (DOM), mescaline, DMT	Oral	Euphoria, dysphoria, hallucinations, confusion, paranoia	Dilated pupils, occasional hypertension, hyperthermia, piloerection	Primarily psychiatric with high risk to individuals with unrecognized or previous psychiatric disorder
Hydrocarbons, fluorocarbons	Glue (toluene)	Inhalant	Euphoria, confusion, general intoxication	Nonspecific	Secondary trauma, asphyxiation from plastic bag used to inhale fumes
	Cleaning fluid (trichloroethylene)	Inhalant	Euphoria, confusion, general intoxication, vomiting, abdominal pain	Oliguria, jaundice	Hepatitis, renal injury
	Aerosol sprays Freon	Inhalant	Euphoria, dysphoria, slurred speech, hallucinations	Nonspecific	Psychiatric
Cannabis	Marijuana, hashish, THC	Smoke, oral	Mild intoxication and simple euphoria to hallucination (dose-related)	Occasional tachycardia, delayed response time, poor coordination	Occasionally psychiatric, with depressive or anxiety reactions

LSD, lysergic acid diethylamide; THC, tetrahydrocannabinol; PCP, phencyclidine piperidine; STP (DOM), 2,5-dimethoxy-4-methylamphetamine; DMT, dimethyltryptamine.

From Vaughan, V., McKay, R., & Behrman, R. (1979). *Nelson's textbook of pediatrics* (11th ed.). Philadelphia: Saunders.

Table 32–2
STREET NAMES FOR COMMONLY ABUSED DRUGS*

Street Name	Drug
A's	Amphetamines
Acid	Lysergic acid diethylamide (LSD)
Angel dust	Dimethyltryptamine (DMT) or phencyclidine piperidine (PCP) sprinkled over parsley or tobacco
Barbs	Barbiturates
Bennies	Benzedrine (amphetamine sulfate)
Black	LSD
Bullets	Secobarbital (Seconal)
Charlie	Cocaine
Coke	Cocaine
Crack	A form of cocaine
Crap	Heroin
Downers	Barbiturates or tranquilizers
Goofballs	Barbiturates
Hash	Hashish
Horse	Heroin
Joint	Marijuana cigarette
Mickey	Combination of alcohol and a hypnotic drug
Pot	Marijuana
PG	Paregoric
Rainbows	Tuinal (secobarbital sodium and amobarbital sodium)
Smack	Heroin
Speed	Methamphetamine
Uppers	Central nervous system stimulants
Yellow jackets	Pentobarbital

*These names change frequently and vary within subcultures.

gateway substances because their use often leads to abuse of stronger drugs (such as cocaine) and drug addiction.

Marijuana. Marijuana is a hemp plant *(Cannabis sativa).* Hashish, a portion of that plant that is most potent, is smoked or ingested and rapidly absorbed by the body and metabolized by the liver. Asthmatic children can have serious reactions to the bronchoconstriction that occurs with smoking this substance. Loss of inhibitions, euphoria, and a loss of coordination and of goal-direction are associated with use of this substance. Users should be referred for professional counseling.

Opiates. Heroin is the most common opiate abused by adolescents. Since opiate users often drop out of school, statistics concerning use by children in school are lacking. The main consequence of heroin abuse is related to the use of unsterile needles, which places the adolescent at risk for HIV infection. Hepatitis and infections are also common among heroin users. Long-term treatment programs are the therapy of choice for adolescents.

Prevention and Nursing Goals. The prevention of substance abuse begins by helping expectant parents to develop good parenting skills. It is imperative that children learn to feel good about themselves very early in life. They need a safe environment and adults whom they can trust and who serve as good role models. As orderly development proceeds, the growing child learns to interact with others and develops a sense of identity (Fig. 32–1). A positive self-image and feelings of self-worth help adolescents to fine-tune their adaptive coping skills. In time they will rely on their own problem-solving abilities and ideally will not need chemicals to manage the complexities of life. Nurses in their various settings can contribute to this process. They can also educate their clients about the seriousness of substance abuse.

Although it is generally true that the problem drinkers cannot be helped unless they want to be, more *intervention* is now being done. Most adolescents involved in substance abuse do not choose to enter treatment but are coerced by family members or the juvenile justice system. Although the issue is controversial, clinical experience in substance abuse treatment settings has shown that many adolescents become interested in treatment and make behavioral changes after they have been required to enter a treatment program (Fig. 32–2).

Children of Alcoholics

Description. Until recently, little attention has been given to children of alcoholics. This trend is changing, and support groups such as Adult Children of Alcoholics are more numerous. This discussion is directed to young children of alcoholics, although unresolved issues are similar in adults.

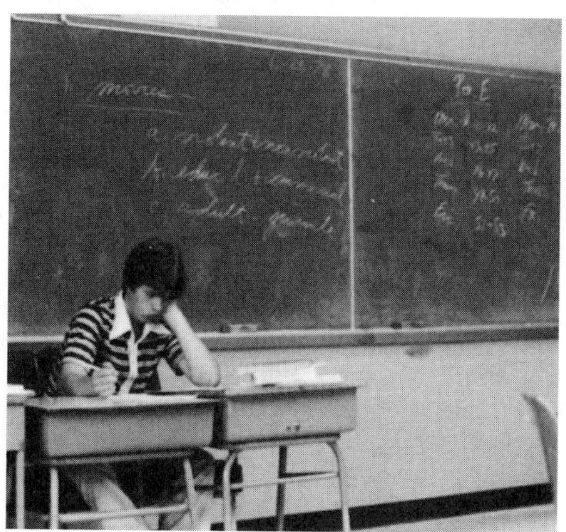

Figure 32–1. • A drop in school grades may be a signal of inner turmoil.

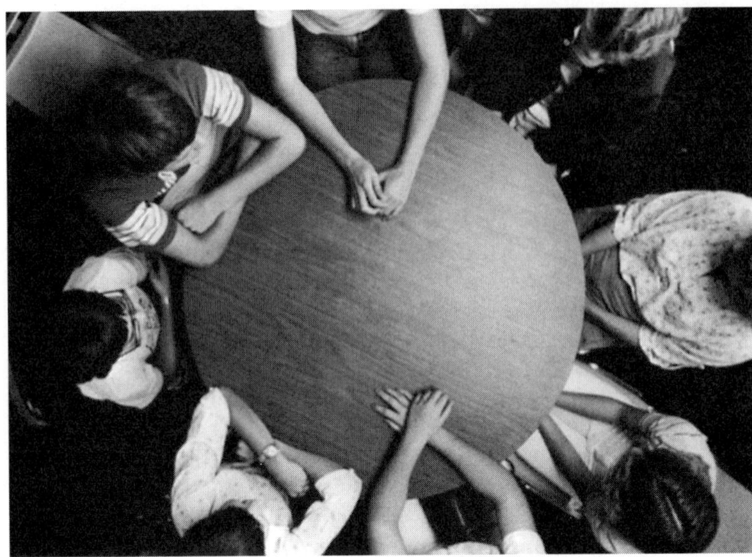

Figure 32–2. • Talking with groups of peers is an important therapeutic modality for adolescents with various addictions or mental health problems.

Pediatric nurses are in an excellent position to recognize and intervene in cases in which physical or emotional neglect exists because of parental alcoholism. These problems stem from the parents' preoccupation with the disease. It is not unusual for both parents to be users.

Children of alcoholics are often confused by the unpredictability of family life. They do not understand why their needs are not being met. In some families, there is a role reversal with the child being forced to act maturely and make decisions ordinarily assumed by a parent. Often these children feel that they are responsible for the disruptive environment. They are at high risk for physical abuse, including sexual abuse. Children of alcoholics are also strong candidates for becoming alcoholics as adults. Role models are distorted or lacking. A parent may try to cover up for the drinking partner by lying to employers and relatives, but may punish the child for the same behavior. The child may become isolated from peers while trying to avoid embarrassment at home. Four predominant coping patterns of these children are flight, fight, the perfect child, and the super coper or family savior (Fig. 32–3).

The child who flees may do so literally or emotionally. The goal is to get away, and as the child grows older, more and more time is spent away from home. Feelings are buried and left unexpressed. The child fighter is aggressive and displays acting-out behavior. The perfect child tries to gain love by never causing any trouble. The child is obedient and generally a good student. The savior or super coper feels overly responsible, often has a job to help out, and tries to do everything perfectly.

Manifestations, Nursing Care, and Treatment. Early recognition of and intervention for children of alcoholics are paramount. The astute nurse with heightened awareness of alcoholism can expand admission observations and nursing history. Some clues that may or may not be related to this problem include refusal to talk about family life, poor school grades or overachievement, unusual need to please, fatigue, passive or acting-out behavior, or maturity beyond the child's years. Treatment is multifold. One immediate priority is to teach the child how to get help in an emergency and to put the youngster in touch with someone from the extended family, school, or other suitable agency. Cultural diversities need to be incorporated into treatment plans.

Attention Deficit Hyperactivity Disorder

Description. The term *attention deficit hyperactivity disorder* (ADHD) refers to a developmentally inappropriate degree of gross motor activity, impulsivity, and inattention in the school or home setting that begins before 7 years of age and lasts more than 6 months and is not related to the existence of any other central nervous system illness. It is more common in boys than in girls. It occurs more frequently in some families, which suggests a genetic connection. The *Diagnostic and Statistical Manual of Mental Disorders IV* (DSM-IV) has defined the condition precisely and established specific criteria for diagnosis.

Learning disability is an educational term; however, learning disabilities occur frequently in children with ADHD. Although these children may have average or above-average intellectual ability, they experience difficulties in such areas as perception, language, comprehension, conceptualization, memory, and control of attention. *Dyslexia* (reading difficulties) and *dysgraphia* (writing difficulties) may be apparent. These children may transpose letters, for example, may read "pot" for "top." They may have difficulty in expressing themselves.

Manifestations. The symptoms of ADHD as defined by the DSM-IV are summarized as follows:

- *Inattention* (at least three). Is easily distracted, needs calm atmosphere in which to work, fails to complete work, does not appear to listen, has difficulty concentrating unless instruction is one-to-one, needs information repeated
- *Impulsivity* (at least three). Is disruptive with other children, talks out in class, is extremely excitable, cannot wait turn, is overtalkative, requires a lot of supervision
- *Hyperactivity* (at least two). Climbs on furniture, fidgets, is always "on the go," cannot stay seated, does things in a loud and noisy way

Nursing Tip

Attention deficit hyperactivity disorder is characterized by inattention, hyperactivity, impulsivity, and distractability.

Assessment history involves a description of the child's behavior and responses, an observation of parenting style and understanding of the existing family stresses. The coping strategies of the child should be observed and input from school teachers sought. Psychologists may interpret behavior rating scales administered to the child.

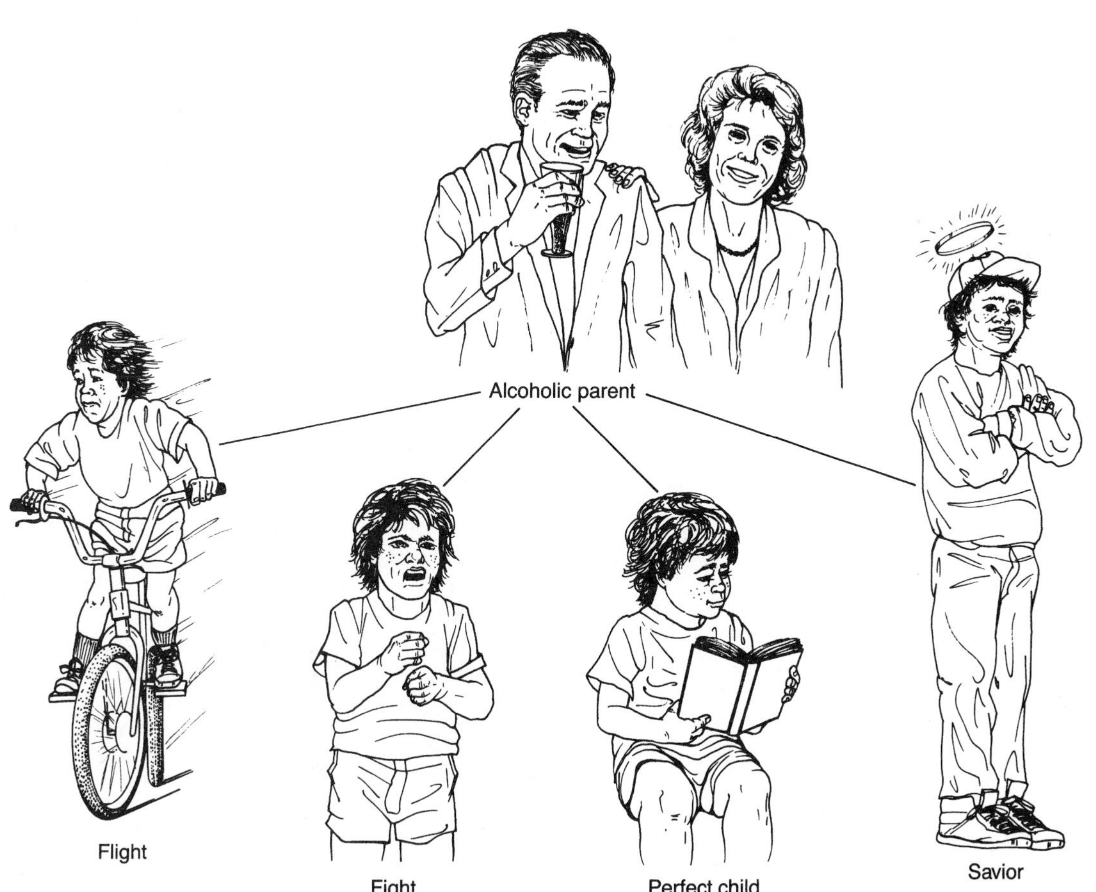

Figure 32–3. • Some defense patterns of children of alcoholics.

Table 32–3

MEDICATIONS USEFUL IN ATTENTION DEFICIT HYPERACTIVITY DISORDER

Drug	Dosage (mg)	Dosage Interval	Side Effects	Nursing Implications
Methylphenidate (Ritalin, Ritalin-SR)	2.5–20 20–40	8 AM, noon 8 AM	Anorexia, weight loss, nervousness, insomnia, occasional dizziness, headache	Frequently used because of rapid and predictable onset, few side effects CBC, differential, and platelet count should routinely be performed during therapy Give 30–45 min before meals Do not give drug in afternoon or evening to avoid insomnia Monitor growth parameters Teach family to avoid tasks that require alertness until response to drug is established Give sugarless gum for dry mouth or sips of water
Dextroamphetamine (Dexedrine)	2.5–20	8 AM, noon	Temporary suppression of weight and height patterns Increased motor activity, talkativeness, mild euphoria, insomnia Dry mouth	Avoid tasks that require alertness, motor skills until response to drug is established
Pemoline (Cylert)	18.75–112.5	8 AM	Anorexia, insomnia, occasional abdominal discomfort, diarrhea	Liver function tests should be performed before therapy begins and periodically during therapy Teach family that the therapeutic response is gradual and may take 3–4 wk Insomnia and anorexia usually disappear during continued therapy Presence of a tic disorder (muscle spasm) or appearance of tics while on stimulant medication is a contraindication to its use or continued use

The management of ADHD is multidisciplinary. Family education to deal with their knowledge deficit about the condition, counseling to help the family and the child to deal with the problems encountered, and medication (see Table 32–3) to help to control some symptoms are the core of therapy. *Emphasizing the strengths of the child rather than the problems is essential.* Various support groups can aid parents in their coping skills. The school nurse can help teachers to develop strategies for managing children with ADHD in the classroom (Box 32–2). Increasing positive interactions, providing tutoring, computer assistance, and behavioral management strategies under the supervision of a professional psychologist are helpful approaches to care. ADHD is a chronic long-term condition that can persist through adulthood. Some children who are "labeled" in school develop low self-esteem and antisocial behavior.

BOX 32–2

STRATEGIES FOR MANAGING CHILDREN WITH ADHD IN THE CLASSROOM

- Seat child in front of classroom to minimize distraction.
- Remind child to focus attention whenever necessary.
- Give clear instructions and repeat instructions often.
- Provide breaks between periods of work or study.

Adapted from Berkowitz, C. (1996). *Pediatrics, a primary care approach.* (p. 407). Philadelphia: Saunders.

Anorexia Nervosa

Description. Anorexia nervosa (*anorexia,* "want of appetite," and *nervosa,* "nervous") is a form of self-starvation seen mostly in adolescent girls. Only 10% of patients with eating disorders are male. The criteria for this disorder are well outlined in the *Diagnostic and Statistical Manual of Mental Disorders IV* (DSM-IV). It is characterized by:

- Failure to maintain minimal normal weight for age and height (less than 85% of expected weight)
- An intense fear of gaining weight
- Excess influence of body weight on self-evaluation
- Amenorrhea

The etiology may have a genetic basis. The adolescents characteristically have average to superior intelligence and are overachievers who expect to be perfect in all areas. For young people with the disorder, their own emerging sexuality is very threatening. They experience anxiety and guilt over imagined or real fear of intimacy. They have low self-esteem, are obedient, are nonassertive and shy.

Families of these young people are often dysfunctional. They may exhibit such behaviors as overprotectiveness, rigidity, lack of privacy, and inability to resolve conflicts. Affluent families may be at high risk when the concept of being thinner rules and the focus is on diet and exercise.

Manifestations. The primary symptom of anorexia nervosa is severe weight loss. Adolescents who wish to be fashion models or actresses or who participate in sports, dance, or gymnastics activities may be at risk for developing an eating disorder. On physical examination, some of the following conditions may be evident: dry skin, amenorrhea, lanugo hair over the back and extremities, cold intolerance, low blood pressure, abdominal pain, and constipation.

Teenagers with anorexia experience feelings of helplessness, lack of control, low self-esteem, and depression. Socialization with peers diminishes. Mealtime becomes a family battleground. The body image becomes increasingly disturbed (Fig. 32–4), and there is a lack of self-identity. The young person remains egocentric and unable to complete normal adolescent tasks. Although eating less, the anorexic individual is preoccupied with food and its preparation. Hunger is denied. The patient complains of bloating and abdominal pain after ingesting small amounts of food.

Treatment and Nursing Care. The treatment of anorexia nervosa is complex and involves several modalities. Some hospitals have eating disorder units. A brief period of hospitalization may be necessary to correct electrolyte imbalance, establish minimum restoration of nutrients, and stabilize the patient's weight. It also provides timeout from a dysfunctional home environment.

Therapies include individual and family psychotherapy, behavioral therapy, and pharmacologic therapy. Antidepressant medications may be helpful. The nurse plays an important role in ensuring that the atmosphere is relaxed and nonpunitive. Follow-up after discharge from the unit is essential. Individual and family therapy are continued.

Nurses working with adolescents in any capacity need to be alert to the symptoms of this condition, a lack of recognition is one of the biggest obstacles to treatment. In the early stages, dissatisfaction with body image, amenorrhea, and social isolation are suspect. Young people need to be educated about the seriousness of the disorder. Educational materials, referral sources, and counseling are available from the National Association of Anorexia Nervosa and Associated Disorders. Encouragement and support from self-help groups are also valuable.

Prognosis. Most patients gain weight in the hospital, regardless of the type of therapy. This may not, however, predict future success. Complications include gastritis, cardiac arrhythmias, inflammation of the intestine, and kidney problems. Fatalities do occur, particularly in untreated persons. Approximately 50% of patients are cured, approximately 30% improve, but continue to have dysfunctional eating problems and a distorted body image, although they function well in school and at work, and approximately 15% remain chronically ill through adulthood.

Bulemia

Bulemia, or compulsive eating, is recognized by the *Diagnostic and Statistical Manual of Mental Disorders IV* (DSM-IV) as a separate eating disorder. It has been estimated that as many as 5% of college women and 1% of college men have this condition. It is characterized by recurrent episodes of uncontrolled binge eating followed by self-induced vomiting and misuse of laxatives and/or diuretics.

Family dysfunctions are usually present in children with bulemia, but unlike anorexia, the mother–daughter relationship is usually distant or strained. Depression and alcoholism may be a family problem. The binge–purge cycle is thought to be a coping mechanism for dealing with guilt, depression, and low self-esteem. Impulsive behaviors are characteristic of bulemic adolescents.

Clinical Pathway 32–1

An Interdisciplinary Plan of Care for the Child with Anorexia

	Patient/Family Intermediate Outcomes					
Nursing Diagnosis	Day 1	Day 2	Day 3	Day 4	Days 5–6	Follow-up/ post discharge
Altered Nutrition: less than body requirements related to eating deficit and excessive exercise	Child will agree to target weight to be reached at end of 1 month. Child will verbalize willingness to follow diet to reach target weight.	Child will follow contract.	→ Child's weight is stabilized.	→ →	→ Child will gain 1 pound before discharge.	→
Knowledge Deficit: related to adequate nutritional needs	Child will verbalize elements of sound nutritional diet.	→	Child will verbalize knowledge of nutritional needs and body requirements.	→	Child will discuss any further concerns or misinformation regarding nutrition.	→
Body Image Disturbance: related to inaccurate messages (self and others)	Child will verbalize statements/beliefs about body image.	Child will engage in self-talk statements that are positive about normal weight.	→	Child will verbalize positive self-statements related to normal weight and self-uniqueness.	→	→
Impared Social Interactions: related to nutritional practices and/or lethargy and introvert type behavior	Child will agree to participate in group therapy.	Child will participate in group therapy.	→	→	→	Child will continue group therapy twice a week until target weight is achieved.
Potential for Noncompliance: related to contract for target weight	Child will adhere to contract.	→	→	→	→	→
	Child will not hide food.	→	→	→	→	→
	Child will not engage in excessive activity.	→	→	→	→	→

(Continued)

Persistent vomiting can cause erosion of the enamel of the teeth and eventual tooth loss. The use of laxatives and self-induced vomiting can cause electrolyte imbalance. If ipecac is routinely used to induce vomiting, muscle weakness will result. The HEADSSS format of interviewing adolescents is helpful in obtaining a detailed assessment (*H*ome, *E*mployment or *E*ducation, *A*ctivities, *D*rugs, *S*exual activity, *S*uicidal ideas, *S*afety).

The nursing role in dealing with adolescents with eating disorders is to educate, prevent, identify, and refer. It is very difficult to identify an adolescent

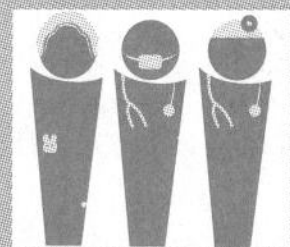

Clinical Pathway 32–1 *(Continued)*

An Interdisciplinary Plan of Care for the Child with Anorexia

Care Intervention Categories

	Day 1	Day 2	Day 3	Day 4	Days 5–6	Follow-up/post discharge
Consults	Psychiatry Nutrition Social work Advanced practice nurse (APN)	School liaison		Family physician		Primary physician 1 week after discharge
Discharge planning		Evaluate family, community and school resources. Coordinate care with school liaison.		Coordinate care with family physician and outpatient services.		
Labs	CBC Electrolytes					
Monitors	Rest, exercise, and eating record	→	→	→	→	
Nutrition/exercise and rest	Contract formulated regarding diet, exercise, and rest.	Contract followed.	→	→	→	→
	Monitor rest periods and adherence to contract.	→	→	→	→	
	Nursing assistant stays with child during mealtimes and snacks.	→	→	→	→	
	Obtain agreement not to hide food.					
Group therapy	Discussion of group therapy and purpose. Obtain agreement to participate.	Begin group therapy.	→	→	→	Group therapy two times a week

(Continued)

with a weight obsession in a society where weight and thinness define beauty. This concept is reinforced in movies and magazines. A supportive, respectful, but firm, manner should be maintained by the nurse. Establishing trust with the adolescent is the first step in education, referral, and treatment. Adolescents with eating disorders must maintain a sense of control in their therapy for success to be achieved. Compromise and contracts must replace authoritative restrictions on diet and activity. Referral to support groups and child and family counseling groups is helpful. A multidisciplinary ap-

Clinical Pathway 32–1 *(Continued)*

An Interdisciplinary Plan of Care for the Child with Anorexia

Care Intervention Categories

	Day 1	Day 2	Day 3	Day 4	Days 5–6	Follow-up/ post discharge
Family therapy		Family session: • Increase family cooperation/ negotiation. • Negotiate family therapy goals.	Participate in family therapy.	→	→	→
Individual therapy	Individual session focused on changing self-talk to positive statements about normal weight and to negative statements about unhealthy current weight.	→	→	→	→	
	Individual and family therapy.	→	→	→	→	
	Reinforce assertive communication skills.	→	→	→	→	
	Help patient identify own strengths.	→	→	→	→	
Teaching	Assess knowledge regarding nutritional needs—individual session.	Individual and family session: etiologic basis of eating disorder	Reevaluate knowledge; correct distortion and misinformation.	→	Answer any remaining questions about diet and normal nutrition.	→
	Teach relaxation skills (music/ meditation).	→	→	→	→	
Vital signs/ baseline parameters	Height Weight Tanner staging Evaluate skin, hair, and mucous membranes.	Weight	→	→	→	→

(Adapted from Bowden, V., Dickey, S., & Greenberg, C. [1998]. *Children and their families: The continuum of care.* Philadelphia: Saunders.)

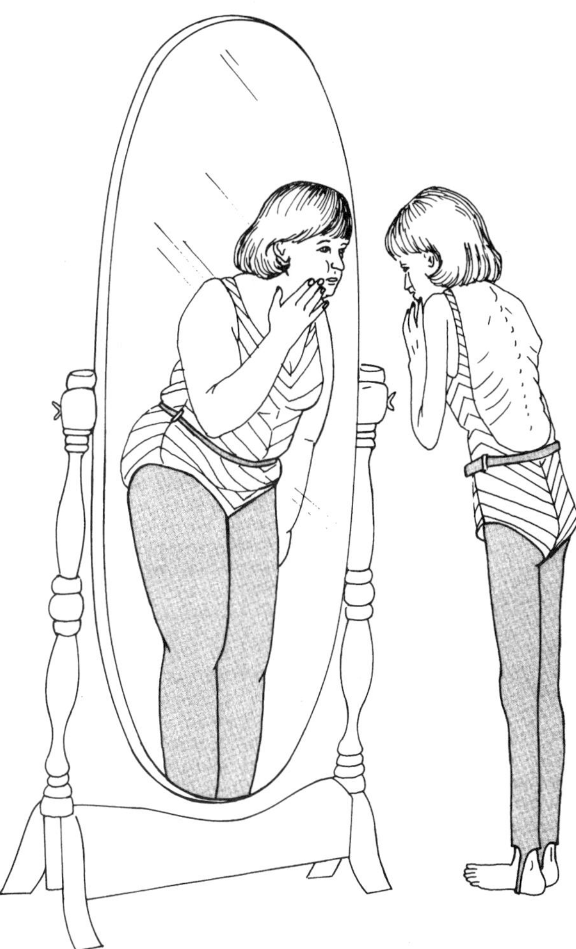

Figure 32–4. • Patients with eating disorders often have a disturbance in self-image.

proach with the nurse, pediatrician, nutritionist, psychiatrist, and social worker helps to achieve a positive outcome.

MINIMIZING THE IMPACT OF BEHAVIOR DISORDERS ON GROWTH AND DEVELOPMENT

Children respond to traumatic events in their life and to stressors within the family as well as in the school and within the peer or social group. The duration and intensity of the stressful event and the child's coping skills will determine the impact on the growth and development process. Knowledge of normal growth and development throughout childhood combined with good observation and listening skills can enable the nurse to play a major role in minimizing the negative impact of behavior problems on growth and development. Because outpatient services play a significant role in health care today, nurses need to be aware of agencies and support groups available to children with behavior disorders and their parents. Prompt, early referral and treatment can improve the prognosis of emotional and behavioral disorders, enabling the children to reach their potential in growth and development.

Children's behavior problems require a total family approach to care. Education of the community (school personnel), family (parents and siblings), and child is an essential nursing responsibility. Patient advocacy with a focus on prevention and long-term management are goals of care. A knowledgeable, caring, understanding, and supportive nature is valuable for any nurse caring for children with behavior disorders.

KEY POINTS

- Early childhood experiences are critical to personality formation.
- The child's environment must be safe, and the child must be able to trust caretakers.
- Nurses play an important role in the mental and emotional assessment of children because they often have the most contact with the hospitalized child and family.
- Talk of suicide must always be taken seriously.
- The risk of suicide increases when there is a definite plan of action, the means are available, and the person has few resources for help and support.
- Substance abuse is the number-one problem of American teenagers.
- Al-Anon and Alateen are two excellent resources for family members of alcoholics.
- The *Diagnostic and Statistical Manual of Mental Disorders IV* (DSM-IV) lists specific criteria for various mental conditions seen in children and adults.

- Attention deficit hyperactivity disorder is characterized by a developmentally inappropriate degree of gross motor activity, impulsivity, distractability, and inattention in school or at home.
- Behavior problems can be caused by the stresses accompanying the transition from childhood to adulthood or genetic or biochemical factors.
- Autistic children do not show interest in other children, do not make eye contact, and do not engage in "pretend" play.
- Obsessive compulsive disorders in children do not involve impaired cognitive functioning. Ritualistic behavior may interfere with daily activities.
- A major depressive disorder is characterized by a prolonged behavioral change from baseline that interferes with school or age-specific activities.
- Substances abused by children and adolescents may be inhaled, injected, or ingested. The use of unsterile needles may lead to HIV infection.
- Emphasizing the strengths of the child rather than the weaknesses is essential when caring for a child with a behavioral disorder.
- Anorexia nervosa can lead to starvation and death.
- Bulemia is an eating disorder that involves binging and purging and can result in deterioration of teeth and electrolyte imbalance.
- Education, prevention, identification, and referral are essential nursing functions in the care of the child with a behavior disorder.

MULTIPLE-CHOICE REVIEW QUESTIONS

Choose the most appropriate answer.

1. The adolescent with anorexia nervosa has a body self-image characteristically expressed by
   a. wearing tight clothing to emphasize thinness.
   b. increasing elation as weight is lost.
   c. feeling "fat" even when appearing thin.
   d. efforts to achieve specific figure measurements.
2. A priority goal in the approach to a child with anorexia nervosa is to
   a. encourage weight gain.
   b. prevent depression.
   c. limit exercise.
   d. correct malnutrition.
3. A child with suspected bulemia should be assessed for
   a. abnormal weight gain.
   b. abnormal weight loss.
   c. erosion of tooth enamel.
   d. amenorrhea.
4. An important approach to the care for a 7-year-old child diagnosed with attention deficit hyperactivity disorder (ADHD) is to encourage
   a. a diet high in processed foods.
   b. regular use of sedatives.
   c. strict discipline.
   d. a structured, one-on-one environment.
5. When assessing an 8-year-old child with obsessive compulsive disorder (OCD), the nurse would expect to find
   a. an intelligence deficit.
   b. ritualistic behavior.
   c. antisocial behavior.
   d. combative behavior.

BIBLIOGRAPHY AND READER REFERENCE

American Psychiatric Association. (1994). *Diagnostic and statistical manual of mental disorders—DSM-IV* (4th ed.). Washington, DC: Author.

Ashoomoff, N. A., Courchesne, E., & Towsend, J. (1997). *The role of the cerebellum and cognition.* New York: Academic Press.

Behrman, R., Kleigman, R., & Arvin, A. (1996). *Nelson's textbook of pediatrics* (15th ed.). Philadelphia: Saunders.

Berkowitz, C. (1996). *Pediatrics, a primary care approach.* Philadelphia: Saunders.

Bolton, P., Murphy, M., MacDonald, H., et al. (1997). Obstetric complications in autism: Consequence or cause of the condition? *Journal of the American Academy of Child and Adolescent Psychiatry, 36*(2), 272–281.

Cavanaugh, R., Licamele, W., & Ovide, C. (1997). What's normal and what's not: Teen mental health. *Patient Care, 31*(11), 82–109.

Courchesne, E. (1997). Brainstem, cerebellar and limbic neuroanatomical abnormalities in autism. *Current Opinion in Neurobiology, 7*(2), 269–278.

Finberg, L. (1998). *Saunders manual of pediatric practice.* Philadelphia: Saunders.

Gilman, J., & Tuchman, R. (1995). Autism and associated behavioral disorders: Pharmacotherapeutic intervention. *Annals of Pharmacotherapy, 29*, 47–54.

Leifer, R. (1997). *The Happiness Project.* New York: Snow Lion Press.

McGee, G., Feldman, R., & Morrier, M. (1997). Benchmarks of social treatment for children with autism. *Journal of Autism and Developmental Disorders, 27*(4), 353–363.

Ollendick, N., King, J., & Yule, W. (Ed.). (1994). *International handbook of phobic and anxiety disorders in children and adolescents.* New York: Plenum Press.

Osterling, J., & Dawson, G. (1994). Early recognition of children with autism. *Journal of Autism & Developmental Disorders, 24*(3), 247–257.

Piven, J., & Arndt, S. (1995). The cerebellum and autism. *Neurology, 45*, 398–399.

Rapoport, J., Leonard, H., Swedo, S., & Lenane, M. (1993). Obsessive compulsive disorder in children and adolescents: Issues in management. *Journal of Clinical Psychiatry, 54*(6), 27–28.

Wong, D. (1997). *Whaley & Wong's essentials of pediatric nursing.* St. Louis, MO: Mosby.

Glossary

abdominal delivery: cesarean birth.

abduction: a movement away from midline of the body.

abortion: end of a pregnancy before the fetus is viable, whether spontaneous or elective.

abruptio placentae: premature separation of a normally implanted placenta.

abuse: to attack or cause injury—physical, sexual, emotional, or spiritual. This term includes nonaccidental injury and neglect.

acme: peak, or period of greatest strength, of a uterine contraction.

acrocyanosis: peripheral blueness of the hands and feet due to reduced peripheral circulation (normal in newborns).

adduction: a movement toward the midline of the body.

adolescence: period of human development beginning with puberty and ending with young adulthood.

advocacy: speaking or acting in support of a person's rights and needs.

afterbirth: placenta and membranes delivered during the third stage of labor.

afterpains: painful contractions of the uterus that occur for several days after delivery; occur most often in multiparas and are more painful during breastfeeding.

AIDS: acquired immunodeficiency syndrome, caused by HIV; characterized by depressed immune system involving deficiency in CD4+ and t-lymphocytes.

airway management: positioning of the head and neck to ensure patency of the airway; may include interventions to ensure adequate oxygenation.

allergy: an abnormal immune response to a substance that causes an inflammatory response resulting in hypersensitivity.

amenorrhea: absence or suppression of menstruation; normal before puberty, during pregnancy and lactation, and after menopause.

amniocentesis: transabdominal puncture of the amniotic sac (fetal membranes) to obtain a sample of amniotic fluid for study.

amnioinfusion: infusion of warmed saline into the uterus to relieve cord compression or to wash meconium out of the cavity to prevent aspiration at birth.

amnion: the inner of the two fetal membranes; thin and transparent; holds fetus suspended in amniotic fluid.

amniotic fluid: transparent, almost colorless fluid contained in the fetal membranes/amnion; protects fetus from injury, maintains even temperature, and allows fetal movement.

amniotic sac: the sac formed by the amnion and chorion that contains fluid and the fetus, commonly known as the "bag of waters."

analgesic: a drug that relieves pain but does not produce unconsciousness.

androgen: a substance that stimulates masculinization, such as the male hormones testosterone and androsterone.

android pelvis: a female pelvis that resembles a masculine size and shape.

anesthesia: partial or complete loss of sensation, especially of pain, with or without loss of consciousness.

angioma: a tumor, usually benign, that is made up chiefly of blood and lymph vessels.

animism: a period of cognitive development in which the child attributes life to inanimate objects.

anomaly: not normal in form, structure, or position; a congenital anomaly is an abnormality present at birth.

anorexia nervosa: a syndrome most often seen in adolescent girls, characterized by an extreme form of self-starvation. Although its onset may be acute, the underlying emotional problem develops over a relatively long time.

antenatal: before birth.

antepartum: before the onset of labor.

anterior: pertaining to front.

anterior fontanel: diamond-shaped area between the two frontal and the two parietal bones of the newborn's head; also called *soft spot.*

anthropoid pelvis: a female pelvis with a transverse diameter that is equal to or smaller than the anteroposterior diameter.

antibody: specific protein substance, formed in the body in response to antigens, that restricts or destroys antigens.

antigen: a substance that precipitates an immune response resulting in the formation of antibodies. Antigen-antibody reactions form the basis for immunity.

Apgar score: an evaluation tool with a maximum score of 10, used to assess a newborn at 1 minute and 5 minutes after delivery. Five factors, scored 0, 1, or 2, are heart rate, color, muscle tone, reflex irritability, and respiratory effort.

apnea: cessation of respirations.

areola: pigmented circle of tissue around the nipple of the breast.

AROM: artificial rupture of (amniotic) membranes with a sterile instrument, such as an Amnihook or Allis clamp.

artificial insemination: mechanical injection of viable semen into the vagina for the purpose of impregnation.

ascariasis: roundworm infestation.

asphyxia: inadequate amount of oxygen or an increased amount of carbon dioxide in the blood and tissues of the body.

asynchrony: lack of concurrence in time. A growing child may look gangling because of asynchrony of growth, i.e., different body parts maturing at different rates.

atelectasis: incomplete expansion of the lungs or a collapse of the alveoli after expansion.

atony: a lack of muscle tone or strength.

attachment: a strong psychological bond of affection between infant and significant other.

augmentation of labor: enhancement of labor after it has begun.

autoimmunity: a condition in which the body produces antibodies against its own tissues.

autonomy: functioning independently; self-control.

bacteriuria: presence of bacteria in the urine.

bag of waters: the membrane containing the amniotic fluid and the fetus.

ballottement: In obstetrics, the fetus, when palpated, floats away and then returns to touch the examiner's fingers.

barrier technique: a method of medical asepsis using various types of isolation precautions or standard precautions recommended by the Centers for Disease Control. In contraception: a method in which sperm are prevented from entering the cervix.

Bartholin's glands: two small mucous glands situated on each side of the vaginal orifice that secrete small amounts of mucus during coitus (intercourse).

bilirubin: orange or yellowish pigment in bile; a breakdown product of hemoglobin carried by the blood to the liver, where it is chemically changed and excreted in bile or is conjugated and excreted in the stools.

biophysical profile (BPP): a system of estimating status of a fetus by evaluating heart rate, respiratory movement, muscle movement and tone, and amniotic fluid volume. Low scores require prompt delivery.

bleb: an irregularly shaped elevation of the epidermis; a blister or bulla.

bloody show: a mixture of blood and mucus from the cervix that often precedes labor.

bonding: attachment; the process whereby a unique relationship is established between two people; used in conjunction with parent–newborn attachment.

bone marrow transplant: transplantation of bone marrow from one person to another; currently used to treat aplastic anemia and leukemia.

booster injection: administration of a substance to renew or increase the effectiveness of a prior immunization injection, e.g., a tetanus booster.

Braxton-Hicks contractions: intermittent contractions of the uterus; they occur more frequently toward the end of pregnancy and are sometimes mistaken for true labor contractions.

breech presentation: a birth in which the buttocks or feet, or both, present instead of the head; occurs in approximately 3% of all deliveries.

Broviac catheter: a central venous line used in small children who require total parenteral or continuous intravenous infusion.

brown fat: also called *brown adipose tissue;* forms in the fetus around the kidneys, adrenals, and neck; between the scapulae; and behind the sternum. Its dark brown hue is due to its density, enriched blood supply, and abundant nerve supply. Its main purpose is heat production in the neonate.

Bryant traction: a type of skin traction apparatus commonly used for toddlers suffering from a fractured femur. Vertical suspension is used.

café-au-lait spots: light brown patch spots on the skin that may be characteristic of neurofibromatosis (condition of tumors of various sizes on peripheral nerves).

caput: the head; the occiput of the fetal head, which appears at the vaginal introitus prior to delivery of the head.

caput succedaneum: swelling or edema occurring in the newborn scalp that crosses the suture lines. Usually simply called *caput.* It is self-limiting and requires no treatment.

cardiac decompensation: heart failure.

cephalic presentation: birth in which the fetal head is presenting against the cervix.

cephalocaudal: the orderly development of muscular control, which proceeds from head to foot.

cephalohematoma: subperiosteal swelling containing blood, found on the head of a newborn. The swelling does not cross suture lines and therefore often appears unilateral. Usually disappears within a few weeks to 2 months without treatment.

cephalopelvic disproportion (CPD): a condition in which the fetus cannot pass through the maternal pelvis. Also called *fetopelvic disproportion.*

certified nurse-midwife (CNM): registered nurse who has completed special training approved by the American College of Nurse Midwives and passed a certification test. The CNM provides care to women who have a normal, uncomplicated pregnancy and delivery.

cerclage: closing the cervix with a suture to prevent early dilitation and spontaneous abortion.

cerumen: ear wax.

cervical os: the small opening of the cervix that dilates during the first stage of labor.

cervix: the lower part of the uterus.

cesarean birth: delivery of the fetus by means of an incision into the abdominal wall and the uterus; abdominal delivery.

Chadwick's sign: violet-bluish color of vaginal mucous membrane caused by increased vascularity; visible about the 4th week of pregnancy.

chignon: newborn scalp edema created by vacuum extractor.

chloasma: yellowish-brownish pigmentation over the bridge of the nose and cheeks during pregnancy and in some women who are taking oral contraceptives; also known as *mask of pregnancy.*

chordee: a congenital anomaly in which a fibrous strand of tissue extends from the scrotum to the penis, preventing urination with the penis in the normal elevated position; commonly associated with hypospadias.

chorion: the fetal membrane closest to the interior uterine wall; it gives rise to the placenta and continues as the outer membrane surrounding the amnion.

chorionic villi: threadlike projections on the chorionic surface of the placenta; they help to form the placenta and secrete human chorionic gonadotropin.

chromosome: structure composed of tightly packed DNA found in the nuclei of plant and animal cells responsible for the transmission of hereditary characteristics.

circumcision: the surgical removal of the foreskin of the penis.

clitoris: female organ homologous to male penis; a small oval body of erectile tissue situated at the anterior junction of the vulva.

coitus: sexual intercourse.

colostrum: secretion from the breast before onset of true lactation; it has a high protein content, provides some immune properties, and cleanses the newborn's intestinal tract of mucus and meconium.

comedo: a skin lesion caused by a plug of keratin, sebum, and bacteria; there are two types, blackheads and whiteheads.

conception: union of male sperm and female ovum; fertilization.

congenital: present at birth.

congenital anomaly: a malformation present at birth.

contraception: prevention of conception or impregnation.

contraction: tightening and shortening of uterine muscles during labor, causing effacement and dilation of the cervix; contributes to downward and outward movement of fetus.

contraction stress test (CST): manual manipulation of the nipple of the breast to stimulate production of oxytoxin and test fetal response to uterine contractions. Used for high risk pregnancies. Also see *oxytocin challenge test* (OCT).

coping: dealing effectively with stress and problems.

couvade: a syndrome in which the father experiences the symptoms of the pregnant partner.

craniosynostosis: premature closure of the cranial sutures that produces a head deformity and damage to the brain and eyes; craniostenosis.

crowning: appearance of presenting fetal part (head) at vaginal orifice during labor.

cystic hygroma: a lymphangioma most frequently seen in the neck and axillae.

culture: symbols, ideas, values, traditions, and practices shared by a group of people. Can also mean growth of organisms in a special medium.

DDST: Denver Developmental Screening Test. Assesses the developmental status of a child during the first 6 years of life in five areas: personal, social, fine motor adaptive, language, and gross motor activities.

deceleration: periodic decrease in baseline fetal heart rate. Can be early, late, or variable.

decidua basalis: the part of the decidua that unites with the chorion to form the placenta. It is shed in lochial discharge after delivery.

deciduous teeth: baby teeth.
decrement: decrease or stage of decline, as of contraction.
delivery: expulsion of infant with placenta and membranes from the woman at birth.
Denis Browne splint: two separate footplates attached to a crossbar and fitted to a child's shoes, used to correct clubfeet.
developmental task: a skill that occurs at a particular time or age range and, when accomplished, provides the basis for future tasks.
diaphoresis: profuse sweating.
diaphragm: a contraceptive device that is used with a spermicide to prevent sperm from entering the uterus.
diploid: containing a set of maternal and a set of paternal chromosomes. In humans, the diploid number of chromosomes is 46.
dizygotic twins: fetuses that develop from two fertilized ova; fraternal twins.
DNA (deoxyribonucleic acid): a complex molecule that is the storehouse of hereditary information. It is present in the chromosomes of cell nuclei.
dyscrasia: a synonym for "disease."
dysfunctional: inadequate, abnormal.
dyspareunia: painful sexual intercourse.
dystocia: difficult labor due to mechanical factors produced by the fetus or the maternal pelvis or due to inadequate uterine or other muscular activity.

eclampsia: pregnancy-induced hypertension complicated by one or more seizures.
ectoderm: outer layer of cells in the developing embryo that give rise to the skin, nails, and hair.
ectopic pregnancy: implantation of fertilized ovum outside uterine cavity; the most common ectopic site is the fallopian tube.
effacement: thinning and shortening of the cervix that occurs late in pregnancy and during labor.
egocentrism: a kind of thinking in which a child has difficulty seeing anyone else's point of view; this self-centering is normal in young children.
ejaculation: expulsion of semen from the penis.
embryo: early stage of development. In humans, the period from about 3 to 8 weeks' gestation.
empowerment: providing tools and knowledge to the family to enable informed participation in decision making about health care.
encephalitis: an inflammation of the brain.
encopresis: the passage of stools in a child's underwear or other inappropriate places after the age of 4 years. Some children display concurrent behavioral problems.
endoderm: inner layer of cells in a developing embryo that give rise to internal organs such as the intestines.
endometrium: the mucous membrane that lines the inner surface of the uterus.
en face: a position where the parent and infant have eye-to-eye contact at no more than a 9- to 10-inch distance.
engagement: entrance of fetal presenting part into the pelvis; e.g., the leading edge of the fetal head is at the level of the maternal ischial spines in a vertex presentation.
engorgement: vascular congestion or distention. In obstetrics, the swelling of breast tissue brought about by an increase in blood and lymph supply to breast, preceding true lactation.
enuresis: abnormal inability to control urine; may be due to organic, allergic, or psychological problems.
epidural block: regional anesthetic block achieved by injecting local anesthetic agent in the space overlying the dura of the spinal cord.
episiotomy: incision of the perineum to facilitate delivery and to avoid laceration of perineum.
epispadias: a congenital anomaly in which the urethral meatus is located on the dorsal surface of the penis.
estimated date of delivery (EDD)—"due date": The date when the fetus is expected to be born.
ethic: a system of moral principles or standards that guides behavior.
ethnic: groups of people within a culture classified according to religious, racial, national, or physical characteristics.
external os: lower cervical opening.

facies: pertaining to the appearance or expression of the face; certain congenital syndromes typically present with specific facial appearance.
fallopian tubes: tubes that extend from the uterus to the ovaries. They serve as a passageway for ova from the ovary to the uterus and for spermatozoa from the uterus toward the ovary; oviducts; uterine tubes.
false labor: contractions of the uterus, regular or irregular, that may be strong enough to be interpreted as true labor but do not dilate the cervix.
family Apgar: screening test that reveals how a member of the family perceives its function.
fertilization: union of an ovum and a sperm.
fetal heart rate (FHR): the number of times the fetal heart beats per minute; normal range is 110 to 160 beats/min at term.
fetal heart tones (FHTs): the fetal heartbeat as heard through the mother's abdominal wall.
fetoscope: a stethoscope specially adapted to facilitate listening to the fetal heart.

fetus: term used for the developing structure from the 8th week after fertilization until birth.

first stage of labor: stage beginning with the first contractions of true labor and completed when the cervix is fully dilated to 10 cm.

flexion: in obstetrics, a situation that occurs when resistance to the descent of the infant down the birth canal causes its head to flex or bend, the chin approaching the chest, thus reducing the diameter of the presenting part.

fontanels: openings at the point of union of skull bones, often referred to as *soft spots.*

footling: a breech presentation in which one foot or both feet present.

forceps: obstetric instruments occasionally used to aid in birth by assisting fetal rotation and/or descent.

foreskin: the fold of loose skin covering the end of the penis; prepuce.

Friedman graph: a method of describing and recording the progress of labor.

fulminating: occurring rapidly; usually said of a disease.

fundus: the upper portion of the uterus between the fallopian tubes.

fourth trimester: the first 12 weeks following birth when family adaptation occurs.

gamete: a mature germ cell; an ovum or sperm.

gavage: feeding the patient by means of a stomach tube or with a tube passed through the nose, pharynx, and esophagus into the stomach.

gene: smallest unit of inheritance; genes are located on the chromosomes.

genetics: the study of heredity.

geographic tongue: unusual patterns of papilla formation and denuded areas on the tongue.

gestation: period of intrauterine development from conception through birth; pregnancy.

glucometer: a meter used to measure blood glucose.

gonad: sex gland; ovaries in the female and testes in the male.

Goodell's sign: softening of cervix that occurs during 2nd month of pregnancy.

graafian follicle: the ovarian cyst containing the ripe ovum; it secretes estrogens.

gravid: pregnant.

gravida: the number of times a woman has been pregnant; a pregnant woman.

Hegar's sign: softening of the lower uterine segment found upon palpation in the 2nd or 3rd month of pregnancy.

hemangioma: a benign tumor of the skin that consists of blood vessels.

holism: an approach to caring for a person that recognizes and adapts to his or her physical, intellectual, emotional, and spiritual nature; a way of relating to the patient as a whole or biopsychosocial individual rather than just a person with an ailment.

hormone: substance produced in an organ or gland and conveyed by blood to another part of the body to exert an effect.

human chorionic gonadotropin (hCG): hormone produced by chorionic villi and found in the urine of pregnant women.

human immunodeficiency virus (HIV): the organism that causes AIDS.

hydramnios: an excess of amniotic fluid, leading to overdistention of the uterus. Frequently seen in diabetic pregnant women even if there is no coexisting fetal anomaly; polyhydramnios.

hydrocele: an abnormal collection of fluid surrounding the testicles, causing the scrotum to swell.

hymen: membranous fold that normally partially covers the entrance to the vagina.

hypercapnia: increased amount of carbon dioxide in the blood.

hyperemesis gravidarum: excessive vomiting during pregnancy, leading to dehydration and starvation.

hypernatremia: excess sodium in the blood.

hypokalemia: potassium deficit in the blood.

hypospadias: a developmental anomaly in which the urethra opens on the lower surface of the penis.

hypoxia: inadequate oxygenation of the tissues.

icterus neonatorum: jaundice in the newborn.

implantation: embedding of fertilized ovum in uterine mucosa 6 or 7 days after fertilization.

impregnate: to make pregnant or to fertilize.

incarcerated: confined, constricted.

incest: sexual activities among family members. Often seen in father–daughter relationships, less frequently in mother–son or sibling relationships.

incompetent cervix: a mechanical defect in the cervix, making it unable to remain closed throughout pregnancy and resulting in spontaneous abortion.

increment: increase or addition; to build up, as of a contraction.

induction: artificial initiation of labor.

infertility: inability to produce offspring.

inlet of the pelvis: the upper opening into the pelvic cavity.

innominate bone: the hip bone, ilium, ischium, and pubis.

in vitro fertilization: test tube fertilization in

which the ripe ovum is collected and fertilized in vitro (in glass) by sperm from the woman's husband. The embryo is then transferred to the woman's uterus.

involution: rolling or turning inward; reduction in the size of the uterus following delivery.

karyotype: the chromosomal makeup of a body cell, arranged from largest to smallest. The normal number of chromosomes in humans is 46.

kernicterus: a grave form of jaundice of the newborn, accompanied by brain damage.

labia: in obstetrics, the external folds of skin on either side of the vulva.

labia majora: the larger outer folds of skin on either side of the vulva.

labia minora: the smaller inner folds of skin on either side of the vulva.

labor: the process by which the fetus is expelled from the uterus; childbirth; confinement; parturition.

laceration: in obstetrics, a tear in the perineum, vagina, or cervix.

lactase: the enzyme that breaks down lactose.

lactation: process of producing and supplying breast milk.

lactiferous ducts: tiny tubes within the breast that conduct milk from the acini cells to the nipple.

lanugo hair: fine, downy hair seen on all parts of the fetus, except the palms of the hands and soles of the feet, by the end of 20 weeks of gestation.

late deceleration: slowing of the fetal heart during a uterine contraction that continues after the contraction ends.

letdown reflex: pattern of stimulation, hormone release, and muscle contraction that forces milk into the lactiferous ducts, making it available to the infant; milk ejection reflex.

L.G.A. (large for gestational age): a newborn who is larger and heavier than expected for gestational age. Associated with diabetes.

lie: position of the fetus described by the relationship of the long axis of the fetus to the long axis of the mother.

lightening: moving of the fetus and uterus downward into the pelvic cavity.

linea nigra: line of darker pigmentation extending from the pubis to the umbilicus noted in some women during the later months of pregnancy.

lochia: maternal discharge of blood, mucus, and tissue from the uterus that may last for several weeks after birth.

lochia alba: white vaginal discharge that follows lochia serosa and that lasts from about the 10th to the 21st day after delivery.

lochia rubra: red, blood-tinged vaginal discharge that occurs following delivery and lasts 2 to 4 days.

lochia serosa: pink, serous, and blood-tinged vaginal discharge that follows lochia rubra and lasts until the 7th to 10th day after delivery.

L/S ratio: the ratio of the phospholipids lecithin and sphingomyelin produced by the fetal lungs; useful in assessing fetal lung maturity.

lunar month: a 28-day cycle corresponding to the phases of the moon. A normal pregnancy lasts 10 lunar months.

luteinizing hormone (LH): anterior pituitary hormone responsible for stimulating ovulation and for development of the corpus luteum.

mammary glands: compound glandular elements of the breast that in the female secrete milk to nourish the infant.

McDonald's sign: a probable sign of pregnancy, in which the examiner can easily flex the body of the uterus against the cervix.

mechanisms (cardinal movements) of labor: the positional changes of the fetus as it moves through the birth canal during labor and delivery.

meconium: the first stool of the newborn; a mixture of amniotic fluid and secretions of the intestinal glands.

meconium ileus: a deficiency of pancreatic enzymes in the intestinal tract in which the meconium of the fetus becomes excessively sticky and adheres to the intestinal wall, causing obstruction. Occasionally seen in babies born with cystic fibrosis.

meconium-stained fluid: amniotic fluid that contains meconium.

megacolon: Hirschsprung's disease a congenital absence of ganglionic cells in a segment of the large bowel that results in massive dilatation of the bowel.

meiosis: cell division to halve number of chromosomes in the ova and sperm to 23.

menarche: beginning of menstrual and reproductive function in girls.

menopause: the permanent cessation of menses.

menstrual cycle: cyclic buildup of uterine lining, ovulation, and sloughing of the lining occurring approximately every 28 days in nonpregnant females.

menstruation (menses): shedding of uterine lining at the end of the menstrual cycle, resulting in a bloody discharge from the vagina.

mesoderm: intermediate layer of germ cells in embryo that gives rise to connective tissue, bone marrow, muscles, blood, lymphoid tissue, and epithelial tissue.

metered dose inhaler (MDI): a device that delivers measured puffs of medication for inhalation.
microcephaly: a congenital anomaly in which the head of the newborn is abnormally small.
miliaria: prickly heat; inflammation of the skin caused by sweating.
miscarriage: lay term for spontaneous abortion.
mitosis: cell division in all body cells other than the gametes (ova and sperm).
molding: shaping of the fetal head to facilitate movement through birth canal during labor.
monozygotic twins: two fetuses that develop from a single divided fertilized ovum; identical twins.
mons veneris: fleshy tissue over the female symphysis pubis, from which hair develops at puberty.
Montgomery's glands: small nodules located around the nipples that enlarge during pregnancy and lactation. They produce moisturizing secretion.
morbidity: pertains to illness, disease.
morning sickness: nausea and vomiting occurring during the 1st trimester of pregnancy; may occur at any time during the day.
Moro reflex: when a newborn is jarred, the legs draw up and the arms fold across the chest.
mortality: pertains to death.
mucous plug: a collection of thick mucus that blocks the cervical canal during pregnancy.
multifetal pregnancy: a pregnancy in which the woman is carrying two or more fetuses; also called *multiple gestation*. Can be twins, triplets, etc.
multigravida: a woman who has been previously pregnant.
multipara: a woman who has had more than one pregnancy in which the fetus(es) was viable (20 weeks' gestation).
murmur: a sound heard when listening to the heart, caused by blood leaking through openings that have not closed before birth, as they should.
mutation: a change in genetic material.

Nägele's rule: a method of determining the estimated date of delivery (EDD): after obtaining the 1st day of the last menstrual period, subtract 3 months and add 7 days.
nevus (pl, nevi): a congenital discoloration of an area of the skin, such as a strawberry mark or mole.
nonnutritive sucking: sucking activity that is not related to intake of nutrients.
NST: nonstress test. An assessment method by which the reaction (or response) of the fetal heart rate to fetal movement is evaluated.
nuchal: pertaining to the neck.
nuclear family: family group consisting of one or more adults and one or more children.
nulligravida: a female who has never been pregnant.
nullipara: a female who has not delivered a live fetus.

obstetrics: the branch of medicine concerned with the care of women during pregnancy, childbirth, and the postpartum period.
occiput: the posterior part of the skull.
oligohydramnios: decreased amount of amniotic fluid.
oliguria: decrease in urine secretion by the kidney.
omphalocele: a herniation of abdominal contents at the umbilicus.
ophthalmia neonatorum: acute conjunctivitis of the newborn, often caused by the gonococci.
orthopnea: a condition in which the patient has to sit up to breathe.
ovulation: normal process of discharging a mature ovum from an ovary approximately 14 days prior to the onset of menses.
ovum: female reproductive cell; egg.
oxytocics: drugs that intensify uterine contractions to hasten birth or control postpartum hemorrhage.
oxytocin challenge test (OCT): a method of assessing fetal response to labor by administering an oxytoxic drug to stimulate a few labor contractions. Used in high risk pregnancies. See *contraction stress test* (CST).

para: a woman who has borne offspring who reached the age of viability (20–24 weeks' gestation).
paraphimosis: impaired circulation of the uncircumcised penis due to improper retraction of the foreskin.
parenteral: a medication route other than the gastrointestinal tract. Can be intravenous, intramuscular, etc.
parity: the condition of having borne offspring who attained the age of viability. The number of pregnancies ending after the age of viability.
parturient: pertaining to the act of childbirth. A woman giving birth.
parturition: the process of giving birth.
pelvis: the lower portion of the trunk of the body, bounded by the hip bones, coccyx, and sacrum.
penis: the male organ of copulation, reproduction, and urination.
perineum: the area of tissue between the anus and the scrotum in males or between the anus and the vagina in females.
phenotype: the whole physical, biochemical, and

physiologic makeup of an individual as determined both genetically and environmentally.

phimosis: a tightening of the prepuce of the uncircumcised penis.

phocomelia: absence of or incomplete formation and development of arms, forearms, thighs, and legs. Hands and feet are present but may be abnormally developed.

phototherapy: the treatment of disease by exposure to light. Used frequently to treat hyperbilirubinemia in the newborn.

pica: the eating of substances not ordinarily considered edible or to have nutritive value.

PIH: pregnancy-induced hypertension, characterized by hypertension, albuminuria, and edema.

pincer grasp: use of index finger and thumb to grasp an object.

placenta: specialized disk-shaped organ that connects the fetus to the uterine wall for gas, nutrient, and waste exchanges; also called *afterbirth.*

placental souffle: soft blowing sounds produced by blood coursing through the placenta; has the same rate as the maternal pulse.

polydactyly: a developmental anomaly characterized by the presence of extra fingers or toes.

postpartum: after childbirth.

precipitate birth: a birth that occurs without a trained attendant present.

precipitate labor: rapid progression of labor that lasts less than 3 hours.

pregnancy: the condition of having a developing embryo or fetus in the body after fertilization of the female egg by the male sperm.

prehension: use of hands to pick up small objects; grasping.

prenatal: before birth.

presentation: the fetal body part that enters the maternal pelvis first.

presenting part: the fetal part that first enters the maternal pelvis.

presumptive signs of pregnancy: symptoms that suggest pregnancy but that do not confirm it, such as cessation of menses, quickening, Chadwick's sign, and morning sickness.

primigravida: a woman who is pregnant for the first time.

primipara: a woman who has given birth to her first child (past the point of viability), whether or not that child is living or was alive at birth.

prodrome: the initial symptoms indicating an approaching disease.

projectile vomiting: vomiting that occurs with force (vomitus landing 2–4 feet away).

prolapsed cord: umbilical cord that becomes trapped between the fetal presenting part and maternal pelvis.

PROM: premature rupture of amniotic membranes. Rupture of the membranes before the onset of labor.

pseudocyesis: a condition in which the woman has symptoms of pregnancy but in which hormonal pregnancy test results are negative; false pregnancy.

psychoprophylaxis: psychophysical training aimed at preparing the expectant parents to cope with the processes of labor and to avoid concentration on the discomforts associated with childbirth.

puberty: the period of time during which the secondary sexual characteristics develop and the ability to procreate is attained.

pudendal block: injection of an anesthetizing agent at the pudendal nerve to produce numbness of the external genitals and the lower one-third of the vagina.

puerperium: the period of time after delivery until involution of the uterus is complete, usually 6 weeks.

pulse oximeter: equipment that determines level of blood oxygen saturation by means of a sensor placed on the skin.

quickening: first fetal movements felt by the pregnant woman, usually between 16 and 18 weeks' gestation.

rapport: harmonious relation.

RDA: recommended dietary allowances—refers to level of specific nutrient intake necessary to maintain optimum health.

reflux: a backward flow of fluid, e.g., vesicoureteral reflux: urine is forced from the bladder into the ureters; gastric reflux: stomach contents flow into the esophagus. It may or may not enter the oral cavity.

regression: behavior that is more appropriate to an earlier stage of development. Often occurs in children as a response to stress.

relaxin: a water-soluble protein secreted by the corpus luteum that causes relaxation of the symphysis pubis and facilitates cervical dilation during birth.

retractions: abnormal "sucking in" of chest wall during inspiration. Can be substernal or intercostal; indicates respiratory distress.

retrolental fibroplasia: blindness usually found in the preterm infant that is associated with oxygen concentrations and in which the blood vessels of the retina become damaged.

Rh factor: antigen present on the surface of blood cells that make the blood cell incompatible with blood cells that do not have the antigen.

rhabdomyosarcoma: extremely malignant neoplasm originating in skeletal muscle.
rickets: a disease of the bones, caused by lack of calcium or vitamin D.
ritualism: a need to maintain strict structure and routine.
ROM: rupture of (amniotic) membranes; also stands for range of motion.
rooting reflex: an infant's tendency to turn the head and open the lips to suck when one side of the mouth or cheek is touched or stroked.

sacrum: five fused vertebrae that form a triangle of bone just beneath the lumbar vertebrae and between the hip bones.
scoliosis: lateral curvature of the spine.
second stage of labor: stage lasting from complete dilation of the cervix to expulsion of the fetus.
semen: thick, whitish fluid ejaculated by the male during orgasm, which contains the spermatozoa and their nutrients.
separation anxiety: distress that occurs when strangers separate infant from parents.
sex chromosomes: the X and Y chromosomes, which are responsible for sex determination; women have two X chromosomes; men have one X and one Y chromosome.
sexually transmitted disease (STD): refers to diseases ordinarily transmitted by direct sexual contact with an infected individual.
shunt: a bypass.
small for gestational age (SGA): inadequate weight or growth for gestational age; birth weight below the 10th percentile.
Snellen alphabet chart: a device used to measure near and far vision; a variation of the Snellen E chart.
spermatogenesis: process by which mature spermatozoa are formed, during which the number of chromosomes is reduced by half.
spermatozoa: mature sperm cells produced by the testes.
spinnbarkeit: elasticity seen in cervical mucus at the time of ovulation.
standard precautions: infection control guidelines established by the Centers for Disease Control to prevent the spread of infection.
station: relationship of the presenting fetal part to an imaginary line drawn between the pelvic ischial spines.
stillbirth: the delivery of a dead fetus.
striae gravidarum: stretch marks; shiny reddish lines that appear on the abdomen, breasts, thighs, and buttocks of pregnant women as a result of stretching the skin.
stridor: a shrill sound heard during respiration caused by air passing through a narrowed portion of the respiratory tract.
surfactant: a surface-active mixture of lipoproteins secreted in the alveoli and air passages that reduces the surface tension of pulmonary fluids and contributes to the elasticity of pulmonary tissue.
surrogate mother: a fertile woman who is impregnated for the purpose of producing a child for another (infertile) couple.
sutures: separation between fetal skull bones that permit molding during the birth process.

taking hold: second phase of maternal adaptation when mother assumes control of self and infant.
taking in: initial maternal adaptation following birth where passive acceptance of care occurs.
talipes equinovarus: clubfoot.
teratogen: a nongenetic factor that can produce malformations of the fetus.
term infant: a live-born infant of 38 to 42 weeks' gestation.
testes: the male gonads, in which sperm and testosterone are produced.
testosterone: the male hormone; responsible for the development of secondary male characteristics.
therapeutic play: guided play that results in physical or psychological well-being.
third stage of labor: the time from the delivery of the fetus to the time when the placenta has been completely expelled.
tissue perfusion: nutrition and oxygenation of tissue resulting from adequate blood flow.
tocodynamometer: external device that can be used to identify the pressure of uterine contractions during labor.
tocolytic: a drug that inhibits uterine contractions.
TORCH: acronym used to describe a group of infections that represent potentially severe fetal problems if infection occurs during pregnancy. TO, toxoplasmosis; R, rubella; C, cytomegalovirus; and H, herpesvirus.
TPN: total parenteral nutrition. Providing for all nutritional needs by administration of liquids into the blood; used in life-threatening conditions; also known as *hyperalimentation.*
transition: the period during labor when the cervix is approximately 8 cm dilated, contractions are very strong, and the laboring woman feels the urge to push.
triage: a process used to determine urgency of illness to prioritize care.
trimester: one-third of the gestational time for pregnancy.
turgor: normal elasticity of the skin.

tympanometry: measurement of mobility of the tympanic membrane of the ear and estimation of middle-ear pressure.

ultrasound: high-frequency sound waves that may be directed, through use of a transducer, into the maternal abdomen. The ultrasonic sound waves reflected by the underlying structures of varying densities allow maternal and fetal tissues, bones, and fluids to be identified.
umbilical cord: the structure connecting the placenta to the umbilicus of the fetus through which nutrients from the woman are exchanged for wastes from the fetus.
uterus: hollow muscular organ in which the fertilized ovum is implanted and the developing fetus is nourished until birth.

vacuum extractor: device to assist birth of fetal head using suction.
vagina: the musculomembranous tube or passageway located between the external female genitals and the uterus.
varicella: chickenpox.
varicose veins: permanently distended veins.
variola: smallpox.
VBAC: an acronym for vaginal birth after cesarean.
vector: a carrier that transmits an infective agent from one host to another.
ventriculography: X-ray examination of the ventricles of the brain following the injection of air into the ventricles.
vernix caseosa: a protective cheeselike whitish substance made up of sebum and desquamated epithelial cells that is present on fetal skin and skin of newborn.
vertex: top or crown of the head.
version: a turning of the position of the fetus in the uterus before birth. Can be spontaneous or manually induced.
viable: capable of living.
volvulus: a twisting of the loops of the small intestine, causing obstruction.
vulva: the external structure of the female genitals, lying between the mons veneris and anus.

Wharton's jelly: yellow-white gelatinous material that surrounds and protects the vessels of the umbilical cord.
wheal: large, slightly raised red or blistered area of skin; may itch.
WIC: woman-infant-children; a subsidized supplemental food program for mothers and children.

X chromosome: female sex chromosome.

Y chromosome: male sex chromosome.

zygote: a fertilized ovum.

Appendix A

Standard Precautions and Body Substance Isolation Precautions

All health care providers must apply Standard Precautions to all their patients regardless of diagnosis, disease, or infection status. The health care provider should perform appropriate barrier precautions to prevent exposure to skin or mucous membranes, especially when contact with blood, body fluids, secretions (except sweat), and excretions is anticipated.

- Wash hands thoroughly before and immediately after performing a task/procedure.
- Clean gloves should be worn whenever touching blood, body fluids, secretions (except sweat), and excretions. They should also be worn when handling items or surfaces soiled with blood or body fluids; and for performing venipuncture/vascular access. *Gloves must be changed and hands washed after contact with each and every patient.*
- Personal protective equipment (PPE), such as face masks, protective eyewear (goggles)/face shields, and fluid-repelling gowns should be worn for procedures that are likely to generate droplets of blood or exposure to body fluids, secretions, and/or excretions. If mouth-to-mouth resuscitation is needed, always use a resuscitation mask or bag to avoid direct contact with the patient's mucous membranes.
- All health care providers should take precautions to prevent injuries that can be caused from inappropriate handling of needles, scalpels, and other sharp instruments. After sharp items are used, they *must* be placed in *PUNCTURE-RESISTANT containers* nearby.
- *Transmission-based precautions* (TBPs) are for those patients with a suspected and/or diagnosed infection by an organism with a high risk of transmission. Standard precautions as well as transmission-based precautions must be used.

There are three types of transmission-based precautions:

1. *Airborne precautions* (5 microns or smaller in size) must be used whenever working with a patient who has tuberculosis (TB), chicken pox (varicella), or measles (rubeola). These infecting organisms can be inhaled by the health care provider or others in the room. Therefore, face masks must be worn, and special ventilation and air-handling protocols must be used to prevent the transmission of the organism. Patients are placed in a private room, and specific air-circulation requirements and/or filtration of air particles must be followed. All health care providers coming in contact with the TB-positive patient *MUST* be fitted for *and* wear a Hepa-Filter or N-95 face masks.
2. *Droplet precautions* (5 microns or larger). The infection is spread through talking, coughing, or sneezing. *Haemophilus influenzae* type B, pertussis (whooping cough), scarlet fever, pneumonia, and rubella fall into this category. Transmission of these large droplets require contact within 3 feet, since the large size does not stay suspended in the air for an extended time. Droplet precautions require a separate room, but do not require special ventilation or air handling. When working within 3 feet of a patient with a droplet infection, Standard Precautions and the wearing of a disposable face mask are recommended.
3. *Contact precautions* are used to reduce the spread of infectious organisms by direct or indirect contact. Contact precautions are to be used when skin-to-skin contact may occur, such as turning or bathing a patient. When possible, place this patient in a private room or in a room with someone who has the *same* infection. On entering the room, the health care providers should wear

clean gloves. While performing care on this patient, change gloves after having any contact with blood, body fluids, secretions, or excretions that may have a high concentration of the infecting organism. Be sure to remove gloves *BEFORE* leaving the patient's room and to wash hands thoroughly and dry them. Be careful not to touch anything in the patient's room as you leave. If the potential for your clothing to be exposed to contaminates is high, wear a cover gown, put it on *BEFORE* you enter the patient's room. Once you have completed your care, *remove your gloves BEFORE you remove your cover gown.*

All patients on TBP should be transported from the room *only* for essential purposes. For airborne precautions the patient should wear a mask during transport.

The Center for Disease Control (CDC) in Atlanta, Georgia provides guidelines for infection control and the Occupational Health and Safety Commission (OSHA) establishes legal requirements for infection control. Employers are mandated to provide equipment and employee protection measures.

Appendix B

National Agencies for Obstetrical and Pediatric Clients

AASK (Aid to the Adoption of Special Kids)
2201 Broadway, Suite 702
Oakland, CA 94612
(510) 451-1748

Acoustic Neuroma Association
PO Box 12402
Atlanta, GA 30355
(404) 237-8023
http://132.183.175.10/ana/www.anausa@aol.com

AD-IN: Attention Deficit Information Network
475 Hillside Ave.
Nudham, MA 02194
(617) 455-9895
http://www.adin@gis.net

Adolescent Resources and Teen Health Program
Laverkin, UT
(800) 400-0900

AIDS Medical Foundation
10 East 13th Street, Suite LD
New York, NY 10003
(212) 206-0670

AMEND
Aiding a Mother Experiencing Neonatal Death
4324 Berrywick Terrace
St. Louis, MO 63141
(314) 487-7582

Alexander Graham Bell Association for the Deaf
3417 Volta Place, NW
Washington, DC 20007-2778
(202) 337-5220 (Voice/TTY)

American Academy of Husband-Coached Childbirth
PO Box 5224
Sherman Oaks, CA 91413
(800) 42-BIRTH (in CA)
(800) 423-2397 (outside CA)

American Academy of Pediatrics
141 Northwest Point Blvd
PO Box 927
Elk Grove, IL 60009
http://www.AAP.org

American Association of Acupuncturists and Oriental Medicine
4104 Lake Boone Trail, Suite 201
Raleigh, NC 27607
(919) 787-5181

American Association for the Deaf-Blind
814 Thayer Ave., Suite 302
Silver Springs, MD 20910
(301) 588-6545 (TTY only)

American Association of Kidney Patients (AAKP)
100 South Ashley Drive, Suite 280
Tampa, FL 33602
(813) 223-7099
(800) 749-AAKP
http://www.AAKPnat@aol.com
http://cybermart.com/aakpaz/aakp.html

American Brain Tumor Association
2710 River Rd., Suite 146
Des Plaines, IL 60018
(800) 886-2282
http://pubweb.acns.nwu.edu/~lberko/abata_html/abta.htm
http://neurosurgery.mgh.harvard.edu/ABTA

American Cancer Society, Inc.
1599 Clifton Rd., NE
Atlanta, GA 30329
(800) ACS-2345
http://www.irpub.com/ca

American Cleft Palate Association
1218 Grandview Ave.
Pittsburgh, PA 15211
(412) 681-1376
(800) 24-CLEFT

American College of Obstetricians and Gynecologists
409 12th St., NW
Washington, DC 20024
(800) 762-2264

American Council of the Blind
1155 15th Street, NW, Suite 1720
Washington, DC 20005
(202) 467-5081
(800) 424-8666
http://www.acb.org

American Diabetes Association Diabetes Information Service Center
1660 Duke St.
Alexandria, VA 22314
(800) ADA-DISC
(800) 232-6733
(800) 806-7801 (to join ADA)
http://www.diabetes.org

American Fertility Foundation
2131 Magnolia Ave., Suite 201
Birmingham, AL 35256
(205) 251-9764

American Foundation for the Blind, Inc.
15 West 16th Street
New York, NY 10011
(212) 620-2000
(800) 232-5463
http://www.afb.org/afb

American Foundation for Maternal and Child Health, Inc.
439 E. 51st St.
New York, NY 10022
(212) 759-5510

American Juvenile Arthritis Organization
1330 W. Peachtree St.
Atlanta, GA 30309
(800) 283-7800
(404) 872-7100
http://www.javstin@arthritis.org

American Kidney Fund
6110 Executive Blvd., Suite 1010
Rockville, MD 20852
(800) 638-8299
http://www.arbon.com/kidney

American Lung Association
1740 Broadway
New York, NY 10019
(800) LUNG USA
http://www.lung.usa.org

American Red Cross
430 17th St., NW
Washington, DC 20036
(800) 368-4404

American Society for Psychoprophylaxis in Obstetrics (ASPO)
1200 19th St., NW., Suite 300
Washington, DC 20036
(800) 368-4404

American Sudden Infant Death Syndrome Institute, National Headquarters
6065 Roswell Rd., Suite 876
Atlanta, GA 30328
(404) 843-1030
(800) 232-SIDS (Nationwide)
(800) 847-SIDS (in GA)

The ARC *(mental retardation)*
500 E. Border St., Suite 300
P.O. Box 1047
Arlington, TX 76010
(800) 433-5255
http://www.thearc.org/welcome.html

Association for Birth Defects in Children
3201 E. Crystal Lake Ave.
Orlando, FL 32806
(407) 245-7035

Association for the Care of Children's Health
7910 Woodmont Ave., Suite 300
Bethesda, MD 20814
(301) 654-6549

Association for Retarded Children
PO Box 1047
Arlington, TX 76004
(817) 588-2000

Association of Voluntary Sterilization, Inc. (VAS)
79 Madison Avenue
New York, NY 10016
(212) 351-2500

Association of Women's Health, Obstetric, and Neonatal Nurses (AWHONN)
700 14th St., NW, Suite 600
Washington, DC 20005
(202) 662-1600

Asthma & Allergy Foundation of America
1125 15th St., NW, Suite 502
Washington, DC 20005
(800) 727-8462
(202) 466-7643
http://www.aafa.org

Autism Society of America
7910 Woodmont Ave., Suite 650
Bethesda, MD 20814
(800) 328-8476
http://www.autism-society.org

Autism Research Institute
4182 Adams Ave.
San Diego, CA 92116
(619) 281-7165

Brain Injury Association
1776 Massachusetts Ave., NW, Suite 100
Washington, DC 20036
(800) 444-6443
(202) 296-6443

Brain Tumor Foundation for Children
2231 Perimeter Pk. Dr., Suite 9
Atlanta, GA 30341
(770) 458-5554

Billy Barty Foundation *(dwarfism)*
929 W. Olive Ave., Suite C
Burbank, CA 91506
(800) 891-4022
(818) 953-5410

Celiac Disease Foundation
13251 Ventura Blvd., Suite 3
Studio City, CA 91604-1838
(818) 990-2354

Celiac Sprue Association
P.O. Box 31700
Omaha, NE 68131
(402) 558-0600
http://www.celiacvsa@aol.com

Centers for Disease Control and Prevention
1600 Clifton Rd., NE
Atlanta, GA 30333
(404) 329-1819
(404) 329-3286

Center for Medical Consumers and Health Care Information
237 Thompson St.
New York, NY 10012
(212) 674-7105

Center for Sickle Cell Disease
2121 Georgia Ave., NW
Washington, DC 20059
(202) 636-7930

CHADD: Children & Adults with Attention Deficit Disorders
499 NW 70th Ave., Suite 101
Plantation, FL 33317
(800) 233-4050
http://www.chadd.org

Children's Defense Fund
25 E St., NW
Washington, DC 20001
(800) 233-1200
http://www.tmn.com/cdf/index.htm

Children's Hospice International
700 Princess St., Lower Level
Alexandria, VA 22314
(800) 242-4453

Children's PKU Network
1520 State St., Suite 240
San Diego, CA 92101
(619) 233-3202

Cleft Palate Foundation
1218 Grandview Ave.
Pittsburgh, PA 15211
(800) 242-5338

Compassionate Friends
(following death of an infant)
P.O. Box 3696
Oak Brook, IL 60522-3696
(312) 990-0010

Cooley's Anemia Foundation, Inc.
12909 26th Ave., Suite 203
Flushing, NY 11354
(800) 522-7222

Crohn's Disease and Colitis Foundation of America
386 Park Ave., S. 17th Fl.
New York, NY 10016
(800) 932-2423
http://www.ccfa.org

Cystic Fibrosis Foundation
6931 Arlington Rd.
Bethesda, MD 20814
(301) 951-4422
(800) FIGHT CF (344-4823)
http://www.cff.org

DB-Links National Information Clearinghouse on Children Who Are Deaf-Blind
345 N. Monmouth Ave.
Monmouth, OR 97361
(800) 438-9376
(800) 854-7013 (TTY)
http://www.tr.wosc.osshe.edu/dblink

DES Action USA
1615 Broadway, Suite 510
Oakland, CA 94612
(510) 465-4011

Dyslexia Research Institute
4745 Centerville Rd
Tallahassee, FL 32308
(904) 893-2216

Eczema Association for Science and Education
1221 SW Yamhill, Suite 303
Portland, OR 97205

Environmental Protection Agency (EPA) Public Information Center
Room PM 211-B
401 M Street, SW
Washington, DC 20460
(202) 382-7550

Epilepsy Foundation of America
4351 Garden City Dr.
Landover, MD 20785
(301) 459-3700
(800) EFA-1000
(800) 332-2070

Equal Rights for Fathers
P.O. Box 90042
San Jose, CA 95109
(408) 848-2323

Family Empowerment Network Supporting Families Affected by FAS/FAE *(fetal alcohol syndrome)*
610 Langdon St., Room 521
Madison, WI 53703
(800) 462-5254

Florence Crittenton Association of America
608 South Dearborn St.
Chicago, IL 60605

Food Allergy Network
4744 Holly Ave.
Fairfax, VA 22030
(703) 691-3179
(800) 929-4040
http://www.foodallergy.org

Glaucoma Research Foundation
490 Post St., Suite 830
San Francisco, CA 94102
(800) 826-6693
http://www.glaucoma.org

Gluten Intolerance Group of N. America
P.O. Box 23053
Seattle, WA 98102
(206) 325-6980

Group B Strep Association
P.O. Box 16515
Chapel Hill, NC 27516
(919) 932-5344 (Voice/Fax)
http://www.groupstrep.org

Hemophilia Health Services, Inc. Disease Management Specialists
(800) 800-6606

Human Growth Foundation *(dwarfism)*
7777 Leesburg Pike, Suite 202S
Falls Church, VA 22043
(800) 451-6434
http://www.medhelp.org/web/hgf.htm

Huntington's Disease Society of America
140 West 22nd St., 6th Fl.
New York, NY 10011
(800) 345-HDSA
http://neuro-www2.mgh.harvard.edu/hdsa/hdsamain.nclk

Hydrocephalus Association
870 Market S., Suite 955
San Francisco, CA 94102
(415) 732-7040 (Voice/Fax)

Hyperbaric Services
(800) 559-6863

International Childbirth Education Association (ICEA)
P.O. Box 20048
Minneapolis, MN 55420
(612) 854-8660

International Foundation for Functional Gastrointestinal Disorders
P.O. Box 17864
Milwaukee, WI 53217
(414) 964-1799
http://www.execpc.com/iffgd

International Lactation Consultant Association
201 Brown Ave.
Evanston, IL 60202-3601
(708) 260-8874

International Polio Network
4207 Lindell Blvd., Suite 110
St. Louis, MO 63108

ITP Society: Children's Blood Foundation *(purpura, idiopathic thrombocytopenia)*
333 E. 38th St.
New York, NY 10016
(800) 487-7010
(212) 297-4340

Juvenile Diabetes Foundation, International
120 Wall Street, 19th floor
New York, NY 10005
(800) 533-2873
http://www.jdscore.com

Lact-AID
P.O. Box 1066
Athens, TN 37303
(614) 744-9090

La Leche League
1400 N. Meacham Rd.
Shaumburg, IL 60173
(800) 525-3243 (24-hour line)

Learning Disabilities Association of America
4156 Library Rd.
Pittsburgh, PA 15234
(412) 341-1515
http://www.idanatl.org

Leukemia Society of America
600 Third Ave., 4th Fl.
New York, NY 10016
(800) 955-4572
http://www.leukemia.org

Make-a-Wish Foundation of America
100 W. Clarendon, Suite 2200
Phoenix, AZ 85013
(800) 722-9474
http://www.wish.org

Medic Alert®
2323 Colorado Ave.
Turlock, CA 95382
(800) 825-3785

Muscular Dystrophy Association
3300 E. Sunrise Dr.
Tucson, AZ 85718
(800) 572-1717
http://www.mdusa.org

National Adoption Center
1500 Walnut St., Suite 701
Philadelphia, PA 19102
(800) 862-3678
http://www.adopt.org/adopt

National Association for Sickle Cell Disease
3345 Wilshire Blvd., Suite 1106
Los Angeles, CA 90010
(213) 736-5455
(800) 421-8453

National Association of Parents and Professionals for Safe Alternatives in Childbirth (NAPSAC)
P.O. Box 267
Marble Hill, MO 63764
(314) 238-2010

National Attention Deficit Disorder
P.O. Box 972
Mentor, OH 44061
(216) 350-9595
(800) 487-2282 (message only)
http://www.add.org

National Breast Cancer Coalition
P.O. Box 66373
Washington, DC 20035
(202) 296-7477
(800) 935-0434

National Cancer Institute
Cancer Information Service
9000 Rockville Pike
Bethesda, MD 20892
(800) 4-CANCER

National Catholic Charities
1346 Connecticut Ave., NW
Washington, DC 20036
(202) 526-4100

National Center for Missing and Exploited Children
(800) THE-LOST
(800) 843-5678

National Center for Stuttering
200 E. 33rd St.
New York, NY 10016
(800) 221-2483
http://www.stuttering.com

The National Center on Women and Family Law
799 Broadway, Room 402
New York, NY 10003
(212) 674-8200

National Child Abuse Hotline
(800) 422-4453

National Coalition against Domestic Violence
P.O. Box 34103
Washington, DC 20043
(202) 638-8638
(800) 333-SAFE (Hotline)

National Coalition against Sexual Assault
912 North 2nd Street
Harrisburg, PA 17102
(717) 232-6771

National Coalition of Feminist and Lesbian Cancer Projects
P.O. Box 90437
Washington, DC 20090
(202) 332-5536

National Congenital Portwine Stain Foundation
125 E. 63rd St.
New York, NY 10021

National Diabetes Information Clearinghouse
Box NDIC
9000 Rockville Pike
Bethesda, MD 20892

National Down Syndrome Congress
1605 Chantilly Dr., Suite 250
Atlanta, GA 30324
(800) 232-6372
http://www.carol.net/~ndsc/

National Down Syndrome Society Hotline
666 Broadway
New York, NY 10012
(800) 221-4602

National Easter Seal Society
230 W. Monroe
Chicago, IL 60606
(800) 221-6827
http://www.seals.com

National Father's Network
The Kindering Center
16120 NE 8th St.
Bellevue, WA 98008
(206) 747-4004

National Foundation/March of Dimes
1275 Mamaroneck Ave.
White Plains, NY 10605
(914) 428-7100

National Foundation for Jewish Genetic Diseases, Inc.
250 Park Ave., Suite 1000
New York, NY 10177
(212) 371-1030

National Hemophilia Foundation
110 Green St., Room 303
New York, NY 10012
(800) 424-2634
http://www.infonhf.org

National Highway Safety Administration
400 7th St. SW
Washington, DC 20590
(800) 424-9393

National Institute of Child Health and Human Development (NICHD)
National Institutes of Health
9000 Rockville Pike
Bldg. 3 1, Room 2A32
Bethesda, MD 20892
(301) 496-4000

National Kidney Foundation
30 E. 33rd St., 11th Fl.
New York, NY 10016
(800) 622-9010
http://www/kidney.org

National Marfan Foundation
382 Main St.
Port Washington, NY 11050
(800) 862-7326
http://www.marfan.org

National Neurofibromatosis Foundation
95 Pine S. 16th St.
New York, NY 10005
(800) 323-7938
http://www.nf.org

National Organization on Fetal Alcohol Syndrome
1819 H . St., NW, Suite 750
Washington, DC 20006
(202) 785-4585
http://www.nofas.org

National Organization of Mothers of Twins Clubs, Inc.
P.O. Box 23188
Albuquerque, NM 87192
(505) 275-0955

National Organization for Women (NOW) Legal Defense and Education Fund
99 Hudson St.
New York, NY 10013
(212) 925-6635

National Parent Network on Disabilities
1727 King St., Suite 305
Alexandria, VA 22314
(703) 684-6763

National Perinatal Association
101 ½ S. Union St.
Alexandria, VA 22315
(703) 549-5523

National Resource Center for Domestic Violence
6400 Flank Dr., Suite 1300
Harrisburg, PA 17112-2778
(800) 537-2238 (Hotline)
tty: (800) 553-2508

National Reye's Syndrome Foundation
426 N. Lewis St.
Bran, OH 43506
(800) 233-7393

National Right to Life Committee
419 7th St., NW, Suite 500
Washington, DC 20004
(202) 626-8800

National Scoliosis Foundation
5 Cabot Place
Stoughton, MA 62072
(800) NSF-MYBACK
http://www.scoliosis@aol.com

The National Tuberous Sclerosis Association
8181 Professional Pl., Suite 110
Landover, MD 20785
(800) 225-6872
(301) 459-9888
(301) 459-0394
http://www.ntsa@capcon.net

Organic Acidemia Association
(metabolic disorders, maple syrup urine disease)
2287 Cypress Ave.
San Pablo, CA 94806
(510) 724-0297

The Orton Dyslexia Society
8600 LaSalle Rd.
Chester Bldg., Suite 382
Baltimore, MD 21286
(800) 222-3123
http://www.pic.org/rds

Osteogenesis Imperfecta Foundation
804 W. Diamond Ave., Suite 210
Gaithersburg, MD 20878
(800) 981-2663
http://members.aol.com/bonelink

Phoenix Society for Burn Survivors
11 Rust Hill Rd
Levittown, PA 19056
(800) 888-2876
(215) 946-2876

Poison Control Center *(Check in local telephone directory for phone number or call local hospital for assistance)*

Ronald McDonald House
1 Kroc Drive
Dept. 014
Oakbrook, IL 60521
(630) 623-7048
(888) 984-8453

Sexuality Information and Education Council of the United States (SIECUS)
20361 Middlebelt Road
Livonea, MI 48152

Sickle Cell Disease Association of America, Inc.
200 Corporate Pointe, Suite 495
Culver City, CA 90230
(800) 421-8453

The Sturge-Weber Foundation
P.O. Box 418
Mt. Freedom, NJ 07970
(800) 627-5482
http://www.inforamp.net/~crs0590/mission.html

Tourette Syndrome Association
42-40 Bell Blvd
Bayside, NY 11361
(718) 224-2999
http://www2.mgh.harvard.edu/tsa/tsamain.nclk

Turner's Syndrome Society of the U.S.
1313 SE 5th St., Suite 327
Minneapolis, MN 55414
(800) 365-9944
http://www.turner__syndrome__us.org

United Cerebral Palsy Association
1660 L St., NW, Suite 700
Washington, DC 20036
(800) 872-5827 (Voice)
(202) 973-7197 (TDD)
http://www.ucpa.org

NOTE: This is a partial listing of agencies and organizations available to the professional and the patient.

Appendix C

NANDA-Approved Nursing Diagnoses

This list represents the NANDA-approved nursing diagnoses for clinical use and testing (1997-1998).

Pattern 1: Exchanging

1.1.2.1	Altered nutrition: more than body requirements
1.1.2.2	Altered nutrition: less than body requirements
1.1.2.3	Altered nutrition: risk for more than body requirements
1.2.1.1	Risk for infection
1.2.2.1	Risk for altered body temperature
1.2.2.2	Hypothermia
1.2.2.3	Hyperthermia
1.2.2.4	Ineffective thermoregulation
1.2.3.1	Dysreflexia
1.3.1.1	Constipation
1.3.1.1.1	Perceived constipation
1.3.1.1.2	Colonic constipation
1.3.1.2	Diarrhea
1.3.1.3	Bowel incontinence
1.3.2	Altered urinary elimination
1.3.2.1.1	Stress incontinence
1.3.2.1.2	Reflex incontinence
1.3.2.1.3	Urge incontinence
1.3.2.1.4	Functional incontinence
1.3.2.1.5	Total incontinence
1.3.2.2	Urinary retention
1.4.1.1	Altered (specify type) tissue perfusion (renal, cerebral, cardiopulmonary, gastrointestinal, peripheral)
1.4.1.2.1	Fluid volume excess
1.4.1.2.2.1	Fluid volume deficit
1.4.1.2.2.2	Risk for fluid volume deficit
1.4.2.1	Decreased cardiac output
1.5.1.1	Impaired gas exchange
1.5.1.2	Ineffective airway clearance
1.5.1.3	Ineffective breathing pattern
1.5.1.3.1	Inability to sustain spontaneous ventilation
1.5.1.3.2	Dysfunctional ventilatory weaning response (DVWR)
1.6.1	Risk for injury
1.6.1.1	Risk for suffocation
1.6.1.2	Risk for poisoning
1.6.1.3	Risk for trauma
1.6.1.4	Risk for aspiration
1.6.1.5	Risk for disuse syndrome
1.6.2	Altered protection
1.6.2.1	Impaired tissue integrity
1.6.2.1.1	Altered oral mucous membrane
1.6.2.1.2.1	Impaired skin integrity
1.6.2.1.2.2	Risk for impaired skin integrity
1.7.1	Decreased adaptive capacity: intracranial
1.8	Energy field disturbance

Pattern 2: Communicating

2.1.1.1	Impaired verbal communication

Pattern 3: Relating

3.1.1	Impaired social interaction
3.1.2	Social isolation
3.1.3	Risk for loneliness
3.2.1	Altered role performance
3.2.1.1.1	Altered parenting
3.2.1.1.2	Risk for altered parenting
3.2.1.1.2.1	Risk for altered parent/infant/child attachment
3.2.1.2.1	Sexual dysfunction
3.2.2	Altered family processes
3.2.2.1	Caregiver role strain
3.2.2.2	Risk for caregiver role strain
3.2.2.3.1	Altered family process: alcoholism
3.2.3.1	Parental role conflict
3.3	Altered sexuality patterns

Pattern 4: Valuing

4.1.1	Spiritual distress (distress of the human spirit)
4.2	Potential for enhanced spiritual well-being

Pattern 5: Choosing

5.1.1.1 Ineffective individual coping
5.1.1.1.1 Impaired adjustment
5.1.1.1.2 Defensive coping
5.1.1.1.3 Ineffective denial
5.1.2.1.1 Ineffective family coping: disabling
5.1.2.1.2 Ineffective family coping: compromised
5.1.2.2 Family coping: potential for growth
5.1.3.1 Potential for enhanced community coping
5.1.3.2 Ineffective community coping
5.2.1 Ineffective management of therapeutic regimen (individuals)
5.2.1.1 Noncompliance (specify)
5.2.2 Ineffective management of therapeutic regimen: families
5.2.3 Ineffective management of therapeutic regimen: community
5.2.4 Ineffective management of therapeutic regimen: individual
5.3.1.1 Decisional conflict (specify)
5.4 Health-seeking behaviors (specify)

Pattern 6: Moving

6.1.1.1 Impaired physical mobility
6.1.1.1.1 Risk for peripheral neurovascular dysfunction
6.1.1.1.2 Risk for perioperative positioning injury
6.1.1.2 Activity intolerance
6.1.1.2.1 Fatigue
6.1.1.3 Risk for activity intolerance
6.2.1 Sleep pattern disturbance
6.3.1.1 Diversional activity deficit
6.4.1.1 Impaired home maintenance management
6.4.2 Altered health maintenance
6.5.1 Feeding self-care deficit
6.5.1.1 Impaired swallowing
6.5.1.2 Ineffective breastfeeding
6.5.1.2.1 Interrupted breastfeeding
6.5.1.3 Effective breastfeeding
6.5.1.4 Ineffective infant feeding pattern
6.5.2 Bathing/hygiene self-care deficit
6.5.3 Dressing/grooming self-care deficit
6.5.4 Toileting self-care deficit
6.6 Altered growth and development
6.7 Relocation stress syndrome
6.8.1 Risk for disorganized infant behavior
6.8.2 Disorganized infant behavior
6.8.3 Potential for enhanced organized infant behavior

Pattern 7: Perceiving

7.1.1 Body image disturbance
7.1.2 Self-esteem disturbance
7.1.2.1 Chronic low self-esteem
7.1.2.2 Situational low self-esteem
7.1.3 Personal identity disturbance
7.2 Sensory/perceptual alterations (specify) (visual, auditory, kinesthetic, gustatory, tactile, olfactory)
7.2.1.1 Unilateral neglect
7.3.1 Hopelessness
7.3.2 Powerlessness

Pattern 8: Knowing

8.1.1 Knowledge deficit (specify)
8.2.1 Impaired environmental interpretation syndrome
8.2.2 Acute confusion
8.2.3 Chronic confusion
8.3 Altered thought processes
8.3.1 Impaired memory

Pattern 9: Feeling

9.1.1 Pain
9.1.1.1 Chronic pain
9.2.1.1 Dysfunctional grieving
9.2.1.2 Anticipatory grieving
9.2.2 Risk for violence: self-directed or directed at others
9.2.2.1 Risk for self-mutilation
9.2.3 Posttrauma response
9.2.3.1 Rape trauma syndrome
9.2.3.1.1 Rape trauma syndrome: compound reaction
9.2.3.1.2 Rape trauma syndrome: silent reaction
9.3.1 Anxiety
9.3.2 Fear

Diagnoses revised by small work groups at the 1994 Biennial Conference on the Classification of Nursing Diagnoses; changes approved and added in 1996.

Appendix D

Conversion of Pounds and Ounces to Grams for Newborn Weights

Pounds	Ounces 0	1	2	3	4	5	6	7	8	9	10	11	12	13	14	15
0	—	28	57	85	113	142	170	198	227	255	283	312	336	369	397	425
1	454	482	510	539	567	595	624	652	680	709	737	765	794	822	850	879
2	907	936	964	992	1021	1049	1077	1106	1134	1162	1191	1219	1247	1276	1304	1332
3	1361	1389	1417	1446	1474	1503	1531	1559	1588	1616	1644	1673	1701	1729	1758	1786
4	1814	1843	1871	1899	1928	1956	1984	2013	2041	2070	2098	2126	2155	2183	2211	2240
5	2268	2296	2325	2353	2381	2410	2438	2466	2495	2523	2551	2580	2608	2637	2665	2693
6	2722	2750	2778	2807	2835	2863	2892	2920	2948	2977	3005	3033	3062	3090	3118	3147
7	3175	3203	3232	3260	3289	3317	3345	3374	3402	3430	3459	3487	3515	3544	3572	3600
8	3629	3657	3685	3714	3742	3770	3799	3827	3856	3884	3912	3941	3969	3997	4026	4054
9	4082	4111	4139	4167	4196	4224	4252	4281	4309	4337	4366	4394	4423	4451	4479	4508
10	4536	4564	4593	4621	4649	4678	4706	4734	4763	4791	4819	4848	4876	4904	4933	4961
11	4990	5018	5046	5075	5103	5131	5160	5188	5216	5245	5273	5301	5330	5358	5386	5415
12	5443	5471	5500	5528	5557	5585	5613	5642	5670	5698	5727	5755	5783	5812	5840	5868
13	5897	5925	5953	5982	6010	6038	6067	6095	6123	6152	6180	6209	6237	6265	6294	6322
14	6350	6379	6407	6435	6464	6492	6520	6549	6577	6605	6634	6662	6690	6719	6747	6776
15	6804	6832	6860	6889	6917	6945	6973	7002	7030	7059	7087	7115	7144	7172	7201	7228
	0	**1**	**2**	**3**	**4**	**5**	**6**	**7**	**8**	**9**	**10**	**11**	**12**	**13**	**14**	**15**
	Ounces															

To convert the weight known in grams to pounds and ounces, for example, of a baby weighing 3717 gm, glance down columns to find the figure closest to 3717, which is 3714. Refer to the number to the far left or right of the column for pounds and the number at the top or bottom for ounces to get 8 pounds, 3 ounces.

Conversion formulas:

__Pounds × 453.6 = grams

__Ounces × 28.35 = grams

__Grams ÷ 453.6 = pounds

__Grams ÷ 28.35 = ounces

Appendix E

Temperature Equivalents

Celsius	Fahrenheit
34.0	93.2
34.2	93.6
34.4	93.9
34.6	94.3
34.8	94.6
35.0	95.0
35.2	95.4
35.4	95.7
35.6	96.1
35.8	96.4
36.0	96.8
36.2	97.1
36.4	97.5
36.6	97.8
36.8	98.2
37.0	98.6
37.2	98.9
37.4	99.3
37.6	99.6
37.8	100.0
38.0	100.4
38.2	100.7
38.4	101.1
38.6	101.4
38.8	101.8
39.0	102.2
39.2	102.5
39.4	102.9
39.6	103.2
39.8	103.6
40.0	104.0
40.2	104.3
40.4	104.7
40.6	105.1
40.8	105.4
41.0	105.8
41.2	106.1
41.4	106.5
41.6	106.8
41.8	107.2
42.0	107.6
42.2	108.0
42.4	108.3
42.6	108.7
42.8	109.0
43.0	109.4

Conversion formulas:

__Fahrenheit to Celsius: $(°F - 32) \times (5/9) = °C$

__Celsius to Fahrenheit: $(°C) \times (9/5) + 32 = °F$

Appendix F

Common Spanish Phrases for Maternity and Pediatric Nurses

Is there someone with you who speaks English?	**¿Hay alguien con usted que hable inglés?** *Ah-ee ahl-gee-ehn kohn oos-tehd keh ah-bleh een-glehs?*
I am the nurse.	**Soy la enfermera.** *Soy lah ehn-fehr-meh-rah.*
Sit down, please.	**Siéntese, por favor.** *See-ehn-the-she, pohr fah-bohr.*
Lie down.	**Asuéstese.** *Ah-kwehs-the-she.*
Turn on your right (left) side.	**Voltéese del lado derecho (izquierdo).** *Bohl-the-eh-she dehl lah-doh deh-reh-choh (ees-kee-her-doh).*
Lie on your back.	**Acuéstese boca arriba.** *Ah-kwehs-the-she boh-kah ah-ree-bah.*
Lie on your stomach.	**Acuéstese boca abajo.** *Ah-kwehs-teh-she boh-kah ah-bah-hoh.*
You need to take medicine/medication.	**Usted necesita tomar medicina.** *Oos-tehd neh-she-see-tah toh-mahr meh-dee-see-nah.*
Show me with one finger where you have the pain.	**Enséñeme con un solo dedo dónde tiene el dolor.** *Ehn-seh-nyeh-meh kohn oon soh-loh deh-doh dohn-deh tee-eh-neh ehl doh-lohr.*
Do you have nausea?	**¿Tiene náusea?** *Tee-eh-neh nah-oo-seh-ah?*
Do you have vomiting?	**¿Tiene vómito?** *Tee-eh-neh boh-mee-toh?*
When was the last time that you ate?	**¿Cuándo fue la últim a vez que comió?** *Kwahn-do fweh lah ool-tee-mah behs keh koh-mee-oh?*
Do you have diarrhea?	**¿Tiene diarrea?** *Tee-eh-neh dee-ah-reh-ah?*
Are you constipated?	**¿Está estreñido/-a?** *Ehs-tah ehs-treh-nyee-doh/-dah?*
Are you passing gas?	**¿Está pasando gas?** *Ehs-tah pah-sahn-doh gahs?*
Does it burn when you urinate?	**¿Le arde cuando orina?** *Leh ahr-deh kwahn-doh oh-ree-nah?*

Bend your knees.	**Doble las rodillas.** *Doh-bleh lahs roh-dee-yahs.*
Do you have pain here?	**¿Tiene dolor aquí?** *Tee-eh-neh doh-lohr ak-kee?*
Breathe deeply.	**Respire profundo.** *Rehs-pee-reh proh-foon-doh.*
Drink clear liquids.	**Tome líquidos claros.** *Toh-meh lee-kee-dohs klah-rahs.*
Can you give us a stool sample?	**¿Puede darnos una muestra de excremento?** *Pweh-deh dahr-nohs oo-nah mwehs-trah deh eks-kreh-mehn-toh?*
When was the last time you had a bowel movement?	**¿Cuándo fue la última vez que obró (que usó el baño)?** *Kwahn-doh fweh lah ool-tee-mah behs keh oh-broh (keh oo-soh ehl bah-nyoh)?*
Drink eight glasses of water a day.	**Tome ocho vasos de agua al día.** *Toh-meh oh-choh bah-sohs deh ah-gwah ahl dee-ah.*
Do you have sexual relations with men (women, prostitutes)?	**¿Tiene usted relaciones sexuales con hombres (mujeres, prostitutas)?** *Tee-eh-neh oos-tehd rel-lah-see-oh-nehs sek-soo-ah-lehs kohn ohm-brehs (moo-heh-rehs, prohs-tee-too-tahs)?*
Are you allergic to any medicine or food?	**¿Es alérgica a alguna medicina o alimento?** *Ehs ah-lehr-hee-kah ah aho-goo-nah meh-dee-see-nah oh ah-lee-mehn-toh?*
Do you take medicine?	**¿Toma usted medicina?** *Toh-mah oos-tehd meh-dee-see-nah?*
Do you have the medicine with you?	**¿Trae la medicina con usted?** *Trah-eh lah meh-dee-see-nak kohn oos-tehd?*
Take your medication.	**Tome su medicina.** *Toh-meh soo meh-dee-see-nah.*
I am going to give you pain medicine.	**Le voy a day medicina para el dolor.** *Leh boh-ee ah dahr med-dee-see-nah pah-rah ehl doh-lohr.*
Do you have shortness of breath?	**¿Tiene falta de aire?** *Tee-ehn-eh fahl-tah deh ah-ee-reh?*
We need a urine sample.	**Necesitamos una muestra de orina.** *Neh-seh-see-tah-mohs oo-nah mwehs-trah deh oh-ree-nah.*
You need a catheter in your bladder.	**Usted necesita una sonda en la vejiga.** *Oos-tehd neh-seh-see-tah oo-nah sohn-dah ehn lah beh-hee-gah.*
Have you lost weight?	**¿Ha perdido peso?** *Ah pehr-dee-doh peh-soh?*
How long have you had the discharge?	**¿Cuánto tiempo tiene con el deshecho/flujo?** *Kwahn-toh tee-ehm-poh tee-eh-neh kohn ehl dehs-eh-choh/floo-hoh?*
What do you use to prevent pregnancy?	**¿Qué clase de anticonceptivo usa para prevenir el embarazo?** *Keh klah-seh heh ahn-tee-kohn-sept-tee-boh oo-sah pah-rah preh-beh-neer ehl ehm-bah-rah-soh?*
When was your last period?	**¿Cuándo fue su última regla/menstruación?** *Kwahn-do fweh soo ool-tee-mah reh-glah/mehns-troo-ah-see-ohn?*

Are your periods regular?	**¿Sus reglas/ menstruaciones son regulares?** *Soos **rehs**-glahs/mehns-troo-ah-see-**oh**-nehs sohn reh-goo-**lah**-rehs?*
Are you pregnant?	**¿Esta embarazada?** *Ehs-**tah** ehm-bah-rah-**sah**-dah?*
How many times have you been pregnant?	**¿Cuántas veces ha esado embarazada?** ***Kwahn**-tahs **beh**-sehs ah ehs-**tah** doh ehm-bah-rah-**sah**-dah?*
How many children do you have?	**¿Cuántos hijos tiene?** ***Kwahn**-tohs **ee**-hohs tee-**eh**-neh?*
Have you received prenatal care?	**¿Ha recibido cuidado prenatal?** *Ah reh-see-**bee**-doh kwih-**dah**-doh preh-nah-**tahl**?*
When was the last time you visited your doctor?	**¿Cuándo fue la última vez que visitó a su médico?** ***Kwahn**-doh fweh lah **ool**-tee-mah behs keh bee-see-**toh** ah soo **meh**-dee koh?*
How long have you had vaginal bleeding?	**¿Por cuánto tiempo ha tenido sangrado vaginal?** *Pohr **kwahn**-toh te-**ehm**-**poh** ah teh-**nee**-doh sahn-**grah**-doh bah-hee-**nahl**?*
How many sanitary pads did you use today?	**¿Cuántas toallas femininas usó hoy?** ***Kwhan**-tahs toh-**ah**-yahs feh-meh-**nee**-nahs oo-**soh** **oh**-ee?*
Are you having contractions?	**¿Tiene contracciones?** *Tee-**eh**-neh kohn-trahk-see-**ohn**-ehs?*
How many minutes do the contractions last?	**¿Cuántos minutos le duran las contracciones?** ***Kwahn**-tohs mee-**noo**-tohs leh **doo**-rahn lahs kohn-trakh-see-**ohn**-ehs?*
Did your bag of water break?	**¿Se le rompió la fuente del agua?** *Seh leh rohm-pee-**oh**lah **fwehn**-teh dehl **ah**-gwah?*
When did your bag of water break?	**¿Cuándo se le reventó la fuente del agua?** ***Kwahn**-doh seh leh reh-behn-**toh** lah **fwehn**-teh dehl **ah**-gwah?*
(Don't) push.	**(No) Empuje.** *(Noh) Ehm-**poo**-heh.*
I am going to listen to the baby's heartbeat.	**Voy a escuchar los latidos del corazón del bebé.** ***Boh**-ee ah ehs-koo-**chahr** lohs lah-**tee**-dohs dehl koh-rah-**sohn** dehl beh-**beh**.*
Do you want me to call a friend or relative for you?	**¿Quiere que yo le llame a una amistad o pariente?** *Kee-**eh**-reh keh yoh leh **yah**-meh ah **oo**-nah ah-mees-**tahd** oh pah-ree-**ehn**-teh?*
I need to comb your hair.	**Necesito peinarle el pelo.** *Neh-seh-**see**-toh peh-ee-**nahr**-leh ehl **peh**-loh.*
Do you know if you have diabetes?	**¿Usted sabe si tiene diabetes?** *Oos-**tehd** **sah**-beh see tee-**eh**-neh dee-ah-**beh**-tehs?*
Do you take insulin (diabetic pills)?	**¿Toma insulina (píldoras para la diabetes)?** ***Toh**-mah een-soo-**lee**-nah (**peel**-doh-rahs **pah**-rah lah dee-ah-**beh**-tehs)?*
What type of insulin do you take? Regular? NPH? Humulin 70/30?	**¿Qué tipo de insulina toma? ¿Regular? ¿NPH? ¿Humulina 70/30?** *Keh **tee**-poh deh een-soo-**lee**-nah **toh**-mah? Reh-goo-**lahr**? **Eh**-neh Peh **Ah**-cheh? Oo-moo-**lee**-nah seh-**tehn**-tah **treh**-een-tah?*

How many unit of insulin do you take in the morning (evening)?

¿Cuántas unidades de insulina toma en la mañana (tarde)?
__Kwahn__-tahs oo-nee-__dah__-dehs deh een-soo-__lee__-nah __toh__-mah ehn lah mah-__nyah__-nah (__tahr__-deh)?

Do you check your blood sugar level at home?

¿Usted revisa en casa el nivel de azúcar de la sangre?
Oos-__tehd__ reh-__bee__-sah ehn __kah__-sah ehl nee-__behl__ deh ah-__soo__-kahr deh lah __sahn__-greh?

What was the blood sugar when you checked it?

¿Cuánto fue el azúcar cuándo lo revisó?
__Kwahn__-toh fweh ehl ah-__soo__-kahr __kwan__-doh loh reh-bee-__soh__?

When was the last time you took your medicine?

¿Cuándo fue la última vez que tomó su medicina?
__Kwahn__-doh fweh lah __ool__-tee-mah behs keh toh-__moh__ soo meh-dee-__see__-nah?

(X) hours (days, weeks) ago.

(X) hora (días, semanas).
(X) __oh__-rahs (__dee__-ahs, seh-__mah__-nahs).

Have you eaten breakfast?

¿Ha desayunado?
Ah dehs-ah-yoo-__nah__-doh?

Have you eaten lunch?

¿Ha almorzado (merendado, tomado el lonche)?
Ah ahl-mohr-__sah__-doh (meh-rehn-__dah__-doh, toh-__mah__-doh ehl __lohn__-cheh)?

Have you eaten dinner/supper?

¿He cenado (tomado la comida)?
Ah seh-__nah__-doh (toh-__mah__-doh lah koh-__mee__-dah)?

When did the accident occur?

¿Cuándo ocurrió el accidente?
__Kwahn__-doh oh-koo-ree-__oh__ ehl ak-see-__dehn__-teh?

Did you lose consciousness?

¿Perdió el conocimiento?
Pehr-dee-__oh__ ehl koh-noh-see-mee-__ehn__-toh?

When was the last time you received a tetanus vaccine?

¿Cuándo fue la última vez que recibió una vacuna del tétano?
__Kwahn__-doh fweh lah __ool__-tee-mah behs keh reh-see-bee-__oh oo__-nah bah-__koo__-nah dehl __teh__-tah-noh?

Does the baby sleep more than usual?

¿El/La bebé duerme más de lo normal?
Ehl/Lah beh-__beh dwehr__-meh mahs deh loh nohr-__mahl__?

Does the baby cry more than usual?

¿El?la bebé llora más de lo normal?
Ehl/Lah be-__beh yoh__-rah mahs deh loh nohr-__mahl__?

Do you have difficulty waking up the child?

¿Tiene dificultad para despertar al niño (a la niña)?
Tee-__eh__-neh dee-fee-kool-__tahd pah__-rah dehs-pehr-__tahr__ ahl nee-nyoh (ah lah __nee__-nyah)?

When was the last time you gave him/her medicine for the fever?

¿Cuándo fue la última vez que le dio medicina para la fiebre?
__Kwahn__-doh fweh lah __ool__-tee-mah behs keh leh dee-__oh__ meh-dee-__see__-nah __pah__-rah lah fee-__eh__-breh?

Be sure he/she drinks plenty of fluids.

Asegure que tome muchos líquidos.
Ah-seh-__goo__-reh keh __toh__-meh __moo__-chohs __lee__-kee-dohs.

Give him/her Tylenol every four hours.

Dele Tylenol cada cuatro horas.
__Deh__-leh __Tay__-leh-nohl __kah__-dah koo-__ah__-troh __oh__-rahs.

Is he/she acting normally?

¿Está actuando normalmente?
Ehs-__tah__ ahk-too-__ahn__-doh nohr-mahl-__mehn__-teh?

When he/she vomits, does the emesis shoot out in projectile form?	**Cuándo vomita, ¿sale disparado el vómito en forma proyectil?** *Kwahn-doh boh-mee-tah, sah-leh dees -pah-rah-doh ehl boh-mee-toh en fohr-mah proh-yek-teel?*
When was the last time he/she vomited?	**¿Cuándo fue la última vez que vomitó?** *Kwahn-doh fweh lah ool-tee-mak behs keh boh-mee-toh?*
Has the baby lost weight?	**¿Ha perdido peso el/la bebé?** *Ah pehr-dee-doh peh-soh ehl/lah beh-beh?*
Have you recently traveled outside the country?	**¿Recientemente ha viajado fuera del país?** *Reh-see-ehn-teh-mehn-teh ah bee-ah-hah-doh fweh-rah dehl pah-ees?*
Have you changed his/her formula?	**¿Le ha cambiado la fórmula?** *Leh ah kahm-bee-ah-doh lah fohr-moo-lah?*
What brand of formula does he/she take?	**¿Qué marca de fórmula toma?** *Keh mahr-kah deh fohr-moo-lah toh-mah?*
Do you give him/her cow's milk?	**¿Le da leche de vaca?** *Leh dah leh-chech deh bah-kah?*
Does the baby vomit only when you give him/her milk?	**¿El/La bebé vomita solamente cuándo le da leche?** *Ehl/Lah beh-beh boh-mee-tah soh-lah-mehn-teh kwahn-doh leh dah leh-cheh?*
Is there another person in the house with the same symptoms?	**¿Hay otra persona en casa con los mismos síntomas?** *Ah-ee oh-trah pehr-soh-nah ehn kah-sah kohn lohs mees-mohs seen-toh-mahs?*
Does he/she have a history of asthma?	**¿Tiene una historia de asma?** *Tee-eh-neh oo-nah ees-toh-ree-ah deh ahs-mah?*
We need to do an X-ray of his/her chest.	**Necesitamos hacerle una radiografia del pecho.** *Neh-seh-see-tah-mohs ah-sehr-leh oo-nah rah-dee-oh-grah-fee-ah dehl peh-choh.*
When did the convulsion occur?	**¿Cuándo le ocurrió la convulsión?** *Kwahn-doh leh oh-koo-ree-oh lah kohn-bool-see-ohn?*
How long did the convulsion last?	**¿Cuánto tiempo duró la convulsión?** *Kwahn-toh tee-ehm-poh doo-roh lah kohn-bool-see-ohn?*
Did the child lose consciousness?	**¿Perdió el ninó/la niná el conocimiento?** *Pehr-dee-oh ehl nee-nyoh/lah nee-nyah ehl koh-noh-see-mee-ehn-toh?*
When did the rash appear?	**¿Cuándo empezó la erupción?** *Kwahn-doh ehm-peh-soh lah eh-roop-see-ohn?*
Do you have a new dog or cat at home?	**¿Tienen un nuevo perro o gato en casa?** *Tee-eh-nehn oon nweh-boh peh-roh oh gah-toh ehn kah-sah?*
Have you used a new soap, shampoo, detergent, or lotion?	**¿Ha usado un nuevo jabón, champú, detergente, o loción?** *Ah oo-sah-doh oon nweh-boh hah-bohn, chahm-poo, deh-tehr-hehn-teh, oh loh-see-ohn?*
Are your child's shots up to date?	**¿Está al corriente con sus vacunas su hijo/-a?** *Ehs-tah ahl koh-ree-ehn-teh kohn soos bah-koo-nahs soo ee-hoh/-hah?*

Is he/she teething?	**¿Le están saliendo los dientes?** *Leh ehs-**than** sah-lee-**ehn**-doh lohs dee-**ehn**-tehs?*	How long has he/she had trouble walking?	**¿Cuánto tiempo lleva con dificultad al caminar?** ***Kwahn**-toh tee-**ehm**-poh **yeh**-bah kohn dee-fee-kool-**thd** ahl kah-mee-**nahr**?*
Does he/she have problems swallowing?	**¿Tiene problemas al tragar?** *Tee-**eh**-neh proh-**bleh**-mahs ahl trah-**gahr**?*	Did he/she fall?	**¿Se cayó?** *Seh kah-**yoh**?*

Adapted from Nasr, I., Cordero, M. (1996). *Medical Spanish: An Instant Translator.* Philadelphia: Saunders.

Appendix G

Commonly Used Abbreviations in Maternity and Pediatric Nursing

Abbreviation	Meaning
ā	before
A/C	antecubital
AC	abdominal circumference
ā ā	ana (of each)
AROM	artificial rupture of membranes
AAROM	active assistive range of motion
AB	abortion
abd	abdomen
ABD	abduction
ABX	antibiotics
a.c.	ante cibum (before meals)
a.d.	right ear
ADD	adduction
ad. lib.	as desired
AGE	acute gastroenteritis
AM	morning (ante meridiem)
AMA	against medical advice
AS	auricle sinister (left ear)
ASA	acetylsalicylic acid (aspirin)
a.u.	both ears
B.S.	breath sounds
bs	blood sugar
b.i.d.	two times a day
BM	bowel movement
BMR	basal metabolic rate
BOM	bilateral otitis media
BOW	bag of waters
BP	blood pressure
Bpd	biparietal diameter
BPD	bronchopulmonary dysplasia (infants)
BPM	beats per minute
BRP	bathroom privileges
BRS	breath sounds
BS	bowel sounds
BSA	body surface area
BSE	breast self-examination
BW	birth weight
c̄	with
C/O	complains of
C/S	cesarean section
CS	chem sticks
C&S	culture and sensitivity
CAN	child abuse and neglect
cc	cubic centimeter
CC	chief complaint
CHO	carbohydrate
CO	carbon monoxide
CO_2	carbon dioxide
cp	cerebral palsy
CP	chest pain
CPD	cephalo-pelvic disproportion
CR	cardiac rate
CRL	crown rump length
CST	contraction stress test
CTA	clear to auscultation
CX	cervix
d/c	discharge
D/C	discontinue
D.C.	day care
D&C	dilitation & curettage
DFA	diet for age
DOB	date of birth
DOE	dyspnea on exertion
DOI	date of injury
DOS	date of surgery
Dx	diagnosis
EBL	estimated blood loss
EDC	estimated date of confinement
EFM	external fetal monitor
EFW	estimated fetal weight
EGA	estimated gestational age
ENT	ear, nose & throat
Ent	enteral
ET	endotracheal
FB	foreign body
FBS	fasting blood sugar
FH	family history
FHR	fetal heart rate

FHT	fetal heart tone
FHS	fetal heart sound
fs	full strength
FTND	full term normal delivery
FTT	failure to thrive
FUO	fever of unknown origin
FX	fracture
GER	gastro esophageal reflux
G	gravida (number of pregnancies)
GI	gastrointestinal
GSW	gunshot wound
GT	gastrostomy tube
gt	(gutta) drop
gtt	drops
GTT	glucose tolerance test
hct	hematocrit
Hgb	hemoglobin
H/H	home health
H/O	history of
H.O.	house officer
H&H	hemoglobin and hematocrit
H&P	history and physical
HBO	hyperbaric oxygen
HC	head circumference
HELLP	hemolysis, elevated liver enzymes, low platelet count
HIB	hemophilus influenza B conjugate vaccine
HOB	head of bed
hr	hour
HR	heart rate
I/O	intake & output
I&D	incision and drainage
ICBG	iliac crest bone graft
IM	intramuscular
IM rod	intramedullary rod
IUD	intrauterine device
IUGR	intrauterine growth retardation
KUB	kidney, ureters, bladder
KVO	keep vein open
l	liter
L	left
L&D	labor & delivery
lmp	last menstrual period
LMP	left mentoposterior
LNMP	last normal menstrual period
LOM	left otitis media
LP	lumbar puncture
MDI	metered dose inhaler
med neb	nebulized medication
min	minute
MIN	minimum
ml	milliliter
ML	midline
mm	millimeter
MM	mucous membrane

N/S	normal saline
n/s	no show
N/V/D/C	nausea, vomiting, diarrhea, constipation
NV	neurovascular
n.a.	not applicable
N.A.	nursing assistant
NCP	nursing care plan
NKDA	no known drug allergies
NPO	nothing by mouth
NSVD	normal spontaneous vaginal delivery
NTT	nasotracheal tube
NWB	non weight bearing
OB	obstetric
od	every day
OD	ocular dexter (right eye)
OE	otitis externa
ORIF	open reduction internal fixation
OTC	over the counter (non prescription drug)
OU	each eye
O.S.	left eye
os	by mouth
Para	birth of a viable infant
P.P.	post prandial (after meals)
PP	postpartum
PAR	post anesthesia recovery
pc	post cibum (after meals)
PEG	percutaneous endoscopic gastrostomy
per	through or by
PERRLA	pupils equal, round, react to light and accommodation
pH	Hydrogen ion concentration (pH of 7 = neutral)
PH	past history
PICC	peripherally inserted central venous catheter
po	per os (by mouth)
PO	postoperative
PPD	tuberculin test
PR	per rectum
PROM	premature rupture of membranes
pt	patient
PT	prothrombin time
PTT	partial thromboplastin time
PTA	prior to admission
q	every
qh	every hour
RO	rule out
R.A.D.	reactive airway disease
Rx	prescription
RX	treatment
$\bar{s}$	without
S/S	signs & symptoms
SAT	saturation
sc	subcutaneous (also sq)

Sl	slight
SL	sublingual (under the tongue)
SOAP	subjective/objective/assessment & planning
SOB	shortness of breath
SPROM	spontaneous premature rupture of membranes
ss	one-half
SS enema	soapsuds enema
STAT	at once
std	standard
STD	sexually transmitted disease
sup	superior
supp	suppository
TAT	tetanus antitoxin
t.i.d.	three times a day
TKO	to keep open
TO	telephone order
TOPV	trivalent oral polio vaccine
TRA	to run at
tsp	teaspoon
TSP	total serum protein
ung.	ointment
V.S.S.	vital signs stable
VO	verbal order
vol	volume
VOL	voluntary
W.C.	wheelchair
W/O	without
W-D	well developed
W/D	wet to dry (dressing)
w.a.	while awake
WIC	women, infants, children
wn	well nourished
WNL	within normal limits
y/o	year old
YOB	year of birth

Symbols

<table>
<tr><td>↑</td><td>increase</td></tr>
<tr><td>↓</td><td>decrease</td></tr>
<tr><td>| | |</td><td>parallel bars</td></tr>
<tr><td>+</td><td>positive, plus</td></tr>
<tr><td><</td><td>less than</td></tr>
<tr><td>></td><td>greater than</td></tr>
<tr><td>~</td><td>approximate</td></tr>
<tr><td>Δ</td><td>change</td></tr>
</table>

Index

Note: Page numbers in *italics* refer to illustrations; those followed by t refer to tables.